Volume 78| **January 2005**

BJR British Journal of Radiology

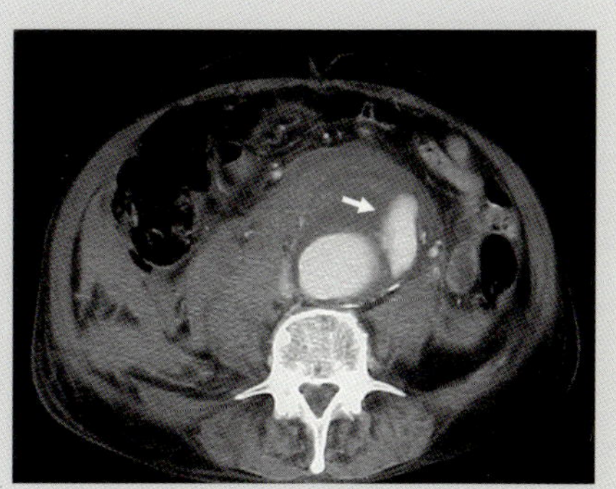

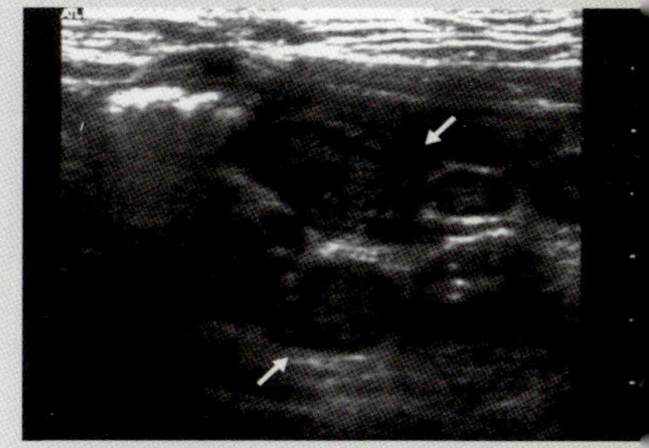

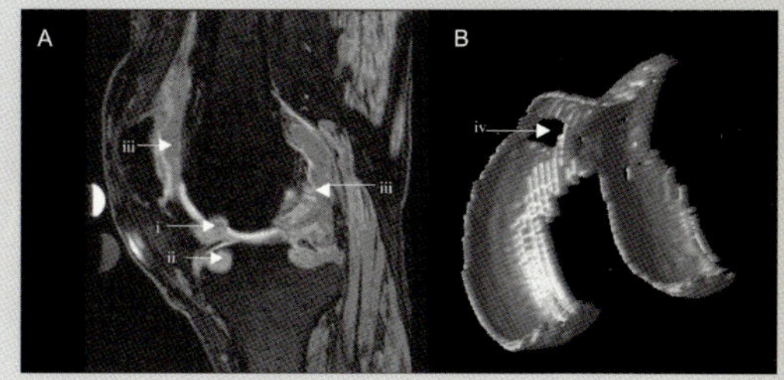

Full papers

Incidental lesions found on CT colonography: their nature and frequency

Enlarged mesenteric lymph nodes in asymptomatic children: the value of the finding in various imaging modalities

Radiation risk and cost-benefit analysis of a paediatric radiology procedure: results from a national study

Measurement of cartilage volumes in rheumatoid arthritis using MRI

Effect of the introduction of helical CT on radiation dose in the investigation of pulmonary embolism

Irradiation with standard tangential breast fields in patients treated with conservative surgery and sentinel node biopsy: using 3D tool to evaluate the first level coverage of the axillary nodes

UKRC 2004 debate
Short communications
Case reports
Pictorial review
Case of the month

Published by

BIR
The British Institute of **Radiology**

http://bjr.birjournals.org

ISSN 0007-1285

BJR

ISSN 0007 1285

THE BRITISH JOURNAL OF RADIOLOGY

Aims and Coverage

The *British Journal of Radiology* is the official peer-reviewed monthly research journal of the British Institute of Radiology. It is a multidisciplinary journal covering all clinical and technical aspects of diagnostic imaging, radiotherapy and oncology, medical physics and radiobiology. BJR is an international journal containing papers both from the UK and overseas, and is circulated to Full Members of the BIR and to libraries worldwide.

Authors are strongly advised to submit manuscripts online using Editorial Manager™, at http://bjr.edmgr.com. Online submission will expedite the peer-review process. Instructions to Authors are available on request from the Refereeing Administrator at the address given below, and are also available on the BIR's website at www.bir.org.uk

Editorial Board

Overseas Advisory Panel

Published by the British Institute of Radiology, 36 Portland Place, London W1B 1AT, UK.
Editorial enquiries: Tel: +44 (0)20 7307 1424; Fax: +44 (0)20 7307 1414
Email: publications@bir.org.uk

www.bir.org.uk **www.birjournals.org** **bjr.edmgr.com**

Subscriptions

Subscriptions fulfilment is carried out by PSP Subscriptions, BMA House, Tavistock Square, London WC1H 9JR, UK (Telephone +44 (0)20 7383 6270; Fax +44 (0)20 7383 6402; email subscriptions@bmjgroup.com). The 2005 annual subscription rate for the printed version of BJR is £524 (includes 12 issues plus two Special Issue). Subscriptions are on a calendar basis only.

Institutional BJR subscribers have free access to both BJR Online and Imaging Online, and are offered a 33% discount on a print subscription to the BJR's quarterly review journal Imaging (see http://imaging.birjournals.org).

US Mailing Agent

The British Journal of Radiology (ISSN 0007 1285) is published monthly by the British Institute of Radiology, c/o Mercury Airfreight Int. Ltd, 365 Blair Road, Avenel, NJ 07001. The Dollar price for US direct subscribers is $786. Periodicals Postage Paid at Rahway NJ. Postmaster: send address corrections to the British Journal of Radiology, c/o Mercury Airfreight Int. Ltd, 365 Blair Road, Avenel, NJ 07001.

Back Issues

Back issues can be ordered from Vine House Distribution, Waldenbury, North Common, Chailey, East Sussex BN8 4DR, UK (Telephone +44 (0)1825 723398; Fax +44 (0)1825 724188). Price is £40 per issue.

BJR Online

BJR Online, produced in association with HighWire Press, is available free of charge to BIR members and Institutional print subscribers: http://bjr.birjournals.org. Enquiries to publications@bir.org.uk

BIR THE BRITISH INSTITUTE OF RADIOLOGY

Founded 1897
Incorporated by Royal Charter
Patron: Her Majesty The Queen

The British Institute of Radiology has as its aim to bring together all the professions in radiology and allied medical and scientific disciplines to share knowledge, and educate the public, thereby improving the prevention and detection of disease and the management and treatment of patients. Particulars of membership and other information can be obtained from the General Secretary, BIR, 36 Portland Place, London W1B 1AT, and from the BIR's website: http://www.bir.org.uk
Telephone: +44 (0)20 7307 1400
Fax: +44 (0)20 7307 1414

Typeset, printed and bound by The Charlesworth Group, Wakefield, UK. Telephone +44 (0)1924 204830.

BJR

VOLUME 78

Number 925

Contents

January 2005

***Front cover:** The illustrations used on the front cover of this issue of BJR can be found on pages 31, 42 and 62. We thank the authors for granting us permission to use their figures.*

Editorial

Page

■ Low dose radiation risk: UKRC 2004 debate — 1
P Dendy

UKRC debate

■ Evidence for beneficial low level radiation effects and radiation hormesis — 3
L E Feinendegen

■ Radiation risk is linear with dose at low doses — 8
K H Chadwick and H P Leenhouts

■ Moderate dose rate ionizing radiation increases longevity — 11
J R Cameron

■ The LNT model provides the best approach for practical implementation of radiation protection — 14
C J Martin

Commentary

■ Public service summit: science & innovation, 2004 — 17
B Jones

■ Incidental lesions found on CT colonography: their nature and frequency — 20
C S Ng and A H Freeman

Full papers

■ Incidental lesions found on CT colonography: their nature and frequency — 22
T Xiong, M Richardson, R Woodroffe, S Halligan, D Morton and R J Lilford

■ Enlarged mesenteric lymph nodes in asymptomatic children: the value of the finding in various imaging modalities — 30
V Rathaus, M Shapiro, M Grunebaum and R Zissin

■ Radiation risk and cost-benefit analysis of a paediatric radiology procedure: results from a national study — 34
H B L Pettersson, K Fälth-Magnusson, J Persliden and M Scott

■ Measurement of cartilage volumes in rheumatoid arthritis using MRI — 39
S J Gandy, A D Brett, P A Dieppe, M C Keen, R A Maciewicz, C J Taylor, J C Waterton and I Watt

■ Effect of the introduction of helical CT on radiation dose in the investigation of pulmonary embolism — 46
J O'Neill, J T Murchison, L Wright and J Williams

■ Irradiation with standard tangential breast fields in patients treated with conservative surgery and sentinel node biopsy: using a three-dimensional tool to evaluate the first level coverage of the axillary nodes 51
R Orecchia, A Huscher, M C Leonardi, R Gennari, V Galimberti, C Garibaldi, E Rondi, L C Bianchi, S Zurrida and S Franzetti

Short communication

■ Training in neonatal cranial ultrasound: a questionnaire survey 55
P J C Davis, R M Cox and J Brooks

Case reports

■ False negative 16 detector multislice CT for scaphoid fracture 57
A M Groves, H K Cheow, K K Balan, H M Courtney, P W P Bearcroft and A K Dixon

■ Renal replacement lipomatosis associated with renal transplantation 60
S D Chang, F V Coakley and R B Goldstein

■ Endovascular repair of a ruptured abdominal aortic aneurysm under local anaesthesia 62
J P Morales, F G Irani, K G Jones, P R Taylor, R Dourado and T Sabharwal

■ Renal cell carcinoma vertebral body metastasis extending into the azygos venous system causing superior vena cava obstruction 65
M Strugnell, M Gibson, R Hopkins, I Lyburn and G McGann

■ Rectus abdominis endometriosis: a report of two cases 68
V Coeman, R Sciot and I Van Breuseghem

■ Uterine lipoma: advantage of MRI over ultrasound 72
L U Lau and R F Thoeni

Pictorial review

■ Neck masses in children 75
J R A Turkington, A Paterson, L E Sweeney and G D Thornbury

Book reviews 86

Case of the month

■ Acute neck swelling 89
B A Kumar, S Chandramohan and N Parasu

Acknowledgment to referees 91

BIR Company Subscribers 94

Meetings and courses 96

The British Journal of Radiology, *78* (2005), 1–2
DOI: 10.1259/bjr/16783587

Editorial

Low dose radiation risk: UKRC 2004 debate

P DENDY

In this issue we reproduce edited versions of the four contributions that were made to the debate on the motion "There is no radiation risk to health at low doses" at the UK Radiological Congress in Manchester in June (UKRC 2004).

The basis of the debate was that the Ionising Radiation (Medical Exposure) Regulations 2000 [1] and associated Guidance Notes [2] constitute wide-ranging legislation controlling the use of ionizing radiation in medicine. Primarily under the headings of Justification and Optimization this has led to the introduction of many new requirements in our procedures and new levels of record keeping. No one can question that this causes a lot of extra work. So what is the experimental basis for these requirements?

In attempting to reduce a complex problem to one simple statement, we might say "Application of the principles of Justification and Optimization to the very low doses usually encountered in diagnostic radiology is based primarily on the advice of the International Commission on Radiological Protection (ICRP) that there is no safe level of ionizing radiation – the so-called linear no threshold (LNT) model.

But how robust is the science underpinning this advice? The problem is that nearly all the hard data on radiation-induced cancer in humans comes from effective doses above 250 mSv. How can we extrapolate over two orders of magnitude to annual background and typical diagnostic radiological doses of 1–2 mSv? ICRP thinking is that after a dose and dose-rate correction factor at higher doses, extrapolation should be linear to zero dose. However, this view is being increasingly challenged by evidence that there may be a threshold or even beneficial effects at low doses. For further detail on extrapolation models see for example Dendy and Dixon [3].

Thus the purpose of the motion was to examine critically currently accepted thinking on this controversial issue.

The motion was proposed by Ludwig Feinendegen under the title "Radiation Hormesis – fact or fiction" [4]. He started by observing that radiation-induced cancer has never been recorded at the doses used in diagnostic radiology and suggested there is now good radiobiological evidence that this is not simply a statistical problem. He pointed out that cells, tissues and organisms are complex adaptive systems and that adaptive protection is continuously being stimulated by reactive oxygen species generated by exogenous and endogenous toxins. From here he went on to develop the argument that the balance between damage and protection generally favours protection at low doses, *i.e.* hormesis.

Ken Chadwick opposed the motion with a lecture entitled "A mechanistic approach to justify the contention that radiation risk is linear with dose from zero dose up" [5]. He pointed out that induction of chromosome aberrations, somatic mutations and cell killing can all be described by a linear-quadratic dose–effect relationship. DNA double strand breakage is regarded as the critical lesion, resulting in a dose–effect curve that is normally linear-quadratic but linear at very low doses from zero dose upwards. On this model there is no threshold dose for radiation risk.

John Cameron spoke third for the motion. Using as his title "Moderate dose rate radiation is good for your health" [6], he presented epidemiological data, some of which is either unpublished or not readily accessible in the literature, to support the hypothesis that we need increased background radiation to improve our health.

Finally, Colin Martin opposed the motion. Taking as his title "The LNT model provides the best approach for practical implementation of radiation protection" [7], he considered both practical and political implications. He explored some of the difficulties of introducing any alternative model for protection and concluded that this is not the right time to abandon the LNT approach to implementation of radiation protection in healthcare.

Another successful innovation at UKRC 2004 was electronic interactive voting. This proved both enjoyable for the audience and informative. Each speaker had been invited to suggest one question based on the theme of their talk. The questions and voting are shown at the end of each lecture. An interesting finding was that, whereas almost 50% of the audience were prepared to question the underlying science of the LNT model, 70% were in favour of retaining it for practical implementation.

The substantive motion "That this house believes there is no radiation risk to health at low doses" was defeated (For the motion 30%; against the motion 54%; abstaining 16%). This was a clear but not overwhelming majority, and was a fairly strong signal that this important question should be kept under review. Although it is politically expedient to retain the LNT model, this should not deter scientific questioning of the model independently of political or practical considerations.

Undoubtedly the most encouraging voting response was that 77% of the audience said the debate had improved their understanding of the issues involved.

References

1. Ionising Radiation (Medical Exposure) Regulations 2000 (Statutory Instrument 2000 No. 1059). London, UK: HMSO, 2000.

2. Institute of Physics and Engineering in Medicine. Medical and dental guidance notes. A good practice guide to implementing ionising radiations legislation in the clinical environment. York, UK: IPEM, 2002.
3. Dendy PP, Dixon B. Effects of human exposure to ionising radiation and risk estimates. In: Medical Imaging and Radiation Protection for Medical Students and Clinical Staff. Martin CJ, Dendy PP, Corbett RH, editors. London: British Institute of Radiology, 2003:103.
4. Feinendegen LE. Evidence for beneficial low level radiation effects and radiation hormesis. Br J Radiol 2005;78:3–7.
5. Chadwick KH, Leenhouts HP. Radiation risk is linear with dose at low doses. Br J Radiol 2005;78:8–10.
6. Cameron JR. Moderate dose rate ionizing radiation increases longevity. Br J Radiol 2005;78:11–13.
7. Martin CJ. The LNT model provides the best approach for practical implementation of radiation protection. Br J Radiol 2005;78:14–16.

The British Journal of Radiology, *78* (2005), 3–7 © 2005 The British Institute of Radiology
DOI: 10.1259/bjr/63353075

UKRC 2004 debate

Evidence for beneficial low level radiation effects and radiation hormesis

L E FEINENDEGEN, MD

Heinrich-Heine-University Düsseldorf, Germany and Brookhaven National Laboratory, Upton, NY, USA

Abstract. Low doses in the mGy range cause a dual effect on cellular DNA. One is a relatively low probability of DNA damage per energy deposition event and increases in proportion to the dose. At background exposures this damage to DNA is orders of magnitude lower than that from endogenous sources, such as reactive oxygen species. The other effect at comparable doses is adaptive protection against DNA damage from many, mainly endogenous, sources, depending on cell type, species and metabolism. Adaptive protection causes DNA damage prevention and repair and immune stimulation. It develops with a delay of hours, may last for days to months, decreases steadily at doses above about 100 mGy to 200 mGy and is not observed any more after acute exposures of more than about 500 mGy. Radiation-induced apoptosis and terminal cell differentiation also occur at higher doses and add to protection by reducing genomic instability and the number of mutated cells in tissues. At low doses reduction of damage from endogenous sources by adaptive protection maybe equal to or outweigh radiogenic damage induction. Thus, the linear-no-threshold (LNT) hypothesis for cancer risk is scientifically unfounded and appears to be invalid in favour of a threshold or hormesis. This is consistent with data both from animal studies and human epidemiological observations on low-dose induced cancer. The LNT hypothesis should be abandoned and be replaced by a hypothesis that is scientifically justified and causes less unreasonable fear and unnecessary expenditure.

Ionizing radiation and endogenous toxins at low doses

Everyone agrees that cellular responses to low values of absorbed doses of ionizing radiation are not readily predictable by extrapolation of responses observed at high doses. One reason for this unpredictability is in the physics of energy distribution in low-dose exposed tissues. For penetrating radiation, particle tracks arise stochastically throughout the exposed tissue with a relatively low density at low doses [1]. These tracks generate unevenly distributed ionizations and excitations of constituent molecules along the track path, as well as bursts of reactive oxygen species (ROS) [2]. In the case of exposure to internal emitters, the distribution of particle tracks is determined by the distribution of the emitter in tissue [3]. The lower the radiation fluence or number of particle emitters in a given tissue mass, the less crowded are the particles in the exposed mass and consequently the more heterogeneous is the distribution of ionized molecules and of ROS bursts.

The other reason stems from various biological confounding factors, especially the abundant and constant metabolic generation of ROS and of other endogenous toxins, on top of which low-dose radiation acts [4, 5]. The average production rate of endogenous DNA double strand breaks (DSB) per cell per day in the body is about 10^3 times higher than that of radiogenic DSB from background irradiation. However, at low-LET (linear energy transfer) irradiation the probability of radiation induced DSB per primary DNA alteration of any type is about 10^5 times higher than that caused endogenously [5].

Ratio of DNA damage and cancer probabilities

Radiation induced DNA damage and genomic instability increases with absorbed dose [2]. Such cellular effects come through direct energy deposition events from traversing particle tracks by which DNA damage rises proportional with dose. Depending on the amount of energy deposited per cell, bystander effects in non-irradiated neighbouring cells may add to this damage in tissue at low doses [6, 7]. By measuring damage in multicellular systems, values of damage per exposed cell or defined micromass are calculated averages. This implies that any bystander phenomenon that may have occurred is coregistered and expressed in the observed values. A dose of 1 mGy of low-LET radiation, such as 100 kVp X-rays, causes on average the following effects per potentially oncogenic stem cell with an average mass of 1 nanogram: 1 particle track; about 150 ROS; 2 DNA alterations of any kind; 10^{-2} DSB; 10^{-4} chromosomal aberrations; and the probability of an oncogenic transformation of the hit cell with lethal outcome is about 10^{-13} to 10^{-14} [8–10]. In other words, the ratio of the probabilities for radiation induced lethal cancer and the corresponding DSB is about 10^{-11} to 10^{-12}. This means the statement that even one DSB poses a risk of causing a lethal cancer to develop from the affected cell is unreal and in fact, scientifically unfounded.

Adaptive responses, protection

A sudden suprabasal yet non-lethal rise of toxin concentration in a biological target tends to elicit stress responses and to stimulate adaptation, usually in terms of protective mechanisms in the sense of hormesis [11]. Increasing evidence in the literature over the past 25 years indicates that adaptive protection responses occur in mammalian cells *in vivo* and *in vitro* after single as well as protracted exposures to X- or γ-radiation at low doses (for reviews [5, 8–10, 12]). There appear to be two principal types of adaptive protection, one is to prevent and repair DNA damage and in doing so to keep cells alive and functioning properly. The other is to remove damaged cells from tissue by inducing apoptosis, terminal differentiation, and immune responses and thus to reduce genomic instability in the tissue system and eliminate mutated cells.

Contrary to the immediate initiation of repair after DNA damage has occurred, adaptive protection develops as a physiological stress response relatively slowly within a few hours and may last for several weeks to months. It reduces accumulation of DNA damage in tissue from many sources such as from metabolically generated or environmental toxins or renewed irradiation [13]. Protective responses occur in various ways. They appear to depend on mammalian species, individual genomes, cell types, cell cycle, and cell metabolism. Adaptive protection categories after single low-dose, low-LET irradiation, are as follows (for reviews [10, 14, 15]):

Damage prevention

Stimulation of detoxification of ROS appears to reach a maximum at about 4 h after irradiation and lasts for several hours or even weeks, depending on tissue and cell type. The process involves a rise of free glutathione and increased levels of superoxide dismutase (SOD) with decreased lipid peroxidation lasting for weeks in some tissues. This response accompanied a change in enzyme activities such as of thymidine kinase in mouse bone marrow *in vivo* to some 70% of control. Moreover, ROS detoxification has been linked to gene activation such as transcriptional regulation of the gamma-glutamylcysteine synthetase gene, predominantly through the AP-1 binding site in its promoter.

Damage repair

Protection against high-dose induced chromosomal aberrations and/or micronuclei formation in human lymphocytes and tissue culture cells increased to a maximum about 4 h after a conditioning low-dose of low-LET irradiation and lasted for about 3 days; the protection also operated against other DNA damaging agents. This protection covered up to about 30% of the damage seen in non-conditioned controls and varied between individuals and cell types; it was absent in some individuals and is probably determined genetically. This adaptive response probably involves a several-fold enhancement of the DNA repair rate. In human fibroblasts, micronuclei formation responded to conditioning doses from 1 mGy to 500 mGy equally effectively. At the lowest dose an energy-deposition event occurred in only about 40% of the cells and bystander effects may have been involved in causing the adaptive protection. Inhibition by a high dose of X-rays of DNA synthesis and cell growth in rat glial cells in culture was only about one quarter to one third at several hours following a conditioning low-dose exposure and this adaptive protection decreased with age of the donor rats. This response involved protein-kinase C (PCK), DNA-dependent protein-kinase (DNA-PK), and phosphatidylinositol 3-kinase (PI3K), as well as the activity of the ataxia-telangiectasia gene (ATM).

Damage removal by apoptosis

Damaged cells may be induced into apoptosis by intracellular and intercellular cellular signalling. Apoptosis may also occur within hours after high-dose irradiation. Low-dose induced apoptosis of pre-damaged cells with replacement by healthy cells may be a major route of *in vivo* removal of oncogenically transformed cells. Low-dose induced apoptosis is also assumed to operate through intercellular signalling from normal cells, which may also be activated by transformed cells in culture. Non-growing human fibroblasts in culture with DSBs from low-dose low-LET irradiation readily lost this damage to the level of DSBs in non-irradiated control cells after induction of proliferation; this damage removal was mainly due to apoptosis. Low-dose induced enhancement of DNA repair may be responsible for the observation in rat thymocytes, where the incidence of radiation-induced apoptosis first declined at low doses and only rose with higher doses. The induction of apoptosis apparently requires a certain level of DNA damage.

Stimulation of immune response

Removal of damaged cells occurred *in vivo* by way of a low-dose induced immune competence. This was, in another study, associated with a reduction in the incidence of cancer metastases to less than one third of control concomitantly with an increased number of circulating cytotoxic lymphocytes. Such response had its maximum *in vivo* at about 0.2 Gy. Low-dose induced immune competence may last for several weeks.

Protection and cell cycle

Damaged cells may also exit the system by premature differentiation and maturation to senescence. The various mechanisms of protection may be linked directly or indirectly to transient changes in the activity of the G_1 cell cycle checkpoint. Another mechanism in this category of damage removal is known to occur in a number of tissue culture cell types by way of hypersensitivity to low-dose radiation that disappears at higher doses. This hypersensitivity in some cells was linked to the cell cycle and disappeared in a number of cultured cells within about 4 h, but not immediately, after a single low-dose, low-LET irradiation. Radiation-induced predisposition to genetic instability in cultured cells also declined following low-dose irradiation. These data indicate prevention of damage removal by way of low-dose induced DNA repair.

Reduction of carcinogenesis

These protective responses, in one form or another, may be responsible for the observation of a reduction of spontaneously occurring cancers also through the action of bystander effects, *in vivo* as well as *in vitro*, where clonogenic transformation was the endpoint of observation. For instance, a single low dose low-LET irradiation of 2 month old mice heterozygous for the Trp-53 gene significantly delayed the appearance of "spontaneous" lymphoma and spinal osteosarcoma later in life. On the other hand, a review of tumour development following low-dose, low-LET irradiation in normal rodents showed the existence of a threshold dose. Several human epidemiological studies also indicate either a threshold or a reduced cancer incidence below control values following a single low-dose irradiation.

Low-dose induced changes in gene expression

The categories of adaptive protection listed above involved changes in gene expression. Thus, exposure of human skin fibroblasts in culture to a single dose of 20 mGy γ-radiation caused more than 100 genes to change their expression within 2 h. This gene group included stress response genes and was different from the group of genes in parallel cultures that concomitantly responded to 500 mGy. A similar pattern of expression amongst a total of 1574 genes developed with a delay of at least 30 min in γ-irradiated mouse brain, with 30% of the genes exclusively affected by 0.1 Gy. Moreover, human fibroblasts in culture showed DNA repair in the course of adaptive protection against micronucleus formation following acute high-dose irradiation; the repair was more effective in the gene-poor chromosome than in the gene-rich chromosome of the cells.

A common pattern

Despite the disparity of the systems examined and the responses, there appears to be a common pattern in the data. Adaptive protection following low doses of low-LET radiation appears to be the consequence of changed cellular signalling and to be ubiquitous. Adaptive protection is a physiological expression of cellular capabilities to maintain integrity of tissue structure and function in the face of various exposures to potentially toxic agents including ROS, whether from endogenous sources or from ionizing radiation [5, 16, 17]. One might speculate that DNA damage accumulation from any source eventually conditions a cell to become susceptible to apoptosis induced by low doses including that from background radiation exposure [4]. In this sense, background radiation exposure comes into focus as a possible trigger for maintaining tissue homeostasis.

Regarding their dependence on absorbed dose, the above listed categories of adaptive protection are summarized schematically in Figure 1. Except for apoptosis and terminal cell differentiation, all protective responses to single exposures tend to be expressed maximally after about 0.1 Gy and very little after more than about 0.5 Gy X- or γ-radiation [8, 18, 19]. Depending on type of adaptive protection in a given cell system, as summarized previously [5, 8–10, 14], in most mammalian cells so far examined, the expression of adaptive protection had a maximum above 5 mGy and below about 200 mGy.

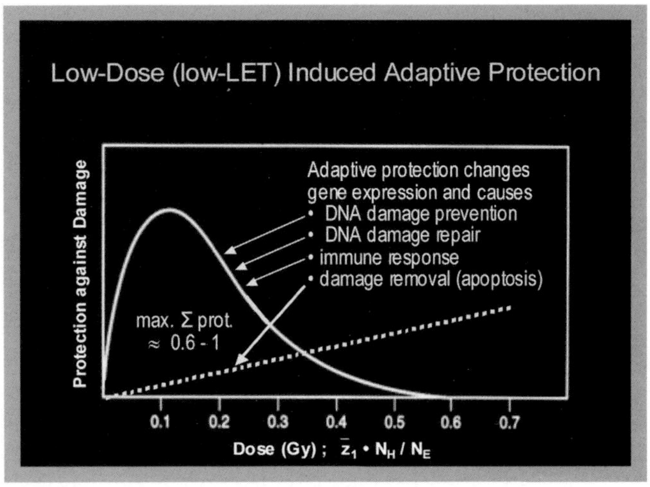

Figure 1. Single low-dose induced adaptive responses have a protecting function through various mechanisms. Note that mechanisms of DNA damage prevention and repair and the immune stimulation decrease after a maximum at doses between 0.1 Gy and 0.2 Gy, in contrast to apoptosis incidence that increases with dose. Absorbed dose is in Gy and also in terms of microdosimetry, in that the mean energy deposition per particle traversal per defined micromass (specific energy $\bar{z}_1$) (ICRU 1983) [1] is multiplied by the number of such events (N_H) in the number of exposed micromasses (N_E).

Regarding the duration of their effectiveness, Figure 2 gives a schematic summary of available published data. The time scales of duration of adaptive protection of various kinds are crucially important for the assessment of dose rate effects [20]. Depending on radiation type and dose rate, energy deposition events per defined micromass such as a cell happen at certain average time intervals. The time interval between repetitive energy deposition events in a defined biological target at a given dose rate may

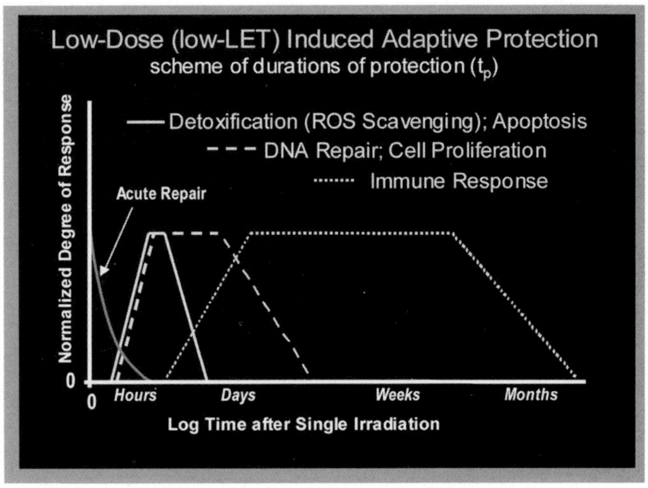

Figure 2. Single low-dose induced adaptive responses have different times of duration depending on protective mechanisms that begin with a delay of several hours and may last for days to weeks – and even up to months for immune response. Note that repair in response to radiation damage begins immediately after damage has occurred.

determine to what degree damage or adaptive protection prevails.

Since DNA damage and cancer in mammals arise mainly from non-radiogenic sources, it is justified to relate the low-dose induced various adaptive protection mechanisms mainly to non-radiogenic, *i.e.* "spontaneous" DNA damage and cancer in addition to their potential effect against radiogenic damage and cancer, as presented in more detail in a model elsewhere [9, 10, 14, 15]. Graphs summarizing the application of the model of risk evaluation after single low-dose irradiation are shown in Figure 3. They illustrate that low-doses induce adaptive protection against DNA damage and its accumulation in tissue, mainly from endogenous, *i.e.* "spontaneous" sources, and that these can counterbalance radiation effects. The net risk of cancer becomes lower than predicted by the LNT-hypothesis, or even negative with more benefit than damage to the low-dose exposed system.

Summary

(1) Ionizing radiation causes DNA damage in mammalian cells proportional to the dose with additional possible bystander effects. (2) At background radiation exposure levels, DNA damage comes overwhelmingly from non-radiation sources. (3) The probability of radiation induced adaptive protection measurably outweighs that of damage from doses well below 200 mGy low-LET radiation. (4) The delayed and temporary adaptive protection at low doses involves damage prevention, damage repair and immune responses. They appear to operate primarily against DNA damage from non-radiation sources. Moreover, apoptosis and terminal cell differentiation also occur at higher doses and tend to remove susceptible damaged cells, as does the low-dose induced stimulation of the immune system. Cell removal reduces genomic instability and mutated cells from tissue. (5) At higher absorbed doses in tissue, cell and DNA damage appear increasingly to overrule, negate, or annihilate the more subtle signalling effects seen after low doses that lead to adaptive protection, whereas apoptosis and terminal cell differentiation continue to function. (6) The linear-dose-risk function appears invalid and should be replaced by a function that includes both linear and non-linear terms. Basic research data and human epidemiological data conform to a threshold or hormesis in the low-dose range.

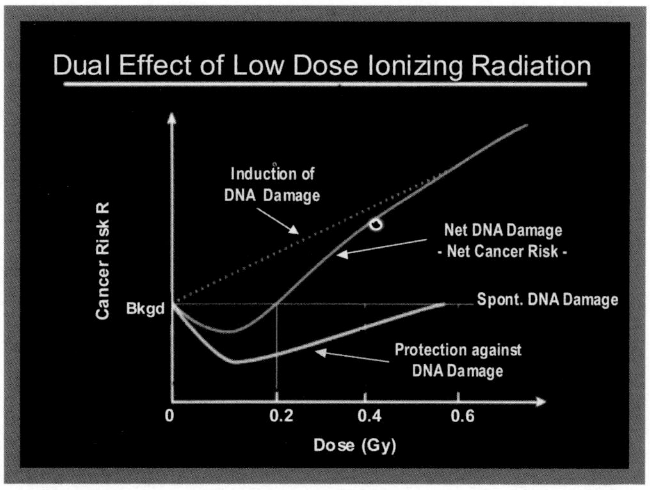

Figure 3. The dual effect of single low dose irradiation is schematically analysed according to a simplified model [10]. The net cancer risk derives from the difference between cancer induction through DNA damage and its prevention at the various dose levels (additional protection against damage accumulation from apoptosis is not shown here).

References

1. ICRU (International Commission on Radiation Units and Measurements). Microdosimetry, ICRU-Report 36, Bethesda, MD, USA, 1983.
2. Hall EJ. Radiobiology for the Radiologist (5th edn), Philadelphia, Baltimore, New York, USA: Lippincott Williams & Wilkins, 2000.
3. ICRU (International Commission on Radiation Units and Measurements). Absorbed-Dose Specification in Nuclear Medicine, ICRU-Report 67, Bethesda, MD, USA, 2002.
4. Feinendegen LE. Reactive oxygen species in cell responses to toxic agents. Human Exper Toxicol 2002;21:85–90.
5. Pollycove M, Feinendegen LE. Radiation-induced versus endogenous DNA damage: possible effect of inducible protective responses in mitigating endogenous damage. Human Exper Toxicol 2003;22:290–306.
6. Little JB. Radiation sensitive tissue: cell volume, bystander effects and genomic instability. In: Fliedner TM, Feinendegen LE, Hopewell JW, editors. Chronic Irradiation: Tolerance and Failure in Complex Biological Systems. Br J Radiol 2002;Suppl 26:15–18.
7. Dendy PP, Brugmans MJP. Low dose radiation risks. Br J Radiol 2003;76:674–7.
8. Feinendegen LE, Loken MK, Booz J, Muehlensiepen H, Sondhaus CA, Bond VP. Cellular mechanisms of protection and repair induced by radiation exposure and their consequences for cell system responses. Stem Cells 1995;13 (Suppl. 1):7–20.
9. Feinendegen LE, Bond VP, Sondhaus CA. The dual response to low-dose irradiation: Induction vs. prevention of DNA damage. In: Yamada T, Mothersill C, Michael BD, Potten C, editors. Biological Effects of Low Dose Radiation. Excerpta Medica. International Congress Serie 1211. Amsterdam, London, New York, USA: Elsevier, 2000:3–17.
10. Feinendegen LE. Relative implications of protective responses versus damage induction at low-dose and low-dose rate exposures, using the microdose approach. Radiat Prot Dosim 2003;104:337–46.
11. Calabrese EJ, Baldwin LA. Toxicology rethinks its central belief. Nature 2003;421:691–2.
12. UNSCEAR. Sources and Effects of Ionizing Radiation, Annex B, Adaptive Responses to Radiation in Cells and Organisms. New York, USA: United Nations, 1994.
13. Wolff S. The adaptive response in radiobiology: evolving insights and implications. Environ Health Perspect 1998;106:277–83.
14. Feinendegen LE. Biological effects of low doses of ionizing radiation: damage versus protection. In: LE Feinendegen, WW Shreeve, W Eckelman, Y-W Bahk, HN Wagner Jr, eds. Molecular Nuclear Medicine; The Challenge of Genomics and Proteomics to Clinical Practice. Heidelberg, New York, Springer Verlag 2003:747–61.
15. Feinendegen LE, Pollycove M, Sondhaus CA. Responses to low doses of ionizing radiation in biological systems. Nonlinearity in Biol Toxicol Med (in press).

16. Wolff S, Afzal V, Wienke JK, Olivieri G, Michaeli A. Human lymphocytes exposed to low doses of ionizing radiations become refractory to high doses of radiation as well as to chemical mutagens that induce double-strand breaks in DNA. Intern J Radiat Biol 1988;53:39–49.
17. Feinendegen LE, Muehlensiepen H, Bond VP, Sondhaus CA. Intracellular stimulation of biochemical control mechanisms by low-dose low-LET irradiation. Health Phys 1987;52:663–9.
18. Shadley JD, Wiencke JK. Induction of the adaptive response by X-rays is dependent on radiation intensity. Intern J Radiat Biol 1989;56:107–18.
19. Feinendegen LE, Bond VP, Sondhaus CA, Muehlensiepen H. Radiation effects induced by low doses in complex tissue and their relation to cellular adaptive responses. Mutation Res 1996;358:199–205.
20. Feinendegen LE, Graessle DH. Energy deposition in tissue during chronic irradiation and the biological consequences. In: Fliedner TM, Feinendegen LE, Hopewell JW, eds. Chronic Irradiation: Tolerance and Failure in Complex Biological Systems. Br J Radiol 2002;Suppl 26:6–14.

Footnote

Owing to the limitation of space, it has not been possible to include a comprehensive list of references. A full list with text orientation may be obtained from the Editorial Office of the BJR.

Audience participation

The question put to the audience based on this contribution was "Does it appear reasonable to accept the experimental evidence of adaptive protection and the lack of epidemiological evidence of cancer following low dose exposure for the purpose of amending radiation protection recommendations?"

Responses: Yes 30%; no 52%; don't know 18%.

The British Journal of Radiology, *78* (2005), 8–10
DOI: 10.1259/bjr/51173413

UKRC 2004 debate
Radiation risk is linear with dose at low doses

[1]K H CHADWICK, PhD and [2]H P LEENHOUTS, PhD

[1]*Ellerbank, Cowan Head, Kendal, Cumbria LA8 9HX, UK and* [2]*FredBantinglaan, 6721 BC Bennekom, The Netherlands*

Abstract. This paper presents a brief argument, based on a mechanistic approach, to show that radiation risk is linear with radiation dose from zero dose up. Similarities in cellular effects lead to the assumption of a common mechanism and the DNA double strand break is identified as the crucial radiation-induced lesion. A cancer model extends the cellular effects to the main radiation risk providing confirmation of the dose effect for cancer at low doses.

The question of radiation risk, *i.e.* radiation induced cancer, and the shape of its dose–effect relationship at very low doses is the subject of intense debate in the radiological protection community, especially because the International Commission on Radiological Protection (ICRP) is currently preparing a revision of its Recommendations [1]. The recent article by Brenner et al [2] makes it very clear that in order to quantify a risk of radiation for doses of lower than 10 mSv, impossibly large epidemiological studies would be necessary and the authors suggest that at lower doses inferences on risk need to be based on an understanding of the mechanisms of radiation action. This paper briefly presents a pathway of linkage using experimentally derived cellular and human data which associates a basic molecular lesion with the occurrence of cancer and which implies, on a mechanistic basis, that radiation risk is linear with dose from zero dose upwards. It is not possible to illustrate all the experimental evidence mentioned and readers should consult the quoted references for confirmation of the claims made [3, 4].

Theoretical background

Cellular effects

The induction of chromosomal aberrations, the induction of somatic mutations and the induction of cell killing can all be described by a linear-quadratic dose–effect relationship *i.e.*

$$\text{Effect} = k(\alpha D + \beta D^2),$$

where "Effect" can be yield of chromosomal aberrations (Y), mutation frequency (M) or the negative of the logarithm of cell survival ($-\ln S$). Indeed, Gillespie et al [5, 6] have shown that the linear-quadratic equation fits cell survival data as well as can be expected.

The three different cellular effects show the same systematic behaviour with dose rate changes and with radiation quality changes. As the dose rate is reduced all three effects decrease reflecting a reduction of the β-coefficient in the linear-quadratic equation and at very low dose rates β becomes zero. As the quality of radiation is increased, *e.g.* from gamma rays to alpha particles the dose–effect relationships for all three effects become more linear and the α-coefficient increases.

The common dose–effect relationship and the similarities in response to changes in exposure conditions imply that a common mechanism may be the origin of the three different cellular effects. If this is the case it may be expected that when different effects are measured in the same experiments direct correlations should be found with relationships such as $-\ln S = KY$ and $-\ln S = qM$ where K and q are constants.

Several examples of these correlations have been determined [7–14] and we conclude that a common radiation induced lesion may be at the origin of each of the three cellular effects. The chromosomal aberrations and mutations imply that the common lesion involves damage to the DNA and we continue by examining correlations between cell survival and the induction of DNA double strand breaks.

The molecular lesion

Radford [15–17] was the first to measure the induction of DNA double strand breaks at doses of radiobiological relevance and make the correlation with cell survival determined in the same experiment using different exposure conditions. The single straight line correlation in accordance with the equation:

$$-\ln S = pN$$

where N is the number of DNA double strand breaks and p is a constant, led him to conclude that the DNA double strand break was the lethal radiation induced lesion. Two other laboratories have also measured the correlation between DNA double strand breaks and cell survival [18–20].

Figure 1 presents, schematically, the way in which DNA double strand breaks might be induced by ionizing radiation.

Radiation may break both strands in the passage of an ionizing particle track or two independent particle tracks may break each strand of the DNA double helix. The number (N) of double strand breaks is:

$$N = \alpha D + \beta D^2$$

and we have a basis for the linear-quadratic equation.

It is important to note that at low doses (and low dose rates) the linear-quadratic equation reduces to $N = \alpha D$,

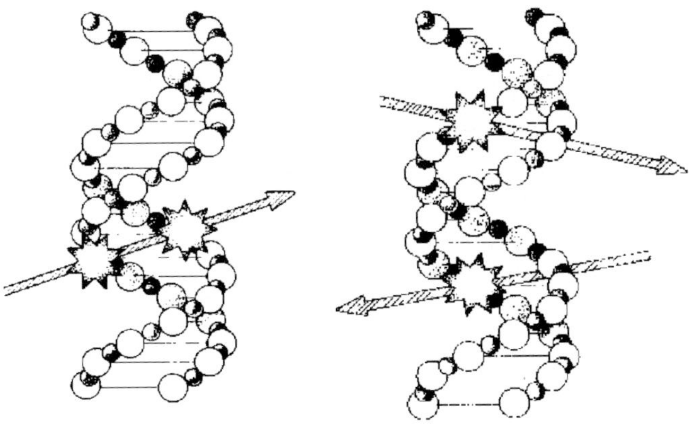

Figure 1. Schematic presentation of the way in which DNA double strand breaks might be induced by ionizing radiation.

which is linear with dose from zero dose up. So we conclude at this point that radiation induced cellular effects can all be ascribed to the induction of DNA double strand breaks and exhibit a dose–effect relationship which is linear with dose from zero dose up.

Cancer

Figure 2 presents a schematic representation of a two mutation clonal expansion model of cancer development.

Briefly, a population of normal stem cells (S) are targets for a mutation (μ_1), which converts the cell to an intermediate state (I). With time the intermediate cell divides (ε) and eventually forms a large population of cells which are targets for a second mutation (μ_2) which converts the cell to a malignant state. The malignant cell divides and in time (t_{lag}) produces a detectable tumour (T). Time, a large part of lifetime, is an important parameter in this model.

It has been possible to fit several sets of human radiation induced cancer data to this cancer model [21–25].

Spontaneous tumours arise from spontaneous mutations, radiation adds to the spontaneous mutations but does not affect clonal expansion, at least at low doses. The model calculates the age dependent increase in cancer for spontaneous cancers and after radiation exposure. It should be obvious that a single acute exposure may affect the first or the second mutation step but not both so that the radiation induced mutation in one of the steps relies on a spontaneous mutation in the other step to make the cell malignant and the radiation effect depends on the spontaneous mutations or the spontaneous cancer incidence. The same situation occurs with a protracted exposure and the radiation induced mutation will usually rely on a spontaneous mutation to create a malignant cell because spontaneous mutations are much more common. Thus the radiation effect on cancer induction reflects the

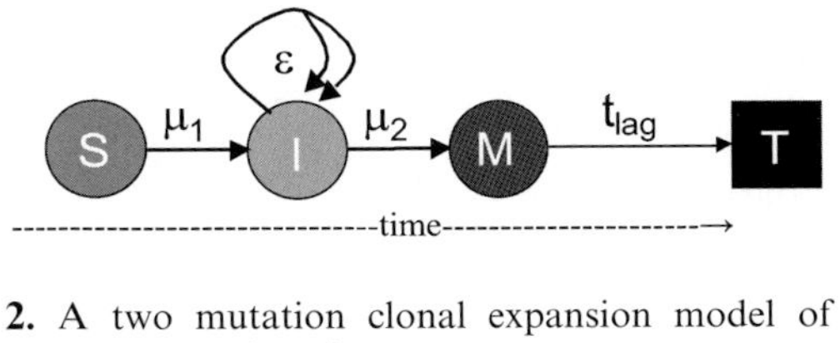

Figure 2. A two mutation clonal expansion model of cancer development. For explanation see text.

radiation induction of mutations which is linear-quadratic, in general, but linear with dose at low doses and dose rates.

Conclusion

We conclude that the DNA double strand break is the critical lesion leading to cellular effects and that a radiation induced mutation or aberration arising from a double strand break can ultimately lead to cancer so that the dose–effect for cancer induction is linear-quadratic, in general, but at low doses and low dose rates it is linear with dose from zero dose up.

References

1. ICRP. The evolution of the current system of radiological protection: the justification for new ICRP recommendations (a memorandum from the International Commission on Radiological Protection). J Radiol Prot 2003;23:129–42.
2. Brenner DJ, Doll R, Goodhead DJ, Hall EJ, Land CE, Little JB, et al. Cancer risks attributable to low doses of ionizing radiation: Assessing what we really know. Proc Natl Acad Sci USA 2003;100:13761–6.
3. Chadwick KH, Leenhouts HP. The molecular theory of radiation biology. Heidelberg: Springer Verlag, 1981.
4. Chadwick KH, Leenhouts HP, Brugmans MJP. A contribution to the linear no-threshold discussion. J Radiol Prot 2003;23:53–78.
5. Gillespie CJ, Chapman JD, Reuvers AP, Dugle DL. The inactivation of Chinese hamster cells by X-rays: synchronized and exponential cell populations. Radiat Res 1975;64:353–64.
6. Gillespie CJ, Chapman JD, Reuvers AP, Dugle DL. Survival of X-irradiated hamster cells: analysis in terms of the Chadwick-Leenhouts model. In: Alper T, editor. Cell survival after low doses of radiation: theoretical and clinical implications. London: IOPP and John Wiley & Sons Ltd, 1975: 25–31.
7. Dewey WC, Furman SC, Miller HH. Comparison of lethality and chromosome damage induced by X-rays in synchronized Chinese hamster cells in vitro. Radiat Res 1970;43:561–81.
8. Dewey WC, Stone LE, Miller HH, Giblak RE. Radiosensitization with 5-bromodeoxyuridine of Chinese hamster cells irradiated during different phases of the cell cycle. Radiat Res 1971;47:672–88.
9. Dewey WC, Miller HH, Leeper DB. Chromosomal aberrations and mortality of X-irradiated mammalian cells; emphasis on repair. Proc Natl Acad Sci USA 1971;68:667–71.
10. Dewey WC, Sapareto SA, Betten DA. Hyperthermic radiosensitization of synchronous Chinese hamster cells: relationship between lethality and chromosomal aberrations. Radiat Res 1978;76:48–59.
11. Bhambhani R, Kuspira J, Giblak RE. A comparison of cell survival and chromosomal damage using CHO cells synchronized with and without colcemid. Can J Genet Cytol 1973;15:605–18.
12. Franken NAP, Ruurs P, Ludwikow G, Van Bree C, Kipp JBA, Darroudi F, et al. Correlation between cell reproductive death and chromosome aberrations assessed by FISH for low and high doses of radiation and sensitization by iododeoxyuridine in human SW-1573 cells. Int J Radiat Biol 1999;75:293–9.
13. Goodhead DT, Thacker J, Cox R. Effectiveness of 0.3 keV carbon ultrasoft X-rays for the inactivation and mutation of cultured mammalian cells. Int J Radiat Biol 1979;36:101–14.

14. Rao BS, Hopwood LE. Modification of mutation frequency in plateau Chinese hamster ovary cells exposed to gamma radiation during recovery from potentially lethal damage. Int J Radiat Biol 1982;42:501–8.
15. Radford IR. The level of induced DNA double-strand breakage correlates with cell killing after X-irradiation. Int J Radiat Biol 1985;48:45–54.
16. Radford IR, Hodgson GS. ^{125}I-induced DNA double strand breaks: use in calibration of the neutral filter elution technique and comparison with X-ray induced breaks. Int J Radiat Biol 1985;48:555–66.
17. Radford IR. Evidence for a general relationship between the induced level of DNA double-strand breakage and cell killing after x-irradiation of mammalian cells. Int J Radiat Biol 1986;49:611–20.
18. Prise KM, Davies S, Michael BD. The relationship between radiation-induced DNA double-strand breaks and cell kill in hamster V79 fibroblasts irradiated with 250 kVp X-rays, 2.3 MeV neutrons or ^{238}Pu α-particles. Int J Radiat Biol 1987;52:893–902.
19. Murray D, Prager A, Miles L. Radioprotection of cultured mammalian cells by amniothiols WR-1065 and WR-255591: correlation between protection against DNA double-strand breaks and cell killing after α-radiation. Radiat Res 1989;120:154–63.
20. Murray D, Prager A, Vanankeren SC, Altschuler EM, Kerr MS, Terry NHA, Milas L. Comparative effect of the thiols dithiothreitol, cysteamine aand WR-151326 on survival and on the induction of DNA damage in cultured Chinese hamster ovary cells exposed to gamma-radiation. Int J Radiat Biol 1990;58:71–91.
21. Leenhouts HP. Radon-induced lung cancer in smokers and non-smokers: risk implications using a two mutation carcinogenesis model. Radiat Environ Biophys 1999;38:57–71.
22. Leenhouts HP, Chadwick KH. A two-mutation model of radiation carcinogenesis: applications to lung tumours in rodents and implications for risk evaluations. J Radiol Prot 1994;14:115–30.
23. Leenhouts HP, Brugmans MJP. An analysis of bone and head sinus cancers in radium dial painters using a two-mutation carcinogenesis model. J Radiol Prot 2000;20:169–88.
24. Leenhouts HP, Brugmans MJP. Calculation of the 1995 lung cancer incidence in the Netherlands and Sweden caused by smoking and radon: risk implications for radon. Radiat Environ Biophys 2001;40:11–21.
25. Leenhouts HP, Brugmans MJP, Chadwick KH. Analysis of thyroid cancer data from the Ukraine after ‘Chernobyl’ using a two-mutation carcinogenesis model. Radiat Environ Biophys 2000;39:89–98.

Audience participation

The question put to the audience based on this contribution was “Taking the spontaneous levels of cancer into account, do you think it will ever be possible to determine low dose radiation effects at doses just above background levels using experimental or epidemiological methods?”

Responses: Yes 21%; no 66%; don’t know 13%.

The British Journal of Radiology, *78* (2005), 11–13
DOI: 10.1259/bjr/62063624

UKRC 2004 debate
Moderate dose rate ionizing radiation increases longevity

J R CAMERON, PhD

Departments of Medical Physics, Radiology and Physics, University of Wisconsin, Madison WI, USA

Abstract. This paper presents little-known data to support the hypothesis that we need increased background radiation to improve our health. Attention will be drawn to results that demonstrate health benefits of ionizing radiation that have been largely ignored by the news media.

Science progresses by interpreting new data not by accepting unfounded assumptions. Arthur Conan Doyle cautioned against making assumptions until one has enough data on which to base the assumption. The International Commission on Radiological Protection failed to follow that advice when it adopted the linear assumption of radiation risk in 1977, primarily to simplify radiation protection regulations. Conan Doyle also pointed out that a premature assumption results in a tendency to interpret data to agree with the assumption. I believe this is one of the reasons the linear assumption has survived for so long.

Few radiologists, or other healthcare workers involved with radiation, are aware that billions of their cells are bombarded daily by natural ionizing radiation, much of it from ~9 kBq of natural radioactivity in their bodies. Nearly all the trillions of cells in our body are hit each year, many more than once. Despite this huge amount of radiation damage, cancer is primarily a disease of the elderly. It is reasonable to assume that our very early ancestors solved the problem of cellular repair billions of years ago and that we now have highly efficient repair mechanisms. Cells beyond repair undergo controlled destruction by lysis (apoptosis). According to Cohen [1] if all cancers were curable, longevity would only be increased by about 3 years. It is illogical to suggest that radiation damage to one cell may cause cancer. The probability of one damaged cell causing cancer is infinitesimal – less than ones chance of winning a World lottery if everyone had a ticket. Scientists should not base health effects on assumptions that cannot be proved or disproved. The linear assumption of radiation risk was made to simplify radiation protection regulations. It is unfortunate that many persons have accepted the assumption as a scientific truth despite the contradictory evidence of lower cancer mortality in high background areas.

Population studies

There is much evidence that radiation induction of cancer is not linear with dose and that a threshold dose rate of the order of 1 Gy $year^{-1}$ must be exceeded to induce cancer. In addition, recent studies of radiation workers show that moderate dose rate radiation produces a very significant reduction in death rate from non-cancer. The increase in longevity in two studies of radiation workers was about 3 years, about equal to the increase in longevity if all cancer were curable [2].

If ionizing radiation is as dangerous as many now believe, it seems impossible for life to have evolved. I have suggested that ionizing radiation may be an "essential trace energy" analogous to the many essential trace elements we need for good health [3].

A report by the US Atomic Energy Commission in 1973 showed that the population in the six US States with the highest radiation background had 15% lower cancer death rates than the average for the 48 States [4]. In 1998 the results of this study were confirmed by a comparison of the cancer mortality and background radiation of three mountain States to those of three Gulf States [5]. The annual level of natural background radiation in the three Rocky Mountain States (Idaho, Colorado and New Mexico) is 3.2 times that in three Gulf Coast States (Louisiana, Mississippi and Alabama), but the overall age-adjusted cancer death rate in the Gulf States is 1.26 times higher. Thus the difference from proportionality is a factor of 4.0.

For lung and bronchus cancer mortality there is a strong negative correlation with natural radon levels (the main cause of the difference in background levels) – factors of 5.7 to 7.0.

In such studies, the possibility of confounding factors must always be considered. However, to quote from Jagger's paper "It is possible that confounding factors such as smoking, poverty or environmental pollution, contribute to the differences in cancer mortality between Rocky Mountain and Gulf Coast States. However, the factor of disproportion is so great (4.0–7.5) that it strains credulity that such confounding factors could reverse this negative correlation".

Although this finding was published in a well-read journal, it attracted no attention from the news media.

The 100-year study of British radiologists (1897–1997) is the most important study of health effects of moderate dose rate radiation ever published [6, 7]. It compared the death rates of British radiologists from cancer, non-cancer and all causes to those of all male non-radiologist physicians in England and Wales, hereafter referred to as controls. The study showed that radiologists who joined a radiological society between 1897–1920 had 75% greater cancer mortality than the controls. It is not possible to make close estimates of doses received by radiologists at that time. Braestrup [8] estimated average accumulated doses to US radiologists in the 1920s and 1930s using non-protective equipment at about 1 Gy $year^{-1}$ (in modern units). 75% of the dose arose from fluoroscopy (assumed at 1 h day^{-1}), the remainder was equally divided between diagnostic radiography and therapy. There is no doubt that the significant cancer increase ($p<0.001$) was due to high radiation doses in those early years of radiology.

The increased radiation had a significant beneficial effect that was not noticed at the time. The radiologists' death rate from non-cancer was 14% lower ($p<0.05$) than the controls. Their deaths from all causes were slightly less than the controls, that is to say the longevity of the earliest radiologists was not reduced despite their 75% increase in cancer death rate. British radiologists who joined a radiological society after 1920 have never shown a statistically significant excess of cancer mortality compared with the controls. This dramatic contradiction of the linear assumption has been largely ignored. The abrupt decrease in cancer deaths after 1920 suggests that X-ray induction of cancer has a threshold as suggested by two earlier studies [9, 10].

With the introduction of beam collimation and personal protection, and much later image intensifiers, doses to radiologists fell dramatically. By the late 1950s the average had fallen to about 0.01 Gy $year^{-1}$ and by the 1990s to about 0.5 mGy $year^{-1}$ [11]. The healthiest British radiologists were those who joined a radiological society between 1955 and 1979. Their death rate from cancer was 29% lower (not significant); from non-cancer was 36% lower ($p<0.001$) and from all causes was 32% lower ($p<0.001$) than the controls. Their increase in longevity over the controls is estimated to be about 3 years.

The best epidemiological study of radiation workers ever done is the US nuclear shipyard worker study – NSWS (1980–1988) – supported by the US Department of Energy [12]. I was a member of the Technical Advisory Panel (TAP) that met twice a year to review progress and to suggest improvements. TAP comprised eight well-qualified scientists who unanimously approved the draft of the final report of the NSWS in early 1988. It is unfortunate that the details of this important study have not yet appeared in a peer reviewed scientific journal. I am sure that if the results had supported the linear hypothesis of radiation risk the details would have been published promptly. I am the co-author of a review article on the NSWS that has not yet been accepted by a journal [13].

The scientists who performed the study selected about 28 000 nuclear shipyard workers with the largest cumulative doses. They had a death rate from cancer 15% lower ($p<0.01$); from non-cancer 31% lower ($p<10^{-16}$) and from all causes 24% lower ($p<10^{-16}$) than 32 500 age-matched and job-matched unexposed shipyard workers. No other study of radiation workers has had the important advantage of job-matched controls. The very significant reduction in non-cancer deaths is in agreement with a similar reduction of deaths from non-cancer of British radiologists who joined a radiological society between 1955 and 1979 referred to earlier [6]. Since the nuclear shipyard worker study had not been published, the authors of the 100-year study were apparently unaware of the striking similarity of the results. Neither the 100-year study of British radiologists nor the nuclear shipyard worker study emphasised the strong evidence that moderate dose radiation stimulates the immune system.

It is a mystery to me why some radiologists and other healthcare workers involved with radiation still believe that diagnostic X-ray doses much lower than annual background radiation carry a risk of inducing cancer. None of the above studies proves that moderate dose radiation increases longevity but they do provide strong evidence that moderate dose radiation is beneficial to the health. I have suggested that valuable information on this question of longevity could be obtained from a double blind study using increased background radiation of about 10 mGy $year^{-1}$ to half of a population of senior citizen volunteers. This dose rate is lower than that to British radiologists in the second quarter of the last century where there was no significant increase in cancer. I have suggested such a double blind might be carried out in the US Gulf States where the population seems to be suffering from "radiation deficiency" [3].

Conclusion

The linear model is often defended as a conservative assumption. It is not conservative if we need a moderate dose rate of radiation to stimulate our immune system. Too little radiation appears to result in an earlier death. The analogy would be to reduce essential trace elements in our diet because they are poisonous in large quantities. The great statistical strength of the studies on the reduction in non-cancer deaths of the British radiologists and the US nuclear shipyard workers should not continue to be ignored.

References

1. Cohen BL. The nuclear energy option. Plenum Press, 1990.
2. Cameron JR. Longevity is the most appropriate measure of health effects of radiation. Radiology 2003;229:14–16. http://www.medphysics.wisc.edu/~jrc/art_longevity.htm
3. Cameron JR. Is radiation an essential trace energy? Physics and Society, October 2001. http://www.aps.org/units/fps/newsletters/2001/october/a5oct01.html
4. Frigerio NA, Eckerman KF, Stowe RS. Carcinogenic hazard from low-level, low-rate radiation, Part I, Rep. ANL/ES-26. Argonne Nat. Lab. 1973. A pdf file of this report may be obtained from the BJR Editorial Office.
5. Jagger J. Natural background radiation and cancer death in Rocky Mountain and Gulf Coast States. Health Phys 1998;75:428–34.
6. Berrington A, Darby SC, Weiss HA, Doll R. 100 years of observation on British radiologists: mortality from cancer and other causes 1897–1997. Br J Radiol 2001;74:507–19.
7. Cameron JR. Radiation increased the longevity of British radiologists. Br J Radiol 2002;75:637.
8. Braestrup CB. Past and present radiation exposure to radiologists from the point of view of life expectancy. Am J Roentgenol Rad Ther Nucl Med 1957;78:988–92.
9. Evans RD. Radium in man. Health Phys 1974;27:497–510.
10. Rossi HH, Zaider M. Radiogenic lung cancer. The effects of low doses of low-LET radiation. Rad Env Biophys 1997;36:85.

11. Hughes JS, O'Riordan MC. Radiation exposure of the UK population 1993 review. Chilton: National Radiological Protection Board, 1993.
12. Matanoski G. Health effects of low-level radiation in shipyard workers final report. 471 pages Baltimore, MD, DOE DE-AC02-79 EV10095, (1991) http://cedr.lbl.gov/shipyard.pdf
13. Sponsler R, Cameron JR. Nuclear shipyard worker study (1980–1988): a large cohort exposed to low dose-rate gamma radiation. http://www.medphysics.wisc.edu/~jrc/art_nsws1.htm (unpublished).

Audience participation

The question put to the audience on the basis of this lecture was "Considering that a typical adult has billions of cells hit each day by ionizing events resulting from background radiation, is it reasonable to conclude that radiation damage to even one cell may initiate cancer, as assumed by the linear, no-threshold hypothesis?"

Responses: Yes 47%; no 44%; don't know 10%.

The British Journal of Radiology, *78* (2005), 14–16
DOI: 10.1259/bjr/31745335

UKRC 2004 debate
The LNT model provides the best approach for practical implementation of radiation protection

C J MARTIN, BSc, PhD

Health Physics, Gartnavel Royal Hospital, Glasgow G12 OXH, UK

Abstract. This contribution argues the case that, at the present time, the linear-no-threshold (LNT) model provides the only rational framework on which practical radiation protection can be organized. Political, practical and healthcare difficulties with attempting to introduce an alternative approach, *e.g.* a threshold model, are discussed.

The current system for radiological protection, which is applied to all practices using ionizing radiation, is robust. It has been developed through a substantial effort by the scientific community made over many decades. However, one of the fundamental precepts, that there is proportionate risk of cancer induction extending down to doses at the level of a few millisievert, is a matter of debate. Epidemiological studies of the Japanese survivors of the atomic bombs and patients receiving high exposures from medical procedures do not show a definite link between radiation dose and cancer incidence below 200–400 mSv [1, 2]. Nevertheless, researchers have concluded that there is no convincing evidence to show that the dose–effect response is not a linear extrapolation to zero dose for solid tumours [3].

It may never be possible to resolve the question of risks at low doses completely through epidemiological studies, because the natural incidence of cancer in the population is so high that the sizes of populations which would have to be studied in order to provide statistical validity are too large. Moreover, there are too many confounding factors, such as smoking habits and the "healthy worker" effect, to enable a large enough matched control population to be found [4]. Thus, it is not surprising that there is little evidence of radiation effects at doses below 200 mSv, as such a link would be almost impossible to prove. However, there is one group which does have a much lower natural incidence of cancer, namely children, and among those radiographed while in the womb there does indeed appear to be an excess number of cancer cases from doses as low as 10 mSv, although interpretation of the results is a matter for debate [5].

Political justification

If science does not provide a definitive answer about the risks from low doses of radiation the choice of precepts on which radiological protection should be based must take account of the political, sociological and practical implications. Any change made to the system of radiological protection should be justified by the weight of evidence available and this can best be judged from the views of experts conversant with results of research in the field. Polls held at the L H Gray conference on "Radiation cancer analysis and low dose risk assessment" give an idea of expert opinion [6]. To the question "Is radiation at low doses acting as an initiator?" 80% of the participants answered "yes", and when asked "Does the dose effect relation for cancer induction have a threshold at low doses?" 79% responded "no". Thus the weight of expert opinion at the conference considered that low doses of radiation may carry risk.

Governments have a duty to protect the public, so their advice should err on the side of safety, and cannot afford to ignore the views of the scientific community. The linear-no-threshold (LNT) dose–effect model is a conservative approach. If current practice is continued, individuals are unlikely to be exposed to unnecessary risks. On the other hand, a relaxation of restrictions on low dose exposures has the potential to expose large numbers of individuals to higher doses. If research confirms that there are indeed effects of radiation at low doses, those who have been exposed as a result of the changes are likely to seek redress. This could place a significant burden of liability on governments involved.

There is a "fear factor" associated with radiation in the minds of the public. This has evolved from its destructive beginnings with nuclear weapons and the arms race, and been reinforced by accidents at nuclear power stations such as Chernobyl where large quantities of radioactive material were released into the environment. There is also concern about potential hazards from releases of radioactivity to people living near nuclear establishments, and this has built up a strong environmental lobby. The nature of the unseen hazard, causing hidden damage, which can lead to development of cancer many years later, contributes to the public perception and experts have been unable to allay these fears. If restrictions on the use of radiation are reduced, then the public will be suspicious. Their approval will be difficult to win over, even if the scientific evidence in support of relaxation is undeniable. Any disagreement between experts about the consequences will undermine confidence and the press will seek out dissenting voices to support theories of government conspiracy. Therefore, any decision to relax radiation protection controls can be implemented only if there is overwhelming support from the scientific establishment and experts in the field.

Practical implementation

Another important aspect that must be considered is the practical implication of setting up an alternative system of radiological protection based on a different precept. There are advantages to the current methodology, which may not be easy to replace. The LNT model assumes that risk is directly proportional to effective dose. Not only that, but the dose is cumulative, so that doses can be summed and risk quantified directly. This is not an unreasonable approach based on current evidence. Since doses received by any individual or group can be assessed by measurement or calculation, this provides a methodology with which risks can readily be determined but with large uncertainties. Risks can therefore be used in justification for a wide range of practices involving radiation, including research proposals, planning radiation facilities, restricting radioactive discharges and medical exposures. They can also provide the basis for guidance setting out radiation protection measures for these diverse practices.

Thus the LNT model provides a solid foundation for determination of radiation protection in practice. The application of a graded scale for protection measures based on the advice of radiation experts is accepted. An alternative system derived from a threshold model would be difficult to develop and the basis for it is unclear. The implication with such a system is that low doses can be ignored. However, this is not appropriate unless it is certain that low doses are safe. Decisions would need to be taken about what constituted a low dose and a new strategy developed for implementation of radiation protection. Considerable effort has gone into the present system and it should be maintained unless there is clear, unambiguous evidence that it is incorrect.

The acceptance of a low dose threshold would imply that there are no risks from low doses of radiation, such as those received from radioactivity in the environment arising from radioactive discharges. Constraints relating to the doses received by workers and members of the public from discharges would no longer make any sense. However, any relaxation of regulation would receive strong opposition from the environmental lobby. Therefore, restrictions on the amounts of radioactivity released would still need to be implemented, but application of the threshold model would remove the basis on which radiological impact on the environment is assessed. The foundation on which a replacement methodology could be built is full of uncertainty.

Medical exposures

It is important for the healthcare profession to consider the potential impact of a threshold dose model on medical exposures. The principle of justification could be relaxed to make radiation examinations more widely available, but is this prudent and would it improve healthcare? A robust system is in place in the UK under the Ionising Radiation (Medical Exposure) Regulations 2000 [7]. Diagnostic medical exposures should only be carried out if they will affect patient management. Relaxation of the principle of justification is more likely to result in an increase in unnecessary investigations than to improve the provision of diagnostic imaging services. X-rays might be taken to keep patients happy, probably many by non-specialists, without the same level of training in image interpretation. Any increase in demand on medical imaging facilities will impose a greater burden on the limited funds available for healthcare services. This is likely to affect adversely the overall standard of service provision and add to the spiralling costs of healthcare.

Protagonists of the low dose threshold theory might argue that whole body CT screening would have tremendous health benefits, but this is unlikely. Screening could be carried out for groups at high risk of lung cancer or coronary artery disease, but would not be cost effective healthcare. Examination of the large amounts of image data provided by CT scans would require significant inputs of radiologist time. If abnormalities were found, many would be benign, but would still need to be followed up. CT screening does not make the best use of the limited imaging resources available and could carry a significant health risk. The UK healthcare system needs more resources to allow it to become more efficient, but not to provide more imaging investigations of questionable value.

It might also be possible to relax the optimization of X-rays, if there is less concern about dose. The current UK system for provision of medical imaging services works well. Every effort is made to optimize the procedures for image quality and radiation dose as part of recognized good practice. If the numbers of investigations and facilities are increased, it is likely that X-rays will be taken by non-specialists, who have less experience in optimization, unless the numbers of radiologists and radiographers are expanded. If optimization is not carried out, the healthcare system could be accused of placing patients at unnecessary risk.

The current system of justification and optimization for medical exposures ensures that a high standard of investigation is provided for all patients that need it. Any relaxation would be unlikely to improve patient care and could increase the demand unnecessarily on an already overstretched service. Thus political and practical considerations provide sufficient reasons to continue current practices for medical exposures.

Conclusion

In conclusion, the scientific evidence does not show that there is no risk from radiation at low doses. It is at best inconclusive. Political justification cannot be given to a system based on a low dose threshold that could lead to increased exposures with greater associated risk. Moreover, it would be hard to convince the public of the wisdom for relaxing controls on the use of radiation, and this would be likely to lead to heavy criticism from the press and the environmental lobby, leading to loss of public confidence. Practical implementation of a threshold model would be more difficult because there would be no simple method with which to assess risk. The basis for risk benefit assessments carried out currently in justifying research proposals, planning radiation facilities, restricting radioactive discharges and justifying all practices using radiation would be removed, without any clear alternative methodology being provided in its place. The time is not yet nigh when the LNT approach to implementation of radiation protection should be abandoned, either in healthcare or in other practices using ionizing radiation.

References

1. United Nations Scientific Committee on the Effects of Radiation (UNSCEAR). Epidemiological evaluation of radiation-induced cancer, In: Sources and effects of ionizing radiation, Vol. 2, Annex I, 297–450, New York: United Nations, 2000.
2. Kellerer AM. Radiation risk – historical perspective and current issues. J Radiol Prot 2002;22:A1–A10.
3. US National Council on Radiation Protection and Measurements. Evaluation of the linear-non-threshold dose-response model for ionizing radiation, NCRP Report 136. Bethesda: NCRP, 2001.
4. Lagarde F. Methodology issues in epidemiological assessment of health effects of low-dose ionizing radition. Radiol Prot Dosim 2003;104:297–314.
5. Doll R, Wakeford R. Risk of childhood cancer from fetal irradiation. Br J Radiol 1997;70:130–9.
6. Proc. 20th L H Gray Conference. Radiation cancer analysis and low dose risk assessment: New developments and perspectives. J Radiol Prot 2002; 22(3A). For details of questions and answers in the interactive voting, visit http://www.rivm.nl/rca – click on "Results".
7. The Ionising Radiation (Medical Exposure) Regulations 2000, SI 2000/1059. London: HMSO, 2000.

Audience participation

The question put to the audience based on this contribution was "Do you believe that, for medical exposures, political and practical considerations provide sufficient reasons to continue the current methods used to implement principles of Justification and Optimization, even in the face of strong scientific evidence for a threshold at low doses?"

Responses: Yes 69%; no 22%; don't know 9%.

The British Journal of Radiology, *78* (2005), 17–19
DOI: 10.1259/bjr/12564924

Commentary

Public service summit: science & innovation, 2004

B JONES, MSc, MD, FRCR

Department of Clinical Oncology, Queen Elizabeth University Hospital, Birmingham B15 2TH, UK

Introduction

The public service summit, held in London on the 24th of September 2004, was designed to announce important changes in Science and Innovation funding within the UK. Attendees were from the various Government Agencies, Universities, NHS and Industry.

Phyllis Starkey MP (Chair of the Parliamentary Office of Science and Technology) provided the formal introduction and reminded the audience that The Chancellor of the Exchequer, Gordon Brown, had announced enhanced spending on basic research in the previous budget statement. The political aim is to increase what is regarded as an existing relatively strong science base as a necessary requirement for future prosperity in view of the increasing scientific development of larger countries, such as China and India. It is envisaged that improved cooperation between Universities, Research Councils and Industry will be modelled on the successful practices of the Pharmaceutical industry.

Individual speakers

Daniel Storey, a senior economist from HM Treasury, provided retrospective data, starting from Renaissance times and modified by wars, that investment in technology leads to benefits in society at large. It was not until the early 1950s that Solow identified prospective causal evidence of this relationship. The formal recognition that investment is insufficient in the UK was made by a group at Sussex University in the mid 1990s. There is to be a 5.75% per year real increase in research spending for 10 successive years (2004–2014), which will bring the overall level to around 2.5% of gross domestic product (GDP). A framework for measuring performance with time is to be developed. It is acknowledged that the entire structure of science education, from schools onwards may require attention. Charities, Regional Development Agencies, Universities and Research Councils are all expected to participate in a positive and constructive way in order to "catch up with the USA". The phrase "virtuous circle" was used, but Keynes was not mentioned, which perhaps reflects modern political correctness rather like the frequent omission of Beveridge and Bevan in health spending debates.

Professor Hugh Clare (Director of the UK Micro and Nanotechnology Network) reviewed the successes and future potential from nanotechnology, with anticipation of a post petrochemical world. The UK had been late to formally acknowledge and actively fund this area, which should transform industrial processes and products. A few years ago, France, Switzerland and Germany were well advanced in terms of a good infrastructure. It was typically necessary for the UK to commission a report (The Taylor Report), but its rapid implementation did lead to substantial improvements. There is now good activity in 12 British Universities and the potential benefits extend from improved health care products to water purification and antiterrorism measures.

Received 30 September 2004, accepted 2 November 2004.

Professor Susan Greenfield (Royal Institution and University of Oxford) impressively covered the topic of how science is funded, with examples from her own field of neuropharmacology. She delivered a rational critique of existing public sector peer review mechanisms, which for a variety of reasons are risk averse, of the vicissitudes of industry (*e.g.* market conditions, take-overs, lack of basic understanding at the top level) and of the frequent discrepant agendas in "spin out" companies and technology transfer companies formed by Universities with Investors: all of these can produce delays in the achievement of successful innovation. Recommendations included better arrangements for secured intellectual property, formation of syndicates of risk taking companies in order to reduce the risk to individual companies, tax breaks on profits related to investment and crucially a better choice of personnel for liaisons between academia and commerce. To solve the latter, the presence of "talent scouts" on University campuses were suggested: perhaps we have something to learn from the Football Association after all!

Professor Julia Goodfellow spoke on behalf of all the Research Councils and explained that the concept of joined up working between the respective Councils is increasing, with development of Networks and longer term projects such as Faraday Partnerships and Follow on Funds. It was emphasised that the "Development Gap" in the UK is huge: development requires approximately 10 times the funding of pure research. Much of British Industry has a notorious reputation in this respect (my words). It is the duty of Government to create more efficient and well regulated pathways for investment in long term projects.

There were two relatively long break-out sessions, separated by lunch, with reasonable times allowed for questions from delegates, mainly about their concerns of excessively complex bureaucracy.

The afternoon session consisted of a more holistic approach. Allan Mayo (Department of Trade and Industry) outlined the wide remit and priorities for areas which require research and development. These included environmental safety, reduction of disease risks, better transport etc., but the number one issue was that of the "ageing society". The increased use of cross-over technologies, design simulation, mathematical modelling, grid computing and nanotechnology are to be encouraged.

The Government is naturally disposed to encourage more social science research within the overall framework of advances in Science. Professor Ian Forbes (Academy of Social Sciences and University of Nottingham), described the increasing use of quantitative methods to enable assessment of improved quality of life. Large scaled investigations of social issues are relatively rare but could have major impacts if integrated within the conduct of science. One interesting problem is that, rather like in subatomic physics, if you measure a social parameter it tends to move and in any case changes with time. Some advanced research groups now include a social scientist in order to better inform scientists as to the potential impact of their discoveries. He made an interesting suggestion that the present antipathy to collective goods, such as nationally owned facilities, must be reversed. This has obvious implications for the NHS and Universities, where very expensive facilities may not be affordable in the private sector particularly if the market opportunities are considered to be too small, as is the case with the investigation and treatment of many rare diseases.

James Wilsdon, from the Demos "think tank" group, gave a superlative exposition of the importance of "see through science", with improved public understanding and anticipation of events that will emerge from the new blue sky approaches, which are now relabelled as an "upstream turn". Mark these new buzz words.

Paul Snaith (Group Director, Science and Engineering, Shell Global Solutions) exemplified how business could interact in science and innovation. His company has an enviable reputation in this respect, with an emphasis on product diversity in energy technology. One interesting fact is that all Shell employees can propose new ideas, which are formally assessed within 1 week.

Christopher Henshall (Office of Science and Technology), described the preparations for co-ordination and monitoring the increased expenditure, which will mostly fall under the wing of his department. There is to be an emphasis on improving what are regarded as the weaker areas of science and technology. This admission is heartening, for not long ago many of our senior politicians were of the view that if the UK was no longer particularly efficient at the production of a commodity, this should cease in order to concentrate activity in our service "industries", heritage and tourism; such policies were always anathema to the scientific community.

Discussion

Most rational persons will applaud the proposals, but some may ask the inevitable question is this too little and too late? The National Debt in the 50 years after World War II arguably precluded these enlightened policies, but in that time there have been numerous misplaced public spending projects. Those employed in the delivery of healthcare will remember that vast human resources, many from social sciences backgrounds, have been committed to a series of conflicting administrative reforms and initiatives since the early 1970s, with marginal changes in outcomes emergent from a sea of confusion. Perhaps, as a result of the collective experience of successive Governments, there is a new dawn where carefully controlled incremental funding into the science base will deliver real advantages, unlike the old faith in the "grand projects" such as Concorde and other prestigious defence related schemes that frequently had to be abandoned because of spiralling costs. The "white heat of technology" promised by Harold Wilson in the early 1960s was never fully realised – apart from the expansion of the Universities – but perhaps this new initiative is the way to achieve this long desired goal. It may be our last chance to maintain our status as a proud industrial nation.

All those involved in the radiological sciences, particularly in the academic units, will be pleased to note these changes and should start thinking of how to become involved in the new framework. For example, the advances in grid computing will be of potential application to both diagnostic and therapeutic radiology, since they will allow more complex analysis, storage, rapid transfer of images for second opinions, national quality assurance systems and also as part of national clinical trials; the use of microbeams (*e.g.* protons, X-rays) to identify pathophysiological changes and aid diagnosis at the subcellular level is another important new area for the radiological sciences; nanoparticles will surely be useful in improved imaging interactions (*e.g.* improved contrast media for functional studies) and applications in targeted radiotherapy.

In "questions", Professor Colin Blakemore (Director, Medical Research Council) acknowledged the huge contribution made by British physicists and engineers in the development of CT and MRI and that further advances are expected in biotechnology and nanotechnology, with a high degree of cooperation expected from the pharmaceutical industry. He also praised the successful expansion of cancer therapy clinical trials, to which the MRC/NCRI remains highly committed.

There is a huge remit for biological research which will clearly include cancer studies, although the disappointments associated with gene therapy were readily admitted by several speakers. Whilst there are significant difficulties with the provision of cure for inherited monogenetic conditions, human cancer is a polygenetic disorder and acquired on a stochastic basis, which represents a much more complex problem.

At present there is no formal inclusion of healthcare within the Accelerator Science division of the Research Councils, despite the fact that over 120 000 patients per year receive therapeutic radiation from linear accelerators in the UK. In terms of therapeutic radiation, there seems to be a lack of integration between the funding agencies, although credit must be given for the new MRC Radiobiology Research facility proposed at Oxford. The prospect of funding a National Centre for Particle Radiotherapy remains a distant prospect under the current funding limits and arrangements, although such a sophisticated project seems ideal in the context of the new emphasis for cross disciplinary working between Research Councils (the Central Laboratories, EPSRC, MRC and DH would need to be involved as a minimum) as well as the suggestion for more national ownership schemes coupled with improved quality of life outcomes. Improvements in biotechnology and molecular imaging will almost certainly produce reliable earlier diagnosis of cancer. These advances will lead to a huge requirement for "smart" applications of atomic and medical physics, such as cyclotron/synchrocyclotron and laser produced particle therapy. The fair and respectable "British" answer to this issue would classically be for the Government to commission a report, as in the example given above that resulted in vastly improved nanotechnology funding; but perhaps the need for more and more expensive reports will diminish due to improved interdisciplinary cooperation and a greater decisiveness in the upper echelons of research about what is really necessary.

Acknowledgments and declarations

The author is a member of the Engineering and Physical Sciences Research Council (UK) funded Medical Applications of Ion Beams Network and a trustee of The Cyclotron Trust (UK). Birmingham University Hospitals Endowment Funds and NHS Trust are thanked for allowing professional leave.

The British Journal of Radiology, *78* (2005), 20–21
DOI: 10.1259/bjr/30856690

Commentary

Incidental lesions found on CT colonography: their nature and frequency

[1]C S NG, MA, MRCP, FRCR and [2]A H FREEMAN, FRCR

[1]*Department of Radiology, Unit 57, MD Anderson Cancer Center, 1515 Holcombe Boulevard, Houston, TX 77030-4009, USA and* [2]*Department of Radiology, Addenbrooke's Hospital, Cambridge CB2 2QQ, UK*

Xiong and colleagues [1] are to be congratulated on an excellent and comprehensive review on the topic of incidental lesions detected in the course of undertaking CT colonography. Their task of summarizing the data should not be underestimated: many of the studies utilized differing patient populations, different CT techniques, and had varying definitions, explicitly or implicitly stated, of what constituted extracolonic findings worthy of reporting. For example, some studies have included simple cysts of the liver and kidneys in their data, while others have not and some considered cardiomegaly an important finding [2]. Their difficulties would have been compounded by inconsistent details in the various papers to enable extraction of these figures.

Nevertheless, a common pattern does appear to emerge, namely, that incidental or "extracolonic" findings in the course of CT colonography are common, averaging 40%. As such, this potentially brings considerable added value to an examination primarily designed to interrogate the colon.

Although the accuracy of CT colonography in the detection of colonic polyps has undergone careful evaluations, the question of the accuracy of the detection of extracolonic findings is less well explored. It is one thing to report or document a finding at CT, but quite another to be right about it. This becomes an increasing consideration in the context of the low dose and unenhanced CT techniques used in the majority of "virtual" colonography studies. This inevitably raises the issue as to how many of the incidental lesions or patients with incidental findings in the studies reported were followed up. It is clearly impossible to evaluate every incidental finding, particularly in those with multiple lesions. In our experience, follow up may occur in less than half the patients, especially in the elderly population. This unfortunately limits validation of the findings, and indeed some findings on further investigation may not be substantiated [3]. It is particularly intriguing that lesions that are considered "important" may not be investigated: patient and physician factors probably have a bearing, but a better understanding of such issues would be enlightening.

It is possible that the false positive rates related to incidental findings may have a substantial impact on the utility of detecting these lesions. A cascade of investigations can ensue following report of such findings, contributing to healthcare costs and patient anxiety. Furthermore, some of these investigations may be invasive and carry their own morbidity. As Xiong and colleagues [1] mention, these consequences need to be carefully evaluated.

Missing or failing to detect lesions (*i.e.* false negative rates) may also be a consideration. It can be extremely difficult to detect pancreatic, renal, or liver tumours with noisy unenhanced CT images. However, documentation of these failures would likely be extremely difficult to obtain. The category of "important incidental lesions found on follow-up" (Table 2 in Xiong et al [1]) may cast some light on this. Such considerations may be more important in some medical practice environments than in others.

In considering which patient populations might best benefit from the technology, Xiong and colleagues [1] importantly recognize that the study populations that have been reported fall into two broad categories: asymptomatic patients, in which the study is closer to a "screening" examination, and symptomatic patients, in whom the study is more of a "diagnostic" evaluation. A small subset of the latter group consists of studies on frail and elderly patients. One might expect a higher incidence of extracolonic findings in the older population partly because of age alone, but also because the patients in these studies were typically symptomatic, and the extracolonic disease detected might have contributed to, or been the dominant factor in, their presenting symptoms. The latter is quite intriguing and there has been some attempt to explore this [3], but it is admittedly extremely challenging to unravel. Interestingly, contrary to expectations, Xiong and colleagues [1] identify that fewer incidental findings have been reported in the frail and elderly group than in the studies with younger patients. Part of this might be due to varying reporting practices and differing thresholds for what constitutes findings worthy of reporting in these study populations and environments. There may also be an important contribution from the differing CT techniques that are typically used between the two groups; the "screening" studies tending towards a more "virtual", thinner collimation, technique.

It is possible that with ever improving CT techniques, smaller and smaller lesions may be detected, increasing the incidental lesion detection rate and compounding already existing difficulties about what should be done with the findings. This is comparable with the situation of finding incidental pulmonary nodules in the course of CT pulmonary angiography. Whether detection of such incidental findings has any impact on patient outcome is unknown. At least in the context of cancer and abdominal aortic aneurysms, one might intuitively expect early detection to do so.

In evaluating the true independent contribution of the technique, it is important to determine if the findings detected are truly incidental, with no preceding knowledge of the abnormality. Evaluation of the extracolonic findings is only one half of the equation when considering the utility of CT colonography as a whole, and when considering to which patient population the technique should be offered. Assessment of the extracolonic detection rate together with the spectrum and relevance of findings, needs to be combined with the colonic performance of the test. Importantly, Xiong and colleagues [1] identify that the incidental early cancer detection rate (0.9%) is comparable with the early colorectal tumour detection rate by this technique, and indeed may be higher than detection rates in other cancer screening programmes. Furthermore, the overall extracolonic cancer detection rate is even higher (2.7%). Thus this paper reinforces the power of CT over barium enema and colonoscopy for the evaluation of colorectal neoplasia, in that, at the same study it can examine multiple organs outside of the colon. Although, whether this is beneficial remains to be seen. The time is perhaps right for a carefully designed prospective study.

References

1. Xiong T, Richardson M, Woodroffe R, Halligan S, Morton D, Lilford RJ. Incidental lesions found on CT colonography: their nature and frequency. Br J Radiol 2005;78:21–8.
2. Hellström M, Svensson MH, Lasson A. Extracolonic and incidental findings on CT colonography (virtual colonoscopy). AJR Am J Roentgenol 2004;182:631–8.
3. Ng CS, Doyle TC, Courtney HM, Campbell GA, Freeman AH, Dixon AK. Extracolonic findings in patients undergoing abdomino-pelvic CT for suspected colorectal carcinoma in the frail and disabled patient. Clin Radiol 2004;59:421–30.

The British Journal of Radiology, *78* (2005), 22–29
DOI: 10.1259/bjr/67998962

Incidental lesions found on CT colonography: their nature and frequency

[1]T XIONG, MCh, [1]M RICHARDSON, BSc (Hons), AMINA, [1]R WOODROFFE, MSc, [2]S HALLIGAN, MD, FRCOG, FRCR, [3]D MORTON and [1]R J LILFORD, PhD, FRCOG, FRCP

[1]Department of Public Health and Epidemiology, Public Health Building, The University of Birmingham, Edgbaston, Birmingham B15 2TT, [2]Department of Intestinal Imaging, St. Mark's Hospital, Watford Road, Northwick Park, London HA1 3UJ and [3]Department of Surgery, The University of Birmingham, Edgbaston, Birmingham B15 2TT, UK

Abstract. CT colonography has been used to detect colonic polyps and cancers, but its effect in practice will also be influenced by the frequency with which extracolonic lesions of various types are detected. We performed a systematic review of the types of incidental lesions found on CT colonography. This is necessary to model the benefits and harms of detecting extracolonic lesions. Primary clinical studies of extracolonic findings on CT colonography were identified from electronic databases, scanning reference lists and hand searches of relevant journals and conference proceedings. A data collection proforma was used to collect information on extracolonic findings. 17 discreet studies were identified, involving 3488 patients. In total 40% of patients were recorded to have abnormalities and many had more than one abnormality. Nearly 14% of patients had further investigations and 0.8% were given immediate treatment. Extracolonic cancers were detected in 2.7% (0.9% had N0M0 cancers) and 0.9% had an aortic aneurysm. The number of extracolonic findings was high in all studies. While only a small population were judged "important", the prevalence of serious lesions outside the colon was nevertheless higher than in many other screening programs.

Introduction

CT colonography uses a combination of helical CT scanning and complex image rendering to image the large bowel and is able to produce images that simulate those seen on conventional video-endoscopy; hence the alternative term "virtual colonoscopy" [1, 2]. The sensitivity and specificity of this new health technology for neoplasia (*i.e.* cancers and polyps) is likely to be superior to the established imaging test, barium enema, and similar to video colonoscopy [2]. The results of studies, which have measured the accuracy of colonography by conducting both this test and colonoscopy sequentially on the same patients, have been reviewed elsewhere [1].

One of the intriguing features of colonography, however, is its ability to detect extracolonic lesions – sometimes referred to as "incidental findings", because the whole abdomen, pelvis and lower lung fields are imaged, as opposed to just the colorectum. These incidental findings have been classified according to their importance: *i.e.* highly important, possibly important and unimportant. An holistic assessment of the benefits and drawbacks of colonography as compared with other diagnostic and screening methods, must include an assessment of the benefits and harms which result from the detection of these lesions. In some cases, lives may be saved by detecting disease at a stage when it is still curable. In others, unnecessary procedures may be performed, with resultant complications, anxiety and use of resources.

Received 21 April 2004 and accepted 19 August 2004.

This study was sponsored by the Health Technology Assessment Programme of the Department of Health in England. The views are those of the authors.

A rational assessment of the "balance sheet", contingent on finding these incidental lesions, must begin with careful enumeration of the frequency and nature of such lesions. We therefore performed a systematic review of studies of incidental lesions found in the course of colonography carried out for the purposes of screening or diagnosis.

Methods

Identification of studies

We included primary clinical studies of extracolonic and incidental findings on CT colonography. According to the guidance from the NHS Centre for Reviews and Dissemination [3], we identified studies by searching electronic databases, scanning reference list of papers and consulting experts in the specialty. No date or language limits were placed on the searches. We also hand searched selected journals. We found no other systematic reviews focusing on extracolonic lesions (see Appendix 1 for full search strategies).

One reviewer (TX) examined titles, abstracts and keywords of citations, as given on electronic databases, and selected those which mentioned the concept of extracolonic lesions. Where possible the full text of all of potentially relevant citations was then obtained. All retrieved references were exported to Reference Manager v 10.0 (Thompson ResearchSoft, Thompson Corp., Berkley, CA).

Data extraction and synthesis

One reviewer (TX) decided whether studies met the inclusion criteria and this was checked by a second reviewer (MR). Using a standardized, piloted, data collection proforma, these two reviewers independently extracted data from papers on extracolonic findings from CT colonography.

We first collected methodological information: *i.e.* whether or not the population was clearly described; whether the author stated that consecutive cases were studied; whether the data collection was prospective or retrospective; and whether the investigations were carried out for diagnostic or screening purposes (Table 1). This process was carried out independently by two investigators (TX and MR) and any differences resolved in a three way meeting (TX, MR and RL).

We then extracted the substantive data from each study. We recorded the total number of incidental lesions and the total number of patients who had an abnormality (since patients could have more than one lesion). The number of lesions classified as "important" by the author was noted. However, different authors had different thresholds for their classification and they tended to classify "important" in terms of the need for a clinical response (*i.e.* before further investigations had been carried out), rather than whether detection was likely to have been beneficial in retrospect (*i.e.* in the light of knowledge gleaned from further investigations). We therefore also recorded the incidence of two specific types of lesion where early detection may be life-saving: "early" (N0M0) cancer and abdominal aortic aneurysm. We also noted the number of further investigations performed and the number of patients who required immediate treatment. Lastly, we recorded the number of incidental lesions found in long-term follow-up, which had not been detected at the original colonography.

We assembled data in three separate tables. First, data from full papers published in peer-reviewed articles dealing with patients given a bowel preparation were included in Table 2 (series 1). We assembled data collected from conference proceedings in Table 3 (series 2), on the grounds that these are generally less comprehensive and had been subject to less stringent quality control than the full articles. In some papers, although the focus was on primary CT diagnosis of colorectal cancers, full bowel preparation was not used since the population investigated was the frail elderly, in whom CT was being requested as an alternative to either barium enema (which has a high technical failure rate in this group) [16, 17] or video colonoscopy (which suffers from an increased rate of adverse events in this group) [6, 16, 17]. This might be expected to decrease sensitivity for colonic neoplasia. However, the incidence of extracolonic findings, might be expected to be increased in this group since they are older and clinical presentation is frequently non-specific. We therefore assembled data from these papers in Table 4 (series 3).

Results

17 studies were identified from the above searches [4–20], including 13 full papers and four conference proceedings, of which only the abstracts were available. We then scrutinized the reference lists of relevant papers and detected one further reference [21]. However, the latter was also a conference proceeding, which was unobtainable through the library.

We describe the features of the 18 studies on which reports could be retrieved in Table 1. Only six of the reports clearly stated that consecutive cases were studied. 14 were clearly prospective studies. Three of the studies dealt with colonography as a screening test, while 14 studied diagnostic colonographies. It was not possible to be clear on this issue in the remaining paper. Most of the studies were rather small: only three included more than 200 patients and one included as few as 37 patients.

We discerned that two full papers [5, 11] emanated from the same centre – the Mayo clinic. The most recent paper [5] did not make it clear whether or not the two series overlapped. We therefore contacted two of the authors, who confirmed that the first paper did indeed contaminate the second (we would like to thank Amy Hara and Joel Fletcher from the Mayo for their help in elucidating this issue). We excluded the earlier paper and did not include it in Table 2.

Findings from full papers, excluding papers dealing specifically with the frail elderly, are given in Table 2. The mean age of patients included was the mid 60s in five studies, with slightly older and younger patients in the remaining studies. As expected, the mean age in papers

Table 1. Description of papers

Author	Do they describe population clearly?	Do they state consecutive cases?	Was it prospective or retrospective study?	Were the cases screening or diagnostic tests?
Hellstrom M, et al, 2004 [20]	Yes	No	Prospective	Diagnostic
Pickhardt PJ, et al, 2003 [13]	Yes	Yes	Prospective	Screening
Ginnerup PB, et al, 2003 [12]	Yes	Yes	Prospective	Diagnostic
Gluecker TM, et al, 2003 [5]	Yes	Yes	Prospective	Screening
Munikrishnan V, et al, 2003 [4]	Yes	No	Prospective	Diagnostic
Pineau BC, et al, 2003 [17]	No	No	Prospective	Diagnostic
Robinson P, et al, 2002 [6]	Yes	Yes	Retrospective	Diagnostic
Rajapaksa R, et al, 2002 [7]	No	No	Prospective	Diagnostic
Hopper KD, et al, 2001 [21]	No	No	?	?
Edwards JT, et al, 2001 [8]	Yes	No	Retrospective	Diagnostic
Miao YM, et al, 2000 [14]	Yes	Yes	Prospective	Diagnostic
Hara A, et al, 2003 [18]	No	No	Prospective	Diagnostic
Hara AK, et al, 2002 [19]	No	No	Prospective	Diagnostic
Hara AK, et al, 2000 [10]	Yes	Yes	Retrospective	Screening
Dachman AH, et al, 1998 [9]	No	No	Prospective	Diagnostic
Morrin MM, et al, 1999 [11]	No	No	Prospective	Diagnostic
Domjan J, et al, 1998 [15]	Yes	No	Prospective	Diagnostic
Day JJ, et al, 1993 [16]	Yes	No	Prospective	Diagnostic

Table 2. Extracolonic findings on CT colonography from primary papers (excluding diagnosis in the frail elderly)

Author	Full text	Number of patients	Age range (median)	Contrast	Abnormalities present		Important present[a]	Confirmed cancers N0M0[b]	All the cancers[b]	Aortic aneurysm[b]	Further investigations	Immediate treatment	Important incidental lesions found in follow-up	Author's estimate of additional cost[c]	Additional comments
					Patients	Total									
Hellstrom M, et al, 2004 [20]	Yes	111	19–86 (66)	No	94	232	37	?	9	6	26	1	?	?	
Pickhardt PJ, et al, 2003 [13]	Yes	1233	40–79 (57.8)	No	223	223	56	5	5	2	?	2	?	?	
Ginnerup PB, et al, 2003 [12]	Yes	75	33–78 (61)	No	49	68	?	0	2	0	8	2	?	?	Nine patients needed further investigation but one refused
Gluecker TM, et al, 2003 [5]	Yes	681	41–80 (64)	No	469	858	88	3	4	4	110	9	3	$23380.59	Average added costs per CT colonography examination $34.33
Munikrishnan V, et al. 2003 [4]	Yes	80	29–83 (68)	Yes	25	25	?	3	8	2	?	?	?	$180	The estimated cost of a multislice CT colonography study was $180
Edwards JT, et al, 2001 [8]	Yes	100	55+ (65)	No	15	15	?	?	1	2	6	2	?	?	The single cancer was an unconfirmed hypernephroma
Miao YM, et al, 2000 [14]	Yes	201	55–91 (71)	No	24	25	?	4	23	1	?	?	?	?	
Morrin MM, et al, 1999 [11]	Yes	40	22–96 (62)	?	5	5	5	0	0	1	?	?	?	?	
Dachman AH, et al, 1998 [9]	Yes	44	41–85 (58)	Yes	26	32	10	0	0	0	?	?	1	?	Two data points (the number of patients with an abnormality and the number of "important" abnormalities) were not included in the paper but were ascertained from another paper by the principal author (reference) in which the index paper was quoted

[a]"Important" as defined by author. In many cases the diagnosis of "important" was prospective (*i.e.* potentially important, *e.g.* large ovary cyst), rather than retrospective (*i.e.* turned out to be important, *e.g.* ovarian carcinoma). These are total lesions found.
[b]Total lesions include any that may have been detected previously by other means. The cancers include 12 liver metastases.
[c]Total cost contingent on discovery of an incidental lesion.

Table 3. Extracolonic findings on CT colonography from conference proceedings

Author	Full text	Number of patients	Age range (median)	Contrast	Abnormalities present		Important present[a]	Confirmed cancers N0M0[b]	All the cancers[b]	Aortic aneurysm[b]	Further investigations	Immediate treatment	Important incidental lesions found in follow-up	Author's estimate of additional cost[c]	Additional comments
					Patients	Total									
Pineau BC, et al, 2003 [17]	No	183	49–71 (60)	No	162	?	39	?	?	?	?	?	?	?	All patients had at least one extracolonic finding
Hara A, et al, 2003[d] [18]	No	40	?	Yes	?	65	?	?	6	3	?	?	?	?	Prone images without IV contrast and supine images with IV contrast
Hara AK, et al, 2002[d] [19]	No	50	?	Yes	?	16	?	?	2	1	?	?	?	?	Prone images without IV contrast and supine images with IV contrast
Rajapaksa R, et al, 2002 [7]	No	200	?	?	64	109	14	?	?	0	5	?	?	?	Two patients with liver lesions suspicious for metastases
Hopper KD, et al, 2001 [21]	No	100	?	?	90	?	10	?	?	1	?	?	?	?	The data shown here were quoted from a reference to a conference proceeding

[a]"Important" as defined by author. In many cases the diagnosis of "important" was prospective (*i.e.* potentially important, *e.g.* large ovary cyst), rather than retrospective (*i.e.* turned out to be important, *e.g.* ovarian carcinoma). These are total lesions found.
[b]Total lesions include any that may have been detected previously by other means.
[c]Total cost contingent on discovery of an incidental lesion.
[d]We have sought clarification from the author about any possible "contamination" between these series, but have received no reply to date.
IV, intravenous.

dealing with the frail elderly (Table 4) was considerably higher. Contrast was used in five of all studies.

The number of abnormalities was high in all three series. In total 40% (1314/3280) of patients were recorded to have abnormalities. The percentage of people with an abnormality was 36% (930/2565), 65% (316/483) and 29% (68/232) in the three series, respectively. The total number of abnormalities was even greater, since many patients had more than one abnormality. The total number of abnormalities as a proportion of people screened was 58% (1483/2565), 66% (190/290) and 26% (90/350), respectively, in the three series. These calculations are based on those authors who provided both the relevant numerator and denominator information (some studies did not record the total number of abnormalities – only the number of patients with at least one abnormality). In addition some other papers did not give the number of patients with a diagnosis – only the total number of incidental lesions found (see Tables 2–4). To sum up, extracolonic abnormalities are common, even when the frail elderly are excluded. Indeed, in six of the studies the total number of abnormalities found was greater than the number of patients entered.

In a number of studies, authors graded the lesions according to their "importance". The total number of "important findings" among 2787 patients was 292 (10.5%). As previously stated, they use different criteria to classify lesions as important and in all cases "importance" was based on clinical relevance in terms of the need for further investigations. For this reason, we also separately abstracted cases with relatively common serious diseases – cancers and abdominal aortic aneurysms. When we did this, the proportion of lesions of confirmed importance was much smaller; a total of 2.7% (81/3005) had cancers and 0.9% (30/3305) had aortic aneurysms. Six studies recorded the size of aortic aneurysms. 16 aneurysms were detected in these studies; 3 (19%) were over 5.5 cm in size and the remainder were between 3 cm and 5.5 cm. A total of 0.9% (24/2549) patients had N0M0 cancers. Again, these calculations are based on those authors who provided both the relevant numerator and denominator information (see Tables 2–4).

The number of further investigations carried out was also quite large – in some case it even exceeded the number of lesions regarded as important by the author. A total of 13.8% (188/1362) of patients had further investigation.

The incidence of immediate treatment was only given in six studies and averaged 0.8% (17/2237).

Two studies gave the incidence of lesions found during long-term follow-up. Among these two studies the probability of finding yet a further lesion on long-term follow-up was 2.7% (3/110).

Eight studies explicitly record the nature of early stage (N0M0) primary extracolonic cancers; Table 5 lists these cancers by their primary organ. Among a total of 2549 patients, 6 kidney cancers (0.24%), 5 ovarian cancers (0.20%), 5 lung cancers (0.20%), 4 pancreatic cancers (0.16%) and 1 liver cancer (0.04%) were found. These prevalence figures are all higher than the 25-year incidence figures recorded, for example, in the Surveillance, Epidemiology and End Results (SEER) database [25].

Discussion

A number of points stand out clearly from this dataset. First, the total incidence of incidental lesions is high; at

Table 4. Extracolonic findings on CT colonography in frail and elderly patients

Author	Full text	Number of patients	Age range (median)	Intravenous contrast	Abnormalities present		Important present[a]	Confirmed cancers N0M0[b]	All the cancers[b]	Aortic aneurysm[b]	Further investigations	Immediate treatment	Important incidental lesions found in follow-up	Author's estimate of additional cost[c]	Additional comments
					Patients	Total									
Robinson P, et al, 2002 [6]	Yes	195	47–96 (76)	No	54	54	33	9	15	4	33	?	?	?	Oral contrast was given
Domjan J, et al, 1998 [15]	Yes	118	73–94 (84)	No	?	22	?	?	2	3	?	?	?	?	Oral contrast was given
Day JJ, et al, 1993 [16]	Yes	37	71–88 (80)	Yes	14	14	?	?	4	0	?	1	?	?	Administrations of intravenous contrast were at the discretion of the radiologist, and the incidence of use is not given

[a]"Important" as defined by author. In many cases the diagnosis of "important" was prospective (*i.e.* potentially important, *e.g.* large ovary cyst), rather than retrospective (*i.e.* turned out to be important, *e.g.* ovarian carcinoma). These are total lesions found.
[b]Total lesions include any that may have been detected previously by other means. The cancers include four liver metastases.
[c]Total cost contingent on discovery of an incidental lesion.

Table 5. Extracolonic early stage cancers found on CT colonography by organ of primary

	Pickhardt PJ, et al, 2003 [13]	Gluecker TM, et al, 2003 [5]	Munikrishnan V, et al, 2003 [4]	Miao YM, et al, 2000 [14]	Robinson P, et al, 2002 [6]	Ginnerup PB, et al, 2003 [12]	Morrin MM, et al, 1999 [11]	Dachman AH, et al, 1998 [9]	Total
Number of patients	1233	681	80	201	195	75	40	44	2549
Ovary	1		2		2				5
Lymphoma	1								1
Lung	2	1			2				5
Kidney	1	2		1	2				6
Liver			1						1
Pancreas				3	1				4
Choloangiocarcinoma					1				1
Bladder					1				1
All N0M0 cancers	5	3	3	4	9	0	0	0	24

least 2015 incidental lesions were found in a total of 3488 patients (58%). Second, the number of lesions requiring further investigation was also rather high; 13.8% among the six studies where this information was given. Moving on to consider serious lesions, we confine our attention in the first instance to Table 2. The incidence of serious diseases was low, relative to the total number of lesions found; 0.8% of all patients needed immediate treatment and 3.7% had either cancer or an aortic aneurysm. Thus, although many lesions are deemed important, in terms of the need for investigation, the actual incidence of serious diseases detected by this diagnostic method is considerably lower. For example, the large study by Gluecker [5], including 681 consecutive cases, found 8 aneurysms and 4 cancers; an incidence of just under 2% for either type of lesion. Late cancers have a high mortality, but 0.4% of patients in Gluecker's series had a N0M0 cancer in this study. Across all studies where these data are recorded, 0.9% of patients had N0M0 cancers. This includes Table 4 – elderly and frail patients – and if these are excluded the percentage of these early lesions was 0.6% (15/2354).

However, a detection rate for "early" cancer of about 6 per 1000 is significant in both clinical and epidemiological terms. For example, the prevalence of breast cancer in breast screening programmes is similar (range from 5.6 to 8.5 per 1000 women) [22], and the prevalence of ovarian cancer in ovarian cancer screening programmes is very much lower (about 1 per 2000 women) [23]. Indeed, the prevalence of "early" colorectal cancer detected by this modality in screening studies is of similar magnitude (0.7% had N0M0 bowel cancer) [24]. It therefore transpires that colonography may be an important method for the detection of early cancers other than colon cancers, although we recognize that this modality also detects colonic lesions in their pre-malignant phase (*i.e.* colonic adenomas).

Nearly half (42%) of cancers detected were of an early stage N0M0. Detection of lesions at this stage is, of course, most likely to result in health gains. From these data we therefore tentatively suggest that CT colonography, even without the use of contrast, may be an important potential modality, net of its effect on detecting colonic lesions. That said, it is important not to extrapolate the potential benefits of detecting early lesions uncritically from the prognoses of such lesions detected in normal clinical practice. This is because the prognoses of lesions detected in early stage may differ systematically according to method of detection. A crucial concept that relates to the effects of detecting early lesions is sojourn time. The fact that the prevalence was higher than the 25-year incidence implies quite long sojourn times and suggests that only once or infrequent screening may be effective in reducing eventual mortality. However, very long sojourn times suggest that the number of years of life gained might be quite modest and some lesions may never progress; at the limit, this must be the case where prevalence exceeds lifetime incidence. Future modelling will have to make assumptions about these variables and incorporate further information that will eventually be obtained, for example from the US Prostate, Lung, Colorectal and Ovarian (PLCO) screening study [26].

We also observe that this is "early" days for this form of diagnosis or screening. The publications which we cite are often based on incomplete data sets. For example, in many cases they do not clearly indicate that consecutive cases were studied. Nevertheless, some of the papers (such as that of Gluecker and colleagues) are of high quality [5]. The data from Gluecker study are very much in line with those from the other studies in Table 2. However, we will be the first to argue that bigger and more comprehensive datasets are required. Lastly, practically all of the studies used symptomatic patients rather than those with a population risk for colorectal cancer. It is therefore possible that the condition that prompted the investigation, was extracolonic (especially in the frail elderly group). If so, the common finding of such lesions would add further weight to arguments for the use of this method for diagnosis, but it would also suggest that lower utility would result from detection of extracolonic lesions in a screening program. However, we think that the incidental lesions revealed by this modality would generally have been "silent", *i.e.* they are truly incidental, except for the frail elderly and we analysed this group separately for this reason. If we are right, the possibility of finding serious lesions outside the colon should be added to the colon related benefits of this screening modality, although the model would need to include the "costs" of investigations and interventions prompted by the method. These costs would have to be broadly defined to include the anxiety and other morbidity associated with investigation of incidental lesions.

References

1. Dachman AH. Diagnostic performance of virtual colonoscopy. Abdom Imaging 2002;27:260–7.
2. Fenlon HM, Nunes DP, Schroy PC 3rd, Barish MA, Clarke PD, Ferrucci JT. A comparison of virtual and conventional colonoscopy for the detection of colorectal polyps. N Engl J Med 1999;341:1496–503.

3. NHS CRD. Undertaking systematic reviews of research on effectiveness: CRD's guidance for those carrying out or commissioning reviews. CRD report number 4 (2nd edn). NHS Centre for Reviews and Dissemination, University of York, 2001.
4. Munikrishnan V, Gillams AR, Lees WR, Vaizey CJ, Boulos PB. Prospective study comparing multislice CT colonography with colonoscopy in the detection of colorectal cancer and polyps. Dis Colon Rectum 2003;46:1384–90.
5. Gluecker TM, Johnson CD, Wilson LA, Maccarty RL, Welch TJ, Vanness DJ, et al. Extracolonic findings at CT colonography: evaluation of prevalence and cost in a screening population. Gastroenterology 2003;124:911–6.
6. Robinson P, Burnett H, Nicholson DA. The use of minimal preparation computed tomography for the primary investigation of colon cancer in frail or elderly patients. Clin Radiol 2002;57:389–92.
7. Rajapaksa R, Macari M, Bini EJ. Prevalence and impact of extracolonic findings in patients undergoing CT colonography. Am J Gastroenterol 2002;97(Suppl. 1):S111–2.
8. Edwards JT, Wood CJ, Mendelson RM, Forbes GM. Extracolonic findings at virtual colonoscopy: implications for screening programs. Am J Gastroenterol 2001;96: 3009–12.
9. Dachman AH, Kuniyoshi JK, Boyle CM, Samara Y, Hoffmann KR, Rubin DT, et al. CT colonography with three-dimensional problem solving for detection of colonic polyps. AJR Am J Roentgenol 1998;171:989–95.
10. Hara AK, Johnson CD, Maccarty RL, Welch TJ. Incidental extracolonic findings at CT colonography. Radiology 2000;215:353–7.
11. Morrin MM, Kruskal JB, Farrell RJ, Goldberg SN, McGee JB, Raptopoulos V. Endoluminal CT colonography after an incomplete endoscopic colonoscopy. AJR Am J Roentgenol 1999;172:913–8.
12. Ginnerup PB, Rosenkilde M, Christiansen TE, Laurberg S. Extracolonic findings at computed tomography colonography are a challenge. Gut 2003;52:1744–7.
13. Pickhardt PJ, Choi JR, Hwang I, Butler JA, Puckett ML, Hildebrandt HA, et al. Computed tomographic virtual colonoscopy to screen for colorectal neoplasia in asymptomatic adults. N Engl J Med 2003;349:2191–200.
14. Miao YM, Amin Z, Healy J, Burn P, Murugan N, Westaby D, et al. A prospective single centre study comparing computed tomography pneumocolon against colonoscopy in the detection of colorectal neoplasms. Gut 2000;47: 832–7.
15. Domjan J, Blaquiere R, Odurny A. Is minimal preparation computed tomography comparable with barium enema in elderly patients with colonic symptoms? Clin Radiol 1998;53:894–8.
16. Day JJ, Freeman AH, Coni NK, Dixon AK. Barium enema or computed tomography for the frail elderly patient? Clin Radiol 1993;48:48–51.
17. Pineau BC, Manus S, Phillips K, Chen GJ, Mikulaninec C, Han P, et al. Prevalence of extracolonic findings at virtual colonoscopy. Am J Gastroenterol 2003;98(Suppl. 1):S117.
18. Hara A, Leighton JA, Sharma V, Heigh RI. CT colonography with IV contrast: colon polyp enhancement and improved evaluation of extracolonic findings. Gastroenterology 2003;124(Suppl.):A114.
19. Hara AK, Leighton JA. CT colonography with IV contrast: Improved evaluation of intra and extracolonic findings. Radiology 2002;225(Suppl.):223.
20. Hellstrom M, Svensson MH, Lasson A. Extracolonic and incidental findings on CT colonography (virtual colonoscopy). AJR Am J Roentgenol 2004;182:631–8.
21. Hopper KD, Khandelwal M, Thompson C. CT colonoscopy: experience of 100 cases using volumetric rendering. Proceedings of SPIE 2001:489–94.
22. The Breast Screening Frequency Trail Group. The frequency of breast cancer screening: results from the UKCCCR Randomised Trial. Eur J Cancer 2002;38:1458–64.
23. Bell R, Petticrew M, Luengo S, Sheldon TA. Screening for ovarian cancer: a systematic review. Health Technol Assessment 1998;2:15–31.
24. Lieberman DA, Weiss DG, Bond JH, Ahnen DJ, Garewal H, Chejfec G, et al. Use of colonoscopy to screen asymptomatic adults for colorectal cancer. N Engl J Med 2000;343:162–8.
25. Ries LAG, Eisner MP, Kosary CL, Hankey BF, Miller BA, Clegg L, et al (editors). SEER Cancer Statistics Review, 1975–2000, National Cancer Institute. Bethesda, MD, 2003. http://seer.cancer.gov/csr/1975_2000/
26. Miller AB, Yurgalevitch S, Weissfeld JL. Prostate, Lung, Colorectal, Ovarian Cancer Screening Trial Project Team. Death review process in the Prostate, Lung, Colorectal and Ovarian (PLCO) Cancer Screening Trial. Control Clin Trials 2000;21(6 Suppl.):400S–6S.

Appendix 1: Search strategy for electronic databases and hand search run in March 2004

Pubmed

• Text terms used and the corresponding number of papers retrieved:

Search	Terms	Result
#1	Colonography	350
#2	Virtual colonoscopy	322
#3	Colography	19
#4	CT colonoscopy	723
#5	Virtual endoscopy	713
#6	CT pneumocolon	10
#7	CT OR computed tomography OR computerized tomography	213591
#8	#1 OR #2 OR #3 OR #4 OR #5 OR #6 OR #7	213960
#9	Extracolonic findings	288
#10	#8 AND #9	35
#11	Extracolonic lesions	82
#12	#8 AND #11	14
#13	Incidental findings	824
#14	Colon OR colonic OR colorectal	145371
#15	#8 AND #13 AND #14	6
#16	Incidental lesions	926
#17	#8 AND #14 AND #16	9

• We obtained in total 64 papers from searches in Pubmed. We then removed the duplicate titles from each search, which resulted in the retrieval of 43 different papers.

Other electronic databases searched

• We also repeated the searches in the following databases:

Databases	Result
ISI Web of Knowledge	23
EMBASE	9
OVID	10
ScienceDirect	9
Cochrane database	0

• Six papers overlapped across the four databases, providing a yield of 36 papers from these searches.

Hand searched following relevant journals

Gastroenterology. Diseases of the Colon and Rectum. The American Journal of Gastroenterology. Radiology. British Journal of Radiology. European Journal of Radiology. European Radiology. (from January 2003 to February 2004).

Conference proceedings handsearched

• Boston Medical Center. Proceedings of the Fourth International Symposium of Virtual Colonoscopy, Boston, USA. 13–15 October 2003.

• American College of Gastroenterology. Proceedings of the 68th Annual Scientific Meeting of the American College of Gastroenterology, Baltimore, USA. 13–15 October 2003.

• American College of Gastroenterology. Proceedings of the 67th Annual Scientific Meeting of the American College of Gastroenterology, Washington, USA. 20–23 October 2002.

• ASCRS. Proceedings of the meeting of the American-Society-of-Colon-and-Rectal-Surgeons, New Orleans, LO, USA. 21–26 June 2003.

• ASCRS. Proceedings of the meeting of the American-Society-of-Colon-and-Rectal-Surgeons, Chicago, IL, USA. 03–09 June 2002.

• AGA. Digestive Disease Week 2003 Meeting. Proceedings of the 104th Annual Meeting of the American-Gastroenterological-Association. Orlando, FL, USA. 17–22 May 2003.

• AGA. Proceedings of the Annual Meeting of the American-Gastroenterological-Association. San Francisco, CA, USA. 19–22 May 2002.

• AGA. Digestive Disease Week 2001 Meeting. Proceedings of the 102nd Annual Meeting of the American-Gastroenterological-Association. Atlanta, GA, USA. 20–23 May 2001.

• RSNA. Proceedings of the 89th Scientific Assembly and Annual Meeting of the Radiological-Society-of-North-America. Chicago, IL, USA. 30 November – 05 December 2003.

• RSNA. Proceedings of the 88th Scientific Assembly and Annual Meeting of the Radiological-Society-of-North-America. Chicago, IL, USA. 01–06 December 2002.

• RSNA. Proceedings of the 87th Scientific Assembly and Annual Meeting of the Radiological-Society-of-North-America. Chicago, IL, USA. 25–30 November 2001.

• RSNA. Proceedings of the 86th Scientific Assembly and Annual Meeting of the Radiological-Society-of-North-America. Chicago, IL, USA. 26 November–01 December 2000.

• European Congress of Radiology. ECR 2003 Conference, Vienna, Austria, 07–11 Mar 2003.

• ECR. Proceedings of the 14th Annual Meeting of the European Congress of Radiology. Vienna, Austria. 01–04 March 2002.

• ECR. Proceedings of the 13th Annual Meeting of the European Congress of Radiology. Vienna, Austria. 02–06 March 2001.

The British Journal of Radiology, *78* (2005), 30–33
DOI: 10.1259/bjr/68274086

Enlarged mesenteric lymph nodes in asymptomatic children: the value of the finding in various imaging modalities

[1]V RATHAUS, MD, [1]M SHAPIRO, MD, [2]M GRUNEBAUM, MD and [1]R ZISSIN, MD

[1]*Department of Diagnostic Imaging, Sapir Medical Center affiliated to Sackler Medical School, Tel-Aviv University, Tel-Aviv and* [2]*Veteran Paediatric Radiologist, Kfar Saba, Israel*

Abstract. The purpose of this study was to determine the prevalence of enlarged mesenteric lymph nodes in asymptomatic children. We prospectively studied 189 consecutive asymptomatic children from the outpatients' nephrological clinics who were referred for abdominal ultrasound. For comparison, we retrospectively reviewed the abdominal CT studies of 99 children, performed following blunt abdominal trauma. The children of both groups were divided into four subgroups according to their ages. The size, the number and the morphology of mesenteric lymph nodes were assessed. On abdominal ultrasound, enlarged mesenteric lymph nodes were detected in 55 of 189 asymptomatic children (29.1%). The longitudinal diameter of the lymph nodes ranged between 5 mm and 19 mm. These lymph nodes were arranged in clusters (three to nine in number in a cluster). All the lymph nodes were oval-shaped, flattened, and without any discomfort following graded transducer compression. On abdominal CT, enlarged mesenteric lymph nodes were diagnosed in 28 of the 99 children (28.3%). These lymph nodes measured more than 5 mm and were arranged in clusters (three or more in number). In seven of these children associated minimal mural thickening of the terminal ileum was seen. The presence of enlarged mesenteric lymph nodes in asymptomatic children of all ages and in both sexes is a common, non-specific finding and should be evaluated only in the appropriated clinical context.

The ultrasound identification of mesenteric lymph nodes (MLNs) in children with acute abdominal trauma is considered an incidental, non-specific finding, especially when the examination is performed with graded compression [1]. Enlarged MLNs are often seen in children with mesenteric lymphadenitis, but may also be found in asymptomatic children [1–4]. The prevalence of such enlarged lymph nodes in asymptomatic children has rarely been assessed [1–3].

We have examined prospectively the prevalence of enlarged MLNs in asymptomatic children, who underwent an abdominal ultrasound examination for follow-up of renal pathologies and we wish to report our experience with these cases. In addition, we reviewed retrospectively the prevalence of enlarged MLNs in children who had abdominal CT examination for abdominal trauma and were otherwise symptom free. The results of these two groups have been compared.

Material and methods

We evaluated two separate groups of children.

Group 1

This group was a prospective cohort of 189 consecutive children from the outpatient nephrological clinics (126 boys and 63 girls), whose ages ranged from 1 month to 16 years (mean age 4.8 years). The children were referred for an elective abdominal ultrasound between 1 January, 2003 and 30 June, 2003 for a variety of urological or developmental conditions. All were asymptomatic at the time of the examination, and had negative urine culture. Indications for the ultrasound examination are summarized in Table 1.

All studies were performed by a paediatric radiologist (VR) with a 7–12 MHz linear transducer HDI 5000 SonoCT ATL (Philips, Israel). Oblique, transverse, and longitudinal scans of the lower abdomen were obtained by means of the graded ultrasound compression technique, described by Puylaert [5]. No fasting was required for the examinations.

Group 2

This group consisted of a cohort of 99 children who underwent an abdominal and pelvic CT after sustaining blunt abdominal trauma between the years 1998 and 2002. This group of otherwise healthy children prior to the examination included 77 boys and 22 girls with an age

Table 1. Indications for ultrasound examination in 189 children

Indication	Number of children
Follow-up of vesicoureteral reflux	73
Follow-up of pre-natal enlargement of the collecting system	48
Kidney anomalies (MCDK, cyst, ectopia, single kidney)	30
Enuresis	15
Miscellaneous (precocious puberty, spina bifida, ear tag, supernumerary nipples, single umbilical artery)	23

MCDK, multicystic dysplastic kidney.

Received 17 March 2003 and in final form 6 August 2004, accepted 17 September 2004.

Table 2. The site of abdominal trauma diagnosed by CT. (In most cases more than one organ was involved)

Site of trauma	Number of cases
Spleen	46
Kidney	24
Liver	18
Intestine	14
Bladder	3
Pancreas	2
Normal	6

ranging between 1 year and 18 years (mean age 9.7 years). Table 2 summarizes the site of the abdominal injuries diagnosed by CT.

The CT studies were performed with one of two scanners: a conventional non-helical (Elscint 2400 Elite; Philips) with a slice collimation ranging from 5 mm to 10 mm and at 5–10 mm interval (depending on the age and the size of the child); or by a helical CT (Picker Mx Twin-flash) using a slice collimation of either 5.5 mm or 8 mm with a reconstruction interval of 5–6 mm, from the diaphragm down to the symphysis pubis. All patients received diluted water-soluble contrast material orally. Intravenous, non-ionic contrast of Ultravist (Iopromide, Schering, Germany) (2–3 ml kg^{-1}) was injected by bolus. All CT examinations were reviewed retrospectively by two radiologists (VR and RZ).

The children of both groups were divided into four subgroups according to their ages and gender at the time of the study: 0–1 years, 2–6 years, 7–10 years, 11–15 years.

The definition of enlarged MLNs was based on the following criteria:

1. On ultrasound: a lymph node with a longitudinal diameter of more than 4 mm and in a cluster of at least 3 nodes [1];
2. On CT: a node measuring 5 mm or more, and appearing in a cluster of three or more glands located in the small bowel mesentery or in the right lower quadrant (RLQ) [6].

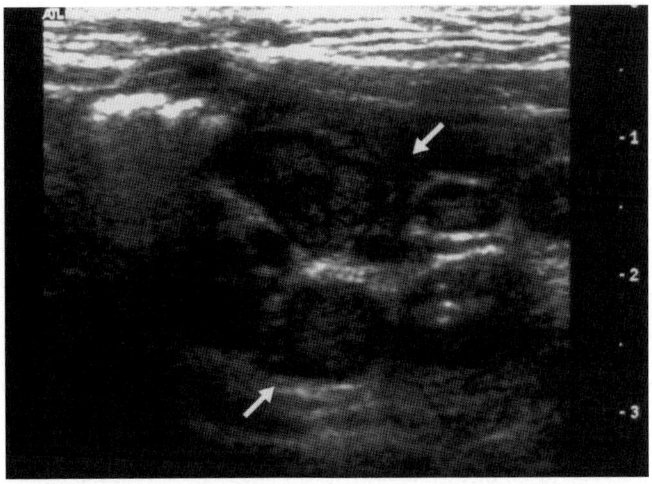

Figure 1. A 9-year-old child referred for an abdominal ultrasound for a single kidney follow-up. An abdominal ultrasound at the right lower quadrant: transverse view shows a cluster of four enlarged lymph nodes (arrows).

Statistical analysis

We analysed the differences of the prevalence of enlarged MLNs between the two groups, and in the different age subgroups using the chi squared test on SPSS for Windows (SPSS Inc., Chicago, IL).

Results

Group 1

Enlarged MLNs were detected in 55 of the 189 asymptomatic children (29.1%), 33 males and 22 females. The longitudinal diameter of the lymph nodes ranged between 5 mm and 19 mm and the number of the enlarged nodes seen in a cluster varied between three and nine (Figure 1). Tables 3 and 4 summarize the number and size of the MLNs detected by ultrasound per age subgroup. All

Table 3. The number of MLNs detected by ultrasound in the age subgroups

Age (years)	No. of children	No. of negative examinations	No. of lymph nodes found in positive examinations		% of the positive examinations
			3–4	>5	
0–1	27	25	2		7.4
2–6	91	61	22	8	33
7–10	39	22	7	10	43.6
11–15	32	26	2	4	29.1

MLNs, mesenteric lymph nodes.

Table 4. Size of MLNs detected by ultrasound in the age subgroups

Age (years)	No. of positive children	Size of lymph nodes				
		<5 mm	5–8 mm	>15 mm	9–11 mm	12–14 mm
0–1	2/27		1	1		
2–6	30/91		20	8	2	
7–10	17/39	2	5	6	3	1
11–15	6/32		2	2		2

MLNs, mesenteric lymph nodes.

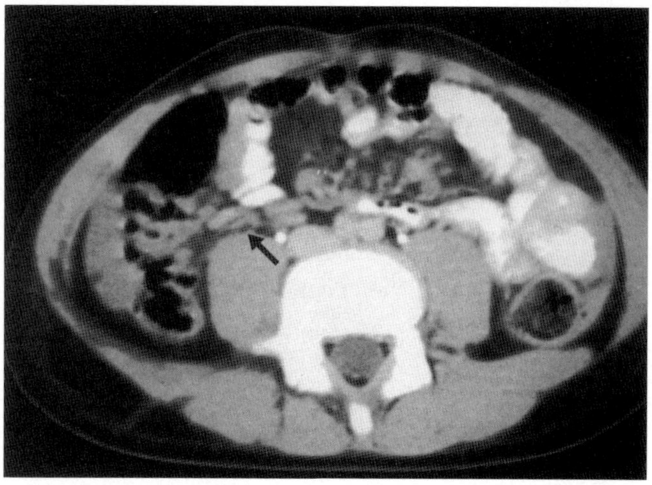

Figure 2. An 8-year-old boy after motor vehicle accident. Contrast-enhanced CT at level of the upper pelvis shows a cluster of lymph nodes (arrows) are seen in right lower quadrant mesentery.

the lymph nodes were oval-shaped and flattened following graded compression. No discomfort was elicited during the transducer compression. The enlarged nodes were mainly located in the RLQ, lateral and/or anterior to the right common iliac vessels or at the level of the inferior vena cava bifurcation. The presence of enlarged MLNs was significantly higher in children aged between 2 years and 10 years (p=0.006). No significant gender difference was noted in the presence, number or size of the detected nodes.

Group 2

Enlarged MLNs were diagnosed in 28 of the 99 children (28.3%) who underwent abdominal CT (Figure 2). 20 were males and 8 females. Table 5 summarizes the number of MLNs per age group detected by CT. In seven children a minimal mural thickening (<5 mm) of the terminal ileum was also seen. In all patients the appendix was normal. In 6 of 99 children no traumatic findings were detected on the CT. In 3 of 6 cases, MLNs were enlarged, and in one of them minimal mural thickening of the terminal ileum was also seen. 14 patients suffered from injury of the intestine and omentum, in five of them enlargement of the MLNs was detected, and in two cases, associated with minimal thickening of the terminal ileum.

Table 5. Numbers of the examinations with enlarged MLNs detected by CT in the age subgroups

Age (years)	No. of children	No. of negative examinations	No. of positive examinations	% of positive examinations
0–1	2	1	1	50%
2–6	24	16	8	30%
7–10	21	12	9	30%
11–15	52	42	10	19%

MLNs, mesenteric lymph nodes.

Discussion

Nowadays, the improvement of the ultrasound equipment has increased the detection rate of MLNs and mesenteric lymphadenopathy is a common ultrasound finding in children with acute, chronic and/or recurrent abdominal pain [1, 2, 4]. Enlargement of MLNs is often related to primary mesenteric adenitis, frequently caused by viral infection, *Yersinia enterocolitica* or *Yersinia pseudotuberculosis* infections [5]. Primary mesenteric adenitis is believed to occur more frequently in children than in adults [6]. This is a clinical entity related to a benign inflammation of the lymph nodes in the bowel mesentery, usually within the RLQ, without an identifiable acute inflammatory process or with mild (<5 mm) mural thickening of the terminal ileum [6, 7]. In these patients the clinical presentation is non-specific including abdominal pain, fever and leukocytosis mimicking a broad spectrum of different clinical diagnoses, such as acute appendicitis, infectious enterocolitis and pyelonephritis [1, 8].

Mesenteric lymphadenopathy may also be secondary to a detectable or known intra-abdominal inflammatory process such as acute appendicitis, Crohns' disease or systemic lupus erythematosis [6].

Enlargement of MLNs, however, may also be detected in asymptomatic children [1–4]. In our series we have found such enlarged nodes in 28.3–29.1% of asymptomatic children examined by CT or ultrasound, respectively, who had neither antecedent abdominal complaints nor tenderness during graded compression on ultrasound. This finding had the greatest prevalence in the age group between 2 years and 10 years old without a gender predilection. These lymph nodes were all smaller than 20 mm, elliptical in shape, and demonstrated no tenderness during compression. When these characteristics were present, it is more feasible to assume that these nodes represent a non-pathological finding [2]. The most common location is around the iliac vessels. Since this region also involves lymphatic drainage from the lower limb, the significance of enlarged lymph nodes in this area may not only be related to abdominal pathology. Watanabe et al [2] also detected enlarged ileocecal lymph nodes in asymptomatic children examined by ultrasound, with a slightly lower incidence (26 of the 122 cases; 21%). In addition, they found that the shape and the size of the detected lymph nodes, as well as their tenderness, during compression, could be used as an imaging criterion for distinguishing normal from pathological lymphadenopathy [2]. Healy and Graham [3] also reported that the size of the lymph nodes and their number appeared to play an important role in differentiating normal from pathological MLNs. Different results were reported by Sivit et al [1], using the same measurement criteria as ourselves, and Vayner et al [4], using the measurement criteria of Puylaert [5], who observed enlarged MLNs only rarely in asymptomatic children (4% and 9%, respectively).

We found enlarged MLNs in 28.3% of the asymptomatic children who underwent abdominal and pelvic CT after sustaining abdominal trauma. These results are in contrast to those reported by Macari et al [6] who found no enlarged MLNs in any of 60 adult patients examinated after abdominal trauma by CT.

In conclusion, our data suggest that the presence of enlarged MLNs with a longitudinal diameter of more than 4 mm but less than 20 mm in children of all ages and both sexes is a relatively common non-specific and usually non-pathological finding.

References

1. Sivit CJ, Newman KD, Chandra RS. Visualization of enlarged lymph nodes at US examination. Pediatr Radiol 1993;23:471–5.
2. Watanabe M, Ishii E, Hirowatari Y, Hayashida Y, Koga T, Akazawa K, et al. Evaluation of abdominal lymphadenopathy in children by ultrasonography. Pediatr Radiol 1997;27:860–4.
3. Healy MV, Graham PM. Assessment of abdominal lymph nodes in a normal paediatric population: an ultrasound study. Australian Radiol 1993;37:171–2.
4. Vayner N, Coret A, Polliack G, Weiss B, Hertz M. Mesenteric lymphadenopathy in children examinated by US for chronic and/or recurrent abdominal pain. Pediatr Radiol 2003;33:864–7.
5. Puylaert JB. Mesenteric adenitis and acute terminal ileitis. US evaluation using graded compression. Radiology 1986;161:691–5.
6. Macari M, Hines J, Balthazar E, Megibow A. Mesenteric adenitis: CT diagnosis of primary versus secondary causes, incidence and clinical significance in pediatric and adult patients. AJR Am J Roentgenol 2002;178:853–8.
7. Rao PM, Rhea JT, Novelline RA. CT diagnosis of mesenteric adenitis. Radiology 1997;202:145–7.
8. Birnbaum BA, Jeffrey RB Jr. CT and sonographic evaluation of acute right lower quadrant pain. AJR Am J Roentgenol 1998;170:361–73.

The British Journal of Radiology, 78 (2005), 34–38
DOI: 10.1259/bjr/79694026

Radiation risk and cost-benefit analysis of a paediatric radiology procedure: results from a national study

[1]H B L PETTERSSON, PhD, [2]K FÄLTH-MAGNUSSON, MD, PhD, [1,3]J PERSLIDEN, PhD and [4]M SCOTT, PhD

[1]*Department of Radiation Physics, IMV and* [2]*Department of Paediatrics, IMK, Faculty of Health Science, University of Linköping, S-581 85 Linköping, Sweden,* [3]*Department of Medical Physics, Örebro University Hospital, S-701 85 Örebro, Sweden and* [4]*Department of Statistics, University of Glasgow, Glasgow G12 8QW, UK*

Abstract. A national study was performed to investigate radiation doses and associated risks to patients during X-ray fluoroscopy-guided small intestinal biopsies in the investigation of coeliac disease. Thermoluminescent dosemeters (TLD) and questionnaires were sent to 42 of the 43 paediatric departments in Sweden performing these biopsies. During the study period (2×3 weeks) 257 biopsies were recorded, representing about 10% of annually performed paediatric investigations. The results show that the absorbed dose during biopsy ranged from 0.04 mGy to 23.8 mGy (mean 1.87 mGy). The fluoroscopy time ranged from 2 s to 663 s (mean 60 s). The collective dose from the procedure amounts to 4.7 manSv year^{-1}. Thus, the annual excess cancer mortality, including severe hereditary effects, can be estimated at 0.6–0.7 cases per year. However, significant dose saving can be obtained by proper choice of sedation and biopsy equipment.

Several studies have been performed on dose and related risk to the patient from different diagnostic radiological procedures. The vast majority of these studies have concerned adult patients. However, the risk of lethal cancer from radiation exposure of children is expected to be 2–4 times higher than for adults per dose unit [1, 2]. The reason for this difference is not fully clear, but greater cell proliferation rate and longer life expectancy for children both result in a higher risk of developing late effects. Therefore, initiatives have been taken among radiation protection authorities [3–5] to give priority to investigations of dose levels and frequencies of X-ray examinations among children. The main objective is to establish recommendations of upper dose limits for various diagnostic procedures and to implement minimum requirements for equipment standards [6].

In a previous study [7] we measured the radiation dose and assessed the associated long-term risk of paediatric small intestinal biopsies performed at our hospital during a 10-year period. In a follow-up study, performed in co-operation with a neighbouring hospital [8], we found considerably lower radiation doses associated with their biopsy investigations. This urged us to extend our investigations to a national study to obtain extensive information on this diagnostic procedure, including information about equipment and the resulting radiation dose to assess the potential for dose reduction. A full report of patient absorbed doses and fluoroscopy times was published elsewhere [9].

In this study we examined parameters such as (i) X–ray equipment; (ii) sedation techniques; (iii) capsule device; (iv) examination frequency, with the purpose of identifying their importance for the dose and associated risk to the patient, and from a cost-benefit point of view to suggest optimal examination conditions.

Received 6 May 2003 and in final form 4 August 2004, accepted 18 August 2004.
This work was supported by grants (#SSI 815/94) from the Swedish Radiation Protection Authority.

Material and methods

Dose measurements

All Swedish paediatric departments that performed small intestinal biopsies were invited to participate in a co-operative study, and 42 out of 43 units accepted. The study was approved by the Paediatric Section of Gastroenterology and Nutrition and performed under the consent of the Swedish Paediatric Association. The dose measurements were carried out during two periods of 3 weeks each in 1992. Dosemeters were sent by mail and returned after each irradiation, and the measurements were performed by $Li_2B_4O_7$ thermoluminescence dosimetry. Two $Li_2B_4O_7$ chips were placed together in thin plastic bags for each dosemeter. Four dosemeters were each placed on the anterior and posterior side of the trunk in the area of irradiation. Reproducible positioning of the dosemeters was ensured by providing dosemeters fixed in plastic bags, with paper backing and pre-cut circles for the umbilicus, and a drawing marked out for the spine. The thickness of each child was measured at the umbilical level, with the child lying supine. This measure is entered in the calculations of the absorbed dose.

The absorbed doses, D [Gy], were calculated as the mean absorbed dose in the irradiated volume from the anterior and posterior dosemeter readings according to methods previously reported [7]. Based on the reported number of biopsies and the calculated average of all absorbed doses, the annual collective effective dose, E_c [Sv] for this procedure in Sweden could be evaluated.

In addition, all participating departments were asked to report the conditions of their examinations, *i.e.* method of sedation, type of biopsy capsule, type of X-ray equipment and exposure conditions (fluoroscopic time, image system sensitivity and age, image memory, grid ratio, distance focus spot–image intensifier surface).

We chose to study the conditions at each paediatric unit, and not ask for the identity of each paediatrician performing the biopsy procedure, since we feared that this would have significantly decreased the participation in the study.

Cancer risk assessment

The cancer risk due to radiation exposure, *e.g.* expressed as the cancer excess lifetime mortality risk (CELMR), is well documented. BEIR-V [2] give estimates of CELMR for exposure of different age groups; the unisex CELMR of radiation exposure at high dose rate at 5 years of age being 0.14 per Sv whole body dose (effective dose).

Fluoroscopy during coeliac biopsy does not correspond to a whole-body exposure situation, *i.e.* it affects only a limited part of the body (lungs, liver, spleen, kidneys, bladder, digestive system). However, if we examine the relative sensitivity of the different organs (using tissue weighting factors, w_t) [1] we find that most of the "high-risk" organs are exposed, which means that the risk factor is not significantly overestimated. One could of course argue that the chosen values of w_t do not explicitly reflect the relative sensitivity of organs in children. However, recent work [10] indicates that significant differences in these factors between children and adults are not to be expected.

Loss of life expectancy

The reduction of life expectancy is the mathematical expectation of the loss of lifetime due to accidents, diseases, exposure of pollutants etc. In this context we use this concept of loss of life expectancy (LLE) to evaluate the effect of radiation exposure [1]. It is calculated from the relationship: $\mathrm{LLE}=R\times Y$, where R is the attributal lifetime probability of death, *i.e.* here equal to CELMR, and Y is the mean loss of lifetime if the radiation exposure is the cause of death. The LLE concept is only applicable to exposure of a cohort to estimate the collective loss of lifetime, *i.e.* for the individual the LLE is either zero or Y. In our assessment, we assume a mean loss of lifetime of 40–70 years if the fluoroscopic radiation causes cancer death, to account for both cancers with relatively short latency period, *i.e.* leukaemia, thyroid cancer and those with longer latency period. This gives the following equation:

$$\mathrm{LLE}=R\times Y=0.14\,\mathrm{Sv}^{-1}\times Y\,(40-70\text{ years})=$$

$$5-10\text{ year per Sv}=2-4\text{ days per mSv.}$$

Generally speaking, when diagnostic radiological procedures are used, the practice should produce a net benefit for the patient, *i.e.* the risk attributed to radiation should be much smaller than the diagnostic benefit for the patient, a concept known as "justification of the practice" [11]. In most situations the net benefit is easily obtained. In addition, all exposures shall be kept as low as reasonably achievable, a radiation protection concept known as the ALARA principle [11]. Thus, for a given procedure, a cost-benefit analysis, which establishes optimum levels of radiation protection for the patient, should be performed. The action taken depends on the exposure situation. In diagnostic radiology it could involve introduction of different radiation shields, proper choice of diagnostic procedure and equipment and adequate training of personnel. The cost to society of a lost life is taken into consideration and could be expressed as a monetary value, α. The actual value of α is not fixed since it depends on decisions made at a national level. For the Nordic countries, the Nordic radiation protection authorities advocate that up to US $100 000 would be a reasonable amount to spend for reducing the collective dose by 1 manSv [12].

Results and discussion

Number of biopsies and age of the children

The total number of biopsies performed during the 6 week study period was 257 (130 in the spring period and 127 in the autumn). This frequency (an average of 43 biopsies per week) corresponds rather well with the information previously received in a national questionnaire, reporting a total of 2500 small intestinal biopsies per year (48 biopsies/week). As both central, regional and university hospitals perform these examinations, the number of biopsies performed per clinic showed great variation; from 0 to 18. This introduces a risk of bias when results from different clinics are compared.

The age of the children ranged from 0.2 years to 18.7 years, showing a skewed distribution. Normality was obtained by log transforming the data, resulting in a mean age of 2.7 years (95% CI: 2.4–3.1 years), compared with a median age of 2.5 years.

Dose results

Figure 1 shows the distribution of the absorbed doses. Large variations in dose, both between different departments and also within the same department, were observed. The departmental median absorbed doses ranged between 0.11 mGy and 14.4 mGy and the individual doses ranged between 0.04 mGy and 23.8 mGy (mean 1.87 mGy, median 0.69 mGy).

The corresponding range of fluoroscopy time was 2–663 s (mean 60 s, median 30 s), *i.e.* more than two orders of magnitude variability.

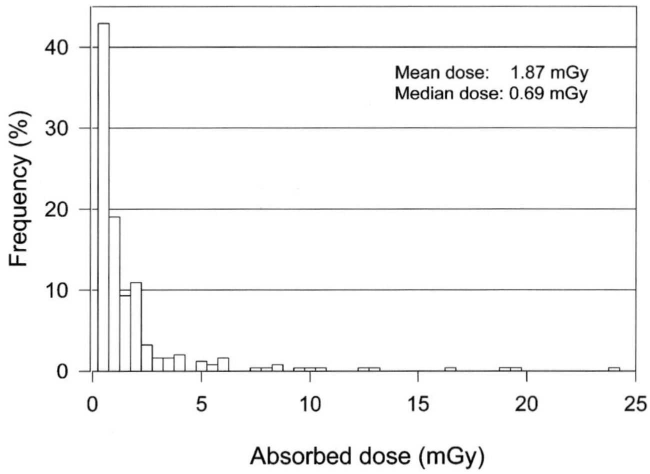

Figure 1. Frequency distribution of absorbed doses.

Cancer risk assessment

Based on the annual number of X-ray examinations for the investigation of paediatric coeliac disease in Sweden (2500), the annual collective dose derived from the individual doses is 2500×1.87 mSv=4.7 manSv. Accordingly, the annual number of excess lethal cancers per year in Sweden due to this procedure is 0.6–0.7 (4.7 Sv $\times$ 0.14 Sv^{-1}) and the collective annual LLE is 20–50 years (4.7 Sv $\times$ 5–10 years Sv^{-1}).

Exposure conditions and cost-benefit analysis

All the results on fluoroscopy time (t) and absorbed dose (D) obtained for the 257 biopsy examinations were tested statistically (standard parametric 1 and 2 sample t-tests, analysis of variance and regression methods) against the different examination conditions, *i.e.* X-ray equipment parameters (image system sensitivity and age, image memory, grid ratio, distance focus spot–image intensifier surface), sedation technique and the departmental experience (number of biopsies performed annually). Both the fluoroscopy time and absorbed dose data displayed clearly skewed and non-normal distributions. However normal distributions were obtained by log-transforming the data, for which parametric statistics were applied. Multiregression analysis was used initially to identify any linear relationships between t and D and the different variables. Only the relation to different sedation techniques was identified as strongly significant. However, due to the large number of variables and the rather limited number of departments (42) the result cannot exclude other significant variables.

Sedation

The paediatric units reported that they used one of three different levels of sedation: full anaesthesia, parenteral sedation or oral/rectal sedation. In full anaesthesia, intubation is used and ventilation is taken over (no spontaneous breathing). In parenteral sedation, the child is under deep sedation but has maintained spontaneous breathing. In oral/rectal sedation, the child is more superficially sedated.

24 of the 257 (9.3%) biopsies were performed with oral/rectal sedation, 188 of 257 (73.2%) by parenteral sedation and 35 of 257 (13.6%) by full anaesthesia. The dose distributions for the three sedation techniques used (Figure 2) were studied by two sample t-test. A significant difference was obtained both for (a) oral *vs* parenteral sedation (p=0.02, D(mean)=3.40 and 1.66 mSv, respectively) and (b) oral sedation *vs* full anaesthesia (p<0.00001, D(mean)=3.40 and 0.81 mSv, respectively), but parenteral sedation *vs* full anaesthesia showed a statistically non significant difference (p=0.15). Using a 95% confidence interval we can conclude that oral sedation results in 0.5–2.9 mSv higher dose than for parenteral sedation and 1.5–3.7 mSv higher dose than for full anaesthesia.

Thus, on a national basis, the collective doses can be reduced by changing sedation techniques. If instead of the oral/rectal sedation technique parenteral sedation or full anaesthesia were to be used, 0.12–0.67 manSv and 0.35–0.86 manSv, respectively, could be saved annually. If full anaesthesia were adopted at all clinics, the net gain would be 1–3 manSv annually. From a cost-benefit point of view, up to $100 000–300 000 US gross could thereby be spent annually to cover costs for changing sedation technique. The full anaesthesia procedure brings additional cost of personnel for surveillance of the patient. Information from the hospitals showed that the calculated additional cost of change of practice from oral sedation to full anaesthesia amounts to at least US $200–250 per patient. Thus, if full anaesthesia is adopted at all clinics, the total additional annual medical cost amounts to about US $500 000.

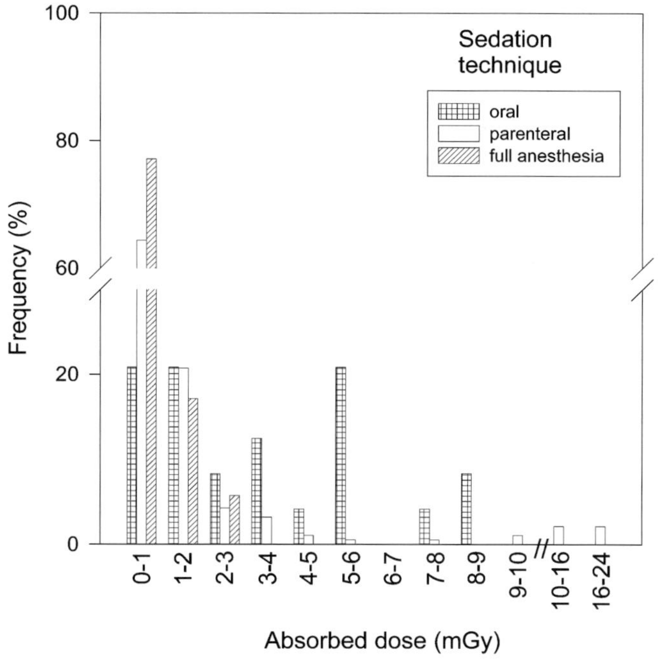

Figure 2. Frequency distributions of absorbed doses with sedation technique as parameter.

Hence, from a cost-benefit point of view, a change of sedation practice is not justified. However, according to the opinion of most paediatricians performing this procedure, full anaesthesia or parenteral sedation is considered far less traumatic for the child, which could justify a change of sedation practice. But, in daily life, the availability of staff at the anaesthetic unit may be a limiting factor for such change.

Image memory

Overall, 48.5% of the biopsy examinations were carried out with X-ray units equipped with image memory. In order to facilitate comparison in dose distribution between the two options, only the cases where parenteral sedation technique was used were considered. Of these investigations, 50% were performed with image memory and 50% without. No significant difference in the two dose distributions (Figure 3) was observed; p=0.90, D(mean)=1.38 and 1.32 mSv, respectively, *i.e.* from a cost-benefit point of view it does not seem worthwhile to change the current practice. However, if for example the investigation is performed in a teaching hospital, our experience is a 30% reduction in fluoroscopy time using image memory in the teaching situation.

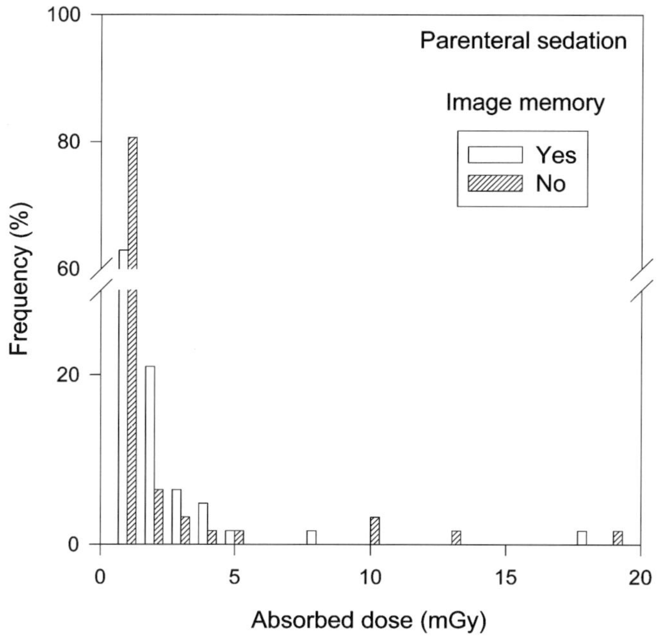

Figure 3. Frequency distribution of absorbed doses for X-ray equipment with and without image memory (only parenteral sedation cases shown).

Choice of biopsy capsule

Three types of biopsy capsule were used. The Crosby and Watson capsules are both one-port devices, giving only one chance to obtain a mucosal specimen, while the Storz capsule enables repeated firing, thereby decreasing the risk of a failure in the sampling. 76% of the investigations were performed with Watson capsule, 16% with Storz capsule and 8% with Crosby capsule. Figure 4 shows the frequency distributions of fluoroscopy times for the three options, clearly displaying skewed distributions. The mean fluoroscopy times, calculated on log-transformed data, and the median fluoroscopy times were: Watson capsule; t(mean)=37 s (95% CI: 32–44 s), and t(median)=36 s, Storz capsule; t(mean)=11 s (95% CI: 6–19 s) and t(median)=12 s, Crosby capsule; t(mean)=12 s (95% CI: 5–29 s) and t(median)=5 s. One-way analysis of variance (ANOVA) showed statistically significant differences ($p<0.001$) between the distributions of fluoroscopy times for Watson *vs* Storz capsule and for Watson *vs* Crosby capsule. The data show that at the 95% confidence level the use of the Crosby capsule results in 0.16 to 0.6 times lower fluoroscopy times compared with using the Watson capsule, and using the Storz capsule results in 0.17 to 0.5 times lower fluoroscopy times compared with using the Watson capsule. These results would suggest significant dose savings by changing from the use of the Watson capsule to the use of either the Crosby or Storz capsule. However, owing to the limited number of cases, 16 cases using the Crosby capsule and 34 cases using the Storz capsule, the risk of bias is clear, which makes an estimate of the cost-benefit uncertain. In recent years there has been a discussion on whether the endoscopic technique to obtain a biopsy is better than the peroral capsule technique [13–16]. The endoscopic technique is becoming more commonly used [15], but the capsule technique is still often used, making it important to optimize the conditions for its use.

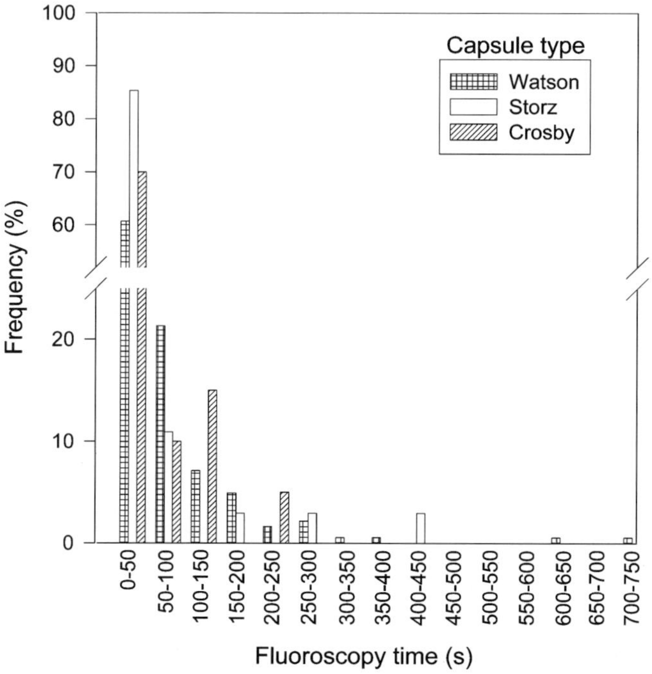

Figure 4. Frequency distribution of fluoroscopy times with biopsy device as parameter.

Age of patient

The age of the child may influence the degree of difficulty experienced in performing the biopsy procedure and thus the time needed for the procedure and the fluoroscopy time. However, analysis of the fluoroscopy and dose data for the different sedation techniques used, did not show any significant correlation with the age of children ($R^2<0.13$). In addition, correlation analysis of fluoroscopy time and child age data from individual hospitals, where the X-ray equipment, sedation technique and biopsy device is fixed, confirmed the lack of correlation ($R^2<0.03$).

Staff experience

The staff experience of the biopsy procedure is likely to influence the fluoroscopy time. The trend outlined in Figure 5 is however rather weak. Even so, one could argue that it could be beneficial to reduce the number of clinics performing this kind of procedure, thereby increasing the number of patients per clinic, *i.e.* maintaining staff experience. However, such changes may increase the cost of transportation and inconvenience for the patient. It was not possible to study the influence of experience at the individual level, *i.e.* how many biopsies per year were performed by each investigator.

X-ray equipment

It is often not possible to choose X-ray equipment at a radiology department. The best equipment should be chosen (low dose, good image quality, easy to operate), especially for paediatric radiology. It has been shown in colon examinations

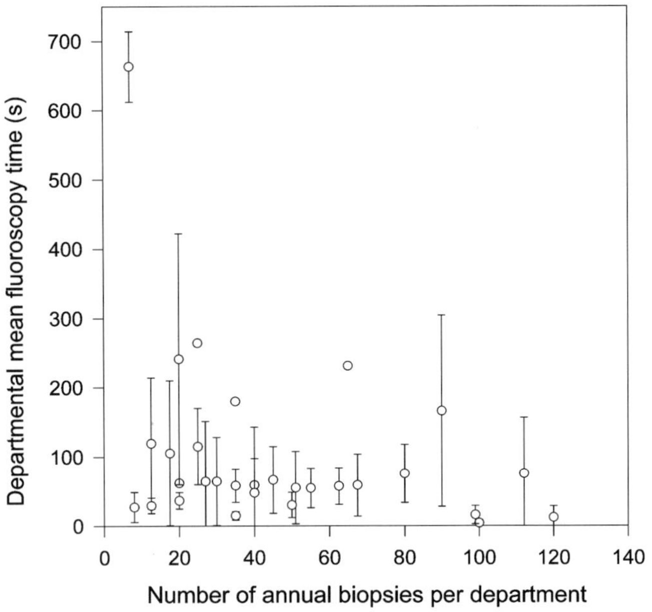

Figure 5. The departmental mean fluoroscopy time (±1 standard deviation) as a function of the number of annually performed biopsies (only parenteral sedation cases shown).

[17] that the KAP-value (kerma–area product=DAP-value (dose–area product)) to patients can be reduced by as much as 60% by a change from analogue fluoroscopy, including screen–film overview images, to digital equipment with pulsed fluoroscopy and exclusion of the large overview images. Pulsed fluoroscopy alone reduced the KAP-value by 30%. Unfortunately, in our study, we were not able to obtain information about the use of pulsed or non-pulsed fluoroscopy by individual radiologists/paediatricians.

Conclusions

Several factors influence the fluoroscopy time in paediatric small intestinal biopsies. X-ray units equipped with image memory represent an obvious advantage in teaching and training situations. The sedation technique was found to be an important aspect of this procedure as well as the choice of capsule. Since the biopsy device is not a part of the X-ray equipment, its importance may be overlooked and not taken into consideration in investigations of patient absorbed doses. The training of staff, reflected in the mean fluoroscopy time versus number of annual biopsies performed, did not have a great influence on patient exposures. However, the identities of the paediatricians were not revealed, which makes it impossible to evaluate the impact of personal experience. It could be hypothesized that it is more beneficial to study and learn the procedure at centres with optimized procedures than to perform many biopsies in a non-optimized manner. Taking the different steps in this X-ray investigation into consideration, it is possible to reduce the absorbed dose to the patient considerably. The general results shown here are likely to be important also in other types of paediatric X-ray examinations.

Acknowledgments

We gratefully acknowledge the cooperation of the staff at paediatric and radiation physics units at the participating hospitals.

References

1. ICRP 60. International Commission on Radiological Protection. 1990 Recommendations of the International Commission on Radiological Protection. Oxford: Pergamon Press, 1990.
2. BEIR-V. Committee on the Biological Effects of Ionizing Radiations. Health effects of exposure to low levels of ionizing radiation. BEIR V Report. Washington: National Academy Press, 1990.
3. Fendel H, Schneider K, Kohn M, Bakowski C. Specific principles for optimization of image quality and patient exposure in paediatric diagnostic imaging. BIR Report 20: Optimization of image quality and patient exposure in diagnostic radiology. London: BIR Press, 1989:91–101.
4. Schneider K, Fendel H, Bakawski C, Stein E, Kohn M, Kellner M, et al. Results of a dosimetry study in the European Community on frequent X-ray examinations in infants. Radiat Prot Dosimetry 1992;43:31–6.
5. Schneider K, Kohn M, Bakowski C, Stein E, Freidhof C, Horwitz AE, et al. Impact of radiographic imaging criteria on dose and image quality in infants in an EC-wide survey. Radiat Prot Dosimetry 1993;49:73–6.
6. European Guidelines on Quality Criteria for Diagnostic Radiographic Images in Paediatrics, EUR 16261. Luxembourg: Office of Official Publications of the European Communities, 1996.
7. Persliden J, Pettersson HBL, Fälth-Magnusson K. Small intestinal biopsy in children with coeliac disease: measurement of radiation dose and analysis of risk. Acta Paediatr 1993;82:296–9.
8. Persliden J, Pettersson HBL, Stenhammar L, Fälth-Magnusson K. Small intestinal biopsy of children with coeliac disease: the influence of X-ray equipment on radiation dose. Eur Radiol 1994;4:458–61.
9. Persliden J, Pettersson HBL, Fälth-Magnusson K. Intestinal biopsy in children with coeliac disease; a Swedish national study of radiation dose and risk. Acta Paediatr 1996;85:1042–6.
10. Almén A. Radiation dose to children in diagnostic radiology. Thesis. Malmö University Hospital, Lund University, 1995.
11. ICRP 42. International Commission on Radiological Protection. A compilation of the major concepts and quantities in use by the ICRP. Oxford: Pergamon Press, 1984.
12. News from SSI. Stockholm: National Radiation Protection Institute (SSI), 1991; 14. ISSN 0280-0357.
13. Branski D, Faber J, Freier S, Gottschalk-Sabag S, Shiner M. Histologic evaluation of endoscopic versus suction biopsies of small intestinal mucosae in children with and without coeliac disease. J Pediatr Gastroenterol Nutr 1998;27:6–11.
14. Magliocca FM, Bonamico M, Petrozza V, Danesi H, Liuzzi M, Velucci O, et al. Usefulness of endoscopic small intestinal biopsies in children with coeliac disease. Ital J Anat Embryol 2001;106 (2 Suppl 1):329–35.
15. Stenhammar L, Ascher H, Daniesson L, Dannaeus A, Hernell O, Ivarsson A, et al. Small bowel biopsy in Swedish paediatric clinics. Acta Paediatr 2002;91:1126–9.
16. Thomson M, Kitching P, Jones A, Walker-Smith JA, Phillips A. Are endoscopic biopsies of small bowel as good as suction biopsies for diagnosis of enteropathy? J Pediatr Gastroenterol Nutr 1999;29:438–41.
17. Sjöholm B, Andersson T, Jonsson B, Persliden P. Does digital radiology increase or decrease the dose to the patient? Svenska Läkarsällskapet Hygiea 1999;108/3:239. (In Swedish.)

The British Journal of Radiology, *78* (2005), 39–45
DOI: 10.1259/bjr/79023662

Measurement of cartilage volumes in rheumatoid arthritis using MRI

[1,2]S J GANDY, PhD, [3]A D BRETT, PhD, [4]P A DIEPPE, MD, FRCP, [1]M C KEEN, PhD, [5]R A MACIEWICZ, PhD, [3]C J TAYLOR, PhD, [6]J C WATERTON, PhD and [7]I WATT, MD, FRCR

[1]Department of Medical Physics & Bioengineering, Bristol General Hospital, Guinea Street, Bristol BS1 6SY, [2]Rheumatology Unit, University of Bristol Division of Medicine, Bristol Royal Infirmary, Bristol BS2 8HW, [3]Division of Imaging Sciences and Biomedical Imaging, University of Manchester, Stopford Building, Oxford Road, Manchester M13 9PT, [4]MRC Health Services Research, Canynge Hall, Whiteladies Road, Bristol BS8 2PR, [5]Respiratory and Inflammation Research, [6]Enabling Science Technology and Information, AstraZeneca, Alderley Park, Macclesfield, Cheshire SK10 4TG and [7]Department of Clinical Radiology, Bristol Royal Infirmary, Bristol BS2 8HW, UK

Abstract. MRI is a valuable imaging modality for assessment of the articular cartilage in rheumatoid arthritis (RA) and is potentially of use in monitoring disease progression and response to therapy. In this study, we investigated the sources of error in volume measurements obtained by segmentation of MR images of knee cartilage in patients with RA and followed cartilage volume in a group of RA patients for 12 months. 23 RA patient volunteers were recruited for knee imaging. Six subjects were imaged at baseline only, six were imaged at baseline and again within an hour in the same imaging session, six subjects were imaged at baseline and 7 days, and 17 subjects were imaged at baseline, 4 ± 2 months and 12 months. Imaging was performed at 1.0 T using a three-dimensional spoiled gradient-echo sequence with fat-suppression. Manual image segmentation was performed once or twice on the lateral tibial, medial tibial, patellar and femoral compartment by either one or two segmenters. Coefficients of variation (CoV) for repeated volume measurement of total cartilage were 2.2% (same segmenter, same scan), 5.2% (different segmenter, same scan), 4.9% (same segmenter, different scan, same session), and 4.4% (same segmenter, different scan, different session). Over the 12 month duration of the study there was no significant change in total cartilage volume, nor were there significant changes in volume in any individual compartment. This measurement technique is reproducible, but any net change in cartilage volume over 1 year is very small.

Rheumatoid arthritis (RA) is characterized by a chronic proliferative synovitis, or pannus, which leads to bone erosions and destruction of the underlying articular hyaline cartilage. Research on strategies to prevent destruction of the articular cartilage in arthritis requires reliable measurement of the clinical effectiveness of intervention. Disease activity in RA has been traditionally investigated by monitoring clinical indices of disease such as C-reactive protein (CRP) or erthyrocyte sedimentation rate (ESR), together with global assessment of joint pain and disability scores (*e.g.* Health assessment questionnaire (HAQ)) and characterization of damage to the tissues by radiographic scoring using Larsen or Sharp scores [1, 2]. The current gold-standard for *in vivo* assessment of change to hyaline cartilage is X-radiographic measurement of the joint space or interbone distance [3] but this technique provides only an indirect assessment of cartilage and lacks precision.

MRI is potentially of value in monitoring cartilage disease progression and response to therapy in arthritis. Considerable work has been published describing the methodology and validation of MRI cartilage volume measurements in healthy subjects [4, 5] and synthetic models [6], and also in models of arthritis in animals [7, 8] and osteoarthritis (OA) patient cohorts [9–12]. In RA, qualitative MRI methods have been employed to classify the stage of disease by clinically scoring the extent of synovial proliferation, together with scoring of cartilage lesions and bony erosions at the wrist and finger joints [13]. Quantitative MRI measurements of synovial joint effusion volumes and synovitis at the knee joint have also been reported [14, 15]. One report has appeared demonstrating a correlation between cartilage volume in RA patients, and Larsen grade, ESR, and CRP [16], however to our knowledge no data on reproducibility or progressive changes in cartilage volume in the knee in RA have been reported.

Volume assessment usually requires precise and accurate identification of the extent of the cartilage via the process of image segmentation. However, segmentation is technically challenging in the articular cartilage, because of the large surface area to volume ratio, the complex patterns of signal intensity variation exhibited even by normal cartilage using typical clinical MRI pulse sequences, and the additional complexity of the images in the presence of

Received 10 May 2004 and in revised form 12 August 2004, accepted 7 September 2004.

Current address for Dr Stephen J Gandy, Medical Physics Department, Ninewells Hospital, Dundee DD1 9SY, UK.

Current address for Dr A D Brett, Image Metrics plc, Regent House, Heaton Lane, Stockport SK4 1BS, UK.

Current address for Dr I Watt, Department of Radiology C2-S, Leids Universitair Medisch Centrum, Postbus 9600, 2300 RC Leiden, The Netherlands.

Grant sponsors: Medical Research Council, AstraZeneca, United Bristol Healthcare NHS Trust.

arthritis pathology. The complexity of cartilage MRI segmentation is further enhanced in RA due to the presence of pathological tissue such as joint effusion and pannus that are commonly found in the vicinity of the cartilage. Furthermore, widespread erosive damage to the cartilage is commonly observed in RA in contrast to other arthritides such as OA where damage to the cartilage is usually more focal.

The objective of this study was to quantify the various factors that influence the reproducibility of cartilage volume measurements in RA using MRI, and to explore the value of MRI in a 1-year follow-up study of RA patients.

Method and materials

Patients and imaging

Following the approval of the United Bristol Healthcare Trust Ethics Committee, 23 fully informed patient volunteers were recruited for imaging after providing written consent. Inclusion criteria were a diagnosis of RA together with knee pain plus one of joint line tenderness, an obvious effusion or soft tissue swelling. A full clinical assessment of each patient was performed by a Consultant Rheumatologist (PAD), and an individual knee was selected for imaging in each case. Imaging was performed on a 1.0 T clinical scanner ('Impact Expert'; Siemens, Erlangen, Germany) using a three-dimensional (3D) spoiled gradient-echo (FLASH) sequence with fat suppression. The imaging parameters used were: TR (sequence repetition time) 50 ms, TE (echo time) 11 ms, 40° nutation angle, and a 100 mm slice selection slab which generated 64 contiguous sagittal slices across the knee, each 1.56 mm thick. The image field-of-view in each case was 140 mm × 140 mm; images were acquired with 192 phase encode steps, and 256 frequency encode steps, and zero-filled to allow display on a 256 × 256 matrix. The displayed in-plane pixel resolution was 0.55 mm × 0.55 mm. An image time of 10 min (one signal average) was chosen, in order to minimize patient movement artefact. Previously, Morgan et al [17] established the reproducibility of this imaging protocol and found no relevant systematic differences in knee cartilage volume measurement from MR images acquired with this protocol using scanners at 1.0 T or 1.5 T.

Five substudies were performed (Table 1). The group in substudy 3 were scanned at baseline and again within an hour after cessation of knee weight-bearing without reimposition of weight-bearing. All patients were scanned during the middle of the day on each occasion.

Knee radiographs were acquired for substudy 5 at baseline and 12 months and were extended weight-bearing views. The precision of the X-ray measurement in this centre has previously been established [18–20]. Joint space narrowing (JSN) was measured at the mid-point of the medial tibiofemoral compartment using the graticule method as described by Lequesne [21].

Image analysis

After data acquisition, an image analysis package (Tosca; IBM, Winchester, UK) was used to segment all four hyaline cartilage compartments (femoral, medial tibial, lateral tibial and patellar) of one knee.

In previous studies with healthy joints [22], we employed a semi-automatic image segmentation technique in which the segmenter placed within the cartilage a seed point, which invoked a region-growing algorithm [23]. However, preliminary experience of segmentation for this patient population (some with advanced RA) using that method proved the semi-automated approach to be unreliable. In many cases the algorithm was incapable of distinguishing between genuine cartilage signal and surrounding soft tissue effusions. Consequently we elected to use a fully manual segmentation procedure. Manual segmentation was performed by two medical physicists familiar with MR images of the knee (SJG: Segmenter A and MCK: Segmenter B, details in Table 1) under the supervision of a musculoskeletal radiologist (IW). Femoral, patellar, medial tibial and lateral tibial cartilage segmentations were generated by enclosing all cartilage pixels within a region-of-interest (ROI) for each 2D image slice. Following careful checking and realignment of the ROI contour where necessary, the process was repeated for each image

Table 1. Study details

Substudy	Timepoints	Patients	Segmentation details
1. Reproducibility same segmenter, same scan	Baseline	N=6 (4M, 2F)	Twice by segmenter A
2. Reproducibility different segmenter, same scan	Baseline	N=6 (4M, 2F)	Once by segmenter A Once by segmenter B
3. Reproducibility same segmenter, same visit, different scan	Baseline $<$1 h	N=6 (3M, 3F)	Once for scan 1 by segmenter A Once for scan 2 by segmenter A
4. Reproducibility same segmenter, different visit, different scan	Baseline 1 week	N=6 (6F)	Once for visit 1 by segmenter A Once for visit 2 by segmenter A
5. Disease progression	Baseline 4$\pm$2 months 12 months	N=17 (8M, 9F)	Once for visit 1 by segmenter A Once for visit 2 by segmenter A Once for visit 3 by segmenter A

M, male; F, female.

slice until a cartilage compartment volume had been fully segmented. The process of segmenting an entire knee (four compartment segmentations) with thorough checking took approximately 4–5 h.

We calculated the volume of each segmentation by finding the area of each 2D ROI and multiplying by the slice thickness over all slices. The Tosca package uses a curve-fitting algorithm in order to interpolate a contour defining each 2D ROI. We found the area of each enclosed 2D ROI by using this curve-fitting algorithm and then re-sampling this interpolated curve with 1000 equally-spaced vertices to produce a dense polygon. The area of a polygon with n vertices (x_i, y_i) $\{i=0..n-1\}$ is then given by:

$$\text{Area}=0.5\sum_{i=0}^{n-1}\{x_i\cdot y_{(i+1)\text{mod}(n)}-y_i\cdot x_{(i+1)\text{mod}(n)}\} \quad (1)$$

In addition to the quantitative volume calculation, 3D volume images were reconstructed and displayed using the data visualization package DX data explorer (IBM, Winchester, UK).

Effect of image quality on reproducibility

Prior to segmentation, in order to assess the effect of image quality on reproducibility, both segmenters studied the quality of all patient images at all timepoints for evidence of movement artefact and "ease of segmentation". A score for movement artefact was recorded on a qualitative 1–5 scale, where 1=very sharp, 2=sharp, 3=fair, 4=blurred and 5=very blurred. Similarly, ease of segmentation was assessed by taking into account features such as cartilage structural integrity, osteophytes, synovitis and joint effusions. Ease of segmentation was scored on a qualitative 1–5 scale, where 1=very easy, 2=easy, 3=fair, 4=difficult and 5=very difficult.

Segmentation rules

In order to provide experimental consistency, both operators agreed upon a segmentation strategy for dealing with any potential pitfalls prior to the study. The common difficulties were agreed to be erosive loss of cartilage and identification of cartilage in regions of rheumatoid effusion or synovitis. During segmentation, care was taken to identify regions of cartilage thinning and lesions, *i.e.* regions of complete (or very nearly complete) loss. Any regions of cartilage associated with damaged bony surfaces were carefully examined before inclusion into (or exclusion from) the segmentation. Similarly, all regions of cartilage in close proximity to rheumatoid tissue were carefully reviewed, in order to ensure that only cartilage was included in the ROI.

Geometrical issues (*e.g.* partial volume effects) were also carefully considered before embarking upon segmentation. To avoid errors due to partial volume effects, each operator only segmented image slices where an articulating surface could be clearly defined. To aid segmenter interpretation of partial volume effects, a 3D model of the knee joint was provided for anatomical reference (Somso NS50; Adam Rouilly, Sittingbourne UK).

Statistical analysis of the data

Errors in measuring cartilage volumes may arise from many different experimental or physiological sources. Such errors can be assessed either through a single experiment with nested analysis of variance in which all possible sources of error are systematically varied, or through a series of experiments with pairwise comparison in which each possible source of error is varied in turn. The latter approach was adopted in this work. The reproducibility of each pairwise comparison was assessed from the test–retest coefficient of variation (CoV). For each subject, s, the CoV is the standard deviation, σ_s, for the two measurements on that subject, divided by the mean volume, μ_s, for the subject. The overall test–retest CoV for a group of N subjects is then

$$\sqrt{\sum_s\left(\frac{\sigma_s}{\mu_s}\right)^2/N} \quad (2)$$

Use of the CoV is most appropriate when σ_s is proportional to μ_s. If σ_s is independent of μ_s, it is appropriate to compare σ_s values directly. In this work it was found that σ_s increased with μ_s (although the dependency was less than linear), so the CoV was employed. Point estimates of CoV are imprecise unless very large numbers of patients are sampled: in the case of a small sample, it is also helpful to quote the upper bound of the 80% confidence interval on the CoV:

$$\text{CoV upper bound}=\sqrt{\frac{(N-1)\cdot(\text{CoV})^2}{X^2_{0.9,N-1}}} \quad (3)$$

Changes between group means were compared using the paired two-tailed Student's t-test. A p-value of less than 0.05 was considered significant.

Results

General observations

All subjects gave analysable data: no datasets were excluded from quantitative analysis. A typical MR image and the corresponding volume segmentation are shown in Figure 1. These images clearly highlight the MRI features of the disease process, and illustrate the difficulties in segmenting. Segmentation was found to be particularly difficult when dealing with the following situations:

- Regions of very thin cartilage, where the "band structure" was lost or altered;
- Regions of "merged" cartilage between two articulating surfaces (*e.g.* central regions of the tibiofemoral joint, and the base of the patellofemoral joint);
- Regions of cartilage above and surrounding bony abnormalities, such as erosions;
- Femoral cartilage at the base of the intercondylar notch, and also in other weight-bearing areas;
- Cartilage associated with rheumatoid synovitis, particularly in central regions of the patella and posterior regions of the femur.

All images showed at least one area of focal cartilage loss. Rheumatoid knees were characterized by cartilage loss and bony erosions commonly found at the femur and

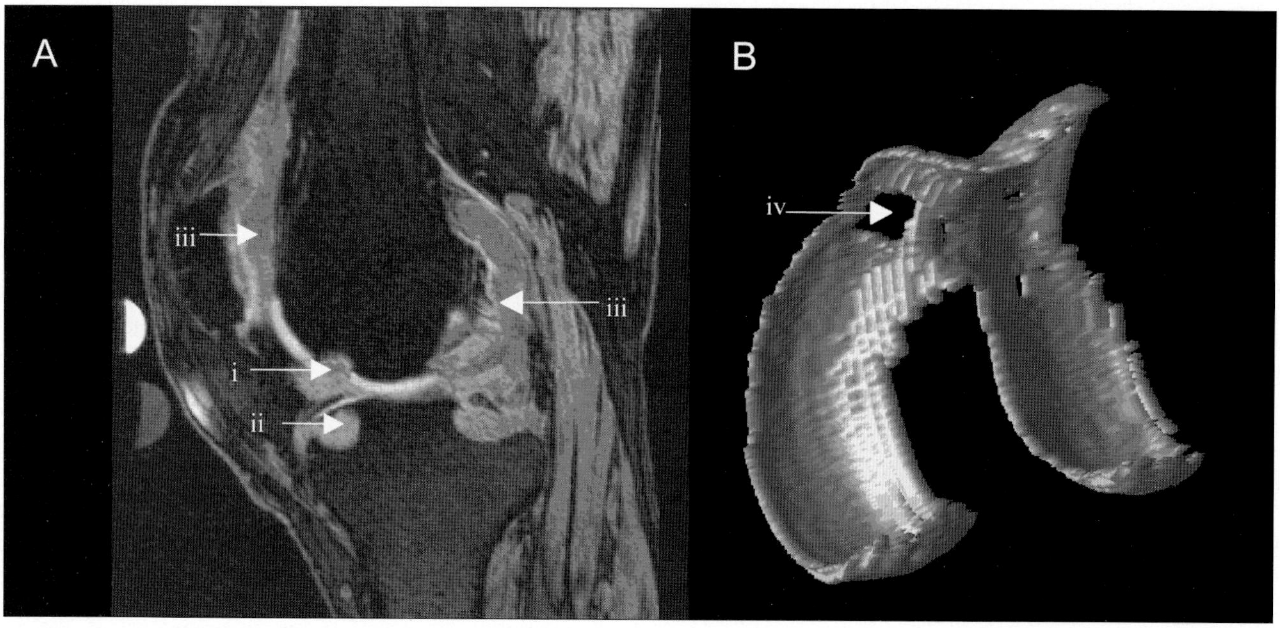

Figure 1. (A) A typical sagittal image slice taken from a patient with rheumatoid arthritis, showing cartilage loss (arrow i), bony erosion (arrow ii) and joint effusion (arrow iii). (B) The resulting three-dimensional (3D) segmentation of the femoral cartilage, showing cartilage loss (arrow iv).

the tibia. Joint effusion and synovitis was also regularly seen, particularly between the femur and the patella and also in posterior regions of the femur. Cartilage volumes (Table 2) tended to be lower than previously seen in normal volunteers [22] or OA patients [9], but were somewhat higher than those reported by Kimura [16].

Reproducibility

Repeat segmentations of the same images demonstrated good reproducibility. In comparison with the first segmentation by segmenter A, total cartilage volume was 1.8% higher at the second segmentation by segmenter A and 0.9% lower when segmented by segmenter B. Table 3 shows the intrasegmenter and intersegmenter CoV obtained. The intersegmenter CoV was substantially larger than the intrasegmenter CoV for all compartments. Volumes tended to be larger, and CoV values were smaller, in males than in females.

There was no apparent trend for a worse image quality score (sum of movement artefact and ease of segmentation scores) to correlate with an increased intrasegmenter or intersegmenter CoV.

Repeat scans of the same patients in the same visit (<1 h interval, substudy 3) or in different visits (1 week interval, substudy 4) also demonstrated good reproducibility, although this was generally inferior to the same-segmenter-same-scan comparison (Table 3). In comparison with the first scan, total cartilage volume was 4% higher in substudy 3 and 0.6% lower in substudy 4 at the second scan. These tiny differences were not statistically significant. A relationship between standard deviation (SD) and mean was found for intrasegmenter, intersegmenter and scan–scan comparisons. CoV tended to decline with increasing volume with approximately two-thirds power relationship consistent with the hypothesis that the errors in this case depend strongly on the surface area characteristics of the segmentation, since the surface area tends to increase with the two-thirds power of volume.

Progression

Table 4 shows the demographic information for the 17 subjects included in substudy 5 (progression over 1 year). All subjects met the inclusion criteria. In addition to pain in the index knee all had swelling (17/17); the majority had knee effusions (12/17) and a few had a tender joint (4/17). Assessment of the X-rays showed that five of the 17 subjects had osteophytes, while six of the 17 had erosions. The mean change in joint space width over the 12 months of the study was −0.26 mm (SD 0.32, n=15).

Table 2. Cartilage volumes

Compartment	Volume (SD) at baseline/ml (N=17)	Mean (SD) % change from volume at baseline	
		4±2 months (N=16)	12 months (N=16)
Femoral	8.8 (3.1)	0 (5)	−1 (7)
Lateral tibial	1.6 (0.7)	−1 (11)	−7 (16)
Medial tibial	1.4 (0.6)	−3 (10)	−2 (16)
Patellar	2.3 (0.8)	4 (12)	3 (11)
Total	14.1 (5.0)	0 (5)	−1 (7)

SD, standard deviation.

Table 3. Coefficients of variation associated with repeated measurements of cartilage volume in each compartment

Substudy (each N=6)	Cartilage compartments – coefficients of variation				
	Femoral	Patellar	Medial tibial	Lateral tibial	Total
1. Reproducibility same segmenter, same scan	3.0 (5.8)	8.5 (17)	7.1 (14)	4.7 (9.0)	2.2 (4.2)
2. Reproducibility different segmenter, same scan	7.0 (14)	6.8 (13)	7.5 (15)	4.7 (9.1)	5.2 (10)
3. Reproducibility same segmenter, same visit, different scan	5.7 (11)	5.4 (11)	6.7 (13)	7.6 (15)	4.9 (9.5)
4. Reproducibility same segmenter, same visit, different scan	5.4 (10)	7.5 (15)	8.0 (15)	8.7 (15)	4.4 (8.5)

In each case, the first figure is the root mean square (rms) coefficient of variation and the second (in parentheses) is the 80% confidence interval upper bound.

Figure 2 shows total cartilage volume over the 1-year duration of the study, while Table 2 shows changes in the individual compartments. There was no statistically significant change in volumes over this time period. When the X-ray and MRI data were correlated on a patient-by-patient basis, there was a suggestion of a weak correlation between the subject's loss of joint space width, and the subject's loss of cartilage (p=0.1, one-sided comparison).

Discussion

At present it is not yet established whether MRI measurement of cartilage volume can provide a useful method for assessment of disease management in RA. However, radiographic joint space (cartilage) narrowing in rheumatoid joints has previously been observed, and a recent study by Kirwan et al [24] reports that the progression of joint space narrowing in RA behaves differently from the progression of erosions and may be more closely related to cumulative development of synovitis in the RA joint. More recently, Kimura [16] has identified a clear correlation between MRI cartilage

Table 4. Demographic information for substudy 5

Patient demographics	Number/total	Mean (SD)	(Range)
Gender (female/total)	9/17		
Age (years)		58.1 (7.6)	(41–67)
BMI		28.4 (4.4)	(21–35)
Duration of disease (years)		15 (11.6)	(0.6–35)
Index knee soft tissue swelling			
None	0/17		
Little	11/17		
Lot	6/17		
Index knee tenderness			
None	13/17		
Little	4/17		
Lot	0/17		
Index knee effusion			
None	5/17		
Little	9/17		
Lot	3/17		
Joint space width [mm]			
Baseline	15/17	4.14 (1.46)	(0.6–6.1)
1 year	15/17	3.88 (1.48)	(0.8–6.1)
Change over 1 year	15/17	−0.26 (0.32)	(0–0.9)
% change over 1 year	15/17	−5.2 (14.3)	(0–33.3)

BMI, body mass index; SD, standard deviation.

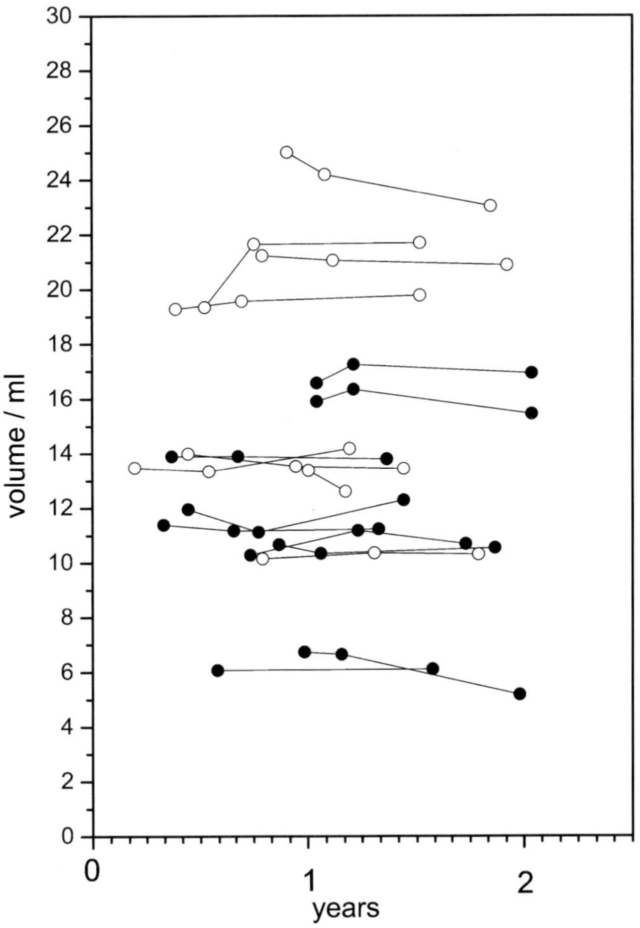

Figure 2. Total cartilage volume in the knee in 17 rheumatoid arthritis patients over 12 months (○ male; ● female).

volume loss and increased Larsen radiographic score at the knee joints of patients with RA, which further validates the use of MRI for knee cartilage investigations in RA populations. Other MRI methods such as measurement of regional bone erosion [25–27] and synovitis volumes [15] also provide encouraging data relative to radiographic assessments. Evidence therefore suggests that the longitudinal measurement of cartilage volumes using MRI may provide an important measure in helping to understanding how to manage RA.

Variations in cartilage volume determined by MRI can be influenced by scan quality, by the choice of segmentation technique, by observer segmentation bias, and by swelling or hydration in response to short term local changes in pressure. Other variations in the measured volume may be attributable to biological change as a result of disease processes.

In this study we adopted a manual segmentation technique, and explored these potential causes of volume variation. This manual method was implemented to extract the cartilage from surrounding tissue with similar MR signal intensities, which was not possible with automated or semi-automated methods. We achieved a "best case" CoV of 2.2% (intrasegmenter measurement, total cartilage volume; Table 3) for our patient cohort, which is similar to measurements made by ourselves and others on healthy joints [22, 28, 29]. This best case CoV was unsurprising, since errors that are made assigning cartilage at the point of articulation to individual compartments are effectively eliminated when the entire knee volume is considered. In virtually all cases, the intersegmenter CoV was larger than the intrasegmenter CoV. This has important implications for clinical studies where longitudinal cartilage volume assessments may be required. This major source of measurement error may be eliminated by using the same segmenter for intrapatient comparisons.

CoVs were generally smaller for measurements made on male joints compared with female joints, which reflects the larger (and therefore simpler to segment) anatomy of the male joints. Further, the CoVs for measurements made on these RA joints were mostly larger than those reported previously on OA joints [30]. This highlights the particular difficulty in RA that can arise when attempting to distinguish cartilage from surrounding diseased tissues such as joint effusion or pannus. However, somewhat surprisingly, reproducibility did not appear to deteriorate when image quality was suboptimal or "segmentation difficulty" increased. Qualitative scoring of "movement artefact" and ease of segmentation was also undertaken for a cohort of 16 OA patients as part of a previously published parallel study [9]. The median movement artefact scores for OA and RA cohorts were identical when compared (the images were deemed sharp), whilst the median ease of segmentation score was, as expected, higher for RA (3, fair) than for OA (2, easy). This demonstrates that the quality of the acquired data is reproducible between studies, but that the ease of segmentation due to the presence of pathological tissue is variable.

Repeated measurement of cartilage volumes within the same scan session (substudy 3) and within 1 week (substudy 4) was also found to be reproducible. The CoVs resulting from these substudies are comparable with those obtained for intrasegmenter measurements made on the same datasets. In other words, short-term volume fluctuations are negligible, and our instrument and measurement techniques are stable.

Baseline cartilage volumes for these patients with RA were found to be smaller than those for normal control subjects or from a similar OA population [9], but comparable with (slightly larger than) the RA volumes reported in the recent study by Kimura [16]. In our study, no significant changes to the cartilage volumes were seen when patients were followed over 12 months. The largest change was observed in the lateral tibial compartment where a loss of 7% was recorded over 12 months. However, the CoV associated with the volume measurement for different scans and different visits (substudy 4) for this compartment was 8.7%, which implies that a 7% loss over 12 months cannot be considered significant. Furthermore, if the total cartilage volume is considered then the net loss over 12 months was only 1%. A weak correlation between cartilage volume and joint space narrowing was evident when a one-sided comparison was implemented, *i.e.* we assumed that a loss in cartilage volume did not correlate with an increase to the joint space width. However, Mazzuca et al [31] have reported that a reduction in joint pain can result in alteration of the positioning of the knee (in particular favouring a better knee full extension), resulting in a change in joint space width that may confound the estimate of JSN. This potential source of error was not evaluated in our study, and as such a two-sided comparison may be considered more appropriate. However we believe that the likelihood of this reciprocal correlation would be extremely low.

Clinical assessment of joint tenderness, effusions and swelling were also recorded for each patient in the study. There was no difference in median score of tenderness or effusions in those individuals who demonstrated no loss of cartilage relative to those who demonstrated a small loss. However there was a trend towards increased swelling in this latter group, but the significance of these results is unknown given the low sample size and the small cartilage volume loss. In summary, whilst we acknowledge that our work has only considered data from a relatively small patient cohort, even with limited patient numbers we are satisfied that the study methodology is robust, and that these volume measurements have remained static over the 12 month duration.

Conclusion

We have considered the main variables that affect reproducibility in measuring cartilage volume changes in RA. The intersegmenter component of volume measurement is clearly the greatest source of variability, which suggests that the same segmenter should be used for any intrapatient longitudinal studies of cartilage volume. We have found that our method of volume measurement is reproducible, even when RA knees are compared over weekly durations. These session-to-session CoVs are comparable with the intrasegmenter measurement CoVs made on the same dataset. The CoV for the entire (total) cartilage is consistently smaller than for any of the individual compartments, which suggests that if cartilage loss is uniform across compartments then the "total" compartment offers the best statistical power. Over the 12 month duration of the study there was no significant change in total cartilage volume, nor were there significant changes in volume in any individual compartment.

Acknowledgments

The authors would like to acknowledge Bristol University Rheumatology Unit staff for their help with patient recruitment and care, and all the MRI Radiography staff at Bristol Royal Infirmary for scanning the patients.

References

1. Larsen A, Dale K, Eek M. Radiographic evaluation of rheumatoid arthritis and related conditions by standard reference films. Acta Radiol Diagn 1977;18:481–91.
2. Sharp JT, Young DY, Bluhm GB, Brook A, Brower AC, Corbett M, et al. How many joints in the hands and wrists should be included in a score of radiologic abnormalities used to assess rheumatoid arthritis? Arthritis Rheum 1985;28:1326–35.
3. Van der Heijde DM. Radiographic imaging: the 'gold standard' for assessment of disease progression in rheumatoid arthritis. Rheumatology (Oxford) 2000;39 Suppl. 1:9–16.
4. Cicuttini FM, Wluka AE, Wang Y, Davis SR, Hankin J, Ebeling P. Compartment differences in knee cartilage volume in healthy adults. J Rheumatol 2002;29:554–6.
5. Stammberger T, Eckstein F, Michaelis M, Englmeier K-H, Reiser M. Inter-observer reproducibility of quantitative cartilage measurements: comparison of B-spline snakes and manual segmentation. Magn Reson Imaging 1999;17:1033–42.
6. Kauffmann C, Gravel P, Godbout B, Gravel A, Beaudoin G, Raynauld JP, et al. Computer-aided method for quantification of cartilage thickness and volume changes using MRI: validation study using a synthetic model. IEEE Trans Biomed Eng 2003;50:978–88.
7. Tessier JJ, Bowyer J, Brownrigg NJ, Peers S, Westwood FR, Waterton JC, et al. Characterisation of the guinea pig model of osteoarthritis by in-vivo three-dimensional magnetic resonance imaging. Osteoarthritis Cartilage 2003;11:845–53.
8. Faure P, Doan BT, Beloeil JC. In-vivo high resolution three-dimensional MRI studies of rat joints at 7 T. NMR Biomed 2003;16:484–93.
9. Gandy SJ, Dieppe PA, Keen MC, Maciewicz RA, Watt I, Waterton JC. No loss of cartilage volume over three years in patients with knee osteoarthritis as assessed by magnetic resonance imaging. Osteoarthritis Cartilage 2002;10:929–37.
10. Vanwanseele B, Eckstein F, Knecht H, Spaepen A, Stussis E. Longitudinal analysis of cartilage atrophy in the knees of patients with spinal cord injury. Arthritis Rheum 2003;48:3377–81.
11. Cicuttini FM, Wluka AE, Wang Y, Stuckey SL. Longitudinal study of changes in tibial and femoral cartilage in knee osteoarthritis. Arthritis Rheum 2004;50:94–7.
12. Peterfy C, White D, Zhao J, VanDijke C, Genant HK. Longitudinal measurement of knee cartilage volume in osteoarthritis (Abstract). Arthritis Rheum 1998;41:S361.
13. McQueen F, Lassere M, Edmonds J, Conaghan P, Peterfy C, Bird P, et al. OMERACT Rheumatoid arthritis magnetic resonance imaging studies. Summary of OMERACT 6 MR imaging module. J Rheumatol 2003;30:1387–92.
14. Gylys-Morin VM, Brent Graham T, Blebea JS, Dardzinski BJ, Laor T, Johnson ND, et al. Knee in early juvenile rheumatoid arthritis: MR imaging findings. Radiology 2001;220:696–706.
15. Ostergaard M, Ejbjerg B, Stoltenberg M, Gideon P, Volck B, Skov K, et al. Quantitative magnetic resonance imaging as a marker of synovial membrane regeneration and recurrence of synovitis after arthroscopic knee joint synovectomy: a one year follow up study. Ann Rheum Dis 2001;60:233–6.
16. Kimura M. Quantification of cartilage volume in the knees of rheumatoid arthritis patients: relationship of physical characteristics and disease conditions to cartilage volume. Teikyo Med J 2003;26:411–23.
17. Morgan SR, Waterton JC, Maciewicz RA, Leadbetter JE, Gandy SJ, Moots RJ, et al. Magnetic resonance imaging measurement of knee cartilage volume in a multicentre study. Rheumatology 2004;43:19–21.
18. Dieppe PA, Cushnaghan J, Young P, Kirwan J. Prediction of the progression of joint space narrowing in osteoarthritis of the knee by bone scintigraphy. Ann Rheum Dis 1993;52:557–63.
19. Dieppe PA, Cushanghan J, Shepstone L. The Bristol 'OA 500' study: progression of osteoarthritis (OA) over 3 years and the relationship between clinical and radiographic changes at the knee joint. Osteoarthritis Cartilage 1997;5:85–97.
20. Mazzuca SA, Brandt KD, Dieppe PA, Doherty M, Katz BP, Lane KA. Effect of alignment of the medial tibial plateau and x-ray beam on apparent progression of osteoarthritis in the standing anterioposterior knee radiograph. Arthritis Rheum 2001;44:1786–94.
21. Lequesne M. Quantitative measurements of joint space during progression of osteoarthritis: chondrometry. In: Kuettner K, Goldberg V, editors. Osteoarthritic disorders. Rosemont, IL: American Academy of Orthopaedic Surgeons, 1995:427–44.
22. Waterton JC, Solloway S, Foster JE, Keen MC, Gandy S, Middleton BJ, et al. Diurnal variation in the articular cartilage of the knee in young adult humans. Magn Reson Med 2000;43:126–32.
23. Sivewright GJ, Elliott PJ. Interactive region and volume growing for segmenting volumes in MR and CT images. Medical Inf (Lond) 1994;19:71–80.
24. Kirwan J, Byron M, Watt I. The relationship between soft tissue swelling, joint space narrowing and erosive damage in hand x-rays of patients with rheumatoid arthritis. Rheumatology 2001;40:297–301.
25. Bird P, Lassere M, Shnier R, Edmonds J. Computerized measurement of magnetic resonance imaging erosion volumes in patients with rheumatoid arthritis: a comparison with existing magnetic resonance imaging scoring systems and standard clinical outcome measures. Arthritis Rheum 2003;48:614–24.
26. Ostergaard M, Hansen M, Stoltenberg M, Jensen KE, Szkudlarek M, Pedersen-Zbinden B, et al. New radiographic bone erosions in the wrists of patients with rheumatoid arthritis are detectable with magnetic resonance imaging a median of two years earlier. Arthritis Rheum 2003;48:2128–31.
27. McQueen FM, Benton N, Perry D, Crabbe J, Robinson E, Yeoman S, et al. Bone edema scored on magnetic resonance imaging scans of the dominant carpus at presentation predicts radiographic joint damage of the hands and feet six years later in patients with rheumatoid arthritis. Arthritis Rheum 2003;48:1814–27.
28. Peterfy CG, van Dijke CF, Janzen DL, Glüer CC, Namba R, Majumdar S, et al. Quantification of articular cartilage in the knee with pulsed saturation transfer subtraction and fat-suppressed MR imaging: optimization and validation. Radiology 1994;192:485–91.
29. Westhoff J, Eckstein F, Sittek H, Lösch A, Faber S, Kolem H, et al. Dreidmensionale dicken- und volumenbestimmung des knie-gelenkknorpels mit der MRT: reproduzierbarkeit am probanden. Fortschr Röntgenstr 1997;167:585–90.
30. Eckstein F, Cicuttini F, Raynauld J-P, Waterton JC, Peterfy C. Magnetic resonance imaging (MRI) of articular cartilage in knee osteoarthritis (OA): morphological assessment. Osteoarthritis Cartilage 2004; (In press).
31. Mazzuca SA, Brandt KD, Lane KA, Katz BP. Knee pain reduces joint space width in conventional standing anteroposterior radiographs of osteoarthritic knees. Arthritis Rheum 2002;46:1223–7.

The British Journal of Radiology, 78 (2005), 46–50 © 2005 The British Institute of Radiology
DOI: 10.1259/bjr/53924376

Effect of the introduction of helical CT on radiation dose in the investigation of pulmonary embolism

[1]J O'NEILL, MB BCh, FRCR, MSc, [2]J T MURCHISON, MBChB, FRCR, FRCP, [2]L WRIGHT, BSc, MSc and [2]J WILLIAMS, MSc, FIPEM

[1]*Radiology Department, St Josephs Hospital, 50 Charlton Ave East, Hamilton, Ontario, Canada and* [2]*Department of Radiology, Royal Infirmary of Edinburgh, Little France Crescent, Edinburgh EH16 4SA, UK*

Abstract. The aim of this study was to assess the change in patient radiation dose in the radiological investigation of pulmonary embolism since the introduction of helical CT pulmonary angiography (CTPA) in a large teaching hospital. All radiological investigations performed as an integral part of the imaging protocol in the investigation of clinically suspected pulmonary embolism (PE) were retrospectively reviewed. The protocol for the investigation of PE changed in our institution after the introduction of CTPA. Protocols 1 and 2 were the protocols in place before and after the introduction of CTPA, respectively. An in-depth evaluation was made of the imaging records and radiation dose for 30 consecutive patients investigated for clinically suspected PE in 1995 (protocol 1) and 2002 (protocol 2). Radiation doses were then extrapolated for the total number of patients investigated in each year. The number of radiological investigations performed per patient decreased from a mean of 1.17 in protocol 1 to 1.06 in protocol 2. There was a 44% increase in the total number of patients investigated. The effective dose per patient increased from 1.30 mSv to 1.35 mSv with the introduction of CTPA into the imaging protocol, an increase of only 4%. First line investigations showed a significant decrease in indeterminate examinations from 25.7% to 8.5%. Two different imaging protocols are reviewed with respect to type and number of procedures required for the investigation of PE and the resulting patient effective dose incurred. Results demonstrate an increase in the number of patients being investigated for suspected PE and a small increase in effective dose per patient since the introduction of helical CTPA. Although CTPA in itself incurs a higher effective dose, this is offset by the significant decrease in the number of non-diagnostic and total number of investigations per patient. In addition the ventilation component of lung scintigraphy was not required in protocol 2, thus reducing the dose further. We believe this small increase in effective dose is justified by the decrease in non-diagnostic studies and the reduction in total number of investigations per patient. We hope this paper will serve as a stimulus for the radiology community to examine current protocols in all areas of diagnostic imaging. We stress the importance of assessing new and established imaging investigative protocols to maximize the benefit and reduce any risk to patients.

The introduction of a new diagnostic imaging test in the investigative protocol for the diagnosis and management of patient pathology requires the fulfilment of several criteria. The predominant criterion is that the benefit of the test outweighs any incurred risks and that this benefit/risk ratio is equal to or greater than for the imaging tests already in place. In the investigation of pulmonary embolism (PE), helical computed tomographic pulmonary angiography (CTPA) and the newer multislice CTPA require both the use of ionizing radiation and intravenous contrast material (IVCM) which can be considered risk factors. The risk of adverse reactions from IVCM is established but to our knowledge there has been no review of the radiation dose incurred in this new investigation as part of a diagnostic imaging protocol with direct comparison with those imaging tests previously available. The purpose of our study is to assess what impact the introduction of helical CTPA in the investigation protocol of PE has had on patient radiation dose. In addition we review the measurement of this radiation dose and if there has been a change, the significance of this to the patient.

Received 7 October 2003 and in revised form 23 August 2004, accepted 17 September 2004.

Address correspondence to John M O'Neill, Radiology Department, St Josephs Hospital, 50 Charlton Ave East, Hamilton, Ontario, Canada.

Pulmonary embolism is a common condition with significant morbidity and mortality, the latter reaching 30% in some series in untreated cases [1, 2]. Appropriate use of anticoagulation or thrombolytic therapy improves outcome with a reduction in mortality to as little as 2.5% [3]. Therapy however is not risk free and serious complications may occur [4]. Identifying the correct patients to treat is therefore essential. Unfortunately the clinical manifestations of PE are variable and lack specificity to diagnose reliably or exclude clinically significant PE [5]. Imaging is mandatory to confirm the diagnosis but conventional strategies have been imprecise [6].

Multiple studies have reviewed CTPA against both formal pulmonary angiography and radionuclide ventilation/perfusion (V/Q) imaging and have consistently demonstrated a high sensitivity and specificity [7–12]. It is only minimally invasive, allows direct visualization of the thrombus and thrombus load. However demonstration of PE beyond segmental artery level is limited at present for single slice CT. Whether subsegmental emboli contribute significantly to morbidity and mortality is debatable [13].

The dosimetric measurement that provides a direct relationship to the radiation hazard is the effective dose (ED). This was introduced in 1990 by the International Commission on Radiological Protection and is defined by the sum of the products of the equivalent organ dose and its relevant organ weighting factor for all tissues and organs within the body. It is therefore not measured directly. Expressing the dose in the form of an effective dose allows the relative biological effect and therefore the relative risk of different radiation doses to be compared directly. It is this latter point that makes it the most appropriate measurement for use in this study due to the use of different imaging modalities.

Materials and method

A retrospective review of imaging protocols for the investigation of PE was performed. Protocol 1 and 2 were assigned to the imaging protocols in place in our centre before and after the introduction of CTPA, respectively (Figures 1 and 2). Imaging records and radiation dose for 30 consecutive patients investigated for clinically suspected PE in 1995 were reviewed. Plain radiographs were a necessary part of both protocols and therefore were excluded from further calculations assessing the change, if any, in effective dose. Radionuclide lung scintigrams (V/Q) and where appropriate lower limb venography and conventional pulmonary angiograms were assessed. The process was repeated in 2002 using the same parameters with the addition of CTPA. Due to the small number of conventional pulmonary angiograms, each of these studies was separately assessed for ED. The same applies to the seven cases of lower limb venography in protocol 2, with 20 cases assessed for protocol 1. Both years were then assessed with respect to the total number of radiological investigations performed for clinically suspected PE and the total effective doses involved.

Patients in protocol 2 had a perfusion scan performed if the chest radiograph was normal and there was no history of chronic pulmonary disease. If the chest radiograph provided an alternative diagnosis, no further imaging was performed with respect to PE unless there was a high clinical suspicion of concurrent PE. Otherwise the remaining patients proceeded to CTPA.

Radionuclide lung scintigrams were obtained using a GE MaxiCamera 400 (Single Head; GE, Milwaukee, WI) gamma camera. 80 MBq technetium-99m macro-aggregated albumin (MAA) was injected via a peripheral intravenous cannula with saline flush. Images were obtained in anterior, posterior, right and left anterior and posterior obliques, with 400 000 counts per image. Those patients requiring ventilation as part of this study, protocol 1, received 160 MBq of xenon-133 via aerosol. Reports were divided into three groups, normal, indeterminate and high probability and assessed in conjunction with the clinical presentation.

CTPA was performed on a GE HiSpeed Advance Single Slice CT machine (Milwaukee, WI, USA). 100 ml non-ionic contrast media (Niopam 300 mg ml^{-1}), was diluted with 40 ml saline and injected via a 16G or 18G needle into the antecubital fossa at a rate of 4 ml s^{-1}. Images

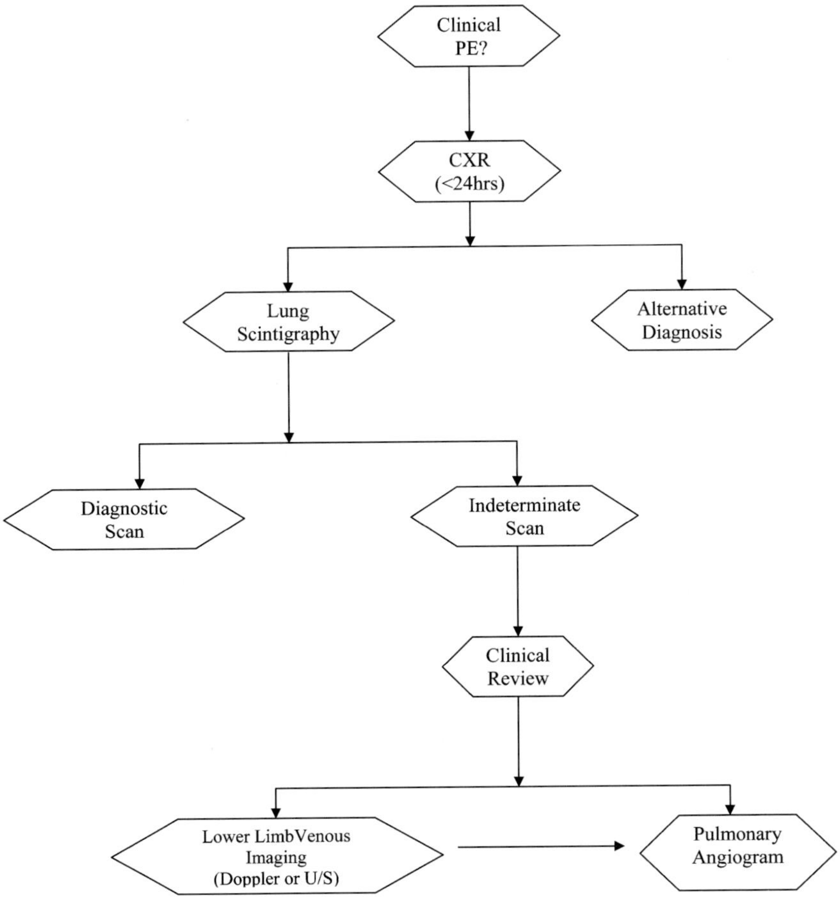

Figure 1. Protocol 1, radiological investigation clinically suspected pulmonary embolism (PE) pre CT pulmonary angiography (CTPA). CXR, chest radiograph; U/S, ultraround.

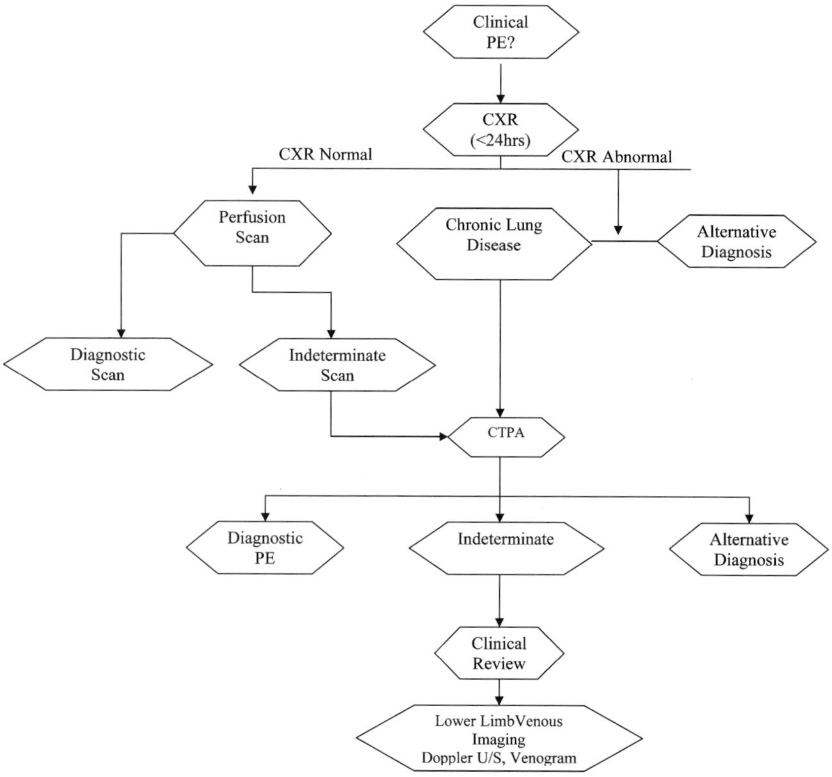

Figure 2. Protocol 2, radiological investigation clinically suspected pulmonary embolism (PE) post CT pulmonary angiography (CTPA). CXR, chest radiograph; U/S, ultraround.

were obtained with a delay of between 10–15 s, depending on the patient's cardiac status, from diaphragm to aortic arch using a pitch of 1.7, 3 mm slice thickness with image reconstruction at 1.5 mm intervals. Tube potential, tube current and the number of slices per examination were noted.

Venography and Doppler examinations are well recognized investigations for deep venous thromboembolic disease and were performed using standard protocols. Conventional pulmonary angiography was performed using a femoral approach and 100 cm 5 F pigtail catheter. Selective right and left main pulmonary artery runs with AP and 30° anterior oblique views were performed. Coned segmental runs were acquired when indicated.

Patient dosimetry

Doses for CT scanning were calculated from the CT dose index measured in air ($CTDI_{air}$) using the matched scanner technique developed by ImPACT [14]. Patient organ doses and thus effective dose are calculated using the NRPB Monte Carlo dose data for CT scanners [18]. The scanning protocol on the single slice scanner used 120 kV and 200 mA with a slice thickness of 3 mm and a pitch of 1.7.

Doses for radionuclide studies were derived from the administered activity using data in the ARSAC Notes for Guidance [15].

For conventional pulmonary angiography and for venography, effective dose was calculated from dose–area product (DAP) using conversion factors taken from Hart et al [16].

All dose calculations assume that the patient has an average build.

Results

The dose for CTPA was calculated for 16 patients. The average ED was 1.6 mSv. The standard scanning protocol was used for all patients with the only variant being the scanned length varying from 78 mm to 108 mm leading to a relatively small range of ED (1.4–1.9 mSv). V/Q (protocol 1) and Q (protocol 2) imaging were associated with doses of 1.2 mSv and 0.8 mSv, respectively, with no variation since the same activity was used for all patients. Doses for lower limb and pelvic venography were assessed for 12 patients. For these patients the average DAP was 3.1 Gy cm^2 (range 1.7 to 7.2) from which it was estimated that the average ED was 0.3 mSv. Doses for conventional pulmonary angiography were assessed for three patients. The average DAP was 21.3 Gy cm^2 from which ED equal to 3.2 mSv was calculated (range 2.3 to 4.1 mSv).

Both years were then reviewed with respect to total investigations and results. In the first year 526 patients were investigated for PE with 617 examinations performed, equivalent to 1.17 per patient. 526 V/Q studies demonstrated a combined positive or normal result in 74.3% with the remaining 25.7% been indeterminate. Additional investigations in the latter group were performed in 63% (Table 1). The average dose was 1.30 mSv per patient with 92% of this average being attributed to the V/Q studies (Table 2).

In the final year of the study 760 patients were investigated for clinically suspected PE, with 805 investigations, equivalent to 1.06 investigations per patient. CTPA was diagnostic in 97.8%, been the primary investigation in 59.3% of patients with Q lung scanning in the remaining 40.7%. The latter examination was diagnostic in 79.3% with 21% indeterminate. Further investigations included CTPA in 48% of the indeterminate group with 26% being positive (Table 3). 2.2% of CTPA

Table 1. Results Protocol 1 investigations

Primary investigation	V/Q (%)	Secondary investigations (indeterminate group)	Pulmonary angiography (%)	VG (%)	Doppler ultrasound (%)
Positive	95(18)		4(40)	18(28)	7(41)
Normal	296(56.3)		6(60)	38(59)	10(59)
Indeterminate	135(25.6)		0	8(12.5) result unavailable	0
Total	526		10	64	17

V/Q, ventilation/perfusion radionuclide imaging; VG venous angiogram.

examinations were indeterminate. In 8.9% of patients in the second protocol further investigations were performed due to discrepancy between the clinical and radiological diagnosis and to assess the presence and extent of peripheral thrombus. The average effective dose was 1.35 mSv per patient with 24% and 75% of this being attributed to Q studies and CTPA, respectively (Table 4).

Discussion

Radiological examinations are required to conform to two principles: justification to ensure that the benefit outweighs any risk, and optimization to ensure that dose is kept as low as reasonably achievable (ALARA) consistent with the clinical imperative for accurate diagnosis. In radiology using ionizing radiations, risk is assumed to be proportional to effective dose. In evaluating any new investigation protocol, it is not only necessary to consider the benefits in terms of diagnostic accuracy and patient acceptability, the risks, including the radiation risks, must also be assessed. Radiation risks are assessed in terms of effective dose and for the general population, the fatal cancer risk has been estimated to be 5% per sievert [17]. In this study we have considered the radiation risks for two protocols. In protocol 1 all patients for whom PE was not excluded by a preliminary chest X-ray, had V/Q scans with an average of 0.16 additional follow up radiology investigations, the average patient dose was 1.3 mSv. More recently (in protocol 2) the chest X-ray has been used to determine whether a perfusion scan or a CT pulmonary angiogram is the most appropriate investigation. For this protocol the number of follow up radiological investigations was reduced (to an average of 0.07 per patient) and the average effective dose per patient (1.35 mSv) was not significantly different. The overall radiological risk for the two protocols is therefore in the range of 6 to 7 fatal cancers per 100 000.

There are significant uncertainties in the estimation of effective dose from the measurable dosimetry quantities, *i.e.* activity, DAP and CTDI. In each case the standard conversion factors from the measured quantity to ED are taken from calculations based on a mathematical phantom representing an average sized person. The inherent uncertainties in the calculation depend on whether it is an internal radiation source, as in radionuclide imaging, or whether it is an external source, CT or conventional angiography. There are additional uncertainties introduced into the CT dose calculation due to the use of the scanner matching method used in the ImPACT dose calculator [14]. There are also patient-to-patient dose variations, the effect of which may have influenced the results of the study due to the relatively low proportion of the full patient cohort for whom doses were assessed. However, the effect

Table 2. Effective dose (ED) (mSv) per examination (Protocol 1)

Investigation	ED	Patient No	Total ED
V/Q	1.2	526	631.2
Pul Angio	3.2	10	32
Venography	0.3	64	19.2
Doppler ultrasound	0.0	17	0.0

Mean ED per patient=1.30 mSv.
V/Q, ventilation/perfusion radionuclide imaging.

Table 4. Effective dose (ED) (mSv) per examination (Protocol 2)

Investigation	ED	Patient No.	Total ED
Q	0.8	309	247.2
Pulmonary angiography	3.2	1	3.2
Venography	0.3	7	2.1
Doppler ultrasound	0.0	6	0.0
CTPA (Total)	1.6	482	772.8

Mean ED per patient=1.35 mSv.
CTPA, CT pulmonary angiography; Q, perfusion radionuclide imaging.

Table 3. Results Protocol 2 investigations

	CTPA (%)	Q (%)	Secondary investigations (indeterminate group)	Pulmonary angiography	VG	Doppler	CTPA (Q indeterminate) (%)	Q (CTPA indeterminate)
Positive	136(30.1)	47(15.3)		0	3	4	8(26)	0
Normal	304(67.4)	198(64)		1	4	2	23(74)	1
Indeterminate	11(2.4)	64(20.7)		0	0	0	0	0
Total	451	309		1	7	6	31	1

CTPA, CT pulmonary angiography; Q, perfusion; VG, venous angiogram.

of these variations was minimized by standardization of the three principal investigations. In protocol 1, 92% of the average patient dose was from the V/Q scan for which a standard activity was administered. In protocol 2, 24% of the dose was from perfusion scans with a standard activity and 75% of the dose from CTPA in which the maximum to minimum dose ratio assessed for 16 patients was 1.36. The much bigger uncertainties in the doses for other examinations (venography and conventional angiography) therefore have little significance in the overall conclusions.

The results are for a particular model of single slice helical scanner used for CTPA in this Hospital at the time of this study. The variation in dose between different models of scanner and between different institutes is known to be very large, *e.g.* by a factor of 8.4 for routine chest CT in an early CT dose survey [19]. It should also be noted that it is increasingly common to use multislice scanners for CTPA studies for which dose might be expected to be higher than reported here due to the use of a lower effective pitch. Notwithstanding these reservations regarding the dose which might be given elsewhere, it has been demonstrated that it is possible to use CTPA in protocol 2 without a significant increase in effective dose and thus in radiation risk.

The new diagnostic protocol that we present has a minimal increase in effective dose. The ED for CTPA is higher than for perfusion or V/Q scans and the role and position of CTPA in other diagnostic protocols must be carefully examined so that the patient receives the optimum benefit while minimizing risk.

In conclusion, our study has reviewed the total effective dose of the diagnostic imaging protocols as outlined above pre and post introduction of CTPA. Although in itself CTPA has a higher ED than the previously used V/Q imaging, the reduction in the number of additional investigations, and performing perfusion only for lung scintigraphy in protocol 2, has limited its impact from an ED viewpoint. With the introduction of CTPA there has been a significant increase in the total number of patients investigated, which is likely due to a multitude of factors including increased awareness of a disease with the advent of a new diagnostic tool, a reduction in the number of non-diagnostic results and the possibility of identifying alternative diagnosis. This has led to a corresponding increase in the total population radiation dose but only a minimal increase in the ED per patient investigated. This must be balanced against the social, economic and patient benefits due to the reduced number of examinations performed per patient with a significant reduction in the number of non-diagnostic examinations of a potentially fatal medical condition. This study will serve as a valuable baseline for the assessment of multislice CT with respect to ED. We hope this paper will serve as a stimulus for the radiology community to examine current protocols in all areas of diagnostic imaging. We stress the importance of assessing new and established imaging investigative protocols to maximize the benefit and reduce any risk to patients.

References

1. Dalen JE, Alpert JS. Natural history of pulmonary embolism. Prog Cardiovasc Dis 1975;17:259–70.
2. Moser KM. State of the art: venous thromboembolism. Am Rev Respir Dis 1990;414:235–49.
3. Carson JL, Kelley MA, Duff A, Weg JG, Fulkerson WJ, Palevesky M, et al. The clinical course of pulmonary embolism. N Engl J Med 1992;326:1240–5.
4. Ginsberg JS. Management of venous thromboembolism. N Engl J Med 1996;335:1817–28.
5. British Thoracic Society. Suspected acute pulmonary embolism: a practical approach. Thorax 1997;52:s1–24.
6. Murchison JT, Gavan DR, Reid JH. Clinical utilization of the non-diagnostic lung scintigram. Clin Radiol 1997;52:295–8.
7. Safriel Y, Zinn H. CT pulmonary angiography in the detection of pulmonary emboli. A meta-analysis of sensitivities and specificities. J Clin Imaging 2002;26:101–5.
8. Hansell DM. Spiral computed tomography and pulmonary embolism: current state. Clin Radiol 1997;52:575–81.
9. Remy-Jardin M, Remy J, Deschildre F, Artaud D, Borgi JP, Hossein-Foucher C, et al. Diagnosis of pulmonary embolism with spiral CT: comparison with pulmonary angiography and scintigraphy. Radiology 1996;200:699–706.
10. Goodman LR, Lipchik RJ, Kuzo RS. Acute pulmonary embolism: the role of computed tomographic imaging. J Thorac Imag 1997;12:83–6.
11. Fennerty T. The diagnosis of pulmonary embolism. BMJ 1997;314:425–9.
12. Teigen CL, Maus TP, Sheedy PF, Stanson AW, Johnson CM, Brear J, et al. Pulmonary embolism: diagnosis with contrast-enhanced electron-beam CT and comparison with pulmonary angiography. Radiology 1995;194:313–9.
13. Remy-Jardin M, Remy J, Wattinne L, Giraud F. Central pulmonary thromboembolism: diagnosis with spiral volumetric CT with the single breath-hold technique—comparison with pulmonary angiography. Radiology 1992;185:381–7.
14. http://www.impactscan.org/ctdosimetry.htm
15. Administration of Radioactive Substances Advisory Committee. Notes for guidance on the clinical administration of radiopharmaceuticals and use of sealed radioactive sources. Chilton: NRPB, 1998.
16. Hart D, Jones DG, Wall BF. Estimation of effective dose in diagnostic radiology from entrance surface dose and dose-area product measurements. NRPB-R262. Chilton: NRPB, 1995.
17. International Commission on Radiological Protection. 1990 Recommendations of the International Commission on Radiological Protection. ICRP pub 60. Oxford: Pergamon, 1991.
18. Jones DG, Shrimpton PC. Normalised organ doses for X-ray computed tomography calculated using Monte Carlo techniques. NRPB software report SR250. Chilton: NRPB, 1993.
19. Shrimpton PC, Jones DG, Hillier MC, Wall BF, Le Heron JC, Faulkner K. Survey of CT practice in the UK Part 2: Dosimetric aspects. NRPB-R249. Chilton: NRPB, 1991.

The British Journal of Radiology, *78* (2005), 51–54
DOI: 10.1259/bjr/29242407

Irradiation with standard tangential breast fields in patients treated with conservative surgery and sentinel node biopsy: using a three-dimensional tool to evaluate the first level coverage of the axillary nodes

[1,4]R ORECCHIA, MD, [1]A HUSCHER, MD, [1]M C LEONARDI, MD, [2]R GENNARI, MD, [2]V GALIMBERTI, MD, [3]C GARIBALDI, PhD, [3]E RONDI, PhD, [1]L C BIANCHI, MD, [2]S ZURRIDA, MD and [1]S FRANZETTI, MD

[1]*Division of Radiotherapy,* [2]*Division of Senology,* [3]*Medical Physic Unit, European Institute of Oncology, Milan and* [4]*University of Milan, Milan, Italy*

Abstract. Recent data show that axillary coverage can be obtained, but only through a selective CT-based treatment planning, as standard tangential fields are inadequate to deliver therapeutic doses. Currently, the replacement of axillary dissection with new techniques, such as sentinel node (SN) biopsy, makes it necessary to re-address the question about the real role of axillary irradiation, complicated by the differences in the anatomy of dissected and undissected axillary regions. The purpose of this paper is the dosimetric analysis of first axillary level coverage in standard irradiation of 15 breast-cancer patients treated with quadrantectomy and SN biopsy (negative finding). During surgery a clip on the site of the SN was positioned, marking the caudal margin of first axillary level. After the breast treatment plan was completed, the first axillary level was contoured on CT scans, from the site of the surgical clip up to the sternal manubrium, for coverage analysis with dose–volume histograms (DVHs) and three-dimensional isodose visualization. The maximum dose mean ranged from 5% to 80% of the prescribed dose (mean value 48.7%). The mean total dose received by the volume of interest was lower than 40 Gy in all but one patient. No patient had total irradiation of first nodal level; only one patient had 35% of the volume enclosed in the 100% isodose. Our analysis lead to the conclusion that therapeutic doses are not really delivered to first level axillary level nodes by a standard tangential field technique, and that specific treatment planning and beam arrangement are required when adequate coverage is necessary.

Adjuvant radiation therapy significantly decreases the incidence of local recurrences in women treated with breast-conserving surgery for early stage breast cancer [1, 2]. The standard clinical approach for patients with none or minimal involvement of regional lymph nodes still uses tangential photons fields to irradiate the whole residual breast parenchyma. Partial breast irradiation, limited to the tumour bed, is still under evaluation and will probably be indicated in selected subgroup of patients not yet reproducibly identified [3–5].

It was generally thought that tangential fields included the lowest part of axilla [6, 7] but there has been no clear demonstration of a coverage of this area by an adequate dose. The role of tangential chest irradiation in eradicating microscopic nodal disease reported in different papers [8, 9] is still unclear. Recent data show that the axillary coverage can be obtained, but only through a selective CT based treatment planning and a three-dimensional (3D) reconstruction of the target volumes, as the standard tangential fields usually fail to deliver therapeutic doses to any of the three axillary levels [10–13]. The coverage of the nodal area with the two-portal tangential irradiation technique can be strongly dependent on different factors, including anatomy of the patient, treatment position (use of the breast board), beam (blocks, wedges) and gantry (angles) arrangement.

Currently, the replacement of the routine axillary dissection with the introduction of new techniques for the examination of the axilla, such as sentinel node (SN) biopsy, makes it necessary to re-address the question of the real role of axillary irradiation, complicated by the differences in the anatomy of dissected and undissected axillary regions [14].

Material and methods

We analysed the treatment plans of 15 consecutive patients with invasive breast cancer (maximum tumour diameter 25 mm) treated with quadrantectomy and SN biopsy (negative finding).

Lymphoscintigraphy

The day before surgery, 5–10 MBq of technetium-99m-labelled human albumin colloidal particles was administered subdermally immediately above the breast lesion. More details on the technique are reported in previous literature [15].

Surgical procedures

A small incision was made over the area previously marked in the regional lymphatic drainage basin, and the

Received 17 October 2003 and in revised form 27 August 2004, accepted 7 September 2004.

Address correspondence to Prof. Roberto Orecchia, Division of Radiotherapy, European Institute of Oncology, Via Ripamonti 435, I-20141 Milan, Italy.

area explored with a gamma-detecting probe (GDP). Once the SN was identified a metallic clip was placed in its site marking the caudal margin of first axillary level.

Radiation therapy simulation

According to our current practices, the patients were lying supine on a tilted breast board (angles from 15° to 30°) placed on the simulator couch. Alignment along the longitudinal axis was ensured using a sagittal laser and fluoroscopy. The ipsilateral arm was extended above with the hand behind the head, at an angle of between 60° and 45° to the body axis. A polyurethane foam cast was used both for the CT scan and the treatment. The reference system was taken as the mid-sternal line and a plane at 90° to this passing through the ipsilateral nipple. In order to assist the set-up for the CT imaging study, radio-opaque markers were placed on the skin at the intersection of the two axes and over the tip of the xiphoid process; metal threads were also positioned along the mid-axillary lines on both sides in such a way as to be parallel to the long axis of the simulator couch. The extension of the clinical target volume (CTV), represented by the whole gland, was first clinically defined for each patient. The superior, inferior, medial and lateral margins of the breast were detected by palpation and metallic marks were used to identify them. On average, the upper margin of the portals has usually placed at the head of the clavicle, the medial margin at less than 1 cm over the meadline, the lateral margin near the midaxillary line, and the inferior margin was drawn 1–2 cm below the inframmammary fold.

A spiral CT scan (CT ProSpeed, GE Medical Systems) with 3 mm thickness and 10 mm sections was then performed, in quiet respiration, from the supraclavicular fossa to 1–2 cm below the inframammary fold. The breast CTV was outlined on each of the selected CT images. The planning target volume (PTV) was manually shaped applying from 1 cm to 1.5 cm margin to the CTV. The dimensions, the orientation of the two opposed, non parallel 6 MV tangential fields, and the characteristic of the wedge filters were defined on the treatment planning system (TPS) (Cadplan; Varian). The deep alignment of beams was used to minimize lung involvement and no collimator rotation was needed because of the breast board. The 100% tumour dose was specified at the isocentre (ICRU point). A correction factor for lung was also used to calculate the dose distribution.

Anatomical definition of the axilla

The nodal areas were identified and contoured on CT images after the preparation of the conventional breast treatment plan. The first axillary level was contoured from the site of the surgical clip up to the sternal manubrium, for the analysis of its coverage with dose–volume histograms (DVHs) and 3D isodose visualization.

Radiation therapy treatment

All patients received whole breast irradiation, 50 Gy delivered in 25 fractions are 5 weeks, and a 10 Gy boost to the tumour bed was given by a direct electron field. Seven patients were treated with a breast board angle of 15° and eight with 30°. Nine patients were treated for superior quadrant lesions while the other six had tumours in the lower part of the breast.

Results

The mean volume of the first axillary level was 28.9 cm^3, ranging from 14.5 cm^3 to 58.6 cm^3 with a standard deviation (SD$\pm$13 cm^3). The mean value of the maximum dose detected in the analysed region was 94.3% of the dose prescribed to the breast (SD$\pm$12.9%), ranging from 55% to 105%. The mean doses delivered ranged from 5% to 80% of the prescribed dose, with a mean value of 48.7% (SD$\pm$21.5%). The mean total dose received was lower than 40 Gy in all but one patient, as shown in Figure 1. Minimum doses inside the volume ranged from 0 to 10% of the prescribed dose, with a mean value of 3.3% (SD$\pm$3.1%). No patient had total irradiation of the first nodal level and only one patient had 35% of the volume enclosed in the 100% isodose. The percentages of first axillary level volume enclosed in the 80% and 100% isodose are shown in Figure 2. The mean volume of the first axillary level receiving at least 80% of the prescribed dose was 30.7%, ranging from 0 to 70% (SD$\pm$22.4%); the volume encompassed by 100% isodose was even smaller: a mean value of 2.5%, ranging from 0 to 35% (SD$\pm$9%). Figure 3 shows the DVHs of the first axillary level for all patients, while in Figure 4 the minimum, maximum and mean DVHs are plotted. These DVHs are obtained by calculating for each dose, the minimum, maximum and the mean values, respectively, of all the observed data. Higher doses of radiation to the lowest part of the axilla were related to a low angle of the breast board, as shown in Table 1, but no statistical significance was detected. The site of the primary lesion did not significantly affect the axillary irradiated volume (Table 2).

Discussion

External beam radiotherapy using standard tangential fields after conservative surgery is the current approach in managing early stage breast cancer [1, 2]. The role of this technique in local control of breast cancer is unquestionable [16]. On the other hand, its effectiveness in reducing axillary recurrence rate is controversial although some

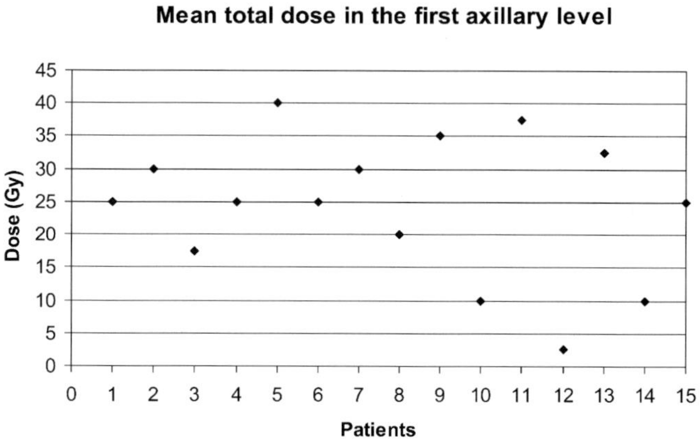

Figure 1. Mean total doses absorbed in the first axillary level, with standard therapy of 50 Gy, in 2 Gy fractions.

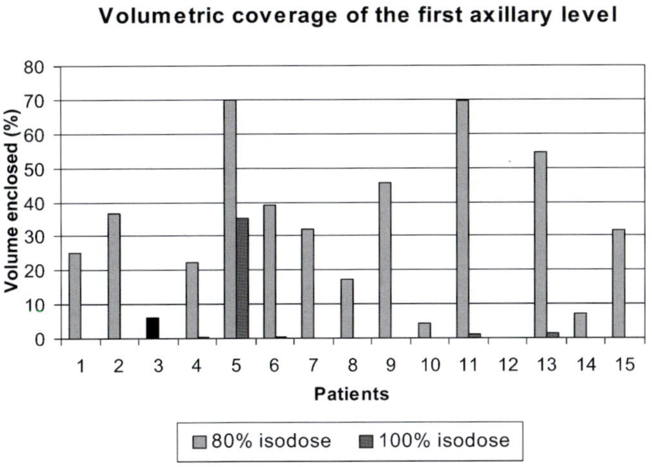

Figure 2. Volumetric coverage of the first axillary level.

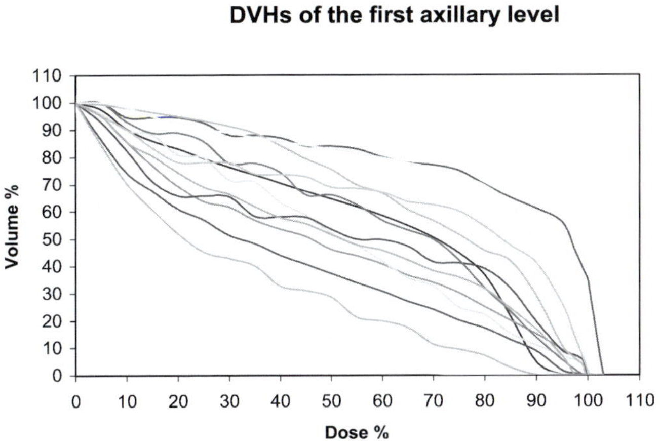

Figure 3. Dose–volume histograms (DVHs) of the first axillary level for all patients.

clinical data show that breast tangential irradiation also resulted in better axillary local control [8, 9]. X-ray simulation film based analysis shows that first axillary levels could be included in the standard tangential fields, although not expressly included in the PTV of breast irradiation [6, 7]. It is commonly thought that the lower part of the axilla often gets a significant dose of radiation that could have a tumoricidal effect. A recent analysis, based on CT scanning and 3D reconstruction, seems to

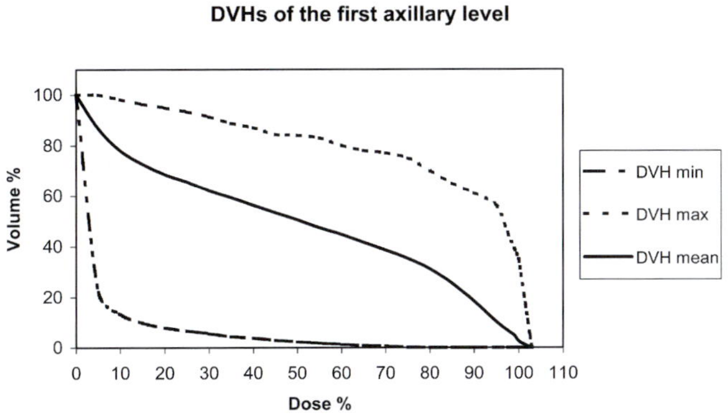

Figure 4. Minimum, maximum and mean dose–volume histograms (DVHs) of the first axillary level.

Table 1. Inclusion of first axillary level in tangential fields for breast cancer

Tilted breast board angle	% Volume in the 80% isodose (Range/Mean)	No. patients
15°	4–69/42	8
30°	0–32/18	7

Table 2. First axillary level inclusion depending on site of the primary lesion

Site of primary lesion	% Volume in the 80% isodose	No. patients
Superior	6–54/30	9
Inferior	0–70/30	5
Midline	70	1

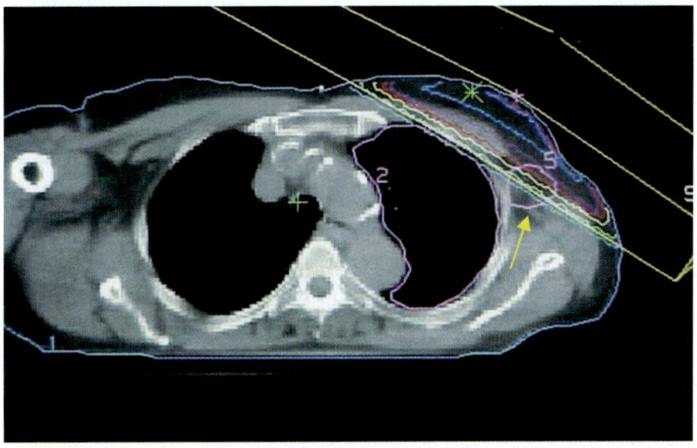

Figure 5. First level axillary lymph nodes contoured on CT slice (arrow) and its relationship to the upper border of planned tangential fields.

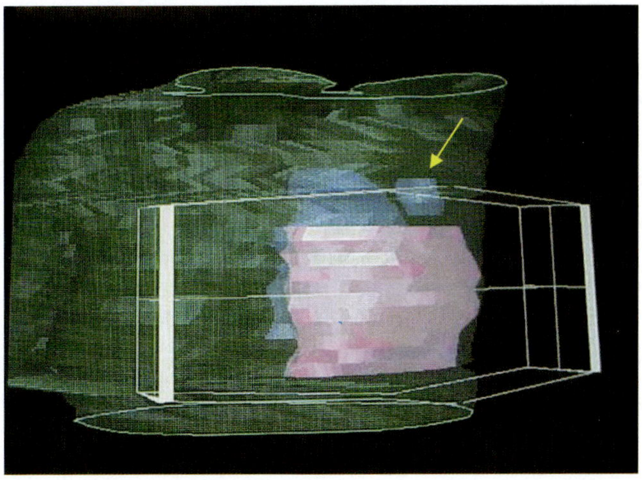

Figure 6. Surface rendered image of tangential portals of a typical patient, showing breast target volume, underlying lung and first axillary node level (arrow). Note that the first level nodes are only partially included within the tangential fields.

demonstrate that effective axillary irradiation through breast tangential fields is not so frequent [12]. The first level nodes were in fact only partially included and more importantly, not at clinically significant doses (Figures 5 and 6). Our work seems to confirm the conclusions of other papers already published [10–13], although the main characteristic of our series was the different management of patients who all had sentinel lymph node biopsy leaving the axilla undissected. As demonstrated also in our cases, only few patients had a consistent dose of radiation to the axilla while most of them received very small doses to part of the volume of interest. The volumes contoured in our patients were smaller than those reported by Krasin et al [12], with a mean value of 28.9 cm^3 (ranging from 4.5 cm^3 to 58.6 cm^3, SD$\pm$11.3 cm^3). This may be due to differences in longitudinal definition of first level on the clip marker and the image definition rather than on anatomical landmarks.

While the longitudinal extension of the third axillary level is almost the same with different positions of the arm, location of first and second level is strictly dependent on arm abduction. In patients with a markedly abducted arm (CT scan position) the first axillary level begins at the aortic arch up to the sternal manubrium. Medially and above this lies the second level. The apex of the axilla (third level) is located below the central part of the clavicle, limited posteriorly and inferiorly by the first rib and anteriorly and superiorly by the clavicle itself.

In our experience the angle of the breast board did not significantly affect axillary coverage. The better volumetric coverage that was detected in patients with a lower angle seems to be related to the physical characteristics of these patients, four of them being obese with large breasts. The site of primary breast tumour also did not affect nodal coverage, as the entire breast was irradiated in all cases and the breast PTV always defined in the same way. Moreover we did not include in the analysis patients with a primary tumour located in the axillary tail.

The analysis of dose distribution shows that the axillary CTV received a mean total dose of about 25 Gy (delivered in 1 Gy fractions), with a SD of $\pm$21.5 Gy, too low to expect that this could affect local control. Our analysis, as has already been reported, led to the conclusion that therapeutic doses are not delivered to the first level axillary nodes by a standard tangential technique and that specific treatment planning and beam arrangements are required to achieve adequate coverage. It is probable that the reduction in axillary recurrences detected in breast irradiated patients derives from sterilization of skip metastasis, as already proposed by Krasin [12]. It is important to remember that all recent papers are based on patients who had undergone axillary dissection, and currently the surgical approach to the axilla is more often discussed and the role of axillary radiotherapy of increasing interest [14]. In order to ensure an adequate coverage of the axillary volume it will be necessary to overcome the limitation of standard irradiation.

References

1. Veronesi U, Cascinelli N, Mariani L, Greco M, Saccozzi R, Luini A, et al. Twenty-year follow-up of a randomized study comparing breast-conserving surgery with radical mastectomy for early breast cancer. N Engl J Med 2002;16:1270–1.
2. Fisher B, Anderson S, Bryant J, Margolesse R, Deutsch M, Fisher E, et al. Twenty-year follow-up of a randomized trial comparing total mastectomy, lumpectomy, and lumpectomy plus irradiation for the teatment of invasive breast cancer. N Engl J Med 2002;16:1233–41.
3. Morrow M, Harris JR, Schnitt SJ. Local control following breast conserving surgery for invasive cancer: results of clinical trials. J Natl Cancer Inst 1995;87:1669–73.
4. Vicini F, Kini VR, Chen P, et al. Irradiation of the tumor bed alone after lumpectomy in selected patients with early-stage breast cancer treated with breast conserving therapy. J Surg Oncol 1999;70:33–40.
5. Veronesi U, Orecchia R, Luini A, Gatti G, Intra M, Zurrida S, et al. A preliminary report of intraoperative radiotherapy (IORT) in limited-stage breast cancers that are conservatively treated. Eur J Cancer 2001;37:2178–83.
6. Wong J, Recht A, Beard C, Busse P, Cady, B, Chaffey J, et al. Treatment outcome after tangential radiation therapy without axillary dissection in patients with early-stage breast cancer and clinically negative axillary nodes. Int J Radiat Oncol Biol Phys 1997;39:915–20.
7. Recht A, Houlihan M. Axillary lymph nodes and breast cancer. Cancer 1995;76:1491–512.
8. Fisher B, Redmond C, Poisson R, Margolese R, Wolmark N, Wickerham L, et al. Eight-year results of a randomized clinical trial comparing total mastectomy and lumpectomy with or without irradiation in the treatment of breast cancer. N Engl J Med 1989;320:822–8.
9. Ribeiro G, Magee B, Swindell R, Harris M, Banerjee SS. The Christie Hospital breast conservation trial: an update at 8 years from inception. Clin Oncol 1993;5:278–83.
10. Smitt M, Goffinet D. Utility of three-dimensional planning for axillary node coverage with breast-conserving radiation therapy: early experience. Radiology 1999;210:221–6.
11. Takeda A, Shigematsu N, Kondo M, Amemiya M, Kawaguchi M, Michinao S, et al. The modified tangential irradiation technique for breast cancer: how to cover the entire axillary region. Int J Radiat Oncol Biol Phys 2000;46:815–22.
12. Krasin M, McCall A, King S, Olson M, Emami B. Evaluation of a standard breast tangent technique: a dose-volume analysis of tangential irradiation using three-dimensional tools. Int J Radiat Oncol Biol Phys 2000;47:327–33.
13. Aristei C, Chionne F, Marsella A, et al. Evaluation of level I and II axillary nodes included in the standard breast tangential fields and calculation of the administered dose: results of a prospective study. Int J Radiat Oncol Biol Phys 2001;51:69–73.
14. Schlembach PJ, Buchholz TA, Ross MI, et al. Relationship of sentinel and axillary level I-II lymph nodes to tangential fields used in breast irradiation. Int J Radiat Oncol Biol Phys 2001;51:671–8.
15. Veronesi U, Paganelli G, Viale G, et al. Sentinel lymph node biopsy and axillary dissection in breast cancer: results in a large series. J Natl Cancer Inst 1999;91:368–73.
16. Early Breast Cancer Trialist's Collaborative Group. Favorable and unfavorable effects on long-term survival of radiotherapy for early breast cancer: an overview of the randonmized trials.Lancet 2000;355:1757–70.

The British Journal of Radiology, 78 (2005), 55–56 © 2005 The British Institute of Radiology
DOI: 10.1259/bjr/63858589

Short communication

Training in neonatal cranial ultrasound: a questionnaire survey

[1]P J C DAVIS, MRCPCH, [2]R M COX, MRCP (Paeds), MA and [3]J BROOKS, MRCPCH, MA

[1]*University Hospitals Coventry and Warwickshire NHS Trust, Clifford Bridge Road, Coventry CV2 2DX,* [2]*Department of Paediatric Oncology, Llandough Hospital, Penlan Road, Llandough, Vale of Glamorgan CF64 2XX and* [3]*Department of Neonatology, Birmingham Women's Hospital, Metchley Park Road, Edgbaston, Birmingham B15 2TG, UK*

Abstract. A questionnaire was sent to every paediatric specialist registrar in the West Midlands to assess the training of paediatric specialist registrars in neonatal cranial ultrasound. 26% had never carried out supervised scans. 51% lacked confidence in performance and 57% in interpretation of scans. The current pattern of training in neonatal cranial ultrasound lacks structure, supervision and assessment of competency.

Background

Neonatal cranial ultrasound is an integral part of neonatal practice. It is used routinely in the investigation of neonates, both pre-term and with neurological pathologies, and plays a significant role in guiding their management [1–3]. Significant decisions regarding continuing or withdrawing care may be based on scan results, which are dependent on both technical performance and interpretation skills.

In the UK, the majority of neonatal cranial ultrasound is performed by consultant neonatologists or middle grade paediatric staff, mainly specialist registrars (SpRs). The SpR grade is attained usually 2–3 years post registration and after successful completion of the membership of the Royal College of Paediatrics and Child Health examinations. There are no formal training guidelines or compulsory training requirements for neonatal cranial ultrasound in the UK [4], although the Royal College of Radiologists (RCR) cite paediatric transcranial ultrasound as a core skill [5] and the British Society of Paediatric Radiologists (BSPR) have a technical standard for neonatal cranial ultrasound scans on their website [6]. Many SpRs move frequently between neonatal units during their training and are therefore exposed to varying practices.

We aimed to assess the current patterns of training of paediatric SpRs in the West Midlands deanery in cranial ultrasound technique and interpretation.

Design

A questionnaire was sent to every paediatric SpR (n=96) in the West Midlands region, including a stamped addressed envelope for return. Each trainee would either have completed core training, or currently be undertaking core training, which includes the neonatal attachment of at least 6 months in a level 3 unit. It asked the trainee to estimate how many supervised and unsupervised cranial ultrasound scans they had performed to date. Details of supervised training in performing and interpreting scans were requested. The respondents were also asked to assess their own level of confidence in performing and interpreting scans. In addition, we asked whether trainees were expected to perform urgent scans and whether they had been trained to use the scanner available to them.

A pilot study involving a group of neonatal senior house officers (SHOs) did not result in any modification to the questionnaire.

Results

73% of the 96 questionnaires were returned.

Figure 1 shows the number of supervised and unsupervised scans performed by SpRs during their training to date. 26% had never performed any supervised scans, whilst 55% had performed <20 supervised scans. Only 18% had performed >50 scans (whether supervised or not). Those who had performed >50 unsupervised scans may not have performed any scans under supervision.

Figure 2 shows those who supervised the SpRs performing cranial ultrasound scans. Supervision may have been on an *ad hoc* or weekly basis.

Similarly, Figure 3 shows which health professionals supervised the interpretation of the scans. Supervision may have taken place on a one-to-one basis, or during a ward round or clinical meeting.

Figure 4 demonstrates the respondents' levels of confidence in performing and interpreting scans. 51% felt unsure or not at all confident in performing scans, whilst 57% felt unsure or not at all confident in interpreting scans. These data represent the respondents' own interpretation of their skills and not their competence, which this study did not assess.

Discussion

Our survey showed that the current pattern of training in neonatal cranial ultrasound in the West Midlands lacks

Received 26 April 2004 and in revised form 27 August 2004, accepted 20 September 2004.

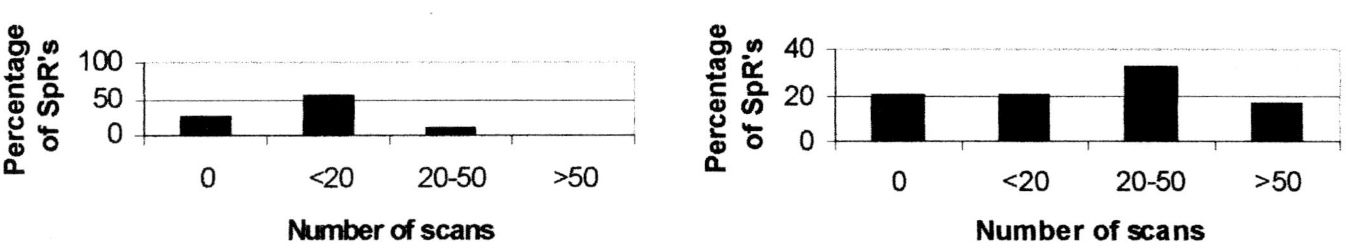

(a) (b)

Figure 1. (a) Number of scans performed with supervision. (b) Number of scans performed without supervision.

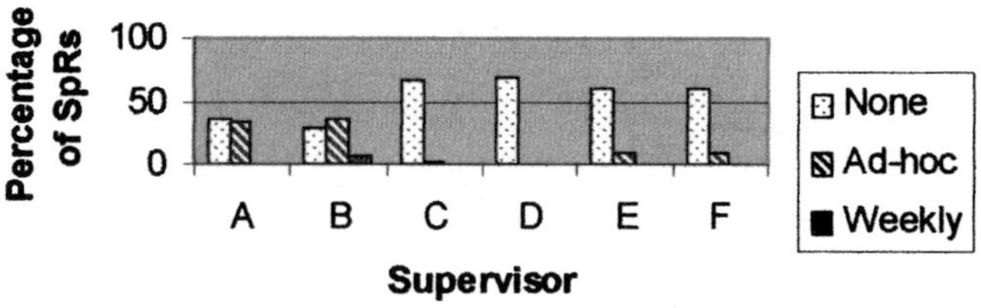

Figure 2. Who supervised specialist registrars (SpRs) performing scans? A, other SpR; B, consultant neonatologist; C, consultant radiologist; D, radiographer; E, nurse practitioner; F, other.

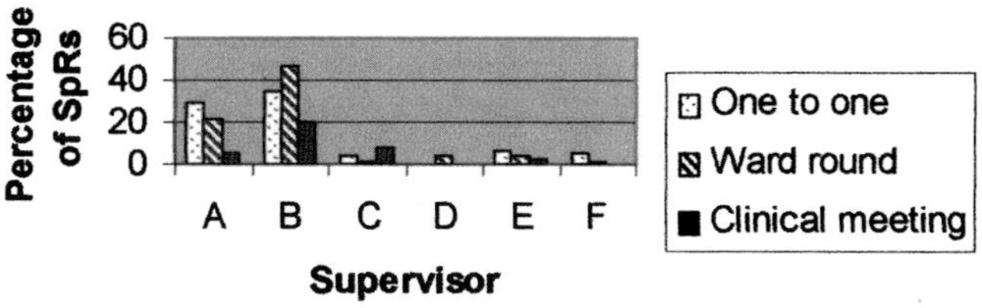

Figure 3. Who supervised specialist registrar (SpRs) interpreting scans? A, other SpR; B, consultant neonatologist; C, consultant radiologist; D, radiographer; E, Nurse practitioner; F, other.

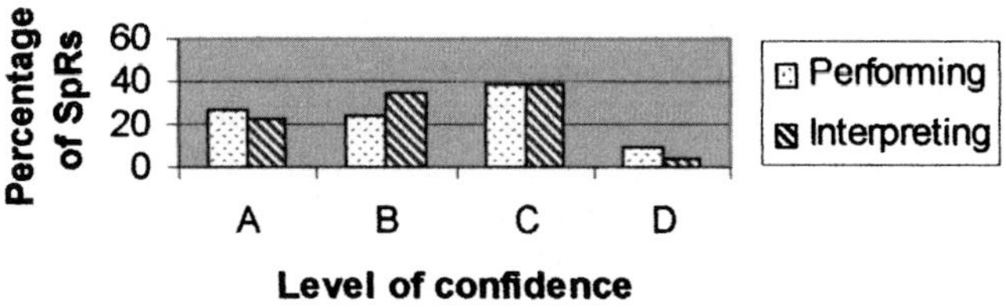

Figure 4. Specialist registrars' level of confidence in cranial ultrasound scanning. A, not at all confident; B, unsure; C, adequate; D, completely confident.

both structure and adequate supervision. Many SpRs are supervised by other trainees. This is reflected in trainees' level of confidence. In addition, there is currently no measure of competency in this field, although the BSPR technical standard suggests a minimum requirement of attendance at a theoretical course plus scanning under direct supervision of a competent sonographer until competent to scan independently [6]. Despite this, trainees are expected to perform and interpret cranial ultrasound scans even during their core training. As Reynolds et al comment, "it [performing cerebral ultrasound] appears to be a skill hastily acquired once the newly appointed specialist registrar starts his/her neonatal placement" [4].

We suggest that consideration is given to the development of formal training to those who are expected to acquire and interpret scans, along with appropriate assessment of competency in this skill. The RCR are expected to issue guidance of requirements for training in the near future.

References

1. Pape KE, Blackwell RJ, Cusick G, Sherwood A, Houang MTW, Thorburn RJ, et al. Ultrasound detection of brain damage in preterm infants. Lancet 1979;1:1261–4.
2. Levene MI, Wigglesworth JS, Dubowitz V. Cerebral structure and intraventricular haemorrhage in the neonate: a real-time ultrasound study. Arch Dis Child 1981;56:416–24.
3. Mercuri E, Dubowitz L, Paterson Brown S, Cowan F. Incidence of cranial ultrasound abnormalities in apparently well neonates on a postnatal ward: correlation with antenatal and perinatal factors and neurological status. Arch Dis Child Neonatal Ed 1998;79:F185–9.
4. Reynolds PE, Dale RC, Cowan FM. Neonatal cranial ultrasound interpretation: a clinical audit. Arch Dis Child Neonatal Ed 2001;84:F92–5.
5. Core training: core skills in Paediatrics. Structured Training in Clinical Radiology (3rd edn). London: Royal College of Radiologists, 2001. www.rcr.ac.uk
6. Technical standard: Neonatal Cranial Ultrasound Scans. www.bspr.org.uk

The British Journal of Radiology, *78* (2005), 57–59
DOI: 10.1259/bjr/55015850

Case report
False negative 16 detector multislice CT for scaphoid fracture

[1]A M GROVES, FRCR, [2]H K CHEOW, FRCR, [2]K K BALAN, FRCPI, [1]H M COURTNEY, DCR, [1]P W P BEARCROFT, FRCR and [1]A K DIXON, FRCR

Departments of [1]Radiology and [2]Nuclear Medicine, Addenbrooke's Hospital and the University of Cambridge, Hills Road, Cambridge CB2 2QQ, UK

Abstract. We discuss a case of a 19-year-old man with scaphoid trauma. We describe the imaging findings on three sets of radiographs, bone scintigraphy, CT and MRI. CT failed to identify a scaphoid fracture, which was present on 6 week radiographs, MRI and scintigraphy. The case illustrates that despite multidetector technology, CT still relies upon cortical and or trabecular displacement to demonstrate fractures.

The scaphoid is the most common carpal bone to fracture [1]. However the incidence, mechanism, natural history and treatment of such fractures remain controversial [1]. The fracture must be identified early, as immediate treatment is required to minimize the chances of non-union and thus avoiding disability [2]. Unfortunately, clinical examination and plain radiographs are unreliable diagnostic tools [2].

We present a case of suspected scaphoid fracture, where multistage radiographs, CT, MRI and bone scintigraphy were all performed. The discordance between imaging modalities shown in this case (Table 1) illustrates that despite multidetector technology, CT relies upon cortical and or trabecular displacement to demonstrate fractures.

Case report

A 19-year-old man presented to the accident and emergency department having fallen on his outstretched left hand. On clinical examination he was found to be tender in the anatomical snuffbox. Radiographs of four views (including a Stretchers/30 degree angled view) of his scaphoid were obtained, but no fracture was demonstrated (Figure 1a). His wrist was splinted and he attended follow up 10 days later. He remained tender in the snuffbox and four further radiographic views of his wrist were performed. Once again no fracture was identified (Figure 1b). On the same day he was referred for conventional $^{99}Tc^{m}$-methylene diphosphonate (MDP) bone scintigraphy of his wrist. The scintigram showed increased MDP uptake in the scaphoid in keeping with a fracture (Figure 2). After scintigraphy the patient underwent 16 detector multislice CT. This was performed with the hand above the head and flat on the table. Images were acquired in the axial plane using 0.75 mm detectors and reconstructed in 0.5 mm slice widths. Images underwent multiplanar reconstruction and were viewed in interactive cine mode, but no fracture could be detected (Figure 3). As a result of these discrepant findings a 1.5 Tesla MRI examination of the wrist was undertaken 3 days later. On T_1 weighted images there was reduced signal seen in the marrow of the proximal scaphoid consistent with oedema (Figure 4a). T_2 weighted fat saturated images showed high signal in the proximal pole of the scaphoid and a suggestion of a linear low signal line transversing the proximal third of the bone (Figure 4b). Although the latter was equivocal it was thought to probably represent a fracture. The patient was treated for a scaphoid fracture and his wrist immobilized for 6 weeks. At this time further radiographs were performed which showed a fracture line at the lower pole (Figure 5).

Received 18 February 2004 and in revised form 18 June 2004, accepted 13 August 2004.

Discussion

The high sensitivity of skeletal scintigraphy in the detection of fractures is well established. For this reason, as well as its widespread availability, many investigators recommend its use in the detection of occult scaphoid fractures [2–4]. In recent years however, the increasing availability of MRI has led to its use in the diagnosis of various traumatic bone injuries, including scaphoid fracture. There are claims of benefit in diagnosis, cost and clinical impact using MRI [5–7].

CT has inherent advantages when examining high attenuation tissues such as bone. However, although methodology for examining the scaphoid successfully on CT has been described for many years [8], the use of CT to diagnose scaphoid fractures is rather limited. This may be the result in part of one early study, which suggested scintigraphy was significantly more sensitive than CT in the diagnosis of scaphoid fractures [4]. Since these early studies, the advent of multidetector technology has revolutionized the CT technique, allowing fine section,

Table 1. Summary of imaging findings

Imaging technique	Findings
Radiograph day of trauma	Normal
Radiograph day 10 after trauma	Normal
Bone scintigram day 10 after trauma	Scaphoid fracture
CT day 10 after trauma	Normal
MR day 14 after MRI	Probable scaphoid fracture
Radiograph day 42 after trauma	Scaphoid fracture

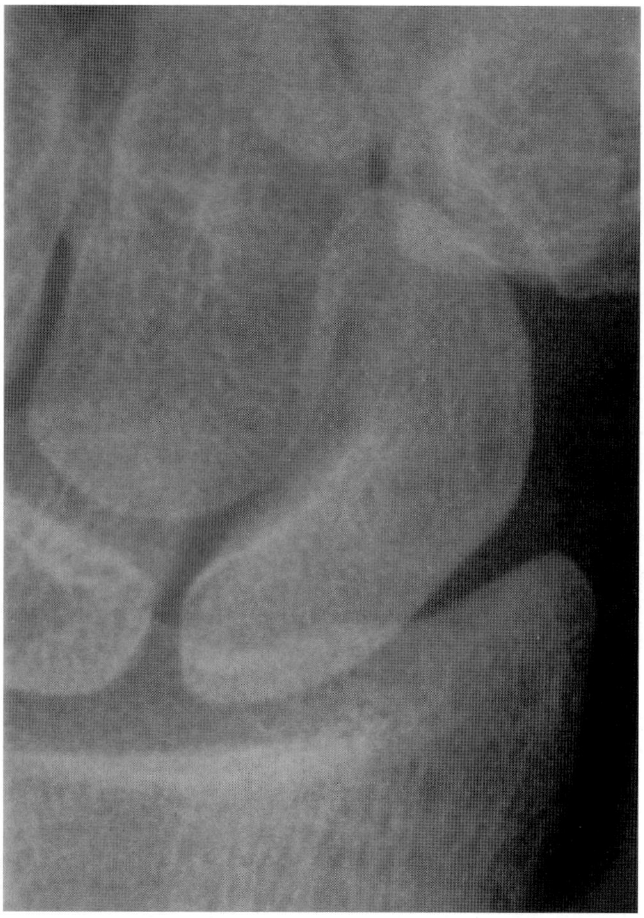

(a)

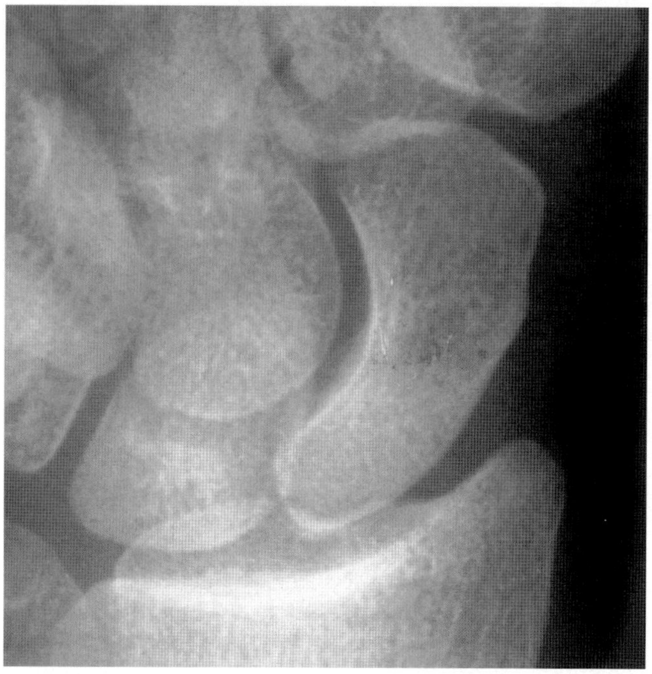

(b)

Figure 1. (a) Dorsopalmar radiograph of the left wrist on the day of injury with no evidence of fracture. (b) Dorsopalmar radiograph of the left wrist 10 days post trauma. No evidence of fracture is seen.

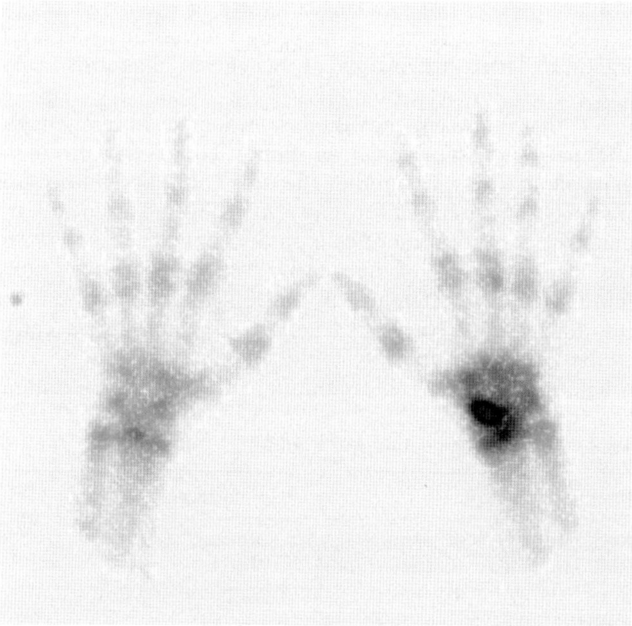

Figure 2. Local view of the hand from a $^{99}Tc^{m}$-methylene diphosphonate labelled bone scintigram showing increased tracer uptake in the region of the left scaphoid.

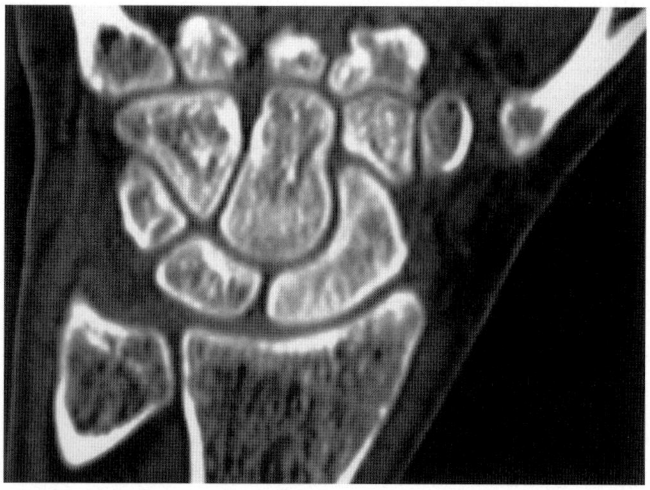

Figure 3. Coronal reconstruction from a 16-detector multi-detector CT of the left wrist 10 days post injury. The image was obtained using the 0.75 mm detectors and reconstructed in 0.5 mm intervals using a hard tissue algorithm. No fracture is identified.

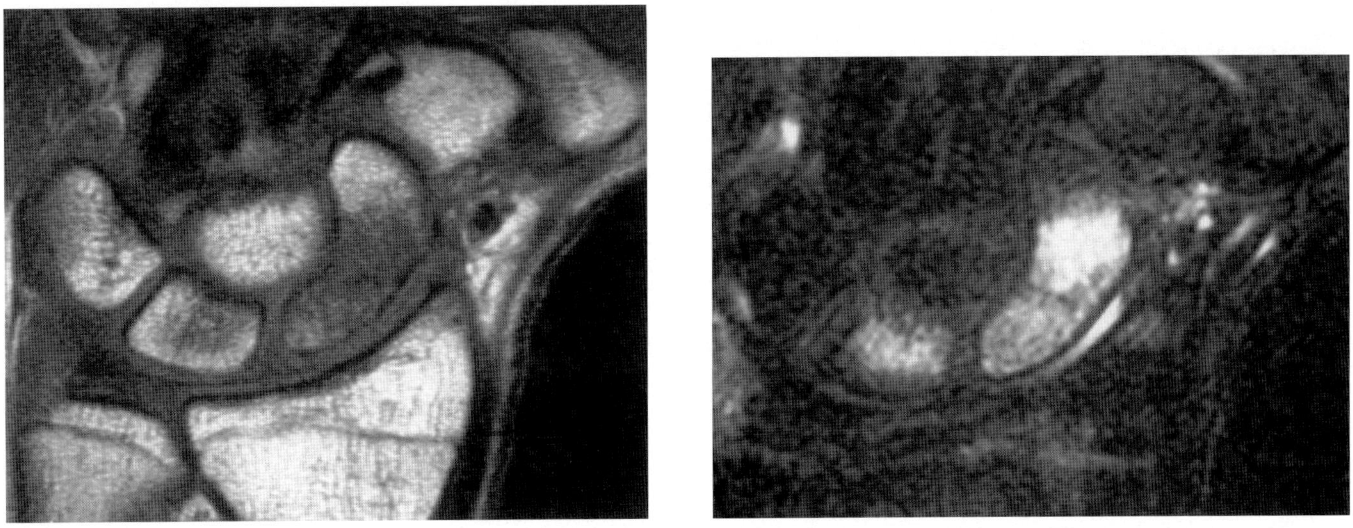

(a) (b)

Figure 4. (a) T_1 weighted coronal MRI of the left wrist performed 13 days post trauma showing reduced signal in scaphoid. (b) Fat saturated T_2 weighted coronal MRI of the left wrist performed 13 days post trauma showing high signal in the scaphoid. There is a suggestion of a fracture line in the proximal one third.

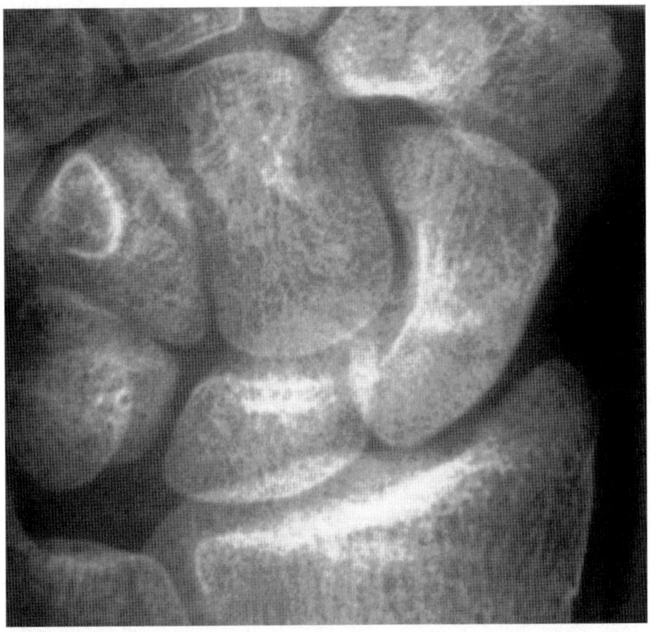

Figure 5. Dorsopalmar radiograph of the left wrist 6 weeks post injury. A fracture is identified affecting the proximal pole of the scaphoid.

multiplanar reconstructions from isometric voxels at subminute examination times. These advances have led CT to exquisitely demonstrate bone cortex and trabecula pattern, which should in theory aid the detection of bone fracture. In this case, the isometric voxels allow multiplanar reconstructions through the long axis of the scaphoid and thus diminishes the necessity to perform true coronal sections of the wrist in ulnar deviation. These advances in CT have led our institution to investigate the potential use of this technology in diagnosing fractures.

Despite the most modern CT machines, with use of 0.5 mm sections and multiplanar examination, this case demonstrates the potential fallibility of the technique against the sensitivity of conventional scintigraphy and MRI. The case illustrates that despite multidetector technology, CT still relies upon cortical and/or trabecular displacement to demonstrate fractures.

References

1. Kozin SH. Incidence, mechanism, and natural history of scaphoid fractures. Hand Clinics 2001;17:515–24.
2. Chakravarty D, Sloan J, Brenchley J. Risk reduction through skeletal scintigraphy as a screening tool in suspected scaphoid fracture: a literature review. Emerg Med J 2002;19:507–9.
3. Tiel-van Buul MM, Roolker W, Broekhuizen AH, van Beek EJ. The diagnostic management of suspected scaphoid fracture. Injury 1997;28:1–8.
4. Tiel-van Buul MM, van Beek EJ, Dijkstra P, Bakker AJ, Broekhuizen TH, van Royen EA. Significance of a hot spot on the bone scan after carpal injury-evaluation by computed tomography. Eur J Nucl Med 1993;20:159–64.
5. Dorsay TA, Major NM, Helms CA. Cost-effectiveness of immediate MR imaging versus traditional follow-up for revealing radiographically occult scaphoid fractures. AJR Am J Roentgenol 2001;177:1257–63.
6. Mack MG, Keim S, Balzer JO, et al. Clinical impact of MRI in acute wrist fractures. Eur Radiol 2003;13:612–7.
7. Brydie A, Raby N. Early MRI in the management of clinical scaphoid fracture. Br J Radiol 2003;76:296–300.
8. Bain GI, Bennett JD, Richards RS, Slethaug GP, Roth JH. Longitudinal computed tomography of the scaphoid; a new technique. Skeletal Radiol 1995;24:271–3.

The British Journal of Radiology, 78 (2005), 60–61
DOI: 10.1259/bjr/31723131

Case report
Renal replacement lipomatosis associated with renal transplantation

[1]S D CHANG, MD, [2]F V COAKLEY, MB BCh and [2]R B GOLDSTEIN, MD

[1]*Department of Radiology, University of British Columbia, Vancouver Hospital & Health Sciences Centre, 899 West 12th Avenue, Vancouver, BC, Canada V5Z 1M9 and* [2]*Department of Radiology, University of California San Francisco, 505 Parnassus Avenue, San Francisco, CA 94143-0628, USA*

Abstract. We report a case of extensive renal replacement lipomatosis demonstrated by ultrasound (US) and computed tomography (CT) in a 57-year-old woman with a history of two cadaveric renal transplants. One transplant was non-functional due to chronic rejection. The second renal transplant is functioning normally and the renal replacement lipomatosis did not cause mass effect on either of the renal transplants.

Renal replacement lipomatosis (RRL) is the benign proliferation of fibrofatty tissue replacing renal parenchyma that has atrophied. In most cases, there is severe destruction of the renal parenchyma with fibrofatty tissue replacement and the extent of the proliferation can involve the renal sinus, renal hilum and perirenal space. However, cases with focal involvement of the renal tissue can also occur. RRL is usually a result of chronic inflammation and in greater than 70% of cases, it is associated with calculus disease [1, 2]. We report a case of extensive renal replacement lipomatosis in a patient who had received two cadaveric renal transplants. Possible aetiological factors are discussed.

Case report

A 57-year-old woman was admitted for evaluation of an enterocutaneous fistula, which had developed as a complication of a right colectomy performed for carcinoma of the colon 3 months previously. Her past medical history was notable for a 21 year history of insulin-dependent diabetes mellitus. Her past surgical history included cadaveric renal transplantation for end-stage urate nephropathy 10 years previously. This transplant failed due to rejection and a second transplant was performed 2 years later. Since transplantation, the patient had been successfully maintained on corticosteroids, Cyclosporin and Imuran, with no evidence of rejection in the second transplant. Findings on physical examination included severe truncal obesity, a right lower quadrant ileostomy and an enterocutaneous fistula.

CT was performed for assessment of the enterocutaneous fistula. Unexpectedly, CT showed fat deposition in the renal sinus and hilum replacing most of the atrophic native kidneys. There was extensive fatty proliferation of the perirenal space with marked anterior and medial displacement of the bowel (Figure 1). A functioning renal allograft was present in the left iliac fossa and an atrophic non-functioning allograft in the right iliac fossa. Both of these renal transplants were not affected by the extensive RRL. A subsequent ultrasound (US) performed to evaluate the renal transplant, also showed extensive retroperitoneal fat. The pancreas and native kidneys were not visible at US owing to the extensive retroperitoneal fat deposition. A follow-up CT performed 1 year later showed no change in the appearance of the extensive renal replacement lipomatosis.

Received 7 April 2004 and in revised form 21 July 2004, accepted 9 September 2004.

Discussion

RRL is a rare condition characterized by the proliferation of the renal sinus, renal hilum and perirenal fatty tissue with replacement of the atrophic renal parenchyma. The extent of this disease is variable. A milder and more common form of this entity involving the renal sinus is referred to as renal sinus lipomatosis. Fibrofatty proliferation of the renal sinus, renal hilum, and/or perirenal space

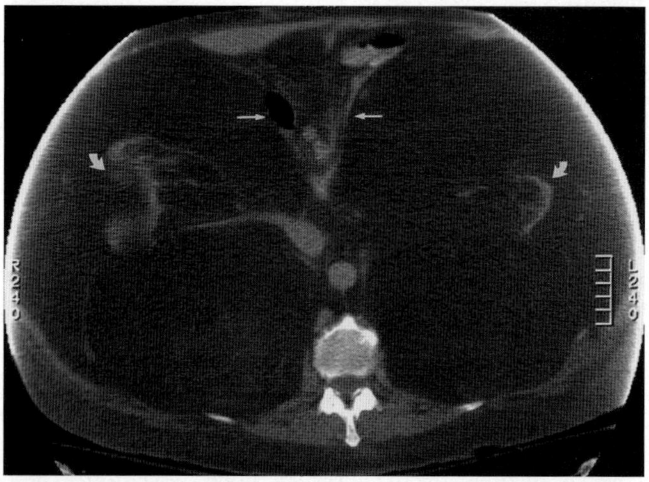

Figure 1. A 57-year-old woman with extensive renal replacement lipomatosis following two cadaveric renal transplants and on long-term steroid therapy. CT shows extensive deposition of fat in the retroperitoneum surrounding and replacing most of the native atrophic kidneys (curved arrows). Mass effect on the bowel loops (straight arrows) is also demonstrated.

can also occur with obesity, Cushing's syndrome, corticosteroid excess or be idiopathic but there is usually preservation of the renal parenchyma which helps to distinguish these entities from RRL [3, 4]. In RRL, there is fatty replacement of the atrophic/destroyed renal tissue and usually a history of chronic inflammation and stone disease [1, 2]. The clinical presentation of RRL is non-specific and variable. Patients may have a history of urinary tract infection, flank pain, weight loss, haematuria, fever or palpable mass [5]. Occasionally, they can be asymptomatic. RRL can simulate a soft tissue neoplasm on plain film and hydronephrosis or xanthogranulomatous pyelonephritis (XGPN) with contrast radiography. The advent of US and particularly CT, allows for direct visualization and can reliably distinguish adipose tissue from other soft tissue masses. CT is the best imaging modality to diagnose RRL and differentiate it from other fat containing lesions such as renal angiomyolipomas, retroperitoneal lipomas and liposarcomas [6]. Angiomyolipomas are usually well-circumscribed, focal intrarenal or extrarenal masses. Lipomas are well circumscribed and encapsulated. Liposarcomas may be well circumscribed or infiltrative, but are characteristically identified by the presence of internal thick soft tissue strands or nodules. And in all three of these entities, renal function is expected to be preserved and they are not usually associated with chronic inflammation and stone disease. CT can also differentiate RRL from XGPN and hydronephrosis. In all three of these conditions, an associated calculus may be seen. In RRL, the kidney is atrophic and replaced with fatty tissue whereas in XGPN, the renal outline is generally preserved and enlarged and true fat density is usually not seen [7, 8].

Our case of extensive fat deposition replacing most of the atrophic native kidneys and extensive proliferation around the native kidneys in a patient with a history of end-stage renal disease is compatible with renal replacement lipomatosis. To our knowledge the severity in this case and the association with renal transplantation has not been previously reported. The extensive involvement also suggests more than one aetiological factor may be involved and are subsequently discussed.

Hypoechogenicity of the perinephric fat has been described in 13.5% of renal transplant recipients [9] and probably reflects reduced water content [10, 11]. These findings suggest the perinephric fat around the native kidneys of renal transplant recipients may be different from adipose tissue elsewhere in the body. While the nature of these differences is unclear, they may account for the extensive distribution of lipomatosis seen in our patient. Long-term steroid administration may also be a factor in the development of lipomatosis, although a perinephric pattern of lipomatosis is not characteristic of the fatty proliferation seen in Cushing's syndrome.

A potential criticism of this report is the lack of pathological correlation. However, the diagnosis of renal replacement lipomatosis is essentially radiographic. Biopsy of lipomatosis demonstrates unremarkable mature adipose tissue and may contain fibrous tissue, and does not contribute to the diagnosis of lipomatosis, which depends on the demonstration of abnormal fatty accumulation by imaging.

In summary, we report a case of extensive renal replacement lipomatosis in a patient with a history of renal transplantation and previous urate nephropathy. This extensive pattern of RRL may be also be attributed by the distinct properties of the perinephric fat after renal transplantation and long term corticosteroid usage.

References

1. Kuthman A. Replacement lipomatosis of the kidney. Surg Gynecol Obstet 1931;52:690–701.
2. Roth LJ, Davidson HB. Fibrous and fatty replacement of renal parenchyma. JAMA 1938;111:233–9.
3. Ambos MA, Bosniak MA, Gordon R, Madaya MA. Replacement lipomatosis of the kidney. AJR Am J Roentgenol 1978;130:1087–91.
4. Hurwitz RS, Benjamin JA, Cooper JF. Excessive proliferation of peripelvic fat of the kidney. Urology 1978;11:448–56.
5. Kullendorff B, Nyman U, Aspelin P. Computed tomography in renal replacement lipomatosis. Acta Radiologica 1987;28:447–50.
6. Waligore MP, Stephens DH, Soule EH, McLeod RA. Lipomatous tumors of the abdominal cavity: CT appearance and pathologic correlation. AJR Am J Roentgenol 1981;137:539–45.
7. Goldman SM, Hartman DS, Fishman EK, Finizio JP, Gatewood OM, Siegalmann SS. CT of xanthogranulomatous pyelonephritis: radiologic-pathologic correlation. AJR Am J Roentgenol 1984;142:963–9.
8. Claes H, Vereecken R, Oyen R, Van Damme B. Xanthogranulomatous pyelonephritis with emphasis on computerized tomography scan. Urology 1987;29:389–93.
9. Heinz-Peer G, Oettl C, Mayer G, Mostbeck GH. Hypoechoic perirenal fat in renal transplant recipients. Radiology 1994;193:717–20.
10. Behan M, Kazam E. The echographic characteristics of fatty tissues and tumors. Radiology 1978;129:143–51.
11. Brammer HM, Smith SW, Lubbers PR. Septated hypoechoic perirenal fat on sonograms: a pitfall in renal ultrasonography. J Ultrasound Med 1992;11:361–3.

The British Journal of Radiology, 78 (2005), 62–64
DOI: 10.1259/bjr/13370263

Case report
Endovascular repair of a ruptured abdominal aortic aneurysm under local anaesthesia

[1]J P MORALES, MD, [1]F G IRANI, MBBS, MD, [2]K G JONES, FRCS, [2]P R TAYLOR, MA, MChir, FRCS, [1]R DOURADO, DCR and [1]T SABHARWAL, MBBCH, FRCSI, FRCR

Departments of [1]Interventional Radiology and [2]Vascular Surgery, Guy's and St Thomas' Hospital, London, UK

Abstract. Abdominal aortic aneurysm (AAA) is a common degenerative condition affecting the elderly population. Rupture carries a high overall mortality. Elective endovascular stent graft repair is well described. We describe a patient with ruptured AAA and co-morbid conditions making him unfit for surgery and general or epidural anaesthesia, who was successfully treated by endovascular stent graft under local anaesthesia.

Abdominal aortic aneurysm (AAA) is a common degenerative condition affecting men three times more frequently than women [1]. There were 6800 deaths in England and Wales in the year 2000 from rupture of AAA [2]. The overall mortality rate from aneurysm rupture is in the order of 65–85% [3]. Of the deaths attributed to ruptured aneurysm, about half occurred before the patient reached hospital [4] and for those who survived the initial period; the mortality rate from emergency open surgical treatment was between 30% and 70% [3, 4].

Endovascular repair of AAA has evolved dramatically since it was first described in 1991 [5]. Elective endovascular repair of AAA is now an established procedure and given the potential to reduce morbidity and mortality associated with open surgical repair, endoluminal stenting offers therapeutic options to patients who are not surgical candidates due to their co-morbidities [6, 7].

Case report

A 71-year-old gentleman was admitted to a District General Hospital with pain in the abdomen and a tender partially irreducible right inguinal hernia. He had previously been diagnosed as having bilateral inguinal herniae and an asymptomatic infrarenal AAA, for which he refused treatment. During admission, the patient developed further abdominal pain, with a hypotensive episode and his haemoglobin fell from 15 gm% to 9 gm%. A clinical diagnosis of aortic aneurysm rupture was made. As he was haemodynamically stable, a CT scan was performed. The scan revealed an infrarenal suprailiac AAA with a maximum anteroposterior dimension of 6.5 cm. There was a large retroperitoneal haematoma extending into the pelvis, right scrotal sac and the right paracolic gutter. Active extravasation of contrast medium was noted from the left side of the aneurysmal sac (Figure 1).

Received 24 May 2004 and in revised form 12 August 2004, accepted 1 October 2004.

Address correspondence to Dr Tarun Sabharwal, Consultant Radiologist, Department of Radiology, 1st Floor Lambeth Wing, St Thomas' Hospital, Lambeth Palace Road, London SE1 7EH, UK.

The patient was a known hypertensive on treatment. He had suffered from rheumatic fever in childhood and now suffered from arrhythmias and atrial fibrillation for which he was receiving Verapamil, Amiloride and Warfarin. He also suffered from chronic obstructive pulmonary disease (COPD) and carbon dioxide retention. In view of his high cardiopulmonary co-morbidities and abnormal coagulation profile, the patient was considered unfit for open surgery and general anaesthesia.

The appearance on CT suggested that the patient was suitable for endoluminal stent grafting (aneurysmal neck length 35 mm and favourable iliac arteries) and he was consequently transferred to our specialist vascular unit.

On arrival, the patient was drowsy, pale with a tender tense abdomen. His pulse rate was 80 beats per minute, blood pressure 108/60 mm Hg, haemoglobin of 9.0 gm%, oxygen saturation 97% on 2 l min^{-1} of oxygen with bilateral basal and right mid-zone crepitations. A coagulation profile revealed an international normalized ratio (INR) of 3.5 and activated partial thromboplastin time of 1.85.

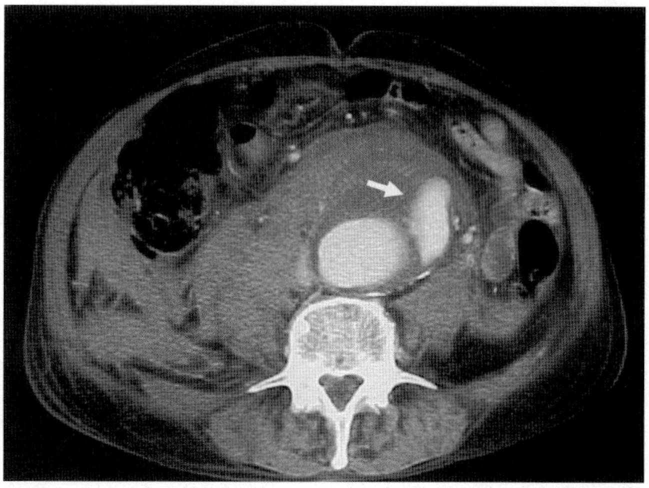

Figure 1. Contrast enhanced CT scan showing an abdominal aortic aneurysm with retroperitoneal, right paracolic gutter haematoma and active extravasation of contrast (arrow).

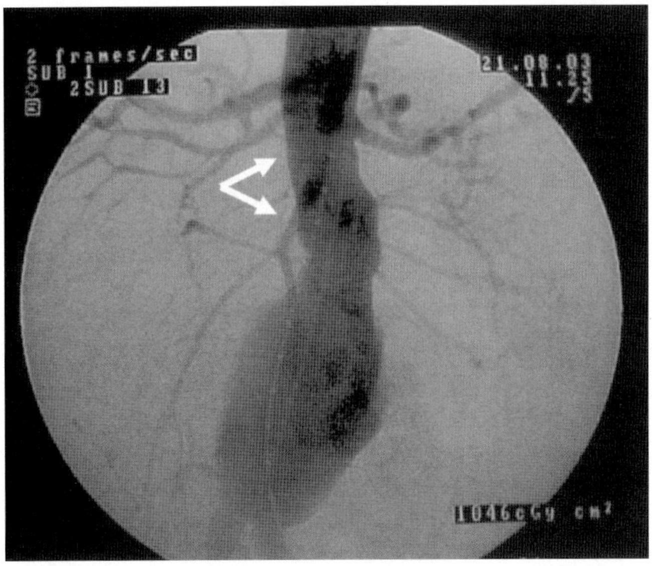

Figure 2. Early phase angiogram showing abdominal aortic aneurysm with a favourable 3.5 cm length infrarenal neck (arrows).

It is our normal practice to insert aortic stent grafts under epidural or general anaesthesia. However in view of his deranged coagulation and co-morbid health state, particularly COPD, after obtaining informed consent, we performed the procedure under local anaesthetic (20 ml of 0.5% Bupivacaine hydrochloride, Astra Zeneca, Kings Langley, UK) and sedo-analgesia (Remifentanyl 10 μg ml^{-1} Ultiva; Glaxo Wellcome, London, UK and Propofol 1% Diprivan; Astra Zeneca). We chose to insert an aorto-bi-iliac endovascular stent graft. Two units of fresh frozen plasma were infused prior to the procedure, which was performed in the operating theatre using a Siemens Siremobil Iso-C Image Intensifier (Siemens AG, Erlangen, Germany).

Access was gained via common femoral arteriotomies. On table angiogram with a measuring catheter (5 F, Royal

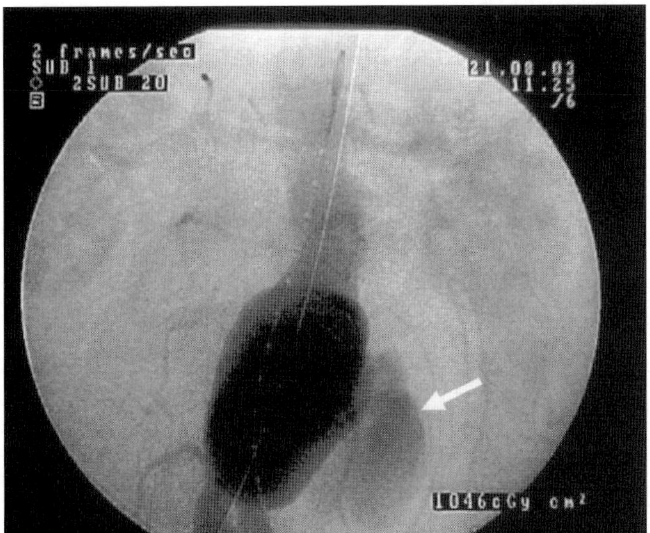

Figure 3. Late phase angiogram showing active extravasation of contrast medium (arrow).

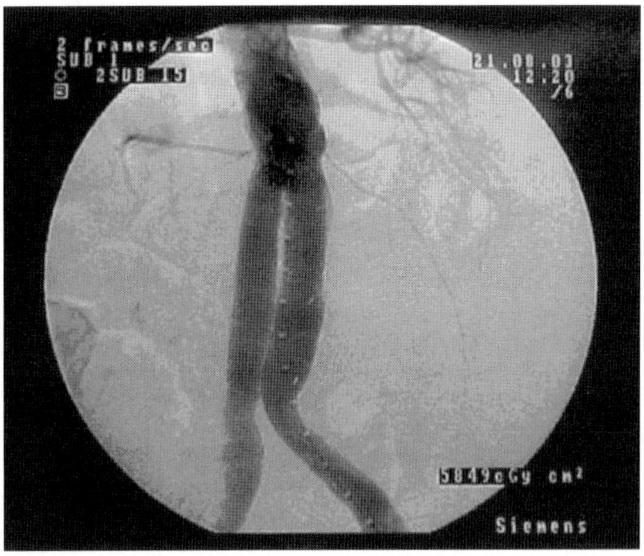

Figure 4. Post deployment angiogram showing stent graft *in situ*, with exclusion of aneurysm sac and leak.

Flush® Plus Beacon® Tip Pigtail Angiographic Catheter; William Cook, Europe, Bjaeverskov) showed an infrarenal AAA without extension into the common iliac arteries (Figure 2) and extravasation of contrast from the sac (Figure 3).

An aorto-bi-iliac bifurcated Excluder endoprosthesis (WL Gore, Flagstaff, AZ) of size 23 mm × 160 mm × 95 mm was positioned and deployed infrarenally under fluoroscopy guidance using standard techniques.

Post deployment angiography showed complete exclusion of the aneurysmal sac, with no further extravasation of contrast medium (Figure 4) and preservation of both internal iliac arteries. Intraprocedurally the patient received 3000 IU of Monoparin® (heparin sodium 1000 units ml^{-1}, CP Pharmacueticals, Wrexham, UK) and 1.2 g of Augmentin® (amoxiclav 1000/200, Glaxo Wellcome) intravenously. No immediate complications were noted and the total procedure time was 125 min.

Following the procedure, the patient with his poor pulmonary reserve decompensated and became acidotic. He was transferred to the high dependency unit where he was closely monitored for 2 days. He received 2 units of packed cells and his haemoglobin remained stable. He was discharged after 3 days on the ward with a haemoglobin of 8.7 gm%.

On 6 month clinical follow up, the patient is alive and doing well, with no complaints related to his AAA.

Discussion

Following rupture of an AAA, only an estimated 38–64% of patients reach hospital alive [1]. Operative repair of ruptured AAA is associated with mortality rates between 25% and 60% [8].

AAA rupture can result in haemodynamic collapse and death before the patient reaches hospital. In slow ongoing contained leaks, the patient presents with abdominal pain, pulsating abdominal mass, falling blood pressure and haemoglobin.

The patient's risk of rupture from their AAA is increased if they also suffer with chronic obstructive airway disease, cardiac disease, stroke and aneurysm of size greater than 5 cm [7]. These same factors, in addition to malignancy, chronic renal failure, Parkinson's disease, dementia, co-existent severe acute pancreatitis and known thoracoabdominal extension of the aneurysm make patients unfit for surgery [8, 9]. The co-morbidities in our patient, not only made the aneurysm prone to rupture but also made him unfit for open surgery and general or epidural anaesthesia.

Endovascular repair of AAA is a minimally invasive procedure with a potentially reduced morbidity and mortality, as it avoids the need for surgical exposure of the aorta and aortic cross clamping [6, 10]. In addition, the use of endoprosthesis can considerably reduce the cardiac strain during the procedure as compared with open surgery and hence is particularly advantageous in high risk surgically unfit patients [11].

During the endovascular repair, the endograft is positioned within the aorta by a transfemoral or transiliac route to exclude the aneurysmal sac from the circulation, the graft being anchored by one or more metallic stents [6].

Experimental studies have shown that covered stents seal off the AAA immediately after stent placement, with gradual obliteration of the aneurysmal sac by collagen resulting in the reduced risk of further aneurysmal expansion and rupture [12].

The Registry of Endovascular Treatment of Abdominal Aortic Aneurysms (RETA) data have shown that only 30–50% of aneurysms are suitable for endovascular repair [10]. The procedure requires an accurate determination of aneurysm morphology with contrast enhanced CT or angiography. In symptomatic and ruptured AAA, a helical CT scan can rapidly assess the feasibility of endovascular treatment [10, 12]. This is provided that the patient is in a haemodynamically stable condition, as in our case.

The use of local anaesthesia with liberal sedation is an acceptable technique for endovascular aneurysmal repair because of its simplicity, reduced haemodynamic manipulation (in particular less vasopressor administration), reduced requirement for both intravenous fluid and subsequent monitoring and usage of ICU and hospital beds [11]. Further it provides a particular advantage in patients at high risk of cardiovascular complications and leaking aortic aneurysm since it does not change the haemodynamic situation in contrast to general anaesthesia [11, 13]. Bettex et al [11] in their study comparing the use of general, epidural and local anaesthesia for endovascular repair successfully used local anaesthesia in 63 of 91 patients, including four patients with ruptured aneurysms. The poor cardiopulmonary reserve in our patient made him unsuitable for general anaesthesia. The high INR made the patient unsuitable for epidural anaesthesia for fear of development of an epidural haematoma. For the moment, endoluminal repair of ruptured AAA, only seems applicable in selected haemodynamically stable unfit patients, as overall health status of patients and burden of co-morbid disease are important predictors of survival after endovascular repair [6, 9].

Whilst open surgical repair still remains the treatment of choice in haemodynamically unstable patients with ruptured AAA, we have demonstrated that endoluminal treatment under local anaesthesia in patients with raised INR can be successfully performed avoiding the complications of laparotomy, general and epidural anaesthesia, long hospital and intensive care stays.

References

1. MacSweeney STM, O'Meara M, Alexander C, O'Malley MK, Powell JT, Greenhalgh RM. High prevalence of unsuspected abdominal aortic aneurysm in patients with confirmed symptomatic peripheral or cerebral arterial disease. Br J Surg 1993;80:582–4.
2. Ashton HA, Buxton MJ, Day NE, Kinn LG, Marteau TM, Scott RAP, et al. The multicenter aneurysm screening study (MASS) into the effect of abdominal aortic aneurysm screening on mortality in men: a randomised control trial. Lancet 2002;360:1531–9.
3. Kniemeyer HW, Kessler T, Reber PU, Ris HB, Hakki H, Widmer MK. Treatment of ruptured aortic aneurysm, a permanent challenge or a waste of resources? Prediction of outcome using multi-organ dysfunction score. Eur J Vasc Endovasc Surg 2000;19:190–6.
4. Wilmink TBM, Quick CRG, Hubbard CS, Day NE. The influence of screening on the incidence of ruptured abdominal aortic aneurysm. J Vasc Surg 1999;30:203–8.
5. Parodi JC, Palmaz JC, Barone HD. Transfemoral intraluminal graft implantation for abdominal aortic aneurysm. Ann Vasc Surg 1991;5:491–9.
6. Thomas SM, Gaines PA, Beard JD. Short term (30 days) outcome of endovascular treatment of abdominal aortic aneurysm: results from the prospective registry endovascular treatment of abdominal aortic aneurysm (RETA). Eur J Vasc Endovasc Surg 2001;21:57–64.
7. Jones A, Cahill D, Gardham R. Outcome in patients with a large abdominal aortic aneurysm considered unfit for surgery. Br J Surg 1998;85:1382–4.
8. Bradbury AW, Makhdoomi KR, Adam DJ, Murie JA, Jenkins AM, Ruckley CV. Twelve year experience in the management of ruptured abdominal aortic aneurysm. Br J Surg 1997;84:1705–7.
9. Laheij RJF, van Marrewijk CJ. Endovascular stenting of abdominal aortic aneurysm in patients unfit for elective open surgery. Lancet 2000;356:832.
10. Benedikt P, Lachat M, Pfammatter T, Stalder N, Schmidli J, von Smekal A, et al. Emergency surgery for abdominal aortic aneurysms — could an endovascular method be considered? Swiss Surg 1999;5:239–42.
11. Bettex DA, Lachat M, Pfammatter T, Schmidlin D, Turina MI, Schmid ER. To compare general, epidural and local anaesthesia for endovascular aneurysm repair (EVAR). Eur J Vasc Endovasc Surg 2001;21:179–84.
12. Ruiz CE, Zheng HP, Whittaker P. Non-surgical treatment of abdominal aortic aneurysms. Cardiologica 1997;42:903–12.
13. Lachat M, Pfammatter T, Bernard E, Jerggy C, Vogt P, Turina M. Successful endovascular repair of leaking abdominal aortic aneurysm under local anaesthesia. Swiss Surg 2001;7:86–9.

The British Journal of Radiology, *78* (2005), 65–67
DOI: 10.1259/bjr/68967544

Case report

Renal cell carcinoma vertebral body metastasis extending into the azygos venous system causing superior vena cava obstruction

M STRUGNELL, MRCS, M GIBSON, FRCR, R HOPKINS, FRCR, I LYBURN, FRCR and G McGANN, FRCR

Cheltenham General Hospital, Sanford Road, Cheltenham GL53 7AN, UK

Abstract. We describe a case of superior vena cava (SVC) obstruction caused by extension of tumour thrombus from a vertebral body metastasis through the azygos system to the SVC. The primary tumour was a renal cell carcinoma.

It is well known that primary renal cell carcinoma (RCC) can involve the inferior vena cava (IVC) by extension of tumour thrombus along the renal vein. Venous involvement is incorporated into the TNM classification system of the International Union Against Cancer (UICC); the tumour being classified as stage T3b if there is involvement of the renal vein alone, T3c if the tumour thrombus extends into the infradiaphragmatic IVC and T4b with extension to the supradiaphragmatic IVC. Tumour thrombus can cause obstruction of the IVC, and there have been reports of tumour thrombus extending as far as the right atrium [1]. We report a case of superior vena cava (SVC) obstruction due to azygos vein tumour

Received 26 April 2004 and in revised form 11 August 2004, accepted 1 October 2004.

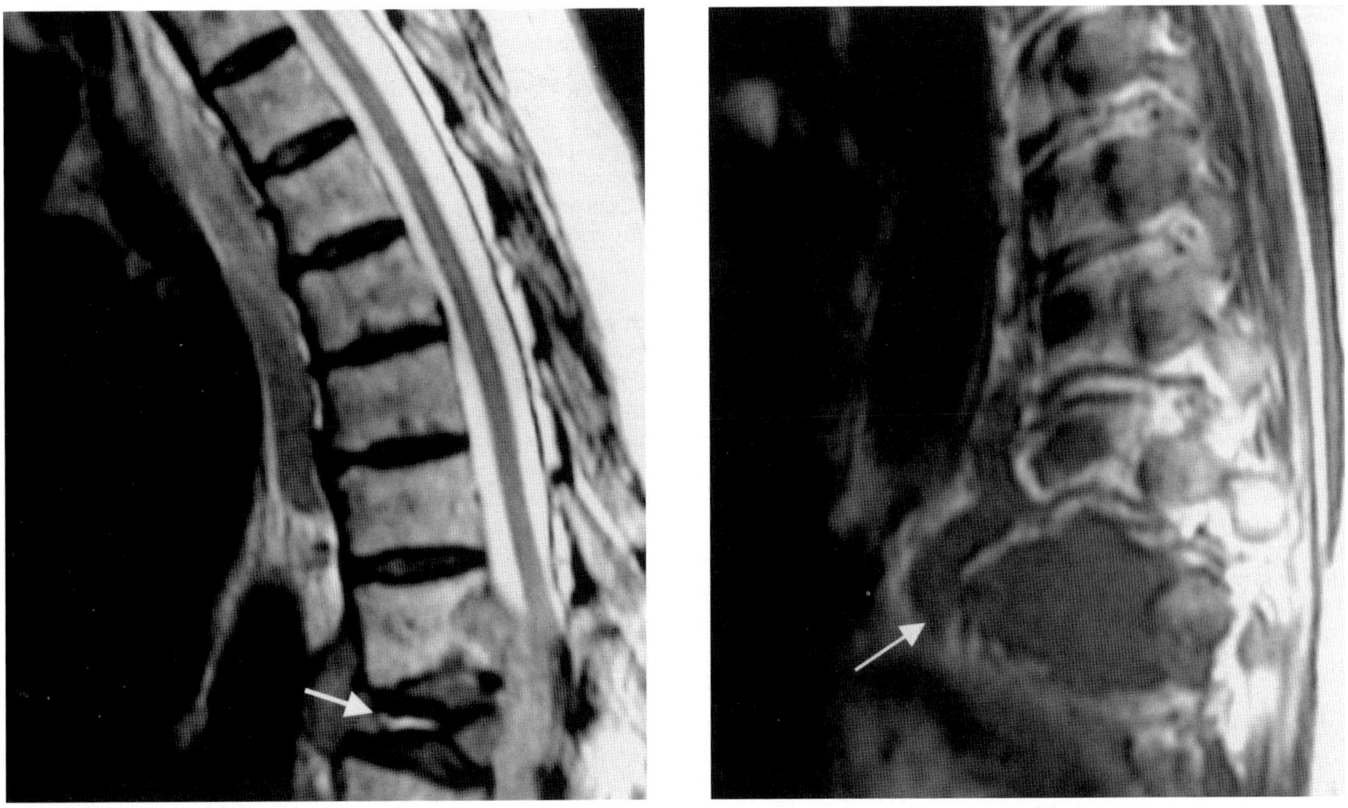

(a) (b)

Figure 1. 66-year-old female with metastatic renal cell carcinoma. (a) Sagittal T_2 weighted MRI (repetition time/echo time (TR/TE) 3500/107.6) of the spine showing collapse of the T11 vertebral body (arrow) and cord compression due to metastatic renal cell carcinoma. (b) T_1 weighted parasagittal MRI (TR/TE 460/10.8) showing metastatic tumour in the vertebral body extending into the azygos venous system anteriorly (arrow).

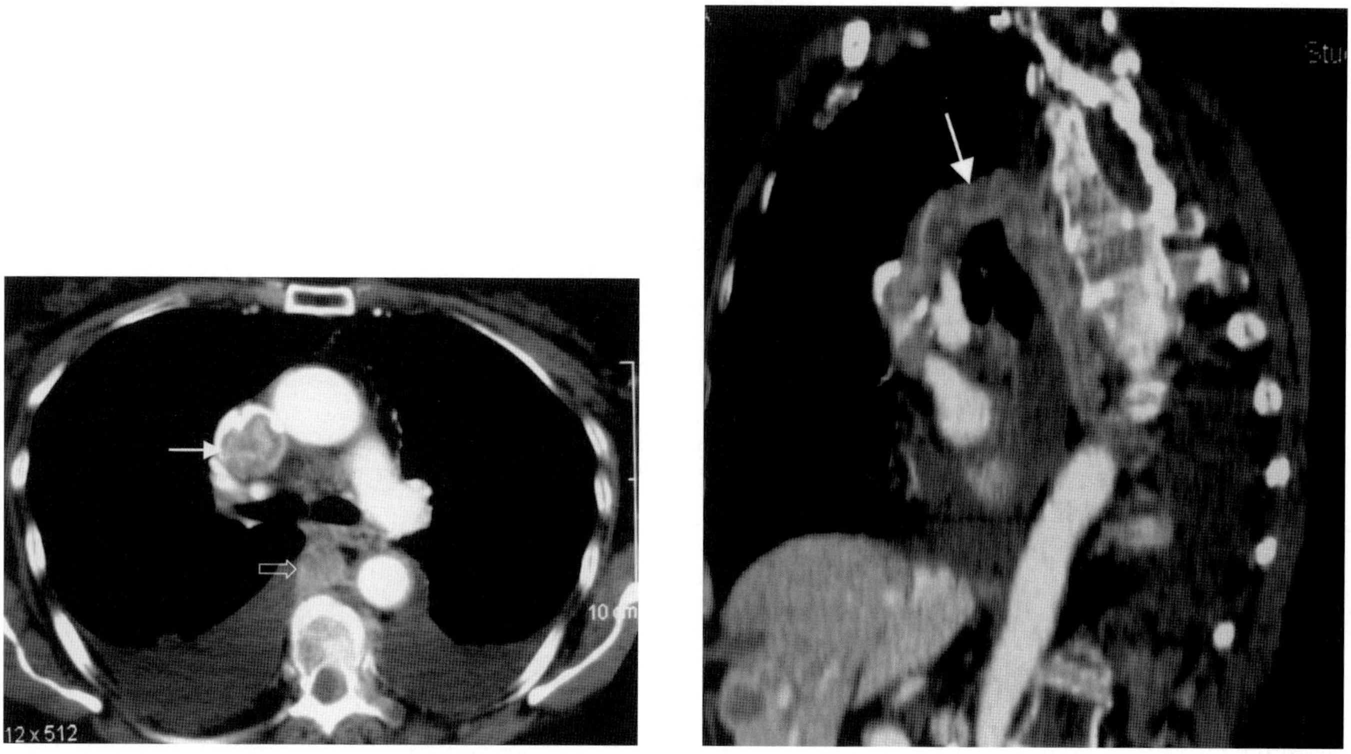

(a) (b)

Figure 2. 66-year-old female with metastatic renal cell carcinoma. Contrast enhanced venous phase CT (120 kV, 150 mAs, 3 mm collimation). (a) Axial image showing tumour thrombus in the superior vena cava (solid arrow) and azygos vein (open arrow). (b) Parasagittal oblique reconstruction showing tumour thrombus in the azygos vein extending into the superior vena cava (arrow).

thrombus arising from a RCC metastasis in a thoracic vertebral body. We can find no previous reports of tumour thrombus causing SVC obstruction.

Case report

A 66-year-old woman presented with a left sided abdominal mass. The initial CT revealed a 16 cm × 11 cm × 10 cm solid left renal mass, which did not extend into the renal vein or IVC and no distant metastases were identified. She consequently had a left nephrectomy. Pathology confirmed a large sarcomatoid renal cell carcinoma, Grade 4, pT3a N0 Stage III. The tumour extended to within 1 mm of the resection margin but the renal vein was not involved and there was no vascular invasion.

The patient re-presented 4 months later with back pain and paraplegia. MRI confirmed cord compression from a destructive soft tissue mass arising from the body of the 11th thoracic vertebral body (Figure 1a). There was also tumour thrombus, with the same signal characteristics as the vertebral metastasis, extending along the hemiazygos vein (Figure 1b). The mass extended anteriorly into the adjacent soft tissue and posteriorly into the spinal canal causing cord compression. She was treated with local radiotherapy. The paraplegia did not resolve.

The patient was re-admitted 5 months later with SVC obstruction syndrome. Contrast enhanced CT showed partially enhancing tumour thrombus distending and obstructing the azygos and hemiazygos veins. The tumour thrombus extended cranially into the SVC, causing obstruction (Figure 2).

Discussion

Primary RCC is well known to extend along the renal vein (20% of cases of RCC) and inferior vena cava (5% of cases) [1]. As such an integral part of the staging system is assessment of venous involvement at this is vital for surgical planning. Although tumour grade is the primary prognostic indicator [2], tumour size also has a relationship with the development of metastases, with 86% of patients with tumours greater than 12 cm in diameter developing metastases [3]. Larger tumours also have a poorer prognosis [2].

In our case, the primary tumour was large, but venous invasion was not demonstrated on either pre-operative imaging or operative pathology and there was no lymph node involvement. However, the patient represented within 4 months with metastatic disease. The vertebral metastasis in this patient was seen to behave in a similar fashion to primary RCC.

The azygos and hemiazygos veins receive venous blood from the posterior intercostal veins of the right and left thoracic wall and vertebrae, respectively [4]. The metastatic tumour in her thoracic vertebra extended via the azygos venous system into the SVC, producing SVC obstruction. This case highlights the ability of a metastatic deposit to behave in a similar fashion to the primary tumour.

References

1. Malcowicz SB. Clinical aspects of renal tumours. Semin Roentgenol 1995;30:102–15.

2. Strohmeyer T, Ackermann R. Classic and modern prognostic indicators in renal cell carcinoma: review of the literature. Urol Int 1991;47:203–12.
3. Fuhrman SA, Lasky LC, Limas C. Prognostic significance of morphologic parameters in renal cell carcinoma. Am J Surg Pathol 1981;6:655–63.
4. Gray H. Grays anatomy (35th edn). Norwich, UK, Longman: Warwick R & Williams L, 1973:701–2.

The British Journal of Radiology, 78 (2005), 68–71
DOI: 10.1259/bjr/28183033

Case report

Rectus abdominis endometriosis: a report of two cases

[1]V COEMAN, MD, [2]R SCIOT, MD, PhD and [1]I VAN BREUSEGHEM, MD

Departments of [1]Radiology and [2]Pathology, University Hospitals, Catholic University Leuven, Leuven, Belgium

Abstract. Endometriosis is characterized by the presence of histological normal endometrial tissue outside the uterine cavity. Most frequently endometriosis occurs within the pelvis. Extrapelvic endometriosis is less common, but can involve nearly every organ. We present two patients in whom endometriosis was found in the rectus abdominis muscle and discuss the imaging findings and pathological correlation.

Endometriosis is classically defined as the presence of functional endometrial glands and stroma outside the uterine cavity (ectopic as opposed to normally located or eutopic endometrium) [1]. Endometriosis is found predominantly in women of childbearing age. Overall prevalence, including both symptomatic and asymptomatic women, is estimated to be 5–10% [2, 3].

Endometriosis presents clinically with menstrual irregularities, dyspareunia, infertility and occasionally symptoms and signs mimicking an acute abdomen. Endometriosis may be located in the pelvis or be extrapelvic, most cases are intrapelvic. The extrapelvic implantation of endometrial tissue has been described in virtually every organ. The abdominal wall is a uncommon site of extrapelvic endometriosis, where it usually develops in an old surgical scar. Endometriosis involving the rectus abdominis muscle is rare. Until now, only 12 such cases have been described in the medical literature [4–11]. We present two cases of endometriosis involving the rectus abdominis muscle.

Case report

Patient 1

A 38-year-old woman presented with right lower quadrant pain, ongoing for 6 months, but worsening the last 2 months. There was a significant prior medical history of a caesarean section and a vaginal hysterectomy. There was no previous history of endometriosis.

Imaging evaluation started with an abdominal CT scan (Figure 1) demonstrating an asymmetric thickening of the most distal part of the right rectus abdominis muscle which homogeneously enhanced, and was interpreted as a desmoid tumour. Subsequently MRI (Intera 1.5 T; Philips, Best, The Netherlands) was performed to further establish the nature of lesion. The intramuscular location of the mass was confirmed and was inhomogeneously hyperintense on T_2 weighted images with fat saturation (Figure 2a), nearly isointense to surrounding muscle on T_1 weighted images with and without fat saturation (Figure 2b,c) and inhomogeneously enhancing after gadolinium contrast medium administration (Figure 2d). The mass was situated lateral to the Pfannenstiel-scar of the caesarean section. The lesion was encircled by very small tubular structures, in contiguity with and isointense to small blood vessels on all performed sequences. We therefore interpreted these structures as small blood vessels. These imaging findings raised the possibility of a desmoid tumour or a pseudotumoral lesion. The patient underwent a CT-guided biopsy of the lesion. Histological examination revealed areas of typical endometrial glands surrounded by stroma and bordered by vessels with occasional foci of haemosiderin-laden macrophages typical of endometriosis (Figure 3).

Patient 2

A 32-year-old woman presented with a painful mass in the right lower abdominal quadrant giving her a vague discomfort. Her relevant past medical history consisted of a laparascopic tubal ligation and an appendectomy. There was no previous history of endometriosis. High resolution ultrasound of the abdominal wall using a 11.4 MHz linear transducer (Sonoline Antares; Siemens, Erlangen, Germany) showed an ill-defined and inhomogeneous,

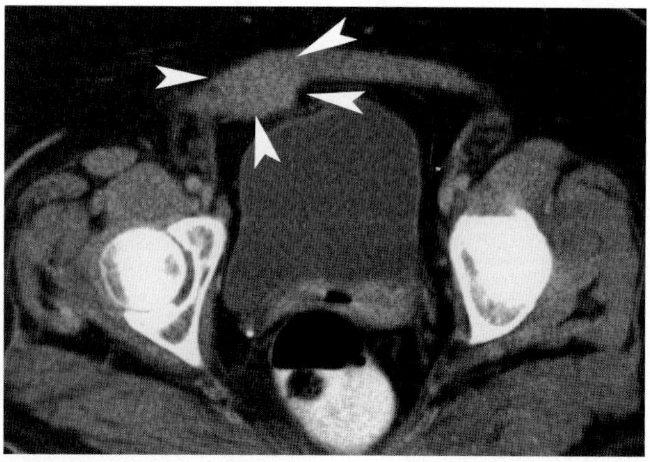

Figure 1. Axial CT-image (W: 400 HU; L: 50 HU) through the lower pelvis after intravenous contrast administration showing the contrast-enhanced mass in the right lower rectus abdominis muscle (arrowheads).

Received 31 March 2004 and in final form 3 September 2004, accepted 1 October 2004.

Address correspondence to Dr Iwan Van Breuseghem, Department of Radiology, University Hospitals Leuven, Herestraat 49, 3000 Leuven, Belgium.

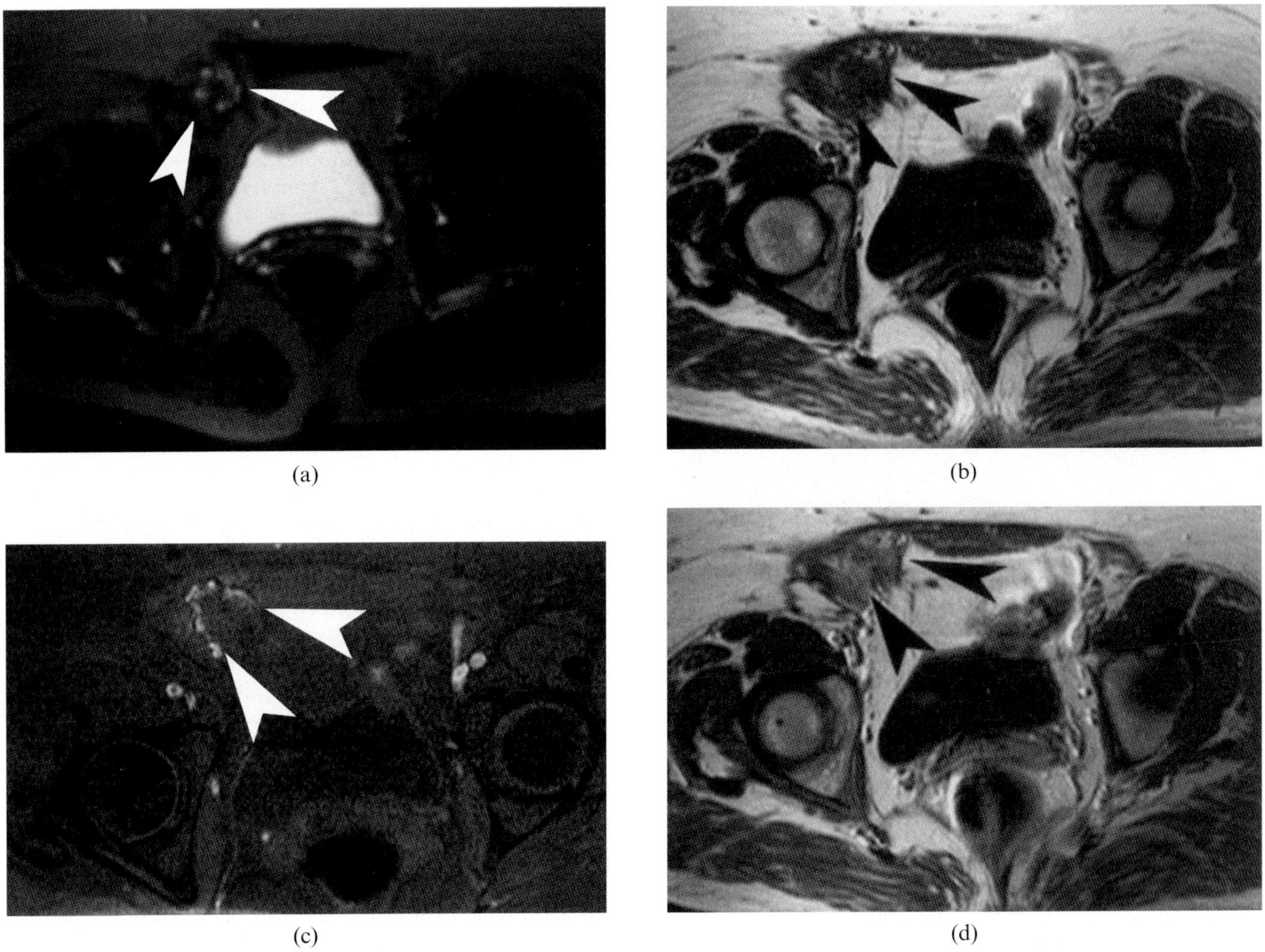

Figure 2. (a) Axial T_2 weighted image with fat saturation (repetition time (TR) 5100 ms; echo time (TE) 60 ms) through the lower pelvic region showing an inhomogeneously multinodular hyperintense mass (white arrowheads) in the lowest segment of the right rectus abdominis muscle. (b) Axial T_1 weighted image (TR 550 ms; TE 17 ms) demonstrating the same mass in the right rectus abdominis muscle (black arrowheads), which is nearly isointense to surrounding normal muscular tissue. (c) Axial T_1 weighted image (TR 550 ms; TE 17 ms) with fat saturation again demonstrating the mass which is isointense to surrounding muscle and splaying surrounding vessels (arrowheads). (d) Axial T_1 weighted image (TR 550 ms; TE 17 ms) after intravenous gadolinium contrast medium administration showing marked but inhomogeneous contrast enhancement of the mass in the right lower rectus abdominis muscle.

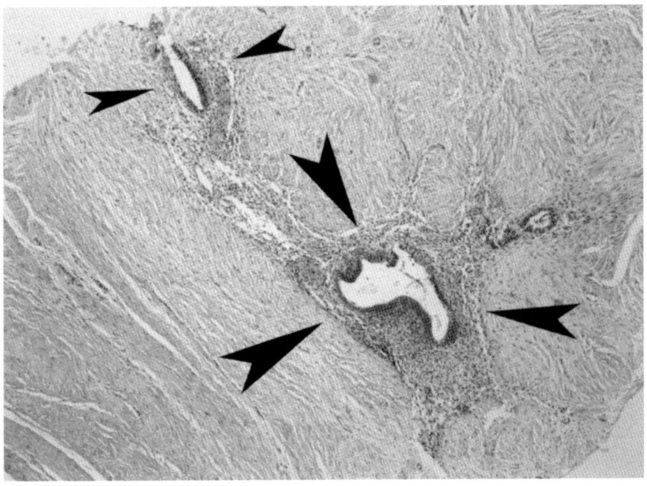

Figure 3. Low power view of the tissue sample of the mass in the rectus abdominis muscle, showing the nests of endometriosis (arrowheads) in a fibrous background.

mainly hyporeflective mass in the distal portion of the right rectus abdominis muscle (Figure 4), which was well vascularized at the periphery of the lesion and with some small vessels running centrally on power Doppler (not shown).

CT-scan (Somatom sensation Volume Zoom; Siemens, Erlangen, Germany) after intravenous and oral contrast administration was performed. This examination demonstrated a vesicular expansion of the distal part of the right rectus abdominis muscle (Figure 5a), which was homogeneously enhancing (Figure 5b). The patient underwent CT-guided biopsy and the tissue samples were confirmed as consistent with endometrial tissue.

Discussion

Endometriosis, a disorder afflicting as many as 5–10% of women of childbearing age, is defined as the presence of functional endometrial glands and stroma outside the uterine cavity [1–3].

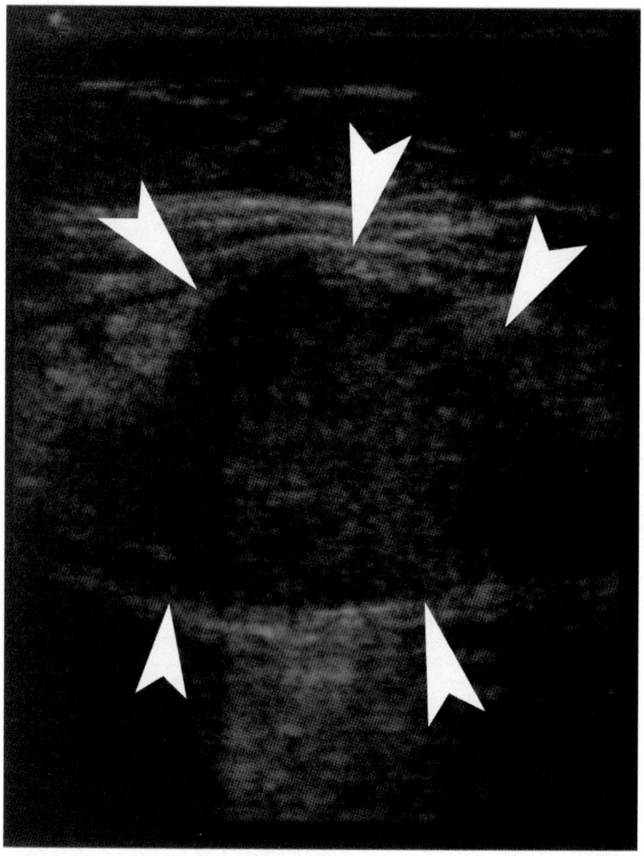

Figure 4. Transverse ultrasound image centred on the mass in the right lower rectus abdominis muscle demonstrating the mass (arrowheads) which is inhomogeneously hyporeflective to surrounding muscle and focally ill-delineated.

Endometriosis is a complex disorder and its causes are probably multifactorial. The most widely accepted theory is that endometriosis results from retrograde menstruation [2, 12]. The theory assumes transportation of endometrial tissue from the uterus in a retrograde fashion into the peritoneal cavity. The endometrial cells remain viable and implant outside the uterus where growth and proliferation of the transplanted cells occurs as well as metaplasia of adjacent cells to endometrial cells [13]. The biological behaviour of ectopic endometrial glands is variable and adds to the complexity of the disease. Ectopic endometriotic implants generally respond to circulating hormones in the same manner as eutopic endometrium (though to a lesser degree). Oestrogen stimulates glandular growth, whereas progesterone inhibits it. However, ectopic endometrium often behaves unpredictably, which leads to difficulties in diagnosis and treatment [13].

Gross pathological findings of endometriosis depend on the duration of the disease and depth of penetration of the lesions. Implants may change in appearance during the menstrual cycle, becoming more swollen and congested during menses and bleeding in some cases. Endometriotic cysts (endometriomas) generally occur within the ovaries and are the result of repeated cyclic haemorrhage within a deep implant. This appearance has been called "chocolate cyst". At microscopic analysis, endometriosis is composed of endometrial glands, stroma, and occasionally smooth muscle fibres. As with eutopic endometrium, the ectopic endometrial foci respond to circulating hormones and may show secretary changes during the second half of the menstrual cycle. Haemorrhage within these foci results in an inflammatory response, with infiltration of histiocytes that become pigment laden with haemosiderin [1]. Although generally confined to intrapelvic sites, such as ovaries, pelvic wall, or peritoneum, endometrial cells have been reported in the pleura, skin, lung, and skeletal muscles of the extremities [14, 15]. Abdominal wall endometriosis is generally found within the skin or subcutaneous tissues of the abdominal wall. The majority of abdominal wall endometriosis is located in surgical scars or tracts resulting from invasive abdominal–pelvic procedures. The aetiology of these foci of endometriosis is thought to be an iatrogenic transfer of endometrial cells into the surgical or procedural wound [16].

Rectus abdominis endometrioma, wherein the endometrial focus is solely confined to within the body of the rectus abdominis muscle is rare and sparsely reported in

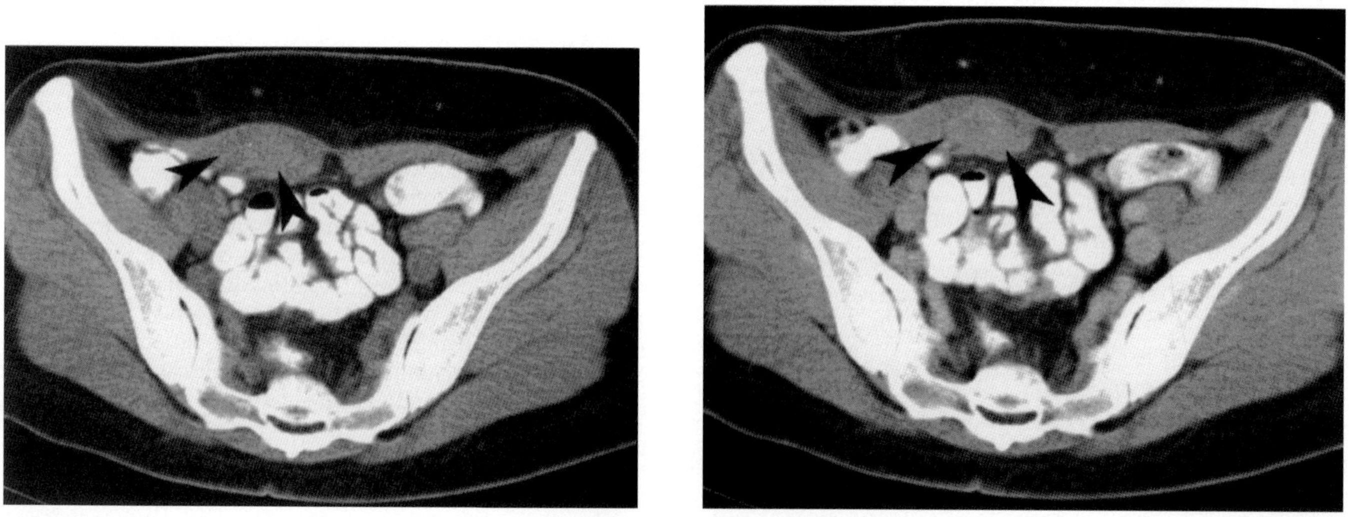

(a)

(b)

Figure 5. Axial CT-image (W: 400 HU; L: 50 HU) through the lower pelvis (a) before and (b) after intravenous contrast administration showing the mass in the right lower rectus abdominis muscle which is slightly enhancing (b).

literature [4–11] with only 11 new cases since it was first described in 1993 by Coley [11].

Endometriosis has no pathognomonic imaging findings on ultrasound, CT nor MRI, as its appearance depends on the phase of the menstrual cycle, the proportion of stromal and glandular elements, the amount of bleeding, and the degree of surrounding inflammatory and fibrotic response [1, 3, 11, 17–19]. The high proportion of glandular tissue versus encysted blood in the endometriomas in both patients might explain the described radiological features. Diffuse low-level internal echoes with septations, as classically described, were absent in our second patient. Classical MRI findings, consisting of multiple cystic structures which appear hyperintense on T_1 weighted images and having different signal intensity patterns on T_2 weighted images [20] were not present in our patients. The high proportion of glandular tissue also might explain the moderate to high contrast enhancement on CT as well as on MRI.

Due to this non-specific presentation, a broad radiological differential diagnosis remains. The differential diagnosis of a solid mass in the rectus abdominis muscle includes abscesses, haematomas, hernia, benign tumours (*e.g.* lipoma, haemangioma, desmoid tumour) and malignancies such as lymphomas and sarcomas [1, 2, 11]. MRI, albeit non-specific, may be useful in distinguishing endometrial tissue from surrounding structures. MR is highly sensitive in detecting very small masses and offers excellent differentiation of endometriomas from neighbouring tissue [10]. The multitude of signal patterns seen in endometriomas is due, in part, to the different stages of blood products found within these implants.

A certain diagnosis can only be accomplished by histological examination of the lesion (fine-needle aspirate or core biopsy obtained under ultrasound or CT-guidance) [21], as was the case in both our patients.

The treatment for endometriotic foci in the rectus abdominis muscle is usually surgically [4], by excision of the mass, or can be expectant depending on the severity of symptoms.

In conclusion, although rare, endometriosis should be part of the differential diagnosis in the work-up of a mass in the abdominal wall in younger women during child-bearing age, especially if there is a history of abdominal or pelvic surgery.

References

1. Woodward PJ, Sohaey R, Mezzetti TP. Endometriosis: radiologic-pathologic correlation. Radiographics 2001;21: 193–216.
2. Olive DL, Schwartz LB. Endometriosis. N Engl J Med 1993;328:1759–69.
3. Lu PY, Ory SJ. Endometriosis: current management. Mayo Clin Proc 1995;70:453–63.
4. Tomas E, Martin A, Garfia C, Gomez FS, Morillas JD, Tortajada GC, et al. Abdominal wall endometriosis in absence of previous surgery. J Ultrasound Med 1999;18: 373–4.
5. Ramsanahie A, Giri SK, Velusamy S, Nessim GT. Endometriosis in a scarless abdominal wall with underlying umbilical hernia. India J Med Sci 2000;169:67.
6. Calbrese L, Delmonte O, Mari R. Endometriosis of the abdominal wall. Clinical case and review of the literature. Acta Biomed Ateneo Parmense 1997;68:35–43.
7. Dell'Acqua A, Colosi E, Angiolillo M, et al. Endometriosis of the abdominal wall after caesarean section. Minerva Ginecol 1993;45:327–31.
8. Toullalan O, Baque P, Benchimol D, et al. Endometriosis of the rectus abdominis muscles. Ann Chir 2000;125:880–3.
9. Ideyi SC, Schein M, Niazi M, Gerst PH. Spontaneous endometriosis of the abdominal wall. Dig Surg 2003;20:246–8.
10. Roberge RJ, Kantor WJ, Scorza L. Rectus abdominis endometrioma. Am J Emerg Med 1999;17:675–7.
11. Coley BD, Casola G. Incisional endometrioma involving the rectus abdominis muscle and subcutaneous tissues: CT appearance. AJR Am J Roentgenol 1993;160:549–50.
12. Wellberry C. Diagnosis and treatment of endometriosis. Am Fam Physician 1999;60:1753–68.
13. Clement PB. Diseases of the peritoneum. In: Kurman RJ, editor. Blaustein's pathology of the female genital tract (4th edn). New York, NY: Springer-Verlag, 1994:660–80.
14. Rychlik DF, Bieber EJ. Thoracic endometriosis syndrome resembling pulmonary embolism. J Am Assoc Gynecol Laparosc 2001;8:445–8.
15. Jubanyik KJ, Comite F. Extrapelvic endometriosis. Obstet Gynecol Clin North Am 1997;24:411–40.
16. Steck WD, Helwig EB. Cutaneous endometriosis. Clin Obstet Gynecol 1966;9:373–83.
17. Wolf C, Obrist P, Ensinger C. Sonographic features of abdominal wall endometriosis. AJR Am J Roentgenol 1997;169:916–7.
18. Miller WB Jr, Melson GL. Abdominal wall endometrioma. AJR Am J Roentgenol 1979;132:467–8.
19. Walsh JW, Taylor KJW, Rosenfield AT. Gray scale ultrasonography in the diagnosis of endometriosis and adenomyosis. AJR Am J Roentgenol 1979;132:87–90.
20. Togashi K, Nishimura K, Kimura I, et al. Endometrial cysts: diagnosis with MR imaging. Radiology 1991;180:73–8.
21. Zwas FR, Lyon DT. Endometriosis: an important condition in clinical gastroenterology. Dig Dis Sci 1991;36:353–64.

The British Journal of Radiology, 78 (2005), 72–74
DOI: 10.1259/bjr/61054799

Case report
Uterine lipoma: advantage of MRI over ultrasound

L U LAU, MD and R F THOENI, MD

University of California, San Francisco, San Francisco General Hospital, Department of Radiology, 1001 Potrero Avenue, 1X55, San Francisco, CA 94110 and University of California, San Francisco, Department of Radiology, P.O. Box 0628, San Francisco, CA 94143-0628, USA

Abstract. Pure fatty tumours of the uterus are exceedingly rare. A case of uterine lipoma demonstrated on ultrasound and MRI with pathological correlation is described. Ultrasound suggested the presence of a uterine lipoma but MRI permitted an unequivocal diagnosis. The usefulness of the various imaging methods is discussed in correctly diagnosing this entity and avoiding unnecessary surgery in the asymptomatic patient.

Lipomatous uterine tumours are rare benign neoplasms. The histological spectrum includes pure lipomas, consisting only of adipose tissue with scanty vascular stroma and mixed lipomas, which may contain smooth muscle tissue, dense fibrous connective tissue, cartilage and abnormal vessels in varying proportions, often called lipoleiomyomas [1]. Most cases described in the literature have been of the mixed type [1–3]. We present a case of a pure uterine lipoma correctly diagnosed pre-operatively by MRI and discuss the utility of ultrasound and MRI in diagnosing this tumour and its differential diagnosis.

Case report

A 62-year-old post-menopausal woman presented with vaginal bleeding. Ultrasound revealed a 7.8 cm well-circumscribed, hyperechoic mass with posterior shadowing and surrounding hypoechoic rim in the fundus of the uterus (Figure 1). This mass could not be separated from the adnexal tissue. On MRI using T_1 weighted gradient recalled echo sequences, a well-circumscribed mass of high signal intensity was demonstrated in the anterior uterine body (Figure 2a). This mass was also high in signal intensity on T_2 weighted images (Figure 2b). Following fat suppression, T_1 weighted images revealed low signal intensity within the tumour (Figure 2c). A few thin septations were noted in the mass, but no solid component or enhancement was present.

The patient underwent a total abdominal hysterectomy and bilateral salpingo-oophorectomy. A 7 cm soft, yellow, well-circumscribed, intramural mass was found within the myometrium (Figure 2d). Histologically, a uterine lipoma with mature adipose tissue interspersed with delicate fibrovascular septa was identified. No smooth muscle tissue was seen within the mass itself.

Discussion

A lipoma is a benign tumour composed of encapsulated adipose tissue, interspersed by thin septa of fibrous tissue [4]. True estimates of the number of cases of pure uterine lipoma are difficult to ascertain given the lack of consensus as to appropriate nomenclature for lipomatous uterine tumours [2]. Willen et al [3] concluded that a pure lipoma should be diagnosed only if smooth muscle cells are confined to the periphery. These criteria were fulfilled in our case.

Most uterine lipomatous tumours occur in post-menopausal women between the ages of 50 years and 70 years [1]. Most patients are asymptomatic but some experience symptoms similar to that of uterine leiomyomas of comparable size, such as pelvic discomfort, heaviness, pressure, or vaginal bleeding [2]. Most of these tumours are associated with uterine fibroids [5]. Most arise in the uterine corpus and are intramural in nature. The lipomas are usually round or oval in configuration, sharply circumscribed and pale yellow [2]. They usually measure 5–10 cm in diameter, although they may range from a few millimetres to as large as 32 cm [1, 5]. Our mass had

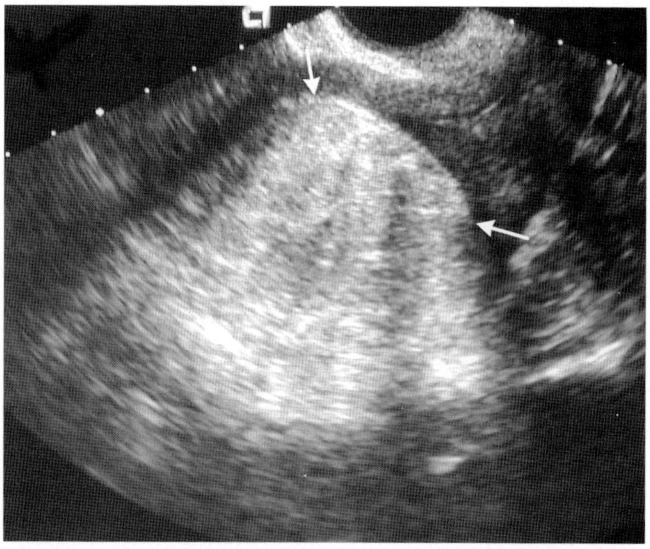

Figure 1. Ultrasound of the pelvis in a 62-year-old post-menopausal woman with vaginal bleeding. Longitudinal, endovaginal ultrasound image of the uterus demonstrates a well-circumscribed, echogenic mass (arrows) with surrounding hypoechoic rim in the fundus of the uterus. The endometrial cavity is seen inferior to the mass.

Received 1 July 2004 and accepted 6 October 2004.

Address correspondence to Dr Ruedi F Thoeni.

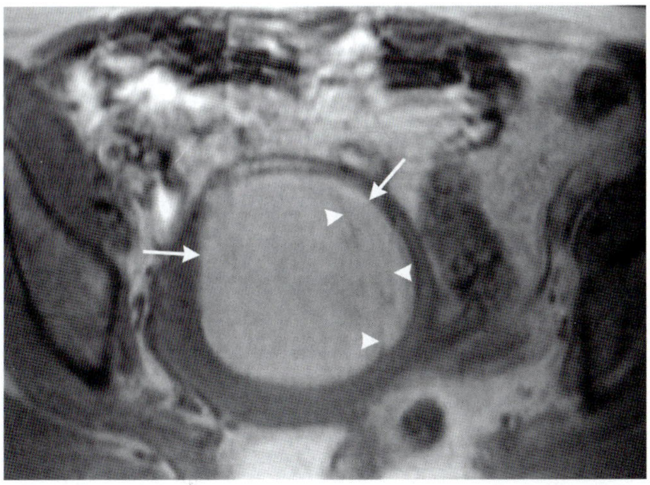

(a)

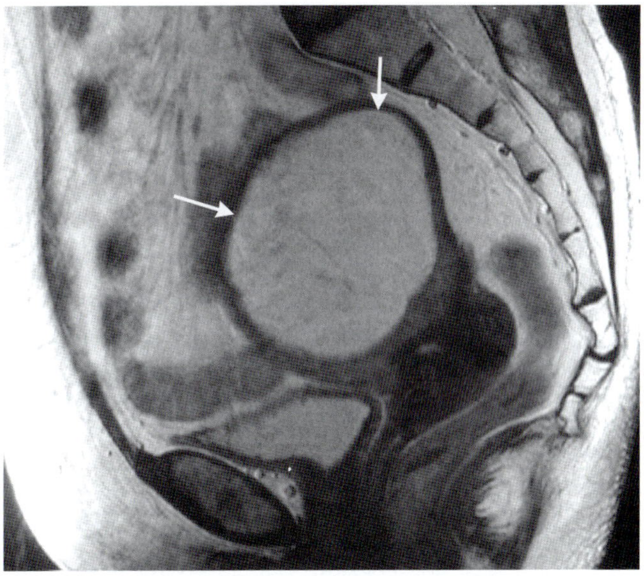

(b)

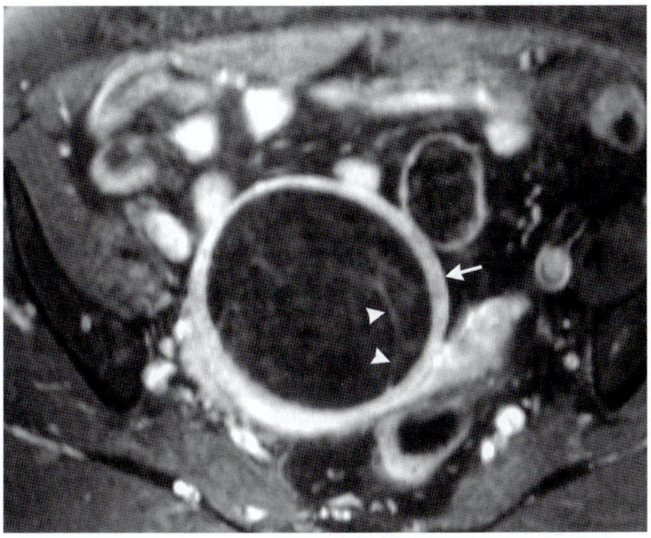

(c)

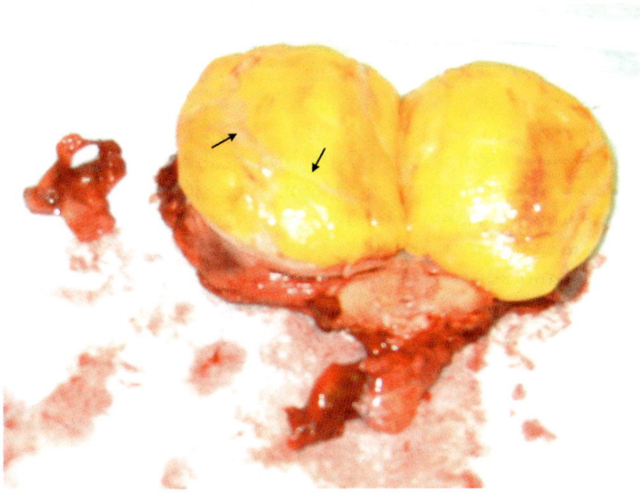

(d)

Figure 2. MR of the pelvis in a 62-year-old post-menopausal woman with vaginal bleeding. (a) The axial T_1 weighted gradient recalled echo sequence (repetition time/echo time (TR/TE)=160 ms/4.2 ms) demonstrates a well-circumscribed mass (arrows) of high signal intensity with thin septations (open arrows). (b) The sagittal T_2 weighted fast spin echo sequence (TR/TE=4000 ms/79.2 ms) shows a high signal intensity mass in the uterus (arrows). (c) The axial, fat suppression T_1 weighted spin echo sequences (TR/TE=550 ms/14 ms) reveals low signal intensity within the tumour (arrows). Thin septations (open arrows) are easily identified with MR within the mass. (d) The gross specimen shows a yellow, well-circumscribed mass within the uterine myometrium. The septations (arrows) clearly can be seen.

similar gross characteristics and associated clinical findings, but no concomitant fibroids were found.

Because fat tissue is not native to the uterus, various theories of histogenesis have been proposed. These include misplaced embryonic fat cells, metaplasia of muscle or connective tissue cells into fat cells, lipocytic differentiation of a specific primitive connective tissue cell, proliferation of perivascular fat cells accompanying the blood vessels into the uterus, inclusion of fat cells into the uterine wall during surgery, or fatty infiltration or degeneration of connective tissue [1, 3].

The correct diagnosis of uterine lipoma was previously made only by surgery or autopsy. With current imaging techniques, the diagnosis can be made without the need for surgery. Identification of fat within these tumours and an origin from the uterus are the key factors in diagnosis. Ultrasound, CT and MRI are methods of diagnosing lipomatous uterine tumours. Because of their benign nature, they require no treatment, unless they are symptomatic. Malignant degeneration of these tumours is extremely rare. To our knowledge, only one case of leiomyosarcoma arising in a uterine lipoleiomyoma has been reported [6].

The ultrasound appearance of a uterine lipoma is that of a highly echogenic mass, corresponding to fatty tissue, with a hypoechoic rim, thought to represent a layer of myometrium surrounding the tumour [2, 5]. The hyperechogenicity depends primarily on the acoustic interfaces between fat and other types of surrounding tissues [8]. Serafini et al [8] also described a lack of colour flow within the lipomatous masses. Even with transabdominal and transvaginal ultrasound imaging, the organ of origin may be difficult to determine. Ovarian masses containing fat and/or calcification, such as dermoids, may appear similar on ultrasound. Pelvic lipomas or liposarcomas may also be considerations. Even if a mass is noted to arise from the uterus, it may be difficult to differentiate a fatty tumour from a degenerating fibroid. In our case, the correct diagnosis was suggested by ultrasound but MRI recommended for confirmation of location and fatty nature of the tumour, and to rule out an associated uterine malignancy.

In cases of lipomatous uterine tumours, CT can be diagnostic when there is a low-density mass with Hounsfield units measuring between -40 to -100 [9]. CT, which was not performed in our patient, has the disadvantages of not demonstrating the various layers of the uterine wall, and at times confusing an adnexal mass with a mass originating from the uterus. Especially when it is exophytic or pedunculated, the location of a lipomatous mass may be difficult to determine, in which case it may be mistaken for an ovarian mass or pelvic lipoma. Multiplanar reformations available with state-of-the-art helical CT may reduce the chance for confusion.

On MRI, the fatty component is high in signal intensity on T_1 weighted images. Fat suppression techniques will confirm macroscopic fat content. Chemical shift artefacts along the frequency-encoding axis may also be seen and will further verify the fatty substance. MRI is the most helpful modality in assessing the organ of origin because of its multiplanar capability, tissue-specific characteristics and ability to discern the various layers within the uterine wall and to distinguish between adnexal tissues, uterus and pelvic fat. MRI also best displays the internal architecture of these fatty tumours. MRI readily enables the detection of thin septations that may be present in a pure uterine lipoma. If MRI demonstrates soft tissue components or enhancement within the uterine mass, a diagnosis of a lipoleiomyoma or other mixed lipoma of the uterus can be made. In our case, MRI enabled an unequivocal diagnosis of a uterine lipoma without other uterine pathology but the patient underwent hysterectomy because of continued vaginal bleeding.

As in our case, ultrasound usually is the first study performed for pelvic symptoms, such as vaginal bleeding. We suggest that if on ultrasound an echogenic mass is seen in the pelvis, MRI is the best modality for determining the presence of fat and the internal architecture within the mass and for localizing the mass within the uterus, ovary or pelvic fatty tissue. Because of the mostly benign nature of lipomatous tumours of the uterus, such an approach can avoid unnecessary surgery in asymptomatic patients.

References

1. Brandfass RT, Everts-Suarez EA. Lipomatous tumors of the uterus: a review of the world's literature with a case report of true lipoma. Am J Obstet Gynecol 1955;70:359–67.
2. Jacobs JE, Markowitz SK. CT Diagnosis of uterine lipoma. AJR Am J Roentgenol 1988;150:1335–6.
3. Willen R, Gad A, Willen H. Lipomatous lesions of the uterus. Virch Archiv A 1978;377:351–61.
4. Robbins SL. Pathologic bases of disease. Philadelphia: WB Saunders Co, 1974:158–9.
5. Dodd GD III, Budzik RF. Lipomatous uterine tumors: diagnosis by ultrasound, CT, and MR. J Comput Assist Tomogr 1990;14:629–32.
6. Scurry J, Hack M. Leiomyosarcoma arising in a lipoleiomyoma. Gynecol Oncol 1990;39:381–3.
7. Tsushima Y, Kita T, Yamamoto K. Uterine lipoleiomyoma: MRI, CT, and ultrasonographic findings. Br J Radiol 1997;70:1068–70.
8. Serafini G, Martinoli C, Quadri P, et al. Lipomatous tumors of the uterus: ultrasonographic findings in 11 cases. J Ultrasound Med 1996;16:195–9.
9. Maebayashi T, Imai K, Takekawa Y, et al. Radiologic features of uterine lipoleiomyoma. J Comput Assist Tomogr 2003;27: 162–5.

The British Journal of Radiology, *78* (2005), 75–85
DOI: 10.1259/bjr/15273006

Pictorial review

Neck masses in children

J R A TURKINGTON, FRCR, A PATERSON, FRCR, L E SWEENEY, FRCR and G D THORNBURY, FRCR

Department of Radiology, Royal Belfast Hospital for Sick Children, 180 Falls Road, Belfast BT12 6BE, UK

Abstract. Infants and children with neck masses frequently present to the radiologist for further evaluation. The role of the radiologist is to differentiate between conditions using imaging modalities such as ultrasound with colour Doppler, CT and MRI. Where appropriate, the radiologist will also stage lesions for management purposes and aid in guiding aspiration or biopsy. This paper presents a pictorial review of paediatric neck masses and their imaging features. Particular emphasis is applied to the anatomical site of the mass to aid in differential diagnosis. It must be emphasised that the radiological findings should always be interpreted in conjunction with the patient's age, the clinical history and the findings on physical examination.

Neck masses are not uncommon in children. The most common aetiologies include congenital lesions and their complications, lymphadenopathy, vascular, inflammatory and malignant lesions. The role of the radiologist is to differentiate between these conditions using imaging modalities such as ultrasound (US) with colour Doppler, CT and MRI. US is useful to determine if a mass is cystic or solid and Doppler tells us if it is vascular. US should be considered as the first-line investigation because it is non invasive, does not require sedation and does not involve ionizing radiation [1]. CT and MRI can then be used to determine the extent of the lesion and whether local invasion is present. Both CT and MRI can provide multiplanar images, however MRI will more effectively demonstrate the soft tissue characteristics of a lesion.

Anatomy

The neck can be divided into the anterior and posterior triangles by the sternocleidomastoid (SCM) muscle (Figure 1). To aid the radiologist, we have divided neck masses into cystic or solid lesions and listed them according to their anatomical location (anterior, posterior or either neck triangle). Lesions arising in the SCM muscle itself are discussed separately.

Anterior triangle masses

Thyroglossal cyst

Thyroglossal cysts usually manifest as an asymptomatic mass during childhood and lie within the anterior triangle [1]. They arise from a remnant of the thyroglossal duct. This extends from the foramen caecum at the base of the tongue to the pyramidal lobe of the thyroid gland, and usually involutes by the 8th week of intrauterine life. Remnants of a portion of the duct may lead to cyst formation or ectopic thyroid tissue. Thyroglossal cysts are midline or just off midline in position, and can be found at any level from the base of the tongue to the isthmus of the thyroid gland. Most (65%) are infrahyoid [5, 9]. On US they appear as a well-defined, thin-walled, anechoic mass with through enhancement (Figure 2). A mass with mixed echogenicity suggests infection of the cyst [5].

Branchial cyst

The branchial apparatus, consisting of six branchial arches separated by five branchial clefts appears by the 15th day of intrauterine life. Incomplete obliteration of the branchial apparatus, predominately the cleft, is postulated to lead to branchial cleft anomalies such as cysts, sinuses or fistulae [1]. Cysts may occur along the course of the first or second branchial clefts, however the majority (75%) arise from remnants of the second branchial cleft [9]. They occur in children and adolescents as a mass situated anterior to the SCM muscle and near to the angle of the mandible. A thin-walled, anechoic fluid-filled cyst is seen on US [5] (Figure 3a). With CT, the centre of the mass will have an attenuation value similar to water and if the cyst is infected, a thickened, enhancing wall will be present [9] (Figure 3b).

Dermoid/teratoma

Developmental anomalies which involve pleuripotent embryonal stem cells result in dermoid cysts and teratomas [1, 7]. Most occur in children less than 3 years of age and are situated in the midline [7]. They are usually suprahyoid, in contrast to thyroglossal cysts. On CT an inhomogenous, multiloculated mass that contains calcification and low attenuation fat enables the diagnosis [1, 7] (Figure 4). MR will show the fat component as high signal on T_1 weighted images.

The thyroid gland

Thyroid masses are uncommon in childhood. They are best evaluated with US and radioisotope imaging. Diffuse enlargement of the gland can occur in thyrotoxicosis and Hashimoto's thyroiditis. The latter shows enlargement with variable echogenicity. In thyrotoxicosis the gland is enlarged, but the echopattern is similar to that of normal thyroid tissue [8]. With a focal thyroid mass US can easily differentiate whether the mass is solid or cystic. Most cystic masses in the region of the thyroid are likely to be

Received 22 December 2003 and in revised form 15 June 2004, accepted 13 August 2004.

thyroglossal cysts. Solid masses all have a similar US appearance of an echogenic mass. An adenoma is characteristically echogenic with a surrounding hypoechoic halo, carcinomas tend to demonstrate heterogeneous echogenicity. The differential diagnosis of a solid mass would also include lymphoma. A focal thyroid mass should be further investigated with an isotope thyroid scan and a "cold" nodule ultimately requires fine needle aspiration (FNA) or biopsy for histological diagnosis (Figure 5).

Salivary gland masses

Most salivary gland calculi occur in the submandibular gland in adolescents. The calculi may be identified on occlusal radiographs or with US. A sialogram will demonstrate a filling defect of a ductal stone and may also show glandular sialectasis due to ductal obstruction. Sialadenitis or inflammation of the salivary gland tends to affect the parotid gland in debilitated patients. The cause is usually due to oral cavity or dental sepsis with *Staphylococcus aureus* the most common pathogen [3]. It can also occur due to the mumps virus. US will demonstrate gland enlargement with abscess formation.

Recurrent parotiditis is rare but may result in unilateral, periodic, parotid swelling. The aetiology is unknown and non-obstructive sialectasis occurs. US shows hypoechoic intraglandular ductal dilatation, which can also be demonstrated with a sialogram or MRI [3] (Figure 6).

Posterior triangle masses

Lymphatic malformations

Congenital vascular and lymphatic malformations of the head and neck can be classified into two groups: vascular and lymphatic malformations and infantile haemangiomas [2]. The latter will be discussed later in this review. Vascular and lymphatic malformations grow in proportion to the child and almost never spontaneously involute. This group includes venous malformations (cavernous haemangiomas), capillary malformations (Port-wine stain) and lymphatic malformations (lymphangiomas and cystic hygromas). The previous terminology is listed in the brackets.

Lymphatic malformations (cystic hygromas) are congenital malformations resulting from blockage of lymphatic channels [6]. They usually present at birth as a painless swelling, and most lesions (90%) appear before the age of 2 years [2, 5, 6]. They are situated posterior to the SCM muscle in the posterior triangle. They tend to insinuate themselves around normal structures and can extend caudad into the superior mediastinum. Most are slow growing; however, sudden enlargement can occur following infection of or haemorrhage into the lesion, and may result in airway compression [2, 5, 6]. On US an anechoic or mixed echogenicity mass with septae of variable thickness will be identified [2, 4, 6]. Haemorrhage can lead to increased echogenicity or fluid–fluid levels being identified [2, 9]. The margins of the mass and the presence of mediastinal extension are better delineated with CT or MRI. CT will show a septated, low density, poorly circumscribed mass. Haemorrhage or infection causes an increase in attenuation. MRI will demonstrate a septated, cystic mass usually of high signal on T_2 and low signal on T_1 weighted images (Figure 7). Any high signal on T_1 weighted images may reflect haemorrhage or a high lipid content. The insinuation around normal structures is well demonstrated on MRI and this can make complete surgical removal of the lesion difficult [6].

Lipoma

This benign tumour of fat most commonly occurs in the posterior triangle of the neck. They are rare in children and appear as a solid, homogeneous mass of similar echogenicity to that of the subcutaneous fat [8]. On CT they will have low attenuation values of between -65 and -125 Hounsfield units indicating fat [1]. They often displace or compress adjacent structures; they are rarely infiltrative.

Lesions of the sternocleidomastoid muscle

Fibromatosis coli

This rare, benign condition presents in the neonatal period as a mass in the SCM muscle. Microscopically muscle is replaced by dense fibrous tissue [4]. A history of birth trauma and resulting torticollis is common. The clinical course is that of spontaneous resolution over a period of 4–8 months, with no treatment or with stretching exercises [4, 9]. US shows a uniformly isoechoic or hypoechoic mass within the muscle [4] (Figure 8). The mass can be seen to move with the muscle on real time ultrasound.

Lesions presenting in either triangle of the neck

Infantile haemangioma

In contrast to congenital vascular and lymphatic malformations, infantile haemangiomas grow faster than the child and then spontaneously involute. Infantile haemangiomas of the head and neck usually occur in children less than 6 months of age, and this term includes the previously classified capillary haemangiomas, strawberry haemangiomas and capillary-cavernous haemangiomas [2]. Infantile haemangiomas usually grow rapidly until 9–10 months of age and then spontaneous regression occurs, which can take up to 10 years. Plain radiographs may show a soft tissue mass with areas of calcification representing phleboliths [9] (Figure 9). US demonstrates a mild to moderately echogenic mass, with echogenic septations that are vascular on colour Doppler interrogation. MRI is better at showing the relationship of the mass to the surrounding normal structures. The well-defined mass will be of high signal on T_2 weighted images and contain flow voids, representing feeding and draining vessels [9] (Figure 9). An involuting haemangioma is less vascular and contains fibrofatty tissue and this is best demonstrated with MRI [2].

Lymphadenitis

Cervical lymphadenitis usually results from a site of infection in the head and neck, such as the tonsils, pharynx or teeth [1]. US identifies numerous, discrete, enlarged, tender, oval masses of reduced echogenicity (Figure 10). Increased, branching vascularity is demonstrated with colour Doppler interrogation [8]. A necrotic lymph node will have a cystic hypoechoic centre [8].

Abscesses

Abscesses can occur in either triangle of the neck and also within the retropharyngeal space. On US a thick-walled, partially or fully fluid-filled mass will be present (Figure 11). Gas forming organisms cause small pockets of hyperechoic air within the collection. Enlarged, hypoechoic lymph nodes may be identified surrounding the abscess. Retropharyngeal abscesses commonly result from tonsillar infection and pre-vertebral soft tissue thickening can be identified on plain radiographs [9] (Figure 11).

Rhabdomyosarcoma

This is the most common childhood soft tissue sarcoma and 40% occur in the head and neck [1, 11]. Embryonal rhabdomyosarcoma is the most common form, accounting for 60% of cases and occurring in the orbit, nasopharynx, middle ear, nasal cavity and paranasal sinuses [11]. Contrast enhanced CT and MRI are the best imaging modalities for diagnosis and staging. CT is valuable in demonstrating associated bony destruction. An enhancing aggressive soft tissue mass that may have foci of necrosis within it, is commonly demonstrated (Figure 12).

Neuroblastoma

Most neuroblastomas arise in the adrenal glands, however they may originate anywhere along the sympathetic chain [9]. Most present before the age of 5 years [10] and those arising in the neck (5%) have a better prognosis than those tumours of adrenal origin [1]. Neuroblastoma can present as an asymptomatic mass, or along with local compressive symptoms, such as dysphagia, hoarseness, airway obstruction, Horner's syndrome or cranial nerve palsies. Imaging findings depend on the histology of the tumour and vary from a homogeneous well defined mass to a heterogeneous one with necrosis and haemorrhage. Calcification can be present, but is less common than in abdominal neuroblastomas [10]. US typically shows an echogenic mass. An unenhanced CT can demonstrate any calcification [1]. Following intravenous contrast medium, the mass of soft tissue density will enhance heterogeneously (Figure 13). MRI shows a tumour of high signal on T_2 weighted sequences and enhancement is seen following the administration of intravenous gadolinium [10].

Lymphoma

Lymphoma accounts for more than 55% of head and neck tumours in children [1]. Upper neck nodes are usually involved. If lower cervical nodes are involved, mediastinal nodes are also usually found. On US or CT large lymphomatous masses are identified and the involved lymph nodes are no longer discrete [1] (Figure 14). Central areas of necrosis within the nodal masses may also be seen.

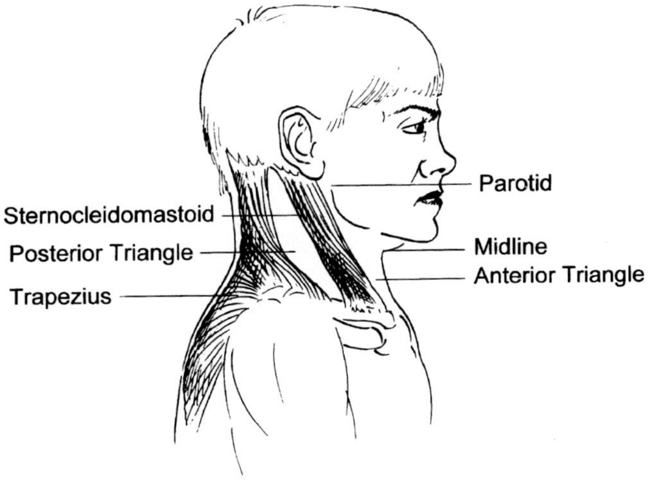

Figure 1. Anatomical diagram illustrating the anterior and posterior triangles of the neck.

Figure 2. Thyroglossal cyst. (a) Ultrasound shows a midline hypoechoic, avascular mass (arrow). (b) Axial short tau inversion recovery MRI confirms a high signal, well defined cyst (arrow).

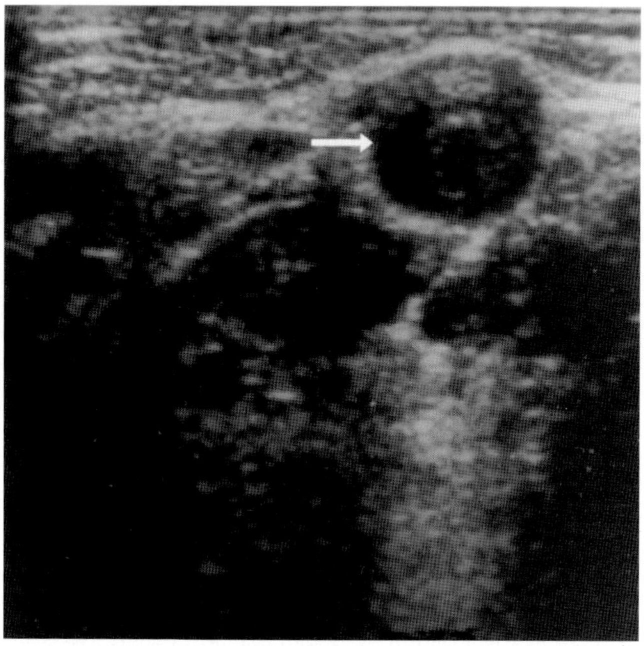

(a)

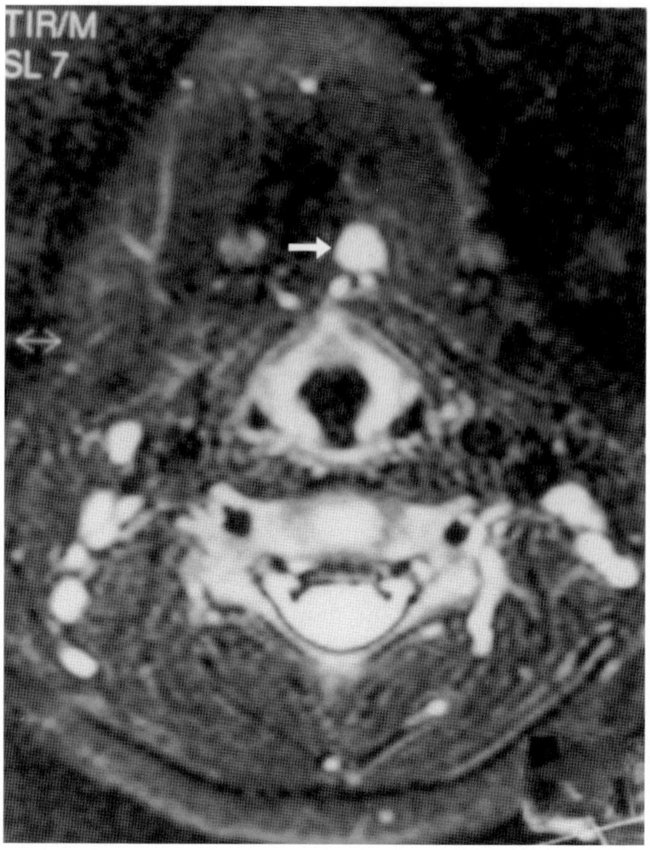

(b)

Figure 3. (a) Ultrasound of an uncomplicated branchial cyst. Note the absence of septations and the through enhancement. (b) Axial contrast enhanced CT showing a right sided low attenuation branchial cyst.

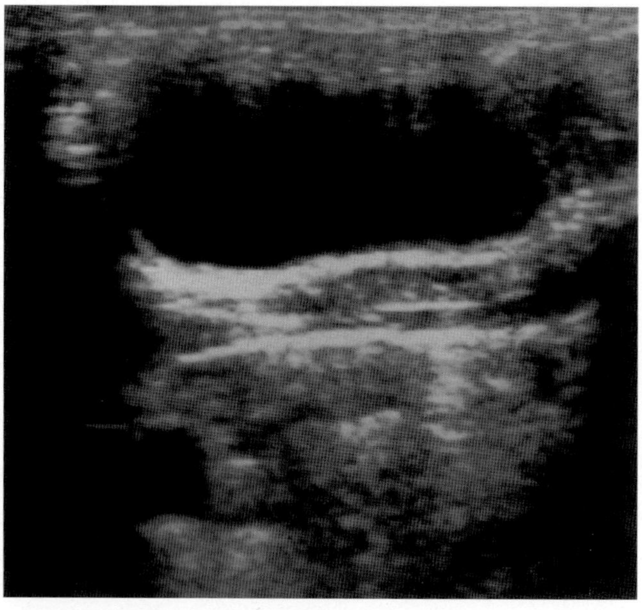

(a)

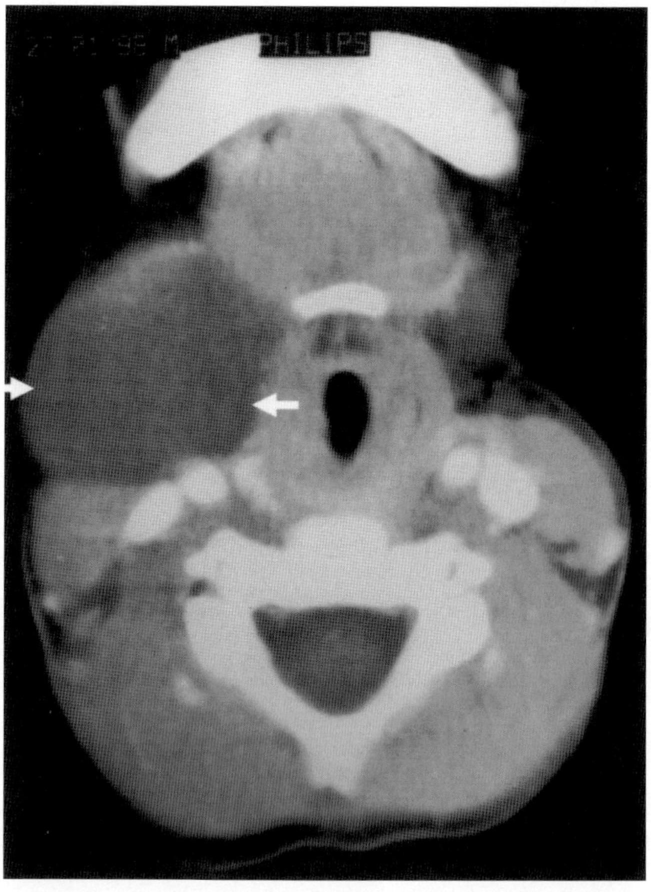

(b)

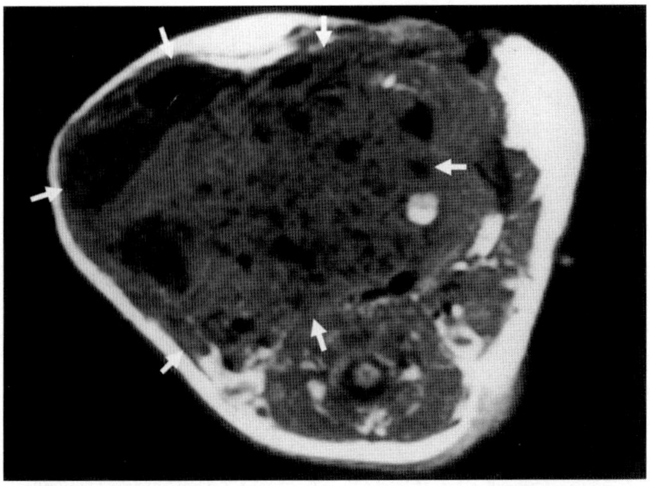

Figure 4. Axial T_1 weighted MRI of a mixed signal, right sided teratoma (arrows). The low signal cystic components and the intermediate signal fat can be identified.

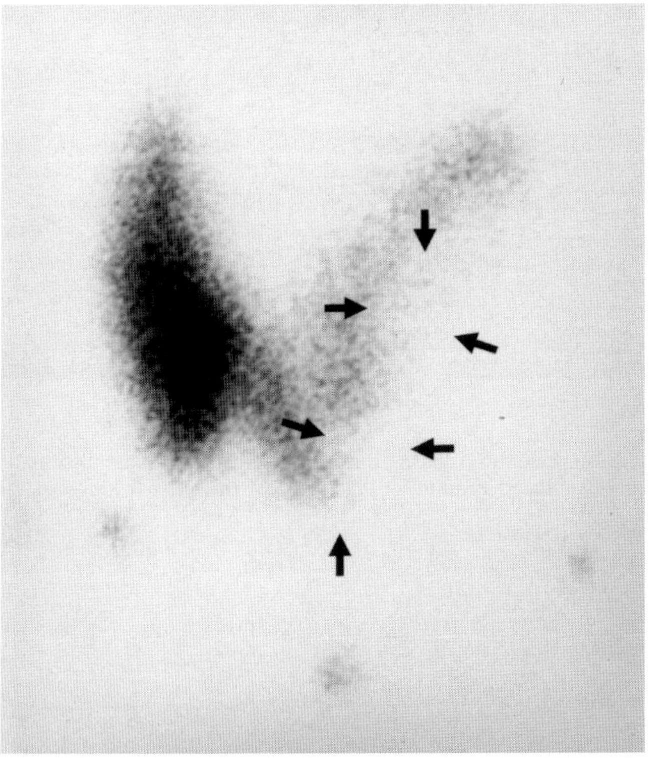

(a)

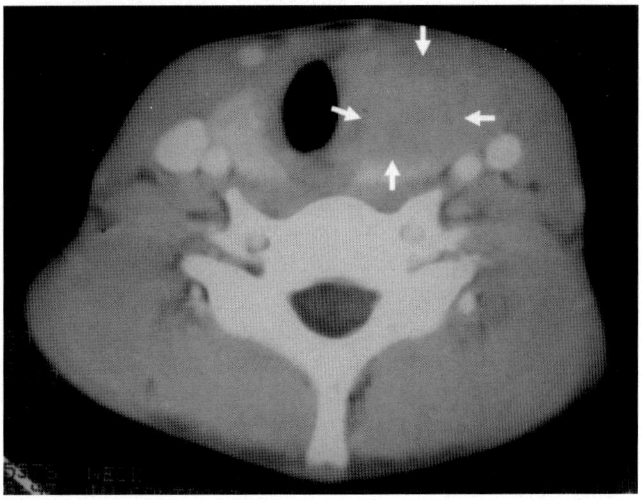

(b)

Figure 5. (a) Isotope scan of thyroid demonstrating a photopenic area within the left lobe. (Reproduced with permission of Springer-Verlag [12]). (b) Axial contrast enhanced CT of the same patient shows a solid mass within left lobe of thyroid (arrows). Lymphoma was proven by biopsy.

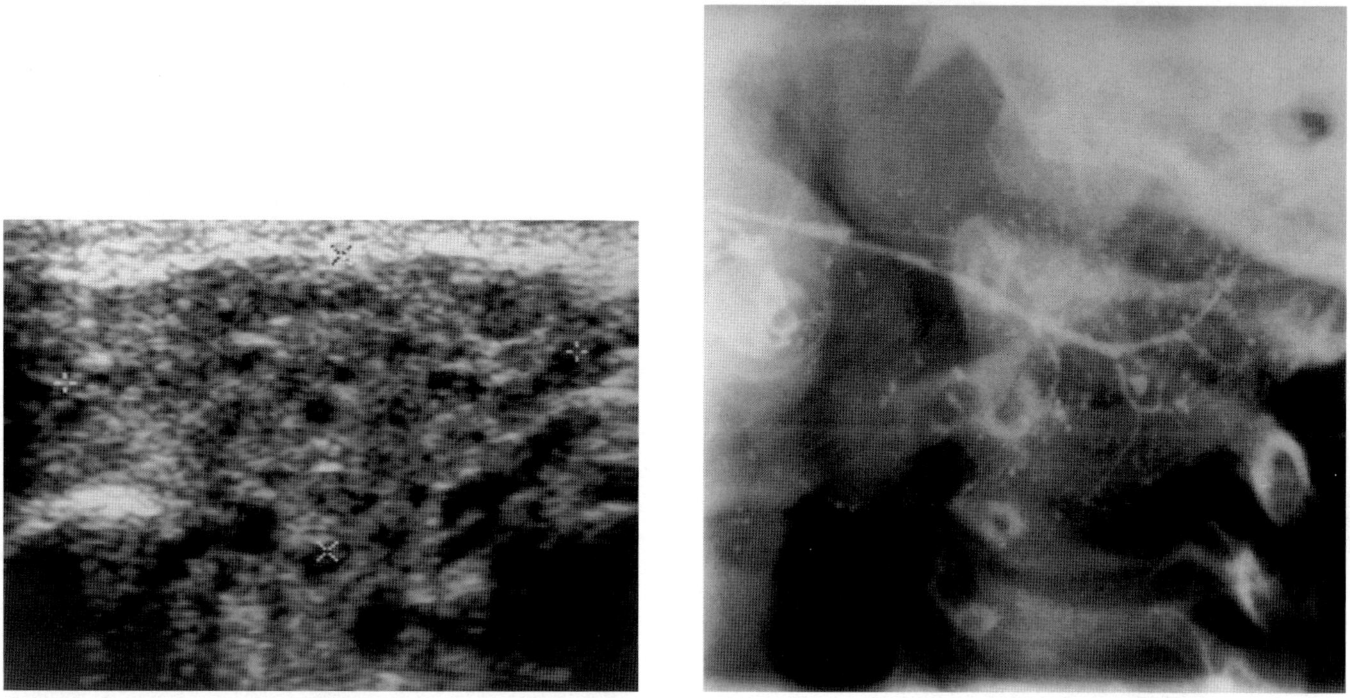

(a) (b)

Figure 6. (a) Parotid ultrasound demonstrating multiple hypoechoic areas representing dilated ducts (reproduced with permission of Springer-Verlag [12]). (b) Sialogram of same patient confirming intraglandular ductal beading of sialectasis of the left parotid gland.

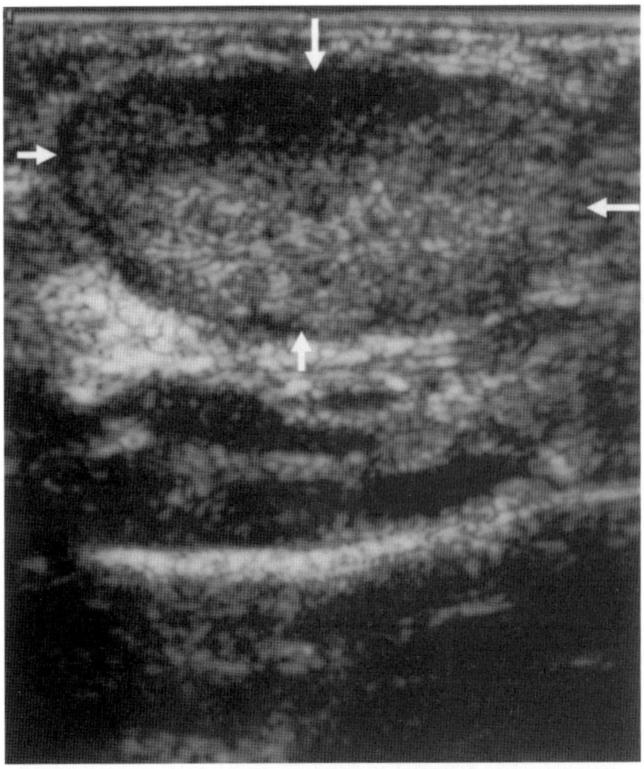

Figure 8. Ultrasound of isoechoic mass (arrows) consistent with fibromatosis coli within the sternocleidomastoid muscle.

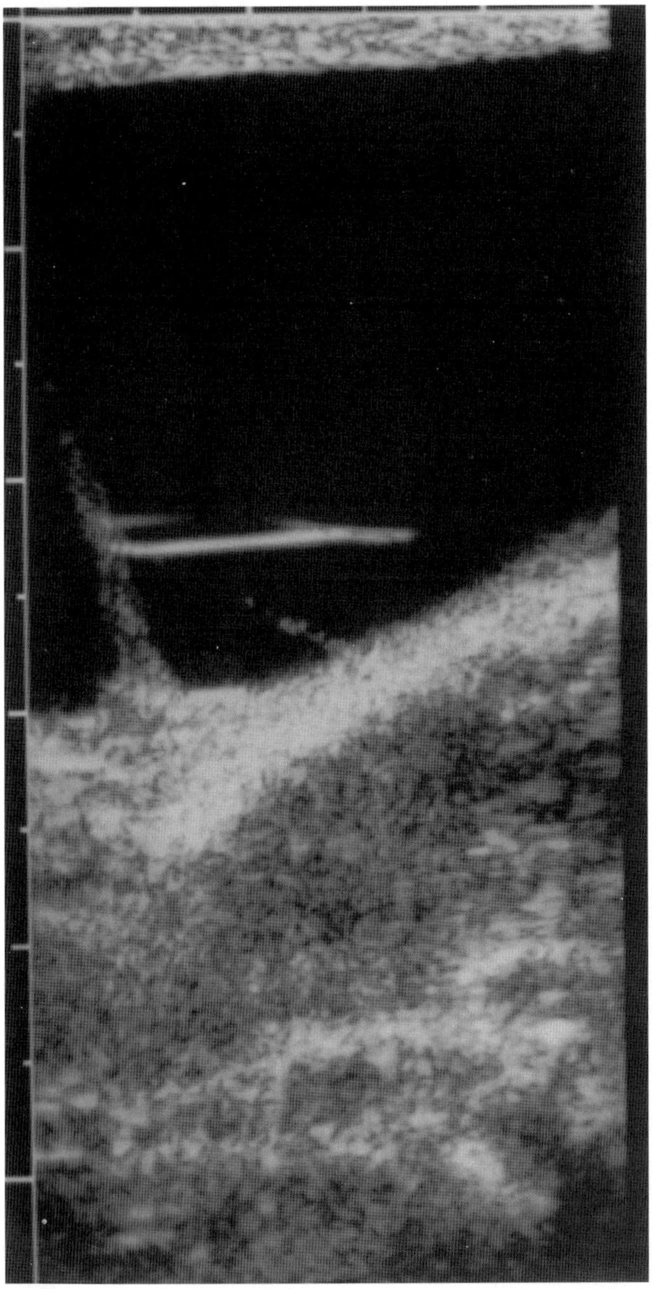

(a)

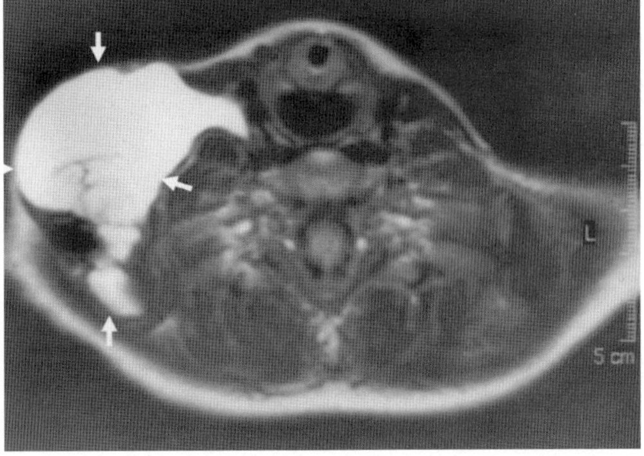

(b)

Figure 7. (a) Ultrasound of a hypoechoic septated cystic hygroma. (b) Axial T_2 weighted MRI of a well defined high signal right sided cystic hygroma (arrows). Note the insinuation around normal structures.

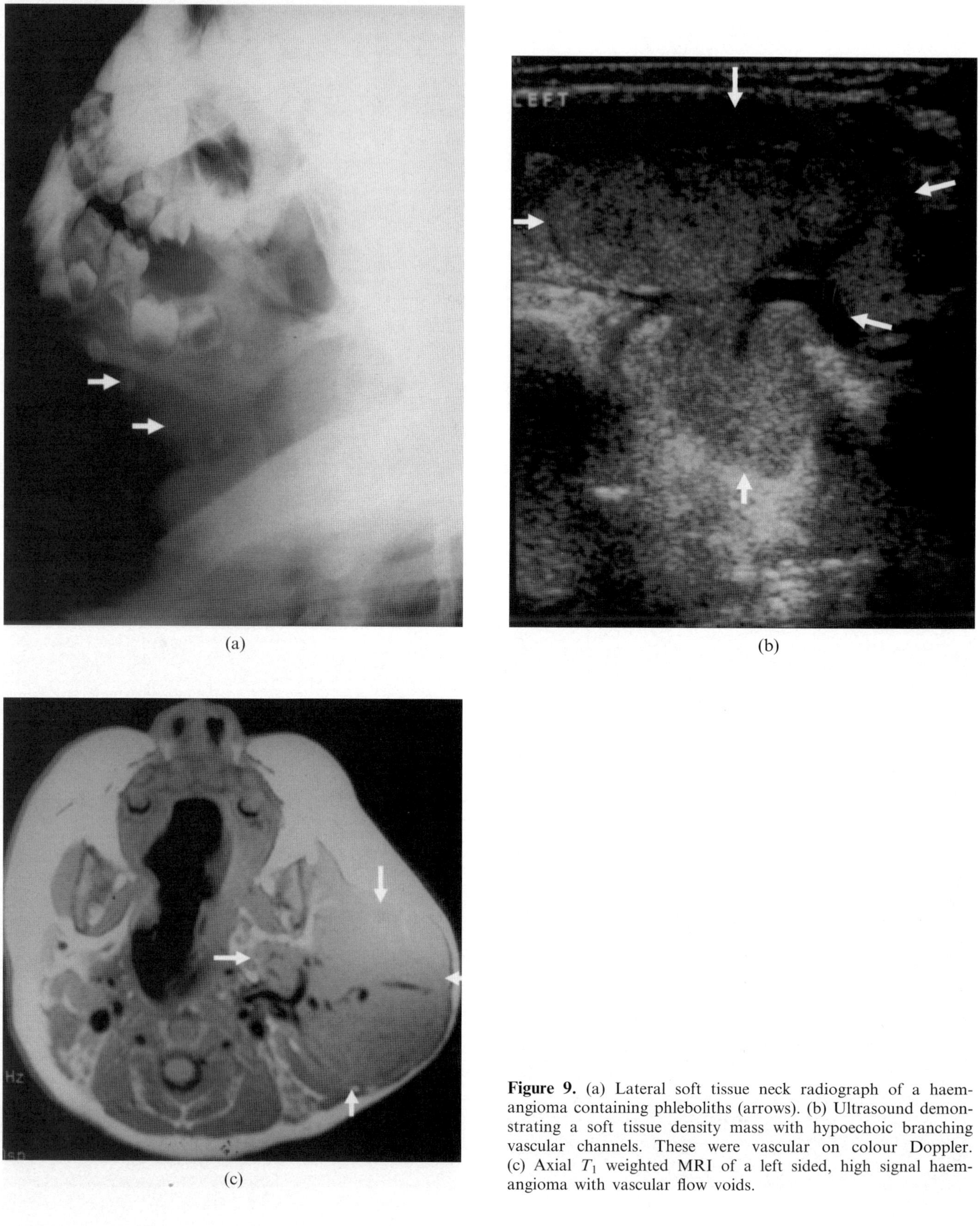

(a) (b) (c)

Figure 9. (a) Lateral soft tissue neck radiograph of a haemangioma containing phleboliths (arrows). (b) Ultrasound demonstrating a soft tissue density mass with hypoechoic branching vascular channels. These were vascular on colour Doppler. (c) Axial T_1 weighted MRI of a left sided, high signal haemangioma with vascular flow voids.

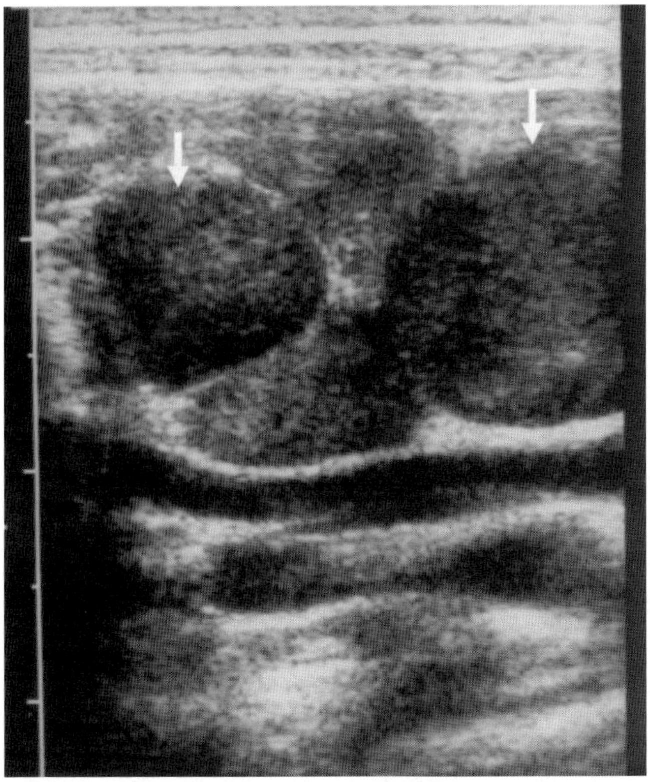

Figure 10. Ultrasound of well defined hypoechoic enlarged lymph nodes (arrows).

Figure 11. (a) Ultrasound of a mixed echogenic, thick walled, ill defined mass with central necrosis consistent with an abscess. (b) Radiograph showing extensive pre-vertebral soft tissue swelling of a retropharyngeal abscess (reproduced with permission of Springer-Verlag [12]).

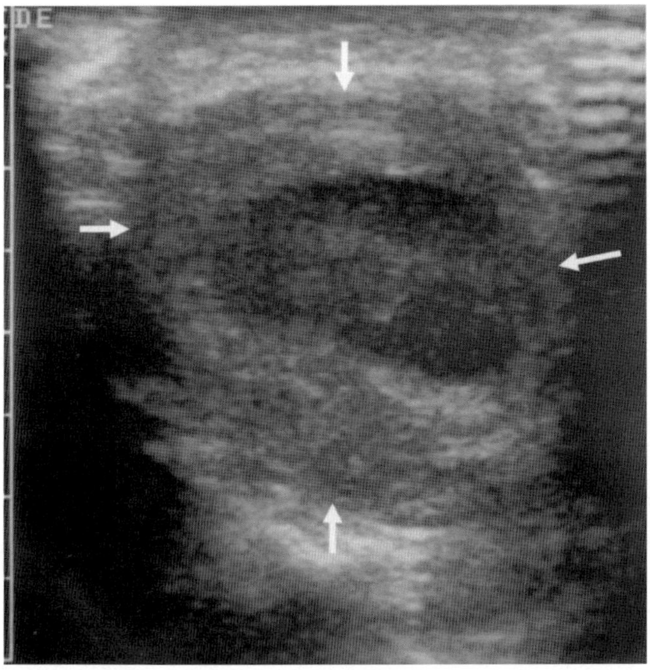

(a)

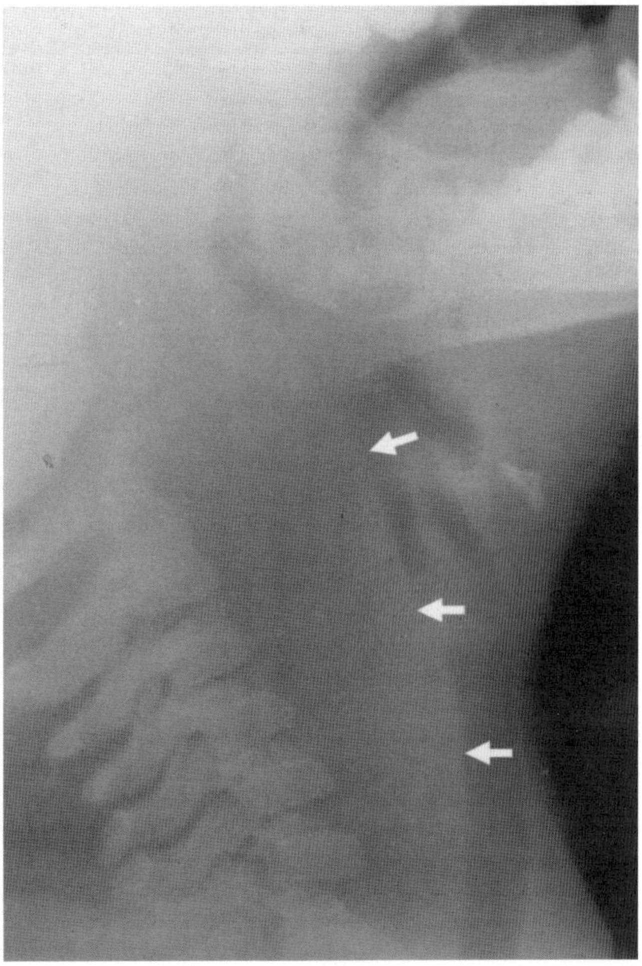

(b)

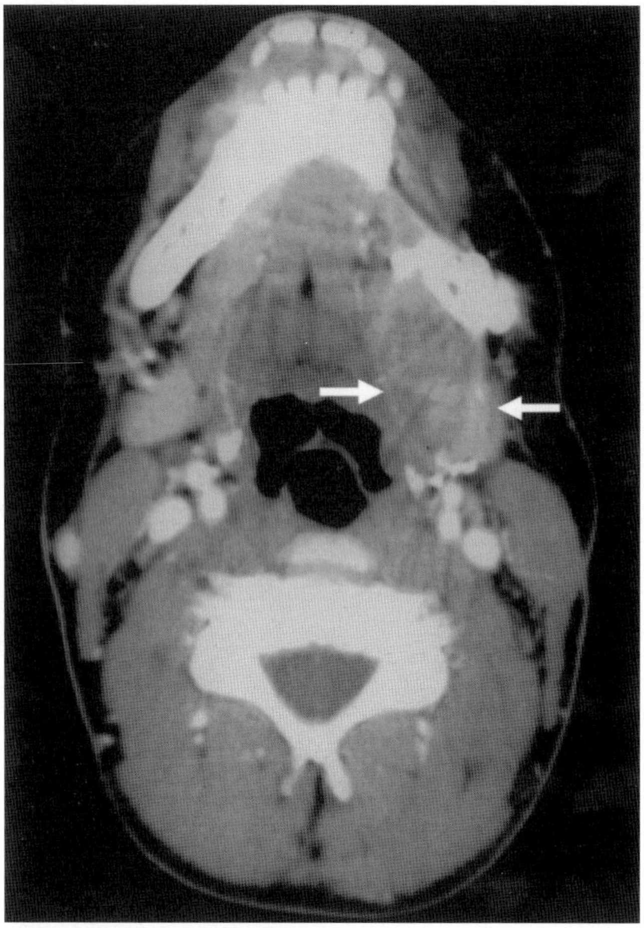

Figure 12. Axial contrast enhanced CT of an inhomogeneous, enhancing, left sided, soft tissue mass within the anterior triangle (arrows). Histological diagnosis was rhabdomyosarcoma.

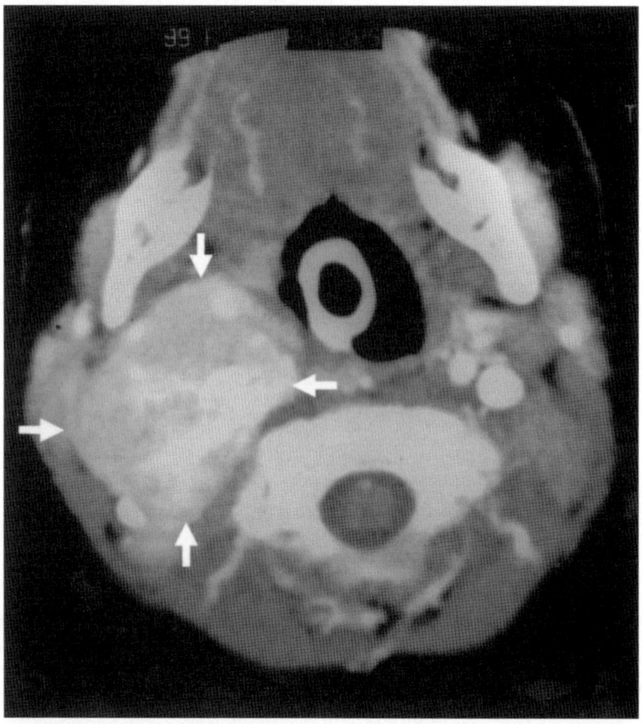

Figure 13. Axial contrast enhanced CT demonstrating an irregular, enhancing right sided, biopsy proven neuroblastoma.

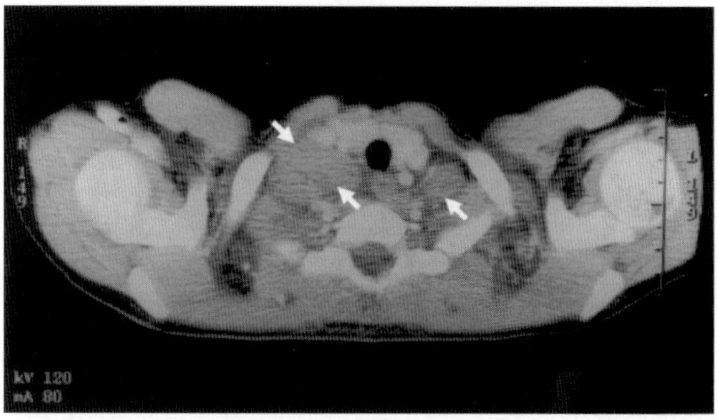

Figure 14. Axial contrast enhanced CT demonstrating multiple left sided lymph nodes and a right sided lymphomatous mass (arrows). Biopsy revealed Hodgkins lymphoma.

Table 1. Classification of soft tissue neck masses by anatomical site and predominant imaging characteristics

	Anterior triangle	Posterior triangle	Either triangle
Solid	Dermoid/ teratoma Thyroid mass	Lipoma	Infantile haemangioma Rhabdomyosarcoma Lymphadenitis Neuroblastoma Lymphoma
Cystic	Thyroglossal cyst Branchial cyst	Lymphatic malformations	
Mixed	Salivary gland Mass		Abscess

Conclusions

Neck masses are common in children and are a frequent cause of attendance in the Emergency Department. They can be classified according to their anatomical position in the neck and their appearance. The details in Table 1 can be used as an "*aide-memoir*" for the radiological differential diagnosis of paediatric soft tissue neck masses. After clinical examination, US should be the first modality used for investigation as it is readily available and does not involve ionizing radiation, unlike CT, and does not require sedation as is often the case with MRI in infants. It is particularly useful in assessing thyroid masses, thyroglossal and branchial cysts and parotid lesions. For other causes of neck masses it should still be the first line of investigation, after which CT and MRI can be used to determine the extent of the mass and better define its tissue characteristics.

References

1. Faerber EN, Swartz JD. Imaging of neck masses in infants and children. Crit Rev Diagn Imaging 1991;31:283–314.

2. Fordham LA, Chung CJ, Donnelly LF. Imaging of congenital vascular and lymphatic anomalies of the head and neck. Neuroimaging Clin North Am 2000;10:117–36.
3. Garcia CJ, Flores PA, Arce JD, Chuaqui B, Schwartz DS. Ultrasonography in the study of salivary gland lesions in children. Pediatr Radiol 1998;28:418–25.
4. Lin JN, Chou ML. Ultrasonographic study of the sternocleidomastoid muscle in the management of congenital muscular torticollis. J Pediatric Surgery 1997;32:1648–51.
5. Malik A, Odita J, Rodriguez J, Hardjasudarma M. Pediatric neck masses: a pictorial review for practicing radiologists. Curr Probl Diagn Radiol 2002;31:146–57.
6. Sheth S, Nussbaum AR, Hutchins GM, Sanders RC. Cystic hygromas in children: sonographic-pathologic correlation. Radiology 1987;162:821–4.
7. Smirniotopoulos JG, Chiechi MV. Teratomas, dermoids and epidermoids of the head and neck. Radiographics 1995;15: 1437–55.
8. Swischuk LE, John SD. Neck masses in infants and children. Radiol Clin North Am 1997;35:1329–40.
9. Vazquez E, Enriquez G, Castellote A, Lucaya J, Creixell S, Aso C, et al. US, CT and MR imaging of neck lesions in children. Radiographics 1995;15:105–22.
10. Weber AL, Montandon C, Robson CD. Neurogenic tumours of the neck. Radiol Clin North Am 2000;38:1077–90.
11. Yang WT, Kwan WH, Li CK, Metreweli C. Imaging of pediatric head and neck rhabdomyosarcomas with emphasis on magnetic resonance imaging and a review of the literature. Peratr Hematol Oncol 1997;14:243–57.
12. Sweeney LE. Emergency pediatric radiology. In: Carty H, editor. Head and neck emergency radiology. Berlin, Heidelberg, New York: Springer-Verlag, 1999:25–29.

Conference paper

Turkington JRA, Sweeney LE, Thornbury G, Paterson A. Neck masses in infants and children: a pictorial review. In: Royal College of Radiologists Annual Scientific Meeting, 10th–12th September 2003, London.

Book reviews

Safety report series No 21. Optimization of radiation protection in the control of occupational exposure. By IAEA, pp. 66, 2502 (IAEA, Vienna, Austria), €19.00 ISBN 92-0-110302-6

This thin book forms part of the valuable IAEA Safety Report Series. Its stated objective is to provide practical information on how to apply optimization in the work-place and it supplements the guidance already available in other international recommendations, *e.g.* from the ICRP. Whilst being aimed at all users of ionizing radiation, its examples are drawn predominantly from the nuclear industry and consequently its application to the medical sector is limited. Its main target audience is managers with responsibility for controlling radiation dose, including those with responsibility for production, finance and regulation, but also accepts that all workers have a role to play in optimization. It covers all aspects of routine work *e.g.* facilities, design, operation and decommissioning but not emergency situations.

Basically, the report provides guidance on the development of an ALARA programme or plan within an organization. It encourages all to ask themselves the question "Have I done everything that I reasonably can to reduce these radiation doses" and points out that ALARA requires significantly more thought than just complying with stated dose limits. It adopts the ICRP concept of dose constraints, which are to be used prospectively and should be set by consultation between management and workers. It also recommends the use of an individual investigation levels and collective dose targets as part of the optimization process.

Section 2 of the report outlines the optimization process in general terms with sections 3 to 6 exploring the different aspects in greater detail and providing examples taken from actual practice. The process is split into the following basic steps: an initial assessment and evaluation of the situation (be it at design stage or of a practice currently undertaken), a review of the possible methods and approaches to achieve ALARA, an evaluation of options and finally the implementation of the ALARA plan and the monitoring of its effectiveness.

The report also contains three annexes providing an overview of decision aiding techniques, a review of the monetary value adopted in different countries for the detriment associated with unit collective dose, and examples of ALARA checklists drawn solely from the nuclear industry.

I have found that reading this report has made me more aware of the need to plan and develop strategy for optimization. The overall principles outlined remain valid, be they applied in the medical sector, nuclear sector or industry. The overview of decision making tools and monetary values for collective dose could provide a useful starting point when presented with the need to evaluate radiation protection options. Consequently, the report will be of use to radiation protection professionals but I doubt whether it contains enough of relevance to clinical mangers to make it widely read within the health sector.

A Walker

Reeder and Felson's gamuts in radiology (4th Edn). Edited by MM Reeder, pp. xxv + 998, 2003 (Springer-Verlag, New York, NY), £104.00 ISBN 0-387-9558-7

I will admit to not using "Gamuts in Radiology" as a reference text for more years than vanity will allow me to admit, but it was my "bible" for the multiple choice section of the FRCR.

This comprehensive, well-referenced and indexed book is primarily written for the American market, hence the use of the American College of Radiology Index for Roentgen Diagnosis. Although the book consists mainly of lists set out alphabetically (I appreciate the reasons for this, but my clinical thought processes are ordered differently), I did welcome the inclusion of a few interesting tables and diagrams *viz.*

- CT characteristics of orbital masses in children;
- Favoured sites of origin of various bone lesions;
- Patterns of bone destruction;
- Features useful in CT identification of various types of intracranial tumours.

However, the table of the international classification of radiographs of the pneumoconioses, only re-affirmed that my decision not to report "HRCT" CT scans was the correct one (for me anyway).

Maurice M Reeder is obviously a generous and "ideal" radiologist (definition of "ideal" from his preface to the 4th edition – The ideal radiologist should combine exceptional visual activity with the intuitiveness of a good detective and the knowledge of odds and probabilities of a smart card player. It is these qualities and attention to detail that set him or her apart from other physicians who "look at" films).

There is serious competition to this text and with the exception of the chapter on MR, other books such as the "green bible" offer more value for money.

However, this book would be useful for all those departments with radiology trainees as it would undoubtedly increase the chance of success in any multiple choice exam.

F Gardner

MRI of the fetal brain: normal development and cerebral pathologies. By C Garcl, pp. xvi+267, 2004 (Springer-Verlag, Berlin, Heidelberg, New York), £115.00 ISBN 3-540-40747-2

Advances in antenatal diagnosis by ultrasound over the last 25 years are well established but the increase in use of magnetic resonance imaging, a much more specialized and less used modality is only now becoming recognized. This book addresses the most important area of fetal brain MRI discussing basic sequences used and their advantages and disadvantages but assumes a basic knowledge of MRI sequences. The first part of the book is concluded with an extensive atlas showing the normal fetal brain appearances from 22 weeks to term presented by slice with details of gyration, myelination and measurement.

The second part of the book deals with pathological lesions and gives a comprehensive atlas of the more common abnormalities as well as some of the rare ones. These are divided into pathology of the midline, abnormalities of proliferation and cortical organization, intracranial space occupying lesions, ventricular dilatation, abnormalities of the posterior cerebral fossa and two shorter sections on antenatal brain infections and ischaemic and haemorrhagic lesions. The quality of the illustrations is exquisite and this reviewer has already found the atlas most useful in the difficult area of assessing brain maturity in the fetus as well as helping to confirm a rare diagnosis.

Fetal MRI will never take over from ultrasound as a screening procedure but certainly now is very important in the further evaluation of suspected brain lesions. This book is a major contribution to the literature and should find a place in all fetal medicine departments and in those undertaking fetal MRI.

D Pilling

Quantitative MRI of the brain: measuring changes caused by disease. By P Tofts, pp. xvi+633, 2003 (John Wiley & Sons Ltd, Chichester, UK) £175.00 ISBN 0-470-84721-2

This is a large multiauthor book with over 600 pages in total which covers effectively all the advanced image analysis techniques currently in clinical research use in cerebral magnetic resonance. The contributors will be well known to workers in the field and the whole thing has been pulled together by Paul Tofts into a well integrated, well written and extremely informative reference book. There are in total 18 chapters split into 3 sections. The first section talks about basic concepts of the measurement process related to the acquisition of magnetic resonance images covering potential sources of variations or unexpected errors in acquired images and potential corrections amongst others. Section B concerns techniques that are designed to try and measure independent parameters within the brain. These range from the direct measurement of proton density, T_1 and T_2 (chapters 4, 5 and 6) through measurement of diffusion and magnetization transfer (chapter 7 and 8), but also include the more biologically directly appropriate methods of spectroscopy, T_1 and T_2 dynamic contrast enhanced MR, functional MRI and arterial spin labelling (chapters 10–13). Section C is a single chapter that reviews the biological significance of measured MR parameters in multiple sclerosis. This chapter stands alone and it might have been nice to see other specific disease-related chapters although I do not think the book suffers significantly for their lack. Finally section D deals with pure "image analysis" techniques including spatial registration of images, measurement of structural volume and detection of atrophy, measurement of shape and texture and statistical methods for measuring subtle changes in diffuse disease.

It should be said that each of these chapters is extraordinarily well written. They are, by the nature of the book, rather technical but despite that are highly accessible even to the relatively non-technical reader in most cases. Each of the chapters starts with a basic conceptual introduction to the technique and then deals in a highly principled way with factors affecting accuracy, precision, reproducibility and potential problems associated with analysis models etc.

I think many of the people who would benefit from this book are those involved in doing MR-based research on the brain in disease and a large number of them will already have the book on the bookshelf. It is quite clear that this is one of the most comprehensive and up to date textbooks of quantitative methodology in cerebral MRI currently available. I would strongly recommend that anybody intending to use one of these quantitative MR techniques who is not already highly familiar in its application should review the appropriate chapters in this book at an early stage to help them avoid making easily avoidable errors which is all too common with the applications of this type of technical methodology.

A Jackson

Practical MR mammography. By U Fischer (Author/Editor), pp. xi+211, 2004 (Georg Thieme Verlag, Stuttgart, Germany) €99.00 ISBN 3-13-132031 1

The author states the goal of this text is to provide an introduction and compendium of MR mammography. The presented text provides a concise summary of the topic, primarily over chapters 7 to 10. A correlation of imaging and pathology is achieved having been preceded by a systematic description of normal findings. The book's strength lies in consistent presentation, avoiding large quantities of prose. For each disease, two to three sentences of pathology, with accompanying microscopy, is followed by bullet points; clinical findings, mammographic findings and ultrasound. It is only then that MR mammography is discussed and illustrated. This approach ensures that MR is appreciated in the appropriate clinical context of the triple assessment. However, since there is only a limited spectrum of breast MR appearances, many of which are none specific, these chapters are challenging to sit and read end to end. They are, as the author intended, a practical reference.

The book begins with brief outlines of the history of MR mammography, patient preparation, and MR physics and then outlines protocols. This leads to chapter five, which in eight uncluttered pages explains and illustrates how to logically analyse morphology and enhancement. In short how to interpret MR mammograms. The brevity and clarity of this section stands out.

Chapters on artefacts and indications cover what would be expected. The only omission being breast imaging of patients previously treated for Hodgkin's Disease.

Chapter 12 is text free. Differential diagnoses are presented as a series of diagrams and tables, which, although not immediately intuitive, provide alternative problem solving algorithms.

Implant imaging is covered with the same consistent presentation as pathology. Additional line drawings are used to keep text to a minimum. Appropriate sequences are discussed. However the MR images used (to good effect) as illustration, lack sequence identification.

The final chapters are a when, why and how of MR intervention, followed by six pages of references – the literature up to 1999.

Overall, this text could be useful for breast imagers, who are starting to add MR mammography to their imaging strategies. Sections and chapters stand-alone, image quality is consistent and good, making this a practical reference.

D J Edwards

Fundamentals of nuclear pharmacy. By G B Saha, pp. xvii+383, 2004 (Springer-Verlag, Berlin, Heidelberg, New York) £57.50

ISBN 0-387-40360-4

This volume is the fifth edition of a very popular text on Radiopharmacy. The author packs a lot of very useful basic information into 383 pages, starting at the atom and progressing through to adverse reactions. I particularly liked the chapter on radioactive decay which was enhanced by several worked problems and calculations.

All the chapters are well augmented by a list of references and suggested books for further reading. Each chapter is also concluded by a number of questions based on the material covered. The answers to questions involving calculations are given at the end of the book.

Apart from the chapters covering radioactivity, radiation detectors, production of radionuclides, generators, radiopharmaceuticals and radiolabelling. This is a comprehensive chapter describing radiopharmaceuticals currently in use, including PET radiopharmaceuticals. Practical aspects such as the operation of a radiopharmacy and quality control are covered, though there is only a very brief mention of the equipment required for maintaining sterility such as laminar flow workstations and isolators.

There is an expanded chapter on internal radiation dosimetry in this new edition. The chapter on regulation is, of course, focused upon US law, however there is an additional page or two briefly reviewing European requirements.

A good range of imaging and non-imaging tests are described, including the "*in vitro*" application radioimmunoassay and "*in vitro*" tests such as red blood cell survival.

This comprehensive text also manages to cover therapeutic applications, including relatively new agents such as Zevalin, and to survey molecular imaging.

Overall the book gives a good and comprehensive coverage of the topic with the exception that the European based reader would need to supplement study with references on Good Manufacturing Practice and European Legislation.

I would recommend it both to newcomers to the topic who wish to gain a rapid grasp of the issues and also to practitioners who require a good reference volume.

L Malone

The British Journal of Radiology, *78* (2005), 89–90
DOI: 10.1259/bjr/16786605

Case of the month

Acute neck swelling

B ANIL KUMAR, MD, FRCR, S CHANDRAMOHAN, MRCS and N PARASU, MRCP

Ninewells Hospital, Ninewells Avenue, Dundee DD1 9SY, UK

A previously well 23-year-old female presented to the accident and emergency department with a 2 week history of left neck swelling, dysphagia and neck pain which was not responding to oral antibiotics. On examination she was tachycardic and had a temperature of 38.8℃. There was an 11 cm × 11 cm firm, tender swelling over the left anterior triangle of the neck. There was also decreased air entry over the left lung base. She had a profound neutrophilia. A chest X-ray was performed (Figure 1) which was followed by a CT scan (Figures 2–4). What is your diagnosis?

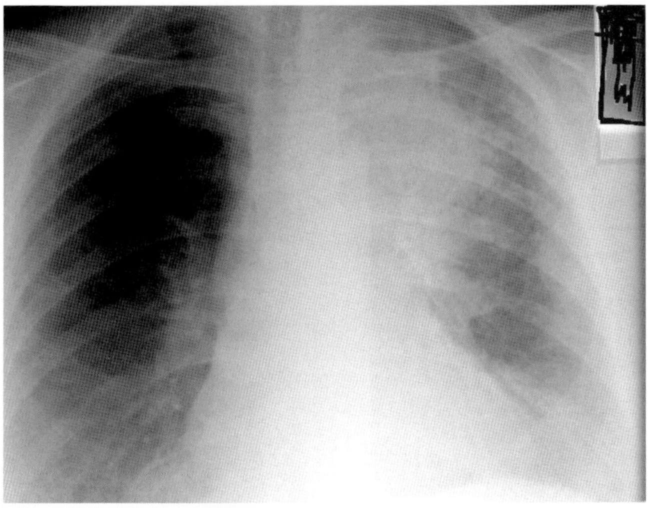

Figure 1. Posteroanterior chest radiograph.

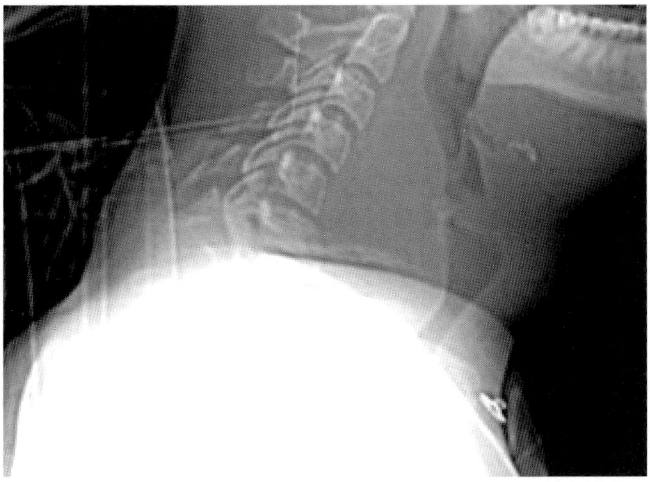

Figure 2. Lateral scanogram of neck.

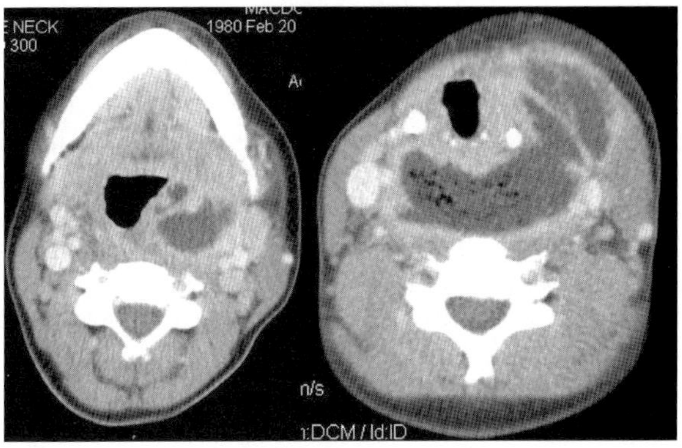

Figure 3. Post contrast CT images of the neck.

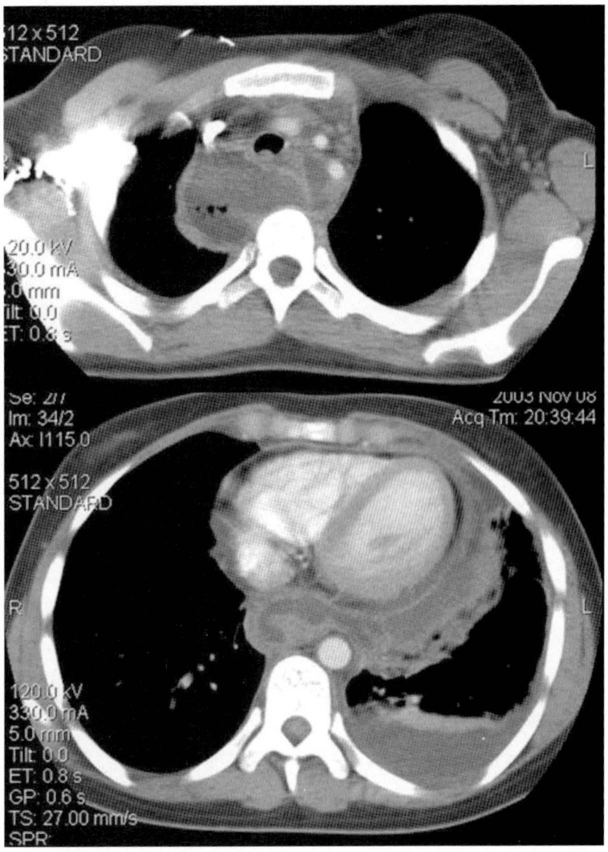

Figure 4. Post contrast CT images of the chest.

Received 12 October 2004 and in revised form 27 October 2004, accepted 1 November 2004

The chest radiograph demonstrates widened mediastinum and left pleural effusion (Figure 1). The lateral scanogram of the neck reveals a large pre-vertebral soft tissue opacity pushing the trachea anteriorly (Figure 2). CT scan shows large retropharyngeal abscess causing narrowing of the trachea and the oesophagus, and extending inferiorly into the thorax. The abscess extends into the left paracardiac and the left pleural space (Figures 3 and 4). A diagnosis of descending thoracic mediastinitis due to retropharyngeal abscess was made. She was transferred to the nearest thoracic centre where she had an emergency drainage of neck abscess and left posterolateral thoracotomy to remove the thoracic collection. She was discharged home with oral antibiotics following 3 weeks of hospital stay.

Descending necrotizing mediastinitis (DNM) is a rare and life-threatening complication of deep neck space infection, which occurs when infection spreads from the deep spaces of the neck, propagating within the soft tissue into the mediastinal spaces [1]. Early diagnosis and early, aggressive surgical treatment are required to improve the poor prognosis of DNM. CT is important in determining the level of infection, showing the presence and extension of fluid collections (with or without gas bubbles) as well as soft-tissue infiltration of the mediastinal fat and indicating the best surgical approach and progress of treatment [1].

The deep layer of the deep cervical fascia has two layers: the alar fascia runs from the base of the skull to the superior mediastinum and has a midline raphe. The pre-vertebral fascia lies directly on the vertebral bodies. A potential space lies between the alar and pre-vertebral fasciae, called danger space [2]. It is patent from the skull base to the diaphragm. Its upper part is the retropharyngeal space, which lies between the pre-vertebral fascia and the buccopharyngeal fascia on the outer surface of the pharynx. The space contains retropharyngeal lymph nodes [2] which drain the adenoids, nasal cavities, nasopharynx, and posterior ethmoid sinuses. Pathological walling-off of infection usually occurs in the retropharyngeal space, but there is no anatomical barrier to the spread of infection downward into the mediastinum. The lower part of this potential space extends behind the oesophagus, through the superior mediastinum, and into the posterior mediastinum. Knowledge of the anatomy is important in the identification and treatment of this potentially fatal condition.

References

1. Pinto A, Scaglione M, Giovine S, Lassandro F, Gagliardi N, Romano L, et al. Regarding three cases of descending necrotizing mediastinitis: spiral CT assessment. Radiol Med (Torino) 2003;105:291–5.
2. Chong VF, Fan YF. Radiology of the retropharyngeal space. Clin Radiol 2000;55:740–8.

Acknowledgment to Referees

The Editors would like to thank all their colleagues who have contributed their valuable time and effort in reviewing manuscripts submitted to *The British Journal of Radiology*. Listed below are the names of referees of papers submitted to BJR between 1 November 2003 and 31 November 2004.

A
Adam, A
Adam, E J
Adam Mitchell, A
A'Hern, R P
Aird, E G A
Allen, G
Alton, H
Amatiello, H
Amin, Z
Anbarasu, A
Anderson, H
Annesley-Williams, D
Antonio, G
Appleton, D
Ardeshna, K
Armstrong, S
Armstrong, P
Arthur, R
Ashleigh, R
Aspelin, P
Atchley, J

B
Barber, J
Barber, C
Barker, C S
Barker, D K
Barker, F
Barr, H
Barrett Lee, P
Barrington, S
Barron, D
Barton, D
Bartram, C
Bathurst, N
Baumann, M
Bearcroft, P W
Beards, S C
Beavis, A W
Beharry, N
Bell, J
Belli, A-M
Bentzen, S
Berry, E
Bessell, E
Biassoni, L
Bidmead, M
Birchall, D
Blake, G M
Blake, P
Blease, S
Blomley, M
Blunt, D
Boggis, C R M
Boivin, C
Bonnett, D E
Brada, M
Bradley, K M
Branson, A N
Breen, D
Brennan, P
Brettle, D
Britton, P
Brookes, J
Brooks, J
Brown, P
Buckingham, S
Budgell, G
Buffa, F M
Burch, A
Burnet, N
Buscombe, J
Byrne, J V

C
Callaway, M P
Campbell, S
Campbell, R
Casey, M
Castellano, I
Castellano, I A
Chalmers, N
Chambers, R J
Chapman, T
Chapple, C-L
Cleveland, T
Coley, S
Collie, D
Collins, D J
Collins, M
Conaghan, P
Cook, G
Cook, P G
Copley, S
Cornes, P
Cosgrove, D
Cowan, N C
Cowling, M
Crabtree, N
Crawley, C
Crellin, A
Curtis, J
Czajka, J

D
Dale, R G
Dance, D R
Darby, M J
Davies, N
Davies, S G
Davies, A M
Dawson, S
Dendy, P P
Denton, E
Desai, S R
Dixon, A
Dobbs, J
Donovan, T
Dowling, A
Drury, A
Duck, F A

E
Elliott, M
Emberton, P
Errington, D
Evans, R

F
Fairbairn, K J
Fenton, D
Finney, L
Fogelman, I
Fong, R Y L
Fowler, R
Fox, B
Francis, R M
Francis, I
Freeman, A
Friedman, E
Frost, R

G
Gallagher, A
Ganatra, R
Garcea, G
George, J
Gibson, M
Giles, J A
Gillams, A
Gillespie, J E
Gillespie, J
Given-Wilson, R
Glendinning, A G
Goh, V
Goldstone, K
Goodman, D A
Gould, D
Grant, D
Greaves, M
Green, R
Green, R A R
Greener, T
Griffiths, P
Grundy, A
Guibelalde, E

H
Hacking, C
Haddaway, M J
Hadley, D M
Hain, S
Hall, E J
Halligan, S
Halliwell, M
Halpin, S
Hancock, J
Hancock, B
Hare, C
Harrison, R M
Hart, D
Hart, G
Hatton, M
Hay, J
Haybittle, J L
Haylock, B
Healy, J
Heinz-Peer, G
Henson, J
Heron, C
Herwadkar, A
Hide, G
Higginson, T
Hill, A R
Hilson, A J W
Hirst, D
Hoggard, N
Hollings, N
Hopkins, K
Horsman, M
Hosie, K
Hoskin, P
Hosking, D
Houghton, S
Hounsell, A
Hourihan, M
Howells, J
Howlett, D C

Hufton, A P
Hughes, S
Hughes, D
Hunter, R D
Hutchinson, C
Hutchinson, C E

J
Jackson, A
Jackson, S
Jackson, S A
Jaspan, T
Jayakrishnan, V
Jefferies, S
Jenkins, J
Johnson, K
Jones, B
Julian, W L
Julian, W

K
Kearney, S
Keat, N
Keeling, F
Kemp, P
Kenny, P
Kessel, D
Khaw, K-T
Khoo, V
Koh, D M
Kotre, C J

L
Laitt, R
Laperriere, N
Larkin, E A
Lecomber, A R
Lee, S H
Leen, E
Lees, W R
Lewis, M A
Lewis-Jones, H G
Liddicoat, A
Lim, A K P
Lindquist, C
Litherland, J
Lomas, D J
Loveday, E
Lowe, S
Lyburn, I

M
MacBeth, F
MacDougall, R H
Mackay, R
Mackenzie, A
MacVicar, D
MacWilliams, R
Mallick, U K
Malone, L A
Manning, D
Marshall, M
Marshall, N
Marshall, N W
Marshall, T
Martin, C J
Martin, D
Maskell, G
Matson, M
Matthews, S
Mayles, P
Mayles, W P
McCafferty, I M
McCall, J
McHugh, K
McJury, M
McLean, A M
McMenamin, A
McNulty, H
Meaney, J
Miller, J
Mitchell, A
Mittal, T
Mittal, T K
Mohan, H K
Mohiaddin, R
Moore, N R
Moore, R
Moores, M
Morgan, A
Morgan, D A L
Morgan, R
Morrison, G D
Moskovic, E
Moss, H
Moussa, S
Murphy, D
Murray, D
Myint, S

N
Nakielny, R
Newman-Sanders, T
Nisbet, A
Nixon, P
Norton, S
Nusslin, F
Nutting, C

O
O'Connor, P
O'Hare, N J
Olliff, J F C
O'Reilly, G
Ostlere, S J
Owens, S E

P
Padayachee, T S
Padhani, A
Padley, S
Padley, S P
Paisley, E
Paley, M
Parker, G
Parkin, A
Parry, J
Partridge, J
Patel, U
Payne, D
Pelling, M
Pelling, M X
Perrin, R
Phelan, N
Phillips-Hughes, J
Pilcher, J
Pilling, D W
Piper, K
Pitcher, E M
Platt, K
Platts, A D
Plowman, P N
Pointon, K
Pope, R
Poynter, A J
Price, A
Price, P
Prvulovich, L
Putney, R

R
Raby, N
Rampling, R
Ramsden, R
Rawlings, D
Reed, N
Reek, C S
Reid, A
Remedios, D J
Reynolds, J
Rezvani, M
Richards, D
Richenberg, J
Ridley, N
Ring, E F G
Ritchie, D
Robertson, I
Robson, K J
Robinson, P J
Robinson, P
Rockall, A
Rodgers, P
Romanowski, C
Roobottom, C A
Rose, J D G
Rostom, A Y
Rothkamm, K
Rottenberg, G T
Rowbottom, C G
Rowell, N
Rubens, M B
Rubin, C
Rust, A G
Ryan, S

S
Sabarwhal, T
Sahdev, A
Sampson, M
Saunders, M I
Schelvan, C
Scott, D
Shaw, A
Shaw, A
Shentall, G
Shoaib, A
Shorvon, P J
Sidhu, P
Silver, D
Sivananthan, M
Sohaib, A
Spittle, M
Sprigg, A
Starritt, H
Steel, J
Sutton, D
Sykes, J R
Symonds, P

T
Tait, D M
Tait, P
Tan, L T
Taylor, A
Taylor, R E
Taylor, S
Taylor, S A
Teh, W
Temperton, D H
Thomas, S
Thomsen, H S
Thorniley, M
Thorogood, S V
Tibballs, J
Travis, S
Trott, K-R
Troughton, A
Turnbull, I
Tutt, A

U
Uberoi, R

V
Varghese, A
Venables, K
Vennart, W
Vinall, A
Vinnicombe, S

W
Wade, J P
Wakeley, C
Wall, B F
Waller, M
Wardman, P
Warren, M
Watkinson, A F
Watson, M
Watt, I
Webb, J A W
Webb, S
Whitehouse, G H
Whitehouse, R W
Wilde, P
Wilkins, J
Wilkinson, L
Williams, C
Williams, H
Williams, J
Williams, M
Wilson, P
Winder, J
Wong, W L
Wood, A M
Wood, B J
Workman, A
Worthy, S
Wright, A
Wright, E G

Y
Yarnold, J
Yates, S
Yates, S J
Young, K C

BIR CORPORATE MEMBER SCHEME

The BIR Corporate Member Scheme is aimed at all companies with an interest in radiology and allied sciences. For an annual subscription member companies are offered an attractive benefits package. To find out why your company should join the leading edge companies listed below, please contact Mr Adrian C Laws, Marketing Manager, British Institute of Radiology, 36 Portland Place, London W1B 1AT. Tel: +44 (0) 20 7307 1404.

Agfa-Gevaert Ltd
Tel: 020 82314900
Contact Mr M Hill, Business Manager Medical Imaging and PACS Systems
Product Code: 1, 2, 3, 4, 6, 9, 10, 12, 13, 14, 15, 20, 22 and 23

Alliance Medical Ltd
Tel: 01295 671223
Contact Mr Charles Fox, Marketing Executive
Product Code: 1, 4, 5, 16, 20 and 21

Amersham Health
Tel: 01494 798666
Contact Mr D G Rothery, Marketing Manager
Product Codes: 1, 2, 3, 4, 5 and 6

Bard Limited
Tel: 01293 606864
Contact Ms T Empson, Product Manager
Product Code: 2

B.M.V.A.
Tel: 01483 689838
Contact Dr R Bowden, Meetings Officer
Product Codes: 1, 3, 4, 9, 10 and 21

Bracco UK Ltd
Tel: 01628 851500
Contact Mr A Quinn, Product Manager
Product Codes: 1, 2 and 5

BVM Medical Ltd
Tel: 01455 614555
Contact Jay Tailor, Managing Director
Product Codes: 2 and 18

Cerner Corporation (UK)
Tel: 01452 831533
Contact Mr C Harrison, Client Executive
Product Codes: 9, 10, 13 and 20

Clinical Press Ltd
Tel: 0117 9420256
Contact Professor Paul Goddard, Chairman
Product Codes: 17 and 21

Cook (UK) Ltd
Tel: 01462 482884
Contact Mr Iain Mackintosh, regional Manager - Diagnostic and Interventional Products
Product Code: 2

Department of Radiography & Imaging Sciences (St Martin's College, Lancaster)
Tel: 01524 384640
Contact Mr Philip Harris, Acting Head of Department
Product Code: 21

Dictaphone International
Tel:020 78785000
Contact Dr F Brabant, Director of Product Management
Product Codes: 9 and 13

E-Z-EM Ltd
Tel: 01869 366900
Contact Mr Martin Suggitt, Product Manager
Product Codes: 1, 2 and 8

Ferrania UK Ltd
Tel: 01344 312100
Contact Mr Alan Budge, General Marketing Manager
Product Codes: 1, 3, 4, 9, 10, 13, 14, 15 and 18

Fuji Photo Film (UK) Ltd
Tel: 01234 326780
Contact Mr R G Brown, Strategic Business Manager
Product Codes: 1, 3, 4, 6, 9, 10, 12, 13, 14, 15, 18 and 22

GE Medical Systems
Tel: 01753 874000
Contact Mr A Trivett, Managing Director
Product Codes: 1, 2, 3, 4, 6, 8, 9, 10, 15, 18 and 22

Guerbet Laboratories Ltd
Tel: 01908 522888
Contact Mr Trevor Furniss, General Manager
Product Code: 1 and 2

Insignia Medical Systems Ltd
Tel: 01420 540206
Contact Mr Richard Dormer, Managing Director
Product Code: 9

Kimal plc
Tel: 01895 270951
Contact Mr S Clarke, Technical Director
Product Code: 2

Kingsmoor Publications Ltd
Tel: 01371 812960
Contact Mr David Roberts, Managing Director
Product Code: 17

Kodak Ltd
Tel: 01442 844473
Contact Mr Chris Wright, Marketing Manager UK and Ireland
Product Codes: 1, 3, 4, 6, 8, 9, 10, 12, 13, 14, 15, 18, 21, 22 and 23

Landauer, Inc.
Tel: 01865 373008
Contact Dr T Finnigan, Director, European Operations
Product Code: 8

Lanmark
Tel: 01494 675535
Contact Mrs Liz Beckmann, Director
Product Codes: 6, 9, 10, 13, 17 and 20

Lodestone Patient Care Limited
Tel: 020 89449630
Contact Mrs J Hill, Director of Operations
Product Code: 1, 3 and 21

Medical Imaging Systems Limited
Tel: 020 82059500
Contact Mr P W Sykes, Director
Product Code: 1

Mirada Solutions Ltd
Tel: 01865 265500
Contact Dr Clare Jones, VP Marketing
Product Codes: 1, 4, 6, 9, 10, 13, 21 and 22

Nucletron UK Ltd
Tel: 018297 71111
Contact Mr J Banks, Managing Director
Product Codes: 6 and 8

Pantak Medical Systems Agfa NDT
Tel: 0118 9310310
Contact Mr R Howton, Managing Director
Product Codes: 1, 6, 7 and 8

Philips Medical Systems
Tel:01737 230400
Contact Ms Anita Littlechild, Marketing Communications Manager
Product Codes: 1, 2, 9, 10, 22 and 23

Samsung SDS Europe Ltd
Tel:020 83807000
Contact Mr G Wheeler, Sales Manager (Medical)
Product Codes: 1, 9, 10, 13, 15, 16 and 20

Schering Health Care Ltd
Tel: 01444 232323
Contact Mr Chris Matthews, Product Manager
Product Codes: 1, 2 and 3

Sectra Ltd
Tel: 020 86106033
Contact Jan Wolfram, Managing Director
Product Codes: 9 and 10

Siemens Medical Solutions
Tel: 01344 396317
Contact Mr Mike Bell, Manager, Advertising and Exhibitions
Product Codes: 1, 2, 3, 4, 6, 9, 15 and 22

Sony Scientific and Medical
Tel: 01932 816267
Contact R Holt, Marketing Manager
Product Code: 14

Sonosite Ltd
Tel: 01767 313117
Contact Ms Gillian Duffy, European Marketing Director
Product Codes: 3

Southern Scientific Ltd
Tel: 01903 604000
Contact Mr Stephen Adams, Sales Manager
Product Codes: 1, 3, 4, 8, 10, 12 and 22

Toshiba Medical Systems UK
Tel: 01293 653700
Contact Mr S M Weeden, Manager X-ray Products
Product Codes: 1, 2, 3, 4, 9, 10 and 15

Varian Oncology Systems
Tel: 01293 531244 (UK)
Contact Mr Rolf Stähelin (Switzerland - tel. 00 41 417498844), Marketing Manager, Europe
Product Code: 6

Vertec Scientific Ltd
Tel: 01734 817431
Contact Mr B Hipgrave, Managing Director
Product Codes: 1, 4, 6, 8 and 12

Wardray Premise Ltd
Tel: 020 83989911
Contact Mr R Beach, Sales Manager
Product Codes: 8, 18 and 20

Wolverson X-Ray
Tel: 01902 637333
Contact Mr N Bacon, Sales Director
Product Codes: 1, 8, 15, 18 and 23

Xograph Imaging Systems
Tel: 01666 501501 or 07000 for X-ray
Contact Mr N Staff, Technical Director
Product Codes: 1, 8, 12, 14, 15, 18, 22 and 23

PRODUCT CODES

1. Diagnostic X-ray including NMR and CT
2. Interventional radiology
3. Ultrasound
4. Nuclear medicine
5. Radiopharmaceuticals
6. Radiotherapy and oncology
7. Radiobiology
8. Radiation protection
9. PACS
10. Image processing
11. Nuclear fuel cycle service
12. Quality assurance
13. Radiology data management computer systems
14. Video printing
15. Equipment leasing
16. Hospital-shared services
17. Medical publishing
18. X-ray consumables distribution
19. Electricity generation
20. Medical reporting systems
21. Education
22. Mammography
23. Dental X-ray

Meetings & Courses

Designing nuclear medicine facilities with special reference to radiation safety
26 January 2005
London, UK
Further details: The British Institute of Radiology, 36 Portland Place, London W1B 1AT.
Tel: 0207 307 1406. Fax: 0207 307 1414.
Email: registrations@bir.org.uk. Visit: www.bir.org.uk

Role of PET scanning within radiotherapy
27 January 2005
London, UK
Further details: The British Institute of Radiology, 36 Portland Place, London W1B 1AT.
Tel: 0207 307 1406. Fax: 0207 307 1414.
Email: registrations@bir.org.uk. Visit: www.bir.org.uk

Radiotherapy in breast cancer
1 February 2005
London, UK
Further details: The British Institute of Radiology, 36 Portland Place, London W1B 1AT.
Tel: 0207 307 1406. Fax: 0207 307 1414.
Email: registrations@bir.org.uk. Visit: www.bir.org.uk

FMRI lung imaging
4 February 2005
London, UK
Further details: The British Institute of Radiology, 36 Portland Place, London W1B 1AT.
Tel: 0207 307 1406. Fax: 0207 307 1414.
Email: registrations@bir.org.uk. Visit: www.bir.org.uk

Computed radiography: image quality and dose issues
23 February 2005
London, UK
Further details: The British Institute of Radiology, 36 Portland Place, London W1B 1AT.
Tel: 0207 307 1406. Fax: 0207 307 1414.
Email: registrations@bir.org.uk. Visit: www.bir.org.uk

Image guided therapy
24 February 2005
London, UK
Further details: The British Institute of Radiology, 36 Portland Place, London W1B 1AT.
Tel: 0207 307 1406. Fax: 0207 307 1414.
Email: registrations@bir.org.uk. Visit: www.bir.org.uk

Nuclear medicine in oncology
17 March 2005
London, UK
Further details: The British Institute of Radiology, 36 Portland Place, London W1B 1AT.
Tel: 0207 307 1406. Fax: 0207 307 1414.
Email: registrations@bir.org.uk. Visit: www.bir.org.uk

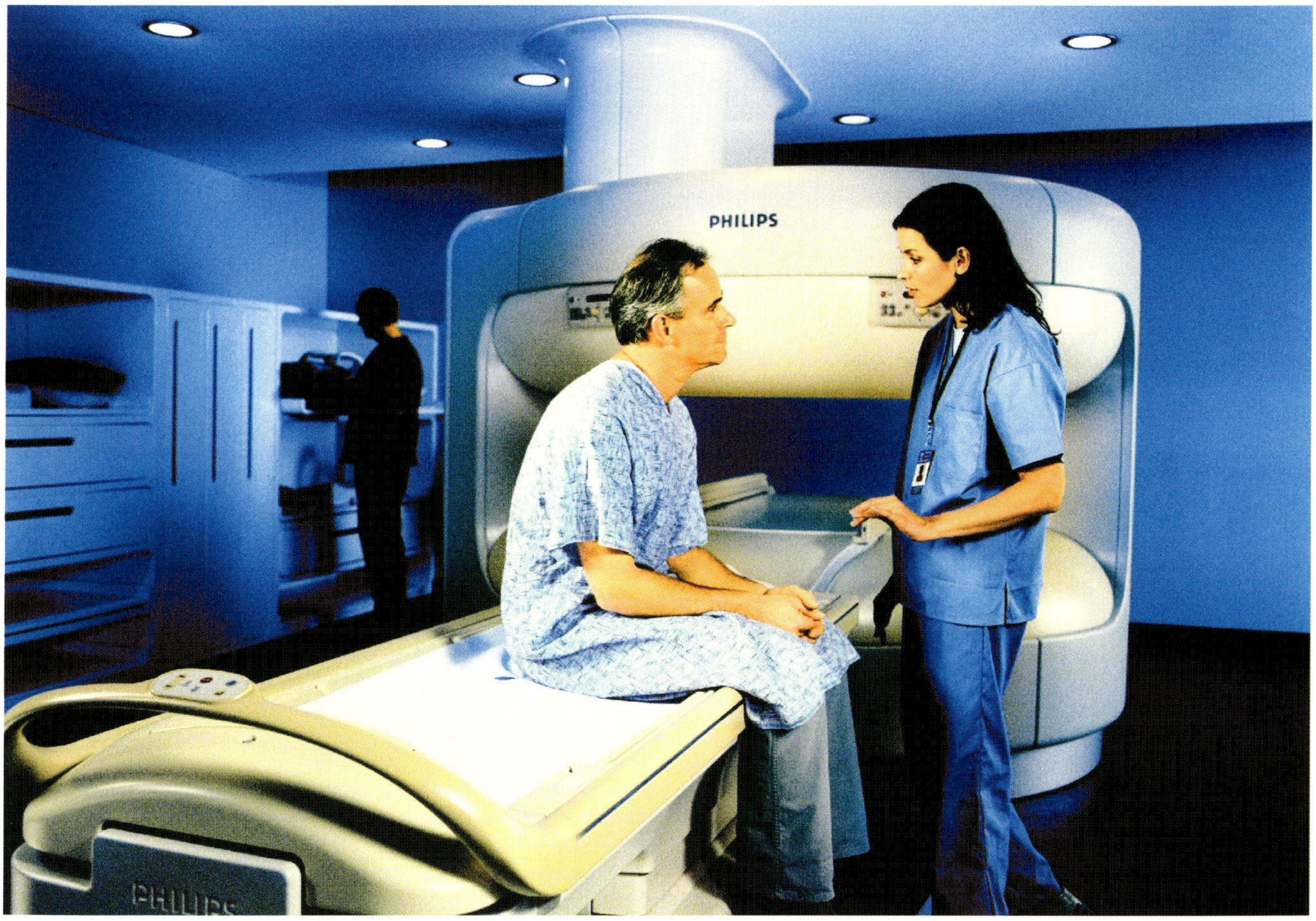
PHILIPS

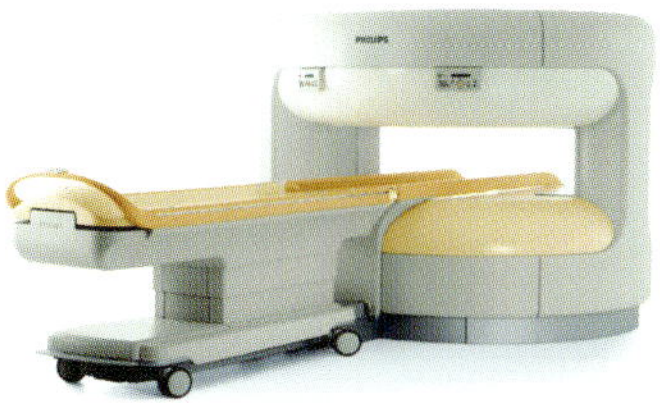

Volume 78| **February 2005**

BJR British Journal of Radiology

Full papers

Comparison of hepatic perfusion index measured with gadolinium-enhanced volumetric MRI in controls and in patients with colorectal cancer

Role of somatostatin receptor scintigraphy in patients with pituitary adenoma or post-surgical recurrent tumours

Magnetic resonance coronary angiography with 3D TrueFISP: breath-hold versus respiratory gated imaging

In vivo validation of a novel semi-automated method for border detection in IVUS images

Dose implications of fluoroscopy guided positioning (FGP) for lumbar spine examinations prior to acquiring plain film radiographs

Effective doses in angiography and interventional radiology: calculation of conversion coefficients for angiography of the lower limbs

The hyfrecator: a treatment for radiation induced telangiectasia in breast cancer patients

Commentaries
Short communications
Case reports
Pictorial review
Case of the month
Book reviews

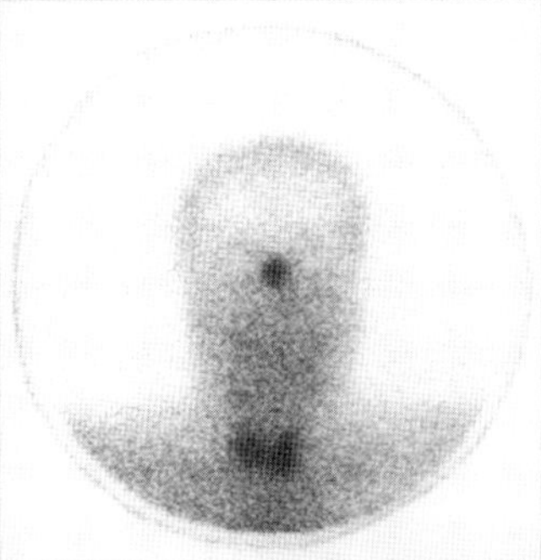

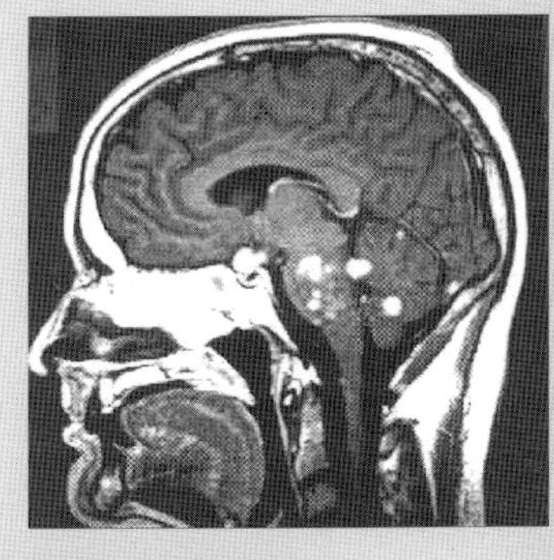

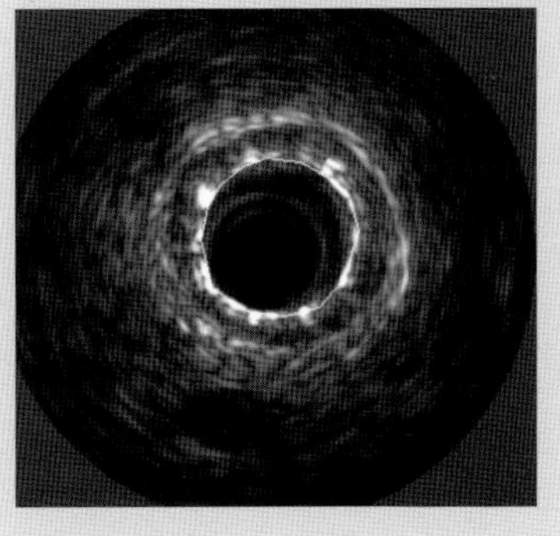

http://bjr.birjournals.org

ISSN 0007-1285

Published by

BIR The British Institute of **Radiology**

BJR

ISSN 0007 1285

THE BRITISH JOURNAL OF RADIOLOGY

Aims and Coverage

The *British Journal of Radiology* is the official peer-reviewed monthly research journal of the British Institute of Radiology. It is a multidisciplinary journal covering all clinical and technical aspects of diagnostic imaging, radiotherapy and oncology, medical physics and radiobiology. BJR is an international journal containing papers both from the UK and overseas, and is circulated to Full Members of the BIR and to libraries worldwide.

Authors are strongly advised to submit manuscripts online using Editorial Manager^{TM}, at http://bjr.edmgr.com. Online submission will expedite the peer-review process. Instructions to Authors are available on request from the Refereeing Administrator at the address given below, and are also available on the BIR's website at www.bir.org.uk

Editorial Board

Overseas Advisory Panel

Published by the British Institute of Radiology, 36 Portland Place, London W1B 1AT, UK.
Editorial enquiries: Tel: +44 (0)20 7307 1424; Fax: +44 (0)20 7307 1414
Email: publications@bir.org.uk
Advertising sales and enquiries: please contact Gareth Liddiatt at McMillan Scott: Tel: +44 (0)20 7878 2313
Email: gareth@mcmslondon.co.uk
www.bir.org.uk www.birjournals.org bjr.edmgr.com

Subscriptions

Subscriptions fulfilment is carried out by PSP Subscriptions, BMA House, Tavistock Square, London WC1H 9JR, UK (Telephone +44 (0)20 7383 6270; Fax +44 (0)20 7383 6402; email subscriptions@bmjgroup.com). The 2005 annual subscription rate for the printed version of BJR is £524 (includes 12 issues plus two Special Issue). Subscriptions are on a calendar basis only.

Institutional BJR subscribers have free access to both BJR Online and Imaging Online, and are offered a 33% discount on a print subscription to the BJR's quarterly review journal Imaging (see http://imaging.birjournals.org).

US Mailing Agent

The British Journal of Radiology (ISSN 0007 1285) is published monthly by the British Institute of Radiology, c/o Mercury Airfreight Int. Ltd, 365 Blair Road, Avenel, NJ 07001. The Dollar price for US direct subscribers is $786. Periodicals Postage Paid at Rahway NJ. Postmaster: send address corrections to the British Journal of Radiology, c/o Mercury Airfreight Int. Ltd, 365 Blair Road, Avenel, NJ 07001.

Back Issues

Back issues can be ordered from Vine House Distribution, Waldenbury, North Common, Chailey, East Sussex BN8 4DR, UK (Telephone +44 (0)1825 723398; Fax +44 (0)1825 724188). Price is £40 per issue.

BJR Online

BJR Online, produced in association with HighWire Press, is available free of charge to BIR members and Institutional print subscribers: http://bjr.birjournals.org. Enquiries to publications@bir.org.uk

Typeset, printed and bound by The Charlesworth Group, Wakefield, UK. Telephone +44 (0)1924 204830.

BJR

VOLUME 78

Number 926

Contents

February 2005

Front cover: *The illustrations used on the front cover of this issue of BJR can be found on pages 112, 128 and 154. We thank the authors for granting us permission to use their figures.*

Editorial

Page

■ X-ray computed tomography – a truly remarkable medical development 97
J Husband and G Dombrowe

Commentaries

■ Particle Therapy Co-operative Oncology Group (PTCOG 40) Meeting, Institute Curie 2004 99
B Jones and I Rosenberg

■ Imaging investigation of liver haemodynamics in patients at risk for hepatic metastatic disease 103
C Harvey and M Blomley

Full papers

■ Comparison of the hepatic perfusion index measured with gadolinium-enhanced volumetric MRI in controls and in patients with colorectal cancer 105
J J Totman, R L O'Gorman, P A Kane and J B Karani

■ The role of somatostatin receptor scintigraphy in patients with pituitary adenoma or post-surgical recurrent tumours 110
M J Acosta-Gómez, M A Muros, J M Llamas-Elvira, A Ramírez, S Ortega, G Sabatel, C Ramos and A de la Riva-Aguilar

■ Magnetic resonance coronary angiography with 3D TrueFISP: breath-hold versus respiratory gated imaging 116
N M C So, W W M Lam, D Li, A K Y Chan, J E Sanderson and C Metreweli

■ *In vivo* validation of a novel semi-automated method for border detection in intravascular ultrasound images 122
C V Bourantas, M E Plissiti, D I Fotiadis, V C Protopappas, G V Mpozios, C S Katsouras, I C Kourtis, M R Rees and L K Michalis

■ Dose implications of fluoroscopy-guided positioning (FGP) for lumbar spine examinations prior to acquiring plain film radiographs 130
M Saunders, A Budden, F MacIver, M Teunis and H Warren-Forward

■ Effective doses in angiography and interventional radiology: calculation of conversion coefficients for angiography of the lower limbs 135
L Struelens, F Vanhavere, H Bosmans and R Van Loon

■ The hyfrecator: a treatment for radiation induced telangiectasia in breast cancer patients 143
C M E Rowland Payne, N Somaiah, A J Neal and J P Glees

Short communications

■ Technical report: use of ultrasound guidance in the removal of tunnelled venous access catheter cuffs 147
A M Barnacle and A W M Mitchell

■ Late effects of radiotherapy: how to assess and improve outcomes 150
D A Power

Case reports

■ Xanthoma disseminatum: a case report and literature review 153
A S Alexander, R Turner, L Uniate and R G Pearcy

■ Visceral leishmaniasis: diagnosis by ultrasound-guided fine needle aspiration of an axillary node 158
M Reus, B García, V Vázquez, D Morales, M Fuster and J Sola

■ Renal artery pseudoaneurysm following partial nephrectomy treated with stent-graft 161
M D Horwitz, D C Hanbury and C M King

■ Ultrasound findings of iodide mumps 164
S J Park, H S Hong, H K Lee, J H Joh, J G Cha and H C Kim

■ Radiological findings of primary retroperitoneal synovial sarcoma 166
S Ulusan, O Kizilkilic, T Yildirim, C Hurcan, N Bal and T Z Nursal

Pictorial review

■ Commonly encountered adrenal pseudotumours on CT 170
T Gokan, Y Ohgiya, H Nobusawa and H Munechika

Case of the month

■ The rapidly enlarging chin mass 175
C Offiah and E Hall

Book review 177

BIR Company Subscribers 178

Meetings and courses 180

The British Journal of Radiology, *78* (2005), 97–98
DOI: 10.1259/bjr/52138043

Editorial

X-ray computed tomography – a truly remarkable medical development

J HUSBAND and G DOMBROWE

Since the death last year of Sir Godfrey Hounsfield there have been many tributes to him. Mostly in the form of obituaries, these have concentrated on the man and his lifetime's work. The *British Journal of Radiology* wishes to pay its own tribute by reminding readers of the extraordinary impact X-ray CT has had, and continues to have, on the diagnosis, treatment and management of disease.

Janet Husband, immediate Past President of the British Institute of Radiology and President of the Royal College of Radiologists writes of the clinical impact:

The advent of computed tomography (CT) in the early 1970s changed the practice of medicine forever. It was like switching on a light in a darkened room, a light which burns ever more brightly as advances in technology have taken us from early generation CT scanners, to single slice and then to multislice machines.

The first clinical results were presented at the Annual Meeting of the British Institute of Radiology in 1972 by Dr Jamie Ambrose, who showed images from the prototype of the very first EMI brain scanner. The atmosphere in the lecture theatre was electric, there was standing room only and I was there as a very junior trainee in radiology. The ability to demonstrate lesions in the brain, tumours, abscesses and haemorrhage directly for the first time caught the imagination of radiologists around the World. It was clear even in those early days that the invention of CT had launched a new era in the detection and evaluation of disease. Professor Isherwood undertook pioneering work at Manchester University on the first commercial EMI scanner and the radiology literature began to reveal the potential impact of CT on the management of patients.

Then, in 1975 Sir Godfrey took the World by storm once more with the announcement of body CT at an international conference in Bermuda. The feverish activity which followed again took radiology to the forefront of medical advance.

I was fortunate to work with Dr Louis Kreel on the prototype of the World's first body scanner, the EMI 5000 in 1976. The UK, together with a few centres in the USA led the World in exploring and evaluating the clinical potential of body CT. Within 5 years most of the major centres throughout the World had installed CT systems and CT had already made a major impact as a first line investigation for staging and follow up of malignant disease. This, of course, has been one of its major applications throughout the decades, but in the early 1980s clinical investigation and further technological development led to much wider applications of CT such as the evaluation of lung disease, musculoskeletal disorders and the assessment of trauma. During the last 20 years major development in CT technology has focused on reduction in scan times and reconstruction times and improvements in image quality. Today it is hard to believe that we began reporting CT from images stored on magnetic tape, and a scan of the chest, abdomen and pelvis took about 45 minutes to review. We scanned a maximum of eight patients a day and now we can perform over 35 whole body examinations a day.

By 1980 the number of CT installations had expanded so rapidly that there was an urgent need to share knowledge, educate each other and train the CT specialists of the future. Teaching courses sprang up in the USA and in other parts of the World and together with Dr Ian Kelsey Fry and other young CT enthusiasts, I set up The Annual London CT Course, which was first held at the Selsdon Park Hotel in Surrey with a total of 50 delegates. We moved to the Gleneagles Hotel in 1985 and here Tiba Seear and I have continued to run and develop the course so that today the programme incorporates multislice CT, MRI and PET scanning. In 2001 we were very proud that Sir Godfrey agreed to give his name to our annual prestigious honorary lecture. This year we are looking forward to celebrating our 25th Anniversary of "The Gleneagles Course". It is astonishing to reflect that, over the years, well over 3500 radiologists from all over the World have participated in the programme. We hope this educational forum in cross-sectional imaging will continue for many years to come.

CT remains the workhorse of cancer imaging and is the investigation of choice in a wide range of other areas. There are literally millions of people throughout the World who have benefited from Sir Godfrey Hounsfield's extraordinary achievement.

Today imaging is at the dawn of another new era, the era of molecular medicine in which we will use imaging to identify early disease, to profile disease more precisely and to observe the effects of specific therapies. I am sure the next 30 years will be just as exciting as the last, but it has been a great privilege to work in radiology at a time of astonishing technological and clinical development.

Günter Dombrowe, President of the British Institute of Radiology, adds a technical dimension:

When rumours of a cross-sectional X-ray imaging technique first emerged during the early 1970s, research and development departments in the traditional X-ray companies were highly sceptical. Most of the technological innovation effort at that time was aimed at improving spatial resolution (typically down to 0.2 mm) and exposure time. A technique that promised an image comprising 80 by 80 pixels which took minutes to acquire and hours to compute seemed decidedly unattractive.

All this changed overnight with the first public demonstration of clinical images by Dr Ambrose, which impressively demonstrated the huge potential of improved contrast resolution, and within weeks all major established companies as well as a number of newcomers had started crash programmes to replicate and improve on the results.

Soon afterwards, there were almost 20 different commercial scanner designs and a fierce debate was raging about the merits of different "generations" of scanning geometry, which in some quarters did not subside until the mid 1990s, although all the basics had been proposed by 1977. Hounsfield and his team initially seemed slow in adopting the more adventurous approaches and continued to rely on the original translate-rotate mechanical scanning principle, until they once again appeared to set the pace with their prototype of a much faster body scanner which was to combine the advantages of "third" and "fourth" generation designs with its unique "nutating" detector ring. Unfortunately it was a step too far for the time and EMI decided to leave the field soon after.

In the meantime, the more traditional X-ray vendors had invested heavily in dedicated CT component design and computing know-how, and with their superior understanding of clinical requirements rapidly achieved great improvements in examination speed, post-processing and user friendliness, thereby turning CT from an esoteric scientific instrument to the workhorse of the modern imaging department. As a secondary effect of Sir Godfrey's work, once these fundamental skills and capabilities, created in the pursuit of CT excellence, existed, they could be utilized as the basis for equally rapid development of later technologies, such as MRI and digital radiography, thereby completely changing the World of medical imaging as we knew it.

25 years later CT is thriving, its R&D and manufacturing is dominated by the "big four" diagnostic imaging companies with an annual segment turnover of several billion pounds. CT technology and clinical application has shown enormous resilience against alternative diagnostic methods and at the moment is stronger than ever. There have been important enhancements of the basic design principles on the way, perhaps most notably the introduction of spiral CT, followed more recently by multislice systems. It is humbling to note how even these recent developments owe something to the genius to Sir Godfrey. The manuscript of the original project proposal written by him in 1967 (!) contains a drawing of a multirow detector which could come straight off one of today's commercial brochures.

X-ray CT has not only stood the test of time, its obvious relevance to cutting edge research such as molecular imaging, its increasing use in radiotherapy treatment planning and the substantial commercial investment in combined imaging modalities such as CT/PET show that it has much more to offer.

We owe Sir Godfrey a deep debt of gratitude.

The British Journal of Radiology, 78 (2005), 99–102 © 2005 The British Institute of Radiology
DOI: 10.1259/bjr/18664944

Commentary

Particle Therapy Co-operative Oncology Group (PTCOG 40) Meeting, Institute Curie 2004

[1]B JONES, MSc, MD, FRCR and [2]I ROSENBERG, MA, PhD, FIPEM

[1]*Department of Clinical Oncology, Queen Elizabeth University Hospital Cancer Centre, Birmingham B15 2TH and* [2]*Department of Radiotherapy Physics, Meyerstein Institute of Oncology, University College London Hospitals, London, UK*

Introduction

The question of whether the UK should commission a new high-energy cyclotron or synchrocyclotron in order to be at the cutting edge of radiation therapy cancer research remains unanswered. At present the only such UK facility, situated at Clatterbridge on the Wirral peninsula, has sufficient energy to treat cancers of the eye; deeper situated targets are not accessible to such sophisticated treatment. This report has been written in order to inform British Oncologists, Physicists, the administrators of the Research Councils and other relevant funding bodies about the latest research and development in particle radiotherapy. Some British children and young adults are referred to the proton therapy Centre in Orsay, near Paris: this fact and the probable increase in future demand for proton and ion beam treatments abroad should also be of interest to our Department of Health.

Over 30 000 patients have by now received proton therapy for cancer, with 3000 treated in the last year. The growth in centres and patients treated follow linear and exponential rates, respectively. There are now 21 treatment centres, with the largest throughput of over 1000 patients per year at the University of Loma Linda facility and nearly 500 patients per year at Massachusetts General Hospital (MGH), where many new techniques are being developed particularly for cancers in children. Dr Janet Sisterson (MGH) presented these facts at the opening of PTCOG40 (Particle Therapy Cooperative Oncology Group) held in Paris (June 16–18, 2004) under the auspices of the Institute Curie. PTCOG has now held two meetings per year for the last 20 years for persons in all disciplines relating to particle therapy. Their website (http://ptcog.web.psi.ch/index.html) lists the worldwide proton and light ion centres with updated figures of patients treated. Further details of the PTCOG40 meeting such as speakers and their institutions will become available in the newsletter section of the website, entitled "Particles".

The pioneering efforts of those involved in particle therapies have provided conventional radiotherapy with many of its more advanced techniques, *e.g.* three-dimensional (3D) treatment planning, respiratory gating, equivalent uniform dose, etc. In parallel with the increased clinical activity, there are now seven industrial companies that manufacture "turn-key" cyclotron centres capable of treating 2000–3000 patients per year in 3–5 treatment rooms. There was a pictorial exhibition of these products at the meeting and it is apparent that installation costs are falling due to the increased competition.

Proton therapy initially developed as radiosurgery and evolved into fractionated therapy for rare cancers that were considered incurable using conventional radiotherapy. At present, an increasing range of common cancers over a wide range of TNM staging are being successfully treated with resultant higher control rates and/or reduced normal tissue complication probabilities. This is possible owing to the excellent dose localization properties of the Bragg peak characteristic of energetic charged particles. A further recent development is the emergence of carbon ion therapies, with participating centres in some cases using mixtures of conventional therapy, in the intensity-modulated radiotherapy (IMRT) mode, and ions. The application of these treatments could not have occurred without the recent improvements in tumour imaging, so that far safer dose escalation and improved patient selection for radical treatment is now possible. Positron emission tomography (PET) imaging has also been used to define patients with minimal numbers of metastatic deposits for treatment by proton or ion extracranial radiosurgery.

Techniques

The technical improvements described at PTCOG40 include: standards of particle dosimetry; fast analytical planning software, for example using Moliere's theory of charged particles and various Monte Carlo programmes all with good fits to measured dose [1]; improved immobilization; analysis of the influence of patient movement [2] and of varying tissue inhomogeneities; detailed and impressive analyses of reliability and accuracy in the entire clinical setting were presented.

Various methods of treatment delivery were discussed, from uniform passively scattered fields with spread out Bragg peaks, modulated using mechanical range shifters and compensators, to individual pencil beams that can "dose paint" a cancer target, using scanning "wobbler" magnets [3]. There are several methods of dose painting such as lateral edge tracking, which is forgiving of uncertainties in Bragg peak position. A technique called double parallel scanning is being developed in Switzerland.

Received 5 July 2004 and in revised form 15 September 2004, accepted 4 October 2004.

Confirmation of regional dose deposition within the patient is possible by PET scanning of beam auto-activation products [4]. Various additional devices such as robotic treatment couches have been utilized to improve the accuracy of patient positioning while maintaining efficiency.

One of the advantages of particle beam therapy is that only one particle source, such as a central cyclotron, is required for treatments in several (*e.g.* 3–5) treatment rooms. The beam can be diverted or "switched" between rooms by the operation of bending magnets. This means that large numbers of patients can be treated from a single source, which is economically advantageous. Throughput issues were discussed, such as the logistics of efficient treatment set-ups using adjacent rooms, with rapid transfer of patients to the actual treatment position. Fast beam switching from room to room is being improved: at Orsay this is now achieved in only 10–20 s. Gantry design is critical – these weigh around 100 tonnes for protons and up to 600 tonnes for carbon ions and need to be able to rotate while keeping to an accuracy of below 1 mm. The use of bending magnets placed at the mouth of the collimator of a fixed horizontal beam, combined with robotic motion of the patient support couch, may reduce costs and tonnage, yet cover 85% of treatment geometries.

Confirmation of the regional dose deposition within a patient is possible by PET scanning of beam auto-activation products.

A separate forum was held for physicians and considered target volume determination and treatment planning exercises for difficult cases of recurrent chordomas and other paraspinal tumours; this successful new development will hopefully be repeated in future meetings.

Treatment results

Protons

Many centres presented descriptions of techniques and of phase 1 and 2 dose escalation studies with outcomes. There is a dearth of phase 3 randomized controlled trials in this area, but these are anticipated when optimum techniques and dose levels have been agreed. For protons, the highlights included head and neck oropharyngeal cancers, where tumour control rates and disease-free survival rates were 84% and 65%, respectively. Re-treatment of nasopharyngeal cancers provides a survival of 50% at 2 years with no brain necrosis to date. Adenoid cystic and other radioresistant cancers such as melanoma are also well controlled. Techniques were also described for acoustic neuromas, T1N0M0 breast cancers, olfactory neuroblastoma, benign meningiomas and lachrymal gland cancers. There were no detailed updates of the base of skull proton therapy experience in the MGH Boston apart from a statement that the 10 year control rate is 98% for chondrosarcomas and 44% for chordomas. Recruitment to the MGH randomized dose escalation trial for chordomas is expected to be complete towards the end of 2004.

The majority of patients treated to date have received proton therapy to the eye using relatively low energy beams. These treatments have become increasingly sophisticated due to the refinement of the indications to include certain sizes of melanoma [6] and hamartomas. A reduction in the usual tumour margins from 2.5 mm to 1 mm where tumours are close to critical structures such as the optic nerve and macula has not been associated with an increased recurrence rate, as correctly predicted by Chauvel and colleagues [7], although some opthalmologists use additional laser therapy if treatment margins are small.

Carbon ions

In the case of carbon ions, very impressive results were presented from Germany and Japan, particularly from the HIMAC centre (National Radiological Sciences Institute) where nearly 1800 patients have been treated with meticulous attention to detail. Despite a relative biological effect (RBE) of three in the spread out Bragg peaks, the safety of therapy is well confirmed with impressive local control rates, although in some instances X-ray IMRT is given as a first phase to minimize potential ion beam overdosage due to organ movement and in the case of large treatment volumes. Examples include large inoperable high-grade osteosarcomas of the pelvis in young adults [8]. Control rates of 77% and survival rates of 45% at 5 years were described after 73.6 Gy eq. in 16 fractions over 1 month, with no neurological or other severe adverse late effects. Small peripheral non-small-cell lung cancers are highly curable [9] without long-term loss of lung function (measured by gas transfer factor) and only minor short-term changes in forced expiratory volume in 1 s (FEV_1) [10]. In such cases single fractions of 28 Gy eq. have recently been found to give the same results as higher doses given in 15–17 fractions (around 60% survival at 5 years with no serious complications). Thus for small cancers, the prospects of carefully conducted radiosurgery is feasible, without the complications that follow radical surgery. Hypofractionation of prostate cancer (stages T1–T3) to 66 Gy in 20 fractions with hormone therapy gives high control rates (79% at 5 years for initial prostate specific antigen (PSA) levels above 20) [11]. Of 201 recently analysed patients, only 2 had rectal bleeding and 6% had grade 2 bladder side effects: the technique continues to be refined. Other applications include pre-sacral rectal recurrences (78.4% control at 2 years) and inoperable melanomas with concomitant chemotherapy. Large hepatic cell cancers are now treated to a dose of 52.8 Gy eq. in only 4 fractions, without significant toxicity and with a local control rate of 90%, a 5 year survival equivalent to surgery but without the attendant morbidity.

Paediatric cancers

For cancer in children, a European Proton Therapy Group is being established and proton therapy is now approved within American paediatric research protocols. It is already evident from Boston that chemo-proton radiotherapy is very well tolerated in children, and the Massachusetts General retain reserved treatment slots for treating children at short notice. For example, in the treatment of orbital rhabdomyosarcoma 88% eye retention has been found after doses of 40–55 Gy in 20–25 fractions. In France, the optimization of posterior fossa radiotherapy in children with medulloblastomas is designed to reduce deafness. In Boston they aim to virtually eliminate the dose to a substantial portion of the vertebral bodies and all other anterior structures during cranio-spinal therapy, in order to reduce growth disorders and the occurrence of second malignancies in later life.

Orsay site visit

The conference included a visit to the Centre de Protontherapie Orsay (CPO) situated on the outskirts of Paris at the University of Orsay campus, where proton therapy is provided for a large range of sites including children and adults with skull base cancers (including some British patients). The last PTCOG meeting held there was in 1993 and the present authors have noted a marked improvement in the general facilities for patients, although the surrounding environment is not that of a hospital. The majority of the treatment is actually given by conventional radiotherapy at the central Paris hospitals, with protons used as a boost. This has all been made possible due to a highly motivated cooperative group of physicians in various Paris hospitals. There is considerable central government support via the Commissariat à l'Energy Atomique, which also supports radiotherapy research. There are already plans to extend the facility and possibly to open another centre in central Paris, as well as the ambitious Etoile project at Lyon [12], which aims to treat 2000 patients per year with carbon ions.

Radiobiology

The radiobiology content was relatively sparse, but included some high linear energy transfer (LET) bio-effect modelling incorporated into treatment planning [13], and unpublished work on the different apoptotic responses in three glioma lines exposed to protons at Clatterbridge. There was an interesting poster follow-up of some recently published work [14] on proton irradiation of DNA plasmids loaded with platinum atoms, which showed that the high ionization cross section of platinum caused more efficient double strand breaks during proton irradiation than for X-rays. This suggests a role for concurrent or sequential chemoradiation in tumours that take up platinum avidly. Only one oral presentation, from Cape Town South Africa, presented their doses as biological effective dose (BED) and concluded that the α/β ratio for acoustic neuromas treated by stereotactic proton therapy is around 1.7 Gy. Surprisingly, there were no presentations of radiobiological comparisons of particle beams situated at different international centres. Such research can provide important quality assurance, although funding across national boundaries can be a restrictive issue.

Discussion

PTCOG meetings consider the highest possible ideals in radiation oncology and we would encourage greater UK participation for a variety of reasons. For the UK to adapt to the inevitable demand for particle therapy abroad [15, 16], it would be sensible to have a rational plan based on the existing Cancer Networks. Designated specialists (clinical oncologists and physicists) could advise patients and their relatives as to the relative merits or unsuitability of therapy abroad. For this to occur, it will be necessary for at least some centres in the UK to obtain appropriate treatment planning software and for the specialists concerned to develop and maintain an interest in this subject. It would be preferable for the UK to possess its own service, based initially on one large facility with equity of access controlled via the existing Cancer Networks.

It is anticipated that very high intensity lasers targeted through plasma at thin metallic foils will eventually allow proton facilities to be located in a single room at relatively low cost [17, 18]. With such methods, we envisage that most of the largest cancer centres in the UK could provide proton therapy. However, as yet there is no such prototype for clinical or biological use, so that such an expansion is at least a decade or more away. In the meantime, a large National Centre with multiple treatment rooms and based on existing cyclotron technology needs to be commissioned so that considerable experience can be acquired before an eventual expansion of smaller units can occur.

Future PTCOG meetings are planned for Bloomington, Indiana (October 2004), Japan (spring 2005) and Munich (October 2005). After 2007 there will only be one such meeting per year. We would encourage specialists not only to attend these meetings but also to visit proton centres abroad: a reasonable start would be to visit the Clatterbridge Cyclotron, used only for eye treatments.

Recent Austrian estimates conclude that around 14% of all radiotherapy treatments would have improved outcomes if given using protons rather than X-rays: this represents a challenge to us all. The UK needs the equivalent of the French Commissariat à l'Energy Atomique or the National Radiological Sciences Institute in Japan, as there seems to be no single arm of the UK Government that can represent the interests of different departments about radiation research and development. Should a UK proton facility either be funded for the delivery of healthcare by the Department of Health or, in order to answer important medical, physics and associated engineering research questions, should funding originate from the two relevant Research Councils, the MRC and EPSRC? The main UK cancer research charity (CRUK) is highly focused and dedicated to improve the control of cancer by biochemical means, with scant resource allocation to radiation research. In the meantime, perhaps the new National Cancer Research Institute should take the lead in this important area and bring the relevant stakeholders together? The UK radiation oncology community could undoubtedly rationalize the indications for particle therapy by performing randomized control trials that compare the best available treatments such as IMRT with protons, and test the use of protons as part of mixed schedules. The prospectus for research alongside such projects is vast and extends into the molecular and genetic fields as well as experimental and clinical radiobiology.

Conclusions

Protons and light ions should not be seen as competitors to existing conventional treatments, but as a complementary force in the fight against cancer. Their precise roles remain to be fully defined, but it is inevitable that there will be increasing indications for their use in cancer therapy here in the UK, either by increased referral of patients abroad or by investment in particle treatment facilities for the eventual benefit of a larger number of UK cancer patients; they deserve the best treatment.

Acknowledgments

The authors are grateful for the financial support of The Cyclotron Trust, their respective NHS Hospital Trusts and NHS endowment funds in order to attend PTCOG40. Owing to space constraints we regret not being able to mention the names and affiliations of all the many excellent speakers that contributed to this meeting.

References

1. Paganetti H, Gottshalk B. Test of Geant3 and Geant4 nuclear models for 160 MeV protons stopping in CH2. Med Phys 2003;30:1926–31.
2. Paganetti H. Four dimensional Monte Carlo simulation of time dependent geometries. Phys Med Biol 2004;49:N75–N81.
3. Kohno R, Kanenatsu N, Yusa K, Kanai T. Experimental evaluation of analytical penumbra calculation model for wobbled beams. Med Phys 2004;31:1153–7.
4. Hishikawa Y, Kagawa K, Murakami M, Sakai H, Akagi T, Abe M. Usefulness of positron emission tomographic images after proton therapy. Int J Radiat Oncol Biol Phys 2002;53:1388–91.
5. Pedroni E, Bearpark R, Bohringer T, Coray A, Duppich E, et al. The PSI gantry 2: a second generation proton scanning gantry. Z Med Phys 2004;14:25–34.
6. Domato B, Lecvonak K. Conservation of eyes with choroidal melanoma by a multimodality approach to treaatment: an audit of 1632 patients. Opthalmology 2004;111:977–83.
7. Courdi A, Caufolle JP, Grange JD, Diallo-Rosier L, Sahel J, et al. Results of proton therapy of uveal melanomas treated in Nice. Int J Radiat Oncol Biol Phys 1999;45:5–11.
8. Kamada T, Tsujii H, Tsuji H, Yanagi T, Mizoe JE, et al. Efficacy of carbon ion radiotherapy in bone and soft tissue sarcomas. J Clin Oncol 2002;20:4466–71.
9. Miyamoto T, Yanamoto N, Nishimura H, Koto M, Tsujii H, et al. Carbon ion radiotherapy for stage 1 non-small cell lung cancer. Radiother Oncol 2003;66:127–40.
10. Kadono K, Homma T, Kamahara K, Nakayama M, Satoh H, Sekizawa K, et al. Effect of heavy-ion radiotherapy on pulmonary function in stage I non-small cell lung cancer patients. Chest 2002;122:1925–32.
11. Akakura K, Tsujii H, Morita S, Tsuji H, Yagishita T, et al. Phase I/II clinical trials of carbon ion therapy for prostate cancer. Prostate 2004;58:252–8.
12. Pommier P, Balosso J, Bolla M, Gerard JP. The French project ETOILE: review of clinical data for light ion hadrontherapy. Cancer Radiother 2002;6:369–78.
13. Wilkens JJ, Oelfke U. A phenomenological model for the relative biological effectiveness in therapeutic proton beams. Phys Med Biol 2004;49:2811–25.
14. Lacombe S, Le Sech C, Esaulov V. DNA strand breaks induced by low keV energy heavy ions. Phys Med Biol 2004;49:N65–N73.
15. Suit H, Goldberg S, Niemerko A, Trofimov A, Adams J, et al. Proton beams to replace photon beams in radical dose treatments. Acta Oncologica 2003;42:800–8.
16. Jagsi R, DeLaney TF, Donelan K, Tarbell NJ. Real time rationing of scarce resources: the Northwest proton Therapy experience. J Clin Oncology 2004;22:2246–50.
17. Malka V, Fritzler S, Lefebvre E, Aleonard M-M, Burgy F, et al. Electron acceleration by a Wake Field forced by an intense ultra short laser pulse. Science 2002;298:1596–600.
18. Fourkal E, Li JS, Ding M, Tajina T, Ma CM. Particle selection for laser accelerated proton therapy feasibility study. Med Phys 2003;30:1660.

The British Journal of Radiology, 78 (2005), 103–104 © 2005 The British Institute of Radiology
DOI: 10.1259/bjr/58764378

Commentary

Imaging investigation of liver haemodynamics in patients at risk for hepatic metastatic disease

C HARVEY, BSc, MRCP, FRCR and M BLOMLEY, MD, MRCP, FRCR

Imaging Sciences Department, Faculty of Medicine, Imperial College, Hammersmith Hospital, Du Cane Road, London W12 0NN, UK

Advances in imaging techniques have provided opportunities to explore tissue haemodynamics and study tissue microvasculature. The development of spiral CT in the 1990s facilitated single level tracking of a bolus injection of contrast medium by rapid sequential imaging of a volume of interest. Since attenuation values, measured in Hounsfield Units, are linearly related to changes in contrast agent concentration, measurement of physiological indices such as perfusion is possible. In the liver, the fact that simultaneous measurement from tissues and vessels is possible means the arterial and portal components of blood flow can be measured [1, 2]. This technique has been applied, with some success, to the study of liver haemodynamics in both diffuse liver disease [3] and in patients with colorectal carcinoma, in both overt and occult metastatic hepatic disease. In this issue Totman et al [4] have adapted the dynamic CT technique and measurements of hepatic perfusion to MR, in controls and in patients with metastatic colorectal carcinoma, with promising preliminary results.

Using currently available imaging techniques metastases of 1 cm or greater can be detected with a sensitivity of approximately 100% using superparamagnetic iron oxide (SPIO) enhanced MR, and a sensitivity of 90–95% using spiral CT [5]. The sensitivity of imaging modalities for the detection of lesions smaller than 1 cm is about 50% using surgery and intraoperative ultrasound as gold standard, although the "true" accuracy of these standards is unknown. However, it is these subcentimetre metastases that account for disease recurrence. Clinical interest in detecting these subcentimetre liver metastases has increased recently as there is a potential role for adjuvant chemotherapy (especially given the advent of newer regimens), angiogenesis inhibitors and segmental resection, which if delivered early may alter disease progression and prognosis. Therefore functional imaging techniques have been applied in an effort to solve this problem. Using radionuclide bolus tracking studies it was shown that patients with liver metastases had a raised arterial/portal ratio (hepatic perfusion index, HPI) [6] and in patients with apparently "clear" livers who developed liver metastases, a significant proportion had an abnormal HPI at presentation [7]. The development of perfusion CT techniques allowed the direct measurement of separate arterial and portal hepatic perfusion using methodology modified from dynamic scintigraphy [1, 2, 8, 9]. Subsequent studies have demonstrated dynamic CT can detect perfusion abnormalities generated by occult metastases [10, 11]. Leen et al [12] developed a Doppler ultrasound perfusion index that was more sensitive than conventional imaging techniques in detecting metastases and had a strong predictive value in identifying patients who were likely to relapse. However, these results have been difficult to reproduce. Using the ultrasound microbubble contrast agent Levovist, Blomley et al [13] studied liver hepatic venous arrival time using spectral Doppler following a bolus intravenous injection. Patients with metastases demonstrated a significantly earlier arrival time and time to peak intensity than controls presumably owing to the increased hepatic arterial component as well as arteriovenous shunting in metastatic liver disease. This technique has also been shown to be a useful predictive index indicating relapse probability [14]. In addition microbubbles improved the conspicuity of metastases significantly increasing the number and smallest detectable lesion compared with baseline grey scale ultrasound and in some cases CT [15, 16].

The application of the CT methology for the derivation of hepatic perfusion to MR to investigate liver haemodynamics in metastatic colorectal carcinoma is innovative. The significantly elevated HPI in the presence of overt metastatic disease reaffirms the findings of other functional imaging modalities. This MR based approach has the obvious advantages of the lack of ionizing radiation, use of a safe contrast agent as well as operator independence. Like CT it can readily be incorporated into a clinical protocol and parametric imaging performed. The acquisition of the entire liver volume is a novel feature allowing parametric imaging to be performed at multiple levels. This is not possible with spiral CT but could be achieved using multidetector CT technology. However, in MR the relationship between signal intensity and contrast concentration is non-linear unlike CT so the absolute tissue perfusion cannot be derived in ml min^{-1} ml^{-1} and only a hepatic perfusion ratio can be calculated. Flow effects may also make measurement of contrast agent concentrations in vessels problematic. Also the authors do not present any data regarding the reproducibility of this technique. Dynamic CT imaging is usually performed during a single breathold whereas the MR technique is acquired during gentle breathing. The effect of this on signal changes requires further investigation. Also the length of extra time incurred in acquisition of the functional and data analysis is comparable with CT methods. Of course these preliminary results in small numbers do not allow us to draw definite conclusions regarding the robustness of

Received 24 November 2004 and accepted 7 December 2004.

this technique and validation in large prospective studies is warranted to assess whether it can become a reliable prognostic index in the detecting micrometastases in colorectal carcinoma.

Acknowledgments

The authors would like to thank Professor Jo Hajnal of the Imaging Sciences Department, Clinical Sciences Centre, Imperial College, London for his advice and comments.

References

1. Blomley MJK, Coulden R, Dawson P, et al. Liver perfusion studied with ultrafast CT. JCAT 1995;19:424–33.
2. Miles KA, Hayball MP, Dixon AK. Functional images of hepatic perfusion obtained with dynamic CT. Radiology 1993;188:405–11.
3. Van Beers BE, Leconte I, Materne R, Smith AM, Jamart J, Horsmans Y. Hepatic perfusion parameters in chronic liver disease: dynamic CT measurements correlated with disease severity. AJR Am J Roentgenol 2001;176:667–73.
4. Totman JJ, O'Gorman RL, Kane PA, Karani JB. Comparison of the hepatic perfusion index measured with gadolinium-enhanced volumetric MRI in controls and in patients with colorectal cancer. Br J Radiol 2005;78:105–9.
5. Robinson PJ. Review article. Imaging liver metastases: current limitations and future prospects. Br J Radiol 2000;73:234–41.
6. Parkin A, Robinson PJ, Baxter P, Leveson SH, Wiggins PA, Giles GR. Liver perfusion scintigraphy- method, normal range, and laparotomy correlation in 100 patients. Nucl Med Commun 1983;4:395–402.
7. Warren HW, Gallagher H, Hemingway DM, Angerson WJ, Bessent RG, Wotherspoon H, et al. Prospective assessment of the hepatic perfusion index in patients with colorectal carcinoma. Br J Surg 1998;85:1708–12.
8. Leggett DA, Kelley BB, Bunce IH, Miles KA. Colorectal cancer: diagnostic potential of CT measurements of hepatic perfusion and implications for contrast enhancement protocols. Radiology 1997;205:716–20.
9. Harvey CJ, Blomley M, Deponte J, et al. Can dynamic CT predict the presence of hepatic micrometastases in colorectal cancer? Radiology 2001;221(P):575.
10. Cuenod CA, Leconte I, Siauve N, Resten A, Dromain C, et al. Early changes in liver perfusion caused by occult metastases in rats: Detection with quantitiative CT. Radiology 2001;218:556–61.
11. Kruskal JB, Thomas P, Kane PA, Goldberg SN. Hepatic perfusion changes in mice livers with developing colorectal cancer metastases. Radiology 2004;231:482–90.
12. Leen E, Angerson WJ, Wotherspoon H, Moule B, Cooke TG, McArdle CS. Comparison of laparotomy, CT, US and DPI in the detection of colorectal metastases. Radiology 1995;195:113–6.
13. Blomley MJK, Albrecht T, Cosgrove DO, et al. Liver vascular transit time analyzed with dynamic hepatic venography with bolus injections of an US contrast agent: early experience in 7 patients with metastases. Radiology 1998;209:862–6.
14. Harvey CJ, Blomley M, Lynch M, et al. Liver vascular transit time measured using the carotid delay time with bolus injections of the microbubble Levovist can predict the presence of occult metastases in colorectal cancer. Radiology 2001;221(P):269.
15. Albrecht T, Blomley MJK, Burns PN, Wilson S, Harvey CJ, et al. Improved detection of hepatic metastases with pulse inversion ultrasonography during the liver-specific phase of SHU 508A (Levovist)– a multicenter study. Radiology 2003;227:361–70.
16. Harvey CJ, Blomley MJK, Eckersley RJ, Cosgrove DO, Patel N, Heckemann RA, et al. Hepatic malignancies: improved detection with pulse inversion US in late phase of enhancement with SHU 508A. Radiology 2000;216:903–8.

The British Journal of Radiology, 78 (2005), 105–109
DOI: 10.1259/bjr/13525061

Comparison of the hepatic perfusion index measured with gadolinium-enhanced volumetric MRI in controls and in patients with colorectal cancer

[1]J J TOTMAN, DCR(R), MSc, [2,3]R L O'GORMAN, MSc, [1]P A KANE, MBBS, MRCP, FRCR and [1]J B KARANI, BSc, MBBS, FRCR

[1]*Departments of Radiology,* [2]*Neuroimaging and* [3]*Medical Engineering and Physics, King's College Hospital, Denmark Hill, London SE5 9RS, UK*

Abstract. The aim of the study was to adapt the methodology established for dynamic CT measurements of the hepatic perfusion index (HPI) to MRI, and to assess the potential role of MRI measurements of the HPI in detecting regional alterations in liver perfusion between patients with colorectal liver metastases and normal controls. The HPI was evaluated from serial T_1 volume acquisitions acquired over the course of a Gd-DTPA bolus injection. Time-course data from regions of interest in the liver, spleen and aorta were used to calculate the HPI; and HPI data from control subjects were compared with data from patients with known colorectal metastases. Significant differences were found between the relative portal perfusion and hepatic perfusion indices calculated for the patient and control groups ($p<0.005$). These results suggest that hepatic perfusion indices can be derived using MRI-based methods, and that these perfusion indices are sensitive to differences in liver perfusion associated with established metastatic liver disease on imaging. This technique may contribute to the early detection of liver metastases, allowing early surgical intervention and improved patient survival.

Colorectal cancer is the second most common cause of death from cancer in the UK. Currently 33 000 new cases are diagnosed each year and the incidence is increasing yearly by 1% in men [1]. For patients with colorectal malignancy, the presence of liver metastases is the most accurate predictor of survival. Following apparently curative surgical resection of the primary tumour, 50% of patients will die within 5 years, the majority from disseminated disease. Hepatic involvement is a feature in 50% of patients, and in almost one-third of cases the liver may be the only site of metastatic disease found at autopsy [2]. Improved survival following liver resection is now achievable with 5-year disease-free survival rates of 20–45% and up to 60% in unifocal disease [3]. Without surgery, the 5-year survival rate for these patients is effectively zero [4].

Detection of focal liver lesions pre-operatively is dependent on fundamental differences in the tissue characteristics of tumour and normal liver: first, an intrinsic difference in tissue density and cellular components; second, differences in vascularity and tissue haemodynamics. Current imaging techniques can reliably demonstrate metastases of 1 cm or larger using superparamagnetic iron oxide (SPIO)-enhanced MRI and multidetector CT. The sensitivity of imaging methods for detection of lesions smaller than 1 cm is in the region of 50% when surgery and intraoperative ultrasound are used as the gold standard, but the accuracy of this reference standard itself cannot be established [5]. Even if detected, the characterization of lesions of 1 cm or less may be suboptimal on pre-operative imaging. It is these undetected, subcentimetre lesions that typically account for early disease recurrence within the liver and failure of surgical cure [5]. It is now established practice in centres carrying out liver resection to use a focused, multimodality approach, using CT, MRI and PET in order to enhance detection of lesions, and intrahepatic and extrahepatic staging.

Received 24 March 2004 and in revised form 6 August 2004, accepted 20 September 2004.

One approach proposed to detect occult metastases is based on the alteration in liver blood flow that develops with metastatic seeding in the liver. The ratio of hepatic arterial to total liver blood flow (hepatic perfusion index, HPI), was first investigated using dynamic scintigraphy, and found to be abnormal in 94% of patients with colorectal liver metastases [6]. Furthermore, of those patients who developed liver metastases within 3 years of their original primary resection, 87% had an abnormal HPI at presentation [7]. The methodology developed for measurement of the HPI with scintigraphy was adapted for use with dynamic CT, with similar results [8, 9]. Doppler ultrasound has also been used to identify flow changes in the afferent vessels, giving rise to a Doppler perfusion index (DPI) [10]. All of the above work has been, by necessity, retrospective, but prospective animal studies by Cuenod et al [11] and Nott et al [12] have indicated a high degree of sensitivity to occult metastases for this technique. The aim of the present study was to adapt the methodology established for dynamic CT measurements of the HPI to MRI, and to assess the potential role of MRI measurements of the HPI in the detection of changes in liver perfusion between patients with colorectal liver metastases and controls.

Materials and methods

The patient group consisted of eight men and four women (mean age 65 years, range 44–78 years), with colorectal primary confirmed on biopsy or resection, and liver metastases evident on imaging. The control group consisted of eight men and six women (mean age 45 years, range 21–70 years), taken from patients referred for routine contrast-enhanced spine imaging, with no history of neoplastic disease. This study was performed with the approval of the local research ethics committee, and informed consent was obtained from all subjects prior to MRI. Imaging was performed with a Siemens 1T Harmony scanner (Siemens, Erlangen, Germany) using a modified volume-interpolated breath-hold examination sequence (VIBE) [13]. A total scan time of 1:15 min covers the necessary extent of the perfusion curves, with a maximum sampling rate of 3 s, which is within the constraints recommended by Henderson et al [14] for the accurate sampling of time course data. The sequence was acquired while the patient breathed gently in order to avoid blood flow variations introduced by changes in intra-abdominal pressure [15]. This can introduce periodic motion-induced signal changes, which although present can be readily identified as artefact. To allow for future parametric analysis, the entire volume of the liver was examined, resulting in 25 volumes of 36, 5 mm thick partitions. The spatial resolution achievable within the constraints imposed by the prescribed temporal resolution and liver size results in a matrix size of 128 × 67, covering a field of view of 400 mm × 300 mm. A repetition time of 2 ms, an echo time of 0.83 ms, and a bandwidth of 1150 Hz were employed to enable fast sampling. Typically a flip angle of 12° is used with the VIBE sequence as this produces maximum sensitivity to contrast enhancement. However, phantom studies investigating the VIBE signal dependence on flip angle and gadolinium concentration demonstrated that a flip angle of 12° yields maximum sensitivity to any variation in flip angle. Since higher flip

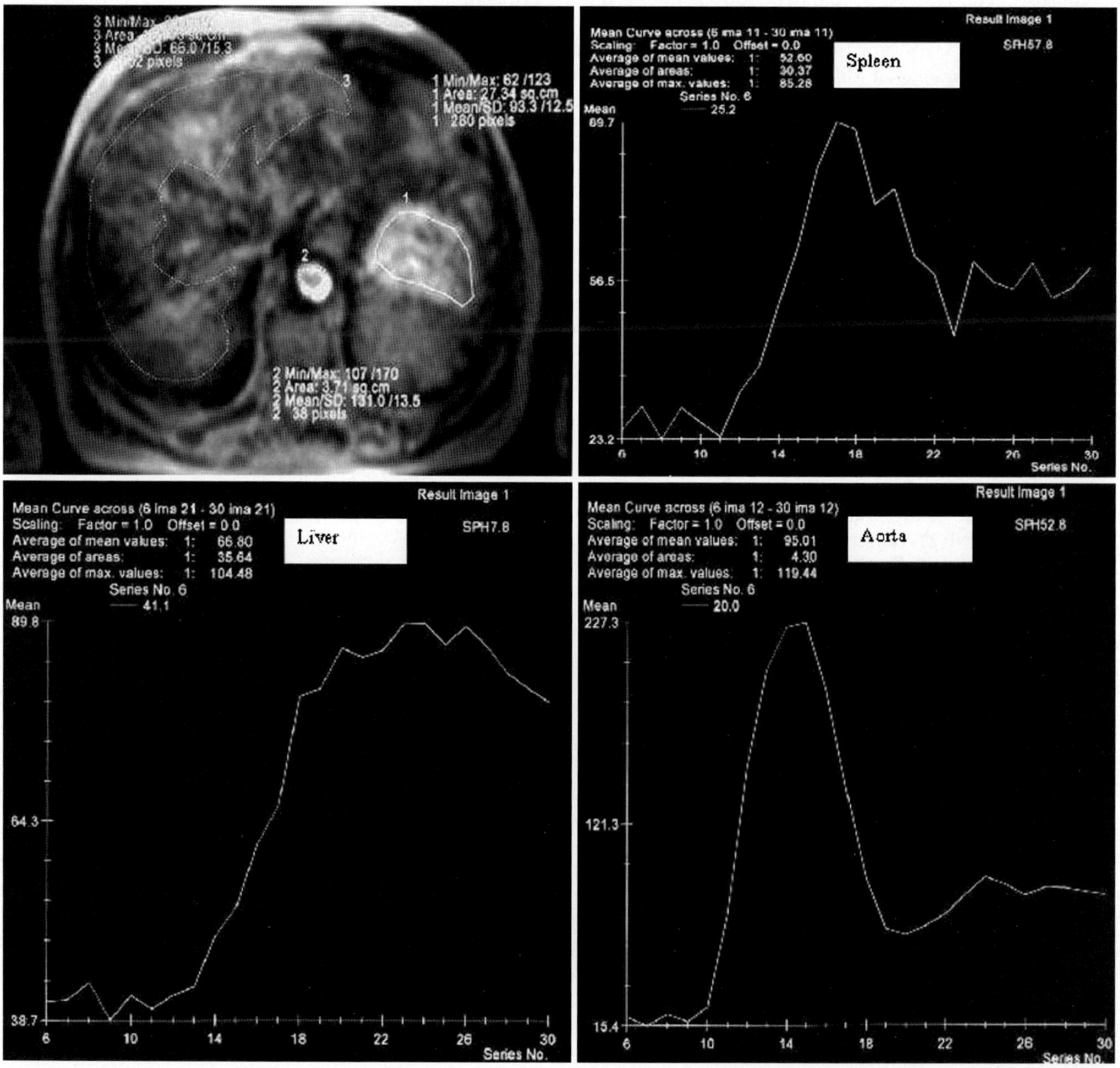

Figure 1. Axial section from one of the colorectal cancer patients showing extracted time-course data for regions of interest in the liver, spleen and aorta. The liver curve demonstrates significant early enhancement prior to the peak of the spleen curve, consistent with an increase in the hepatic component of perfusion and a corresponding decrease in the portal component.

angles demonstrated a much reduced sensitivity to changes in flip angle whilst retaining a linear relationship with contrast enhancement, a flip angle of 90° was selected in order to reduce the impact of B1 and B0 field variations.

The patients were cannulated with a 22-gauge venflon in an antecubital vein, which was flushed with saline and connected to a MRI-compatible injection kit (Medex, Annecy-Le-Vieux, France). The bolus injection of the manufacturer's recommended dose of 0.2 ml kg^{-1} Gd-DTPA (Magnavist, Schering Germany), typically 16 ml, was manually administered and timed to produce an injection rate of 4 ml s^{-1} at the start of the perfusion sequence; and followed immediately by a 20 ml saline flush, similarly timed. The injection duration was in the order of 4 s, plus an additional 5 s for a saline flush. Overall the total examination time was only slightly increased from the examination times associated with conventional contrast-enhanced imaging, since the necessary increase in preparation time is counterbalanced by the need to bring the patient out of the scanner for their contrast injection.

A single central slice was selected where both the liver and spleen were visible, and time intensity curves were derived from regions of interest (ROI) drawn manually by a single clinical specialist Radiographer, and then checked by an experienced Consultant Hepatobiliary Radiologist in the aorta, liver and spleen (Figure 1). The ROIs in the liver were drawn to encompass the parenchyma and metastases, if present, but no major vessels. The HPI was evaluated using a semi-automated program written locally in MATLAB (MathWorks Inc., Natick, MA), following the methodology established for CT by Blomley et al [8]. With this approach, the relative hepatic perfusion is calculated by dividing the maximal slope of the liver curve prior to the time of peak splenic attenuation by the maximal aortic enhancement. The relative portal perfusion is calculated based on the assumption that the liver and spleen receive a similar arterial bolus. Using this model, the hepatic arterial contribution is removed from the liver curve by subtracting a scaled version of the spleen curve (scaled by the ratio of hepatic/splenic perfusion), to yield a curve approximating to the portal contribution to the liver perfusion. The relative portal perfusion is then calculated as the peak up-slope of this curve divided by the peak rise in the splenic or portal vein signal, and the HPI is calculated as the ratio of the apparent hepatic arterial perfusion to the total liver perfusion [8]. In total the data processing requires approximately 15 min per patient, since at present the time-course data must be entered manually.

The statistical analysis was performed after importing the perfusion data into SPSS version 10.1 for Windows (SPSS Inc., Chicago, IL). Levene's test was used to assess the equality of variances between the patient and control groups, and differences in relative hepatic perfusion, relative portal perfusion, and HPI between the two groups were evaluated with an unpaired 2-tailed t-test.

Results

Significant differences were seen between the relative portal perfusion and hepatic perfusion indices calculated for the patient and control groups ($p<0.005$), with patients demonstrating reduced portal perfusion and increased HPI relative to controls. These results are in good agreement with data reported from previous CT and Doppler ultrasound studies [8–10, 16]. In addition, the patients demonstrated increased hepatic perfusion relative to the controls, although this trend did not reach significance ($p=0.063$). The distribution of calculated perfusion indices is shown in Figure 2, and the distribution of relative portal perfusion values is given in Figure 3. (Boxplots show median and interquartile ranges.)

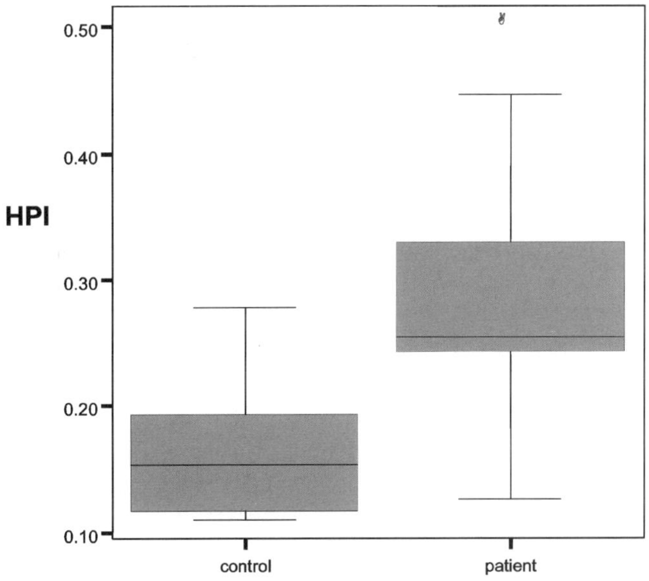

Figure 2. Median and interquartile ranges for the hepatic perfusion index (HPI) measured in patients with colorectal metastases and control subjects ($p<0.005$, unpaired t-test).

Discussion

Dynamic scintigraphy, CT and Doppler ultrasound have been used to develop equivalent marker indices, though all three techniques have recognized drawbacks. Both CT and

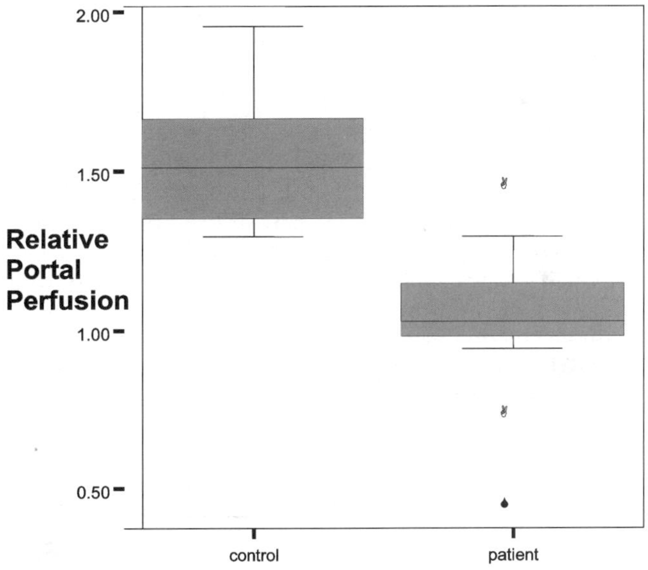

Figure 3. Median and interquartile ranges for the relative portal perfusion measured in patients with colorectal metastases and control subjects ($p<0.005$, unpaired t-test).

scintigraphy involve exposure to ionizing radiation and are "stand alone" procedures, which cannot be easily incorporated into routine diagnostic scanning. In CT, iodinated contrast administration has the attendant risk of anaphylaxis and to date, HPI has only been demonstrated on a single slice, although advances in CT may now allow improved coverage. Doppler ultrasound DPI data is obtained during an extended ultrasound examination, but is operator-dependent, with significant interobserver and intraobserver variability [17]. Furthermore, DPI does not provide any information regarding the anatomical distribution of occult lesions, and relies upon "normal" hepatic arterial anatomy, but only 70% of the population exhibit such anatomy [17].

An MRI-based approach has several perceived advantages over CT and the equivalent marker indices developed for scintigraphy and Doppler ultrasound, including the lack of ionizing radiation and operator dependence. Gadolinium DTPA is also considered an inherently safer contrast agent than those used in CT, and the gadolinium volume used is small, allowing a more compact bolus to be achieved, which aids data processing. The technique can be used with abnormal hepatic anatomy, and can assess the whole liver volume rather than a single slice. This MR-based technique also offers increased spatial and temporal resolution (particularly in comparison with ultrasound and radionuclide based methods), and can be performed in conjunction with high-resolution structural MRI, enabling a more extensive evaluation of tissue morphology and function to be performed.

The linear relationship between concentration of contrast and attenuation of signal in CT allows the perfusion values obtained from CT measurements by this method to be expressed in ml min^{-1} ml^{-1}. With MRI, the relationship between signal intensity and contrast concentration is non-linear and so this type of quantification is much more complex [18]. Nonetheless, as a ratio, the HPI can be calculated from MRI data, and in this preliminary study appears to represent a valid physiological indicator of abnormal perfusion, yielding results consistent with findings reported from previous dynamic CT, Doppler ultrasound and scintigraphy studies [8–10, 16]. However our preliminary observations have not determined the potential modulation of perfusion by other liver tumours, either benign or malignant, or the effects of pre-existing liver disease or chemotherapy.

Follow-up imaging studies will be required in order to assess the temporal consistency and intrasubject variability of the HPI measurements. However, this technique can potentially enable the early identification of patients with multiple areas of abnormal perfusion but no correlative anatomical lesions, likely to demonstrate early recurrence. Analysis of ROIs in various slices and positions throughout the entire liver volume demonstrate comparable results with those observed on the central slice, but fully automated parametric analysis of the HPI MRI data could offer further information regarding regional variations in perfusion throughout the liver. Intuitively, if these regional perfusion changes can be mapped onto the standard axial images, then the multiplanar visualization of these will allow segmental localization within the liver. These patients can then be managed more effectively with increased surveillance, in order to facilitate early detection on anatomical imaging and avoid porto-portal spread. This will need to be examined in a long-term follow-up study, with a large cohort of patients, following excision of their primary tumour. Conversely, a normal perfusion study would allow an extended interval of surveillance, and provide a further marker of continued remission in long-term follow-up. Such a pathway would be potentially more reproducible than ultrasound and avoid the cumulative radiation risk of CT. In addition, it would improve efficacy with resection, cryoablation and chemotherapy with small volume disease, and prevent further dissemination through the portal venous system.

Conclusions

Surgical resection of colorectal metastases may be curative in appropriately selected patients, but appropriate selection of these patients is dependent on accurate radiological detection and staging of these tumours preoperatively. We propose a MRI-based technique for measuring the HPI, and demonstrate that the perfusion indices measured using this technique can distinguish differences in the HPI and portal perfusion associated with metastatic seeding in the liver. This technique has the potential to provide a valuable method for early detection of "occult lesions", prompting early surgical or radiological intervention.

Acknowledgments

We express our deep gratitude to the MRI Radiographers at King's College Hospital, and Dr P E Summers PhD (Institute of Neuroradiology University Hospital, Zurich), and Dr Adam Waldman (Department of Radiology, Charing Cross Hospital, London, UK) for their valuable advice regarding this study.

References

1. www.cancerscreening.nhs.uk NHS Cancer Screening Programmes, The Manor House, 260 Ecclesall Road South, Sheffield S11 9PS.
2. Abrahams HL, Spiro R, Goldstein N. Metastases in carcinoma. Cancer 1950;3:74–85.
3. McArdle CS, Hole DJ. Outcome following surgery for colorectal cancer: an analysis by hospital after adjustment for case mix and deprivation. Br J Cancer 2002;86:331–5.
4. Stangl R, Altendorf-Hofman A, Charnley RM, Scheele J. Factors influencing the natural history of colorectal liver metastases. Lancet 1994;343:1405–10.
5. Ward J, Naik KS, Guthrie JA, Wilson D, Robinson PJ. Hepatic lesion detection: comparison of MR imaging after the administration of superparamagnetic iron oxide with dual-phase CT by using alternative-free response receiver operating characteristic analysis. Radiology 1999;210:459–66.
6. Breedis C, Young G. The blood supply of neoplasms in the liver. Am J Pathol 1954;30:969–85.
7. Cooke DA, Parkin A, Wiggins P, Robinson PJ, Giles GR. Hepatic perfusion index and the evolution of liver metastases. Nucl Med Commun 1987;8:970–4.
8. Blomley MJ, Coulden R, Dawson P, Kormano M, Donlan P, Bufkin C, et al. Liver perfusion studied with ultrafast CT. J Comput Assist Tomogr 1995;19:424–33.

9. Miles KA, Hayball MP, Dixon AK. Functional images of hepatic perfusion obtained with dynamic CT. Radiology 1993;188:405–11.
10. Leen E, Angerson WG, Cooke TG, McArdle CS. Prognostic power of Doppler perfusion index in colorectal cancer. Correlation with survival. Ann Surg 1996;223:199–203.
11. Cuenod CA, Leconte I, Siauve N, Resten A, Dromain C, Poulet B, et al. Early changes in liver perfusion caused by occult metastases in rats: detection with quantitative CT. Radiology 2001;218:556–61.
12. Nott DM, Grime SJ, Yates J, Day DW, Baxter JN, Jenkins SA, et al. Changes in the hepatic perfusion index during the development of experimental hepatic tumours. Br J Surg 1989;76:259–63.
13. Lee VS, Lavelle MT, Rofsky NM, Laub G, Thomasson DM, Krinsky GA, et al. Hepatic MR imaging with dynamic contrast enhanced isotropic volumetric breath hold examination: feasibility, reproducibility and technical quality. Radiology 2000;215:365–72.
14. Henderson E, Rutt BK, Lee TY. Temporal sampling requirements for the tracer kinetics modelling of breast disease. Magn Reson Imaging 1998;16:1057–73.
15. Sadek AG, Mohamed FB, Outwater EK, El-Essawy SS, Mitchel DG. Respiratory and postprandial changes in portal flow rate: assessment of phase contrast MR imaging. J Magn Reson Imaging 1996;1:90–3.
16. Shuman WP. Liver metastases from colorectal carcinoma: detection with Doppler US-guided measurements of liver blood flow – past, present, future. Radiology 1995;195:9–10.
17. Fowler RC, Harris KM, Swift SE, Ward M, Greenwood DC. Hepatic Doppler perfusion index: measurement in nine healthy volunteers. Radiology 1998;209:867–71.
18. Materne R, Smith AM, Peeters F, Dehoux JP, Keyeux A, Horsmans Y, et al. Assessment of hepatic perfusion parameters with dynamic MRI. Magn Reson Med 2002;47:135–42.

The British Journal of Radiology, 78 (2005), 110–115
DOI: 10.1259/bjr/51245688

The role of somatostatin receptor scintigraphy in patients with pituitary adenoma or post-surgical recurrent tumours

[1]M J ACOSTA-GÓMEZ, MD, [1]M A MUROS, MD, PhD, [1]J M LLAMAS-ELVIRA, MD, PhD, [1]A RAMíREZ, MD, PhD, [1]S ORTEGA, MD, [1]G SABATEL, MD, [1]C RAMOS, MD and [2]A DE LA RIVA-AGUILAR, MD, PhD

[1]*Department of Nuclear Medicine, Virgen de las Nieves Hospital, Avda. de las Fuerzas Armadas 2, 18014 Granada and* [2]*Department of Neurosurgery, University Hospital "Reina Sofía", Córdoba, Spain*

Abstract. To assess the role of scintigraphy with 111In-DTPA-D-Phe-octreotide (111In-octreotide) in the diagnosis of pituitary adenomas and in the evaluation of post-surgical recurrent or residual tumours, we performed scintigraphy with 111In-DTPA-D-Phe-octreotide (SRS) in 35 patients: 14 patients with confirmed pituitary tumours and 15 with confirmed recurrent tumours. Clinical, biochemical and histological analyses, conventional images (CT/MRI), and follow-up assessments during a period of 1 year to 4 years were recorded in all patients. In the present study, scintigraphy with 111In-octreotide showed positive uptake in 10 out of 14 patients with confirmed pituitary tumour and in 13 out of 15 patients with confirmed recurrent tumour, with an overall sensitivity of 79%. SRS showed better results in growth hormone (GH)- and prolactin (PRL)-secreting tumours (7/8 patients correctly identified) than in other adenomas (3/9). SRS detected recurrence of adenocorticotrophic hormone (ACTH)-secreting tumours (4/5 patients correctly identified) and non-secreting tumours (5/7 patients correctly identified). 111In-octreotide scintigraphy, in combination with other imaging modalities, is useful in the diagnosis and follow-up of pituitary tumours. It allows scar tissue to be differentiated from tumour recurrence after surgical treatment and ensures better selection of patients who will benefit from medical treatment with somatostatin analogues.

The *in vivo* visualization of somatostatin receptors is becoming more widely used to diagnose neuroendocrine tumours and to assess the therapeutic effects of somatostatin analogues in these patients [1]. Somatostatin receptors have been demonstrated *in vitro* in most cases of growth hormone (GH)-secreting adenomas and in some cases of thyroid stimulating hormone (TSH)-secreting adenomas and prolactinomas. Controversial results have been reported in other types of pituitary adenomas, such as non-secreting adenomas [2–5]. GH-secreting tumours express somatostatin receptor subtypes 2, 3 and 5, whereas non-secreting adenomas mainly express subtype 3 [6].

In the diagnostic work-up of patients with pituitary adenomas, CT and MRI play a principal role in defining the localization and tumour size, as in all brain tumours, but histological diagnosis can only be performed post-operatively. MRI is now the investigation of choice in diagnosis of pituitary adenomas. Micro-adenomas are defined as being smaller than 10 mm in size and usually present because of endocrine dysfunction (the most common is prolactinoma). 80–85% of micro-adenomas are visible on unenhanced T_1 weighted MR images and 33–50% are seen as areas of hyperintensity on T_2 weighted images, and enhancement with dynamic scanning is only necessary in a minority of cases. Macro-adenomas are more likely to be non-functioning and present because of mass effect on adjacent structures such as the optic chiasm. MRI signal characteristics do not necessarily assess the consistency of the tumour accurately but the superior and inferior extent of tumour is well demonstrated by MRI.

It is not easy to distinguish between recurrent/residual tumour and scar/necrotic tissue after surgery [7]. The scintigraphic visualization of hypophyseal tumours may be of value for predicting the response to somatostatin analogue treatment and for the post-surgical detection of small or residual tumours that are undetectable on MRI. Although some authors have reported that somatostatin receptor scintigraphy (SRS) did not permit visualization of post-surgical tumours that were not visible on MRI [8], other authors have described its utility to detect minimal post-surgical residual tumours [9].

The present study aimed to assess the utility of SRS in the diagnosis of pituitary adenomas and in the evaluation of post-surgical recurrent or residual tumours.

Patients and methods

Patients

We performed a prospective study of 35 patients referred to our Department of Nuclear Medicine for suspicion of pituitary tumour or suspicion of pituitary tumour recurrence over 5 years (1997–2001). 35 patients (23 females, 12 males) aged between 9 years and 77 years (mean age 43 years) were referred by the Departments of Neurosurgery, Endocrinology and Radiotherapy. All patients gave their informed consent to undergo the scintigraphy. The Ministry of Health approved the

Received 6 April 2004 and in revised form 23 August 2004, accepted 27 September 2004.

Address correspondence to Dr Maria Angustias Muros, Servicio de Medicina Nuclear, Hospital Virgen de las Nieves, Avda. Fuerzas Armadas, 2, 18014 Granada, Spain.

compassionate use of the radiopharmaceutical in all cases. 18 of the patients were referred for suspected tumour recurrence due to the persistence or post-surgical onset of clinical symptoms (n=9) or elevated levels of hormone markers (n=9). Tumour types in these patients included: adenocorticotrophic hormone (ACTH)-secreting (n=5), GH-secreting (n=3), prolactin (PRL)-secreting (n=2), follicle stimulating hormone (FSH)-secreting adenomas (n=1) and non-secreting adenomas (n=7). The remaining 17 patients were referred for suspicion of pituitary adenomas, presenting with PRL-secreting (n=4), GH-secreting (n=4), ACTH-secreting (n=3) adenomas, non-secreting adenomas (n=3), and thyroid stimulating hormone (TSH)- (n=1), FSH- (n=1), and leutinizing hormone (LH)- (n=1) secreting adenomas. None of 18 patients referred for suspected tumour recurrence were included in the primary tumours group.

Clinical data and biochemical determinations were recorded for all patients prior to the scintigraphic examination. The analytical findings included levels of GH, somatomedin C, insulin-like growth factor-1 (IGF1) growth factor, prolactin, TSH, ACTH, FSH, and LH, and the results of stimulation and inhibition tests of these hormones. CT or MRI and ophthalmological (visual field) studies were carried out in all cases. The mean follow-up period was 2.5 years (range 1–4 years).

A tailored therapeutic approach was developed for each patient, using somatostatin analogues, radiosurgery, medical treatment or surgery as appropriate. Five patients (three with pituitary adenomas and two with tumour recurrence) underwent surgery and the pathological report confirmed the presence of pituitary adenoma or tumour recurrence. The diagnosis was confirmed in the remainder by imaging tests (CT or MRI) in conjunction with analytical results and clinical findings.

[111In-DTPA-D-Phe]-octreotide scintigraphy

The scintigraphy was performed with 185–220 MBq (5–6 mCi) of 111In-chloride-DTPA-D-Phe-octreotide (Octreoscan) obtained from a simple Mallinckrodt kit (Mallinckrodt Ibérica S.A. Spain), which was intravenously administered to all patients. No post-administration adverse reactions or side effects were detected in any patient. Image acquisition was with single-head (Siemens Orbiter; Gammasonics, IL) and double-head (AXIS2; Picker International, Nuclear Medicine Division, Cleveland, OH) gamma cameras with medium energy collimator. Planar images were obtained 4 h, 24 h and 48 h post-injection in all patients, with at least 500 000 counts/acquired per image or 10 min image^{-1}. Tomographic images (SPECT) were obtained 4 h and 24 h post-injection, if using the double-head camera, through a 360° orbit, acquiring 60 steps at 40 s step^{-1}, using a 64×64 matrix. The image analysis was performed by two nuclear medicine specialists according to a qualitative evaluation system visually comparing the tracer uptake in the suspected tumour with that in the skull [10–12]. The grades were defined as follows:

- Grade 0: absence of tracer uptake, no visualization of tumour activity, considered negative;
- Grade I: slight tracer uptake, similar to that in skull;
- Grade II: moderate tracer uptake with good visualization of tumour; uptake slightly greater than that in skull;
- Grade III: intense tracer uptake; uptake clearly greater than that in skull.

MRI

MRI was performed using a 0.5-T scanner (GE Max Medical System, Milwaukee, WI). T_1 weighted gradient echo imaging (without contrast) was performed with a repetition time (TR) of 380 ms and echo time (TE) of 12 ms. T_2 weighted and proton density variable echo (VE) imaging was performed with a TR of 2600 ms, TE of 40–120 ms, and T_1 weighted spin-echo (SE) with a TR of 600 ms, and TE of 25 ms. Studies were also performed with paramagnetic contrast: T_1 weighted SE imaging, using sections of 3 mm thickness with 4 mm section interval. Images were obtained in the coronal and axial planes.

CT

CT scan was carried out before and after intravenous infusion of contrast medium using a third generation Siemens Somatom CR scanner. Section thickness was 4 mm.

Analytical studies: hormone determinations

The following hypophyseal hormones were determined in all patients: GH, ACTH, PRL, TSH, FSH, and LH. IGF1 growth factor was also measured. The determinations were made by radioimmunoanalytical techniques for FSH, LH and PRL (Diagnostic System Laboratories, Inc., TX), GH (IRMA, Immunotech, France), TSH (IRMA, Immunodiagnostic Systems Ltd., UK), and ACTH (Nichols Institute, CA, USA). Hormone inhibition and stimulation tests were carried out: inhibition test with dexamethasone for ACTH-secreting tumours and oral glucose overload test for GH-secreting tumours.

Follow-up

All patients were followed up every 6 months, provided no clinical situations occurred requiring more urgent assessment or admission. The follow-up consisted of: MRI examinations, which were always compared with previous images, hormonal analytical determinations, and clinical examinations.

Complete remission was defined as normalization of all clinical sings with normal tumour markers (including basal and dynamic responses of hypophyseal hormones) at 1 year after therapy with no evidence of residual tumour on CT or MRI. The patient was considered to have tumour recurrence if clinical, biochemical and/or neuroradiological signs of tumour activity were detected after therapy.

Results

Among the 17 patients referred for suspicion of pituitary tumour, SRS was positive in 10 patients (Table 1, Figure 1). The MRI was positive in all 10 patients. Two

Table 1. Data of patients with suspected pituitary adenoma

N°	Sex/age	Tumour type	SRS	MRI	Size (cm)	Treatment	Follow up
1	F/55	PRL-secreting	Positive-III	Positive	3.3	Somatostatin analogues	Size reduction, clinical improvement (TP)
2	M/52	PRL-secreting	Positive-III	Positive	6	Somatostatin analogues	Complete remission (TP)
3	F/14	PRL-secreting	Positive-II	Positive	2.5	Radiosurgery	Size reduction (TP)
4	M/64	PRL-secreting	Negative	Positive	1.6	Radiosurgery	Size reduction (FN)
5	F/67	GH-secreting	Positive-I	Positive	0.8	Somatostatin analogues	Size reduction (TP)
6	F/42	GH-secreting	Positive-II	Positive	1.2	Somatostatin analogues	Size reduction, clinical improvement (TP)
7	M/40	GH-secreting	Positive-I	Positive	0.3	Radiosurgery	Complete remission (TP)
8	F/44	GH-secreting	Positive-III	Positive	2.5	Surgery	Complete remission (TP)
9	M/57	Non-secreting	Positive-II	Positive	2.5	Surgery	Complete remission (TP)
10	F/67	Non-secreting	Negative	Positive	2.7	Medical	Clinical improvement (FN)
11	F/66	Non-secreting	Negative	Positive	2	None	Stable (FN)
12	F/65	ACTH-secreting	Negative	Positive	0.9	Surgery	Complete remission (FN)
13	F/76	ACTH-secreting	Negative	Negative	no mass	None	Without symptom, MRI (-) (TN)
14	F/42	ACTH-secreting	Negative	Negative	no mass	None	Without symptom, MRI (-) (TN)
15	F/14	FSH-secreting	Negative	Positive (FP)	1	None	Without symptom, MRI (-) (TN)
16	F/9	LH-secreting	Positive-II	Positive	0.2	Medical	Clinical improvement (TP)
17	M/68	TSH-secreting	Positive-III	Positive	2.5	Somatostatin analogues	Clinical improvement (TP)

SRS, somatostatin receptor scintigraphy; PRL, prolactin; GH, growth hormone; ACTH, adenocorticotrophic hormone; FSH, follicle stimulating hormone; LH, leutinizing hormone; TSH, thyroid stimulating hormone; TP, true positive; TN, true negative; FN, false negative; FN, false positive.

of these 10 patients underwent surgery and the pathological report confirmed the presence of pituitary adenoma; six patients were treated with somatostatin analogues, and the remaining two patients (with smaller tumour size) received radiosurgery or medical treatment. In follow-up studies, all 10 patients showed clinical, biochemical and/or radiographic improvements after therapy. According to their tracer uptake, eight patients were scored with Grades II or III and two patients with Grade I. Each patient with Grade I had GH-secreting adenoma less than 1 cm in size.

SRS was negative in seven patients. In three of these, the absence of the disease was confirmed by conventional imaging studies, biochemical findings, and clinical follow-up. The initial MRI examination was positive in one case (N° 15), but subsequent biochemical and clinical follow-up ruled out the presence of adenoma in this patient.

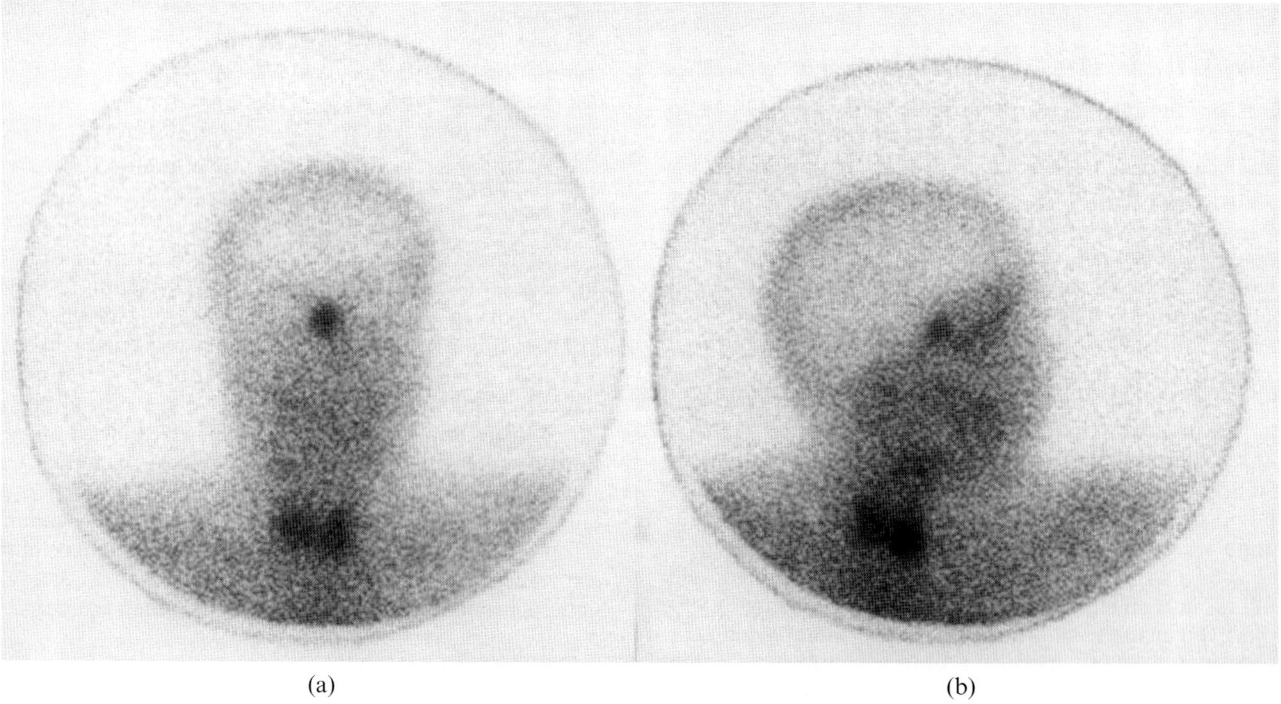

(a) (b)

Figure 1. (a) Anterior and (b) lateral images of 111In-chloride-DTPA-D-Phe-octreotide accumulation in the tumour site in a patient (N° 17) with thyroid stimulating hormone (TSH)-secreting adenoma. The images were taken in a Siemens single-head gamma camera 24 h after tracer administration.

Table 2. Data of patients with suspected recurrent pituitary adenoma

N°	Sex/age	Tumour type	SRS	MRI	Size (cm)	Treatment	Follow up
18	M/32	ACTH-secreting	Positive-III	Positive	small nodule	Somatostatin analogues/Surgery	Complete remission (TP)
19	F/51	ACTH-secreting	Positive-II	Negative	2.5	Radiosurgery and Radiotherapy	Complete remission (TP)
20	F/66	ACTH-secreting	Positive-I	Positive	2.5	Radiosurgery	Size reduction (TP)
21	F/37	ACTH-secreting	Positive-II	Positive	small nodule	Medical	Size reduction (TP)
22	F/34	ACTH-secreting	Negative	Positive	small nodule	Medical	Without symptom, MRI (-) (TN)
23	M/56	Non-secreting	Positive-II	Positive	scant remains	Somatostatin analogues	Clinical improvement (TP)
24	M/54	Non-secreting	Positive-II	Positive	3.8	Somatostatin analogues	Clinical improvement (TP)
25	M/36	Non-secreting	Positive-I	Negative	no mass	Medical	Clinical improvement, MRI (+) (TP)
26	M/66	Non-secreting	Negative	Negative	no mass	None	Without symptom, MRI (-) (TN)
27	M/56	Non-secreting	Positive-I	Positive	2.9	None	Stable (TP)
28	F/40	Non-secreting	Positive-I	Positive	2	Somatostatin analogues/Radiotherapy	Clinical improvement (TP)
29	F/46	Non-secreting	Negative	Positive	1.6	Radiosurgery	Clinical improvement (FN)
30	F/50	GH-secreting	Positive-II	Positive	2	Somatostatin analogue	Complete remission (TP)
31	F/45	GH-secreting	Negative	Negative	no mass	None	Without symptom, MRI (-) (TN)
32	F/33	GH-secreting	Negative	Positive	1	Radiotherapy	Clinical improvement (FN)
33	F/77	PRL-secreting	Positive-II	Positive	5	Surgery	Clinical improvement (TP)
34	M/47	PRL-secreting	Positive-I	Positive	2	Medical	Complete remission (TP)
35	F/32	FSH-secreting	Positive-III	Positive	4.6	Somatostatin analogues	Size reduction (TP)

ACTH, adenocorticotrophic hormone; GH, growth hormone; PRL, prolactin; FSH, follicle stimulating hormone; SRS, somatostatin receptor scintigraphy; TP, true positive; TN, true negative; FN, false negative; FN, false positive.

Scintigraphy failed to detect the presence of tumour in four patients: two with non-secreting adenomas, one with an ACTH-secreting adenoma of less than 1 cm, and one with a prolactinoma.

SRS showed better results in GH- and PRL-secreting tumours (7/8 patients correctly identified) than in other adenomas (3/9).

Among the 18 patients examined for recurrent/residual pituitary tumour, SRS was positive in 13 patients (Table 2). Of these, one (with largest tumour size) underwent repeat surgery, five (with highest uptake grades, II and III) were treated with somatostatin analogues, two with radiosurgery, three underwent medical treatment and one patient was treated with

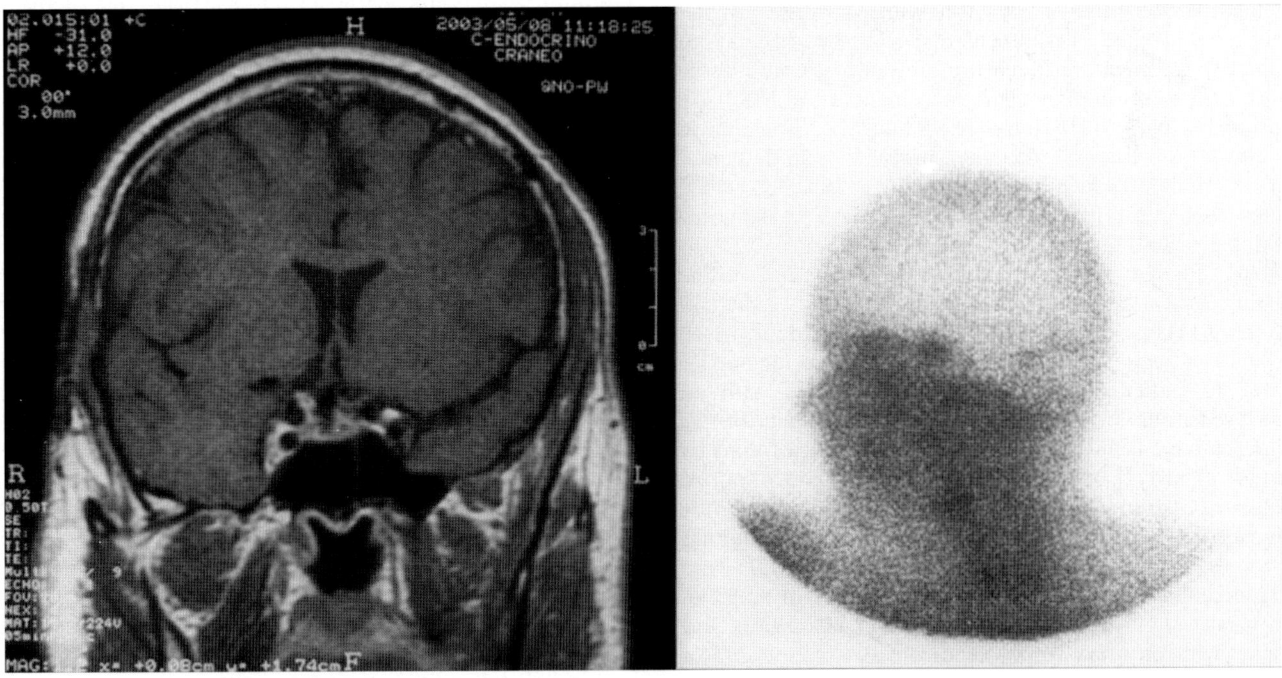

(a) (b)

Figure 2. (a) MRI in the patient N° 21. Represent a study in a coronal view showing a small recurrent tumour in contact with right optic nerve. (b) Lateral images of 111In-chloride-DTPA-D-Phe-octreotide accumulation in the recurrent tumour site in a patient (N° 21) with recurrent adenocorticotrophic hormone (ACTH)-secreting adenoma. The images were taken in a Siemens single-head gamma camera 24 h after tracer administration.

radiotherapy and somatostatin analogues. The remaining patient (N° 27) refused treatment. In all 13 patients, the recurrence was confirmed by clinical and biochemical data and MRI results. In two of the patients (N° 19 and 25) with positive SRS, the MRI gave a negative result (Figure 2), and the recurrence was demonstrated by clinical and biochemical results in follow-up. SRS was negative in five patients: the absence of recurrence was demonstrated by imaging tests and follow-up in three cases, whereas in the remaining two patients, recurrence was confirmed by imaging (MRI and CT) and the evaluation of post-treatment improvements. MRI was negative for recurrence in four patients. The absence of recurrence was confirmed in two of them (N° 26 and 31).

SRS correctly diagnosed 16 of the 18 patients with suspected recurrence, whereas MRI correctly diagnosed 14 of the 17 patients who had MRI (one patient refused MRI).

According to our results, SRS showed the best results in cases of recurrence of ACTH-secreting tumours (4/5 patients correctly identified) and non-secreting tumours (5/7 patients correctly identified).

In the present study, scintigraphy with 111In-octreotide showed uptake in 10 out of 14 patients with confirmed pituitary tumour and in 13 out of 15 patients with confirmed recurrence, with an overall sensitivity of 79%.

Discussion

The presence of high-affinity somatostatin receptors in most neuroendocrine tumour cells allows the *in vivo* scintigraphic visualization of neuroendocrine tumours after the intravenous administration of a radiolabelled somatostatin analogue. The diagnosis of suspected cases of pituitary tumour or pituitary tumour recurrence can be based on CT and MRI but the definitive diagnosis depends on histopathological study following surgery. When tumour recurrence is suspected, it can be difficult to distinguish between residual tumour and scarring associated with post-surgical changes using CT or MRI [7]. Scintigraphy with 111In-octreotide allows the visualization of pituitary tumours on the basis of fundamental characteristics of membrane receptors. Initially, these studies used 123I-Tyr3-octreotide to radiolabel somatostatin analogues [1, 13–15]. Subsequently, the use of 111In-DTPA-D-Phe-Octreotide became widespread and iodine labelling was abandoned. In the present study, scintigraphy with 111In-octreotide showed positive uptake in 10 out of 14 patients with confirmed pituitary tumour and 13 out of 15 patients with confirmed recurrence, with an overall sensitivity of 79%. Reports on the sensitivity of this technique have been variable, ranging from 37% found by Schmidt et al [12], who studied 24 patients and obtained positive uptake in only nine (9/24), to 88.5% described by Colao et al [16] in a study of 38 patients with pituitary adenomas. In our study, the best results were for GH- and PRL-secreting tumours (7/8), similar to the findings of Legovini et al [17] and Oppizzi et al [18]. Among our five patients with pituitary tumour that did not secrete GH or PRL, three showed tracer uptake (1 TSH-secreting adenoma, 1 LH-secreting adenoma and 1 non-secreting adenoma). Van Royen et al [19] showed uptake in five out of six patients with non-GH-secreting pituitary adenoma (2 non-functioning, 2 TSH-secreting, 1 prolactinoma and 1 Nelson's syndrome). In our study, two patients with suspicion of FSH- and LH-secreting tumours were correctly diagnosed using SRS. The utility of SRS was less for non-secreting adenomas in our study, with uptake in one out of the three patients who showed grade II uptake and underwent surgical treatment. Oppizzi et al [18] found uptake in 14 out of 22 patients and Schmidt et al [12] detected uptake in six out of 14 such patients. On the other hand, Duet et al [5] found uptake in five out of five patients with non-secreting adenoma. We studied one patient diagnosed with ACTH-secreting adenoma and detected no uptake, in keeping with several other studies. De Herder and coworkers detected no uptake in eight patients with ACTH-secreting adenoma and Stalla et al suggested that the elevated cortisol levels in patients with ACTH-secreting adenoma may inhibit the expression of somatostatin receptors [20–22].

Among the patients with confirmed tumour recurrence, SRS correctly detected 13 out of 15 patients. Plökinger et al [8] studied 10 patients after surgery for GH-secreting pituitary adenoma. Seven of them with tumours associated with persistent elevation of GH levels were not detected by scintigraphy. They concluded that SRS is not useful in detecting tumour recurrence in cases with a negative MRI result. In our study, tumour recurrence was diagnosed by SRS in 13 patients and two of them had a negative MRI. The diagnosis of recurrence was subsequently confirmed in all cases. Lauriero et al [9] showed uptake in eight of 10 patients (4 GH-secreting and 6 PRL-secreting adenomas) diagnosed with tumour recurrence. Both patients in our study with suspected recurrence of PRL-secreting tumour showed positive uptake. Out of seven patients in our study with recurrence of non-secreting adenoma, five had positive uptake of octretide, with no false positive cases.

In the present study, scintigraphy showed good results in patients with suspected recurrence of ACTH-secreting pituitary adenoma, with detection in four out of the five patients. Various authors have studied the presence of somatostatin receptors in pituitary adenomas and the inhibitory effects of somatostatin, including on ACTH-secreting adenomas, with very variable results [23]. Spada et al [24] studied the inhibitory effects of somatostatin *in vivo* in six patients with ACTH-secreting pituitary adenoma who underwent transesphenoidal surgery, and all showed positive results, implying that these tumours must have somatostatin receptors. In contrast, no uptake was shown by receptor scintigraphy in any of the 19 patients with Cushing's disease or eight patients with ACTH-secreting pituitary adenoma in a prospective *in vivo* study by De Herder et al, although uptake was present in eight out of 10 patients with ectopic secretion of ACTH [20]. This discrepancy may be due to the long-term exposure of patients with ACTH-secreting adenoma to excessive levels of circulating cortisol. This exposure could negatively influence the expression of somatostatin receptors [20], whose presence in these tumours has been confirmed by *in vitro* studies [6, 22, 24]. The present study demonstrates there may be a use for SRS in patients with suspected recurrence of ACTH-secreting pituitary adenoma, although the sample size was small.

Conclusions

SRS, in combination with other imaging modalities, is a useful tool in the diagnosis and follow-up of pituitary tumours. This method allows scar tissue to be differentiated from tumour recurrence after the surgical treatment of pituitary adenomas and showed good results in the detection of recurrence of ACTH-secreting adenoma, although a larger sample size is required to verify this finding. SRS identifies patients with presence of positive receptors for somatostatin, who can then be selected for medical treatment with analogues of somatostatin.

References

1. Lamberts SWJ, Krenning EP, Reubi JC. The role of somatostatin and its analogues in the diagnosis and treatment of tumors. Endocrinol Rev 1991;12:450–82.
2. Peillon F, LeDafniet M, Brandi AM. Receptor studies in endocrine diseases with special reference to pituitary tumors. In: Kovacs K, Asa SL, editors. Functional endocrine pathology. Boston: Blackwell, 1991:877–88.
3. Ikuyama S, Nawata H, Kato K, Karashima T, Ibayashi H, Nakagaki H. Specific somatostatin receptors on human pituitary adenoma cells membrane. J Clin Endocrinol Metab 1985;61:666.
4. Reubi JC, Heitz PU, Landolt AM. Visualization of somatostatin receptor and correlation with immunoreactive growth hormone and prolactin in human pituitary adenomas: evidence for different tumor subclasses. J Clin Endocrinol Metab 1987;65:65.
5. Duet M, Mundler O, Ajzenberg C, Berolatti B, Chendin P, Duranteau, et al. Somatostatin receptor imaging in non-functioning pituitary adenomas: value of an uptake index. Eur J Nucl Med 1994;21:647–50.
6. Greenman Y, Melmed S. Expression of three somatostatin receptor subtypes in pituitary adenomas: evidence for preferential SSTR5 expression in the mammosomatotroph lineage. J Clin Endocrinol Metab 1994;79:724–9.
7. Britton J, Evanson J. Primary tumours of the central nervous system. In: Husband JES, Reznek H, editors. Imaging in oncology. Oxford: Isis Medical Media Ltd, 1998:515–80.
8. Plöckinger U, Bäder M, Hopfenmüller W, Saeger W, Quabbe HJ. Results of somatostatin receptor scintigraphy do not predict pituitary tumor volume- and hormone-response to octreotide therapy and do not correlate with tumor histology. Eur J Endocrinol 1997;136:369–76.
9. Lauriero F, Pierangeli E, Rubini G, Resta M, D'Addabbo A. The role of 111-In-DTPA-octreotide SPET in the detection of minimal post-surgical residues. Nucl Med Commun 1998;19:1127–34.
10. Haldemann AR, Rösler H, Barth A, Waser B, Geiger L, Godoy N, et al. Somatostatin receptor scintigraphy in central nervous system tumors: role of blood-brain barrier permeability. J Nucl Med 1995;36:403–10.
11. Lee JD, Kim DI, Lee JT, Chang JW, Park CY. Indium-111-pentetreotide imaging in intra-axial brain tumors: comparison with Thalium-201 SPET and MRI. J Nucl Med 1995;36:537–41.
12. Schmidt M, Scheidhauer K, Luyken C, Voth E, Hildebrant G, Klung N, et al. Somatostatin receptor imaging in intracranial tumours. Eur J Nucl Med 1998;25:675–86.
13. Krenning EP, Bakker WH, Breeman WA, Koper JW, Kooij PP, Ausema L, et al. Localization of endocrine related tumors with radioionated analogue of somatostatin. Lancet 1989;I:242–5.
14. Flaglia G, Bazzoni N, Spada A, Arosio M, Ambrosi B, Spinelli F, et al. In vivo detection of somatostatin receptors in patients with functionless pituitary adenomas by means of a radioiodinated analog of somatostatin ([123I]SDZ 204-090). J Clin Endocrinol Metab 1991;73:850–6.
15. Ur E, Mather SJ, Bomanji J, Ellison D, Britton KE, Grossman AB, et al. Pituitary imaging using a labelled somatostatin analogue in acromegaly. Clin Endocrinol 1992;36:147–50.
16. Colao A, Lastoria S, Ferone D, Varrella P, Marzullo P, Pivonello R, et al. The pituitary uptake of 111In-DTPA-D-Phe1-octreotide in the normal pituitary and in pituitary adenomas. J Endocrinol Invest 1999;22:176–83.
17. Legovini P, De Menis E, Billeci D, Conti B, Zoli P, Conte N. 111Indium-pentetreotide pituitary scintigraphy and hormonal responses to octreotide in acromegalic patients. J Endocrinol Invest 1997;20:424–8.
18. Oppizzi G, Cozzi R, Dallabonzana D, Orlandi P, Benini Z, Petroncini M, et al. Scintigraphic imaging of pituitary adenomas: an in vivo evaluation of somatostatin receptors. J Endocrinol Invest 1998;21:512–9.
19. van Royen EA, Verhoeff NPLG, Meylaerts SAG, Miedema AR. Indium-111-DTPA-Octreotide uptake measured in normal and abnormal pituitary glands. J Nucl Med 1996;37:1449–51.
20. De Herder WW, Krenning EP, Malchof CD, Hofland LJ, Reubi JC, Kwekkeboom DJ, et al. Somatostatin receptor scintigraphy: its value in tumor localization in patients with Cushing's syndrome caused by ectopic corticotropin or corticotropin-releasing hormone secretion. Am J Med 1994;96:305–12.
21. Lamberts SW, de Herder WW, Krenning EP, Reubi JC. Editorial: a role of (labelled) somatostatin analogs in the differential diagnosis and treatment of Cushing's syndrome. J Clin Endocrinol Metab 1994;78:17–9.
22. Stalla GK, Brokmeier SJ, Renner U, Newton C, Buchfalder M, Stalla J, et al. Octreotide exerts different effects in vivo and in vitro in Cushing disease. Eur J Endocrinol 1994;130:125–31.
23. Moulik PK, Varma TRK, Vora JP, Vinjamuri S. The role of somatostin receptor scintigraphy in the management of pituitary tumours. Nucl Med Commun 2002;23:117–20.
24. Spada A, Reza-Elahi F, Lania A, Bassetti M, Atti E. Inhibition of basal and corticotropin-releasing hormone-stimulated adenylate cyclase activity and cytosolic Ca2+ levels by somatostatin in human corticotropin-secreting pituitary adenomas. J Clin Endocrinol Metab 1990;70:1262–8.

The British Journal of Radiology, 78 (2005), 116–121 © 2005 The British Institute of Radiology
DOI: 10.1259/bjr/66677575

Magnetic resonance coronary angiography with 3D TrueFISP: breath-hold versus respiratory gated imaging

[1]N M C SO, MBBS, FRCR, FHKCR, [1]W W M LAM, MBBS, FRCR, FHKCR, [3]D LI, MD, [2]A K Y CHAN, MBChB, [2]J E SANDERSON, MD, FRCP, FACC and [1]C METREWELI, FRCR, FRCP

[1]*Department of Diagnostic Radiology and Organ Imaging,* [2]*Department of Medicine and Therapeutics, The Chinese University of Hong Kong, Hong Kong, China and* [3]*Department of Radiology, Northwestern University, Chicago, Illinois, USA*

Abstract. To compare the diagnostic accuracy of coronary magnetic resonance angiography with three-dimensional (3D) trueFISP breath-hold and respiratory gated techniques for the detection of significant coronary artery stenosis. 15 patients who recently underwent elective coronary angiogram were studied and a total of 60 arteries and 48 arteries were assessed by breath-hold and respiratory gated 3D trueFISP techniques, respectively. The image quality, length of artery visualized and the presence or absence of significant coronary artery stenosis were recorded. 83.3% and 81.7% of the arteries obtained with the respiratory gated and the breath-hold techniques, respectively, had an image quality suitable for further analysis. There was no significant difference in the length of artery visualized. Sensitivity and specificity of 80%, 100% and 75% and 100%, respectively, were obtained with the breath-hold and respiratory gated techniques in detecting significant stenosis in the coronary arteries. Both techniques have moderate sensitivity and high specificity in detection of significant stenosis in the visualized segments of the major coronary arteries. However, they cannot replace conventional coronary angiogram for diagnosing coronary artery disease at present. Further studies are required to evaluate whether breath-hold approach is more efficient, therefore should be performed first and respiratory gated approach reserved for those who cannot breath-hold.

MR coronary angiography can be used to identify anomalous origin of the coronary arteries. It is potentially useful in screening, diagnosis and monitoring of the progress of coronary artery disease. Different methods and pulse sequences have been used to suppress the pericardial fat, enhance the coronary artery to myocardium signal-to-noise ratio (SNR) and contrast-to-noise ratio, as well as compensate for respiratory and cardiac motions [1]. Recently true-FISP (true fast imaging with steady state precession) technique has emerged as a new MR angiographic technique [2, 3]. We compared the use of breath-hold and respiratory gated true-FISP techniques in assessing coronary artery stenosis.

Methods and materials

Patients

15 patients with suspected coronary artery disease, who had a diagnostic coronary angiogram recently were included in the study. Patients were excluded if they had contraindications to MRI, claustrophobic, had non-sinus rhythm or had interventional procedures to the coronary arteries. There were 9 men and 6 women with mean age of 63.8 years (range 42–82 years). Informed written consent was obtained from all patients.

Received 5 January 2004 and in final form 26 August 2004, accepted 4 October 2004.

Address correspondence to Dr W W M Lam, Department of Diagnostic Radiology and Organ Imaging, Prince of Wales Hospital, Ngan Shing Street, Shatin. N.T., Hong Kong.

MRI

All subjects were imaged in the supine position, with a four-channel body array coil placed over the thorax, in a 1.5 T whole body MRI system (Sonata; Siemens Medical Solutions, Erlangen, Germany). Consecutive axial HASTE images (repetition time/echo time (TR/TE) 600/24; flip angle 160°; field of view (FOV) 340 mm; rectangular FOV varied according to patient's body habitus; matrix 256×108; acquisition time, 7 s; number of excitations 1; slice thickness 4 mm) were obtained from the aortic arch to the diaphragm. These images allowed the identification of the course of the major right and left coronary arteries. With the use of the three-point planscan tool on the scanner, a plane through the major axis of the proximal and middle segments of the right coronary artery was prescribed.

The position of the artery was confirmed by a double oblique scout using a three-dimensional (3D) breath-hold fat-suppressed, segmented true-FISP sequence (TR/TE 3.1/1.3; flip angle 60°; bandwidth per pixel 610 Hz; FOV 350 mm, rectangular FOV varied according to patient's body habitus; matrix 130×256; number of lines per cardiac cycle 35; slices reconstructed per volume after sinc interpolation 16; slice thickness after sinc interpolation 2 mm; voxel size 2.7 mm $\times$ 1.4 mm $\times$ 2 mm; acquisition time per breath-hold scan, ~16 s).

Double oblique 3D volumes were then acquired with a 3D fat-suppressed segmented True-FISP sequence. The breath-hold sequence was performed first, followed by the navigator triggering respiratory gated sequence, with the navigator column positioned in right hemidiaphragm. The parameters used were as follows: (a) breath-hold sequence (TR/TE 3.8/1.6; flip angle 60°; bandwidth per pixel 610 Hz;

FOV 350 mm, rectangular FOV varied according to patient's body habitus; matrix 161 × 512; number of lines per cardiac cycle 35–43; slices reconstructed per volume after sinc interpolation 12; slice thickness after sinc interpolation 1.8 mm; voxel size: 2.1 mm × 0.7 mm × 1.6 mm; acquisition time: 14–27 s; (b) respiratory gated sequence (TR/TE 3.8/1.62; flip angle 60°; bandwidth per pixel 610 Hz; FOV 350 mm, rectangular FOV varied according to patient's body habitus; matrix 163 × 512; number of lines per cardiac cycle 31–35; slices reconstructed per volume after sinc interpolation 12; slice thickness after sinc interpolation 1.3 mm; voxel size: 2.1 mm × 0.7 mm × 1.3 mm; acceptance window: ±3 mm; acquisition time: 53 s–11 min 33 s, imaging efficiency 23–75%.

Interpretation of MR coronary angiograms

Two assessors blinded to the clinical data and coronary arteriogram results reviewed the images and a result was reached by consensus.

The left main coronary artery (LM), right coronary artery (RCA), left anterior descending artery (LAD), and left circumflex artery (LCx) were assessed. The image quality of the scan were graded qualitatively on a three point scale: 1, non-interpretable (artery obscured by pericardial fat and myocardium); 2, good (artery can be distinguished from the pericardial fat and myocardium); 3, excellent (sharp margin of artery, good suppression of pericardial fat and myocardium). The reasons for the non-interpretable images were recorded. The length of each assessable artery was measured with the standard linear measurement tool on the scanner. Presence of signal void segment or marked narrowing of luminal diameter on the assessable arteries (proximal and mid for RCA and LAD, proximal and distal for LM and LCx) was regarded as positive for significant stenosis. The branch arteries were not evaluated.

Conventional coronary angiography

Conventional coronary angiograms were performed with multiple projections. The intervals between the conventional coronary angiograms and the MR examination were between 1 day and 14 days (mean 4 days). All patients had the MR examination after the conventional coronary angiogram. The cardiologist, who was blinded to the MRI results, interpreted the conventional coronary angiograms visually. The presence of significant disease was defined as >50% diameter narrowing of the lumen.

Statistics

The selective coronary angiogram of the patient served as the gold standard for determining the diagnostic value of the non-invasive coronary angiogram. Analysis was carried out on arteries that had an image quality score of >1. The assessable arteries were divided into groups according to their location. The length of each group of arteries was expressed as mean ± standard deviation (SD) cm. The mean lengths of each group of arteries obtained by each technique were compared by the Mann-Whitney's test. The image quality for the arteries obtained with each technique was compared by the Wilcoxon Signed Ranks test. Significance test were 2-tailed and a p-value of <0.05 was considered statistically significant.

The diagnostic accuracy of MR coronary angiography for detecting significant stenosis in a per artery basis was limited to the most distal segment of the coronary artery visualized on the MRA. The sensitivity, specificity, accuracy, positive predictive value, negative predictive value for the detection of significant stenosis were calculated. Statistical values for breath-hold and respiratory gated techniques in detecting stenosis were compared by McNemar's test.

Results

All patients underwent the MRA without any complication. A total of 60 arteries were imaged with breath-hold technique, 48 arteries were imaged with respiratory gated technique as some of the patients refused further investigation after one or two arteries had been imaged by respiratory gated technique. Eleven (18.3%) arteries imaged with the breath-hold technique and eight (16.7%) arteries imaged with the respiratory technique had an image quality score of 1 were excluded from further analysis. 25 arteries obtained with the breath-hold technique had an image quality score of 2 and 24 arteries had an image quality score of 3. 29 arteries obtained with the respiratory gated technique had an image quality score of 2 and 11 had an image quality score of 3 (Table 1). A significantly higher number of arteries obtained with the breath-hold technique had an image quality of ⩾2 (p=0.049). For the 10 arteries that had an image quality score of 1 using the breath-hold technique, 5 were due to motion artefacts, three were due to suboptimal image plane (one vessel was outside the image volume, another due to tortuousity, the third obscured by the right ventricle), two were affected by technical problems with poor SNR and artefacts. For the 8 arteries that had an image quality score of 1 on the respiratory gated technique, 7 had motion artefacts and one was obscured by the right ventricle.

The average length of artery visualized using the breath-hold technique were: left main 1.1 ± 0.3 cm (range

Table 1. Image quality score of coronary artery by breath-hold and respiratory gated technique MR angiography, score 1 refers non interpretable, score 2 refers to good image quality, score 3 refers to excellent image quality

Artery	Image quality score					
	Breath-hold			Respiratory gated		
	1	2	3	1	2	3
LM	1	7	7	1	6	5
LCx	3	7	6	2	8	3
LAD	2	6	7	2	8	1
RCA	5	5	4	3	7	2

LM, left main coronary artery; LCx, circumflex artery; LAD, left anterior descending artery; RCA, right coronary artery.

0.6–1.7 cm); left anterior descending 6.9 ± 1.9 cm (range 2.8–10.6 cm); left circumflex 4.0 ± 1.7 cm (range 1.9–6.9 cm); right coronary 8.8 ± 1.6 cm (range 4.5–10.1 cm).

The average length of artery visualized using the respiratory gated technique were: left main 1.2 ± 0.4 cm (range 0.7–1.8 cm); left anterior descending 6.7 ± 2.1 cm (range 3.7–11.5 cm); left circumflex 4.5 ± 2.1 cm (range 2.3–7.7 cm); right coronary 7.8 ± 2.5 cm (range 3.8–10.7 cm). There is no statistically significant difference between the length of the left main, left anterior descending, left circumflex and right coronary arteries visualized with the two techniques ($p>0.05$).

On the conventional coronary angiogram, 10 arteries showed significant stenosis: left circumflex arteries (four, 70–100%), left anterior descending arteries (three, 70–90%), and right coronary arteries (three, 70–80%).

Of the 49 arteries that were analysed using the breath-hold technique, there were 5 arteries with >50% stenosis on the conventional coronary angiogram. MRA correctly identified 4 of them. Of the 40 arteries that were analysed using the respiratory gated technique, there were 4 arteries with >50% stenosis on the conventional coronary angiogram. MRA correctly identified three of them (Table 2).

Compared with the conventional coronary angiogram, the sensitivity, specificity, accuracy, positive and negative predictive values for the detection of significant coronary artery stenosis for the segments of arteries that could be visualized were 80%, 100%, 98%, 100% and 98% for the breath-hold technique, 75%, 100%, 97%, 100% and 97% for the respiratory gated technique, respectively. There was no statistically significant difference in the detection of stenosis by both techniques compared with the conventional angiogram ($p=1$) (Figures 1 and 2). There was only one false negative case in both techniques. It was from the proximal left anterior descending artery of the same patient, who had a 90% stenosis on the conventional angiogram.

When all 60 arteries were considered the breath-hold technique had a sensitivity of 40% specificity of 100%, positive predictive value of 100% and negative predictive value of 89% in detection of significant coronary artery stenosis. The respiratory gated technique had a sensitivity of 30%, specificity of 100%, positive predictive value of 100% and negative predictive value of 88%.

Table 2. Comparison of MR angiography (MRA) and conventional coronary angiogram for the detection of significant coronary artery stenosis (a total of 49 arteries and 40 arteries were assessed breath-hold and respiratory gated technique, respectively)

	Conventional angiogram		Significant stenosis detected by MRA			
			Breath-hold		Respiratory gated	
	stenosis	no stenosis	stenosis	no stenosis	stenosis	no stenosis
LM	0	14	0	14	0	11
LAD	1	12	0	13	0	11
LCx	3	10	3	10	2	7
RCA	1	8	1	8	1	8
Total	49		49		40	

LM, left main coronary artery; LCx, circumflex artery; LAD, left anterior descending artery; RCA, right coronary artery.

Discussion

Both breath-hold and navigator-echo techniques have been used to reduce respiratory motion for coronary artery imaging using 3D TrueFISP. Each technique has its own advantages and limitations. A larger volume of data or higher resolution can be acquired with the respiratory gated technique. However, it requires a longer imaging time and is sensitive to irregular breathing patterns. Breath-hold imaging, on the other hand, could more completely eliminate respiratory motion with cooperative patients and can be repeated more easily because of the short imaging time. Nevertheless, the spatial coverage and resolution are limited by the short breath-hold time. A direct comparison of the two techniques for detecting significant coronary stenoses on patients has not been performed before.

The proximal and mid segments of the arteries could be consistently visualized with both approaches. This makes the trueFISP technique valuable in assessing the anatomy of the coronary arteries and useful in cases with suspected anomalous origin of the coronary arteries and/or surgical planning. Inadequate image quality was seen more often in the RCA than the other arteries and one reason for this could be that the right coronary artery moves faster in diastole [4]. Acquiring cine images of the mid segment of the artery at a plane perpendicular to the segment may help to define the period in diastole when the artery is relatively stationary.

Our study shows that there were fewer vessels with adequate image quality for analysis using the respiratory gated technique compared with the breath-hold technique. This is consistent with the 40–75% success rate found in other studies [5, 6] with respiratory gating. Most of the arteries with poor image quality using the respiratory gated approach were due to motion artefact. The breath-hold images were acquired before the free breathing images, and some patients might be tired after the first part of the exam, resulting in irregular breathing patterns. The latter may improve with additional coaching and practice prior to the examination. For those who failed both approaches, 2D imaging with contrast and adaptive vessel tracking [7] or recently developed real-time imaging techniques are potential alternatives [8]. However, real-time imaging has lower resolution with pixel size >2.5 mm [9–11]. As there are now several approaches available to image the coronary arteries, a patient tailored approach depending on the patient's unique physical ability and respiratory attributes may be a viable option [12]. As blood in the artery and the vein both show relatively high signal intensity in trueFISP images, it was not possible to differentiate between the two in one case. The application of contrast agent, either intravascular or extracellular, combined with first pass technique may help to resolve the problem [13, 14].

The limitations of the study include a small number of patients, low prevalence of stenosis (10%), inability to visualize the distal arterial segments and that no major branches were evaluated. Despite the small number of patients recruited in this study, this is the first study that

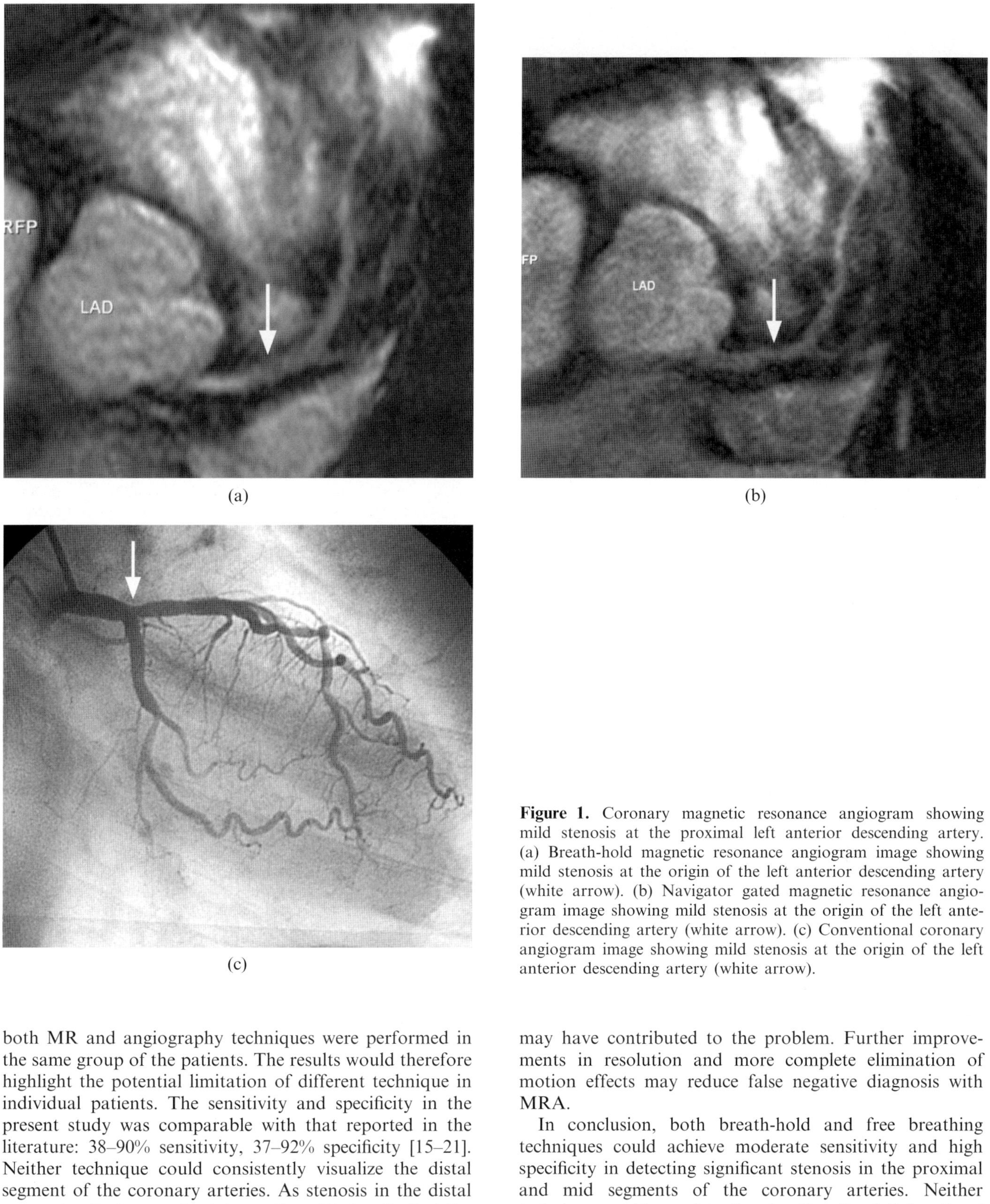

Figure 1. Coronary magnetic resonance angiogram showing mild stenosis at the proximal left anterior descending artery. (a) Breath-hold magnetic resonance angiogram image showing mild stenosis at the origin of the left anterior descending artery (white arrow). (b) Navigator gated magnetic resonance angiogram image showing mild stenosis at the origin of the left anterior descending artery (white arrow). (c) Conventional coronary angiogram image showing mild stenosis at the origin of the left anterior descending artery (white arrow).

both MR and angiography techniques were performed in the same group of the patients. The results would therefore highlight the potential limitation of different technique in individual patients. The sensitivity and specificity in the present study was comparable with that reported in the literature: 38–90% sensitivity, 37–92% specificity [15–21]. Neither technique could consistently visualize the distal segment of the coronary arteries. As stenosis in the distal segment will also require intervention, this has limited the clinical use of coronary MRA. Combining coronary MRA with MR perfusion imaging has been advocated for a more comprehensive assessment of coronary artery disease [22].

A focal 90% stenosis in the proximal LAD was missed in the MRA images. Image blur caused by residual motion and overlapping ventricular myocardium may have contributed to the problem. Further improvements in resolution and more complete elimination of motion effects may reduce false negative diagnosis with MRA.

In conclusion, both breath-hold and free breathing techniques could achieve moderate sensitivity and high specificity in detecting significant stenosis in the proximal and mid segments of the coronary arteries. Neither technique could consistently visualize the full length of all arteries and replace the conventional coronary angiogram for diagnosing coronary artery disease at present. In our small series, more images with adequate image quality could be obtained with the breath-hold than the free breathing technique. Further studies, preferably multicentre studies are required for further evaluation of the most effective and efficient approach.

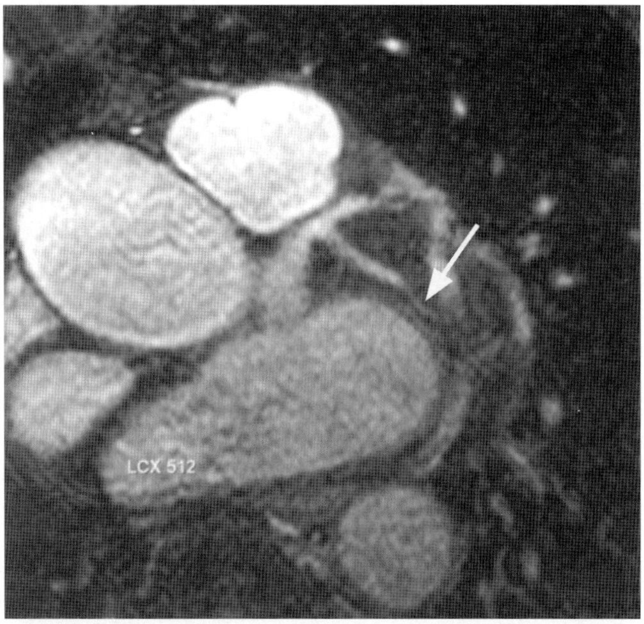

(a)

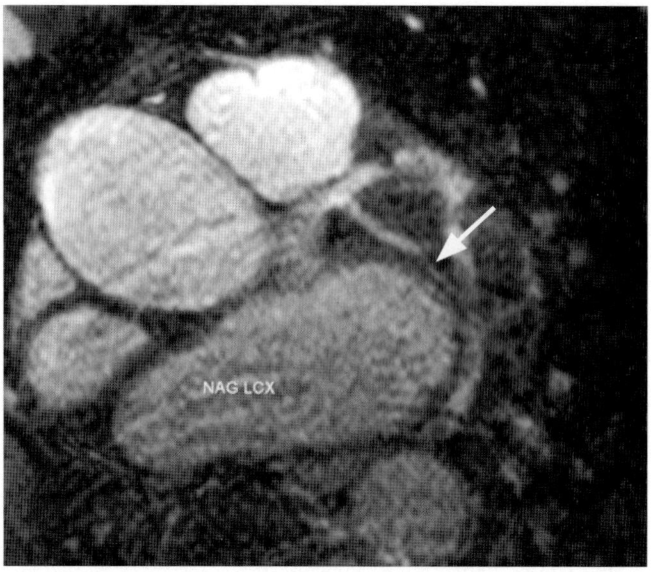

(b)

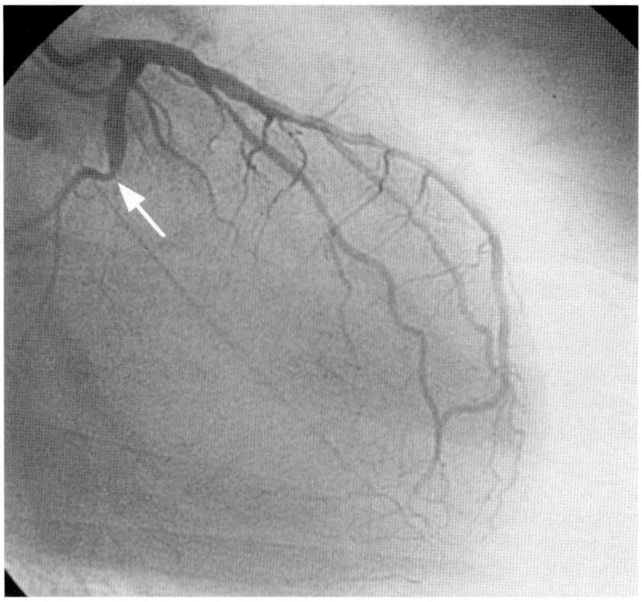

(c)

Figure 2. True positive case with > 50% luminal narrowing in the left circumflex artery. (a) Breath-hold magnetic resonance angiogram image showing significant stenosis at the proximal left circumflex artery (white arrow). (b) Navigator gated magnetic resonance angiogram image showing significant stenosis at the proximal left circumflex artery (white arrow). (c) Conventional coronary angiogram image showing >50% luminal narrowing at the proximal left circumflex artery (white arrow).

References

1. Li D, Deshpande V. Magnetic resonance imaging of coronary arteries. Top Magn Reson Imaging 2001;12:337–47.
2. Spuentrup E, Bornert P, Botnar RM, Groen JP, Manning WJ, Stuber M. Navigator-gated free-breathing three-dimensional balanced fast field echo (TrueFISP) coronary magnetic resonance angiography. Invest Radiol 2002;37:637–42.
3. Deshpande V, Shea SM, Laub G, Simonetti OP, Finn JP, Li D. 3D magnetization-prepared true-FISP: A new technique for imaging coronary arteries. Magn Reson Med 2001;46:494–502.
4. Hofman MB, Wickline SA, Lorenz CH. Quantification of in-plane motion of the coronary arteries during the cardiac cycle: implications for acquisition window duration for MR flow quantification. J Magn Res Imaging 1998;8:568–76.
5. Foo TKF, Ho VB, King KF, editors. Three-dimensional double-oblique coronary artery MR imaging using real-time respiratory navigator and linear phase shift: 1998. Proceedings of the 6th Annual Meeting, International Society for Magnetic Resonance in Medicine; 1998 April 18–24; Berkeley, CA. Sydney: International Society for Magnetic Resonance in Medicine, 1998.
6. Ikonen AE, Manninen HI, Vainio P, Hirvonen TP, Vanninen RL, Matsi PJ, et al. Repeated 3D coronary MR angiography with navigator echo gating. Technical quality and consistency of image interpretation. J Comput Assist Tomogr 2000;24:375–81.
7. Saranathan M, Ho VB, Hood MN, Foo TK, Hardy CJ. Adaptive vessel tracking: automated computation of vessel trajectories for improved efficiency in 2D coronary MR angiography. J Magn Res Imaging 2001;14:368–73.

8. Bogaert J, Kuzo R, Dymarkowski S, Beckers R, Piessens J, Rademakers FE. Coronary artery imaging with real-time navigator three-dimensional turbo-field-echo MR coronary angiography: initial experience. Radiology 2003;226:707–16.
9. Hardy CJ, Darrow RD, Pauly JM, Kerr AB, Dumoulin CL, Hu BS, et al. Interactive coronary MRI. Magn Reson Med 1998;40:105–11.
10. Hardy CJ, Darrow RD, Nieters EJ, Roemer PB, Watkins RD, Adams WJ, et al. Real-time acquisition display, and interactive graphic control of NMR cardiac profiles and images. Magn Reson Med 1993;29:667–73.
11. Kerr AB, Pauly JM, Hu BS, Li KC, Hardy CJ, Meyer CH, et al. Real-time interactive MRI on a conventional scanner. Magn Reson Med 1997;38:355–67.
12. Foo TKF, Saranathan M, Hardy CJ, Ho VB. Coronary artery magnetic resonance imaging. A patient-tailored approach. Top Magn Reson Imaging 2000;11:406–16.
13. Goldfrab JW, Edelman RR. Coronary arteries: breath-hold, gadolinium-enhanced, three-dimensional MR angioraphy. Radiology 1998;206:830–4.
14. Taylor AM, Panting JR, Keegan J, Gatehouse PD, Amin D, Jhooti P, et al. Safety and preliminary findings with the intravascular contrast agent NC100150 injection for MR coronary angiography. J Magn Reson Imaging 1999;9:220–7.
15. Manning WJ, Li W, Edelman RR. A preliminary report comparing magnetic resonance coronary angiography with conventional angiography. N Engl J Med 1993;328:828–32.
16. Duerinckx AJ, Urman MK. Two dimensional coronary MR angiography: analysis of initial clinical results. Radiology 1994;193:731–8.
17. Muller MF, Fleisch M, Kroeker R, Chatterjee T, Meier B, Vock R. Proximal coronary artery stenosis: three dimensional MRI with fat saturation and navigator echo. J Magn Res Imaging 1997;7:644–51.
18. Pennell DJ, Bogren HG, Keegan J, Firmin DN, Underwood SR. Assessment of coronary artery stenosis by magnetic resonance imaging. Heart 1996;75:127–33.
19. Post JC, van Rossum AC, Hofman MBM, Valk J, Visser CA. Three-dimensional, respiratory gated MR angiography of coronary anteries: comparison with conventional coronary angiography. AJR Am J Roentgenol 1996;166:1399–404.
20. Woodard PK, Li D, Haacke EM, Dhawale PJ, Kaushikkar S, Barzilai B, et al. Detection of coronary stenosis on source and projection images using three-dimensional MR angiography with retrospective respiratory gating: preliminary experience. AJR Am J Roentgenol 1998;170:883–8.
21. Kim WY, Danias PG, Stuber M, Flamm SC, Plein S, Nagel E, et al. Coronary magnetic resonance angiography for the detection of coronary stenoses. N Engl J Med 2001;345: 1863–9.
22. Plein S, Ridgway JP, Jones TR, Bloomer TN, Sivananthan MU. Coronary artery disease: assessment with a comprehensive MR imaging protocol – initial results. Radiology 2002;225:300–7.

The British Journal of Radiology, 78 (2005), 122–129
DOI: 10.1259/bjr/30866348

In vivo validation of a novel semi-automated method for border detection in intravascular ultrasound images

[1,3]C V BOURANTAS, MD, [2]M E PLISSITI, MSc, [2,3]D I FOTIADIS, PhD, [2]V C PROTOPAPPAS, MSc, [1,3]G V MPOZIOS, PhD, [1,3]C S KATSOURAS, MD, [2]I C KOURTIS, BSc, [4]M R REES, FRCP, FRCR and [1,3]L K MICHALIS, MD, MRCP

[1]Department of Cardiology, Medical School, [2]Unit of Medical Technology and Intelligent Information Systems, Department of Computer Science, University of Ioannina, [3]Michailideion Cardiology Center, GR 45110 Ioannina, Greece and [4]University Department of Clinical Radiology, Bristol Royal Infirmary, Bristol BS2 8HW, UK

Abstract. The aim of this work was to evaluate a new semi-automated intravascular ultrasound (IVUS) border detection method. The method was used to identify the lumen and the external elastic membrane or the borders of stents in 80 IVUS images, randomly selected from 10 consecutive human coronary arteries. These semi-automated results were compared with observations of two experts. Several indices in each case were obtained in order fully to evaluate the method. The time required for identification of the borders was also recorded. The interobserver variability of the method ranged from 1.21% to 5.61%, the correlation coefficient from 0.98 to 0.99, the slope was close to unity (0.94–1.03), the y intercept close to zero and the Williams index value was close to unity (range 0.67–0.91). The time (mean $\pm$ SD) required for the method to identify the borders of the different vessel layers for the whole IVUS sequence was 5.2 ± 0.2 min. The results demonstrate that the method is reliable and capable of identifying rapidly and accurately the different vessel layers depicted in IVUS images.

Intravascular ultrasound (IVUS) generates cross-sectional images of the coronary arteries with high temporal and spatial resolution. IVUS has been used for the evaluation of vessel wall morphology and dimensions [1–5] and has become an important method in many clinical and research applications [6–10].

IVUS cross-sectional images are generated by detecting the scattered waves of the ultrasound signal while this is passing through the vessel wall. A sequence of IVUS images is acquired during the withdrawal of an IVUS catheter through the artery. In each image, lumen, external elastic membrane, atheroma, calcium, stent and remodelling measurements can be performed [11].

The clinical applications of IVUS have been restricted because IVUS artefacts (*e.g.* non-uniform rotational distortion, guide wire shadow artefacts, ring-down effect and blood speckle artefacts) can reduce the ability to identify vessel wall layers and influence the accuracy of the obtained measurements. Manual border detection in IVUS images is laborious, time consuming and can be unreliable in the hands of an inexperienced operator [12]. To overcome these problems, automatic boundary detection methods have been reported. However these methods have not been able to resolve all issues related to reliability and speed [13–17]. In order to overcome some of the problems related to the usage of these previously reported automated methods we have developed a novel semi-automated method, which identifies accurately and quickly the different layers of the vessel wall [18].

The objective of this study was to evaluate this novel locally developed semi-automated method of IVUS border detection in a clinical setting.

Received 10 February 2004 and in revised form 26 June 2004, accepted 27 August 2004.

Materials and methods

Study group

The study group consisted of 10 consecutive patients (6 male, age range 52–72 years), who underwent IVUS examination for clinical purposes. The segments analysed were located in the left anterior descending artery (3), right coronary artery (5) and left circumflex coronary artery (2). Arterial segments with side branches were excluded for the purpose of this study, while segments with calcified plaques were included. In five out of the 10 coronary arteries assessed, stent implantation preceded the IVUS examination.

From each IVUS examination eight randomly selected IVUS images, spaced >1.5 mm apart from each other, were used for the validation of the method.

Intravascular ultrasound

The IVUS images were obtained using a 2.9 F, 30 MHz catheter (Avanar F/X, Endosonics, USA; catheter size 2.9 F, length 150 cm, maximum guide wire 0.014″, minimum guide catheter 5 F, tapered tip 0.022″). Sequential imaging was obtained with the IVUS catheter connected to a motorized pullback device operating at a speed of 0.5 mm s^{-1}. IVUS images were acquired at a standard rate of 10 frames s^{-1} and were digitized in a DICOM format. From each IVUS examination 60 s was digitized. The calibration markers, displayed on the digitized images, were used to derive the pixel size of 0.027 mm, which was used to calculate the cross-sectional areas and the perimeters of the different regions of interest.

Automated contour detection method

The lumen and external elastic membrane borders in each IVUS frame were extracted using the method described by Plissiti et al [18]. The method is based on the principles of deformable models, and as a consequence, an initial estimation of the borders is required. However, the user's interaction is limited to only the first frame of the IVUS sequence, where an initial estimation for the lumen and the external elastic membrane borders must be provided. The method processes all frames automatically in a sequence using the borders detected in the previous frame as the initial parameters.

For each frame, initially a 3×3 median filter is applied to reduce artefacts and blood speckle. A linear filter is used for image enhancement. The initial estimation of the desired border constitutes the deformable model, which deforms finally to detect the border. In our model, the searching space is limited using perpendicular line segments to the initial contours, at even intervals. Pre-defined points of the line segments are candidate points for the desired border. The deformation of the model is based on the minimization of its energy function. The points corresponding to a global minimum of the energy function constitute the detected border.

The position of each point of the deformable model is given by the cartesian coordinates (x_i, y_i). The energy function, E_{snake}, is given as the sum of two terms,

$$\begin{aligned} E_{\text{snake}} &= \sum_{i=1}^{N}\{E_{\text{int}}(x_i,y_i)+E_{\text{image}}(x_i,y_i)\} \\ &= \sum_{i=1}^{N}\{a\left[(x_i-x_{i-1})^2+(y_i-y_{i-1})^2\right] \\ &\quad + b\left[(x_{i-1}-2x_i+x_{i+1})^2+(y_{i-1}-2y_i+y_{i+1})^2\right]-\gamma g_i\} \end{aligned}$$

where E_{int} represents the internal energy of the model due to bending and E_{image} is derived from image data. Factors a, b and γ are weights that regulate the contribution of each term and g_i is the image gradient of the (x_i, y_i) point. The energy function is minimized using a Hopfield neural network, combined with a simulated annealing schema [18]. The nodes of the network correspond to image pixels.

The convergence of the network might result in points that do not accurately describe the desired boundary, due to the complexity of IVUS images. To detect smooth edges that separate large regions of pixels having similar intensity, the gradient of the image at a specific pixel, which is incorporated in the image energy, is calculated using the mean intensity value of four adjacent square areas (windows) of fixed size. In this way, pixels with a large image gradient corresponding to noise speckle, which may have attracted the contour towards their position and entailed an incorrect identification of the borders, are excluded. We found that small distortions in the shape of the final contour may cause abnormalities in the specification of the searching area for the next frame. For this reason, we look for smooth initial estimations for the external elastic membrane border. From this the convex hull of the extracted border points is calculated, using the plane sweep approach [18].

In the images where calcified plaques exist, our method is capable of overcoming this problem using knowledge from previous frames [18]. The image segmentation method is applied twice on the entire sequence of IVUS frames. The first application results in the detection of the media/adventitia border and the second in the detection of the lumen border. The first border imposes the limitations in the searching space of the second border.

Validation of the proposed method

This new method was validated with regard to its ability to detect the borders of the lumen, the external elastic membrane and the stent against a gold standard. In order to produce the gold standard, two expert observers performed detection of the borders of the above layers in each IVUS frame twice with a month's interval between the two examinations. The mean estimation of the four total estimations was regarded as the gold standard. The mean estimation was extracted using an interpolation method [19].

The reproducibility of manual tracing was assessed by computing the interobserver and intraobserver variability for the area and perimeter of the regions of interest (lumen, external elastic membrane and stent).

Several ways were used to evaluate the performance of the method:

(a) The values of the areas and perimeters estimated by the automated border detection and those that had been detected by the two experts were compared (interobserver variability), correlated (linear regression analysis [20]) and finally their differences were estimated and compared (Williams index [21]).
(b) The surfaces of the regions of interest (lumen, external elastic membrane and stent) estimated by the automated border detection method were superimposed with the ones estimated using the interpolation method and the fit between the two corresponding surfaces was estimated (non-overlapping area analysis [17], Williams index for non-overlapping areas and Williams index for Hausdorff and mean distance).
(c) The time needed in order for the proposed method to detect the borders of the different layers in each IVUS sequence was reported.

Statistical analysis

The interobserver variability of the two observers for the values of area and perimeter was assessed by computing the mean and the standard deviation (SD) of the differences between the two observers' estimations. The intraobserver variability of each observer for the values of area and perimeter was estimated by computing the mean and the SD of the differences between the first and second tracing of each observer. The interobserver variability of our method was computed by assessing the mean and SD of the differences between our method and the mean estimation of the two observers.

For the linear regression analysis purposes, correlation coefficients, slope and y interception were computed.

The Williams index (WI) was calculated according to the following equation:

$$\mathrm{WI}=\frac{\frac{1}{n}\sum_{j=1}^{n}\frac{1}{D_{0,j}}}{\frac{2}{n-1}\sum_{j}\sum_{j'\neq j}\frac{1}{D_{j,j'}}} \tag{1}$$

where n is the number of observers, $D_{j,j'}$ is the average difference between observers and $D_{0,j'}$ is the disagreement between our method and each observer. The Williams index confidence interval was estimated using a jack knife technique [21].

Williams index values close to unity imply that the difference between the results produced by an under evaluation method and the ones obtained by the observers is not larger than the difference between the observers. This suggests that the under evaluation method can be considered equally accurate with the expert observers. The non-overlapping area analysis in percentage was defined as the ratio of the non-overlapping areas (X regions in Figure 1) to the mean areas as they were extracted by the interpolation method. The intraobserver variability of each observer, the interobserver variability between the two observers and the interobserver variability of our method *vs* the expert observers were re-estimated using the non-overlapping area analysis.

The intraobserver variability (V_{intra}) was estimated by the equation [17]:

$$V_{\text{intra}} = \frac{1}{N} 100 \sum^{N} \frac{|A_1 - A_2|}{\frac{A_1 + A_2}{2}}, \quad (2)$$

where $A_1 - A_2$ represents the value of the non-overlapping areas, $\frac{A_1+A_2}{2}$ is the area value of the mean estimation of an expert observer, and N is the number of IVUS images.

The interobserver variability (V_{inter}) between the two observers was estimated by the equation:

$$V_{\text{inter}} = \frac{1}{N} 100 \sum^{N} \frac{|A - B|}{\frac{A + B}{2}}, \quad (3)$$

where $A = \frac{A_1+A_2}{2}$ and $B = \frac{B_1+B_2}{2}$. A, B are the values of the mean estimation obtained from the first and second observer, respectively, using the interpolation method,

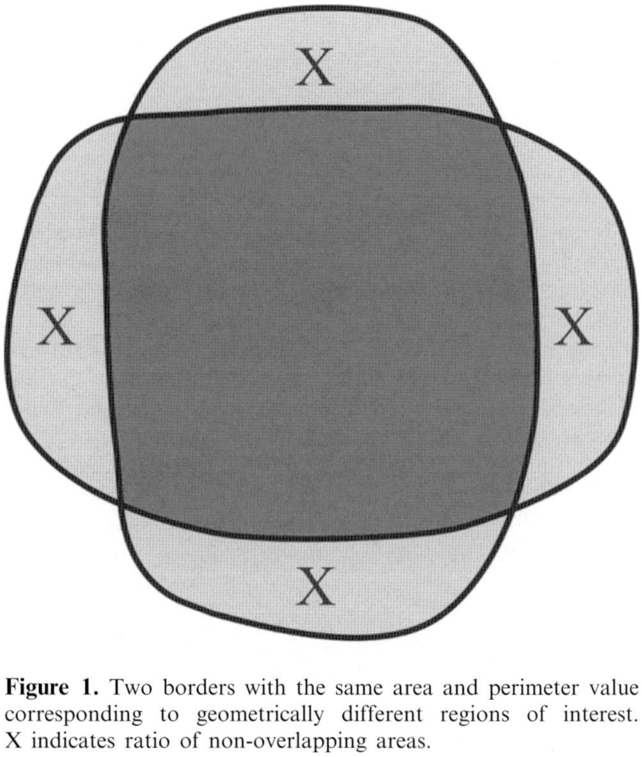

Figure 1. Two borders with the same area and perimeter value corresponding to geometrically different regions of interest. X indicates ratio of non-overlapping areas.

$A - B$ represents the value of the non-overlapping areas between the mean estimations, $\frac{A+B}{2}$ is the value of the mean estimation of the two observers and N is the number of IVUS images.

The interobserver variability ($V_{a\lg}$) of our method was estimated by the equation:

$$V_{a\lg} = \frac{1}{N} 100 \sum^{N} \frac{|C_{a\lg} - (\frac{A+B}{2})|}{\frac{A+B}{2}}$$

where $|C_{a\lg} - (\frac{A+B}{2})|$ represents the value of the non-overlapping areas between our method and the mean estimation of the two observers. The term $C_{a\lg}$ is the estimation of our method.

The Hausdorff and mean distances were estimated after the definition of corresponding points in the borders, which had been detected by the observers and the automated method. In order for the corresponding points to be defined an "object-based" method was used [19]. The Hausdorff distance was defined as the maximum distance between the corresponding points of two contours and the mean distance as the average distance between the corresponding points of two contours. A Hausdorff distance value close to the mean distance implies similarity of the two detected contours, whereas a high difference value between these two distances implies dissimilarity (Figure 2).

Results

80 randomly selected frames were used for the validation of our method. 40 of the examined images were obtained from stented coronary artery segments. In these segments the experts, while being able to trace the stent, were not able to detect the external elastic membrane borders in 22 of the segments. In total, the method was evaluated for its ability to detect the borders of: (a) the lumen in 80 frames; (b) the external elastic membrane in 58 frames; and (c) the stent in 40 frames.

The interobserver and intraobserver variability of the two experts for the lumen, external elastic membrane and stent border based on the values of area and perimeter are shown in Tables 1 and 2, respectively.

The interobserver variability between our method and the two experts for the lumen area, the external elastic membrane and the stent is shown in Figures 3–5, respectively. Moreover the interobserver variability between the proposed method and the two observers was $-1.03\% \pm 2.26$ for the lumen perimeter, $0.04\% \pm 1.47$ for the external elastic membrane perimeter and -1.05 ± 1.63 for the stent perimeter.

The linear regression analyses between our method and the two expert observers for the lumen area, the external elastic membrane area and the stent area are illustrated in Figures 6–8, respectively. Moreover, for lumen perimeter, external elastic membrane perimeter and the stent perimeter the linear regression analysis produced slopes of 1.03, 0.97 and 0.94, respectively, with y intercepts of -0.22 mm, 0.47 mm, and 0.43 mm. The correlation coefficients, between our method and the two observers, for the lumen perimeter, the external elastic membrane perimeter and the stent perimeter were 0.99, 0.99 and 0.98, respectively.

The Williams index for area and perimeter values is shown in Table 3.

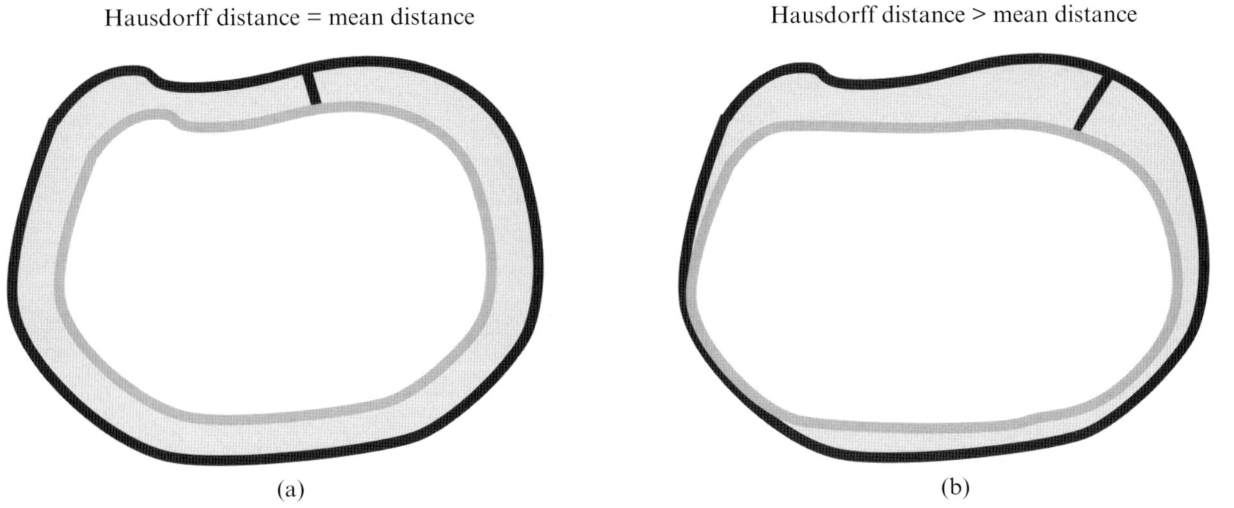

Figure 2. In figures (a) and (b) the non-overlapping areas are the same. The similarity in two border estimations is higher in figure (a) where the Hausdorff and the mean distance have the same value than in figure (b) where Hausdorff is larger than mean distance.

Table 1. Lumen, external elastic membrane and stent area variability. Results are presented as mean ± standard deviation

Variability	Lumen N=80	External elastic membrane N=58	Stent N=40
Intraobserver (1) variability (%)	1.92±4.77	0.34±2.65	0.16±3.57
Intraobserver (2) variability (%)	0.60±3.84	0.15±1.87	0.87±3.64
Interobserver variability (%)	0.97±4.38	0.85±2.07	1.10±2.94

The non-overlapping area analysis is outlined in Table 4. The interobserver variability between our method and the two observers for the non-overlapping areas for the lumen, external elastic membrane and stent is illustrated in Figures 9–11, respectively. The Williams index for non-overlapping areas is given in Table 5. Finally the Williams index for Hausdorff and mean distances are shown in Table 6. The computer time required for the extraction of the regions of interest in a sequence of 600 IVUS images was 5.2±0.2 min using a Pentium 4 computer with a 1.2 GHz processor and a 256 KB RAM memory.

Table 2. Lumen, external elastic membrane and stent perimeter variability. Results are presented as mean ± standard deviation

Variability	Lumen N=80	External elastic membrane N=58	Stent N=40
Intraobserver (1) variability (%)	0.89±2.74	0.37±1.67	0.2±2.36
Intraobserver (2) variability (%)	0.57±2.31	0.02±1.40	0.62±2.19
Interobserver variability (%)	0.54±2.57	0.47±0.71	0.51±1.52

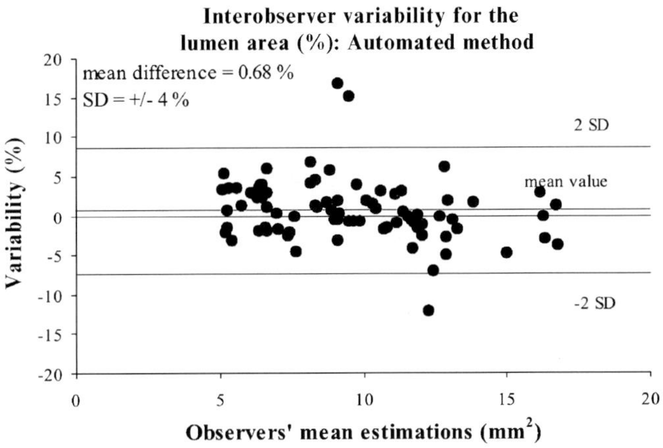

Figure 3. The interobserver variability between the contour detection method and the two observers for the lumen area. SD, standard deviation.

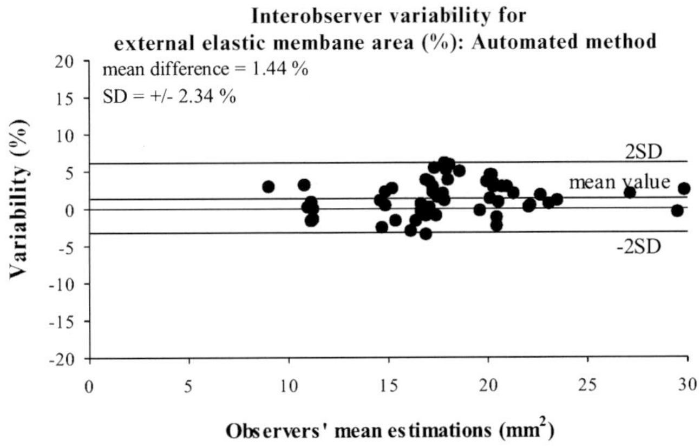

Figure 4. The interobserver variability between the contour detection method and the two observers for the external elastic membrane area. SD, standard deviation.

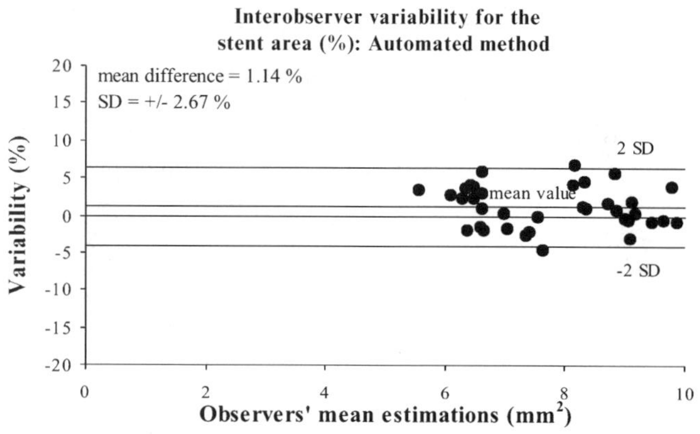

Figure 5. The interobserver variability between the contour detection method and the two observers for the stent area. SD, standard deviation.

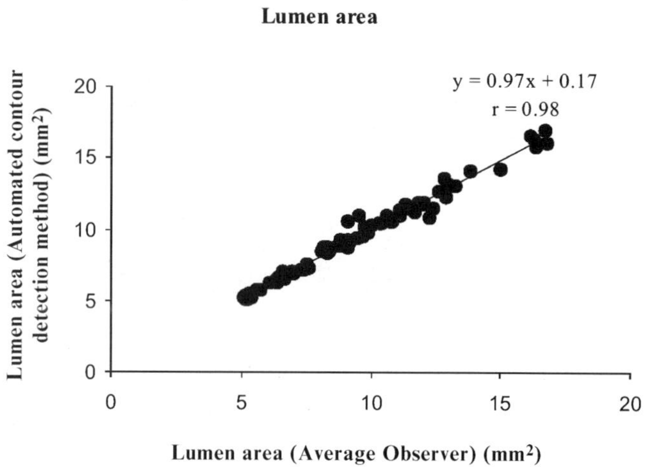

Figure 6. Linear regression analysis of the automatic lumen area *vs* manual tracing.

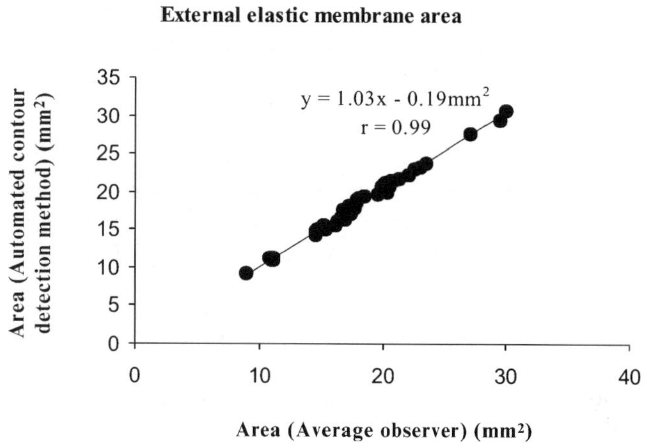

Figure 7. Linear regression analysis for the external elastic membrane area between the automatic and manual tracing.

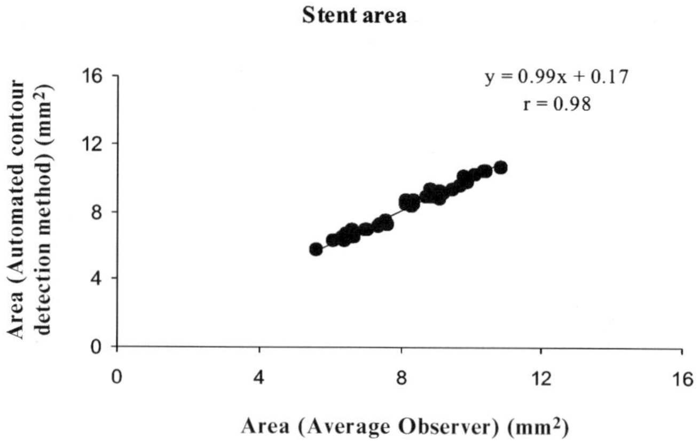

Figure 8. Linear regression analysis of the automatic stent area *vs* manual tracing.

Table 3. Williams index (WI) and 95% confidence intervals (CI) for areas and perimeters

	WI	CI (95%)
Lumen (area)	0.91	(0.89, 0.93)
Lumen (perimeter)	0.84	(0.82, 0.86)
External elastic membrane (area)	0.67	(0.64, 0.70)
External elastic membrane (perimeter)	0.81	(0.78, 0.84)
Stent (area)	0.82	(0.78, 0.86)
Stent (perimeter)	0.73	(0.69, 0.77)

Table 4. Interobserver and intraobserver variability for non-overlapping areas. Results are presented as mean $\pm$ standard deviation

Variability	Lumen N=80	External elastic membrane N=58	Stent N=40
Intraobserver (1) variability (%)	6.64 $\pm$ 3.88	3.88 $\pm$ 1.38	5.16 $\pm$ 2.16
Intraobserver (2) variability (%)	5.95 $\pm$ 2.47	3.62 $\pm$ 0.92	5.58 $\pm$ 2.12
Interobserver variability (%)	5.40 $\pm$ 2.86	3.29 $\pm$ 1.39	4.23 $\pm$ 1.36
Interobserver variability (automated method)	5.61 $\pm$ 2.79	3.75 $\pm$ 1.05	4.99 $\pm$ 1.39

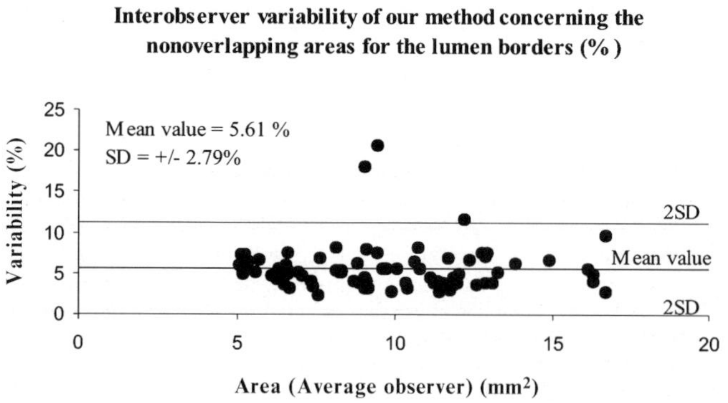

Figure 9. The interobserver variability between our method and the two observers concerning the non-overlapping areas for the lumen borders. SD, standard deviation.

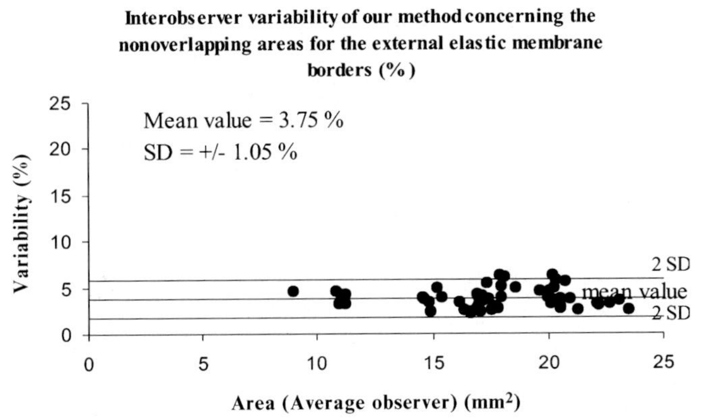

Figure 10. The interobserver variability between our method and the two observers concerning the non-overlapping areas for the external elastic membrane borders. SD, standard deviation.

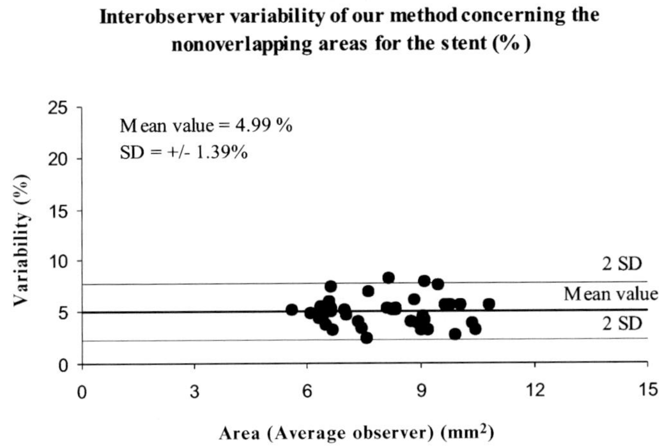

Figure 11. The interobserver variability between our method and the two observers concerning the non-overlapping areas for the stent borders. SD, standard deviation.

Table 5. Williams index (WI) and 95% confidence intervals (CI) for the non-overlapping areas

	WI	CI (95%)
Lumen	0.91	(0.90, 0.92)
External elastic membrane	0.79	(0.77, 0.81)
Stent	0.82	(0.81, 0.83)

Table 6. Williams index (WI) and 95% confidence interval (CI) for Hausdorff distance and mean distance

	WI	CI (95%)
Lumen (Hausdorff distance)	0.88	(0.87, 0.89)
External elastic membrane (Hausdorff distance)	0.88	(0.87, 0.89)
Stent (Hausdorff distance)	0.90	(0.88, 0.92)
Lumen (Mean distance)	0.90	(0.89, 0.91)
External elastic membrane (Mean distance)	0.89	(0.88, 0.90)
Stent (Mean distance)	0.82	(0.81, 0.83)

Discussion

IVUS depicts cross-sectional images of coronary arteries which provide accurate information of coronary artery morphology. Processing of such images by manual segmentation of IVUS has restricted its clinical applicability because manual processing is a tedious, difficult to reproduce and time-consuming procedure and requires considerable expertise. There has been considerable research effort to develop accurate automated methods for the detection of tissue and stent borders in IVUS images. These methods have several limitations due to the lack of homogeneity of tissue, and the high intensity variation that occurs in sampled regions of interest in IVUS images.

In an attempt to increase the clinical applicability of IVUS we have developed a novel semi-automated contour detection method. This method is based on the basic principles of deformable models and involves the incorporation of *a priori* knowledge, provided by an expert observer. The use of a Hopfield neural network makes the application of our method in individual frames fast and efficient. The method addresses common problems in IVUS segmentation such as the computation of the external elastic membrane in images where calcified lesions are present. In addition, our method overcomes the blood speckle artefacts and the guide wire shadow artefact, which have been previously described [18].

Several indices have been used for the validation of the fully automated method (*e.g.* automated method interobserver variability, Williams Index for area and perimeter, Hausdorff and mean distance to the detected borders). This has been achieved by applying direct comparison, linear regression analysis and non-overlapping area analysis. Our results indicate that the accuracy and the reliability of our method is high.

The reliability of the two observers is assessed using interobserver and intraobserver variability. Interobserver variability for area ranges from 0.85% to 1.1%, for perimeter from 0.47% to 0.54% and for non-overlapping areas from 3.29% to 5.4%. The above values confirm the accuracy and the reproducibility of the two observers and compare well with others reported in the literature [12]. The results demonstrate that the variability of the two observers is higher for the lumen borders. The difficulty in detecting the lumen border is probably caused by the speckle artefacts and by the irregularities of the lumen shape.

Linear regression analysis results indicate that the method is accurate. The slopes are close to unity, the y intercept always close to zero and the correlation coefficient is higher than 0.98 in all cases. The worst performance according to linear regression is obtained for the perimeter of the stent. This is due to the fact that the segmentation algorithm placed the stent borders at the pixels with the maximum image gradient and not at the stent struts as the observers did (Figure 12).

For non-overlapping areas, the Williams index ranges from 0.79 to 0.91. The obtained Williams index for the lumen is higher than the Williams index for the stent, although the interobserver variability (between the method and the mean manual estimation) exhibits a lower value for the stent. This discrepancy can be attributed to the low interobserver variability (between experts) for the stent, which decreases the value of the Williams index.

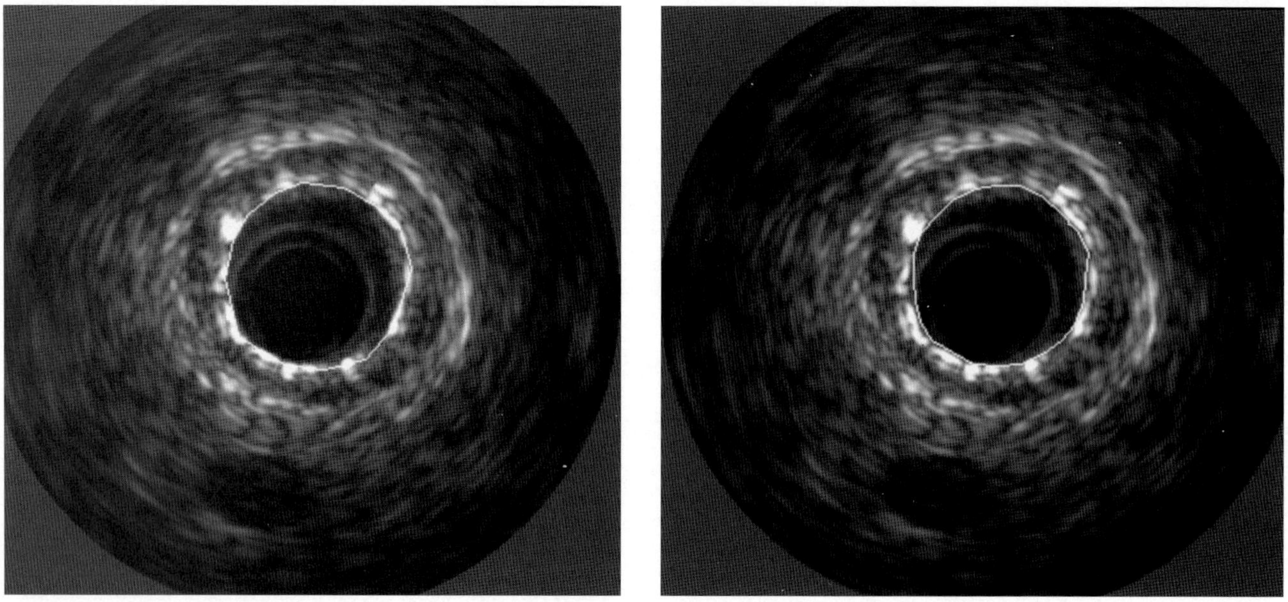

(a) (b)

Figure 12. Stent border detection in an intravascular ultrasound frame by (a) an expert observer and by (b) our automated segmentation method.

The influence of the interobserver variability (between the experts), according to the non-overlapping areas, on the Williams index can be also demonstrated in the external elastic membrane border. In this case the relatively low value of the Williams index (0.79) stems from the high agreement between the two observers and not from the poor performance of our method. The above remarks show that the interobserver variability must be taken into account, when discussing values of the Williams index.

Finally, the Williams indices for the Hausdorff distance and values for mean distance are close to unity (range from 0.88 to 0.90 and from 0.82 to 0.90, respectively). The above results demonstrate that the borders detected by our method have similar shape to those detected by the expert observers.

The task of identifying the regions of interest in IVUS images is a challenging one. Several algorithms have been developed in order to trace automatically the lumen and external elastic membrane borders and several methodologies have been used in order to assess their reliability [12, 14–17, 22–24]. Our method has certain advantages. By exploiting the similarity of sequential frames, user interaction is required only in the first frame of a sequence. The modification of the energy function of the deformable model makes the use of a Hopfield neural network feasible for the minimization of the energy function, which results in the reduction of the processing time for each frame. The introduction of a new expression for the image energy makes the method robust, resulting in accurate boundaries for all images. Our validation methodology is a systematic quantitative validation which employs additional quantitative metrics in addition to the metrics introduced by other researchers [12, 14–15, 17, 23–24]. These quantitative metrics describe further characteristics of the algorithm such as the shape similarity between the borders detected by our method and those detected by the expert observers.

However, our method has certain limitations. First, some tuning of the parameters must be carried out, in order to obtain acceptable values for the weight factors of our deformable model's energy function. In addition, the proposed method cannot accurately extract the region of interest in IVUS images where side branches exist. The energy function is re-instated without manual intervention in the following IVUS images, where no side branches exist.

In conclusion, this new semi-automated method for border detection in IVUS images is able to determine efficiently and quickly the lumen, external elastic membrane and stent borders, overcoming previously reported difficulties and thus extending the clinical applicability of IVUS imaging.

References

1. Nishimura RA, Edwards WD, Warnes CA, Reeder GS, Holmes DR, Tajik AJ, et al. Intravascular ultrasound imaging: in vitro validation and pathologic correlation. J Am Coll Cardiol 1990;16:145–54.
2. Potkin BN, Bartorelli AL, Gessert JM, Neville RF, Almagor Y, Roberts WC, et al. Coronary artery imaging with intravascular high-frequency ultrasound. Circulation 1990;81:1575–85.
3. Mallery JA, Tobis JM, Griffith J, Gessert J, McRay M, Moussabeck O, et al. Assessment of normal and atherosclerotic arterial wall thickness with an intravascular ultrasound imaging catheter. Am Heart J 1990;119:1392–400.
4. Nissen SE, Gurley JC, Grines CL, Booth DC, McClure R, Berk M, et al. Intravascular ultrasound assessment of lumen size and wall morphology in normal subjects and patients with coronary artery disease. Circulation 1991;84:1087–99.
5. De Feyter PJ, Serruys PW, Davies MJ, Richardson P, Lubsen J, Oliver MF. Quantitative coronary angiography to measure progression and regression of coronary atherosclerosis. Value, limitations, and implications for clinical trials. Circulation 1991;84:412–23.
6. Von Birgelen C, Airiian SG, Mintz GS, van der Giessen WJ, Foley DP, Roelandt JR, et al. Variations of remodeling in response to left main atherosclerosis assessed with intravascular ultrasound in vivo. Am J Cardiol 1997;80:1408–13.

7. Lansky AJ, Mintz GS, Popma JJ, Pichard AD, Kent KM, Satler LF, et al. Remodeling after directional coronary atherectomy (with and without adjunct percutaneous transluminal coronary angioplasty): a serial angiographic and intravascular ultrasound analysis from the optimal atherectomy restenosis study. J Am Coll Cardiol 1998;32:329–37.
8. Mehran R, Dangas G, Mintz GS, Lansky AJ, Pichard AD, Satler LF, et al. Atherosclerotic plaque burden and CK-MB enzyme elevation after coronary interventions: intravascular ultrasound study in 2256 patients. Circulation 2000;101:604–10.
9. Von Birgelen C, Mintz GS, Eggebrecht H, Herrmann J, Matthias J, Brinkoff J, et al. Preintervention arterial remodeling affects vessel stretch and plaque extrusion during coronary stent deployment as demonstrated by three dimensional intravascular ultrasound. Am J Cardiol 2003;92:130–5.
10. Nissen SE, Tsunoda T, Tuzcu EM, Schoenhagen P, Cooper CJ, Yasin M, et al. Effect of recombinant ApoA-I Milano on coronary atherosclerosis in patients with acute coronary syndromes: a randomized controlled trial. JAMA 2003;290:2292–300.
11. Mintz GS, Nissen SE, Anderson WD, Bailey SR, Elber R, Fitzgerald PJ, et al. American College of Cardiology clinical expert consensus document on standards for acquisition, measurement and reporting of intravascular ultrasound studies: a report of the American College of Cardiology task force on clinical expert consensus documents (committee to develop a clinical expert consensus on standards for acquisition, measurement and reporting of intravascular ultrasound studies [IVUS]). J Am Coll Cardiol 2001;37:1478–92.
12. Meier DS, Cothren RM, Vince DG, Cornhill JF. Automated morphometry of coronary arteries with digital image analysis of intravascular ultrasound. Am Heart J 1997;133:681–90.
13. Li W, von Birgelen C, Di Mario C, Boersma E, Gussenhoven E, var der Putten N, et al. Semi automatic contour detection for volumetric quantification of intracoronary ultrasound. In: Computers in Cardiology 1994. Los Alamitos, CA: IEEE Computer Society Press, 1994:277–280.
14. Mojsilovic A, Popovic M, Amodaj N, Babic R, Ostojic M. Automatic segmentation of intravascular ultrasound images: a texture-based approach. Ann Biomed Eng 1997;25:1059–71.
15. Zhang X, McKay C, Sonka M. Tissue catheterization in intravascular ultasound images. IEEE Trans Med Imaging 1998;17:889–99.
16. Shekhar R, Cothern RM, Vince DG, Chandra S, Thomas JD, Cornhill JF. Three-dimensional segmentation of luminal and adventitial borders in serial intravascular ultrasound images. Comput Med Imaging Graphics 1999;23:299–309.
17. Kovalski G, Beyear R, Shofti R, Azhari H. Three-dimensional automatic quantitative analysis of intravascular ultrasound images. Ultrasound Med Biol 2000;26:527–37.
18. Plissiti ME, Fotiadis DI, Michalis LK, Mpozios GM. An automated method for lumen and media/adventitia borders detection in a sequence of IVUS frames. IEEE Trans Inf Technol Biomed 2004;8:131–41.
19. Goshtasby A, Turner DA, Ackermann LV. Matching of tomographic slices for interpolation. IEEE Trans Med Imaging 1992;11:507–16.
20. Bland JM, Altman DG. Statistical methods for assessing agreement between two methods of clinical measurement. The Lancet 1986;1:307–10.
21. Chalana V, Kim Y. A methology for evaluation of boundary detection algorithm on medical images. IEEE Trans Med Imaging 1997;16:642–52.
22. Klingensmith JD, Sheknar R, Vince DG. Evaluation of three-dimensional segmentation algorithms for the identification of luminal and medial-adventitial borders in intravascular ultrasound images. IEEE Trans Med Imaging 2000;19:996–1011.
23. Von Birgelen C, Di Mario C, Li W, Schuurbiers CH, Slager CJ, de Feyter PJ, et al. Morphometric analysis in tree-dimensional intracoronary ultrasound: an in vitro and in vivo study performed with a novel system for the contour detection of lumen and plaque. Am Heart J 1996;132:516–27.
24. Koning G, Dijkstra J, Von Birgelen C, Tuinenburg JC, Brunette J, Tardif JC, et al. Advanced contour detection for three-dimensional intracoronary ultrasound: a validation in vitro and in vivo. Int J Cardiovasc Imag 2002;18:235–48.

The British Journal of Radiology, 78 (2005), 130–134 © 2005 The British Institute of Radiology
DOI: 10.1259/bjr/50195548

Dose implications of fluoroscopy-guided positioning (FGP) for lumbar spine examinations prior to acquiring plain film radiographs

M SAUNDERS, BMRS, A BUDDEN, BMRS, F MACIVER, BMRS, M TEUNIS, BMRS and H WARREN-FORWARD, BSc, PhD

Medical Radiation Science, University of Newcastle, Newcastle, NSW, Australia

Abstract. Fluoroscopy is increasingly being used as a positioning device prior to obtaining plain film radiographs. This is particularly true for those examinations where the type of projection and habitus of the patient present difficulties. An example is the examination of the lumbar spine; especially the L5/S1 projection. The purpose of this study was to determine the effect of fluoroscopy-guided positioning (FGP) on patient dose. The study assessed the difference in dose–area product (DAP) between conventional film–screen radiography (FSR) and a FGP assisted series of the lumbar spine. DAP values were monitored on 102 patients (50 FSR, 52 FGP) over 7 (4 FSR, 3 FGP) study sites. The median values for all FGP and FSR procedures were 8.3 Gy cm^2 and 12.5 Gy cm^2, respectively. The differences in doses were attributed to lower mAs and tighter collimation used in FGP assisted procedures. The study has demonstrated that it is possible to achieve lower DAP values using FGP. What now has to be asked is whether FGP should be acknowledged and further introduced into clinical practice. If so, there is a need for careful monitoring and reporting of dose so that strict protocols can be set in place to ensure the ALARA principle is enforced.

Advanced technology and demand for procedures that require fluoroscopy has allowed the introduction of screening units to be affiliated with conventional X-ray tubes within the general X-ray room. Observations at radiology sites have shown that fluoroscopy is being used to aid positioning of the patient, particularly in lumbar spine examinations, prior to conventional film–screen radiography (FSR).

Medical radiation, in the form of X-rays has long been recognized as a benefit to the community. The risk of biological effects following irradiation has also been well established. It is the professional and ethical responsibility of those administering ionizing radiation to the community, to follow the professional guidelines of justification, optimization and limitation set by the International Commission on Radiological Protection (ICRP) to reduce the risk of radiation induced effects [1].

In the past, large accumulated doses have been the result of repeated projections associated with positioning and patient habitus. It has been suggested that fluoroscopy-guided positioning (FGP), prior to plain radiographs, will reduce these repeat examinations, and reduce patient dose. Observation at radiology centres which use FGP techniques have given the subjective impression that exposure factors, and more importantly the time used in screening, do not produce lower patient doses.

Compared with other common X-ray examinations, *i.e.* extremities, chest or abdomen X-ray procedures, lumbar spine examinations result in comparatively larger radiation doses. Lumbar spine examinations contribute approximately 15% of the collective dose of all medical radiation exposure received by the community [2]. The lateral L5–S1 projection gives one of the highest radiation doses to the patient for a given single radiograph [3] and is frequently repeated due to positioning inaccuracies and variations in patient habitus, adding to patient dose. Martin et al conducted a study comparing the doses produced by medical imaging departments to the reference levels set by the National Radiological Protection Board (NRPB) [4]. They reported that thoracic and lumbar spine examinations were of most concern, with doses from 20–30% of units above the reference level. The projection of the L5–S1 joint space was particularly poor, with more than 50% of departments exceeding the reference level of 40 mGy. It is therefore important to reduce the dose from lumbar spine examinations.

The implications of reduced patient dose through the reduction of repeat rates formed the basis of this study. The amount of research previously done in the use of fluoroscopy to guide positioning of a patient for a plain film radiographic examination is very limited. This is probably due to the use of FGP being forbidden in a number of countries. A study in Belgium evaluated the justification of using an ultrashort fluoroscopic pulse to aid patient positioning [5]. It was noted that in difficult examinations, a short fluoroscopic pulse, to guide the radiographer in positioning before the exposure is made, could result in an overall reduction in dose to the patient.

The aim of this pilot study was to determine the effect of FGP techniques, prior to conventional FSR of the lumbar spine on patient dose in comparison with standard FSR techniques.

Methods

Following ethics clearance, a letter of invitation was sent to 35 radiology departments in the Sydney, Central Coast and Hunter regions of New South Wales. Included with

Received 19 August 2002 and in final form 5 July 2004, accepted 24 September 2004.

Address correspondence to Dr Helen Warren-Forward.

the initial letter was an information request form for the radiographic technique used. This requested information on the number and type of projections routinely taken and whether the department used screening for positioning.

Patient selection

Patient selection included all adult patients (>18 years) who required routine lumbar spine examination as specified by the departments. Patients requiring additional projections were excluded, as their resultant DAP could not be compared with the DAP from a routine series of projections. The study included three categories to determine a weight distribution of the patients. These were 50–60 kg, 61–80 kg and 81–90 kg.

Equipment and calibration

The measurement of radiation dose in fluoroscopy is more difficult than the measurement of the radiation dose for plain film examinations. Technique factors are under automatic control and the area being exposed changes continually during the examination. As such, the dosemeter of choice for both FSR and fluoroscopy examinations was the dose–area product (DAP) meter. The DAP meter was individually calibrated on each X-ray unit [6] and each tube underwent a full quality control (QC) assessment as recommended in the radiation guidelines published by the Environment Protection Authority, NSW, Australia [7].

Completion of patient data sheets

Each centre was given data sheets for recording patient age, body habitus, exposure factors for each projection and the total DAP values for the whole examination. The data sheets for FGP also recorded screening time. Instructions on how to fill in data sheets were positioned near the electrometer for ease of use for the radiographer. Repeat views for the examinations were also recorded.

Results

Four sites replied indicating that FGP techniques were used for lumbar spine examinations. It was known that a number of other sites routinely used FGP practice, but failed to indicate its use. The reason for this is that the practice is unacceptable to some members of the radiography profession. Only three of these sites were selected; the fourth centre used the technique too infrequently. There were 11 replies from centres using conventional FSR. Of these sites, four sites were selected. The selected centres consisted of a country private practice, an outer suburb private practice, an inner suburb private practice and a public hospital. These centres were selected to offer a range different clinical sites and potential techniques.

Results for 106 patients undergoing lumbar spine examination were examined. Four patients were excluded from analysis: three due to incomplete datasets and one for being too young. In total, analysis was performed on 50 patients examined with FSR (represented by sites A–D) and 52 patients were examined using FGP (represented by sites E–G).

Table 1. The table shows summary dose–area product (DAP) values and coefficient of variation (CV%) for the whole examination by each study site. Summary values have been given for all conventional film–screen techniques (FSR) and fluoroscopy-guided positioning techniques (FGP)

Study site	*N*	DAP (Gy cm^2)				Range	CV (%)
		Min	Mean	Median	Max		
A	11	5.9	20.7	12.0	66.2	11.3	9
B	10	5.5	14.1	14.8	29.1	5.3	54
C	11	8.3	16.7	12.5	42.8	5.2	61
D	18	5.4	13.9	11.8	34.7	6.5	58
E	13	5.8	9.0	8.3	13.5	2.3	30
F	19	3.6	12.5	12.3	32.1	9.1	54
G	20	2.2	8.2	6.2	21.8	10	69
FSR (A–D)	50	5.4	16.2	12.5	66.2	12.3	72
FGP (E–G)	52	2.2	9.9	8.3	32.1	14.8	58

N, Number of patients; CV, coefficient of variation.

Patient doses

Summary DAP values for each study site are given in Table 1. The DAP values received by patients ranged from 2.2 Gy cm^2, recorded by an FGP site, to 66.2 Gy cm^2, which was recorded by an FSR site. Thus the patient with the highest DAP value received 30 times more radiation than the patient who received the lowest DAP value.

The aim of the study was to investigate the differences in dose between patients investigated with FSR and FGP procedures. Plotting a frequency distribution of all DAP values received by patients for both FSR and FGP techniques resulted in a positively skewed distribution, as expected (Figure 1). The distribution shows the majority of FGP examinations were conducted with lower DAP values (solid line). The median DAP value for FSR (12.5 Gy cm^2) was higher than the FGP (8.3 Gy cm^2) value. A graphical distribution of median DAP value per site (Figure 2) shows values ranging from 6.2 Gy cm^2 to 14.8 Gy cm^2.

Patient parameter

Differences in DAP can be attributed to differences in patient habitus. It is important to ensure the same types of

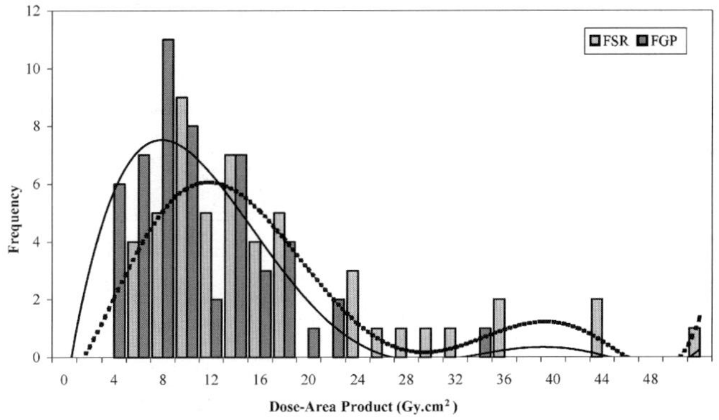

Figure 1. Double histogram of dose–area product (DAP) values for conventional film–screen radiography (FSR) and fluoroscopy guided positioning (FGP). The best line of fit shows that the peak for FGP (solid line) is higher and to the left (lower dose) of the peak of the FSR (dotted line).

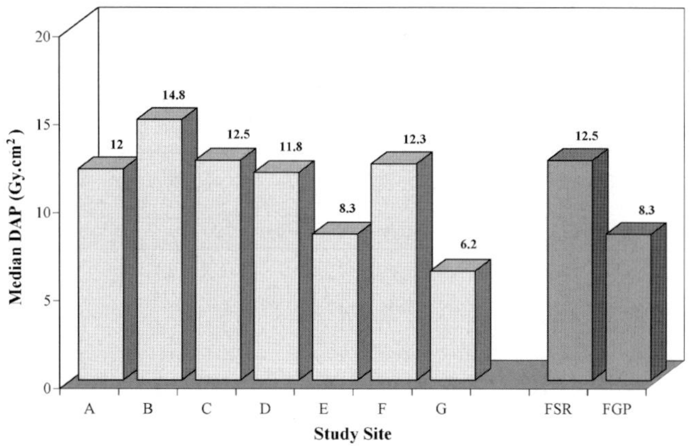

Figure 2. Median dose–area product (DAP) value for each study site. Sites A–D used the conventional film–screen (FSR) technique; sites (E–G) used the fluoroscopy-guided positioning (FGP) technique. The median value for each technique has also been included.

patients are being assessed by each technique. The distribution in genders (45% male and 55% female) was similar for both techniques. There was a slight difference in weight distribution between the two techniques. The patients in the FSR group had a smaller average weight than the patients in the FGP group. This difference was small and not significant enough ($\chi^2=0.87$, $p=0.65$) to contribute to differences in patient dose.

Radiographic technique and projections

There was a difference in the number of projections used for the two techniques. Three projections (AP, Lat, L5/S1) were commonly used in FSR and four (AP, Lat, L5/S1, AP axial) in the FGP series. The reported film–screen sensitivity for each department was 400; however this was not independently assessed nor was the effect of processing, thus the actual sensitivities were not known. Applied potential (kVp) and mAs change according to the habitus of the patient and different radiographic projections depending on the thickness of the body region being examined. High kVp techniques are also used to reduce dose. Applied potential was recorded for all patients in the study, while mAs was only recorded for 72 patients. Median results of applied potential and mAs are given in Table 2.

Repeat rates

Another reason for the lower DAP values in FGP is a smaller repeat rate compared with the FSR procedures. The repeat rates are shown in Table 2. It must be appreciated that these repeat rates are obtained from small sample sizes and may not accurately represent the repeat rates obtained over a longer period of time. The largest repeat rates are seen for the L5/S1 examination, as this is the most difficult to obtain radiographically. While there were differences between the individual sites for the lateral projection, there was no difference between the two procedures (2% compared with 1.9%). The same cannot be said for the L5/S1 projection where the repeat rate for the FSR (10%) was nearly double that of the FGP procedure (5.8%).

Screening time

The median screening time for FGP sites E, F and G were 18 s, 24 s and 12 s, respectively. These values were well correlated ($r=0.99$) with the median DAP values. The variation in screening times and DAP for all patients within one site gave a correlation coefficient of $r=0.50$, while expanding this analysis over the three FGP study sites resulted in a correlation coefficient of $r=0.21$. This correlation coefficient is lower as it incorporates the effect of other influencing factors such as variations in field collimation.

Analysis and discussion

The average DAP was 36% lower for patients undergoing the FGP procedure. This was unexpected as the FGP procedures included screening time and an additional radiographic view. A *t*-test was applied to a logarithmic transformed dataset to test for significance. The calculated *t*-statistic was 3.97 representing a highly significant difference ($p<0.0001$) in the DAP values between the two techniques.

Radiographic technique

Analysis of the radiographic techniques showed that the tube potential used in FSR and FGP sites was almost equal. A more significant difference was seen in mAs values. The mAs used in the FSR sites were on average nearly 20% higher than those used in FGP sites. The

Table 2. The table shows the median applied potential (kVp) and time–current product (mAs) used by each study site. The number of patients (N) examined per site is given together with the repeat rates (RR%) for each projection and each site

Study site	N	AP projection			Lateral projection			L5/S1			AP axial		
		kVp	mAs	RR(%)	kVp	mAs	RR(%)	kVp	mAs	RR(%)	kVp	mAs	RR(%)
A	11	77	50.8	0	85	110	0	109	92	16.7	—	—	—
B	10	70	81.5	0	70	135	0	76	367	10	—	—	—
C	11	71.5	—	0	85	—	9.1	96	—	9.1	—	—	—
D	18	70	—	0	81	—	0	85	—	5.6	—	—	—
E	13	71	104	0	84	111	0	85	254	0	71	102	0
F	19	70	55	0	80	63	0	80	170	10.5	70	66	0
G	20	70	78	0	80	70	5	90	76.8	5	75	61	0

N, number of patients; RR, repeat rate; AP, anteroposterior.

lateral and L5/S1 projections resulted in considerably larger differences.

Comparing individual FSR sites, site A consistently used the highest median tube potential, whilst site B used the lowest. Site A had the lowest median mAs and site B had the highest values. These findings correlated well with the median DAP values for the sites, with site A having the lowest value and site B the highest. Similar comparisons can be made for sites that employed the FGP technique; however the dose readings do not appear as well correlated with the exposure factors.

Screening time

An explanation for the low correlation between tube potential, mAs and DAP values in the FGP procedure is differences in screening time. Site F had the highest screening time and the highest DAP measurement. Similarly, site G had the lowest total screening time and the lowest mean DAP reading. Image display systems varied between clinical sites using FGP techniques. In site G, the spot image taken remained on freeze frame after screening stopped. This image was used as a guide if an alteration of position was required. In sites E and F, there was no freeze frame facility, and the radiographer was required to re-screen to verify an alteration of position. These observations correlated with analysis of screening times (Figure 3a), where the site with the lowest median screening time (site G) used freeze frame and produced the lowest median DAP value (Figure 3b).

The study aim was to determine if FGP techniques produced higher doses in comparison with FSR techniques, as such data were only collected on the total DAP value for each examination. A continuation of this study will monitor DAP due individually to fluoroscopy and radiographic modes, as well as the DAP value for each projection.

Repeat rates

It has been reported that approximately 19% of repeat radiographs are repeated due to incorrect positioning [8]. This implies that the use of FGP would reduce patient dose if FGP techniques were used instead of blind positioning. In this study, the use of FGP did not significantly reduce the repeat rate for the whole examination; the only difference was for the L5/S1 projection, where FSR produced nearly double the repeat rate.

Field size and effective dose

The use of smaller collimated fields used with FGP is another reason for the difference in DAP values. The collimation can be adjusted after the initial fluoroscopy spot film is displayed on the monitor, reducing the overall area of exposure in the subsequent FSR film. The reduction in field size demonstrates the reduction in energy imparted to the patient from a lumbar spine series. Depending on the anatomical area under investigation, there may be greater reductions in effective dose, as beam collimation will limit the amount of primary radiation and scattered radiation reaching the gonads. A more detailed analysis needs to be performed to draw more definite conclusions, and this was beyond the scope of the present study.

Comparison with the reference levels and other studies

The NRPB DAP reference level for a complete lumbar spine examination is 15 Gy cm^2 [2]. The median value for the FGP techniques was 45% lower than this and the median value for FSR techniques 17% lower. Shrimpton et al reported the mean DAP reading for a lumbar spine series as 11.7 Gy cm^2 [9]. A study in Western Australia measured a mean DAP of 11.4 Gy cm^2 for the lumbar spine [10]. A study performed by Warren-Forward et al measured the mean DAP for a lumbar spine as 7.92 Gy cm^2 [11]. The NRPB 2000 Review reports a third quartile level of 7.3 Gy cm^2 for measurements on over 1000 patients and 50 hospitals [12]. This level was calculated from individual projections of the three common projections (AP, LAT, LSJ) used in the UK. If

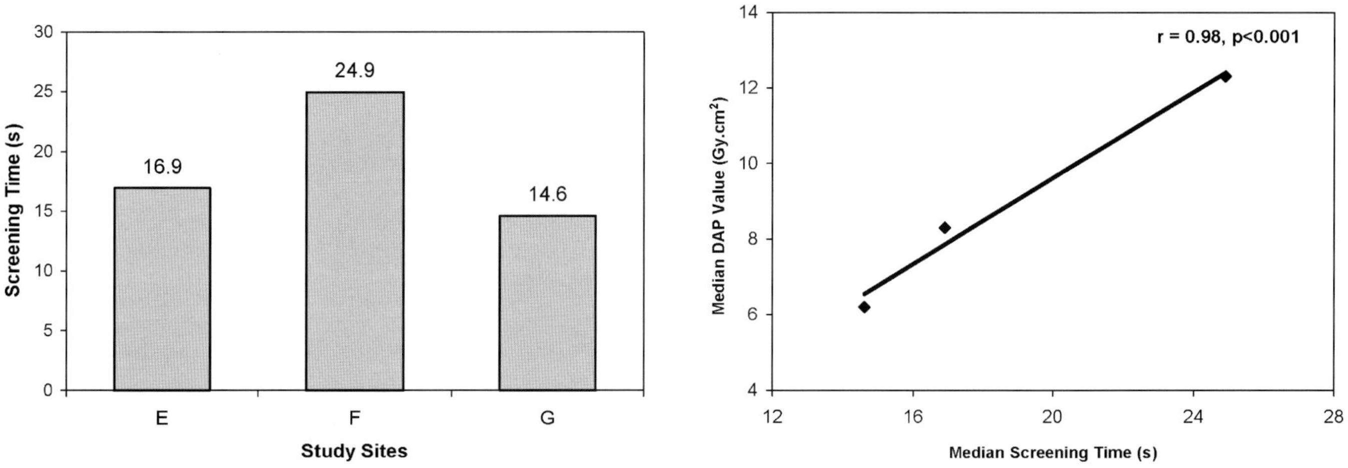

(a) (b)

Figure 3. The median screening times illustrated in (a) correlate with the use of freeze-frame in site G, which displays the lowest median screening time of the three units. There is excellent correlation between median screening time and median dose–area product (DAP) values (b), indicating the importance of minimizing screening time.

the results from the current study are to be compared with this new value, then only one centre produced a lower median dose (noting that three sites used four projections). For over a decade there has been a drive to assess and optimize radiation doses in the UK and Europe while there has been very little assessment in Australia. Doses can thus be expected to be higher in Australia as there has been no basis upon which to change practice.

Additionally, the current study included a large cohort of patients above 80 kg, while the latest NRPB figures are based on a weight range of 50–90 kg. Another explanation is the difference in applied potential. The range of applied potentials in this study (Table 1) are at the low end or even lower than Commission of the European Community (CEC) recommendations [13]. The CEC recommends between 75 kVp and 90 kVp for AP projections, between 80 kVp and 95 kVp for lateral and between 80 kVp and 100 kVp for L5/S1 projections. For the AP projections, six out of the seven departments used median values lower than the recommended value, with a mean value of 71 kVp compared with 76 kVp in the NRPB report. For the lateral projection the mean value (80.7 kVp) was 6 kVp lower than the NRPB mean value (87 kVp). Similarly, for the L5/S1 projection the mean value was 88 kVp compared with 95 kVp, with over half the departments using less than the CEC recommendation. Correspondingly the values of the mean mAs's were significantly higher in our study: AP (47% higher); LAT (53% higher) and L5/S1 (90% higher).

Conclusion

The FGP technique for lumbar spine examinations produced an overall lower median DAP than an FSR technique. This is in agreement with the findings of Deprez et al [5]. This has potential implications for the future of radiographic practice, as the use of FGP has been discouraged in a number of countries. There is a presumption that FGP produces higher levels of radiation dose. What now has to be asked is "should FGP be further introduced into clinical practice for specific examinations?"

Before a definitive answer can be given, a more extensive study is needed involving a wider range of clinical sites both within and outside Australia and data collection incorporating other factors affecting DAP values and repeat rates, such as the use of automatic exposure control. One area of concern is the complacency that may develop if FGP is incorporated into routine clinical practice. The radiographers involved in the study may have been conscious of being "monitored" and thus may have reduced their screening times and deliberately have used tighter collimation than in usual practice. It is known that FGP is being introduced in a number of sites, so it is pertinent that its effect on patient dose is carefully monitored and reported so that strict protocols can be set in place.

References

1. International Commission on Radiological Protection. Recommendations of the International Commission on Radiological Protection. Report 60. Annals of the ICRP 21. Oxford: Pergamon Press, 1990.
2. National Radiation Protection Board. Patient dose reduction in diagnostic radiology. Report by the Royal College of Radiologists and the NRPB. Documents of the NRPB. 1(3). Chilton: NRPB, 1990.
3. Harrison RM, Clayton CB, Day MJ, Owen JP, York MF. A survey of radiation doses to patients in five common diagnostic examinations. Br J Radiol 1983;56:383–95.
4. Martin CJ, Darragh CL, McKenzie GA, Bayliss AP. Implementation of a programme for reduction of radiographic doses and results achieved through increases in tube potential. Br J Radiol 1993;66:228–33.
5. Deprez T, Schrijver L, Pauwels H, Bosmans H, Marchal G. Can patient positioning using an ultrashort fluoroscopic pulse be justified. IAEA International Conference on Radiological Protection of patients in diagnostic and interventional radiology, nuclear medicine & radiotherapy, Malaga, Spain 26–30 March 2001.
6. Faulkner K, Busch HP, Cooney P, Malone JF, Marshall NW, Rawlings DJ. An international intercomparison of dose-area product meters. Radiat Prot Dosim 1992;43:193–5.
7. Environment Protection Agency. Registration requirements and industry best practice for ionizing radiation apparatus used in diagnostic imaging, Radiation Guideline 6: Part 2, Fluoroscopy and Radiography. Environment Protection Agency, Sydney, Australia, 1999.
8. Hill SJ. Reject Analysis in ERPET training course for medical physicist, "Quality Assurance and patient radiation protection in diagnostic radiolgy", Passau. 1996.
9. Shrimpton PC, Wall BF, Jones DG, Fisher ES, Hillier MC, Kendall GM, et al. Doses to patients from routine diagnostic X-ray examinations in England. Br J Radiol 1986;59:749–58.
10. Gray N, Rafferty MW, Black JL, Hartley BM, Thompson RI, Stock B. A patient dose survey for three common diagnostic radiographic examinations using a dose-area product meter. Aust Phys Eng Sci Med 1994;17:79–83.
11. Warren-Forward HM, Haddaway MJ, Temperton DH, McCall IW. Dose-area product readings for fluoroscopic and plain film examinations, including an analysis of the source of variation for barium enema examination. Br J Radiol 1998;71:961–7.
12. Hart D, Hillier MC, Wall BF. Doses to patients from medical x-ray examinations in the UK - 2000 Review. NRPB-W14. Chilton: NRPB, 2002.
13. Commission of the European Communities. Quality Criteria for Diagnostic Radiographic Images. Document XII/221/93 CEC, Brussels, 1990.

The British Journal of Radiology, 78 (2005), 135–142 © 2005 The British Institute of Radiology
DOI: 10.1259/bjr/48072262

Effective doses in angiography and interventional radiology: calculation of conversion coefficients for angiography of the lower limbs

[1]L STRUELENS, [1]F VANHAVERE, ^{2}H BOSMANS and [3]R VAN LOON

[1]*SCK-CEN, Belgian Nuclear Research Centre, Boeretang 200, 2400 Mol,* [2]*Department of Radiology, University Hospitals of the KU Leuven, Herestraat 49, 3000 Leuven and* [3]*Free University of Brussels, Pleinlaan 2, 1050 Brussels, Belgium*

Abstract. The present study reports on investigations that we have performed to allow the calculation of effective doses (E) in interventional radiology. The use of published conversion tables might not allow sufficient guidance for the establishment of optimization strategies for procedures in interventional radiology. With the Monte Carlo N-Particle transport code (MCNP4B), conversion coefficients, linking dose–area product (DAP) measurements with E, are calculated for angiography of the lower limbs in six hospitals. The influence of various parameters on the calculation of these conversion coefficients is studied in a systematic way using the 2^n factorial design. In this design the effect of different parameters and their pair-wise interactions on a certain variable is explored. In our study, the relevant parameters are tube potential, total filtration and field size and position. We concluded that the influence of radiation spectrum (kVp + filtration) is large and that the effect of field position and size is moderate, except when differences are observed in respect of the gonads. In that case, the variation in conversion coefficients is large. The results of this statistical analysis are then applied to the differences observed between the conversion coefficients, calculated for angiography of the lower limbs in the six hospitals. Recommendations for optimization of patient doses are given.

Interventional radiological procedures aim to diagnose or treat percutaneously particular diseases of the vasculature. In recent years there has been an increase in the number, type and complexity of these procedures. These radiological examinations are characterized by extended fluoroscopy times and they require many radiographic images of different areas of the body. As a consequence, the X-ray doses to patients may be high and both stochastic and deterministic effects have to be considered [1]. The Euratom 97/43 directive on health protection of individuals against the dangers of ionizing radiation in relation to medical exposure, requires special attention for these examinations. The directive, as implemented recently in the Belgian national legislation, lists general measures to ensure the application of the ALARA principle, *i.e.* the use of a dose as low as reasonably achievable, for these types of investigations. This study was performed within the framework of the preparation of an auditing structure, as foreseen in the legislation, for dose and image quality specifically for angiographic procedures. We report on a series of investigations we have performed to allow the calculation of effective doses from a particular interventional procedure. We focused on the diagnostic procedure "angiography of the lower limbs" as this is the most frequently performed interventional procedure in X-ray departments.

The effective dose E, a measure for stochastic risk, cannot be measured directly. A practical approach starts from entrance surface dose (ESD) or dose–area product (DAP) measurements and uses dedicated conversion coefficients.

Received 22 December 2003 and in final form 2 September 2004, accepted 29 September 2004.

Different organizations determined conversion coefficients that link ESD or DAP measurements with E. Previously, DAP values for successive projections of angiographic procedures of the lower limbs were multiplied by published conversion coefficients for simple radiographs of corresponding anatomical regions [2, 3]. The following limitations were observed:

- Hart et al [2] did not establish conversion coefficients for the pelvis right-posterior-oblique (RPO) and left-posterior-oblique (LPO) projections and for exposures of the legs;
- There is a large difference in field size used by Hart et al [2] and Drexler et al [3] in comparison with the field sizes used for angiography;
- Drexler et al [3] tabulated mainly conversion coefficients for anterior–posterior (AP) projections, while it is common practice to use also posterior–anterior (PA) projections;
- We observed average differences of the order of 20% between the results using the ESD-conversion factors in the two publications. Also large differences, up to 35%, were found using on the one hand the DAP-related and on the other hand the ESD-related conversion factors in the work of Hart et al [2].

We concluded that the use of these conversion tables might not provide sufficient guidance for establishing optimization strategies for angiographic procedures. As the quantity effective dose (E) is likely to be a useful parameter for the optimization of a technique, more dedicated conversion coefficients seemed necessary.

This paper deals with the calculation of the conversion coefficients and the influence of different parameters on these coefficients.

Material and methods

Characteristics of equipment and examination protocols

During diagnostic angiographic procedures of the lower limbs, particular arteries are visualized by the local injection of a contrast agent using a catheter. The injection of the contrast agent allows high resolution visualization and documentation of the vessels under study. For angiography of the lower limbs, we considered six adjoining standard regions: abdomen, pelvis, upper legs, knees, lower legs and feet.

In six different hospitals, the following parameters were registered for this type of examination: radiation quality, anatomical area irradiated, beam projection and the use of extra absorption filters.

Two hospitals (C and D) have an overcouch configuration, *i.e.* the X-ray tube is above the patient support table. The four other hospitals (A, B, E and F) have an undercouch configuration.

Questionnaires regarding working procedure were completed by all the radiologists in all hospitals. For every exposure, the projections of the beam and the exposed area of the body were clearly documented (Table 1). In Figure 1 the field positions for exposure of the abdomen and pelvis are shown for hospitals A–F, respectively. However, it is very probable that the exact field position will vary not only between the centres, but also between the patients from the same centre. In hospital C, the AP projection of the pelvis (Figure 1c, bold line) does not adjoin the AP projection of the abdomen. It starts much lower, at the bladder height. The adjoining pelvis projections are the RPO and LPO projections. Therefore, in this hospital the AP projection only partly overlaps the LPO and RPO projections of the pelvis. Consequently, the exposure of the upper legs, adjoining the pelvis AP projection, also starts lower compared with the other centres. In hospital D, there is no exposure of the abdomen.

Monte Carlo calculations

Monte Carlo calculations were set-up to calculate the conversion coefficients between DAP and *E*. For these calculations, field size, field position and X-ray spectrum are the input parameters.

The radiation spectra were characterized by the total filtration and the tube potential value. With a PMX-3 solid state dosemeter (RTI Electronics, Sweden) the half value layer (HVL) was determined for every tube in the different hospitals, by measuring dose rate for different thicknesses of aluminium. From these measurements, the total filtration is determined using the conversion tables in the application note of RTI electronics [4]. These filtrations, in terms of equivalent aluminium, comprising X-ray tube and patient support table for the undercouch configurations, are shown in Table 2, together with possible additional copper filtration and the average peak voltage used for every projection. With the "Catalogue of Diagnostic X-ray Spectra and other Data" of IPEM [5] the different spectra in the hospitals were determined for every projection separately, based on the total filtration of the beam and the tube potential.

The Monte Carlo calculations were performed with MCNP4B [6]. MCNP is a computer code in which the tracks of individual particles (photons, neutrons and electrons) are simulated through a well-defined geometry and problem-specific calculations can be done, concerning energy, absorbed dose, fluence, etc. As a model for the patient, the mathematical phantom Bodybuilder [7] was used. Bodybuilder is a computer program for the generation of human anthropomorphic phantoms of arbitrary age, from infant to adult. The human models as represented by Bodybuilder are based on the descriptions for several ages given in a report by Cristy and Eckerman [8].

The phantom's sex and age has to be chosen, as well as the organs to be included in the model. For both sexes, the adult phantom is chosen (21 years for male and 15 years for female model).

For one specific spectrum, projection and exposed body area, MCNP calculates doses in every organ of the phantom. With these organ doses and the tissue weighting factors specified by ICRP [2], effective doses were calculated. The theoretical DAP values associated with a given number of simulated X-ray photons were calculated from the average fluence through a surface at 20 cm from the source. Dividing the calculated effective dose by the theoretical DAP value gives the conversion coefficient for one specific exposure.

Calculation and comparative study of the conversion coefficients

Conversion coefficients were calculated for every specific projection in each hospital and for male and female patients separately. For every hospital the radiation fields are chosen as illustrated in Figure 1 and radiation quality chosen as in Table 2. The difference between the coefficients will be studied in more detail. The mean

Table 1. Different projections[a] used in the six hospitals for angiography of the lower limbs

Hospital A	Hospital B	Hospital C	Hospital D	Hospital E	Hospital F
Abdomen PA	Abdomen PA	Abdomen AP	Lower abdomen+Pelvis AP	Abdomen PA	Abdomen PA
Pelvis PA	Pelvis PA	Pelvis AP		Pelvis PA	Pelvis PA
Pelvis RAO/LAO		Pelvis RPO/LPO		Pelvis RAO/LAO	Pelvis LAO
Legs PA	Legs PA	Legs AP	Legs AP	Legs PA	Legs PA

[a]Terminology used for the projections are according to those used in NRPB-R262.

PA, posteroanterior; AP, anteroposterior; RPO, right posterior oblique; LPO, left posterior oblique; LAO, left anterior oblique; RAO, right anterior oblique.

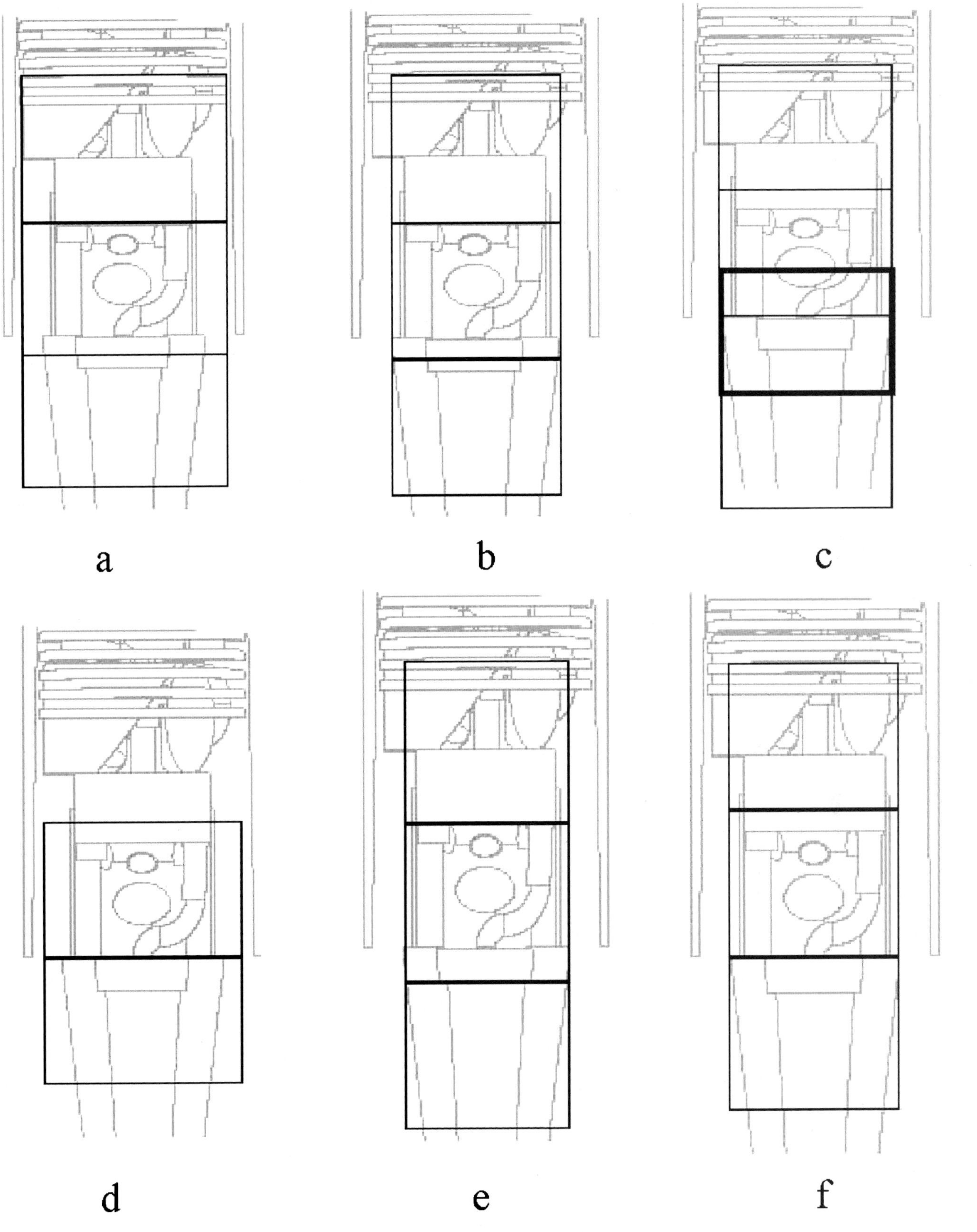

Figure 1. Radiation fields for exposure of the abdomen, pelvis and upper legs in the six hospitals. The anteroposterior (AP)-projection of the pelvis in hospital C is illustrated by the bold rectangle. The field for exposure of the upper legs, adjoins the AP projection of the pelvis.

Table 2. Total filtration and average tube potential value per projection in the six hospitals for angiography of the lower limbs

	Filtration		kVp			
	mm Al	mm Cu	Abdomen AP/PA	Pelvis AP/PA	Pelvis oblique	Legs AP/PA
Hospital A	6.5	0.1	75	75	75	75
Hospital B	5.1	0	70	70	—	65
Hospital C	4.2	0	75	75	75	65
Hospital D	4.1	0	65	65	65	65
Hospital E	4.6	0	80	80	80	70
Hospital F	4.9	0	85	85	85	75

AP, anteroposterior; PA, posteroanterior.

difference between conversion coefficients for men and women is calculated for each anatomical region. The factorial experiment is used to explain the differences in conversion coefficients between the centres, caused by various parameters.

Factorial experiments

Several parameters, such as field size, field position, patient thickness and radiation spectrum (kVp and filtration) are known to affect the conversion coefficients for estimating the effective dose. Ideally, the influence of each parameter would be independent, so that an estimate of a conversion coefficient is the product of several parameters [9]:

$$CF = v\phi_i\phi_j \ldots \phi_n \quad (1)$$

where v is a representative value of the coefficient and ϕ_i, ϕ_j... ϕ_n are the factors which take into account the effect of the variations of the n parameters. It is important not only to determine if the parameters have an influence on the conversion coefficients, but also if there is a significant interaction between the parameters. This means that Equation (1) has to be expanded to:

$$CF = v\phi_i\phi_j \ldots \phi_n\psi_{ij} \ldots \psi_{in} \ldots \psi_{jn} \quad (2)$$

where ψ_{ij}... ψ_{in}... ψ_{jn}... are correction factors which include the additional effect of interaction between the parameters. In general, higher-order interactions do not contribute significantly to the observed variations. This model converts into a linear model if natural logarithms are taken of Equation (2) and resembles the additive effect model with interactions by Snedecor and Cochran [10]. To explore the effects of the different parameters and their interactions in a systematic and efficient way, the 2^n factorial experiment is used [10]. For every parameter, one "low" and one "high" level is given, even though this notation might be arbitrary in the case of qualitative parameters. The complete factorial experiment requires that each level of every parameter occurs with each level of every other parameter, giving a total of 2^n combinations, with n being the number of parameters involved in the analysis.

In our experiment, the effect of the following parameters on the calculation of conversion coefficients for the effective dose were considered:

- Tube voltage (kVp)
- Beam filtration
- Field position and size

The low and high level values chosen for the parameters are determined from our detailed observations for several interventional procedures in different hospitals. We believe that these ranges are representative values for the parameters considered in interventional radiology for the exposure of abdomen and pelvis. For tube voltage (65–85 kVp) and for filtration (4.1 mm Al–6.5 mm Al+0.1 mm Cu). In Figure 2, the low and high levels for the field position are illustrated.

Using MCNP, conversion coefficients (*E*/DAP) are calculated for the $2^3=8$ possible combinations of the 3 parameters. This is done for 4 different projections: (1) abdomen AP, (2) abdomen PA, (3) pelvis AP and (4) pelvis PA. The mathematical phantom in these calculations is androgynous.

Statistical analysis is performed for each of the projections on the logarithms of (*E*/DAP) – conversion coefficients and the main factorial effects and all pair-wise interactions were investigated. These analyses were done using the generalized linear model of the computer package STATISTICA.

The results of the factorial experiment are applied to the differences between the conversion coefficients, calculated for angiography of the lower limbs for the six specific hospitals.

Results

In Table 3 the conversion coefficients are shown that link measured DAP values to the effective dose, both for men and women and for the six hospitals. The statistical error of all these factors is less than 0.1%. This was calculated from the relative errors given on the MCNP output files for every calculated dose.

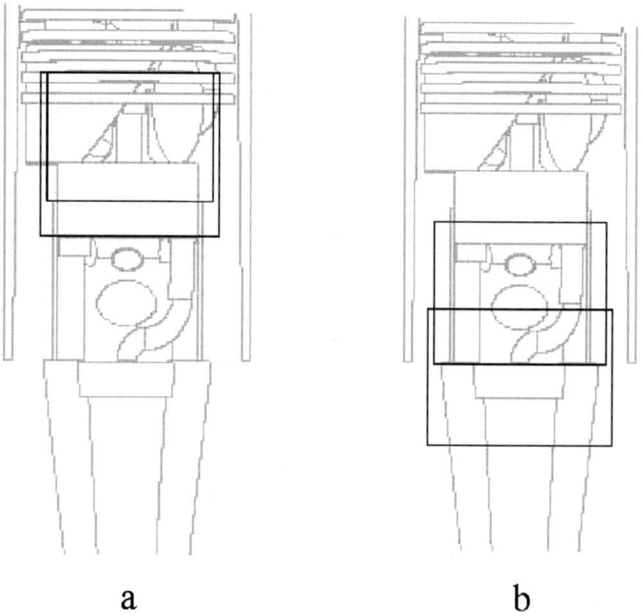

a b

Figure 2. Low and high level for (a) the abdomen and (b) the pelvis exposure in the factorial experiment. In practice, the fields have the same horizontal dimensions. In the figures they are offset to illustrate the different fields more clearly.

Table 3. Conversion coefficients linking dose–area product-measurements (Gy.cm^2) with the effective dose (mSv) for angiography of the lower limbs, for men and women in six hospitals (A–F)

(mSv Gy^{-1} cm^{-2})	Men						Women					
	A	B	C	D	E	F	A	B	C	D	E	F
Abdomen AP/PA	0.134	0.096	0.202	0.130	0.111	0.121	0.195	0.140	0.218	0.185	0.163	0.171
Pelvis AP/PA	0.131	0.103	0.469		0.115	0.130	0.214	0.170	0.089		0.183	0.229
Pelvis RAO/RPO	0.127	—	0.108	—	0.091	—	0.233	—	0.168	—	0.167	—
Pelvis LAO/LPO	0.142	—	0.156	—	0.098	0.121	0.252	—	0.245	—	0.178	0.233
Upper leg AP/PA	0.095	0.046	0.009	0.235	0.032	0.064	0.024	0.013	0.005	0.013	0.011	0.028
Lower leg AP/PA	0.007	0.004	0.003	0.004	0.004	0.005	0.006	0.004	0.003	0.004	0.004	0.004

AP, anteroposterior; PA, posteroanterior; RAO, right anterior oblique; RPO, right posterior oblique; LAO, left anterior oblique; LPO, left posterior oblique.

The conversion coefficients are compared between male and female patients, the difference between two numbers a and b being calculated as $(a-b)/a$. For the abdomen and pelvis projections the mean difference between all hospitals is about 61%. For the upper leg projection the mean difference is 68% and for the lower leg projection the difference is much lower (6%). From Table 3, we can also see that for both genders the conversion coefficients differ between the centres. These variations are evaluated from the results of the factorial experiment.

Effective doses can be calculated for the full procedure by multiplying the conversion coefficients in Table 3 by the measured DAP values per projection in all of the six hospitals: $E = \sum_i \mathrm{CF}_i \times \mathrm{DAP}_i$ with i the different projections.

In Table 4, the average DAP data from each hospital is given for each projection. This results in average effective doses of 8.0 mSv for hospital A (15 patients), 15.5 mSv for hospital B (16 patients), 8.0 mSv for hospital C (20 patients), 3.9 mSv for hospital D (13 patients), 16.8 mSv for hospital E (18 patients) and 11.3 mSv for hospital F (12 patients).

Factorial experiments

The conversion coefficients are calculated for the eight possible combinations of the three parameters per projection and the factorial experiment is applied on these coefficients.

The results of the factorial analysis are given in Table 5. The first value is a representative value for the conversion coefficient and corresponds to the geometrical mean of the eight possible combinations. The main and interaction effects are expressed as multipliers, illustrating how big the effects of the different parameters and their pair-wise interactions are on the mean value of the conversion coefficients. In Table 5, the multipliers are given for the low level of every parameter and their interactions. According to the constraints in the statistical analysis [9], the multiplier for the high level is the reciprocal of the

Table 4. Average dose–area product (DAP)-data (Gy.cm^2) for every projection for angiography of the lower limbs, for men and women in 6 hospitals (A–F)

(Gy.cm^2)	Men/Women					
	A	B	C	D	E	F
Abdomen AP/PA	15.2/13.2	89.7/44.1	11.0/8.1	20.8/9.3	31.8/48.8	31.7/22.5
Pelvis AP/PA	11.7/7.6	81.4/41.1	6.6/6.0		39.0/58.6	21.9/20.5
Pelvis RAO/RPO	11.1/10.3	/	12.0/6.1	/	24.3/23.9	/
Pelvis LAO/LPO	10.5/18.9	/	12.2/8.5	/	25.6/28.0	3.0/5.7
Upper leg AP/PA	1.4/1.1	26.4/9.8	3.9/4.1	8.0/3.3	10.5/24.9	11.6/9.0
Lower leg AP/PA	2.2/1.1	13.5/13.2	9.0/7.9	2.7/2.2	9.7/16.4	5.7/5.0

AP, anteroposterior; PA, posteroanterior; RAO, right anterior oblique; RPO, right posterior oblique; LAO, left anterior oblique; LPO, left posterior oblique.

Table 5. Representative value for the conversion coefficients from dose–area product (DAP) to effective dose (E) and the multipliers, representing the effect of the parameters and their pairwise interactions for the diffferent projections.

	CC (mSv Gy^{-1} cm^{-2})	Multipliers					
		kVp	mmAl	field	kVp × mmAl	kVp × field	mmAl × field
Abdomen AP	0.283	0.884	0.851	0.922	0.988	1.005	0.997
Abdomen PA	0.170	0.842	0.834	0.914	0.986	0.995	0.998
Pelvis AP	0.318	0.896	0.871	1.157	0.988	1.039	1.036
Pelvis PA	0.119	0.817	0.816	0.745	0.982	1.007	1.003

CC, conversion coefficients; AP, anteroposterior; PA, posteroanterior.

multiplier for the low level. For multipliers <1, the conversion coefficient increases and for multipliers >1, the coefficient decreases when the parameter changes from the low to the high level. By analogy with West et al [9], variations between the low and high value of less than 2% are described as "insignificant", of 2–5% as "small", of 5–15% as "moderate" and of over 15% as "large".

Concerning the main effects, the variations for tube potential and filtration parameters can be considered as large for every projection. The field position has a moderate effect (~15%) for the abdomen AP and PA projection, but a very large effect (31–51%) for the pelvis AP and PA projection. For every projection, the pair-wise interactions between the three parameters can be categorised as insignificant, except for the interaction between tube potential and filtration, which should be categorised as small. Moreover, for the pelvis AP projection variations of 7.5% are observed, where the interactions with the parameter "field position" is involved. This tells us that the effect on the conversion coefficients of changing the tube potential or the filtration will depend on the field position for the pelvis AP projection. The effect is moderate.

Conversion coefficients for every combination of the three parameters can be calculated per projection, following Equation (2).

For example, for an abdomen PA exposure at 65 kVp and 6.5 mm Al+0.1 mm Cu with a high field position, the conversion coefficient can be calculated from Table 5 as:

$$\mathrm{CF}=0.170\times 0.842\times(1/0.834)\times(1/0.914)\times(1/0.986)\times(1/0.995)\times 0.998=0.191$$

Since for the abdomen PA projection most interactions are insignificant, they can be omitted. For other levels of a specific parameter, the multiplier can be determined from an interpolation between the low and the high multiplier of that parameter.

Discussion

Male versus female patients

In Hart et al [2], no difference is made between conversion coefficients for male and female patients. From Table 3, however, we see that there is a significant difference in conversion coefficients for both sexes. The position of the gonads is crucial here. For the abdomen and pelvis projection, the conversion coefficients for the female patients are higher than those for the male patients. From Figure 1, we can see that the female gonads are near or in the radiation fields for both projections. For the pelvis projection, the male gonads are also near or in the radiation field. However for the hospitals with tube-undertable configuration, the female gonads are exposed more directly than the male gonads. The conversion coefficients for the upper legs are larger for the male patients, because the male gonads are much closer to the field than the female gonads.

Overcouch versus undercouch configurations

The position of the different radiation sensitive organs in the human body determines the difference in conversion coefficients between the anterior and posterior projections. For the anterior projection of the abdomen, radiation sensitive organs like the liver, stomach and lower large intestine (LLI) have larger doses compared with the posterior projection. For the latter projection, the doses to the mineral bone surface and the red bone marrow are larger compared with the anterior projection. However, they contribute less to the effective dose, because their doses are lower compared with those of the liver, stomach and LLI.

Abdomen projection

From the statistical analysis we can see that the maximum variation in conversion coefficients for the change in field position for the AP and PA exposure of the abdomen is around 15%. The difference between the conversion coefficients in Table 3, for this projection, is therefore mainly due to differences in tube configuration and radiation spectrum. The variation for these projections due to tube potential and filtration is large. This explains why hospitals A and F have larger conversion coefficients for the abdomen exposure. From Table 2, we observed the largest filtration for hospital A and the highest tube potential value for hospital F. The conversion coefficient in hospital C is larger due to the anterior projection, as explained in the previous paragraph.

Pelvis projection

The influence of the field position is much larger for the pelvis exposure: 31% for the AP-projection and 51% for the PA-projection. As mentioned before, this is caused by the difference in exposure of the gonads. This explains the high conversion coefficient for male patients in hospital C in Table 3: the inclusion of the gonads in the radiation field and the direct exposure due to the anterior projection. For the female patients, the conversion coefficient for the pelvis exposure in hospital C is much smaller compared with the other hospitals. The ovaries are far away from the radiation field in this hospital (Figure 1). Again for the pelvis exposure, we observe from the statistical analysis that tube potential and filtration have a large influence for the PA and AP projections, respectively. This explains the difference between the conversion coefficients in the hospitals where the difference in field position with respect to the gonads is small.

Upper leg projection

For the upper leg projection, the conversion coefficient for the male patients in hospital D is much larger than in other hospitals. Again, this can be explained by the inclusion of the gonads in the radiation field and by the anterior projection. In hospital C, the conversion coefficient for the upper leg for men is lower than in any other centre. Because of the lower position of the radiation field for this projection (Figure 1c), the gonads are more distant from the field. We can also observe a difference in conversion coefficients for the hospitals with tube-undertable configuration: for hospital E (0.032 mSv $\mathrm{Gy^{-1}cm^{-2}}$) where the gonads are not in the radiation field, for hospital

B (0.046 mSv $Gy^{-1}cm^{-2}$) with gonads partly exposed and for hospital F (0.064 mSv $Gy^{-1}cm^{-2}$) with gonads completely exposed. The higher conversion coefficient in hospital A (0.095 mSv $Gy^{-1}cm^{-2}$) is mainly caused by the larger filtration.

Patient thickness

The calculation of conversion coefficients for the six hospitals is made for standard-sized patients. In practice, this will not be the case. For the same tube potential and filtration, thicker patients will have smaller conversion coefficients because the organ doses are smaller compared with the standard patient. In practice, however, thicker patients could have larger tube potential values, implying a higher conversion coefficient. However, this will not necessarily mean a larger effective dose to the patient. A higher tube potential might imply a lower mAs value, depending on the tube potential curve and the dose level set in the system. Consequently, the DAP value could decrease. The steeper the tube potential curve, the smaller will be the mAs and the DAP.

Optimization guidelines

When minimizing effective doses for patients, the doses to the gonads play an important role. For procedures such as angiography of the lower limbs, exposure of the gonads is inevitable. In all hospitals the gonads for both genders are often exposed completely or partly in the pelvis projection. However, due to the possible additional oblique views, the pelvis is often more exposed than the other body regions. Therefore, it would be preferable for male patients to expose the gonads with the upper legs projection. Moreover, the beam path through the upper legs is smaller than through the pelvis. This results in lower tube potential and/or mAs values and consequently in lower DAP values. The higher conversion coefficient for the upper legs projection (due to the presence of the gonads) will contribute less to the effective dose, because of the lower associated DAP value.

For the female patients, the ovaries could be exposed with the abdomen projection to avoid the extra exposure from the oblique projections of the pelvis. The ovaries, however, are situated at that point where the abdominal artery splits into the two arteries leading to the legs. As it is mainly for this position of the arterial system that the oblique projections are performed for angiography of the lower limbs, it is not possible to include the ovaries in the abdominal exposure from a medical point of view.

Kicken [11] reported (*E*/DAP)-conversion coefficients for an abdomen PA projection. They were 0.102 mSv $Gy^{-1}cm^{-2}$ for the male patients for 80 kVp and 0.171 mSv $Gy^{-1}cm^{-2}$ for the female patients for 75 kVp, both with a total filtration of 6.0 mm Al_{eq}. They are comparable with the conversion coefficients in our study.

The conversion coefficients in NRPB-R262 [2, 12] are interpolated for 75 kVp and 5 mm Al_{eq} as 0.240, 0.149, 0.268 and 0.112 for the abdomen and pelvis AP and PA projections, respectively. These values, averaged over male and female patients, are comparable with the average values given in Table 5.

The conversion coefficients in this study are for the procedure of angiography of the lower limbs in several hospitals. However, they can also be used for similar projections in other procedures. For example, the conversion coefficients for the pelvis projections can be used in an iliac stenting procedure or the conversion coefficient for the abdomen irradiation can be used in a stent procedure of the kidneys or for a TIPS (transjugular portosystem shunt) procedure, provided that filtration and tube potential are known and that DAP values for each of these projections in the specific procedure are available.

One of the limitations of the study is the small number of participating hospitals. Also, an accurate calculation of effective dose requires a separate DAP value for every projection. This is not routinely available yet.

Conclusions

For the six hospitals in this study, conversion coefficients were calculated for every specific field position and radiation spectrum. This is possible but not routinely very practical. We investigated which parameters have an important influence on the calculation of conversion coefficients in order to limit the set necessary to calculate effective dose in angiography and interventional radiology. From the statistical analysis and the interpretation of the conversion coefficients for the six hospitals, we can conclude that:

(1) X-ray systems with a tube-over-table configuration give higher conversion coefficients and therefore higher effective doses than systems with tube-under-table configuration;
(2) The influence of tube potential and filtration on the conversion coefficients is large (~30%). It is recommended to establish a set of conversion coefficients for the entire range of tube potential and filtration in angiography and interventional radiology;
(3) Radiation fields are small in interventional radiology, compared with other standard radiographic measurement. This means that male- or female-specific organs are not necessarily irradiated by the same radiation fields. Hence, it is recommended to calculate separate conversion coefficients for male and female patients;
(4) The influence of field position on the calculation of conversion coefficients is large (31–51%) whenever variations are observed in respect of the gonads. For an accurate calculation of effective dose in an angio room, one should investigate if there are large deviations between the actual position of the radiation field and the reference field for which the conversion coefficients were calculated in respect to the gonads. If necessary, a new coefficient should be calculated specific for the radiation field used.

In order of priority, we propose to treat separately undercouch and overcouch set ups, to account then for male versus female patients, to adjust conversion coefficients in terms of radiation quality and finally, if necessary, to fine tune for differences in radiation field. If the position of the radiation field is close to or involves the gonads, greater attention should be given to the calculation.

References

1. Faulkner K. Radiation protection in interventional radiology. Br J Radiol 1997;70:325–6.
2. Hart D, Jones DG, Wall BF. Estimation of effective dose in diagnostic radiology from entrance surface dose and dose-area product measurements. NRPB-R262. Chilton: NRPB, 1994.
3. Drexler G, Panzer W, Widenmann L, Williams G, Zankl M. The calculation of dose from external photon exposures using reference human phantoms and monte carlo methods, part III: organ doses in X-ray diagnosis. GSF-Bericht 11/90, 1990.
4. HVL measurements with PMX-III and the PMX detector on units with tungsten target. Application note No. 03-008/01, RTI electronics AB, Sweden, February 1994.
5. Catalogue of Diagnostic X-Ray Spectra and other Data, IPEM-R78, York, UK 1997, ISBN 0 904181 88 X (CD-ROM).
6. Briestmeister JF. "A General Monte Carlo N-Particle Transport Code", Version 4B (LA-12625-M, March 1997).
7. Van Riper KA. Bodybuilder software for Windows, version 1.21, White Rock Science, Los Alamos, USA, 1997-2001.
8. Cristy M, Eckerman KF. Specific absorbed fractions of energy at various ages from internal photon sources. I. Methods. Oak Ridge National Laboratory Report ORNL/TM-8381/VI, 1987.
9. West KN, Sandborg M, Persliden J, Alm Carlsson G. Sensitivity of coefficients for converting entrance surface dose and kerma-area product to effective dose and energy imparted to the patient. Phys Med Biol 1999;44:1937–54.
10. Snedecor GW, Cochran WG. Statistical methods, 7th edn. Iowa: Iowa State University Press, 1980.
11. Kicken PJH. Radiation dosimetry in vascular radiology – organ and effective dose to patients and staff. Chapter 8: Quantitative data about patient exposure conditions and dose estimates for selected procedures in the University Hospital Maastricht. 1996:p140 ISBN 90 5278 217 2.
12. Hart D, et al. Authors' reply. Br J Radiol 1998;71:995.

The British Journal of Radiology, 78 (2005), 143–146
DOI: 10.1259/bjr/20164607

The hyfrecator: a treatment for radiation induced telangiectasia in breast cancer patients

[1,4]C M E ROWLAND PAYNE, MBBS, MRCP, [2,4]N SOMAIAH, MBBS, MD, [3]A J NEAL, MD, MRCP, FRCR and [2,4,5]J P GLEES, MD, DMRT, FRCR

[1]*The London Clinic, London,* [2]*St. George's Hospital, London,* [3]*The Royal Surrey County Hospital, Guildford,* [4]*The Royal Marsden Hospital, Sutton, Surrey and* [5]*University of London, London, UK*

Abstract. Radiation induced telangiectasia is a common problem in breast cancer survivors. By interfering with choice of clothing and acting as an unpleasant visible reminder of their disease, it negatively affects quality of life. The hyfrecator, based on the principles of electrosurgery, is a standard treatment modality for facial telangiectasia. This study aims to demonstrate the efficacy and tolerability of the hyfrecator as a treatment for radiation induced telangiectasia. Patients with radiation induced telangiectasia of breast or chest wall were prospectively identified from the breast cancer follow up clinic and offered treatment with the hyfrecator (sessions at 8 weekly intervals). Pre- and post-treatment photographs were obtained in a standardized manner and two blinded physician observers evaluated response. A linear analogue scale (LAS) was used by the patients to evaluate treatment response and any discomfort. At the end of treatment, patients completed a quality of life questionnaire. Of 16 patients enrolled, 15 completed the study. Treatment benefited all patients with severe or marked telangiectasia. Complete disappearance of telangiectasia was achieved in the majority (88%) of patients by the end of treatment. A median of six sessions (range 3–9) was required. All but one (93%) considered the treatment worthwhile. The majority (69%) judged the treatment to be painless or only mildly painful. 73% reported an improvement in self-confidence. The treatment was well tolerated by all the patients. All patients showed a remarkable clearance of vessels with a high degree of satisfaction with the results. Treatment with the hyfrecator is very effective for radiation induced telangiectasia. Three to four sessions achieve a substantial objective and subjective reduction in telangiectasia with a concomitant improvement in quality of life. It is a cost effective, ambulant out patient procedure requiring no local anaesthesia.

Approximately 30 000 women in the UK are diagnosed with invasive breast cancer each year. Radiotherapy is an accepted part of the local treatment of breast cancer following both breast conserving surgery and in selected cases, mastectomy. The total number of women being treated with radiotherapy is increasing since implementation of the National Breast Screening Programme. With higher patient expectations, the cosmetic result following breast conserving surgery and radiotherapy is an important consideration [1]. Although current technology has reduced the frequency and severity of late radiation morbidity, telangiectasia is still a significant problem.

Radiation induced telangiectasia is a well recognized manifestation of late cutaneous radiation damage [2]. It is usually confined to the site of highest dose (*e.g.* site of radiation boost), and can be very unsightly depending on its site, size and extent. It usually becomes apparent at 1–2 years after completion of treatment, and may slowly progress over subsequent years. In some cases it is the most obvious reminder to the patient of their illness and its treatment. However, most radiation oncologists do not offer any treatment for this condition.

The hyfrecator is a surgical diathermy unit, which uses an electrical discharge to coagulate the dilated small blood vessels that are telangiectasia. This electrosurgical device has been used for decades by dermatologists on the face, as a cosmetic procedure, and is very effective with minimal side effects [3]. One of us (CRP) has had previous experience of good results with this technique in a number of patients with radiation induced telangiectasia over the last decade. It was the reluctance of a radiotherapy colleague, fearful that this procedure would cause a necrotic ulcer that prompted us to undertake this prospective study.

Received 15 December 2003 and in revised form 10 September 2004, accepted 19 October 2004.

Address correspondence to Dr Navita Somaiah, Department of Radiotherapy, The Royal Marsden Hospital, Downs Road, Sutton, Surrey SM2 5PT, UK.

Source of funding: The Dr John Glees Cancer Research fund.

Patients and methods

This prospective study was conducted in the Department of Clinical Oncology (Breast Unit) at The Royal Marsden Hospital (RMH), Surrey Branch. It was approved by the ethics committee of The Royal Marsden NHS Trust/The Institute of Cancer Research (Ethics No. 1419).

Patients with radiation induced telangiectasia of breast or chest wall were identified from the breast cancer follow-up clinic and invited to participate. Those who had participated in the RMH breast fractionation study [4] and those with a cardiac pacemaker or hearing aid were excluded from the study. Informed consent was obtained. Patients were recalled at a convenient date for treatment with the hyfrecator.

The Conmed hyfrecator (Conmed, Utica, NY; Figure 1) was set at low power, 2.4–3.2 W (usually 2.6 W). No skin preparation was required. The skin was gently stretched and an epilation electrode was applied lightly every 2 mm

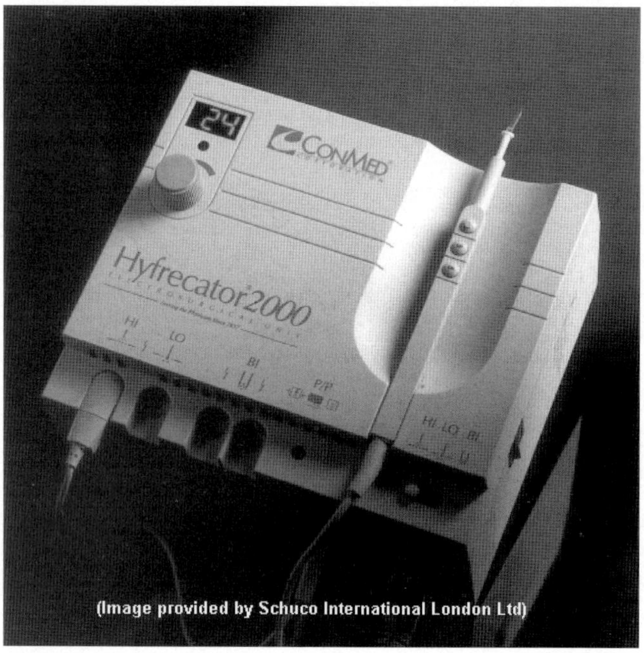

Figure 1. The hyfrecator. A versatile office-based electrosurgical instrument (courtesy of Schuco International, London Ltd).

to 3 mm along the telangiectatic vessels with passage of a controlled electrical discharge by a foot switch, with each application. Pulse frequency was approximately 50–80 pulses per minute with pulse duration of approximately 0.25 s. The entire area was treated at each session. Typically, each session lasted 3–8 min. The sessions were at 8 weekly intervals.

Close up serial photographs were taken by the same medical photographer before each treatment and 8 weeks after the final treatment using colour slide film. For each patient, photographic field, camera settings, lighting and distance from subject were constant.

Before the first and 8 weeks after the last treatment session, patients completed a 10 cm LAS self assessment of telangiectasia severity. After each session, patients were asked (after reaching home) to complete another 10 cm LAS to record any discomfort felt during the session and a further one 48 h afterwards (0, "completely painless" to 10, "the worst pain imaginable"). 8 weeks after the final session, patients were also given a quality of life questionnaire to complete.

Physician-based assessments of colour photography were undertaken after the end of treatment. Three serial colour slides (pre treatment, after 3 sessions and 8 weeks after the final session) of each of the 15 patients (45 slides) were mixed together and presented randomly for independent assessment by the two blinded physician observers. Assessment was according to the following descriptive scale [5]:

Grade 0	No telangiectasia
Grade I	Minimal telangiectasia
Grade II	Moderate telangiectasia
Grade III	Severe telangiectasia

Results

16 caucasian females, aged 43–72 years (mean 57 years), 2–10 years (median 5 years) post-radiation, were enrolled. One dropped out after one session (because of the travelling distance). 15 patients were treated every 8 weeks until their telangiectasia cleared or they were satisfied (range of 3–9 sessions, median 6 sessions).

All (14/15) patients with severe or marked telangiectasia benefited from treatment (Figures 2 and 3). In 88% of patients telangiectasia had completely disappeared by the end of treatment, as judged by the physicians. The treatment was well tolerated by all the patients. Discomfort was usually scored as zero (range 0–8). The majority of sessions (69%, 66/96 sessions) were scored as painless or mildly painful (LAS 0–2). A LAS $\geqslant$5 was recorded in only 18% (17/96) of sessions (session defined as each hospital visit per patient for treatment with the hyfrecator). Only two patients complained of mild pain (LAS 1) 48 h after treatment, the rest (87%) were symptomless. After the final treatment slight skin atrophy was noted by the dermatologist in two patients but was not noticeable to the patients. In some patients, minimal transient pinpoint bleeding was noted which ceased spontaneously or with minimal pressure and was no more than the slightest inconvenience. No other adverse effects occurred. In particular, no necrosis as a result of the treatment was observed during the study and subsequent follow-up (median 4.5 years). Also, there was no recurrence of telangiectasia in the treated vessels.

At the end of treatment, the quality of life questionnaires showed that 93% (14/15) of patients felt the treatment was worthwhile and were very satisfied with the results (Table 1). Compared with before the skin treatment began, the majority of patients (73%, 11/15) reported an improvement in their self confidence, while 60% (9/15) said that they were much less embarrassed or self conscious. Several volunteered that they were pleased to be able to wear lower cut clothes again. One patient felt confident to return to topless sunbathing.

Discussion

Radiation induced telangiectasia is a well recognized manifestation of late cutaneous radiation damage after radiation therapy for breast carcinoma. Univariate and multivariate analyses for the development of skin telangiectasia have shown 5-year and 7-year actuarial rates of telangiectasia to be 59% and 72%, respectively [2]. Patients who have been given an additional boost to the surgical scar are more likely to develop skin telangiectasia.

Morbidity assessments after a median follow-up time of 6.6 years, in the Danish randomized DBCG-82TM breast conservation trial, showed that skin telangiectasia, breast fibrosis and breast retraction were significantly associated with a less satisfactory cosmetic result [1]. Impaired body perception was found to be significantly associated with breast retraction and skin telangiectasia. Patients are distressed because clothing habits are compromised as a consequence of adverse skin reactions and breast retraction. In some cases it is the most obvious reminder to the patient of their previous treatment. However, unfortunately, most oncologists have to date not offered any treatment for this condition.

The hyfrecator has been, for more than half a century, the most popular electrosurgical accessory for outpatient and office-based dermatological surgery (Figure 1). It is a low power (maximum output of 35 W) surgical diathermy

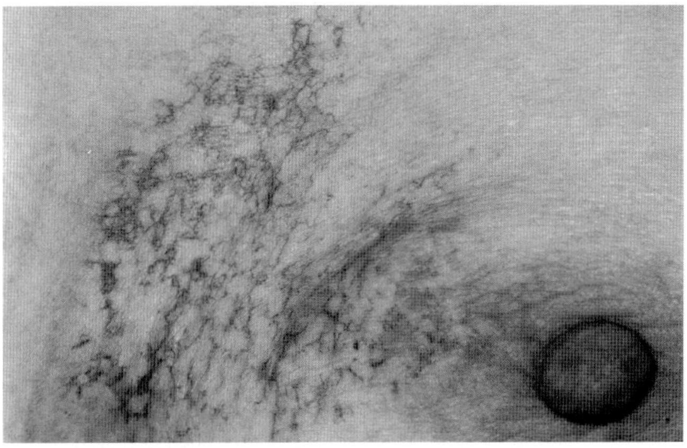

(a)

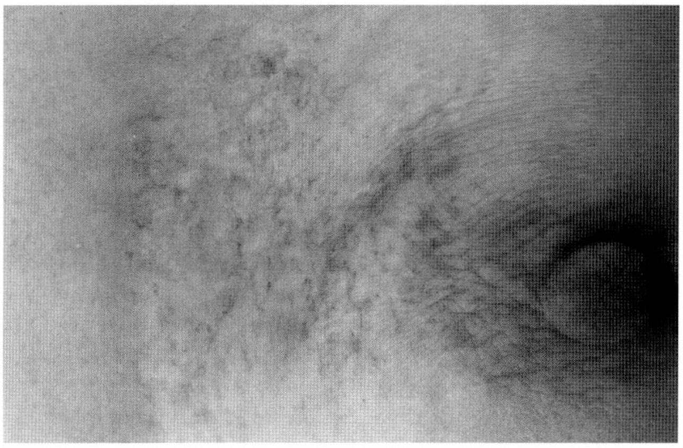

(b)

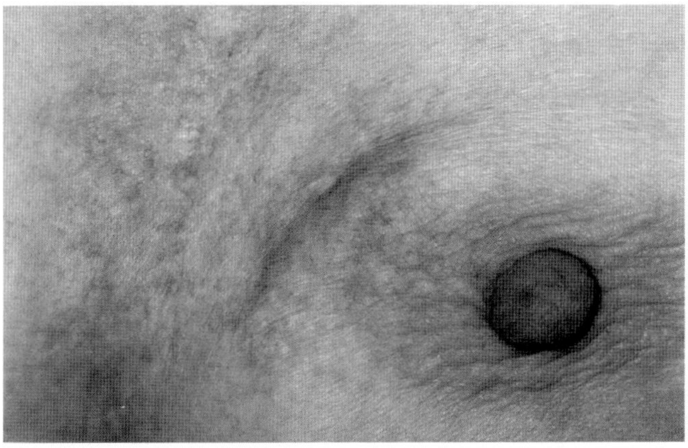

(b)

Figure 2. (a) Pre-treatment. Extensive telangiectasia (grade III) in the radiation boost area after breast cancer treatment. (b) During treatment. After three sessions, telangiectasia (now grade I) has reduced by about 70% (same patient). (c) End of treatment. After seven sessions, telangiectasia has completely disappeared (grade 0) (same patient).

unit, which produces a controlled electrical discharge of high frequency and high voltage, destroying tissue by the passage of electric current. For treatment of telangiectasias it is commonly used at a setting of 0 to 5 W. By comparison, electrocautery (typical power output of 200 W) destroys tissue through heat conduction using an electrically heated metal "burner". The hyfrecator is a compact, portable and versatile instrument (costing approximately £1000), which allows rapid and precise destruction of all types of cutaneous lesions, including telangiectasia [3]. However, until now there has been no controlled data or publication documenting its efficacy and tolerability in the treatment of post radiation telangiectasia in breast cancer patients. With the hyfrecator, three different forms of tissue destruction are possible: fulguration, desiccation and coagulation. In this study, electrodesiccation was used to treat fine telangiectasia.

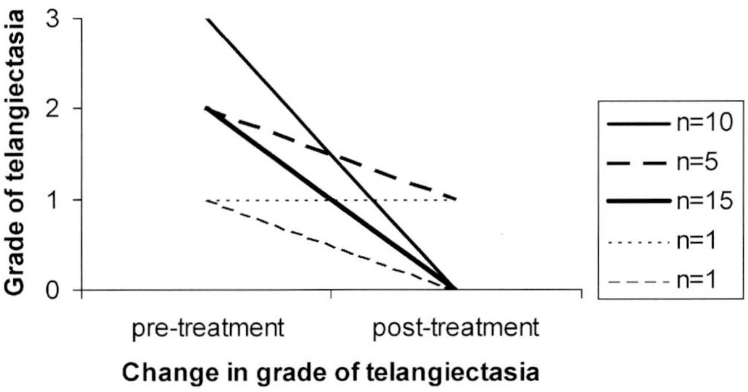

Figure 3. The hyfrecator for radiation induced telangiectasia. Change in severity of telangiectasia, judged photographically by two blinded physician observers (in one patient two separate sites were treated, making a total of 32 observations).

Table 1. Hyphrecation for radiation-induced telangiectasia. Quality of life assessment

Quality of life measure	Very much or a lot	A little or not at all
1. Has the skin treatment been worthwhile?	93%	7%
2. Compared with before the skin treatment began, has your self confidence improved?	73%	27%
3. Compared with before the skin treatment began, how much less embarrassed or self conscious are you because of your skin?	60%	40%
4. Compared with before the skin treatment began, how much does your skin affect the clothes you wear now?	33%	67%
5. Compared with before the skin treatment began, how much does your skin affect any social or leisure activities?	27%	73%
6. How much of a problem has the skin treatment been, for example by taking up your time?	20%	80%

Other effective treatments for post radiation telangiectasia include sclerotherapy and laser [6, 7]. Pulsed dye laser is better than the hyfrecator when erythema, rather than telangiectasia, predominates (a situation very rare after radiotherapy). In terms of efficiency and cost-effectiveness, the hyfrecator is far more advantageous (a laser usually costs tens of thousands of pounds). It is easy to use, has minimal adverse effects compared with other techniques [8, 9] and does not require special training. The treatment does not require anaesthesia or skin preparation or any of the safety procedures needed with laser therapy. Caution is required in patients with implanted cardiac pacemakers.

This study demonstrates that the hyfrecator is an effective treatment for radiation induced telangiectasia. It is well tolerated and well accepted by patients. Women, who are disturbed by post radiation telangiectasia of the breast or chest wall, will achieve a substantial objective reduction in telangiectasia and an improvement in quality of life with 3–4 sessions alone. The hyfrecator is therefore recommended as an efficient and cost-effective treatment for this distressing condition.

Acknowledgments

We thank Professor Peter Mortimer, Professor of Dermatology, and Mr Dennis Underwood and Mr Ray Stucky from the Medical Photography Department at the Royal Marsden Hospital, Sutton, Surrey Branch, London for their help and support in this study. We also thank Schuco International, London Ltd for their help and The Dr John Glees Cancer Research fund for financial support.

References

1. Johansen J, Overgaard J, Rose C, Engelholm SA, Gadeberg CC, Kjaer M, et al. Danish Breast Cancer Cooperative Group (DBCG) and the DBCG Radiotherapy Committee. Cosmetic outcome and breast morbidity in breast-conserving treatment--results from the Danish DBCG-82TM National Randomized Trial in Breast Cancer. Acta Oncol 2002;41:369–80.
2. Huang EY. Predictive factors for skin telangiectasia following post-mastectomy electron beam irradiation. Br J Radiol 2002;75:444–7.
3. Hainer BL. Electrosurgery for the skin. Am Fam Physician 2002;66:1259–66.
4. Yarnold JR, Owen JR, Ashton A, Regan J, Broad B, Jackson C, et al. Fractionation sensitivity of change in breast appearance after radiotherapy for early breast cancer: long-term results of a randomised trial. Radiother Oncol 2002;64(Suppl.):S25, abstract 77.
5. Turesson I, Notter G. The influence of fraction size in radiotherapy on the late normal tissue reaction--I: Comparison of the effects of daily and once-a-week fractionation on human skin. Int J Radiat Oncol Biol Phys 1984;10:593–8.
6. Lanigan SW, Joannides T. Pulsed dye laser treatment of telangiectasia after radiotherapy for carcinoma of the breast. Br J Dermatol 2003;148:77–9.
7. Gordan AB, Harmer CL, O'Sullivan M. Treatment of post-radiotherapy telangiectasia by injection sclerotherapy. Clin Radiol 1987;38:25–6.
8. Mcburney EI. Side effects and complications of laser therapy. Dermatol Clinics 2002;20:165–76.
9. Bihari I, Magyar E. Reasons for ulceration after injection treatment of telangiectasia. Dermatol Surg 2001;27:133–6.

The British Journal of Radiology, 78 (2005), 147–149
DOI: 10.1259/bjr/13913517

Short communication

Technical report: use of ultrasound guidance in the removal of tunnelled venous access catheter cuffs

A M BARNACLE, MRCP, FRCR and A W M MITCHELL, FRCS, FRCR

Department of Radiology, Charing Cross Hospital, Fulham Palace Road, London W6 8RF, UK

Abstract. Venous access catheters are employed for a wide variety of reasons. On removal of the catheter, the subcutaneous catheter cuff can be difficult to extract; retention of the cuff has recognized complications. We describe a simple ultrasound technique that assists in the identification of the cuff within the subcutaneous tissues, simplifying subsequent cuff removal. This may lead to a reduction in associated complications.

Venous access catheters are used to deliver long-term intravenous therapy such as haemodialysis, plasmapheresis, parenteral nutrition and chemotherapy, and enable venous sampling in patients with poor venous access. The majority of tunnelled devices have a short polyester cuff attached to the catheter that encourages fibrosis and therefore anchorage within the subcutaneous tissues. Similar cuffs are employed in some peritoneal dialysis catheters. This cuff can be difficult to localize and extract from the soft tissues when the catheter is removed. In some cases, this may be due to failure to localize the cuff within the soft tissues during manual traction, particularly in large or oedematous patients. We describe a new technique that aids in the identification of the subcutaneous catheter cuff both prior to catheter removal and following cuff retention.

Background

Catheter removal can be achieved by manual traction or by cutdown. Simple manual traction is the preferred technique in many centres, but results in retention of the cuff in 10–50% of cases [1, 2]. In some instances, a surgical cutdown is performed on to the cuff, under local anaesthetic, at the time of catheter removal [3]. This technique is straightforward when the subcutaneous cuff is palpable or is easily localized during traction. In obese or oedematous patients, identification of the cuff is often difficult and a cutdown procedure in such cases is not without risk.

In the majority of cases, cuff retention is regarded as unfortunate but likely to be inconsequential and the cuff is left within the subcutaneous tissues. However, current guidance by catheter manufacturers states that all catheter cuffs should be removed. The sequelae of retained catheter cuffs are uncommon but well documented. The most common complication is infection, leading to cellulitis, abscess formation or delayed healing [1–4]. Retained venous catheter cuffs have been mistaken for metastatic nodules on chest CT [5] and can cause a wide range of abnormal appearances on mammographic studies [6].

Technique for cuff visualization

The polyester cuff surrounding the catheter or retained within the soft tissues is easily visualized on ultrasound, even in overweight or oedematous individuals. In our practice, we use either a L38/10-5 MHz linear array transducer (portable SonoSite 180Plus, SonoSite Ltd, Herts, UK) or a L12-5 MHz linear array transducer (HDI 5000; Philips, Croyden, UK). The venous access catheter itself appears as a linear echogenic structure easily differentiated from the surrounding soft tissues (Figure 1). At the site of the cuff, the walls of the catheter become ill defined (Figure 2) and attenuation of the ultrasound beam leads to marked shadowing within the tissues deep to the cuff (Figure 3). These findings are reliable and allow for greater accuracy in cutdown procedures on to the cuff.

Following recent recommendations regarding the use of ultrasound guidance in the insertion of central venous lines, including the NICE guidelines [7], ultrasound equipment should be available in an increasing number of medical departments. The use of ultrasound guidance in selected medical procedures is invaluable and familiarity with ultrasound of the soft tissues should be encouraged. This report illustrates a simple, useful technique for visualization of catheter cuffs both prior to cutdown procedures in obese or oedematous patients in whom cuff localization is not possible and following episodes of cuff retention. This may lead to quicker and easier removal of catheters and a reduction in associated complications. Given the simplicity of the technique and the increasing availability of ultrasound equipment, any technique that has little cost or time implications should be utilized to prevent potential complications.

Received 22 March 2004 and in revised form 2 August 2004, accepted 1 October 2004.

Current address for Dr A M Barnacle, Department of Radiology, Great Ormond Street Hospital for Children, Great Ormond Street, London WC1N 3JH, UK.

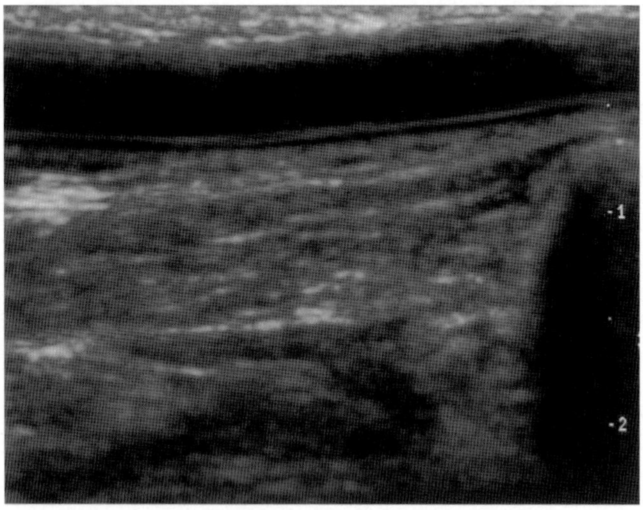

Figure 1. Longitudinal ultrasound image demonstrating the central venous catheter within the subcutaneous tissues of the anterior chest wall, before crossing the clavicle. The echogenic walls of the catheter are well defined and do not cast an acoustic shadow deep to the catheter.

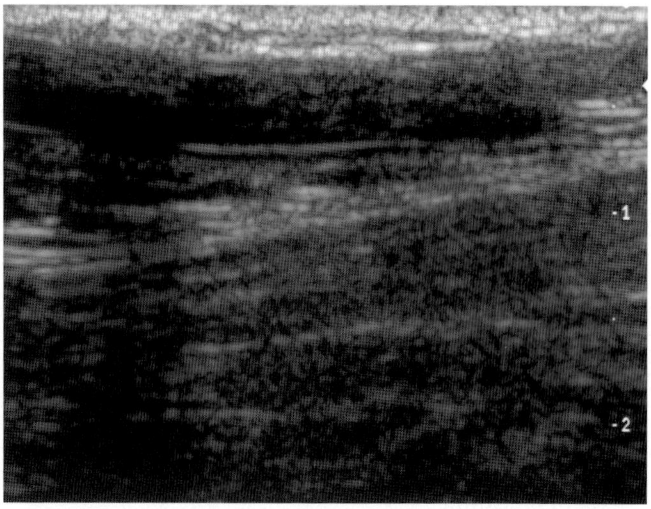

Figure 2. Longitudinal ultrasound image of the catheter demonstrates focal loss of continuity of the well-defined walls at the site of the catheter cuff and marked acoustic shadowing within the soft tissues deep to the cuff.

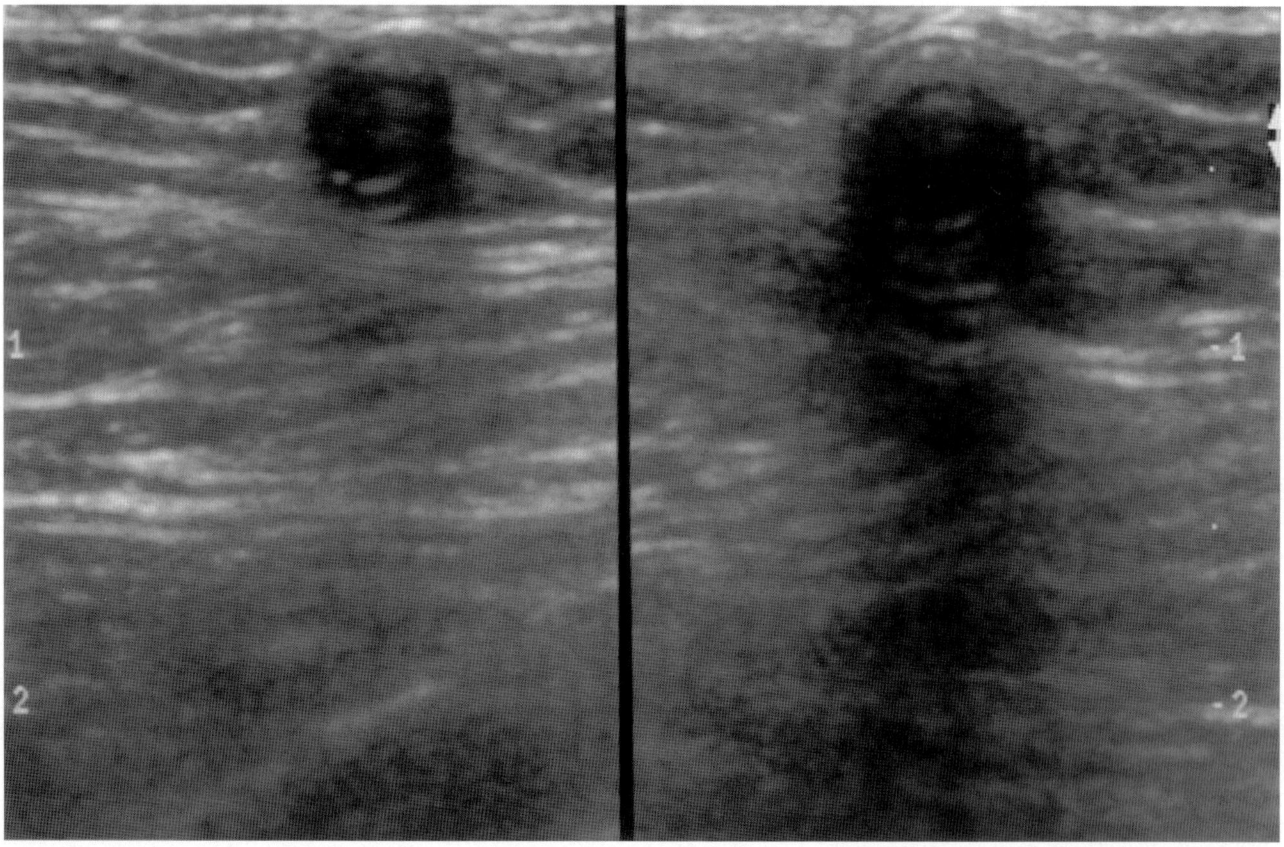

(a) (b)

Figure 3. Transverse ultrasound imaging of (a) the catheter and (b) the cuff shows poor definition and apparent thickening of the walls at the site of the cuff, with dense acoustic shadowing present.

References

1. Kohli MD, Trerotola SO, Namyslowski J, Stecker MS, McLennan G, Patel NH, et al. Outcome of polyester cuff retention following traction removal of tunnelled central venous catheters. Radiology 2001;219:651–4.
2. Fisher WB. Complication of a Hickman line: cutaneous erosion of the Dacron cuff. JAMA 1985;254:2934.
3. Galloway S, Bodenham A. Safe removal of long-term cuffed Hickman-type catheters. Hospital Med 2003;64:20–3.
4. Elkabir JJ, Riaz AA, Agarwal SK, Williams G. Delayed complications following Tenckhoff catheter removal. Nephrol Dial Transplant 1999;14:1550–2.
5. Fernandez GG, Coblentz CL, Cooper C, Sallee DSS. Hickman nodule: a mimic of metastatic disease. Radiology 1989;171:401–2.
6. Ellis RL, Dempsey PJ, Rubin E, Pile NS, Bernreuter WK. Mammography of breasts in which catheter cuffs have been retained: normal, infected and post-operative appearances. AJR Am J Roentgenol 1997;169:713–5.
7. NICE technology appraisal guidance No 49: guidance on the use of ultrasound locating devices for placing central venous catheters. September 2002.

The British Journal of Radiology, 78 (2005), 150–152
DOI: 10.1259/bjr/76700674

Short communication

Late effects of radiotherapy: how to assess and improve outcomes

D A POWER, MRCP, FRCR

Clinical Oncology Department, Charing Cross Hospital, Fulham Palace Road, Hammersmith W6 8RF, UK

The British Institute of Radiology was the venue in May 2004 for an excellent conference addressing issues regarding the recording and analysis of late effects of radiotherapy treatments. Currently there is increasing interest in radiotherapy dose escalation using conformal treatments and novel therapies such as intensity-modulated radiotherapy. In view of the steep dose–response relationship with radiotherapy, dose escalation can be dangerous unless undertaken carefully with accurate reporting of late serious adverse effects, so that the therapeutic ratio of treatments can be determined. The meeting attempted to address issues around assessment of treatment outcomes with a view to consensus regarding current and future practice.

Professor Anne Barrett outlined some of the work in this area achieved by the Recording, Education and Amelioration of the Consequences of Treatment group (REACT). REACT was set up under the auspices of the European ESQUIRE Project [1]. ESQUIRE is co-ordinated by the European Society for Therapeutic Radiology and Oncology with the objective of improving treatment outcomes for cancer patients by addressing various facets of radiotherapy implementation and training. Currently there are a variety of systems in place for the recording of late effects of treatment, including from the RTOG/EORTC, NCI-CTC3 (Common Toxicity Criteria) and the Anglo-Franco system, in addition to inhouse non-validated approaches. Professor Barrett also presented results of an audit undertaken of follow-up practice in Europe. Four centres in the UK were involved in this study. In over 50% of visits patients and doctors reported disease or treatment related problems. There was an attribution bias in patients who, compared with doctors, were more likely to consider their problems related to disease than treatment. The use of a short scale to assess late morbidity of treatment, developed by Professors Dische and Saunders (Table 1), increased the recording of side effects from 23% before the study, to 90% [2]. Grade 3 or 4 late morbidity was reported to be in the range of 4–9%.

Detailed recording of late effects is difficult, given the complexity and time pressures existing in clinics. The LENT SOMA system is one of the most common systems for recording late effects [3]. It is recognized as being an extremely useful tool, as it includes both subjective as well as objective scoring measures, but is cumbersome and difficult to use in daily practice. Dr Susan Davidson from the Christie Hospital, Manchester, discussed their experience of the use of the LENT SOMA system for analysing late effects of radiotherapy treatment. There remain problems in defining what "acceptable toxicity" is, and this varies depending on whether it is a medical or patient view. Validated systems for assessing late effects need to be sensitive, reproducible, feasible and convenient. Although the LENT SOMA system has many of these features, it still could be improved further. The Christie Hospital has developed patient questionnaires based on the LENT SOMA for certain tumour sites, and suggest these could be developed into more useful tools. Details of these questionnaires can be found at: www.christie.nhs.uk/proinfo/departments/clinical_oncology/lent_soma.htm

What was clear is that the use of different reporting systems across the UK, Europe and worldwide makes cross comparisons of differing treatments difficult. This lack of a standardized approach was a theme throughout the conference, as was the need to simplify data collection and educate regarding the importance of recording late effects.

Dr Catharine West, from the Christie Hospital, tried to address the question of whether it is possible to predict normal tissue effects of radiotherapy in advance of treatment. She provided an excellent historical overview of the development of radiobiology understanding through the 20th century to the modern day. Recent developments make the possibility of predictive assays tangible, although as yet not practicable. In the post genomic

Table 1. Influence of the adverse effects due to cancer treatment upon the patient's life: a simple recording system [2]

0	No effect that can be related to cancer treatment or an effect so mild that it requires no regular medication or other healthcare intervention and does not interfere with normal life
1	Mild effects related to cancer treatment that are entirely or almost entirely controlled by medicine and/or other healthcare intervention and do not lead to anything more that a minor alteration in lifestyle
2	Moderate adverse effects related to cancer treatment, that requires continued use of medicine and/or health care intervention. The patient remains able to lead an independent existence although some modifications in activity and in style of living are necessary
3	Severe adverse effects. The patient's life is considerably affected by the adverse effects related to cancer treatment with a considerable and continued restriction of activities. Inpatient care and major surgery may have been required

Received 29 June 2004, accepted 8 October 2004.

era, the concept of radiosensitivity is changing. Rather than mutations in a few DNA damage recognition and repair genes being responsible for intrinsic radiosensitivity, it is recognized that single gene inherent variation has more of a role to play (single nucleotide pleomorphisms). Identifying these variations and their implications on treatment related morbidity depends critically on the presence of a universally accepted tool for recording these late effects.

Sara Faithfull, from the European Institute of Health and Medical Sciences, and Dr Jane Maher from Mount Vernon Hospital, reflected on the current state of follow-up practice in the UK and the future challenges of developing patient care pathways. Different institutions have varying strategies with no consensus as to best practice. Follow-up places a large burden on limited resources. With growing cohorts of long-term surviving cancer patients, this burden is increasing. There are several traditional "medical" aims of follow-up. Specifically we aim to detect tumour recurrence early, assess effectiveness of treatment and record late morbidity of a treatment regimen. Patient expectations of follow-up can differ. They wish to define what is "normal" following treatment, to manage chronic health problems, to deal with psychosocial issues and social consequences of diagnosis and treatment. There are problems with our current practice and we need to consider service redesign and innovative strategies to encompass the aims of follow-up in the challenging new consumer driven environment. Nurse or radiographer led follow-up may be one of these approaches. Future follow-up may rely more on patient self-assessment and reporting of symptoms, with less emphasis on "routine" investigations. Particularly as there is little consensus or evidence as to which tests to do when, except in a minority of tumour sites. Technology, such as using the Internet for patient self reporting, may become routine. New care pathways need also to be seen in a different context. With an ageing population, and increased cancer survival, follow-up will not simply be about assessing the impact of radiotherapy treatments, but dealing with complex medical problems. "Chronically ill people have multiple diagnoses, none of which are particularly revealing about the aggregate severity of illness" (Lyn, 2003). Traditional models of follow-up will have to change.

Dr Jervoise Andreyev from Chelsea and Westminster Hospital and Imperial College, highlighted the importance of multidisciplinary approaches to the management of late effects, from the perspective of a gastroenterologist with specialist interest in this area. The most common symptoms precipitating referral for further investigation are rectal bleeding, urgency and frequency, and tenesmus causing significant problems impacting on quality of life. Faecal incontinence or leakage is a common symptom, frequently under-reported by patients and rarely an indication from clinicians for referral. Current late effect symptom measures are poor in assessing this particular side effect. While often these symptoms are automatically assumed to be due to prior radiotherapy, there is frequently another unrelated diagnosis, which may be amenable to treatment. In his personal experience of managing 257 patients, 12% had underlying neoplasia on further investigation, either disease recurrence or a new secondary tumour. Another diagnosis was made in 38% of patients. There may be simple measures that can be undertaken which may provide symptomatic relief. The input of specialists with in interest in the management of the late effects of radiotherapy will facilitate the development of new treatments, for example, in the management of faecal incontinence.

Professor Andrew Trotti, from the H Lee Moffitt Cancer Centre, USA, gave us a view of the recording and analysis of late effects from an American perspective. He has been in involved in the development of the National Cancer Institutes' Common Toxicity Criteria for grading side effects. The evolution of the multiplicity of grading systems was outlined culminating in the latest NCI common toxicity criteria system version 3 [4]. This latest version is the most comprehensive grading system to date, with 570 items, covering both acute and late effects. These systems generate plentiful data, but several issues arise with respect to further processing of this information. There are computer software systems in development to facilitate data collection. Even once the data are collected, the methodology of data presentation to allow cross comparison of treatments still has to be clarified. As we have CONSORT guidelines for reporting of studies, the aim is to develop similar standards for the reporting of late effects. The Adverse Events in Radiation Oncology Group (AERO) is one group attempting to address this issue. Another initiative is to develop a method for classifying treatment risks, analogous to the UICC TNM classification system used for tumour staging. "TAME" would aim to reflect aggregate risk of treatment by defining T, acute toxicity; A, adverse late effects; M, mortality; and E, end results. This information would help to standardize discussion with patients regarding treatment risk and benefit. It will be interesting to see how this initiative develops.

Ultimately there is further need for international consensus as to the best methods of data collection, which should be validated, sensitive, reproducible and user friendly. While the consensus is being defined, it is still essential we continue to collect data on late effects to assess the therapeutic ratio of our treatments. The Dische and Saunders short scale for toxicity assessment may be a useful initial tool for routine clinic follow-up given the current burdens on time and resources [2]. The LENT SOMA system is a comprehensive system and provides much information, but is difficult to implement in routine practice outside of clinical studies. Information technology certainly will facilitate future data collection, but there are cost implications of new software development and implementation. It is important to continue to push for co-ordinated approaches to late toxicity data collection at a National and International Level. The National Cancer Research Network is one of the forums to take these issues further. Patient care pathways will also need to develop and change in the context of an ageing population and increased numbers of patients on "follow-up". Novel strategies will be required for the recording of toxicity data as the "traditional" mode of follow-up changes. Projects such as REACT are aiming to develop international consensus on the recording and of reporting radiotherapy treatment outcome and will hopefully help to clarify these issues further.

References

1. http://www.estro.be/estro/Index.html (ESQUIRE)
2. Dische S, Saunders MI. Complexity and simplicity in the measurement and recording of adverse effects of cancer treatment. Radiother Oncol 2003;66:249–51.
3. Pavy JJ, Denekamp J, Letschert J, et al. EORTC late effects working group. Late effects toxicity scoring: the SOMA scale. Radiother Oncol 1995;35:11–60.
4. http://www.ctep.cancer.gov/reporting/ctc.html

The British Journal of Radiology, *78* (2005), 153–157
DOI: 10.1259/bjr/27500851

Case report
Xanthoma disseminatum: a case report and literature review

[1]A S ALEXANDER, MD, [2]R TURNER, MDCM, FRCP(C), [3]L UNIATE, MD, FRCS(C) and [1]R G PEARCY, MBBS, FRCP(C)

[1]*Department of Oncology, Division of Radiaion Oncology and* [2]*Department of Oncology, Division of Medical Oncology, Cross Cancer Institute, University of Alberta, 11560 Univerisity Avenue, Edmonton, Alberta T6G 1Z1 and* [3]*Department of Ophthamology, University of Alberta, Edmonton, Alberta, Canada*

Abstract. This case report describes the neuro-opthalmologic and respiratory manifestations of xanthoma disseminatum, a rare histiocytosis syndrome characterized by disseminated lesions in a young male adult. Multimodality management of this disease, including the role of local radiotherapy, is discussed accompanied by a review of the literature.

Xanthoma disseminatum (XD) is a rare, benign proliferative disorder in children and adults characterized by disseminated xanthomatous lesions [1]. Since this condition was first described in 1938 by Montgomery and Osterberg [2], only approximately 100 cases have been reported in the literature [3]. Categorised as a histiocytosis syndrome, XD shares the common feature of mononuclear phagocyte proliferation [4–7]. XD typically involves the skin, particularly the flexor skin folds and eyelids [8]. XD may also manifest in the central nervous system (CNS), ocular structures, and respiratory and gastrointestinal tracts [9].

While the natural history of XD is usually benign with spontaneous resolution of cutaneous lesions over 2–40 years [8, 10], lesions in critical anatomical locations may result in morbidity and mortality [1, 11]. Curative therapy for XD is lacking. While symptomatic lesions may be managed with conservative surgery, the roles of radiotherapy (RT) and chemotherapy are unclear [12–16].

We report a complex case of XD in a young male subject that illustrates the neuro-ophthalmologic and respiratory manifestations of the disease. The case highlights the importance of a multimodality approach in supportive management and describes the use of RT in stabilizing symptomatic lesions.

A review of the published literature on XD is also included; a medline search was conducted to find all articles, in all languages on XD, from 1966 to 2003. Medical subject headings (MeSH) used to search the medline database included histiocytosis syndromes, including subheadings of pathophysiology, drug therapy, radiotherapy and surgery, as well as keyword search using "xanthoma disseminatum". A total of 591 articles were originally identified. Limiting the findings to human data and English language reduced the number of publications to 448. Titles and abstracts of potentially relevant articles were reviewed by a single author. To be accepted in the review, publications had to include data on the pathophysiology of XD, patients with CNS XD lesions, or case reports/case series involving the therapeutic management of the condition.

Received 15 March 2004 and in revised form 13 August 2004, accepted 11 October 2004.

Methods of diagnosis

The patient was diagnosed with XD on September 1999 at the age of 18 years after an initial presentation with vision loss, polyuria, polydipsia, and yellow-brown papules involving the face, eyelids, neck and trunk. MRI of the brain revealed multiple foci of abnormally high signal lesions measuring <1 cm involving the pons, cerebellum, temporal horns, pituitary fossa and right optic nerve (Figure 1). Laboratory studies confirmed the presence of central diabetes insipidus (DI), a blunted luteinizing hormone response, but otherwise normal pituitary hormone levels. Biopsy of a cutaneous chest wall lesion revealed benign dermal histiocytes. Touton and foreign body giant cells were identified causing nodular expansion of the dermis. Langerhans cell histiocytosis (LCH) was ruled out in the absence of Birbeck granules on electron microscopy. Immunohistochemistry was positive for CD68 and negative for S-100. Based on these clinical and pathological findings, a diagnosis of XD was established.

Case

Prior to the XD diagnosis, the patient's past medical history was significant for tibial osteogenic sarcoma diagnosed at age 13 years, treated on a trial protocol with pre- and post-operative chemotherapy (etoposide, cisplatin, adriamycin, ifosfamide) in conjunction with surgery. Complete clinical and radiographic response was achieved with no evidence of recurrent sarcoma at subsequent follow-up.

After the diagnosis of XD, the patient received DDAVP nasal spray therapy with improvement of his DI but a trial of high dose prednisone failed to improve his vision. In the spring of 2001, he was referred to the Radiation Oncology Department at the Cross Cancer Institute with bilateral central vision loss, confirmed on visual field (VF) testing. MRI of May 2001 revealed displacement of the optic chiasm inferiorly by a mass arising from the optic pathway and foreshortening of both optic nerves. Multiple

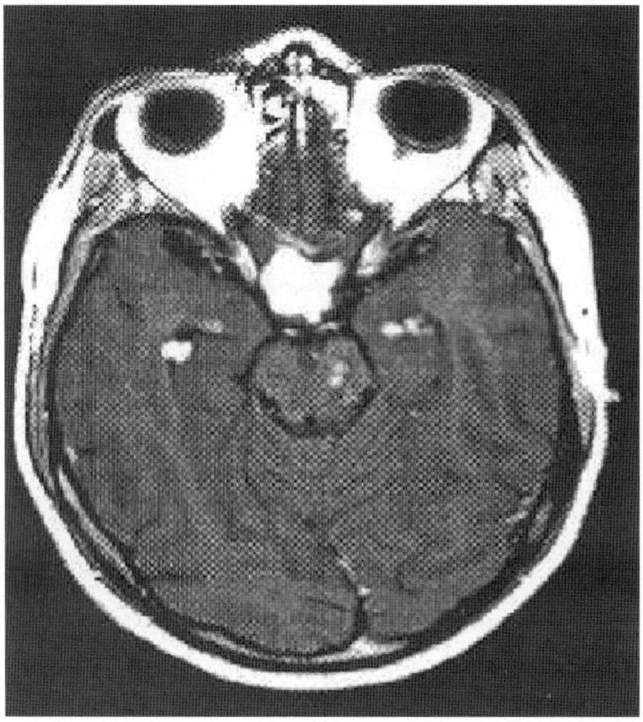

(a)

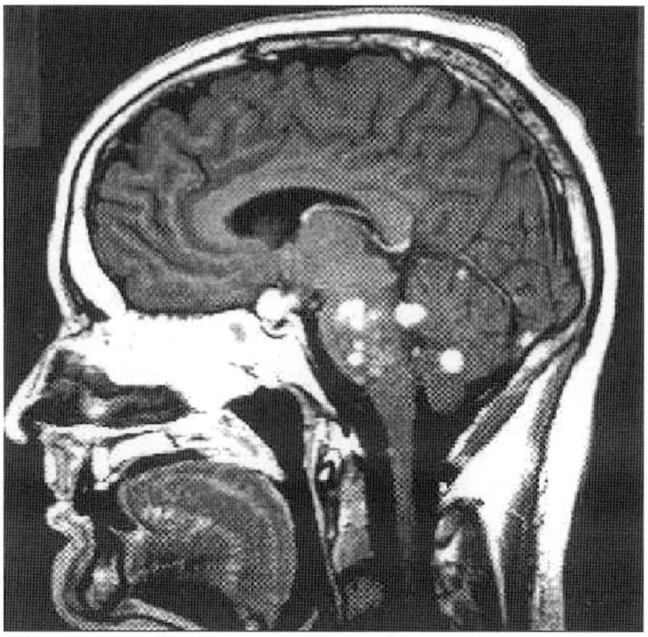

(b)

Figure 1. (a) Transverse and (b) sagittal spin echo MRI images of the brain demonstrating multiple lesions in the pons, cerebellum, temporal horns, pituitary fossa and right optic nerve.

enhancing foci were noted in the pons, the cerebellar hemispheres, and the lateral ventricles. Repeat MRI of the brain 1 month later showed disease progression, accompanied by worsened vision, right hearing loss, and ataxia. A 1 week trial of intravenous cladribine was administered resulting in slight clinical improvement in vision. Given the severe, progressive vision loss and a neurosurgical opinion that resection was not feasible, the decision was made to manage the chiasm mass with radiotherapy. The patient was started on dexamethasone 4 mg po TID to prevent acute RT-induced cerebral oedema. He then underwent pre-treatment CT planning in the supine position with Perspex shell immobilization. The RT course was delivered in two phases using a 6 MV linear accelerator. Phase I consisted of a pair of parallel opposed (POP) fields encompassing the chiasm, the suprachiasmatic mass and pituitary contents, plus a 2 cm margin. The prescribed dose was 16 Gy in 8 daily fractions over 1½ weeks. Phase II consisted of a reduced field boost to the chiasm and suprachiasmatic mass with a 1 cm margin, using a 3-field beam arrangement, for an additional 14 Gy in 9 fractions over 2 weeks. VF testing early in therapy showed only a small island of vision in the right eye, and worsening of the temporal field in the left eye (Figure 2a). Following RT completion, vision in the left eye stabilized, with mild improvement in the right eye (Figure 2b) Over the subsequent 4 months, continued objective improvement was demonstrated on VF testing (Figure 2c,d) accompanied by subjective improvement in vision. Although the patient's vision stabilized, his driver's license was revoked due to the lack of 120° of peripheral vision.

Later that year the patient developed back pain, leg weakness and altered sensation. An intramedullary lesion from T6–T9 was demonstrated on MRI and was surgically treated with resection and laminectomy which restored motor and sensory function In the spring of 2001 the patient developed dyspnoea and stridor confirmed on endoscopy and biopsy to be secondary to XD causing subglottic stenosis. The stenosis was managed with surgical dilatation with symptomatic relief but the patient required further repeated dilatations for recurrent airway symptoms in the subsequent months.

5 months after RT to the chiasm, the patient experienced neurological deterioration with worsening ataxia from cerebellar disease progression. A trial of intrathecal cytarbine, prednisone and etoposide was unsuccessful. Beginning in May 2002 the patient underwent RT to the posterior fossa with lateral photon fields, 21 Gy in 15 daily fractions. MRI after RT demonstrated stabilization of the brainstem and cerebellar disease with continued local control of the pituitary mass.

In November 2002, the patient developed further bronchial lesions, not amenable to surgical management. Palliative RT was again used to treat the larynx, trachea, carina, and main stem bronchi with 15 Gy in 10 daily fractions. 2 months later, although the respiratory disease was stable clinically and radiologically, the pituitary lesion progressed after 1½ years of control. The patient died in March 2003, of presumed respiratory failure. No autopsy was performed. The likely causes of death include airway obstruction or pulmonary embolus.

Discussion

The present report illustrates a devastating course of XD in a young adult, characterized by progressive CNS and airway disease leading to numerous clinical problems. Chemotherapeutic agents and steroids produced little

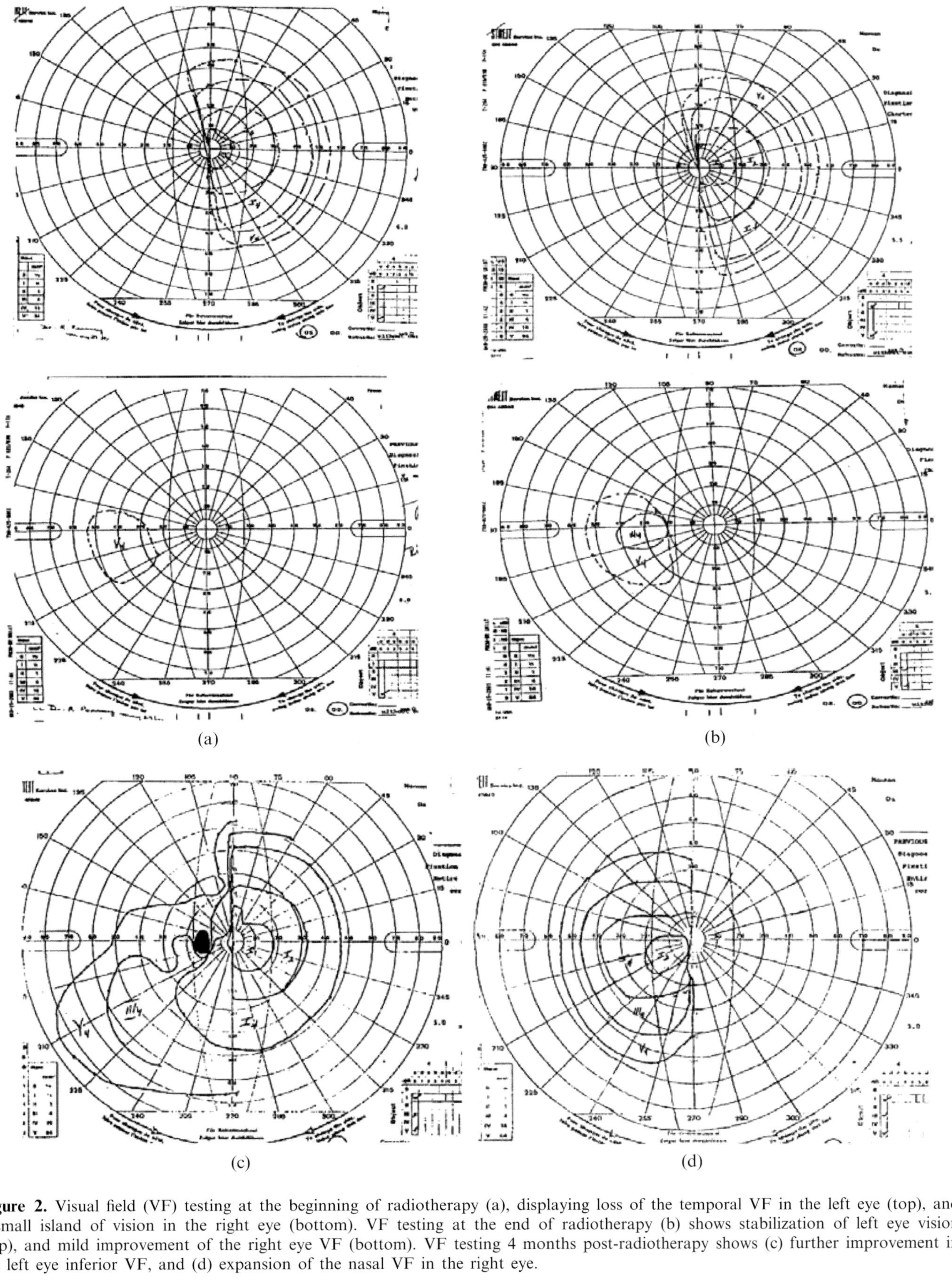

(a) (b)

(c) (d)

Figure 2. Visual field (VF) testing at the beginning of radiotherapy (a), displaying loss of the temporal VF in the left eye (top), and a small island of vision in the right eye (bottom). VF testing at the end of radiotherapy (b) shows stabilization of left eye vision (top), and mild improvement of the right eye VF (bottom). VF testing 4 months post-radiotherapy shows (c) further improvement in the left eye inferior VF, and (d) expansion of the nasal VF in the right eye.

Table 1. Summary of the results of treatment of symptomatic xanthoma disseminatum lesions with various modalities from published case series and reports

	CR	PR	SD	PD	Reference
Chemotherapy (*n*=8)	1/8	2/8	1/8	4/8	[8], [9], [25], [26], [31]
Clofibrate (*n*=3)	—	1/3	1/3	1/3	[8], [22], [28]
Radiotherapy (*n*=4)	—	2/4	—	2/4	[9], [10], [27], [32]
Steroids only (*n*=2)	—	1/2	—	1/2	[8], [25]
Surgery (*n*=4)	1/4	3/4	—	—	[8], [24], [33], [34]
Surgery + chemotherapy (*n*=1)	1/1	—	—	—	[35]

CR, complete response (complete resolution of lesion); PR, partial response (measurable decrease in lesion size); SD, stable disease (no change in size of lesion); PD, progressive disease (measurable increase in lesion size).

objective response. Surgical dilatation was useful to relieve respiratory tract obstruction. For lesions involving critical structures including the CNS and respiratory tract that were not amenable to surgical intervention, local RT temporarily provided symptom control and stabilization of disease progression.

The diagnosis of XD is based on pathological and clinical grounds. Biopsy findings of histiocytic proliferation suggest a histiocytic disorder. Immunophenotyping and ultrastructural studies are required to establish the diagnosis. CD68 positivity supports a histiocytic origin [17]. Absence of S-100 binding and Birbeck granules on electron microscopy rules out LCH [4, 18–20], an important diagnostic consideration since LCH is responsive to cytostatic therapy [17]. Touton giant cells represent an exaggerated xanthomatoid reaction pattern [21] are typical of xanthomatous histiocytoses and are absent in LCH [9, 22, 23]. These pathological findings, along with the clinical manifestations involving the skin, CNS, eyes, and respiratory tract are all consistent with a diagnosis of XD.

Numerous systemic modalities have been utilized in attempts to manage the disease, but none have proven particularly successful. Table 1 summarizes the results of published case series and reports utilizing various treatment modalities. While corticosteroids may produce rare responses [24], most reports utilize steroids in combination with other therapies; the efficacy of steroid monotherapy appears dubious [8, 25–27]. Occasional responses have been observed with the anti-lipemic agent clofibrate [22, 25, 28]. Antineoplastic agents including vinca alkaloids, alkylating agent, and anti-metabolites generally produce little objective responses in the limited number of reported cases [9, 10, 16, 29, 30]. Stojkovic [31] reported symptomatic improvement in a young female with non-LCH CNS lesions treated with combined corticosteroid and chemotherapy.

Reports of local management for XD are also characterized by diverse approaches with various results [9, 10, 29]. Cryotherapy for single lesions has not been successful [26]. Surgery appears to give the best results for readily accessible lesions [8, 24, 33, 34]. The effectiveness of RT is unclear due to the limited number of cases reporting conflicting results. Mahrel et al [27] found no improvement in pituitary XD lesions in an adult male using an RT dose of 18 Gy combined with steroids. Another report described a lack of response after external beam RT to cutaneous XD lesions involving the face and neck [32]. In contrast, Moloney [9] reported one case where airway disease control was achieved after Cobalt irradiation to a dose of 34 Gy over 22 days. Additionally, RT has shown promise in the treatment of juvenile xanthogranuloma, a non-LCH condition pathologically similar to XD [30]. It is important to note that for all therapeutic modalities, the duration of response is extremely variable.

The present report suggests that RT has a role in palliating local symptoms caused by unresectable lesions invading critical structures in the CNS and respiratory tract. An objective response to RT, as illustrated by serial visual field testing, was demonstrated in this case. However, reports of clinical responses must be interpreted with caution since XD has the potential to undergo spontaneous resolution. Caputo et al [8] reported three classifications of XD characterized by their evolution and prognosis: a self-healing form, which typically regresses without intervention, a persistent form and a progressive form. From the clinical course and pattern of spread, our patient most likely suffered the progressive form, thus it is unlikely that spontaneous regression was responsible for the observed clinical response to radiotherapy.

Acknowledging the difficulty in defining the optimal RT dose and fractionation for XD due its rarity, given the benign histology and potential for a prolonged clinical course, relatively low dose fractionated courses to symptomatic lesions would be reasonable to minimize the risks of late normal tissue toxicities. The objective and subjective clinical response achieved in the present case employing contemporary radiotherapy equipment and techniques suggests that targeted RT to doses of 20–30 Gy in 1.4–1.8 Gy per fraction is safe, well-tolerated, and capable of disease stablization and symptom control.

References

1. Giller R, et al. Xanthoma disseminatum: an unusual histiocytosis syndrome. Am J Pediatric Hematology/Oncology 1988;10:252–7.
2. Montgomery H, Osterberg A. Xanthomatous correlation of clinical, histopathalogical, and chemical studies of cutaneous xanthoma. Arch Dermatol Syphilol 1938;37:373–402.
3. Zeleger B, Cerio R, Orchard G, et al. Histologic and immunohistochmical study comparing xanthoma disseminatum and histiocytosis X. Arch Dermatol 1992;128:1207–12.
4. Casset F, Nezlof C, Ferrans V. The histiocytosis. Pathol Ann 1982;27–78.
5. Crocker A. The histiocytoses syndromes. In: Fitzpatrick TB, Eisen AZ, Wolff R, Freedberg IM, Austen FF, editors. Dermatology in general medicine. New York: McGraw-Hill, 1987:1937–46.

6. Favara B. The pathology of the histiocytoses. Am J Pediatric Hematology/Oncology 1981;3:45–56.
7. Roper SS, Spraker MK. Cutaneous histiocytosis syndromes. Pediatric Dermatology 1985;3:19–30.
8. Caputo R, et al. The various clinical patterns of xanthoma disseminatum: consideration of 7 cases and review of the literature. Dermatology 1995;190:19–24.
9. Moloney JR. Xanthoma disseminatum: its otolaryngological manifestations. J Laryngol Otology 1979;93:201–10.
10. Flach DB, Winkleman RK. Juvenile xanthogranuloma with CNS lesions. J Am Acad Dermatol 1986;14:405–11.
11. Davies CWE, Juniper MC, Wojnorowka F, Benson MK. Xanthoma disseminatum with respiratory involvement and fatal outcome. Thorax 2000;55:170–2.
12. Greenberger JS, et al. Radiation therapy in patients with histiocytosis: management of diabetes insipidus and bone lesions. Int J Radiat Oncol Biol Phys 1979;5:1749–55.
13. Greenberger JS, et al. Results of the treatment of 127 patients with systemic histiocytosis. Medicine 1981;60: 311–38.
14. Lahey ME. Histiocytosis X: comparison of 3 treatment regimens. J Pediatr 1975;87:179–83.
15. Urbano-Marquez A, et al. Etoposide in the treatment of multifocal eosinophillic granuloma. Cancer Treatment Rep 1985;69:238–9.
16. Burgdorf WHC, Duray P, Rosai J. Immunohistochemical identification of lysozyme in cutaneous lesions of alleged histiocytic nature. Am J Clin Path 1981;75:162–7.
17. Weiss N, Keller C. Xanthoma disseminatum: a rare normolipemic xanthomatosis. Clinical Investigator 1993;71: 233–8.
18. Writing group of the histiocytosis society. Histiocytosis syndromes in children. Lancet 1987;1:208–9.
19. McMillan EM, et al. Analysis of histiocytosis X infiltrates with monoclonal antibodies directed against cells of histiocytic, lymphoid, and myeliod lineage. Clin Immunol Immunopath 1986;38:295–301.
20. Harrist TJ, et al. Histiocytosis X: in situ characterization of cutanwous infiltrates with monclonal antibodies. Am J Clin Path 1983;70:204–300.
21. Zelger B, Sidoroff A, Orchard G, Cerio R. Non-Langerhans cell histiocytoses: a new unifying concept. Am J Dermatopathol 1996;18:490–504.
22. Kumakiri M, et al. Xanthoma disseminatum: report of a case with histologic and ultrastructural studies of skin lesions. J Am Acad Dermatol 1983;4:291–9.
23. Blobstein SH, Caldwell D, Carter M. Bone lesions in xanthoma disseminatum. Arch Dermatol 1985;121:1313–7.
24. Kalz F, Hoffman MM, Lafrance A. Xanthoma disseminatum – clinical & laboratory observations over a ten year period. Dermatologica 1970;140:129–41.
25. Nanda A, et al. Xanthoma disseminatum. Int J Dermatology 1990;29:727–8.
26. Kuligowski M, et al. Xanthoma disseminatum. Int J Derm 1992;31:281–3.
27. Manhrel R, et al. Problems in the differential diagnosis of non-Langerhans cell histiocytosis with pituitary involvment: case report and review of the literature. Endocrine Pathology 2002;13:363–8.
28. Miskel MA, Cocksott P, Nazir DJ, et al. Xanthoma disseminatum: clinical, metabolic, pathologic, and radiologic aspects. Arch Dermatol 1977;113:1094–100.
29. Leibman SD, et al. Corneal xanthomas in childhood. Arch Ophthalmol 1966;76:221–9.
30. Aristizabal S, Runyon T. Radiotherapy for unusual benign disease. Int J Radiat Oncol Biol Phys 1983;7:1437–40.
31. Stojkovic T, et al. Atypical form of non-Langerhans histiocytosis with disseminated brain and leptomeningeal lesions. J Neurol Neurosurg Psychiatry 2000;69:675–8.
32. Finney W, Montgomery H, New GB. Xanthoma multiplex: two cases in volving the larynx and trachea and associated with diabetes insipidus. JAMA 1932;99:1071–4.
33. Hammond RR, Mackenzie IR. Xanthoma disseminatum with massive intracranial involvement. Clin Neuropathol 1995;14: 314–21.
34. Cauro F, Houtteville JP, Mesnil JL, Guarnieri J. Cerebellar, pulmonary, and cutaneous localizations of juvenile xanthogranuloma. Ann Dematol Venereol 2002;129:307–10.
35. Rampini P, et al. Isolated cervival juvenile xanthogranuloma in childhood. Spine 2001;26:1392–5.

The British Journal of Radiology, 78 (2005), 158–160
DOI: 10.1259/bjr/33263789

Case report

Visceral leishmaniasis: diagnosis by ultrasound-guided fine needle aspiration of an axillary node

[1]M REUS, MD, PhD, [2]B GARCÍA, MD, PhD, [1]V VÁZQUEZ, MD, [1]D MORALES, MD, [1]M FUSTER, MD and [3]J SOLA, MD

Departments of [1]Radiology, [2]Internal Medicine and [3]Cytology, Hospital Universitario "Virgen de la Arrixaca", 30120 El Palmar (Murcia), Spain

Abstract. A 77-year-old woman presented with fever up to 39°C and acute pain in the left upper quadrant and renal fossa. Full blood count and biochemical screen revealed a haemoglobin (Hb) of 9.8 g dl^{-1}, an increased erythrocyte sedimentation rate and an elevated lactate dehydrogenase, all other parameters were normal. Thoracic and abdominal CT demonstrated two enlarged lymph nodes in the left axilla, and splenic infarcts. Ultrasound-guided fine needle aspiration of one of the axillary lymph nodes revealed macrophages filled with leishmanias.

Visceral leishmaniasis (VL), known also as Kala-azar, is a chronic infectious disease caused by a protozoan parasite of the genus leishmania; it is transmitted by fly bite [1]. It is endemic in the Indian subcontinent, East Africa, South America, South Texas and in the Mediterranean region. Commonly, patients with VL present with fever, abdominal pain, splenomegaly, hepatomegaly, cachexia, and pancytopenia [2]. We present a case of VL with multiple splenic infarcts, left axillary lymphadenopathy, without pancytopenia, diagnosed by means of ultrasound-guided (US-guided) fine needle aspiration cytology of the axillary lymph nodes.

Case report

A 77-year-old woman presented with an 11 day history of shivering, fever up to 39°C, and pain in the left upper quadrant and renal fossa. Despite treatment with cefixime, 400 mg day^{-1}, and ciproxine, 500 mg/12 hourly, the patient remained unwell. On physical examination, she had pale skin and mucus membranes and painless splenomegaly. Her full blood count showed a haemoglobin (Hb) of 9.8 g dl^{-1}, with an increased erythrocyte sedimentation rate and an elevated lactate dehydrogenase. All other laboratory studies were normal.

An abdominal ultrasound demonstrated splenomegaly, and an upper pole triangular hypoechoic area. Thoracic CT (Figure 1) showed two enlarged lymph nodes with maximum transverse diameters of 1.5 cm in the left axilla. Abdominal CT (Figure 2) demonstrated a hypodense triangular segment in the spleen suggestive of ischaemic infarction. A diagnosis of lymphoma was suspected. Aspiration using US-guidance was performed on the axillary lymphadenopathy (Figure 3). This revealed macrophages filled with leishmanias (Figure 4), confirmed using an antileishmania antibody immunofluorescence test. Treatment was initiated with intravenous liposomal amphotericin B, 150 mg day^{-1}, for 10 days. On review at 2 months the patient remained asymptomatic.

Received 21 January 2004 and in final form 4 October 2004, accepted 26 October 2004.

Discussion

VL (Kala-azar) is a protozoal infection common in underdeveloped countries; there are an estimated 500 000 new cases every year and there were 41 000 recorded deaths in the year 2000 [2].

Leishmania infantum is the main cause of VL in the Mediterranean region [2–4]. Infected animals – mainly dogs – are the carriers of the disease in the Mediterranean [5]. An insect bite is the vector of transmission. People from unaffected areas, may contract the disease [6, 7] after visiting endemic areas. Cases of leishmaniasis in overseas travellers and US Gulf War veterans has prompted growing interest in this disease [3, 8]. Factors increasing the risk of clinical development of the disease include malnutrition, immunosuppression, and most importantly, HIV infection [2].

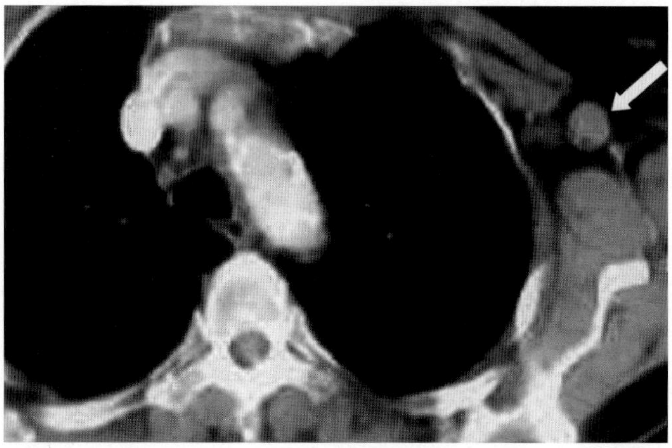

Figure 1. Contrast enhanced thoracic CT showing in the left axillary an enlarged lymph node (arrow).

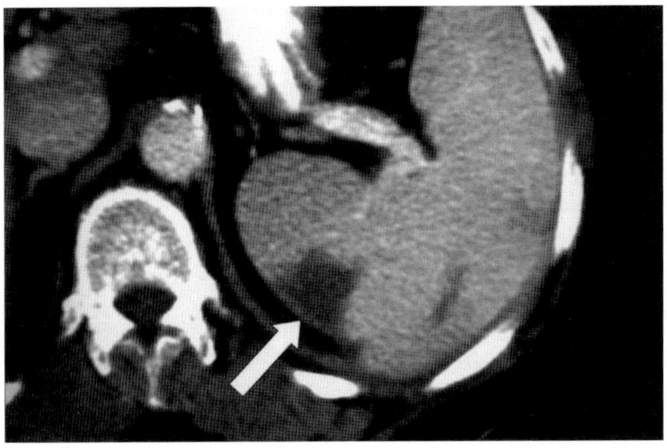

Figure 2. Contrast enhanced abdominal CT scan of the left upper quadrant demonstrated a wedge-shaped area of decreased attenuation in the surface of the spleen (arrow).

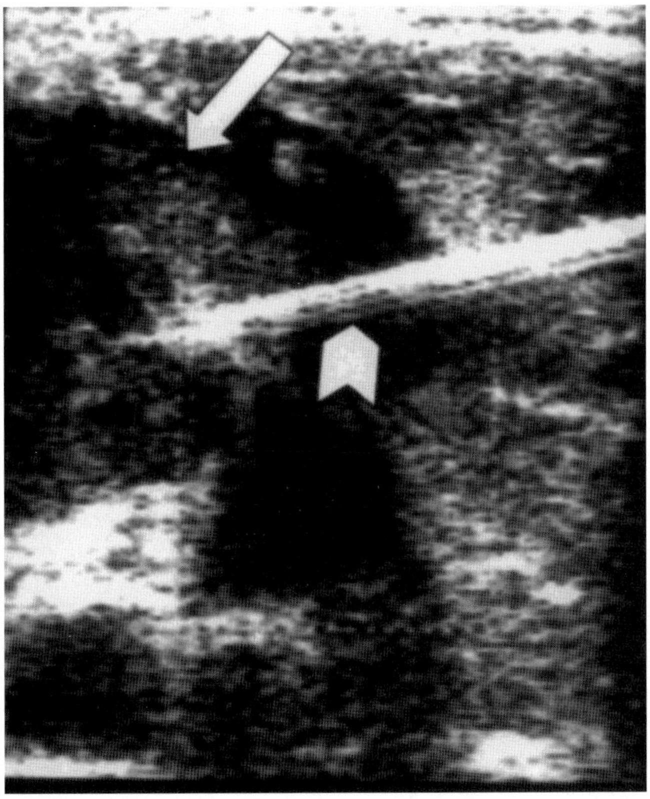

Figure 3. Ultrasound-guided aspiration showing the tip of the needle (arrowhead) inside lymphatic nodule (arrow).

Delay and difficulty in diagnosis are common especially in the early stage of the disease, due to non-specific symptomatology and difficulty in demonstrating intracellular protozoa in tissue aspirates [9]. Intracellular leishmania can be identified from aspirates of spleen, bone marrow, lymph node, or liver [2].

The CT findings of hepatosplenomegaly, and abdominal lymphadenopathy secondary to visceral leishmaniasis has been previously reported [9, 10].

Patients with advanced Kala-azar die without treatment: pentavalent antimony is the main therapeutic agent, but resistance has been reported and there are complications

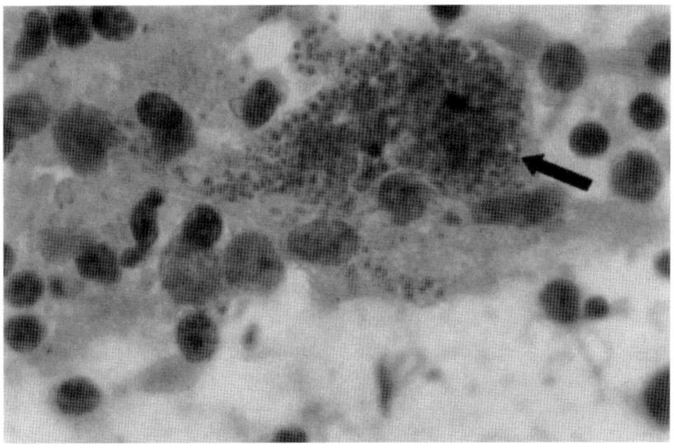

Figure 4. Macrophages containing intracellular leishmanias (black arrow) found in the axyllare lymphadenopathy aspirate (haematoxylin-eosin ×400).

associated with treatment; particularly in cases of associated HIV infection. Liposomal amphotericin B is highly effective against Visceral leishmaniasis [11], even in immunosuppressed patients, but it is expensive [1, 3].

Our case is of interest as presenting with multiple splenic infarcts in VL has not previously been reported [12, 13]. The absence of pancytopenia was also atypical. US-guided aspiration of the axillary lymph nodes was chosen as it is minimally invasive and has a lower risk than aspiration of bone marrow or spleen. Although splenic aspiration is reported to have a sensitivity of 98% [2] in VL.

In conclusion, we suggest that US-guided aspiration of a peripheral lymph node should be considered as a technique to obtain a tissue sample in a patient with suspected VL and peripheral lymphodenopathy, in order to avoid the complications of spleen puncture.

Acknowledgments

The authors thank Lee Boyes, Richard Barbosa, Dolores Abellán and Sally Toft for their review of the English in this manuscript.

References

1. Desjeux P. Human leishmaniases: epidemiology and public health aspect. World Health Stat Q 1992;45:267–75.
2. Guerin PJ, Olliaro P, Sundar S, et al. Visceral leishamniasis: current status of control, diagnosis, and treatment, and a proposed research and development agenda. Lancet lnfect Dis 2002;2:494–501.
3. Herwaldt BL. Leishmaniasis. Lancet 1999;354:1191–9.
4. Berman JD. Human leishmaniasis: clinical, diagnostic, and chemotherapeutic developments in the last 10 years. Clin Infes Dis 1997;16:251–5.
5. Murray HW. Kala-azar—progress against a neglected disease. N Engl J Med 2002;347:1793–4.
6. Granert C, Elinder G, Ost A, Henter JI. Kala-azar in a one year-old Swedish child. Diagnostic difficulties because of active hemophagocytosis. Acta Paediatr 1993;82:794–6.
7. Büyükaşik Y, Ileri NŞ, Haznedaroğlu IC, Demiroğlu H, Dündar S. Fever hepatosplenomegaly, pancytopenia in a patient living in the Mediterreanean region. Postgrad Med J 1998;74:237–41.

8. Pantsan MW, Coleman TA. Images in clinical medicine. Kala-azar. N Engl J Med 2003;349:e13.
9. Cohen D, Fields S. CT findings in visceral leishmaniasis mimichking lymphoma. Comput Med Imaging Graph 1988;12:325–7.
10. Deutch SJ, Sandles MA, Alpern MB. Abdominal lymphadenopathy in benign disease: CT detection. Radiology 1987;163:335–8.
11. Gaeta GB, Maisto A, Di Caprio D, et al. Efficacy of amphotericin B colloidal dispersion in the treatment of Mediterranean visceral leishmaniasis in immunocompetent adult patients. Scand J Infect Dis 2000;32:675–7.
12. Nores M, Phillips EH, Morngestern L, Hiatt JR. The clinical spectrum of splenic infarction. Am Surg 1998;64:182–8.
13. Jaroch MT, Broughan TA, Hermann RE. The natural history of splenic infarction. Surgery 1986;100:743–9.

The British Journal of Radiology, *78* (2005), 161–163
DOI: 10.1259/bjr/68507140

Case report

Renal artery pseudoaneurysm following partial nephrectomy treated with stent-graft

[1]M D HORWITZ, MRCS, [1]D C HANBURY, MS, FRCS (Urol) and [2]C M KING, MRCP, FRCR

Departments of [1]Urology and [2]Radiology, Lister Hospital, Stevenage, Hertfordshire SG1 4AB, UK

Abstract. Haemorrhagic complications due to pseudoaneurysms of branch arteries can be treated by selective embolisation. Injuries to the main renal artery cannot be treated in this way without sacrificing the kidney. We report the successful percutaneous treatment of a main renal artery pseudoaneurysm with a stent-graft in a patient with a solitary kidney.

A 58-year-old man presented with frank haematuria and left sided flank pain. Renal ultrasound and CT showed bilateral 6 cm solid renal tumours; upper pole on the right and mid pole on the left (Figure 1). Pre-operative arteriography demonstrated a single right renal artery bifurcating approximately 3 cm from the aorta. The position of the left sided tumour made nephron sparing surgery impossible. An immediate left radical nephrectomy was therefore performed.

7 weeks later the patient underwent a right upper pole partial nephrectomy. The tumour was found to be adherent to the adrenal gland, main hilar vessels and a disc of peritoneum. The calices and vessels were oversewn and the renal defect closed in a standard manner using haemacell rolls tied over with 2/0 monocryl.

Histology confirmed moderately differentiated clear cell carcinoma on both sides with no capsular or vascular invasion and clear resection margins. The patient made an uneventful recovery, going home on the 9th day with a creatinine of 200 μmol l^{-1} indicating a significant degree of renal impairment consistent with resection of three-quarters of his functioning renal tissue.

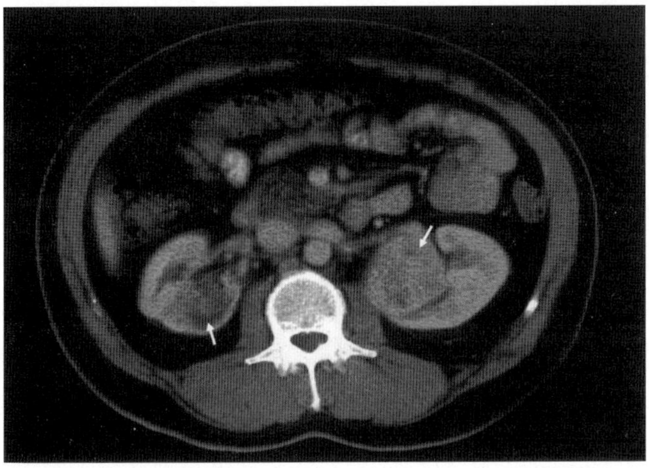

Figure 1. CT of the kidneys following intravenous contrast showing bilateral renal carcinomas.

Received 11 February 2004 and in final form 4 October 2004, accepted 26 October 2004.

On the 11th post-operative day he developed right flank pain, the side of the partial nephrectomy. He was found to be hypotensive by the attending paramedics and was resuscitated with intravenous fluids. On admission his blood pressure was normal and stable and there was a tender mass palpable in the right flank. Ultrasound demonstrated a 13 cm haematoma in this region. As the patient was stable he was initially managed conservatively. His pain resolved and a follow up ultrasound showed no increase in the size of the haematoma. However 5 days later he had further pain and his haemoglobin fell from 10 g dl^{-1} to 8 g dl^{-1} despite a two-unit blood transfusion.

An emergency arteriogram demonstrated a pseudoaneurysm arising from the superior aspect of the main right renal artery, the site of origin of the previous upper pole branch (Figure 2). Embolisation of the main renal artery would have destroyed the remaining kidney so a decision was made to exclude the leak with a covered stent. A 17 mm Jostent peripheral stent graft (Jomed; Abbot Vascular Instruments, Rangendingenn, Germany) was

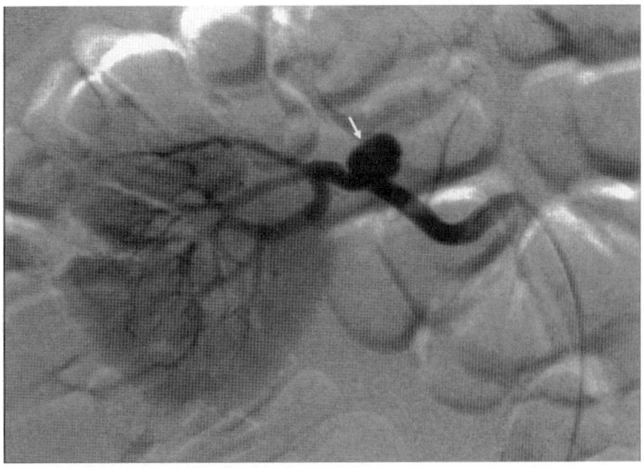

Figure 2. Selective right renal arteriogram (20°C left anterior oblique) showing a pseudoaneurysm arising from the main renal artery. The patient's only remaining renal tissue is demonstrated.

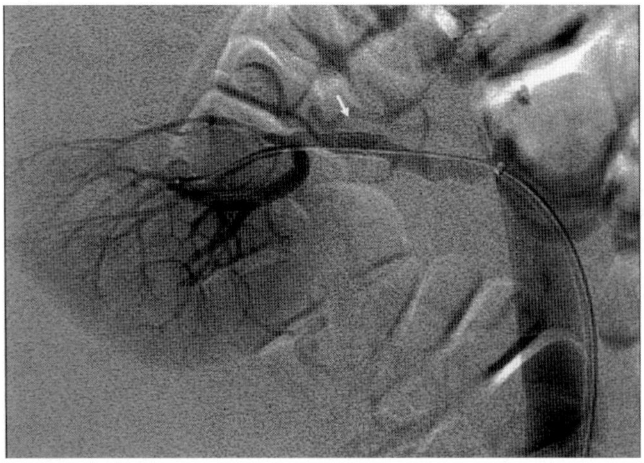

Figure 3. Following deployment of a stent graft, the pseudoaneurysm no longer fills and renal perfusion is maintained (same projection as Figure 2).

hand-crimped onto a 5 mm × 2 cm Cordis Opta-Pro angioplasty balloon (Cordis Europa N.V., Roden, The Netherlands). It was positioned across the defect via a 7 French 40 cm Balkin Introducer Sheath (William Cook Europe, Bjaeverskov). Following deployment the pseudoaneurysm no longer filled but renal perfusion was maintained (Figure 3).

Following the procedure, the patient had no further clinical episodes of bleeding and the haematoma slowly resolved. His creatinine level stabilized and at discharge was 270 μmol l^{-1}. A CT scan at 4 months showed a cystic collection at the site of the previous haematoma with some mural calcification, but no evidence of pseudoaneurysm or tumour recurrence. The patient has remained asymptomatic for 15 months and has a creatinine of 230 μmol l^{-1} indicating stable but suboptimal renal function.

Discussion

The incidence of haemorrhage after partial nephrectomy is between 1% and 2% [1, 2] and may occur into the perirenal tissues or into the collecting system thereby causing haematuria. It is usually self-resolving and treatment is expectant and includes supportive therapies such as blood transfusion and bed rest. Haemorrhage in this particular case may have been due to an arterial injury at resection that was not identified because of vessel spasm at the ice cooling stage of the operation.

Pre-operative arteriography was performed in our case because the patient had bilateral tumours and a knowledge of the vascular anatomy was particularly important for planning the feasibility of nephron sparing surgery. It is also important in larger lesions and those that occupy a more central position close to the renal hilum, especially in a solitary kidney. Less invasive modalities such as multidetector array CT are now of sufficient accuracy that most urologists do not now routinely request arteriography before partial nephrectomy. In patients with suspected haemorrhage post partial nephrectomy the timing and method of investigation must be tailored to the patients' clinical condition. In our case angiography with contrast was initially avoided in an attempt to reduce possible contrast toxicity as he had impaired renal function. If a bleeding source is identified a variety of techniques, such as temporary balloon occlusion and embolisation with detachable coils may then be employed [3, 4].

Bleeding following partial nephrectomy is usually from a branch artery [5], which can be identified angiographically and embolised super-selectively with coils. This technique is well established for haemorrhage following renal biopsy. Where the main renal artery is involved, embolisation would devascularize the entire kidney. In our case the only alternative to this procedure would have been an open re-exploration, and would almost certainly have resulted in an emergency nephrectomy.

The literature reports more frequent use of covered stents for the treatment of renal artery aneurysm [6, 7]. As this case shows, it is possible to safely and effectively treat such a lesion with a covered stent (stent graft). The Jostent® used combines a balloon-expandable steel stent with an expandable PTFE (polytetrafluoroethylene) graft material [8, 9]. The Jomed stent has the advantage that it can be hand crimped onto the appropriate size balloon within the size range given, and is short enough to overcome any rigidity problems that may be encountered in an angulated renal artery.

Other causes of pseudoaneursym that may be amenable to similar treatment include: percutaneous renal biopsy, sharp trauma to the kidney and more rarely infection and atherosclerosis. It must however be noted that the majority of pseudoaneursyms developing after renal biopsy are either asymptomatic or show only transient symptoms [10] and resolve spontaneously.

There is no evidence regarding long-term patency of stent-grafts with respect to the treatment of pseudoaneurysm in the renal vasculature. The risk of stent stenosis due to intimal hypertrophy is unknown and these patients may need reviewing in the future. A previous study using stent grafts to preserve renal function in patients with renal artery stenosis and solitary functioning kidneys showed good patency results as well as good renal function at 24 months [11].

Most departments performing angioplasty keep similar stent grafts in stock in case of arterial rupture during angioplasty. The non-surgical treatment of acute iatrogenic renal artery injuries after stenting has been shown to be very successful [12]. Radiologists should be prepared to treat both main trunk and branch vessel injuries where haemorrhage occurs after nephron-sparing surgery [13].

References

1. Ghavamian R, Cheville J, Lohse CM. Renal cell carcinoma in the solitary kidney: an analysis of complications and outcome after nephron sparing surgery. Clin Urol 2002;168:454–9.
2. Corman JM, Penson DF, Hur K. Comparison of complications after radical and partial nephrectomy: results from the National Veterans Administration Surgical Quality Improvement Program. Br J Urol 2000;86:782–9.
3. Yamamoto N, Ishihara S, Yoshimura S, et al. Endovascular embolisation of a renal artery aneursym using interlocking detachable coils. Scand J Urol Nephrol 1998;32:143–1.
4. Centera LV, Hirsch JA, Choi IS. Wide necked sacular renal artery aneurysm: endovascular embolisation with the Guglielmi detachable coil and temporary balloon occlusion of the aneurysm neck. J Vasc Intervent Radiol 1998;9:513–6.

5. Albani JM, Novick AC. Renal artery pseudoaneurysm after partial nephrectomy: three case reports and a literature review. Urology 2003;62:227–31.
6. Pershad A, Heuser R. Renal artery aneursym: successful exclusion with a stent graft. Cather Cardiovasc Intervent 2004;61:314–6.
7. Tan WA, Chough S, Saito J. Covered stent for renal artery aneurysm. Catheter Cardiovasc Interv 2001;52:106–9.
8. Gaxotte V, et al. Multicenter trial of the Jostent balloon-expandable stent graft for renal and iliac artery lesions. J Endovasc Ther 2003;10:361–5.
9. Schneidereit NP, Lee S, Morris DC, Chen JC. Endovascular repair of a ruptured renal artery aneurysm. J Endovasc Ther 2003;10:71–4.
10. Ilmay B, Izzet R, Bulent A. Endovascular treatment of arteriovenous fistulas complicating percutaneous renal biopsy in three paediatric cases. Nephrology Dialysis Transplantation 1999;14:2726–30.
11. Cioni R, Vignali C, Petruzzi P. Renal artery stenting in patients with a solitary functioning kidney. Cardiovasc Intervent Radiol 2000;24:372–7.
12. Morris CS, Bonnevie GJ, Najarian KE. Non-surgical treatment of acute iatrogenic renal artery injuries occuring after renal artery angioplasty and stenting. Am J Roentgenol 2001;177:1353–7.
13. Parsons JK, Schoenberg MP. Renal artery pseudoaneurysm occurring after partial nephrectomy. Urology 2001;58:105.

The British Journal of Radiology, 78 (2005), 164–165 © 2005 The British Institute of Radiology
DOI: 10.1259/bjr/96432211

Case report
Ultrasound findings of iodide mumps

[1]S J PARK, MD, PhD, [1]H S HONG, MD, [1]H K LEE, MD, [1]J H JOH, MD, [1]J G CHA, MD and [2]H C KIM, MD

[1]*Department of Radiology, Soonchunhyang University Bucheon Hospital, 1174, Jung-dong, Wonmi-gu, Bucheon-shi Gyeonggi-do, 420-021 and* [2]*Department of Diagnostic Radiology, Soonchunhyang University, Cheonan Hospital, 23-20, Bongmyungdong, Cheonan, Choongnam 330-721, Republic of Korea*

Abstract. Iodide mumps, swelling of salivary glands after contrast medium injection, is a rare adverse reaction. We present a case in a 73-year-old man with advanced gastric cancer. About 10 min after a CT scan performed with intravenous injection of 140 ml of the low osmolality contrast agent Ioxaglate (Hexabrix 320, Guerbet, France), he complained of progressive swelling of the submandibular area. Ultrasound showed diffuse swelling and internal low echoic thick septa in the submandibular glands bilaterally. Approximately 1 h afterwards, the swelling of his submandibular glands started to regress and returned to normal within a day.

Iodide mumps, swelling of salivary glands after contrast medium injection, is a rare adverse reaction [1]. The cause remains unclear, but the reaction seems to be idiosyncratic or related to toxic accumulation of iodide in the ductal system of the salivary glands [2]. Even though non-ionic contrast agents result in fewer adverse reactions than ionic contrast agents, iodide mumps may result from any iodinated contrast agent [1]. To our knowledge, reports of ultrasound findings of iodide mumps have been rare in English literature.

Case report

A 73-year-old man with advanced gastric cancer was referred for CT staging. The patient had no past history of allergy and had previously never received iodinated compounds. CT was performed after intravenous injection of 140 ml of the low osmolality contrast agent Ioxaglate (Hexabrix 320, Guerbet, France). Within 10 min of the CT scan, he complained of progressive swelling of the submandibular area. Physical examination revealed bilateral tender swelling of his submandibular glands. Ultrasound of the neck was performed with a GE LOGIQ 700MR ultrasound system with 7–10 MHz linear array transducer (GE Medical System, Wisconsin). Greyscale ultrasound showed diffuse bilateral swelling of his submandibular glands and internal low echoic thick septa. Colour Doppler ultrasound showed no significant increase of vascular flow in the swollen glands (Figure 1). The parotid and thyroid glands were not swollen. Approximately 1 h after contrast medium administration, the swelling of his submandibular glands started to regress and returned to normal size within a day.

Discussion

Iodide mumps is referred to as abnormal swelling of the salivary glands associated with intravascular administration of iodine containing contrast material. This reaction is rare. Use of low-osmolality agents reduces the incidence of adverse reactions, but the incidence of iodism, including iodide mumps, is the same for low and high osmolar contrast agents [1]. The high concentration of iodide appears to induce inflammation of the salivary glands in the form of oedematous swelling of the mucosa. It leads to ductal obstruction with consequent inflammatory swelling of the salivary glands [2–4]. 98% of injected iodide is eliminated by the kidneys and only 2% is excreted from other organs, such as salivary, sweat and lacrimal glands. In normal subjects, the injected dose of contrast medium does not usually reach a sufficiently high iodide concentration to cause iodide mumps [4]. Impaired renal excretion of contrast material results in *in vivo* liberation of iodide and enables the salivary glands to concentrate inorganic iodide [4]. The prognosis of iodide mumps is relatively benign. The onset varies from within a few minutes to up to 5 days after contrast medium administration [2]. Associated adverse reactions with iodide mumps are facial nerve paralysis, severe allergic vasculitis, skin erythema, enlargement of the thyroid and lacrimal glands. However, no life threatening reaction has been reported [2]. The current management of iodide mumps is supportive therapy using analgesics and dialysis [5]. In almost half of reported cases recovery occurred without treatment [2]. In our case, swelling of the submandibular glands started to regress approximately 1 h after contrast medium injection, and returned to normal size within a day. Subsequent episodes of iodide mumps following repeated exposure to contrast media have also been observed [2]. To our knowledge, this is the first reported case in the English language literature of the ultrasound findings of iodide mumps. In our case, ultrasound findings of iodide mumps were diffuse swelling with prominent internal low echoic septa in the submandibular glands bilaterally without increase in vascularity. Although iodide mumps is a rare adverse reaction to the administration of iodine containing contrast material, knowledge of the entity and ultrasound findings should facilitate the diagnosis in patients with neck swelling after administration of iodine containing contrast material.

Received 14 June 2004 and in revised form 17 September 2004, accepted 26 October 2004.

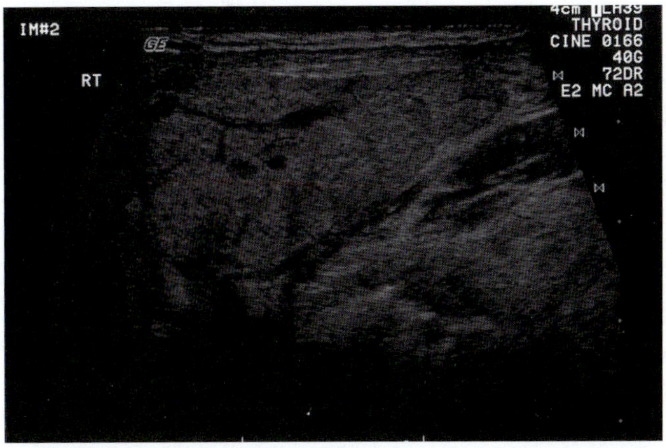

(a)

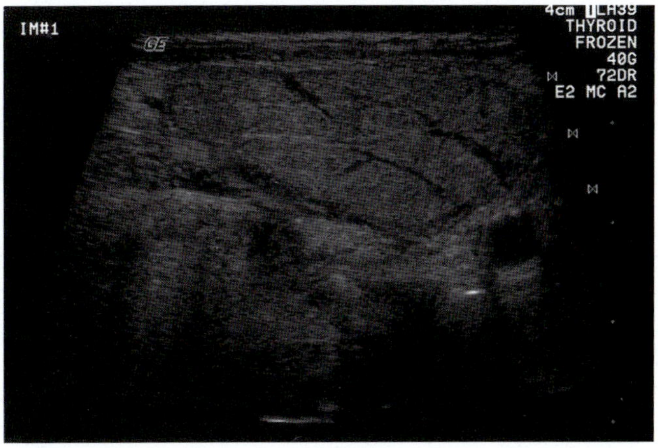

(b)

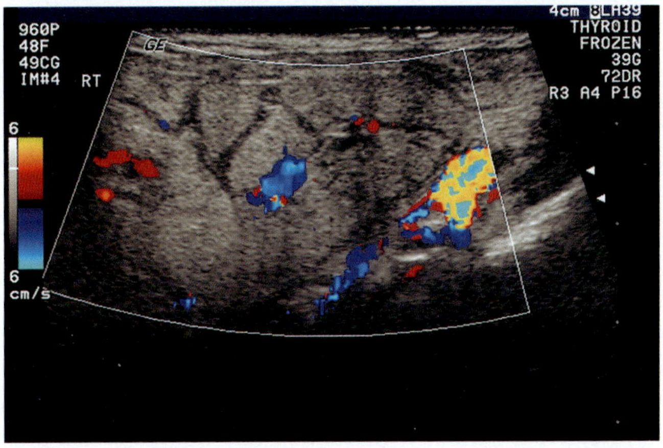

(c)

Figure 1. A 73-year-old man with advanced gastric cancer. (a, b) Greyscale ultrasound images show diffuse swelling of right and left submandibular glands with internal septal thickening. (c) Colour Doppler ultrasound shows no significant increase of vascular flow in the swollen gland.

References

1. Berman HL, Delaney V. Iodide mumps due to low-osmolality contrast material. AJR Am J Roentgenol 1992;159:1099–100.
2. Christensen J. Iodide mumps after intravascular administration of a nonionic contrast medium. Acta Radiol 1995;36:82–4.
3. Kuwatsuru R, Katayama H, Minowa O, Tsukada K. Iodide mumps after contrast enhanced CT with Iopamidol: a case report. Radiat Med 1995;13:147–8.
4. Kohri K, Miyoshi S, Nagahara A, Ohtani M. Bilateral parotid enlargement ("Iodide mumps") following excretory urography. Radiology 1977;122:654.
5. Kalaria VG, Porsche R, Ong LS. Iodide mumps: acute sialadenitis after contrast administration for angioplasty. Circulation 2001;104:2384.

The British Journal of Radiology, *78* (2005), 166–169
DOI: 10.1259/bjr/67990800

Case report

Radiological findings of primary retroperitoneal synovial sarcoma

[1]S ULUSAN, MD, [1]O KIZILKILIC, MD, [1]T YILDIRIM, MD, [1]C HURCAN, MD, [2]N BAL, MD and [3]T Z NURSAL, MD

[1]Department of Radiology, [2]Department of Pathology and [3]Department of Surgery, Baskent University Adana Teaching and Medical Research Center, Dadaloglu Mah Serinevler Adana-Turkey

Abstract. Synovial sarcomas are most commonly localized in the extremities, especially the lower thigh and knee areas. Retroperitoneal synovial sarcoma is very rare. We describe the radiological and pathological findings of an adult retroperitoneal synovial sarcoma.

In general, retroperitoneal soft-tissue sarcomas are relatively rare and the radiological diagnosis is often difficult. Most are malignant and frequently invade contiguous retroperitoneal organs. Surgical resection is often difficult or impossible. Retroperitoneal synovial sarcomas do not have specific imaging features differentiating it from other mesenchymal tumours. Despite the rarity of mesenchymal tumours of the retroperitoneum, synovial sarcoma should be included in the differential diagnosis of a retroperitoneal soft tissue mass detected in adults.

In this report, we present the radiological and pathological findings of an adult case of retroperitoneal synovial sarcoma examination. Although there a few papers describing the surgical and pathological features, this is the first report specifically addressing the imaging features.

Case report

A 38-year old man was admitted to hospital complaining of bilateral paresis in his feet, weight loss and non-specific pain of the upper abdomen. Physical examination revealed a palpable right sided upper abdominal mass. The results of routine blood and urine chemical analysis were within normal limits.

Abdominal ultrasound (US) demonstrated a well-defined hypoechoic mass with a diameter of 8 cm anterior to the inferior vena cava. Colour Doppler US of the retroperitoneal mass showed uniform hypovascularity. The mass was encircled by the vessels and gave off centripetal branches that passed into the parenchyma of the lesion (Figure 1).

CT demonstrated a large spherical, well-defined soft tissue 8 cm mass containing punctate calcification in the right retroperitoneal region. The mass compressed the psoas muscle, inferior vena cava and right ureter resulting in a minor hydroureteronephrosis (Figure 2a). There was marked homogeneous enhancement of the mass post intravenous contrast (Figure 2b).

Received 15 March 2004 and in final form 10 August 2004, accepted 11 November 2004.

MRI confirmed the retroperitoneal mass to have higher signal intensity than that of skeletal muscle on spin-echo T_1 weighted image (WI) (repetition time (TR) 144 ms, echo time (TE) 4.1 ms) moderately higher signal than that of skeletal muscle on turbo-spin-echo T_2WI (TR 5700 ms, TE 120 ms) (Figure 3a,b), and after administration of gadolinium contrast medium (0.1 ml kg^{-1} bw) T_1WI (TR 144 ms, TE 4.1 ms) showed marked, homogeneous enhancement (Figure 3c).

A phaeochromocytoma was excluded by the absence of hypertension, cardiac arrhythmias, and normal serum and urine levels of catecholamine and vanillylmandelic acid and metanephrine.

At surgery, invasion of the inferior vena cava and compression of the right ureter by the mass was seen. Complete resection of the tumour was performed, with repair of the inferior vena cava. In the post operative period, bilateral lower extremity venous thrombosis developed and was treated medically. Post-operatively, the patient received adjuvant chemotherapy.

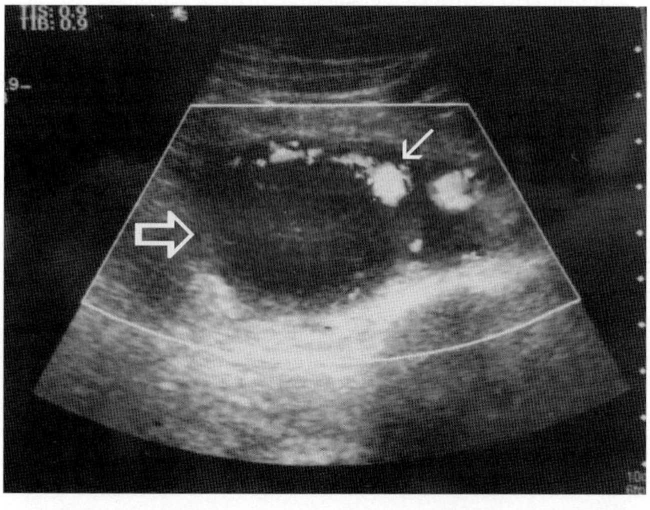

Figure 1. Abdominal Doppler ultrasound image shows a hypoechoic and hypovascular mass (thick open arrow) anterior to the inferior vena cava, encircled by the vessels. The common iliac arteries are seen medial to the mass (thin arrow).

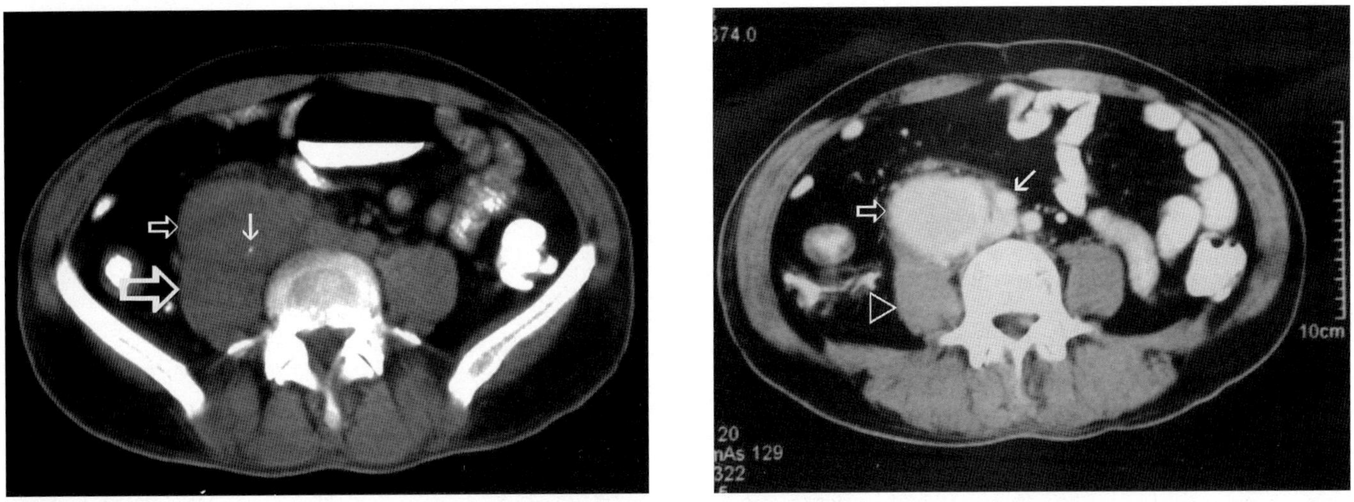

(a) (b)

Figure 2. (a) Non-contrast enhanced abdominal CT image shows a large spherical, well defined soft tissue mass (small open arrow) and punctuate calcification (arrow) and the psoas muscle behind the mass (big open arrow). (b) Post-contrast CT image demonstrates marked and homogeneous enhancement of the mass (open arrow), right common iliac artery just medial to the mass (thin arrow) and psoas muscle position to the mass (arrowhead).

On microscopic examination the tumour was well demarcated. The tumour cells were large, oval, with large round hyperchromatic nuclei and eosinophilic cytoplasm, and had marked nuclear pleomorphism. Bizarre and multinuclear giant cells and stromal lymphocytes were seen. Immunohistochemically epithelial membrane antigen (EMA), (Dako, N 1504, E29) was diffusely positive and S-100 (Doka, N1519) was focally positive. Leukocyte common antigen (LCA) (Neomarkers, CD 45 Ab-3, Mause, Mab, MS-413-R7, 413R301) was positive in lymphocytes and Desmin, HMB-45, CD 20, CD 34, CD99 were negative. The histological and immunohistochemical findings described the tumour as a synovial sarcoma of the monophasic pattern (Figure 4).

Discussion

Synovial sarcoma is a well-recognized soft-tissue malignancy that typically arises in young adults. It is a relatively common primary soft tissue sarcoma and accounts for approximately 5–10% of all malignant mesenchymal neoplasms [1, 2].

The majority (80–95%) of synovial sarcomas occur in the extremities, with approximately 60–70% in the lower limbs [1, 3, 4]. It is the most common malignancy of the foot and ankle in patients aged between 6 years and 45 years old and the most common malignancy of the lower extremity between the ages of 6 years and 35 years [2]. Other rare sites of involvement include the neck, pharynx, larynx, precoccygeal and paravertebral regions, thoracic and abdominal wall, and heart [1, 5].

The retroperitoneal region is a most uncommon place of occurrence. In 1954, Pack and Tabah [6] reported the first retroperitoneal synovial sarcoma. Since then 18 cases have been described. Synovial sarcomas derived from extremities occur more often in males and young adults [7], and the average age of retroperitoneal synovial sarcomas is similar. However, it occurs with an approximately equal sex distribution [7–10]. Since the retroperitoneal space is highly expandable and deeply hidden, early detection of retroperitoneal synovial sarcoma is difficult. The tumour has no special imaging features that distinguish it from other abdominal and retroperitoneal tumours [7]. We considered phaeochromocytoma in the differential diagnosis, as the radiological findings of phaeochromocytoma are those of hypervascular neoplasms that may show central necrosis, and the mass detected in our patient was hypovascular and contained punctuate calcification. Although the presence of calcification is uncommon in phaeochromocytoma, when present, it may have an egg-shell pattern [8]. Our patients' biochemical findings were not suggestive of a phaeochromocytoma.

Although the diagnosis of a retroperitoneal synovial sarcoma is based on the pathological characteristics of the specimen obtained by needle or surgical resection [7], radiographic studies suggest pre-operative diagnosis of synovial sarcoma. CT may identify soft tissue calcifications [11], especially those that are subtle or are located in areas where the anatomy is complex. It may also show areas of haemorrhage, necrosis, or cyst formation within the tumour [12]. CT defines the mass, and readily confirms bone involvement [11, 12]. Intravenous contrast may help in differentiating the mass from the adjacent muscle and neurovascular complex [11, 12].

On MRI, the findings are of a lesion that is usually a non-specific heterogeneous mass with signal intensity approximately equal to that of skeletal muscle on T_1W and higher than that of subcutaneous fat on T_2W MR images [13, 14]. Signal intensity changes compatible with previous haemorrhage and fluid–fluid levels have been reported [4, 13, 15]. The soft tissue calcifications frequently seen on radiographs and CT may not be detected on MRI [13, 14] although larger calcifications may be identified as areas of decreased signal intensity on all pulse sequences.

Scintigraphy may be normal or may show significantly increased uptake of $^{99}Tc^{m}$ methylene diphosphonate due to mineralization within the tumour which may not be apparent on radiographs [16, 17].

Metastases or local recurrence is seen in approximately 80% of patients [18]. Metastases are present at the time of

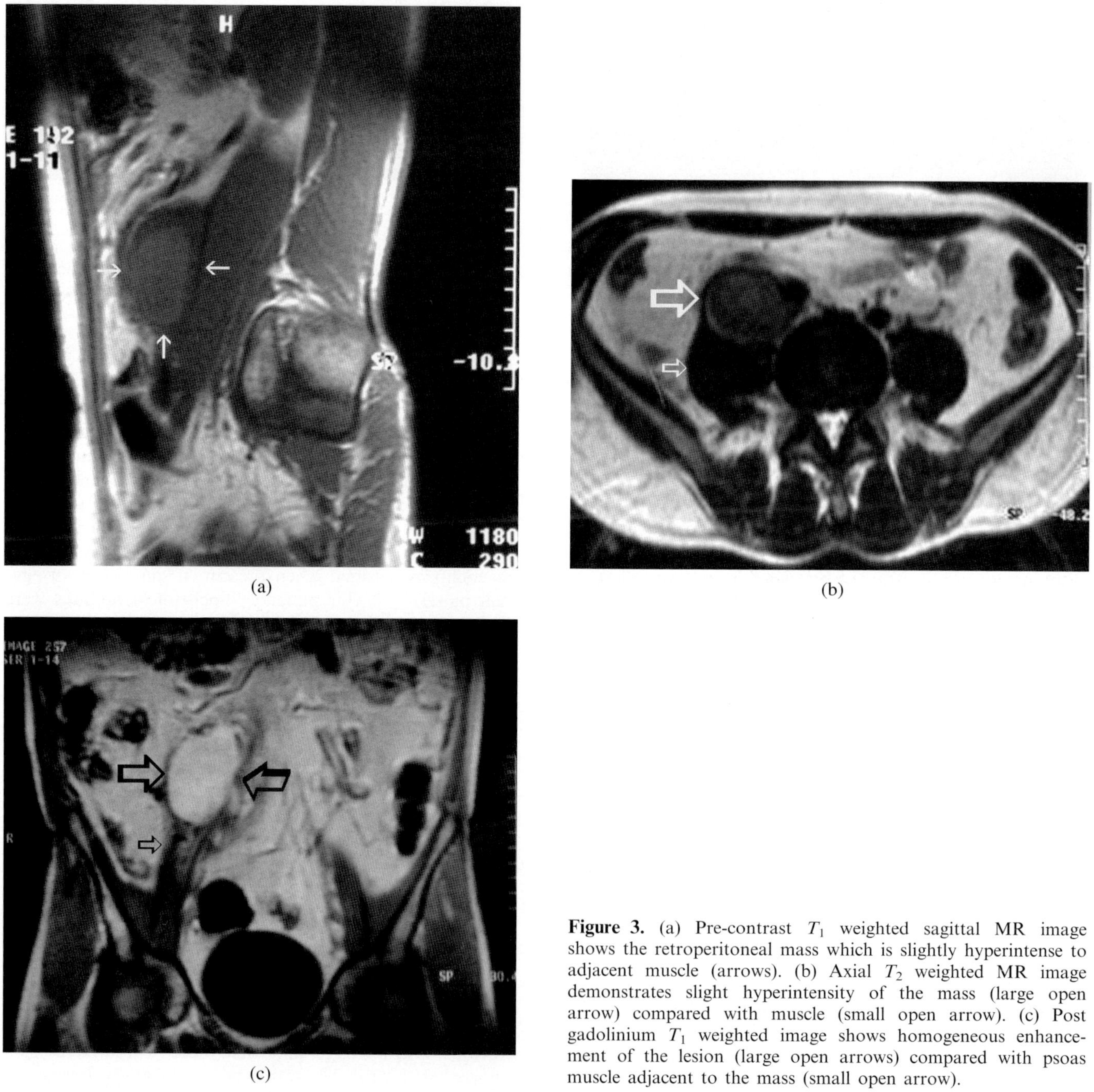

Figure 3. (a) Pre-contrast T_1 weighted sagittal MR image shows the retroperitoneal mass which is slightly hyperintense to adjacent muscle (arrows). (b) Axial T_2 weighted MR image demonstrates slight hyperintensity of the mass (large open arrow) compared with muscle (small open arrow). (c) Post gadolinium T_1 weighted image shows homogeneous enhancement of the lesion (large open arrows) compared with psoas muscle adjacent to the mass (small open arrow).

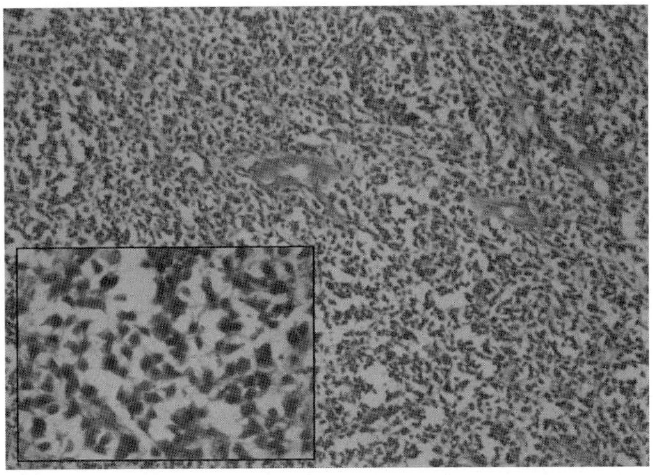

Figure 4. Pathological section of the tumour showing tumour cells consisting of oval, rounded cells with hyperchromatic nuclei and eosinophilic cytoplasms (haematoxylin and eosin (HE) × 100), with high power inset (HE × 400).

initial diagnosis in about one quarter of patients [18] but have been reported with a latency of 35 years following initial diagnosis [1]. Metastases may be to multiple sites but are predominantly pulmonary [4, 18, 19]. Local recurrence is frequent, occurring in the excision scar or the amputation stump, often within 2 years of the initial presentation.

Conclusions

Synovial sarcomas can be classified into four histopathological types: (1) biphasic; (2) monophasic fibrous; (3) monophasic epithelial; and (4) poorly differentiated. Immunohistochemistry is helpful in differential diagnosis. This case was confirmed to be a synovial sarcoma of monophasic epithelial type based on its immunohistochemical features. Primary retroperitoneal sarcomas may be biphasic as well as monophasic. Monophasic synovial sarcomas behave more aggressively and metastasize earlier then do biphasic tumours [20, 21]. No imaging differences have been reported between the monophasic and biphasic variants [22]. To our knowledge, this is the first case of primary retroperitoneal synovial sarcoma, reported with CT, MRI and colour Doppler ultrasound findings.

References

1. Kransdorf MJ, Murphey MD. Synovial tumors. In: Kransdorf MJ, Murphey MD, editors. Imaging of soft tissue tumours. Philadelphia: WB Saunders 1997:275–317.
2. Kransdorf MJ. Malignant soft-tissue tumors in a large referral population: distribution of diagnoses by age, sex, and location. AJR Am J Roentgenol 1995;164:129–34.
3. Cadman NL, Soule EH, Kelly PJ. Synovial sarcoma: an analysis of 34 tumors. Cancer 1965;18:613–27.
4. Wright PH, Sim FH, Soule EH, Taylor WF. Synovial sarcoma. J Bone Joint Surg Am 1982;64:112–22.
5. Genest P, Kim TH, Katsarkas A, Jothy S. Calcified synovial sarcoma of the oropharynx. Br J Radiol 1983;56:580–2.
6. Pack GT, Tabah EJ. Primary retroperitoneal tumours: a study of 120 cases. Int Abstr Surg 1954;99:313–41.
7. Miyashita T, Imamura T, Ishikawa Y, Okinaga K, Kunii O, Miyashita H. Primary retroperitoneal synovial sarcoma. Intern Med 1994;33:692–6.
8. Lee JK, Sagel SS, Stanley RJ, Heiken JP. Computed body tomography with MRI correlation. Philadelphia- New York: Lippincott-Raven 1998;1185–7.
9. Ziran BH, Makley JT, Carter JR. Primary retroperitoneal sarcomas: common symptoms, common diagnoses, uncommon disease. Clin Orthop 1996;331:277–82.
10. Prokopchuk OL, Zemskov SV, Susak YM. Ukrain treatment of a patient with retroperitoneal synovial sarcoma. Case report. Drugs Exp Clin Res 2000;26:255–6.
11. Treu EB, de Slegte RG, Golding RP, Sperber M, van Zanten TE, Valk J. CT findings in paravertebral synovial sarcoma. J Comput Assist Tomogr 1986;10:460–2.
12. Israels SJ, Chan HS, Daneman A, Weitzman SS. Synovial sarcoma in childhood. AJR Am J Roentgenol 1984;142:803–6.
13. Mahajan H, Lorigan JG, Shirkhoda A. Synovial sarcoma: MR imaging. Magn Reson Imaging 1989;7:211–6.
14. Morton MJ, Berquist TH, McLeod RA, Unni KK, Sim FH. MR imaging of synovial sarcoma. AJR Am J Roentgenol 1991;156:337–40.
15. Jones BC, Sundaram M, Kransdorf MJ. Synovial sarcoma: MR imaging findings in 34 patients. AJR Am J Roentgenol 1993;161:827–30.
16. Braeuning MP, Park HM. Three-phase Tc-99 m MDP scan findings of soft tissue sarcoma. Clin Nucl Med 1990;15:572–3.
17. Rice S, Stewart CA. Synovial sarcoma seen on bone scan. Clin Nucl Med 1990;15:445–6.
18. Ryan JR, Baker LH, Benjamin RS. The natural history of metastatic synovial sarcoma: experience of the Southwest Oncology group. Clin Orthop 1982;164:257–60.
19. Vezeridis MP, Moore R, Karakousis CP. Metastatic patterns in soft tissue sarcomas. Arch Surg 1983;118:915–8.
20. Evans HL. Synovial sarcoma. A study of 23 biphasic and 17 probable monophasic examples. Pathol Annu 1980;15:309–31.
21. Hajdu SI, Shiu MH, Fortner JG. Tendosynovial sarcoma: a clinicopathological study of 136 cases. Cancer 1977;39:1201–17.
22. Shmookler BM. Retroperitoneal synovial sarcoma. A report of four cases. Am J Clin Pathol 1982;77:686–91.

The British Journal of Radiology, *78* (2005), 170–174
DOI: 10.1259/bjr/18362306

Pictorial review

Commonly encountered adrenal pseudotumours on CT

T GOKAN, MD, Y OHGIYA, MD, H NOBUSAWA, MD and H MUNECHIKA, MD

Department of Radiology, Showa University School of Medicine, 1-5-8 Hatanodai, Shinagawa-ku, Tokyo 142-8666, Japan

Abstract. There are a variety of causes of adrenal pseudotumours on CT, including gastric diverticulum, prominent splenic lobulation, upper-pole renal mass, pancreatic mass, hepatic mass and periadrenal varices. These adrenal pseudotumours can be elucidated by multiplanar reconstruction using CT and MRI as well as from the axial images.

Introduction

Various adrenal pseudotumours have been previously described on CT. The causes of these pseudotumours include duodenum, colon, gastric diverticulum, hepatic tumour, renal mass, pancreatic mass, and periadrenal varices. With meticulous CT technique, it is usually possible to distinguish adrenal pseudotumours from true adrenal tumours. Cases may be elucidated using multiplanar images of CT or MRI. We present CT images of a variety of adrenal pseudotumours with emphasis on the usefulness of three-dimensional (3D) reconstructions of CT and MRI.

The adrenal glands are surrounded by a variety of anatomical structures. Certain anatomical structures and extra-adrenal pathological conditions may produce CT images suggesting adrenal pathology where none actually exists [1–8] (Table 1). We review and illustrate commonly encountered adrenal pseudotumours.

Prominent lobation of the hepatic lobe, or hepatic tumour

Exophitic right hepatic tumour may simulate a right adrenal tumour (Figure 1). The renal fascia is usually fused superiorly and inserts into the diaphragm. However, it may be open superiorly and communicate with the bare area of the liver. Exophitic hepatic tumour adjacent to the bare area may extend into the perirenal space and be confused with a right adrenal tumour (Figure 2) [1].

Gastric diverticulum and redundant gastric fundus

A fluid-filled gastric fundus, which has not been opacified by orally administered contrast material, may, on occasion, produce a mass-like density in the expected region of the left adrenal gland [3]. A diverticulum of the gastric cardia may simulate a left adrenal mass (Figure 3). A diverticulum of the posterior wall of the gastric cardia may herniate through an area of dorsal mesentery before its fusion with the left posterior body wall. Initially, the diverticulum would lie superior to the pancreas but the inferior aspect of the diverticulum may then lie adjacent to Gerota's fascia and the left adrenal gland. If migration of the diverticulum occurs before renal ascent, the diverticulum could indent Gerota's fascia and interdigitate itself between the left kidney and the left adrenal gland. A diverticulum forming after fusion of the dorsal mesentery might be expected to lie within the lesser sac [4].

Fluid-filled colon

A fluid-filled colon between the kidney and the adrenal gland may simulate an adrenal mass (Figure 4). If the gas is seen in the colon, correct diagnosis is easily made [4]. Intraluminal contrast and thin sections may also be useful.

Splenic lobulation

Prominent splenic lobulation projecting toward the region of the left adrenal gland may simulate an adrenal mass (Figure 5). The fetal spleen is lobulated, but these lobules normally disappear before birth. Splenic lobulations may persist along the medial part of the spleen [2, 5, 6].

Tortuous or dilated splenic arteries and veins

Periadrenal and adrenal portosystemic collaterals may be a cause of adrenal pseudotumour, which may not be anatomically distinguishable from the adrenal tumour on CT. Patients with portal hypertension with suspected adrenal tumour may require dynamic CT or MRI to discriminate between left adrenal gland and splenic vessels (Figure 6) [6–8].

Table 1. Possible causes of the adrenal pseudotumour

Prominent lobation of the hepatic lobe, or hepatic tumour
Gastric diverticulum and redundant gastric fundus
Fluid filled duodenum/colon
Splenic lobulation
Tortuous or dilated splenic arteries and veins
Pancreatic tail in an unusual location, or pancreas tail mass
Exophitic upper pole renal mass
Abundant suprarenal fat
Focal thickening of adjacent diaphragmatic crus
Retroperitoneal tumour localized in the area of adrenal gland

Received 15 September 2003 and in final form 18 May 2004, accepted 18 July 2004.

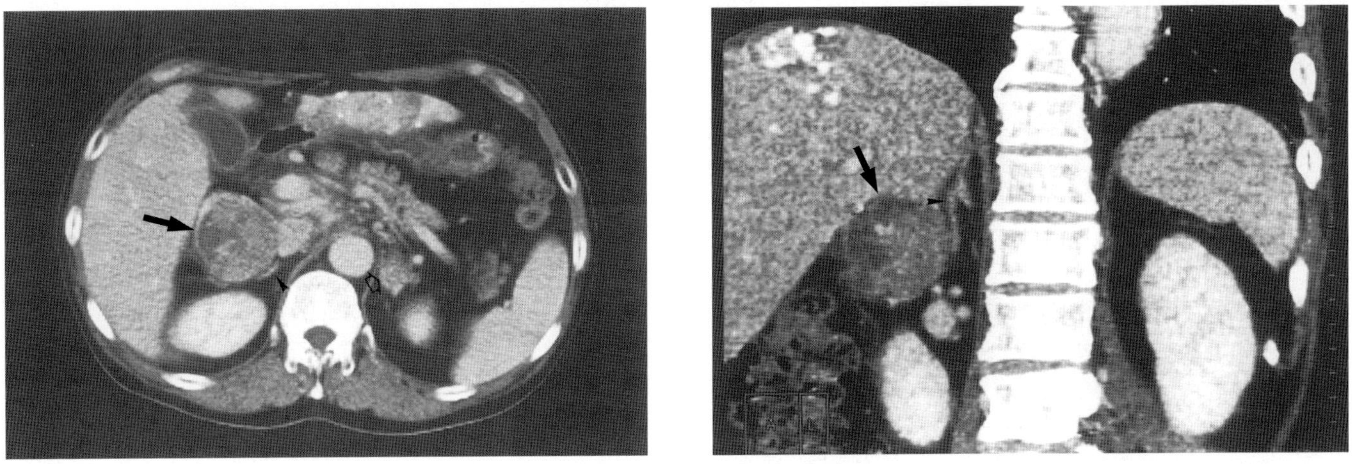

(a) (b)

Figure 1. Right adrenal pseudotumour in a 60-year-old man with hepatocellular carcinoma. (a) Axial multidetector CT (MDCT) shows a low density (arrow) mass anterior to the upper pole of the right kidney. A small linear structure (arrowheads) suggesting adrenal gland is seen. Left adrenal metastasis (open arrow) is demonstrated. (b) Coronal reformatted MDCT image clearly demonstrates an exophitic hepatic tumour (arrow) and normal right adrenal gland (arrowhead).

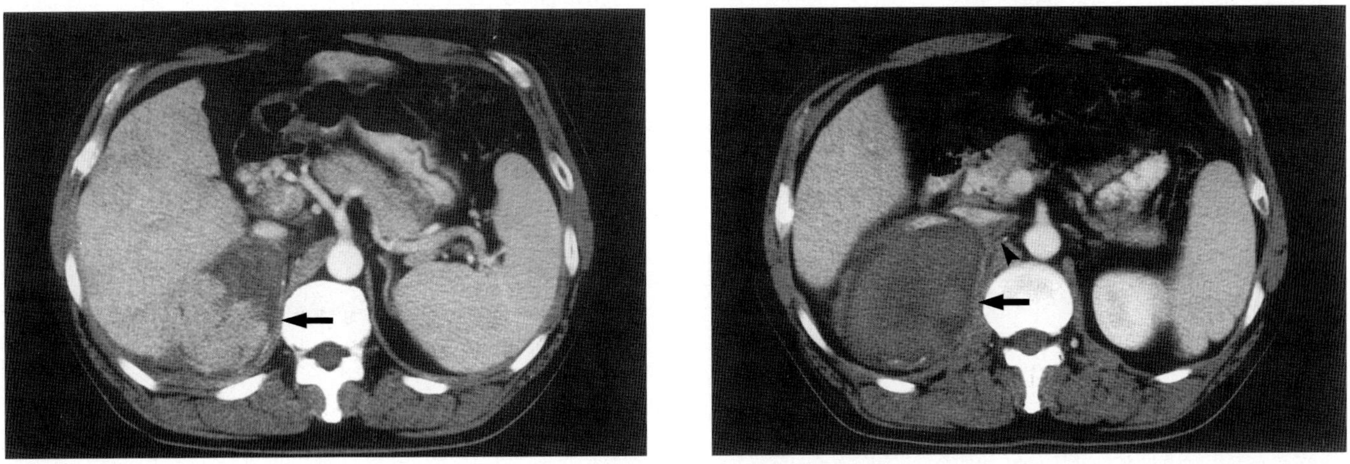

(a) (b)

Figure 2. Ruptured hepatocellular carcinoma with extension to the retroperitoneum simulating right adrenal tumour in a 46-year-old man with right upper quadrant pain. (a) Enhanced CT shows tumour in the region of the adrenal gland that simulates an adrenal tumour (arrow). (b) Enhanced CT obtained 2 cm caudal to (a) shows a large perinephric haematoma (arrow). A compressed right adrenal gland (arrowhead) is seen in the medial aspect of the haematoma.

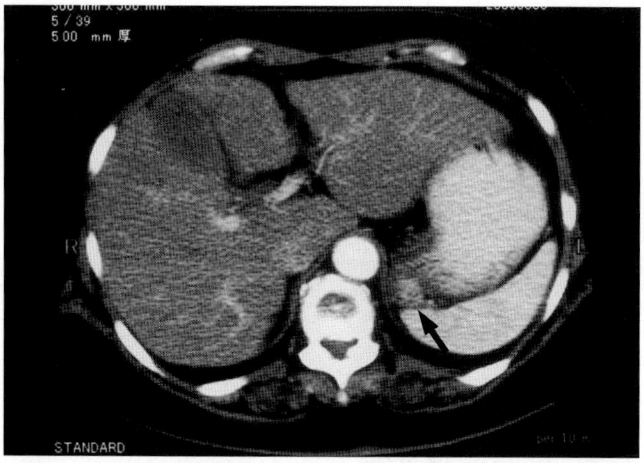

(a)

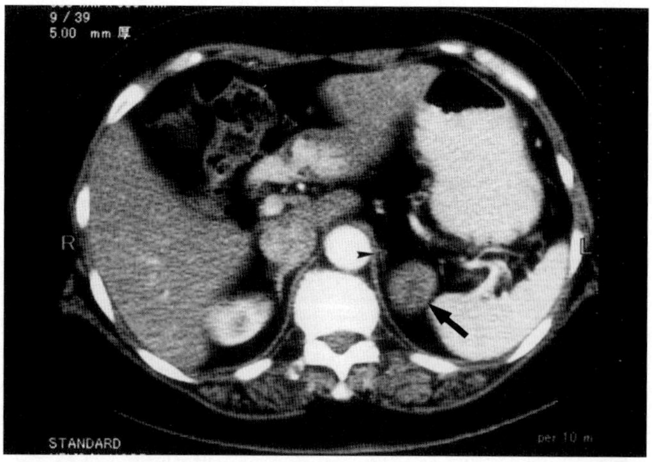

(b)

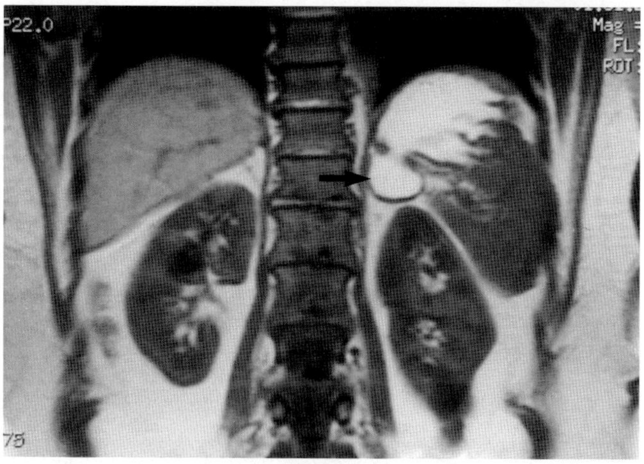

(c)

Figure 3. Gastric diverticulum simulating left adrenal tumour in a 43-year-old man with hypertension. (a, b) Axial images of enhanced multidetector CT (MDCT) with oral contrast shows a mass (arrow) of heterogeneous attenuation in the left supra renal region. A linear structure (arrowhead) suggesting left adrenal gland is demonstrated in the lowest cut of the mass. (c) Coronal T_1 weighted MR image with positive oral contrast clearly demonstrates diverticulum of the gastric fundus (arrow).

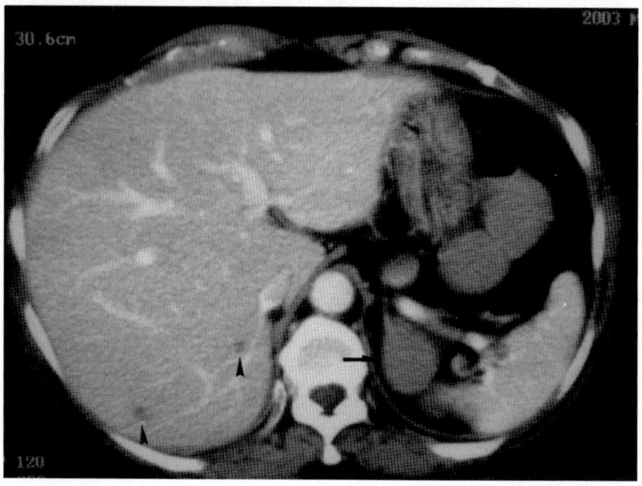

(a)

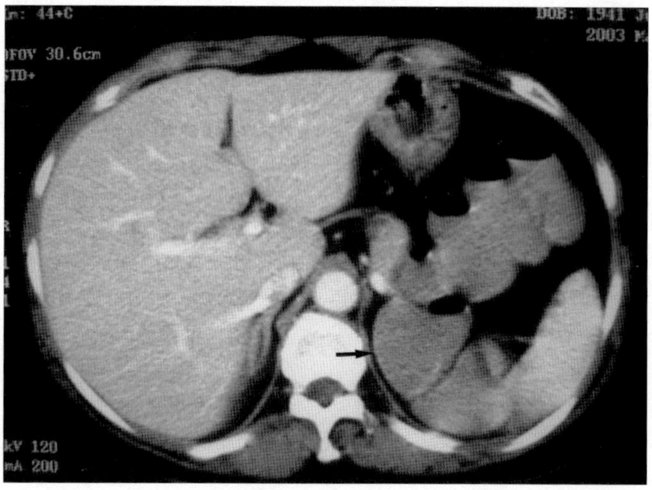

(b)

Figure 4. Dilated colon simulates left adrenal tumour in a 65-year-old man with rectal carcinoma. (a) Axial multidetector CT (MDCT) shows low density mass (arrow) in a left suprarenal region suggesting adrenal tumour. Of note is low density liver metastases (arrowheads). (b) Axial MDCT obtained caudally to (a) demonstrates that the low density mass is a part of the dilated fluid-filled colon (arrow).

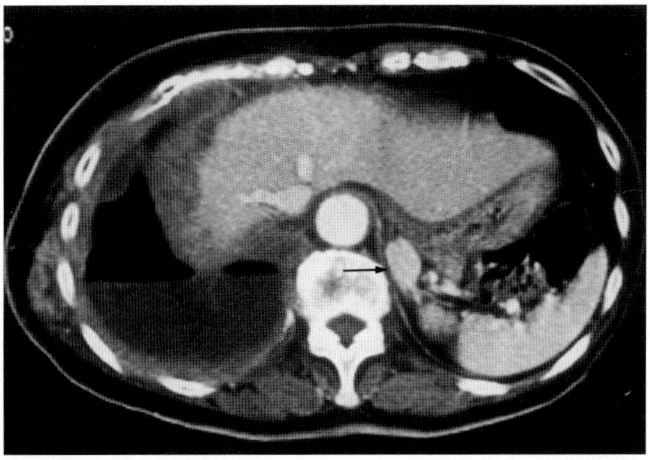

(a)

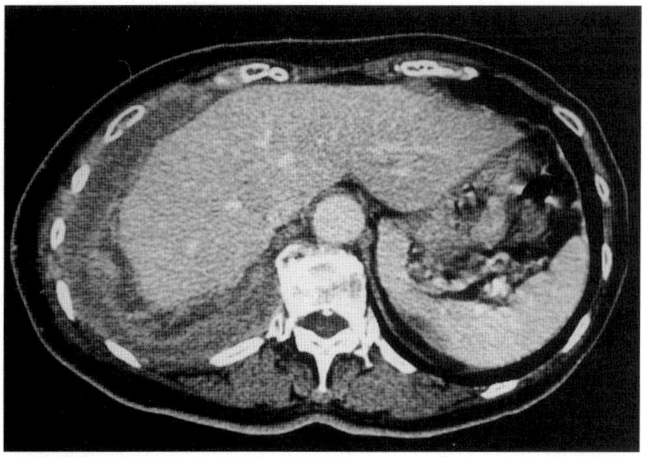

(b)

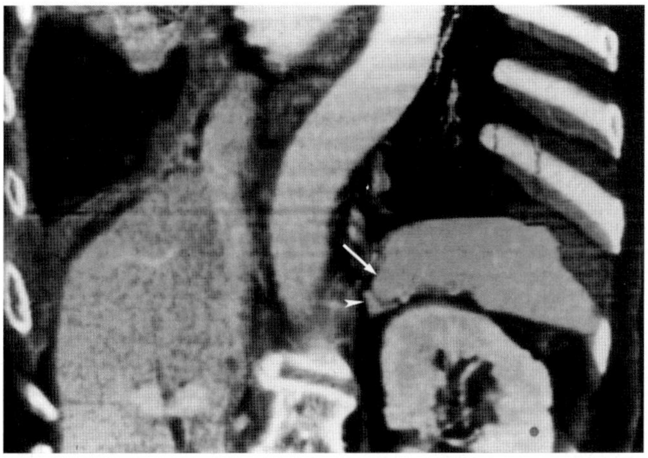

(c)

Figure 5. Left adrenal pseudotumour due to splenic lobulation in a 72-year-old woman with right pleural mesothelioma. (a) Axial CT image suggests a mass of the left adrenal gland (arrow). (b) Axial thin slice (3 mm) images demonstrate the mass is a part of the lobulated spleen (arrow). (c) Oblique coronal volume rendered image of CT clearly demonstrates the lobulated spleen (arrow) close to the left adrenal gland (arrowhead).

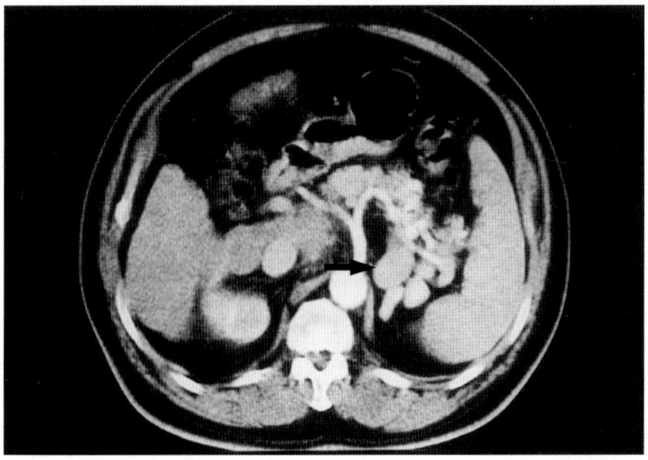

(a)

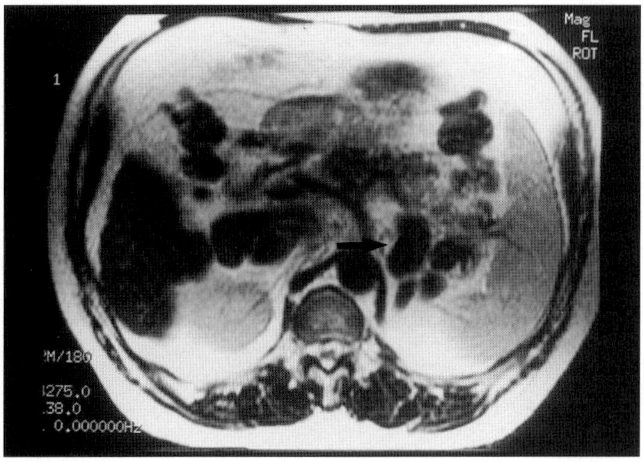

(b)

Figure 6. Left adrenal pseudotumour due to dilated portosystemic veins in a 54-year-old man with portal hypertension due to cirrhosis. (a) Axial CT image shows large tubular varix in left suprarenal region. There is a possible left adrenal mass (arrow) that shows slightly less intense enhancement than the surrounding varices. (b) T_2 weighted MR image demonstrate "flow void" in the mass (arrow) as well as surrounding varix, indicating flowing blood in the varix.

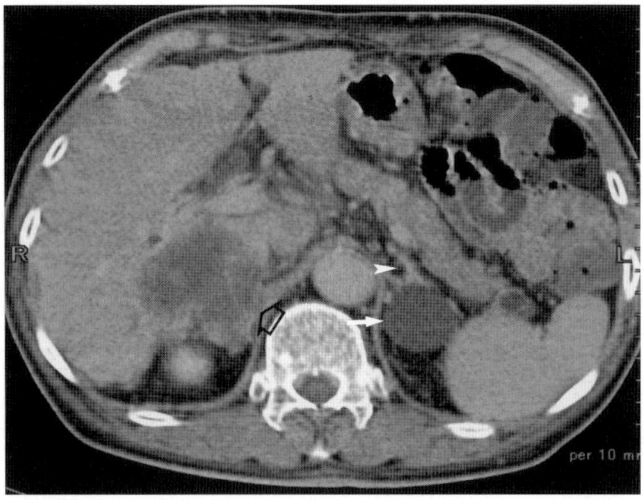

(a)

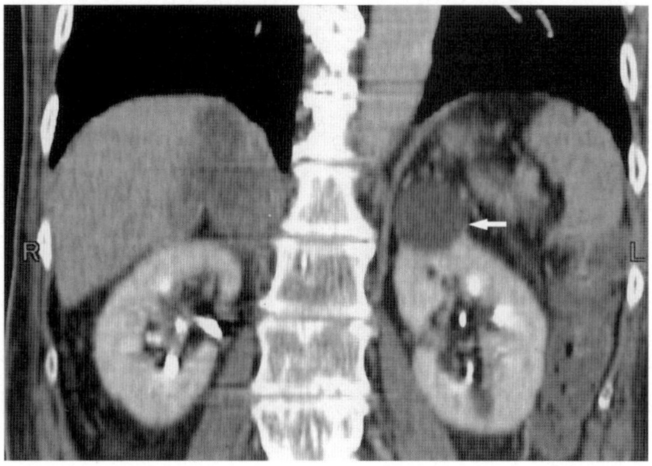

(b)

Figure 7. Pseudotumour of the left adrenal gland due to left upper pole renal cyst in a 56-year-old woman with liver and right adrenal gland metastasis. (a) Axial CT image suggests a cyst (arrow) in the suprarenal area in the posterior aspect of the left adrenal gland (arrowhead). Hepatic metastasis from breast carcinoma invades the right adrenal gland (open arrow). (b) Coronal reformatted CT image demonstrates the cyst of the upper pole of the left kidney with beak sign (arrow).

Pancreatic tail masses

Neoplastic, inflammatory, and/or cystic masses arising in the tail of the pancreas may be difficult to differentiate from an adrenal mass [5].

Exophitic upper pole renal masses

A mass arising in the upper pole of either kidney may be difficult to differentiate from an adrenal mass [3, 5]. Sagittal or coronal reconstructions may be useful to demonstrate the origin of the mass (Figure 7). The usefulness of thin-section CT has been reported previously [3].

References

1. Kim KW, Auh YH, Chi HS, Lee SI. CT of retroperitoneal extension of hepatoma mimicking adrenal tumor. J Comput Assist Tomogr 1993;17:599–602.
2. Berliner L, Bosniak MA, Megibow A. Adrenal pseudotumor on computed tomography. J Comput Assist Tomogr 1982;6:281–5.
3. Schwartz AN, Goiney RC, Graney DO. Gastric diverticulum simulating an adrenal mass: CT appearance and embryogenesis. AJR Am J Roentgenol 1986;146:553–4.
4. Schwartz JM, Bosniak MA, Megibow AJ, Hulnick DH. Right adrenal pseudotumor caused by colon: CT demonstration. J Comput Assist Tomogr 1988;12:153–4.
5. Gayer G, Zissin R, Apter S, Atar E, Portnoy O, Itzchak Y. CT findings in congenital anomalies of the spleen. Br J Radiol 2001;74:767–72.
6. Shirkhoda A. Diagnostic pitfalls in abdominal CT. Radiographics 1991;11:969–1002.
7. Mitty HA, Cohen BA, Sprayregen S, Schwartz K. Adrenal pseudotumors on CT due to dilated portosystemic veins. AJR Am J Roentgenol 1983;141:727–30.
8. Brady TM, Barry HG, Glazer GM, Williams DM. Adrenal pseudomasses due to varices: angiographic-CT-MRI pathologic correlations. AJR Am J Roentgenol 1985;145:301–4.

The British Journal of Radiology, *78* (2005), 175–176
DOI: 10.1259/bjr/72810248

Case of the month
The rapidly enlarging chin mass

C OFFIAH, BSc, FRCS, FRCR and E HALL, MBChB

Department of Neuroradiology, Hope Hospital, Salford, Manchester, UK

A 25-year-old gentleman of Asian origin presented to the department of oral and maxillofacial surgery with a hard immobile well-defined pea-sized swelling overlying the left and midline body of the mandible. He denied any pain associated with the lesion. He did however remark upon what was interpreted clinically as paraesthesia over the mental region of the chin. The lower right anterior and lateral incisors (4 1 and 4 2) were noted to be mobile. Over the course of 6 weeks the mass enlarged to the size of a golf ball.

Plain film radiography in the form of a panoramic projection (Figure 1) and right lower periapical projections (Figure 2) were performed at the initial presentation followed by further plain films – panoramic, periapical and occlusal projections – and a CT examination (Figure 3) 6 weeks later. What is the differential diagnosis given the clinical history and radiological appearances?

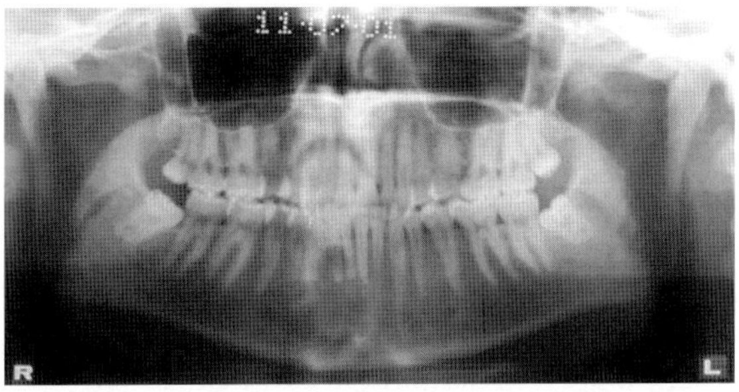

Figure 1. Orthopantomograph demonstrating a cystic lesion in the right side of the body of the mandible causing thinning of the cortex and destruction of the lamina dura of the adjacent incisor and canine teeth. There is no evidence of periosteal reaction.

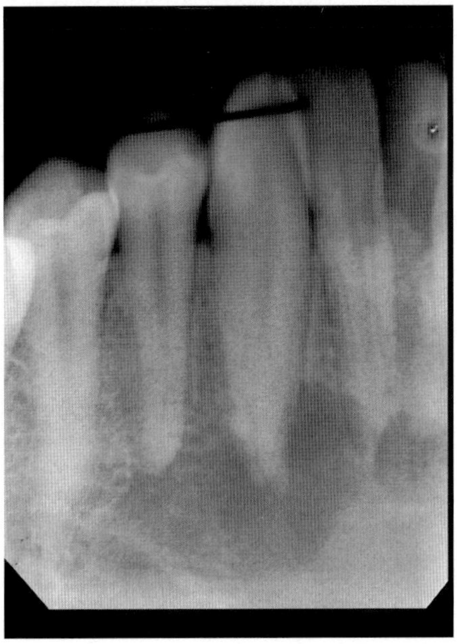

Figure 2. Lower right periapical projection demonstrating root erosion of the right lower canine tooth by the mandibular mass.

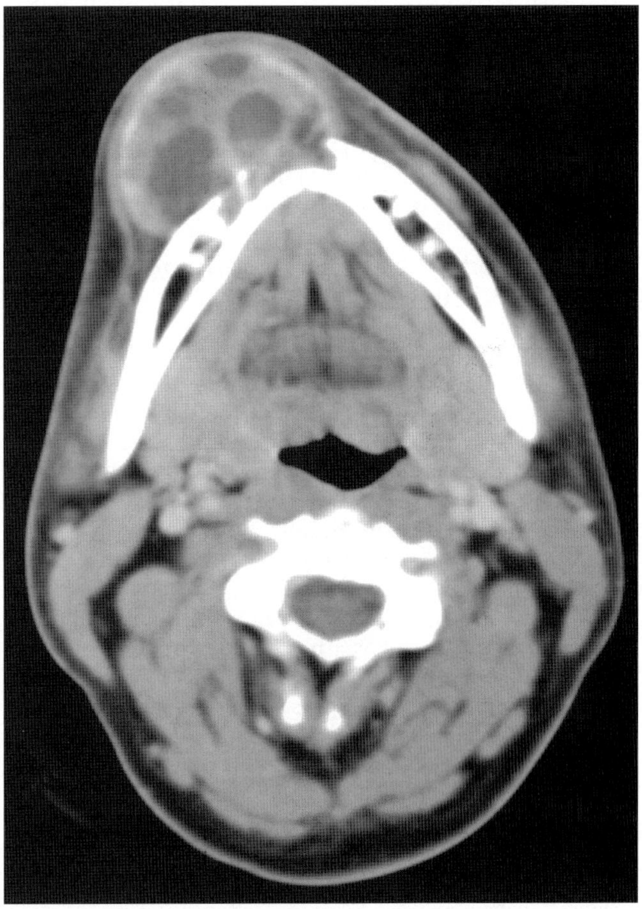

Figure 3. Post-contrast CT images of the mandibular lesion demonstrating its cystic nature with evidence of cortical breakthrough and extension into the overlying soft tissues anteriorly but no evidence of periosteal reaction.

Received 14 May 2004 and in revised form 5 November 2004, accepted 25 November 2004.

Figure 1 is of the initial panoramic projection obtained at presentation and shows a radiolucent lesion with a distinct narrow sclerotic-appearing margin located in the body of the mandible on the right close to the symphysis menti. There is no distinct septation within the lesion suggesting that it is unilocular and there is no discernible periosteal reaction. The lesion has destroyed the periapical lamina dura of the lower right incisors and canine (4 1, 4 2 and 4 3). Figure 2 is a right lower periapical projection, which confirms the destruction of the lamina dura of these teeth but also demonstrates partial resorption of the root of the lower right canine (4 3). Figure 3 shows axial post-contrast CT image through the mandible, which demonstrate destruction of the anterior cortex of the body of the right side of the mandible but no evidence of periosteal reaction. There is marked soft tissue extension anteriorly centred on the involved region of the mandible. The soft tissue component does not enhance avidly and contains areas of fluid attenuation. The overall radiological appearances are of a non-malignant lesion but the history of rapid growth and facial paraesthesia suggests a diagnosis to the contrary. Surgical excision and histological analysis yielded a diagnosis of juvenile active ossifying fibroma.

Juvenile active ossifying fibroma (JAOF) is rare. It is seen most often in patients between the ages of 5 years and 15 years (60% to 80% of cases) [1]. Cases have however been reported in both older and younger patients [2], some authors suggesting an age range of presentation from 3 months to 72 years [3, 4]. There is no clearly defined racial or sexual predilection. With its diverse histopathology, no clear-cut criteria exist for separating JAOF from the more common forms of ossifying fibroma but its behaviour is markedly different [3]. The tumour can increase rapidly in size in a relatively short time as in our case study. The most common site of involvement for JAOF is the craniofacial skeleton – primarily the maxilla, paranasal sinuses, orbital and frontoethmoid bones [1, 2]. Among the 85% of facial lesions, 90% occur in the paranasal sinuses; most commonly the ethmoid sinuses [3, 4]. The remaining 10% arise from the mandible. Extracranial sites of JAOF account for 4% [4–6].

Clinical manifestations usually begin with swelling of the affected site. The patient may have neurosensory disturbances ranging from pain to paraesthesia in the involved area as in our case. Tumour in the maxilla may produce symptoms of nasal blockage and epiphora [1, 4]. Visual disturbances and blindness from compression of orbital contents and the optic nerve can also occur [4]. Skull base erosion via an involved paranasal sinus can lead to meningitis [4]. A case of stenosis of the supraclinoid portion of the internal carotid artery and associated cerebral ischaemic symptoms due to compression by a JAOF has even been reported [4].

The radiographic appearance of JAOF is of a unilocular, oval or spherical lesion with a distinct osteolytic density delineating it from normal bone. As the lesion enlarges, it can become increasingly radiodense, although still remaining less dense than the adjacent normal bone. Tooth displacement and partial destruction of the roots of teeth is well reported. The main radiological differential diagnoses for JAOF are osteogenic sarcoma, osteoblastoma, fibrous dysplasia and aneurysmal bone cyst (ABC). JAOF is a fibro-osseous tumour and can therefore demonstrate osteogenic elements (absent in our case however) making it difficult to distinguish from osteogenic sarcoma on imaging; the lack of periosteal reaction may be helpful in differentiating this tumour from osteogenic sarcoma however often malignant tumours of the craniofacial bones do not exhibit periosteal reaction. Despite the rapid increase in size that JAOF can demonstrate there is a relative lack of destruction, which is particularly apparent on CT examination. The craniofacial skeleton is a very uncommon site for osteoblastoma (another bone-forming tumour) and ABC. Areas of ABC formation can however sometimes be demonstrated histologically within JAOF [5] complicating differentiation of these two entities. Distinction of JAOF from fibrous dysplasia is more difficult but fibrous dysplasia tends to have relatively indistinct borders blending into surrounding bone compared with the typically well-defined demarcation from surrounding, healthy bone demonstrated by JAOF. In addition, root resorption is not a common feature of fibrous dysplasia in contrast to JAOF [3–6].

The painless rapid growth demonstrated by this juvenile form of ossifying fibroma and the tendency to a locally aggressive growth pattern has justified the prefix "active" or "aggressive" in reference to these tumours. Histologically, JAOF shows some variance but typical features include a highly cellular stroma containing calcified components, which is usually fibroblastic and relatively avascular accounting for the lack of enhancement on imaging; woven and interconnecting lamellar bone with numerous eccentric rims of osteoblasts are also demonstrated. The highly cellular nature of the stroma reflects the aggressive nature of these tumours [3, 5, 6].

Complete surgical excision is necessary to obviate local recurrence. This can usually be achieved by local excision and curettage [2, 5]. Adjunctive treatment is not required. Malignant transformation has never been recorded.

JAOF, although a rare lesion, is worthy of inclusion in the radiological differential diagnosis of a rapidly expanding lesion affecting the craniofacial skeleton of an adolescent or young adult. Differentiation from other benign and malignant neoplasms is important in the correct therapeutic management of this tumour.

References

1. Waldron CA. Fibro-osseous lesions of the jaw. J Oral Maxillofac Surg 1993;51:828–35.
2. Wiedenfeld KR, Neville BW, Hutchins AR, Bell RA, Brock TR. Juvenile ossifying fibroma of the maxilla in a 6-year-old male: case report. Pediatr Den 1995;17:365–8.
3. Leimola-Virtanen R, Vahatalo K, Syrjanen S. Juvenile active ossifying fibroma of the mandible: a report of 2 cases. J Oral Maxillofac Surg 2001;59:439–44.
4. Lawton MT, Heiserman JE, Coons SW, Ragsdale BD, Spetzler RF. Juvenile active ossifying fibroma: report of four cases. J Neurosurg 1997;86:279–85.
5. Noffke CEE. Juvenile ossifying fibroma of the mandible. An 8 year radiological follow-up. Dentomaxillofac Radiol 1998;27:363–6.
6. Javadzadeh B, Means CR, Park K. Pathological quiz case: rapidly growing expansile lesion of the left jaw in a 15-year-old boy. Arch Pathol Lab Med 2001;125:1117–9.

Book review

Standards and codes of practice in medical radiation dosimetry. Proceedings of an International Symposium, Vienna, 25–28 November 2002. Volumes 1–2. pp ii + 483, 497, 2003 (IAEA, Vienna, Austria). €130. ISBN 92-0-111403-6

To its credit, the International Atomic Energy Agency takes on many tasks in addition to its role in inspecting and controlling the use of atomic energy for peaceful (and not so peaceful) purposes. One of these tasks is its sponsorship, in collaboration with other international organizations, of meetings to discuss developments in radiation metrology for medical applications. The latest symposium took place over 4 days in December 2002, and this book is the proceedings. There were 58 verbal presentations and 27 poster presentations, the two being indistinguishable when printed.

The scope of the symposium was wider than implied by its title. It is impossible to review the 85 papers in detail, but what any prospective purchaser of this book wants to know is some idea of its scope. So here goes. The papers discuss the following range of methods for measuring radiation: unsealed cylindrical and plane-parallel ionization chambers, extrapolation chambers, 4π chambers, liquid ionization chambers, calorimeters, thermoluminescence, radiochromic film, polymer gel, alanine, optical fibre luminescence, diodes and scintillators. A whole session of seven papers is devoted to calorimetry. The following applications of these methods of measurement are discussed: low and medium energy X-ray beams, gamma-ray beams, megavoltage X-ray and electron beams, intensity-modulated radiotherapy, proton and light ion beams, gamma-ray and beta-ray brachytherapy, nuclear medicine for diagnostic, palliative and therapeutic purposes, diagnostic and interventional radiology, and CT.

There are also papers on the results of audits, quality control, phantoms and treatment planning systems. In the middle of this specialized symposium was a session of four papers on the needs of developing countries, discussing cancer epidemiology, the most suitable radiotherapeutic apparatus, health economics, and the availability (or not) of modern medical imaging equipment.

All the papers were written by experts in their respective fields, and are of a high standard. This is not a teaching manual, as it assumes that readers already possess a good basic knowledge of practical and theoretical radiation dosimetry. Unlike present day medical imaging, for which a book may be out of date within a year or two after its publication, radiation dosimetry does not advance at such a hectic rate, so this book should not suffer that fate for at least 10 years.

Complaints? Well, perhaps just one. There is no subject index: if you happen to come across a new or useful idea, make a careful note of the volume and page number, otherwise you may have difficulty in finding it again hiding somewhere in its 980 pages.

J E Burns

BIR CORPORATE MEMBER SCHEME

The BIR Corporate Member Scheme is aimed at all companies with an interest in radiology and allied sciences. For an annual subscription member companies are offered an attractive benefits package. To find out why your company should join the leading edge companies listed below, please contact Mr Adrian C Laws, Marketing Manager, British Institute of Radiology, 36 Portland Place, London W1B 1AT. Tel: +44 (0) 20 7307 1404.

Agfa-Gevaert Ltd
Tel: 020 82314900
Contact Mr M Hill, Business Manager Medical Imaging and PACS Systems
Product Code: 1, 2, 3, 4, 6, 9, 10, 12, 13, 14, 15, 20, 22 and 23

Alliance Medical Ltd
Tel: 01295 671223
Contact Mr Charles Fox, Marketing Executive
Product Code: 1, 4, 5, 16, 20 and 21

Amersham Health
Tel: 01494 798666
Contact Mr D G Rothery, Marketing Manager
Product Codes: 1, 2, 3, 4, 5 and 6

Bard Limited
Tel: 01293 606864
Contact Ms T Empson, Product Manager
Product Code: 2

B.M.V.A.
Tel: 01483 689838
Contact Dr R Bowden, Meetings Officer
Product Codes: 1, 3, 4, 9, 10 and 21

Bracco UK Ltd
Tel: 01628 851500
Contact Mr A Quinn, Product Manager
Product Codes: 1, 2 and 5

BVM Medical Ltd
Tel: 01455 614555
Contact Jay Tailor, Managing Director
Product Codes: 2 and 18

Cerner Corporation (UK)
Tel: 01452 831533
Contact Mr C Harrison, Client Executive
Product Codes: 9, 10, 13 and 20

Clinical Press Ltd
Tel: 0117 9420256
Contact Professor Paul Goddard, Chairman
Product Codes: 17 and 21

Cook (UK) Ltd
Tel: 01462 482884
Contact Mr Iain Mackintosh, regional Manager - Diagnostic and Interventional Products
Product Code: 2

Department of Radiography & Imaging Sciences (St Martin's College, Lancaster)
Tel: 01524 384640
Contact Mr Philip Harris, Acting Head of Department
Product Code: 21

Dictaphone International
Tel:020 78785000
Contact Dr F Brabant, Director of Product Management
Product Codes: 9 and 13

E-Z-EM Ltd
Tel: 01869 366900
Contact Mr Martin Suggitt, Product Manager
Product Codes: 1, 2 and 8

Ferrania UK Ltd
Tel: 01344 312100
Contact Mr Alan Budge, General Marketing Manager
Product Codes: 1, 3, 4, 9, 10, 13, 14, 15 and 18

Fuji Photo Film (UK) Ltd
Tel: 01234 326780
Contact Mr R G Brown, Strategic Business Manager
Product Codes: 1, 3, 4, 6, 9, 10, 12, 13, 14, 15, 18 and 22

GE Medical Systems
Tel: 01753 874000
Contact Mr A Trivett, Managing Director
Product Codes: 1, 2, 3, 4, 6, 8, 9, 10, 15, 18 and 22

Guerbet Laboratories Ltd
Tel: 01908 522888
Contact Mr Trevor Furniss, General Manager
Product Code: 1 and 2

Insignia Medical Systems Ltd
Tel: 01420 540206
Contact Mr Richard Dormer, Managing Director
Product Code: 9

Kimal plc
Tel: 01895 270951
Contact Mr S Clarke, Technical Director
Product Code: 2

Kingsmoor Publications Ltd
Tel: 01371 812960
Contact Mr David Roberts, Managing Director
Product Code: 17

Kodak Ltd
Tel: 01442 844473
Contact Mr Chris Wright, Marketing Manager UK and Ireland
Product Codes: 1, 3, 4, 6, 8, 9, 10, 12, 13, 14, 15, 18, 21, 22 and 23

Landauer, Inc.
Tel: 01865 373008
Contact Dr T Finnigan, Director, European Operations
Product Code: 8

Lanmark
Tel: 01494 675535
Contact Mrs Liz Beckmann, Director
Product Codes: 6, 9, 10, 13, 17 and 20

Lodestone Patient Care Limited
Tel: 020 89449630
Contact Mrs J Hill, Director of Operations
Product Code: 1, 3 and 21

Medical Imaging Systems Limited
Tel: 020 82059500
Contact Mr P W Sykes, Director
Product Code: 1

Mirada Solutions Ltd
Tel: 01865 265500
Contact Dr Clare Jones, VP Marketing
Product Codes: 1, 4, 6, 9, 10, 13, 21 and 22

Nucletron UK Ltd
Tel: 018297 71111
Contact Mr J Banks, Managing Director
Product Codes: 6 and 8

Pantak Medical Systems Agfa NDT
Tel: 0118 9310310
Contact Mr R Howton, Managing Director
Product Codes: 1, 6, 7 and 8

Philips Medical Systems
Tel:01737 230400
Contact Ms Anita Littlechild, Marketing Communications Manager
Product Codes: 1, 2, 9, 10, 22 and 23

Samsung SDS Europe Ltd
Tel:020 83807000
Contact Mr G Wheeler, Sales Manager (Medical)
Product Codes: 1, 9, 10, 13, 15, 16 and 20

Schering Health Care Ltd
Tel: 01444 232323
Contact Mr Chris Matthews, Product Manager
Product Codes: 1, 2 and 3

Sectra Ltd
Tel: 020 86106033
Contact Jan Wolfram, Managing Director
Product Codes: 9 and 10

Siemens Medical Solutions
Tel: 01344 396317
Contact Mr Mike Bell, Manager, Advertising and Exhibitions
Product Codes: 1, 2, 3, 4, 6, 9, 15 and 22

Sony Scientific and Medical
Tel: 01932 816267
Contact R Holt, Marketing Manager
Product Code: 14

Sonosite Ltd
Tel: 01767 313117
Contact Ms Gillian Duffy, European Marketing Director
Product Codes: 3

Southern Scientific Ltd
Tel: 01903 604000
Contact Mr Stephen Adams, Sales Manager
Product Codes: 1, 3, 4, 8, 10, 12 and 22

Toshiba Medical Systems UK
Tel: 01293 653700
Contact Mr S M Weeden, Manager X-ray Products
Product Codes: 1, 2, 3, 4, 9, 10 and 15

Varian Oncology Systems
Tel: 01293 531244 (UK)
Contact Mr Rolf Stähelin (Switzerland - tel. 00 41 417498844), Marketing Manager, Europe
Product Code: 6

Vertec Scientific Ltd
Tel: 01734 817431
Contact Mr B Hipgrave, Managing Director
Product Codes: 1, 4, 6, 8 and 12

Wardray Premise Ltd
Tel: 020 83989911
Contact Mr R Beach, Sales Manager
Product Codes: 8, 18 and 20

Wolverson X-Ray
Tel: 01902 637333
Contact Mr N Bacon, Sales Director
Product Codes: 1, 8, 15, 18 and 23

Xograph Imaging Systems
Tel: 01666 501501 or 07000 for X-ray
Contact Mr N Staff, Technical Director
Product Codes: 1, 8, 12, 14, 15, 18, 22 and 23

PRODUCT CODES

1. Diagnostic X-ray including NMR and CT
2. Interventional radiology
3. Ultrasound
4. Nuclear medicine
5. Radiopharmaceuticals
6. Radiotherapy and oncology
7. Radiobiology
8. Radiation protection
9. PACS
10. Image processing
11. Nuclear fuel cycle service
12. Quality assurance
13. Radiology data management computer systems
14. Video printing
15. Equipment leasing
16. Hospital-shared services
17. Medical publishing
18. X-ray consumables distribution
19. Electricity generation
20. Medical reporting systems
21. Education
22. Mammography
23. Dental X-ray

Meetings & Courses

Radiotherapy in breast cancer
1 February 2005
London, UK
Further details: The British Institute of Radiology, 36 Portland Place, London W1B 1AT.
Tel: 0207 307 1406. Fax: 0207 307 1414.
Email: registrations@bir.org.uk. Visit: www.bir.org.uk

FMRI lung imaging
4 February 2005
London, UK
Further details: The British Institute of Radiology, 36 Portland Place, London W1B 1AT.
Tel: 0207 307 1406. Fax: 0207 307 1414.
Email: registrations@bir.org.uk. Visit: www.bir.org.uk

Computed radiography: image quality and dose issues
23 February 2005
London, UK
Further details: The British Institute of Radiology, 36 Portland Place, London W1B 1AT.
Tel: 0207 307 1406. Fax: 0207 307 1414.
Email: registrations@bir.org.uk. Visit: www.bir.org.uk

Image guided therapy
24 February 2005
London, UK
Further details: The British Institute of Radiology, 36 Portland Place, London W1B 1AT.
Tel: 0207 307 1406. Fax: 0207 307 1414.
Email: registrations@bir.org.uk. Visit: www.bir.org.uk

Nuclear medicine in oncology
17 March 2005
London, UK
Further details: The British Institute of Radiology, 36 Portland Place, London W1B 1AT.
Tel: 0207 307 1406. Fax: 0207 307 1414.
Email: registrations@bir.org.uk. Visit: www.bir.org.uk

Image display workstations
12 April 2005
London, UK
Further details: The British Institute of Radiology, 36 Portland Place, London W1B 1AT.
Tel: 0207 307 1406. Fax: 0207 307 1414.
Email: registrations@bir.org.uk. Visit: www.bir.org.uk

MR angiography
15 April 2005
London, UK
Further details: The British Institute of Radiology, 36 Portland Place, London W1B 1AT.
Tel: 0207 307 1406. Fax: 0207 307 1414.
Email: registrations@bir.org.uk. Visit: www.bir.org.uk

Volume 78| **March 2005**

BJR British Journal of Radiology

Full papers

Ultrasound-guided drainage of breast abscesses: results in 151 patients

Ultrasound evaluation of the fibrosis stage in chronic liver disease by the simultaneous use of low and high frequency probes

A comparative study of evaluation radiographs, CT and 3D reformatted CT in facial trauma: what is the role of 3D?

MR colonography: baseline appearance of the unprepared rectosigmoid

Radiation doses received in the UK Breast Screening Programme in 2001 and 2002

A study of the distribution of dose across the hands of interventional radiologists and cardiologists

Treatment outcomes and prognostic factors in patients with supratentorial low-grade gliomas

Daytime pulsed dose rate brachytherapy as a new treatment option for previously irradiated patients with recurrent oesophageal cancer

Short communications
Case reports
Pictorial review
Case of the month
Book reviews
Correspondence

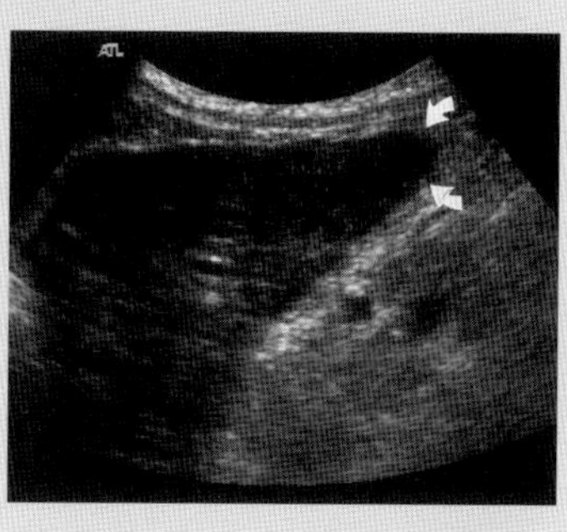

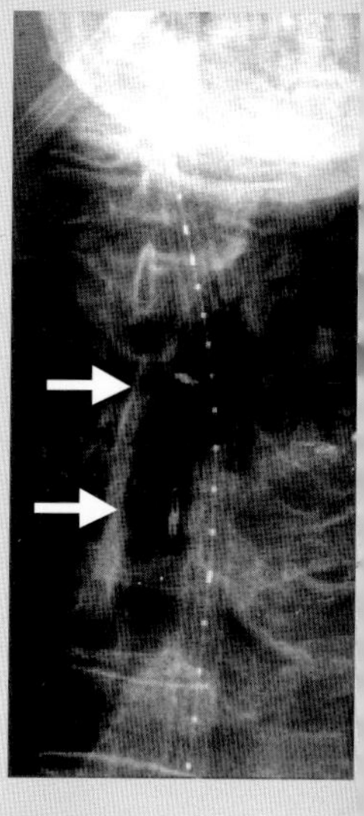

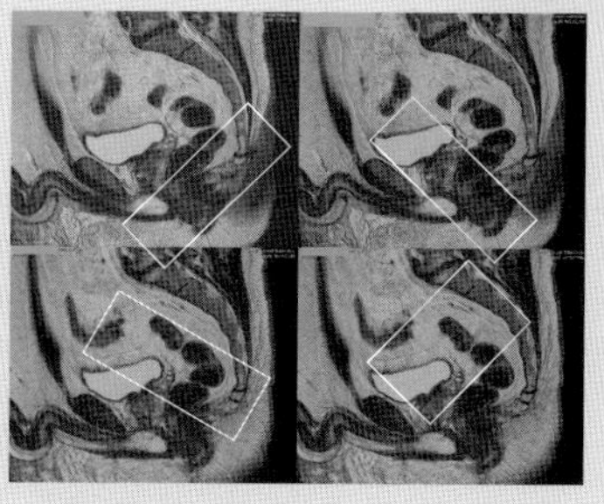

http://bjr.birjournals.org

ISSN 0007-1285

Published by

BIR The British Institute of **Radiology**

BJR

ISSN 0007 1285

THE BRITISH JOURNAL OF RADIOLOGY

Aims and Coverage

The *British Journal of Radiology* is the official peer-reviewed monthly research journal of the British Institute of Radiology. It is a multidisciplinary journal covering all clinical and technical aspects of diagnostic imaging, radiotherapy and oncology, medical physics and radiobiology. BJR is an international journal containing papers both from the UK and overseas, and is circulated to Full Members of the BIR and to libraries worldwide.

Authors are strongly advised to submit manuscripts online using Editorial Manager™, at http://bjr.edmgr.com. Online submission will expedite the peer-review process. Instructions to Authors are available on request from the Refereeing Administrator at the address given below, and are also available on the BIR's website at www.bir.org.uk

Published by the British Institute of Radiology, 36 Portland Place, London W1B 1AT, UK.
Editorial enquiries: Tel: +44 (0)20 7307 1424; Fax: +44 (0)20 7307 1414
Email: publications@bir.org.uk
Advertising sales and enquiries: please contact Gareth Liddiatt at McMillan Scott: Tel: +44 (0)20 7878 2313
Email: gareth@mcmslondon.co.uk
www.bir.org.uk www.birjournals.org bjr.edmgr.com

Subscriptions

Subscriptions fulfilment is carried out by PSP Subscriptions, BMA House, Tavistock Square, London WC1H 9JR, UK (Telephone +44 (0)20 7383 6270; Fax +44 (0)20 7383 6402; email subscriptions@bmjgroup.com). The 2005 annual subscription rate for the printed version of BJR is £524 (includes 12 issues plus two Special Issue). Subscriptions are on a calendar basis only.

Institutional BJR subscribers have free access to both BJR Online and Imaging Online, and are offered a 33% discount on a print subscription to the BJR's quarterly review journal Imaging (see http://imaging.birjournals.org).

US Mailing Agent

The British Journal of Radiology (ISSN 0007 1285) is published monthly by the British Institute of Radiology, c/o Mercury Airfreight Int. Ltd, 365 Blair Road, Avenel, NJ 07001. The Dollar price for US direct subscribers is $786. Periodicals Postage Paid at Rahway NJ. Postmaster: send address corrections to the British Journal of Radiology, c/o Mercury Airfreight Int. Ltd, 365 Blair Road, Avenel, NJ 07001.

Back Issues

Back issues can be ordered from Vine House Distribution, Waldenbury, North Common, Chailey, East Sussex BN8 4DR, UK (Telephone +44 (0)1825 723398; Fax +44 (0)1825 724188). Price is £40 per issue.

BJR Online

BJR Online, produced in association with HighWire Press, is available free of charge to BIR members and Institutional print subscribers: http://bjr.birjournals.org. Enquiries to publications@bir.org.uk

BIR THE BRITISH INSTITUTE OF RADIOLOGY

Founded 1897
Incorporated by Royal Charter
Patron: Her Majesty The Queen

The British Institute of Radiology has as its aim to bring together all the professions in radiology and allied medical and scientific disciplines to share knowledge, and educate the public, thereby improving the prevention and detection of disease and the management and treatment of patients. Particulars of membership and other information can be obtained from the General Secretary, BIR, 36 Portland Place, London W1B 1AT, and from the BIR's website: http://www.bir.org.uk
Telephone: +44 (0)20 7307 1400
Fax: +44 (0)20 7307 1414

Typeset, printed and bound by The Charlesworth Group, Wakefield, UK. Telephone +44 (0)1924 204830.

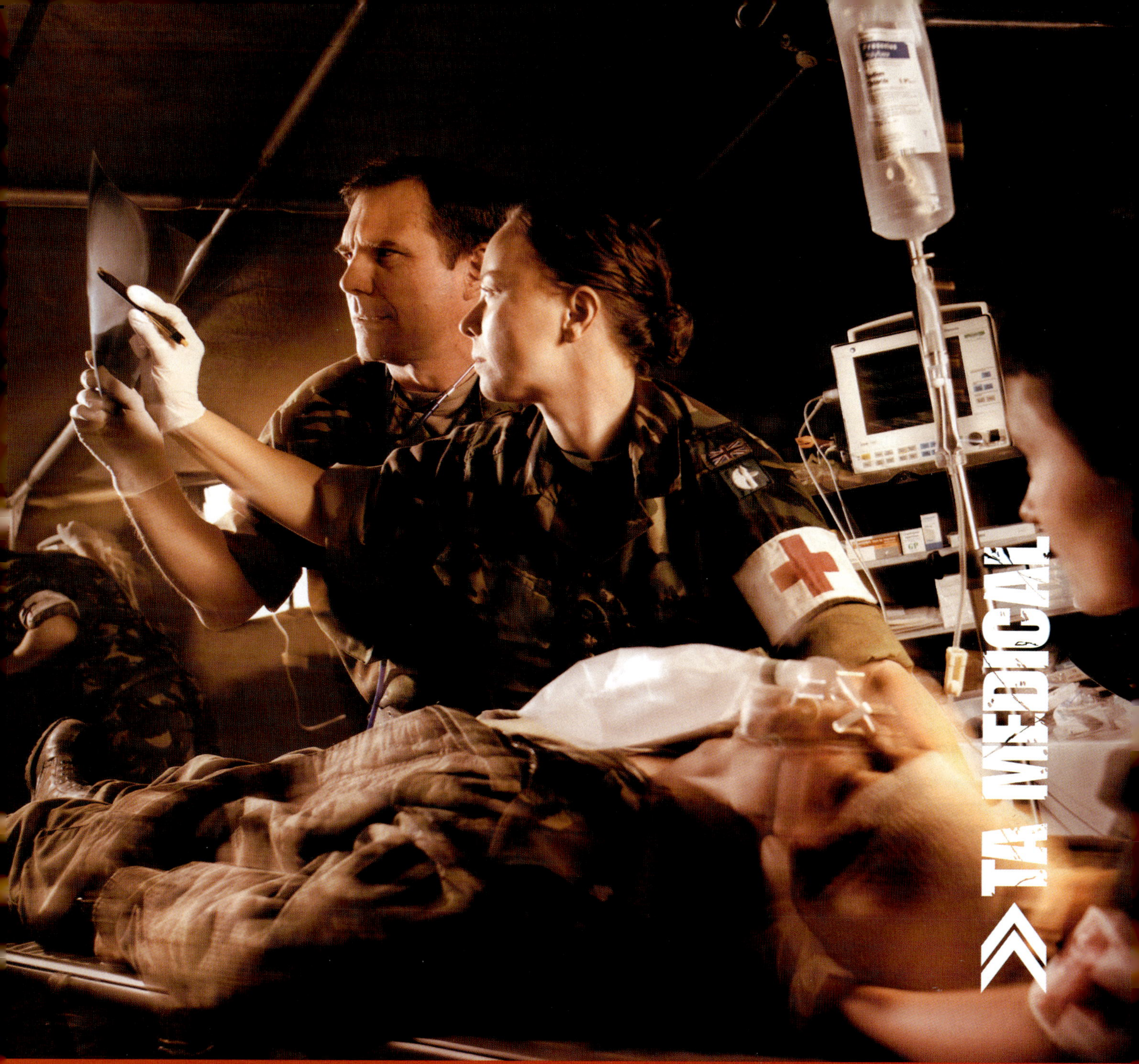
TA MEDICAL

ANNOUNCEMENT

The British Journal of Radiology Young Investigator Award

The British Institute of Radiology is pleased to announce the introduction of a new Award to encourage young workers in the general areas of diagnostic imaging, radiotherapy and related topics to carry out research and publish it. It will be known as the BJR Young Investigator Award and the winner will receive a prize to be known as the Editors' Prize.

Terms and conditions

1. The Award is made annually to the author of the best paper by a younger investigator published in the British Journal of Radiology during the calendar year.
2. The paper must be a "Full Paper" according to the Journal's criteria – not a technical note, short communication etc.
3. The sole author, or first-named author of a multi-author paper, must be under the age of 35 when the paper is first submitted.
4. First-named authors under the age of 35 are asked to indicate that they are eligible for the Award when the paper is submitted.
5. Only papers that are accepted by both referees at the first submission, either without change or with only minimal changes (AccMin) will be eligible for consideration.
6. Short listing is by the Members of the BIR Publications Committee. The definitive choice for the award is made by the Honorary Editors, whose decision is final.
7. The value of the Award is £250. There will also be a certificate.
8. The presentation will be made at the BIR Annual General Meeting and the winner will be invited to be a guest of the Institute at the dinner which follows in the evening.

Interim arrangements

For the 2005 Award, the authors of all papers already published or provisionally accepted that meet the AccMin criterion (see paragraph 5) will be contacted with respect to the age criterion.

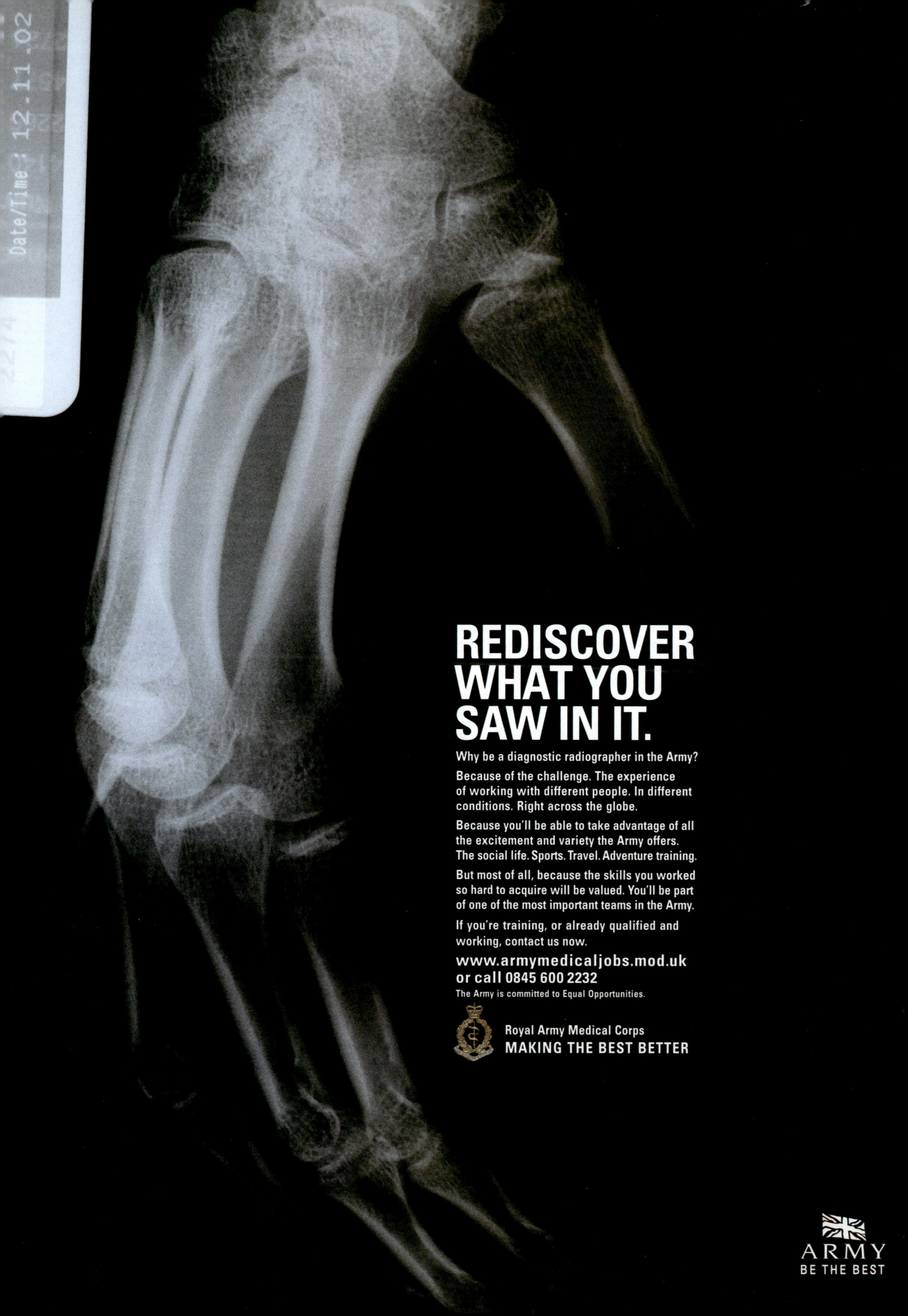
Date/Time: 12.11.02
REDISCOVER WHAT YOU SAW IN IT.
Why be a diagnostic radiographer in the Army?
Because of the challenge. The experience of working with different people. In different conditions. Right across the globe.
Because you'll be able to take advantage of all the excitement and variety the Army offers. The social life. Sports. Travel. Adventure training.
But most of all, because the skills you worked so hard to acquire will be valued. You'll be part of one of the most important teams in the Army.
If you're training, or already qualified and working, contact us now.
www.armymedicaljobs.mod.uk
or call 0845 600 2232
The Army is committed to Equal Opportunities.
Royal Army Medical Corps
MAKING THE BEST BETTER
ARMY
BE THE BEST

BJR

VOLUME 78

Number 927

Contents

March 2005

Front cover: *The illustrations used on the front cover of this issue of BJR can be found on pages 191, 238 and 247. We thank the authors for granting us permission to use their figures.*

Editorial

Page

- BJR Review of the Year – 2004 181

Full papers

- Ultrasound-guided drainage of breast abscesses: results in 151 patients 186
  A F Christensen, N Al-Suliman, K R Nielsen, I Vejborg, N Severinsen, H Christensen and M B Nielsen
- Ultrasound evaluation of the fibrosis stage in chronic liver disease by the simultaneous use of low and high frequency probes 189
  T Nishiura, H Watanabe, M Ito, Y Matsuoka, K Yano, M Daikoku, H Yatsuhashi, K Dohmen and H Ishibashi
- A comparative study of evaluation of radiographs, CT and 3D reformatted CT in facial trauma: what is the role of 3D? 198
  A D Reuben, S R Watt-Smith, D Dobson and S J Golding
- MR colonography: baseline appearance of the unprepared rectosigmoid 202
  V L Jardine, E Sala and D J Lomas
- Radiation doses received in the UK Breast Screening Programme in 2001 and 2002 207
  K C Young, A Burch and J M Oduko
- A study of the distribution of dose across the hands of interventional radiologists and cardiologists 219
  M Whitby and C J Martin
- Treatment outcomes and prognostic factors in patients with supratentorial low-grade gliomas 230
  S-A Yeh, J-T Ho, C-C Lui, Y-J Huang, C-Y Hsiung and E-Y Huang
- Daytime pulsed dose rate brachytherapy as a new treatment option for previously irradiated patients with recurrent oesophageal cancer 236
  W Harms, R Krempien, C Grehn, C Berns, F W Hensley and J Debus

Short communications

- Abnormal hepatic vein Doppler waveform in patients without liver disease 242
  J F Pedersen, A Z Dakhil, D B Jensen, B Søndergaard and P Bytzer

■ Techniques and trouble-shooting in high spatial resolution thin slice MRI for rectal cancer 245
G Brown, I R Daniels, C Richardson, P Revell, D Peppercorn and M Bourne

Case reports

■ Selective conformal radiotherapy for arteriovenous malformation involving the spinal cord 252
K Kishi, S Shirai, T Sonomura and M Sato

■ Small cell carcinoma of the colon: barium study and CT findings 255
H C Kim, S I Park, S J Park, H C Shin, M-H Oh, H H Kim, W K Bae and I Y Kim

■ Pilomatrix carcinoma of the axilla: CT and MRI features 257
T Niwa, T Yoshida, T Doiuchi, T Hiruma, K Kushida, A Mitsuda, Y Kameda, H Hayashi, K Fujii and T Inoue

■ Successful treatment of a chronic post-traumatic 5-year-old osteoporotic vertebral compression fracture by percutaneous vertebroplasty 261
F G Irani, J P Morales, T Sabharwal, R Dourado, A Gangi and A Adam

■ Pseudocyst rupture into the portal vein diagnosed with MRI 265
A Riddell, K Jhaveri and M Haider

■ Erythropoietin-producing renal cell carcinoma arising from autosomal dominant polycystic kidney disease 269
Y Hama, T Kaji, K Ito, M Hayakawa, M Tobe and S Kosuda

Pictorial review

■ Non-infectious manifestations of stem cell transplantation 272
D Beckett and J Olliff

Book reviews

282

Case of the month

■ Whispering enigma 283
H Ansari, T Patankar and A Jackson

Correspondence

■ Posterior fossa treatment 285
B Jones

■ Author's reply 285
P N Plowman and C Usher

BIR Company Subscribers

286

Meetings and courses

288

The British Journal of Radiology, *78* (2005), 181–185 © 2005 The British Institute of Radiology
DOI: 10.1259/bjr/16888100

Editorial

BJR Review of the Year – 2004

One of the ideas put forward during appraisal of the Journal a couple of years ago was that the BJR should introduce a "Review of the Year". The intention would be to identify papers which readers might have overlooked and which, in the opinion of the Editors, best illustrated both the objectives of the British Institute of Radiology and the diverse interests of the readers of its Journal.

The selection has been made by the current Honorary Editors and Deputy Editors but we would also like to acknowledge the hard work, carried out quietly, unassumingly and efficiently, by David MacVicar (Honorary Editor – Medical) and Victor Barley (Deputy Editor – Oncology) who both stood down at the end of September.

It would be presumptuous to suggest that we have necessarily chosen the "best" papers during the year. However, we believe the selection illustrates the multidisciplinary nature of the Journal, contains material of interest for all our readers and draws attention to many points of general importance.

If the "Review" is judged a success, our intention is that it will become a regular feature. Therefore this is something of a trial run and we shall welcome feed-back on the merits or otherwise of this initiative.

Radiology

The choice of a paper on a technique that to many radiologists has already been consigned to historical interest may seem surprising, but the paper from McLean et al [1] has perhaps a greater significance than may first be apparent. They highlight the need for critical appraisal of published papers when the results suggest that either new tests or a change in practice should be implemented locally.

McLean et al [1] reviewed four methods of reporting lung scintigraphy and then prospectively assessed their use on a cohort of 238 patients undergoing lung scintigraphy for suspected pulmonary embolic disease in their own hospital. The PIOPED criteria – locally modified [2], McMaster clinical criteria [3], PisaPED scintigraphic grading [4], and Miettinen logistic regression analysis [5] were all applied to the 238 patients and the results compared. The frequencies for differing levels of probability of pulmonary embolism varied widely between the different algorithms, with cross-referencing revealing correlation only between the modified PIOPED criteria and Miettinen logistic regression analysis. This led the authors to conclude that new diagnostic algorithms and tests are not automatically transferable to new environments.

They suggest that this is not an infrequent finding when new technologies, either diagnostic or therapeutic, are introduced locally, with the results appearing less impressive than the published data. There are clearly many reasons for this, not least the local "learning curve" set against the expertise of the published authors. Other reasons such as referral bias during the study, and underlying prevalence of disease – often high in the study population, will also have an effect, and it is these factors that may to some extent result in the local radiologists' inability to reproduce the published data.

This paper may "strengthen the hands" of those who already use one of the two methods of reporting lung scintigraphy that correlated. More generally it should serve as a lesson to all radiologists that it is essential to critically appraise published data and compare performance with already established techniques when a procedure is implemented locally.

Radiation protection in radiology

Not surprisingly, papers relating to doses to patients dominated these contributions to the Journal in 2004 and scarcely an X-ray technique or a part of the body escaped attention.

Barium examinations of the gastrointestinal system make up about 16% of the collective dose from radiological examinations in the UK [6] and Martin [7] has reported on a review undertaken to assess the impact of dose reduction facilities incorporated into fluoroscopic X-ray equipment in the last 5 years.

Substantial reductions in entrance doses were recorded. For barium enemas monitored in 11 hospitals, the median dose–area product (DAP) was 16.3 Gy cm^2 (range 4.3–30.4 Gy cm^2) compared with 26 Gy cm^2 (range 9.3–48.9 Gy cm^2) in 1994. However, mean screening times were the same (to within 1%) in the two studies and fewer images had been taken in 1994. Therefore some of the dose reduction could be linked to new X-ray equipment that has been installed in nine of the 11 hospitals in the intervening period with dose-saving facilities such as low dose pulsed fluoroscopy and digital imaging.

Additional copper filtration (0.2 mm) reduced DAP values substantially (about 44–50%) but it is important to remember that effective dose is reduced by much less (12–22%) because the beam has been substantially hardened before entering the body. Decubitus films contribute a substantial proportion of the dose for barium enema examinations and the ability to use the image intensifier in C-arm units gives a substantial dose advantage.

Another technique in which there have been significant technological changes is CT with the introduction of multidetector, multislice scanners. Between 1999 and 2002, nine of the 14 scanners assessed in the East Anglian region had been replaced by multislice technology. Carrying out dose audit to a strictly defined protocol allowed meaningful comparison to be made between the 2002 audit and previous audits in 1996 and 1999 [8].

Averaged across a broad spread of 10 routine examinations, regional mean effective doses had increased by 34% between 1999 and 2002. On average the multislice scanners gave 35% more effective dose than the single slice scanners and as would be expected from simple consideration of geometric efficiencies, the difference between single slice and multislice effective doses was greatest for examinations using narrow slice widths, where the effect of beam collimation in multislice CT is most severe.

These findings, combined with the known rapid increase in the frequency of CT examinations, highlights the importance of dose optimization, both in respect of technical improvements such as automatic tube current modulation and examination protocols.

Both of the preceding papers addressed the question of diagnostic reference levels (DRLs) and these were also the subject of an Editorial by Walker in the May issue [9].

DRLs are now a very clear, legally backed requirement placed on each radiology department in the UK to take ownership of patient dose and to set, monitor and use their own DRLs as an aid to patient dose optimization. Therefore the publication of guidance providing a pragmatic methodology for setting local DRLs for procedures carried out in radiology departments is to be welcomed [10]. The report also explains the difference between the setting and use of local DRLs, as opposed to national DRLs, outlines the actions necessary when local DRLs are consistently exceeded and provides a summary of data that can be used for setting national DRLs.

There is considerable benefit to be gained from a unified, national approach to both the setting up of DRLs and their use to optimize patient dose.

Teaching and image interpretation

Extended roles for both radiographers and nurses are an integral part of the UK Government's plans to create more flexibility in the National Health Service (NHS) and break down professional boundaries [11]. One of the areas in which non-medical healthcare professionals have had an extended role has been in the radiographic interpretation of trauma radiographs.

Hardy and Barrett [12] have looked critically at the differences in reporting arrangements in Accident and Emergency (A & E) Departments across a range of NHS hospitals in the UK. They found marked differences in the education provided for radiographers and nurses to support radiographic interpretation and in the range of examinations each staff group was permitted to interpret. A worrying finding was that, whereas the clinical gold standard for radiographer reporting was reporting by consultant radiologists, nurses have tended to compare their ability to interpret radiographic images with that of SHOs.

Overall, the authors concluded that a review of current service delivery strategies was required to ensure that reporting of radiology films in A & E departments is optimized.

Also in this section we note a thought-provoking paper by Manning et al [13] on the reasons for missing lung cancer from the posteroanterior (PA) chest radiograph. Basically the aim of the work was to determine whether observer error in reporting early lung cancer from PA chest radiographs is due to failure of detection or failure of interpretation.

Using a set of digital images containing a variety of pulmonary nodules, a group of radiologists as expert observers, eye tracking procedures to analyse dwell time and alternate free response operating characteristic (AFROC) techniques [14], the authors found that 65% of the false negative decisions were due to failures of interpretation, not failures of detection. As a consequence they question the widely-held assumption that technological changes to improve contrast, image resolution and detective quantum efficiency will naturally and always result in improved diagnostic outcome.

Such a finding is important because, if confirmed, it may add a new dimension to the way image interpretation is taught and may influence the way in which artificial intelligence should be used to assist the radiologist.

Oncology

For the radiation oncologist reading the BJR, this has been the year of intensity-modulated radiation therapy (IMRT). We have had a major, two-part, review article [15, 16]; a review of an alternative approach using helical tomotherapy, discussed in the next section [17]; an account of radiographers' reactions to the introduction of IMRT [18]; an account of the practicalities of setting up IMRT from scratch [19]. Several papers dealt with the comparisons between IMRT and more conventional techniques: in medulloblastoma [20]; in prostate cancer [21, 22]; and in oesophageal cancer [23]. A summary of the conclusions might be: IMRT is more demanding, in terms of both expertise and time, than more conventional techniques, but may have some minor advantages. These dosimetric advantages have not yet been translated into clinical results.

The other strand running through the year's publications has been the question of concomitant dose in patients treated with radiotherapy. Concomitant dose is that dose, additional to the prescribed dose, that is delivered as a result of the simulation and verification procedures performed during a course of radiotherapy [24–26]. The issue is important, not least because it arises when IR(ME)R is applied to clinical radiotherapy [27]. We might ask whether or not radiotherapy requires its own set of IR(ME)R regulations.

The risks posed by concomitant exposures may pale into insignificance, however, when compared with some of the problems raised by IMRT. IMRT uses multiple beams and there may be problems with exit dose [20], and also, compared with conventional treatments, with the increased volume of tissue treated to low dose. This has consequences both for bystander effects and radiation-induced genomic instability, including the induction of second cancers. In a short, but chilling, paragraph Guerrero and Nutting [16] mention that the whole body equivalent dose is nearly 2000 mSv for IMRT and less than 250 mSv for conventional treatment. This could translate into an eightfold increase in radiation-induced cancers. For advanced, otherwise incurable, tumours this might be a risk worth taking, but there is a serious concern for adjuvant radiotherapy where, as in breast cancer, for example, the majority of patients are already cured before they start their radiotherapy.

These are important issues and the BJR, with its multidisciplinary portfolio of authors and readers (physicists, epidemiologists, statisticians, radiation biologists, radiologists, oncologists) is in a unique position to address them. Our Britishness also helps. The NHS insulates us from many of the commercial pressures that, in other countries, may influence the evaluation and adoption of new technologies. We should be the masters of technology, not its servants. We need to know whether, in every sense, IMRT is worth the cost. Publications in the BJR have made major contributions to this debate, and will continue to do so.

Imaging in radiotherapy

Several papers in BJR in 2004 have highlighted the rapid developments in conformal radiotherapy and the integrated imaging systems which are essential to their success. In particular, Beavis [17] reviewed the emergence of helical tomotherapy [28], a radiotherapy technique which draws equally on both linear accelerator and CT technology to produce a design which moves significantly away from conventional linear accelerator concepts. A 6 MV linac waveguide and multileaf collimator produce a fan beam which is used to build up the required conformal dose distribution as the patient is translated through the gantry aperture. A bank of xenon ion chamber CT detectors mounted on the gantry intercepts the transmitted beam and allows volumetric CT imaging of the patient during treatment delivery. This makes possible modification of target volumes and the avoidance of critical structures on a fraction-by-fraction basis, so called adaptive radiotherapy. Moreover, margins to allow for patient movement should be reduced, leading to higher target doses. Helical tomotherapy is not uniquely required for this strategy and other systems have been proposed [29–31], but the integration of dose planning, image fusion facilities, treatment delivery and volumetric imaging within the same system may indicate the way ahead.

Increasing conformance of the dose distribution to a target volume, made possible by these recent developments in radiotherapy, raises the question of how the target volume should be defined in the first place, and what confidence should be ascribed to current imaging techniques in identifying it. Given the known difficulties in defining the planning target volume (PTV) [32, 33], we cannot assume that better *in vitro* dose distributions automatically guarantee better results *in vivo*.

It seems highly likely that the developing field of molecular imaging will be crucial to the understanding of the molecular basis of disease, including cancer. It was therefore timely to see the publication of a BJR Special Issue devoted to these developments [34], including MRI, MRS, PET, SPECT, ultrasound and optical methodologies. It may not be too long before the integration of molecular imaging modalities with radiotherapy planning and delivery is as commonplace as conventional CT is today, making radiotherapy a biologically, as well as geometrically, targeted technique.

Radiobiology/cancer biology

The role of the vasculature in tumour and normal tissue response to therapy has been a significant theme of articles published in the BJR recently.

It has long been suspected that damage to the vasculature is a major contributor to late injury to normal tissues following radiotherapy [35, 36], but direct evidence for this relationship has been lacking. A study published this year in the BJR offers compelling evidence for this in the central nervous system of rats: the use of a radioprotector that does not cross the blood–brain barrier, predictably inhibited vascular damage, but it also completely prevented the brain necrosis seen in non drug-treated animals [37]. While these data might suggest a means of protecting brain tissue against late radiation damage, it may also have the undesirable consequence of protecting against vascular-mediated damage to brain tumours. Recent evidence suggests, however, that tumours release anti-apoptotic factors that inhibit death of their supplying vasculature such that tumour endothelium may be protected anyway [38].

There is much recent evidence for the potential efficacy of agents directed against aspects of tumour vasculature, including direct, specific toxicity against the tumour endothelium and anti-angiogenesis [39–42]. Specific measurement *in vivo* of vascular changes associated with this therapy has been made possible by recent developments in imaging technology. The Special Issue, Angiogenesis Imaging, edited by Dr Padhani, contained articles addressing the key issues of how we might identify the activity of both anti-angiogenic and anti-vascular therapies in the clinic using a variety of modalities. Of particular note were the articles summarizing recommendations for appropriate methodology and endpoints for MRI studies [43, 44]. This information should help to maximize the quality of data obtainable from clinical trials using such agents.

Technical developments

An important technical contribution to the Journal was the Commentary by Visvikis et al on current trends and future developments in PET technology [45]. Bearing in mind the interests of many BJR readers, the article focused on applications in oncology. In this area the goals for developments in PET technology will continue to be improved (faster) patient throughput coupled with improved image quality and quantification. All of these advancements would be assisted by higher sensitivity devices and the authors reviewed some of the ways in which these might be achieved.

High quality PET imaging places stringent demands on the scintillation detectors – high density and atomic number for efficient capture of high energy photons; high yield of scintillation photons to improve positional resolution and scatter rejection; short scintillation decay times to improve dead time characteristics. Two new scintillators, lutetium oxyorthosilicate and gadolinium oxyorthosilicate, have been used in clinical PET scanners with significant reduction in the detection of scatter and random coincidences by comparison with the standard scintillation detectors in PET scanners (bismuth germanate). Further along the imaging chain there is active research to improve the photodetector system and overall photodetector design. For example a continuous light guide coupling the individual crystal elements to the photomultiplier tubes can minimize variations in light collection and improve energy resolution.

Scatter coincidences and random coincidences seriously degrade the information contained in the true coincidences detected and their effect on image quality must be minimized. For large fields of view, where scatter is high, this has generally been achieved by "collimating" the detectors using septa in the imaging field of view (so called two-dimensional PET). Uncollimated systems (three-dimensional (3D) PET) have difficulty handling the large amount of spurious data collected. However, "collimation" leads to a serious loss in sensitivity so work is continuing to try to refine the inherently more sensitive 3D design.

Finally the poor resolution of PET (4–5 mm) has stimulated work on image fusion to combine images from different techniques. This also provides an opportunity to combine anatomical and functional imaging. Since the use of non-linear registration techniques for sets of data acquired in separate systems is inherently more flexible than a combined system (see below) and considerably less expensive, further important developments can be expected in this area.

Notwithstanding, combined PET/CT systems are probably one of the fastest growing hardware developments in imaging technology. Apart from the obvious benefits of rapid and accurate image registration, the CT component provides a simple, quick facility for generating a body-tissue attenuation map that is essential for accurate quantitation of the PET image. Future developments of PET/CT systems will include the use of state-of-the-art multislice CT scanners and increasing use of combined systems in radiotherapy treatment planning. The potential for developing combined PET/MRI devices also must not be overlooked.

References

1. McLean RG, Carolan M, Bui C, Arvela O, Ford JC, Chew M, et al. Comparison of new clinical and scintigraphic algorithms for the diagnosis of pulmonary embolism. Br J Radiol 2004;77:372–6.
2. PIOPED Investigators. Value of the ventilation perfusion scan in acute pulmonary embolism. JAMA 1990;263:2753–9.
3. Wells PS, Ginsberg JS, Anderson DR, et al. Use of a clinical model for safe management of patients with suspected pulmonary embolism. Ann Intern Med 1998;129:997–1005.
4. Miniati M, Pistolesi M, Marini C, et al. Value of perfusion lung scan in the diagnosis of pulmonary embolism: results of the prospective investigative study of acute pulmonary embolism diagnosis (PisaPED). Am J Resp Critical Care Med 1996;154:1387–93.
5. Miettinen OS, Henschke CI, Yankelevitz DF. Evaluation of diagnostic imaging tests: diagnostic probability estimation. J Clin Epidemiol 1998;51:1293–8.
6. United Nations Scientific Committee on the Effects of atomic radiation. Sources and effects of ionising radiation. Volume 1 – Sources. New York: United Nations, 2000.
7. Martin CJ. A review of factors affecting patient doses for barium enemas and meals. Br J Radiol 2004;77:864–8.
8. Yates SJ, Pike LC, Goldstone KE. Effect of multislice scanners on patient dose from routine CT examinations in East Anglia. Br J Radiol 2004;77:472–8.
9. Walker A. A uniform approach to setting and using DRLs? Br J Radiol 2004;77:369.
10. Guidance on the establishment and use of diagnostic reference levels for medical X-ray examinations. Joint Working Party Report 88. London: IPEM, 2004.
11. Department of Health. A health service of all talents; developing the NHS work force. London: Department of Health, 2000.
12. Hardy M, Barrett C. Interpretation of trauma radiographs by radiographers and nurses in the UK; a comparative study. Br J Radiol 2004;77:657–61.
13. Manning DJ, Ethell SC, Donovan T. Detection or decision errors? Missed lung cancer from the posteroanterior chest radiograph. Br J Radiol 2004;77:231–5.
14. Chakraborty DP, Winter LHL. free response methodology: alternate analysis and a new observer performance experiment. Radiology 1990;174:873–81.
15. Guerrero Urbano MT, Nutting CM. Clinical use of intensity-modulated radiotherapy: part I. Br J Radiol 2004;77:88–96.
16. Guerrero Urbano MT, Nutting CM. Clinical use of intensity-modulated radiotherapy: part II. Br J Radiol 2004;77:177–82.
17. Beavis AW. Is tomotherapy the future of IMRT? Br J Radiol 2004;77:285–95.
18. McNair HA, Francis G, Balyckyi J. Clinical implementation of dynamic intensity-modulated radiotherapy: radiographers' perspectives. Br J Radiol 2004;77:493–8.
19. James HV, Scrase CD, Poynter AJ. Practical experience with intensity-modulated radiotherapy. Br J Radiol 2004;77:3–14.
20. Breen SL, Kehagioglou P, Usher C, Plowman PN. A comparison of conventional, conformal and intensity-modulated coplanar radiotherapy plans for posterior fossa treatment. Br J Radiol 2004;77:768–74.
21. Kao J, Turian J, Meyers A, Hamilton RJ, Smith B, Vijayakumar S, et al. Sparing of the penile bulb and proximal penile structures with intensity-modulated radiation therapy for prostate cancer. Br J Radiol 2004;77:129–36.
22. Mott JH, Livsey JE, Logue JP. Development of a simultaneous boost IMRT class solution for a hypofractionated prostate cancer protocol. Br J Radiol 2004;77:377–86.
23. Wu VW, Sham JS, Kwong DL. Inverse planning in three-dimensional conformal and intensity-modulated radiotherapy of mid-thoracic oesophageal cancer. Br J Radiol 2004;77:568–72.
24. Aird EG. Second cancer risk, concomitant exposures and IRMER(2000). Br J Radiol 2004;77:983–5.
25. Harrison RM. Second cancers following radiotherapy: a suggested common dosimetry framework for therapeutic and concomitant exposures. Br J Radiol 2004;77:986–90.
26. Waddington SP, McKenzie AL. Assessment of effective dose from concomitant exposures required in verification of the target volume in radiotherapy. Br J Radiol 2004;77:557–61.
27. Nisbet A, Cocker M. Experiences of a proactive IR(ME)R inspection in radiotherapy. Br J Radiol 2004;77:329–32.
28. Mackie TR, Holmes T, Swerdloff S, Reckwerdt P, Deasy JO, Yang J, et al. Tomotherapy: a new concept for the delivery of dynamic conformal radiotherapy. Med Phys 1993;20:1709–19.
29. Cheng CW, Wong J, Grimm L, Chow M, Uematsu M, Fung A. Commissioning and clinical implementation of a sliding gantry CT scanner installed in an existing treatment room and early clinical experience for precise tumor localization. Am J Clin Oncol 2003;26:e28–36.
30. Court L, Rosen I, Mohan, Dong L. Evaluation of mechanical precision and alignment uncertainties for an integrated CT/LINAC system. Med Phys 2003;30:1198–210.
31. Jaffray DA, Siewerdsen JH, Wong JW, Martinez AA. Flat-panel cone-beam computed tomography for image-guided radiation therapy. Int J Radiat Oncol Biol Phys 2002;53:1337–49.
32. Sidhu K, Cooper P, Ramani R, Schwartz M, Franssen E, Davey P. Delineation of brain metastases on CT images for planning radiosurgery: concerns regarding accuracy. Br J Radiol 2004;77:39–42.

33. Wilkinson JM. Geometric uncertainties in radiotherapy. Br J Radiol 2004;77:86–7.
34. Dzik-Jurasz A, editor. Molecular imaging. Br J Radiol 2003;76 Spec No 2.
35. Sindelar WF, Kinsella TJ. Normal tissue tolerance to intraoperative radiotherapy. Surg Oncol Clin N Am 2003;12:925–42.
36. Hopewell JW, van der Kogel AJ. Pathophysiological mechanisms leading to the development of late radiation-induced damage to the central nervous system. Front Radiat Ther Oncol 1999;33:265–75.
37. Lyubimova N, Hopewell JW. Experimental evidence to support the hypothesis that damage to vascularendothelium plays the primary role in the development of late radiation-induced CNS injury. Br J Radiol 2004;77:488–92.
38. Moeller BJ, Cao Y, Li CY, Dewhirst MW. Radiation activates HIF-1 to regulate vascular radiosensitivity in tumors: role of reoxygenation, free radicals, and stress granules. Cancer Cell 2004;5:429–41.
39. Purow B, Fine HA. Progress report on the potential of angiogenesis inhibitors for neuro-oncology. Cancer Invest 2004;22:577–87.
40. Tozer GM, Bicknell R. Therapeutic targeting of the tumor vasculature. Semin Radiat Oncol 2004;14:222–32.
41. Straubinger RM, Arnold RD, Zhou R, Mazurchuk R, Slack JE. Antivascular and antitumor activities of liposome-associated drugs. Anticancer Res 2004;24:397–404.
42. Kerbel RS. Antiangiogenic drugs and current strategies for the treatment of lung cancer. Semin Oncol 2004; 31(1 Suppl. 1):54–60.
43. Leach MO, Brindle KM, Evelhoch JL, Griffiths JR, Horsman MR, Jackson A, et al. Assessment of antiangiogenic and antivascular therapeutics using MRI: recommendations for appropriate methodology for clinical trials. Br J Radiol 2003;76 Spec No 1:S87–91.
44. Padhani AR. MRI for assessing antivascular cancer treatments. Br J Radiol2003;76 Spec No 1:S60–80.
45. Visvikis D, Chese-le Rest C, Jarrett P. PET technology: current trends and future developments. Br J Radiol 2004;77:906–910.

The British Journal of Radiology, 78 (2005), 186–188
DOI: 10.1259/bjr/26372381

Ultrasound-guided drainage of breast abscesses: results in 151 patients

[1]A F CHRISTENSEN, MD, [2]N AL-SULIMAN, MD, [1]K R NIELSEN, MD, [1]I VEJBORG, MD, [2]N SEVERINSEN, MD, ^{3}H CHRISTENSEN, MD, PhD and [1]M B NIELSEN, MD, PhD, DMSc

[1]*Department of Radiology and* [2]*Department of Surgery CE, Rigshospitalet, and* [3]*Department of Neurology, Bispebjerg Hospital, University of Copenhagen, Denmark*

Abstract. The aim of this paper is to describe the efficacy of ultrasound-guided drainage of breast abscesses with special attention to the risk of recurrence and the need for surgical treatment in a consecutive patient population. 151 patients, 89 with puerperal and 62 with non-puerperal breast abscesses, were treated with ultrasound-guided drainage, by needle or catheter under local anaesthesia. Follow-up punctures were performed at 2 or 3 day intervals until the clinical condition and ultrasound findings had improved. All patients were treated with oral antibiotics. Mammography was performed to search for underlying cancer. 86 (97%) out of 89 patients with puerperal abscesses and 50 (81%) out of 62 with non-puerperal abscesses recovered after the first round of ultrasound-guided drainage. One patient in each group had recurrence in loco but recovered after further ultrasound-guided drainage. 13 patients, 11 with non-puerperal and two with puerperal abscesses, underwent surgical excision of the abscess cavity or fistulas. Breastfeeding continued and 117 patients were treated as outpatients. The median number of follow up examinations in the ultrasound-department was four (range 1–10) for the group of patients with puerperal abscess and three (range 1–7) in the group of patients with non-puerperal abscess. The corresponding figure for the median number of punctures was for both groups one (range 1–6 and 1–4). There were no reports of newly diagnosed breast cancer in the 2 year follow-up period. This study supports the use of ultrasound-guided drainage in puerperal and non-puerperal breast abscesses. The method is less invasive than traditional surgery and has a high rate of success.

Ultrasound-guided drainage has been described in smaller series as a treatment for breast abscesses, the treatment for which has traditionally been surgery or less frequently puncture without imaging guidance [1–5]. Ultrasound guided drainage is now widely accepted as first-line treatment. The aim of this study was to describe the efficacy of ultrasound guided drainage with special attention to resolution and to the risk of recurrence as well as the need for surgical treatment in a consecutive patient population.

Materials and methods

From 1 January 1998 to 31 December 2001, 248 patients were referred to the ultrasound department with clinical suspicion of new-developed breast abscess. In 87 (35%) of these patients breast abscess was excluded by ultrasound examination. The remaining 161 patients had a breast abscess. 10 of these 161 patients were not treated by ultrasound-guided drainage: five patients had abscesses which perforated spontaneously before treatment, three patients underwent surgery because the abscesses were too superficial and not suited for ultrasound-drainage with skin changes which required surgery for healing, one patient refused puncture under local anaesthesia and one 87-year-old patient had syncope before treatment was initiated and no further treatment was undertaken. The remaining 151 patients were treated with ultrasound-guided drainage of an abscess. They form the basis of the study.

Received 22 March 2004 and in revised form 27 August 2004, accepted 4 October 2004.

The 151 patients that underwent ultrasound-guided drainage were all female, 89 had puerperal breast abscesses (median age 32 years, range 15–42 years), and 62 had non-puerperal abscesses (median age 42 years, range 15–72 years). None of the patients were undergoing treatment for other breast pathology.

Rigshospitalet is the centre for breast disease in central Copenhagen, covering a population of approximately 600 000 individuals. All patients with breast disease are referred to the clinic for breast surgery. If breast abscess is clinically suspected patients are referred to ultrasound for diagnosis and if possible for ultrasound-guided drainage with either a 0.8–1.2 mm needle or, if the cavity is larger than 3 cm, a 5.7 F (2 mm) one-step catheter. All punctures are performed under local anaesthesia. The procedure can be performed at any time in our institution when clinically indicated.

Follow-up ultrasound examinations are performed at 2–3 day intervals and if the abscess is still present, another puncture is performed or the catheter is left in place. Ultrasound follow-up ends when the clinical condition improves and two consecutive examinations have shown no residual abscess. The final examination is performed after the final puncture or removal of the catheter in the examination before. The catheter is cared for by the patient herself after instruction is given on the ward. The removal of a catheter requires clinical improvement of the local symptoms and no residual undrained fluid in the abscess visualized by ultrasound. All patients received oral antibiotic treatment; dicloxacillin 1 g three times a day in all patients and additionally metronidazole 0.5 g three times a day for non-puerperal abscesses. Patients allergic to penicillin receive erythromycin 500 mg three times a day. All 151 patients in this study followed this procedure.

In 2003 and 2004 the hospital case records were retrospectively reviewed. The following parameters were registered: patient data, details about drainage procedure and punctures, bacteriology and surgical data and possible recurrent abscess within 24 months. Clinical examination and mammography, ultrasound and where indicated ultrasound-guided biopsy, were performed within 3 months after the resolution of the abscess, mainly in the group of patients with non-puerperal breast abscesses. In January 2004 all 151 patients were followed in the register of the Danish Breast Cancer Group to see if any had been diagnosed with breast cancer within 24 months.

Statistical analyses were performed with SPSS for Windows 9.0 (SPSS Inc., Chicago, IL). Descriptives included numbers, percentage and range. Logistic regression analysis was first performed by univariate testing, where variables were tested based on literature and clinical experience. We planned to include variables reaching a significance level of <0.1 in univariate testing in a final multivariate logistic regression model. The outcome variable used was resolution after ultrasound-guided drainage, being defined as no recurrent abscess and no need for surgery.

Results

Patient data are given in Tables 1 and 2. 136 patients, 86 (97%) of the 89 patients with puerperal breast abscess and 50 (81%) of the 62 patients with non-puerperal breast abscess had no signs of remaining infection in the breasts after the first ultrasound-guided drainage treatment. 77 (87%) of the patients with puerperal breast abscess were treated as outpatients despite catheter drainage treatment. The catheters were cared for by the patients themselves after instruction and removed at the hospital after (median) 4 days (range 2–6 days).

After successful ultrasound-guided treatment of the abscess, three of these patients underwent surgery based solely upon an unconfirmed suspicion of cancer: the findings of a solid nodule in one patient, atypical cells in a biopsy in another patient and an abscess in an atypical cyst.

Two patients, one patient in each group had a recurrent abscess (after 5 months and 10 months, respectively) but recovered after further ultrasound-guided drainage.

13 patients, two with puerperal and 11 with non-puerperal abscesses, underwent surgical excision of the abscess cavity. Two patients preferred surgery to ultrasound-guided drainage, one had pain after the abscess resolved and two other patients had an abscess that perforated during treatment. In six cases surgery was for a complicating fistula, one puerperal and five non-puerperal – two of the non-puerperal fistulae were present prior to commencement of treatment. One patient was not effectively treated with ultrasound-drainage, and one had pus in ectatic ducts and was difficult to treat with ultrasound-guided drainage.

The median number of follow up examinations in the ultrasound department was four (range 1–10) for the group of patients with puerperal abscess and three (range 1–7) in the group of patients with non-puerperal abscess. The corresponding figure for the median number of punctures was for both groups one (range 1–6 and 1–4). The two patients who had the most extensive treatment without reference to surgery needed six punctures and 10 ultrasound examinations each. Both patients had continuous improvement in both clinical condition and ultrasound findings which was why surgery was not performed.

The results of the univariate logistic regression analysis are presented in Table 3. Recovery was seen in 135 out of the 151 patients (87%). In this analysis only a puerperal history reached significance. A multivariate analysis was therefore not performed.

Table 1. Clinical characteristics of 151 patients with breast abscesses

	Puerperal abscess	Non-puerperal abscess
No. of patients	89	62
Age (years)	32 (15–42)	42 (15–72)
Days from symptom onset to diagnosis and treatment	7 (2–70)	7 (1–30)
Needle puncture/catheter drainage	23 (26%)/66 (74%)	46 (74%)/16 (26%)
Hospital admittance/outpatients	12 (13%)/77 (87%)	22 (36%)/40 (64%)
Median no. of follow-up ultrasound examinations (range)	4 (1–10)	3 (1–7)
Central *vs* peripheral localization of abscess	34.5%/65.5%	43.5%/56.5%
Median size of abscess (in cm) (range)	3.5 (1.0–8.0)	2.0 (0.5–8.0)
No. of punctures	1 (1–6)	1 (1–4)

Data are given as median (range) except where indicated otherwise.

Table 2. The outcome of the treatment in the 151 patients

Outcome of the treatment	Breast abscesses	
	Puerperal no. of patients	Non-puerperal no. of patients
Recovered after the first round of ultrasound-guided drainage	86 (97%)	50 (81%)
Had recurrent abscess after end ultrasound-guided drainage	1 (1%)	1 (1%)
Underwent surgery (see results for details)	2 (2%)	11 (18%)

Table 3. Univariate logistic regression analyses of factors possibly affecting breast abscess resolution in 151 females treated with ultrasound-guided drainage of breast abscesses

	OR	CI 95%	*p*-value
Puerperal *vs* non-puerperal	4.1	1.02–16.7	0.0471
Age+10 years	0.8	0.5–1.4	0.504
Delay from symptom onset to treatment	1.0	0.9–1.1	0.6531
Total number of abscesses	0.9	0.1–6.8	0.896
Largest diameter+10 mm	1.6	0.8–3.0	0.175
Central *vs* peripheral localization	1.5	0.5–4.1	0.477
Catheter drainage *vs* only puncture	0.6	0.1–2.9	0.515

OR, odds ratio; CI, confidence interval.

26 patients with puerperal and 51 patients with non-puerperal abscess were referred for clinical evaluation and mammography. All of the 26 patients with puerperal abscess had palpation findings as the basis for referral for mammography. The patients with non-puerperal abscess were referred for mammography unless the abscess was situated centrally and subareolar (only three patients with lateral abscesses were not referred). In the follow-up period there were no reports of cases of *de novo* diagnosed breast cancer in the two patient groups.

Discussion

Ultrasound-guided drainage in combination with oral antibiotics was shown to be an effective treatment for breast abscess, especially for the group with puerperal abscesses. No other factors, including whether treatment was conducted using needle puncture and aspiration or catheter drainage, had any independent effect on the recovery rate.

The high rates of recovery found in this study confirm previous studies, where recovery rates exceeding 90% using ultrasound-guided drainage have been reported [1, 4–6]. To our knowledge no previous study has included more than 30 patients. Treatment failure using ultrasound-guided drainage has been reported in cases where either the abscess has been larger than 3 cm in diameter or it was placed centrally in a subareolar position [1]. This study did not support these findings since neither size nor localization showed any independent effect on the recovery rate.

In some institutions the standard treatment still remains early incision under general anaesthesia combined with drainage tube insertion [7]. The side effects of this treatment include scarring and termination of breast-feeding [3]. Ultrasound-guided drainage causes less scarring, does not affect breast-feeding and does not require general anaesthesia or hospitalization [3]. Ultrasound-guided drainage is a less expensive procedure than surgery [9]. Based on our findings, ultrasound-guided drainage treatment should replace surgery as the first line of treatment in uncomplicated puerperal or non-puerperal breast abscess. Furthermore this technique is not difficult to master and the service can be provided on a 24 h basis.

In treatment resistant cases, where the abscess is unresponsive to the combination of repeated drainage and oral antibiotics, surgical treatment still has a role. It is unclear why some abscesses are unresponsive to treatment. Surgery is also needed in cases with superficial abscesses with skin changes. This can make a surgical excision necessary for healing. Surgery can also be necessary in special cases where other concerns such as suspicion of malignancy or the need for focus excision are important factors. Carcinoma of the breast may be confused with inflammatory conditions and thus pose a diagnostic problem [8]. We use early follow-up mammography within 3 months and when appropriate ultrasound-guided biopsy to exclude this diagnosis. In this study no patients had diagnosed breast cancer in the follow-up period. The number of patients included in this study is in our opinion not large enough to substantiate any statement about whether clinical mammography should be routinely undertaken. Likewise we have not found any reason to alter indications for mammography.

Needle puncture of lactating breasts has previously been associated with fistula formation [10]. In this study, six patients had a fistula in connection with a breast abscess. However only four of the 151 patients receiving ultrasound-guided drainage developed a fistula, of which only one had a puerperal abscess. Two of the six patients had a fistula before treatment started. These data indicate that ultrasound-guided drainage does not cause more fistula formation in puerperal than in non-puerperal abscesses.

In conclusion, this study supports the use of ultrasound-guided drainage in both puerperal and non-puerperal breast abscesses. The method is less invasive than traditional surgery and has a high rate of success.

References

1. Hook GW, Ikeda DM. Treatment of breast abscesses with US-guided percutaneous needle drainage without indwelling catheter placement. Radiology 1999;213:579–82.
2. Tan SM, Low SC. Non-operative treatment of breast abscesses. Aust N Z J Surg 1998;68:423–4.
3. Schwarz RJ, Shrestha R. Needle aspiration of breast abscesses. Am J Surg 2001;182:117–9.
4. Karstrup S, Solvig J, Nolsoe CP, et al. Acute puerperal breast abscesses: US-guided drainage. Radiology 1993;188:807–9.
5. Blaivas M. Ultrasound-guided breast abscess aspiration in a difficult case. Acad Emerg Med 2001;8:398–401.
6. Karstrup S, Nolsoe C, Brabrand K, Nielsen KR. Ultrasonically guided percutaneous drainage of breast abscesses. Acta Radiol 1990;31:157–9.
7. Marchant DJ. Inflammation of the breast. Obstet Gynecol Clin North Am 2002;29:89–102.
8. Das DK, Sodhani P, Kashyap V, Parkash S, Pant JN, Bhatnagar P. Inflammatory lesions of the breast: diagnosis by fine needle aspiration. Cytopathology 1992;3:281–9.
9. Imperiale A, Zandriono F, Calabrese M, Parodi G, Massa T. Abscesses of the breast: US-guided serial percutaneous aspiration and local antibiotic therapy after unsuccessful systemic antibiotic therapy. Acta Radiologica 2001;42:161.
10. Barker P. Milk fistula. An unusual complication of breast biopsy. J RC Surg Edinburgh 1988;106.

The British Journal of Radiology, 78 (2005), 189–197 © 2005 The British Institute of Radiology
DOI: 10.1259/bjr/75208448

Ultrasound evaluation of the fibrosis stage in chronic liver disease by the simultaneous use of low and high frequency probes

[1]T NISHIURA, RMS, ^{1}H WATANABE, RMS, [1,2]M ITO, MD, [3]Y MATSUOKA, MD, [4]K YANO, MD, [4]M DAIKOKU, MD, [4]H YATSUHASHI, MD, [4]K DOHMEN, MD, FACP, SJSUM and [4]H ISHIBASHI, MD, FACP, SJSUM

[1]*Clinical Laboratory,* [2]*Department of Pathology,* [3]*Deartment of Radiology and* [4]*Clinical Research Centre, NHO National Nagasaki Medical Centre, Omura, Nagasaki, 856-8562 Japan*

Abstract. A liver biopsy is currently considered the definitive diagnostic modality for establishing the severity of hepatic fibrosis. We analysed the diagnostic sensitivity and accuracy of ultrasound (US) using both low frequency and high frequency probes as a repeatable, inexpensive, and reliable method to determine the fibrosis stage in chronic liver disease and then compared our results with the histological findings. A total of 103 patients with chronic liver disease (60 males and 43 females, average age 51 years old) who had undergone both a liver biopsy and US with 2–5 MHz frequency and 5–12 MHz frequency probes were prospectively evaluated in this study. An US scoring system using both the low frequency and high frequency probes was performed by evaluating the edge, surface and parenchymal texture of the liver. Each score was obtained by evaluating three parameters; the bluntness of the liver edge, the irregularity of the surface and the coarseness of the parenchymal texture were evaluated and then compared with the histological findings. The US scores of the liver edge (rs: 0.6668), liver surface (rs: 0.9007) and liver parenchymal texture (rs: 0.8853) correlated significantly with the fibrosis stage obtained based on the biopsy findings. The accumulated US scores of these three parameters, however, was found to be the most reliable indicator (rs: 0.9524). Patients with an accumulated score of 6.5 or more were all found to have fibrosis stage 4 in which the accuracy of our scoring system for correctly predicting cirrhosis was found to be 100% sensitive. When an accumulated US score of 3 was interpreted to indicate mild fibrosis (a fibrosis score of 0 or 1), all 42 patients with stage 0 or 1 fibrosis were found to have an accumulated US score of 3 or less (a probability of 100%) and 42 of 53 patients with a score of 3 or less were found to have stage 0 or 1 fibrosis (specificity of 79.2%). An ultrasound evaluation of the liver fibrosis stage based on the scoring system using both low and high frequency probes was found to be a reliable and effective alternative to the histological staging in chronic liver diseases.

The liver fibrosis stage in patients with chronic liver diseases due to an infection with hepatitis B virus (HBV) or C virus (HCV) is a pivotal factor regarding both the therapeutic options and for predicting the prognosis. A liver biopsy is considered to be the gold standard for diagnosing the liver fibrosis stage and predicting the outcome of the diseases. Although a percutaneous liver biopsy is relatively safe, it is still associated with a risk of complications, patient discomfort and a high cost. In addition, liver biopsy examinations may lead to false negative results due to inadequate liver tissue sampling. Therefore, there is a need to develop a simple, reliable and non-invasive modality in order to assess the liver fibrosis stage [1].

Ultrasound (US) is a non-invasive, inexpensive and repeatable modality and has been used as the most important and valuable diagnostic tool for detecting hepatocellular carcinoma (HCC) during the follow-up of patients with viral hepatitis [2, 3]. US is also used for monitoring the response of HCC to treatment.

Received 22 July 2003 and in final form 31 August 2004, accepted 5 October 2004.

Address correspondence to Dr Koji Yano, Clinical Research Centre, NHO National Nagasaki Medical Centre, Kubara 2-1001-1 Omura, Nagasaki 856-8562 Japan.

An ultrasound evaluation of the liver fibrosis stage of chronic liver disease has been performed by assessing various ultrasound factors such as the liver size, the bluntness of the liver edge, the coarseness of the liver parenchyma, nodularity of the liver surface, the size of the lymph nodes around the hepatic artery, the irregularity and narrowness of the inferior vena cava, portal vein velocity or spleen size [1, 4–8]. However, the conventional definition of the fibrosis stage of the liver based on evaluation of these ultrasound factors is imperfect and lacks accuracy and reliability. Furthermore, these findings also depend largely on the equipment used [8]. Indeed, a few reports have demonstrated no consistent correlation between the grey scale ultrasound findings and the histological findings, thus claiming that grey scale US is unreliable for grading and staging the degree of liver damage [9]. However, recent advances in US technology have improved the diagnostic accuracy for fibrosis in patients with chronic liver disease. Therefore, we carried out a study to evaluate the accuracy of the liver fibrosis stage by utilizing the techniques of advanced ultrasound performance in 103 patients with chronic liver disease and compared the results obtained with the histological findings.

Patients and methods

Patients

This study was prospectively designed. 103 consecutive patients, consisting of 60 males and 43 females with a diagnosis of chronic liver disease including liver cirrhosis at National Nagasaki Medical Centre between October 2001 and February 2003 were included. The mean age of the patients was 51 years old, with a range of from 38 years to 75 years. The inclusion criteria were as follows: (a) history of chronic liver disease, based on the detection of persistently high levels of aminotransferase; (b) an absence of clinical and/or biochemical signs of decompensated liver diseases (jaundice, ascites or encephalopathy); and (c) no previous histopathological diagnosis. Regarding the hepatitis virus, 22 patients were infected with HBV, 64 with HCV, 5 with both HBV and HCV and 12 with neither HBV nor HCV. Both ultrasound and histological examination obtained based on a liver biopsy were performed for all patients.

US system

The patients were studied ultrasonically using a real-time apparatus (HDI 5000 Sono CT, ATL, USA) with a 2–5 MHz convex array transducer C5–2 (low frequency probe) and a 5–12 MHz convex array transducer L12–5 (high frequency probe).

US findings and the scoring system (Table 1)

The US examination was performed within an interval of no more than 15 days prior to the biopsy examination. The US examiners (TN, HW) were unaware of the clinical details of the patients, and the US findings were interpreted by two specialists (KY, HI) who had no knowledge of either the biochemical or biopsy results. The ultrasound examinations were recorded on static B-mode imaging. The US examiners were both certified by the Japan Society of Ultrasonics in Medicine. The US score was determined from the right and left lobes and the average score for each parameter was calculated as follows: (1) liver edge (Figure 1): score 0 for sharp; score 1 for mildly blunted; score 2 for blunted; (2) liver surface (Figure 2): score 0 for smooth; score 1 for mildly irregular; score 2 for irregular; score 3 for highly irregular; and (3) liver parenchymal texture (Figure 3) [5, 10]: score 0 for fine; score 1 for mildly coarse; score 2 for coarse; score 3 for highly coarse. A score of 0 was given when no abnormality was observed by a high frequency probe, score 1 was given when a mild abnormality was detected by a high frequency probe while it was undetected by the low frequency probe, a score of 2 was given when a moderate abnormality was detected by the low frequency probe, and a score of 3 was given when a severe abnormality was detected by the low frequency probe. A score of 2 was given for a blunted edge and a score 3 for severe irregular surface or a highly coarse texture when these characteristics were clearly confirmed by the low frequency probe. In cases in which three parameters such as the edge, surface and parenchymal texture could not be determined to be either mild or severe using a low frequency probe, then the high frequency probe was used to determine whether they were mild or severe. The high frequency probe was used to obtain a score 0 or 1 because the sensitivity obtained by the high frequency probe was superior to the one by the low frequency probe regarding mildly abnormal changes such as a score 0 or 1. Conversely, regarding such advanced changes as a score of 2 or 3, the low frequency probe was more useful because the probability obtained by the low frequency probe was superior to that by the high frequency probe. As a result, the fibrosis stage predicted from the accumulated scores of the liver edge, surface and parenchymal texture by US were considerably more reliable than the individual scores of these three parameters when they were compared with the histological findings.

Histological findings

Liver biopsy specimens were obtained from the anterior segment of the right lobe in each patient, using a 16-gauge Sonopsy-C1 biopsy needle (Hakko Co., Tokyo, Japan). All of the histological slides were reviewed by an experienced pathologist without any knowledge of the clinical details or the US findings. The New Inuyama scoring system for chronic hepatitis was proposed by the Japanese Liver Study Group in 1994 [11], which is similar to the classification of chronic hepatitis determined by the USA-European Liver Study Group [12]. The New Inuyama scoring system was used to assess the fibrosis stage as follows; score 0: no fibrosis, score 1: fibrous portal expansion, score 2: bridging fibrosis, score 3: bridging fibrosis with lobular degeneration, and score 4: cirrhosis.

Statistics

The Spearman's correlation test was used to assess any correlations between the liver fibrosis stage and the US scoring system. The sensitivity, specificity and positive predictive values of the US scoring system were calculated and compared with the results of the liver fibrosis stages.

Results

US scoring system and fibrosis stage

The relationship between the liver edge and fibrosis (Figure 4)

Of 11 patients with a sharp liver edge (edge score 0), 6 patients (55%) were found to have stage 0 fibrosis and 5 (45%) in stage 1 fibrosis. The liver edge score of 34 patients

Table 1. Findings for the ultrasound features of the edge, surface and parenchymal texture of the liver

	Score 0	Score 1	Score 2	Score 3
Edge	sharp	mildly blunted edge	blunted edge	
Surface	smooth	mildly irregular	irregular	highly irregular
Parenchymal texture	fine	mildly coarse	coarse	highly coarse

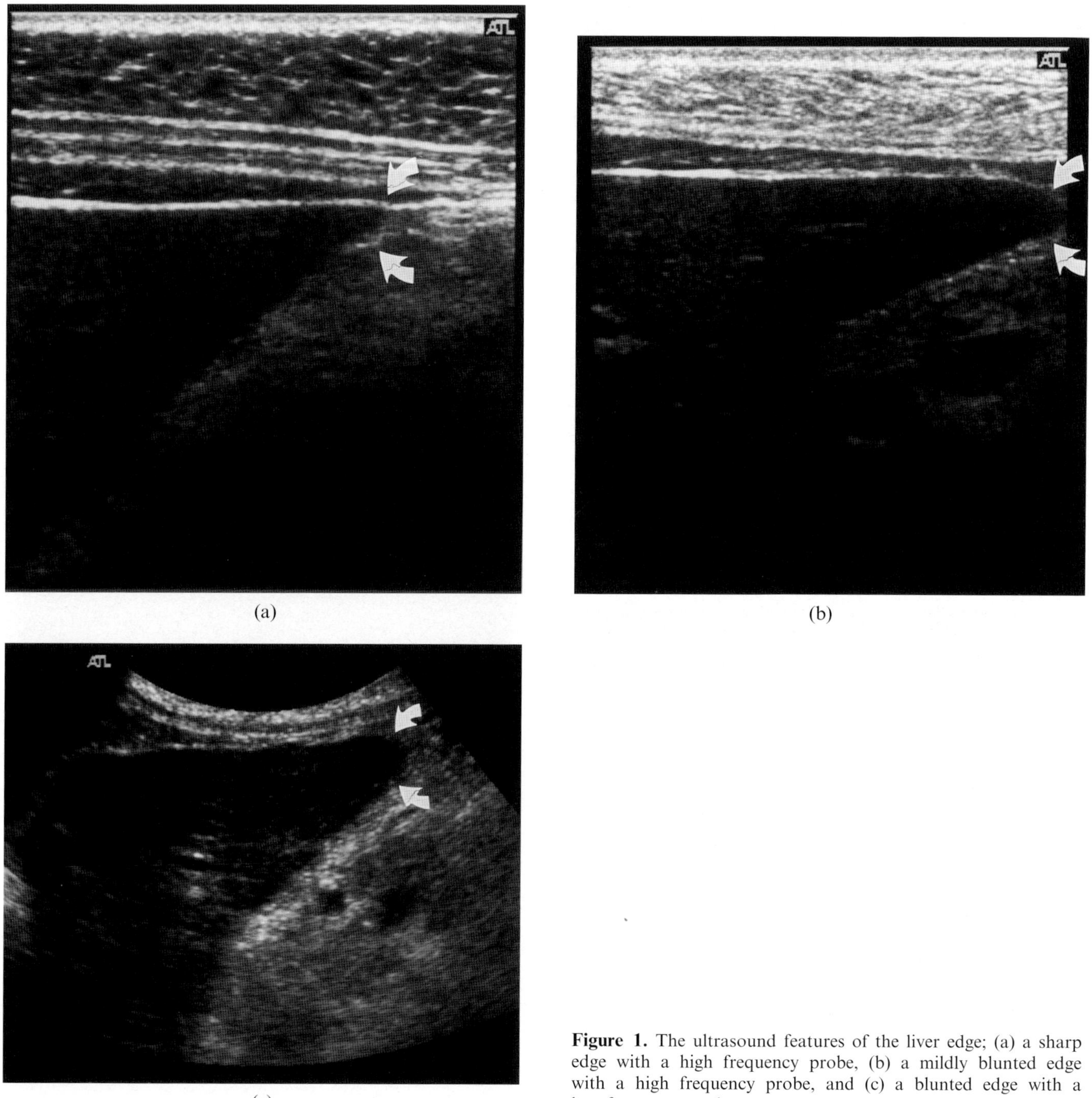

(a) (b) (c)

Figure 1. The ultrasound features of the liver edge; (a) a sharp edge with a high frequency probe, (b) a mildly blunted edge with a high frequency probe, and (c) a blunted edge with a low frequency probe.

in an early fibrosis stage (stage 1) showed various results; 5 patients had a score of 0, 6 a score 0.5, 9 a score of 1, 5 a score of 1.5 and 9 a score of 2. On the other hand, the patients with stage 2, 3 and 4 fibrosis correlated well with the edge score and were categorized into a blunted edge (score 2); 26 of 26 patients with stage 2 fibrosis, 12 of 13 patients with stage 3 fibrosis, 22 of 22 patients with stage 4 fibrosis. The liver edge and the fibrosis score thus showed a statistically significant correlation (rs: 0.6668).

The relationship between the liver surface and fibrosis (Figure 5)

Eight patients with stage 0 fibrosis were all put into the smooth liver surface group (surface score 0), and 34 patients with the fibrosis stage 1 were all found to have a score of 1 or less. 26 patients with the fibrosis stage 2 had different results regarding the surface score, *i.e.* 3 patients had a surface score of 0, 7 a score of 0.5, 9 a score of 1, 4 a score of 1.5 and 3 a score of 2, respectively. 12 of 13 patients with stage 3 fibrosis were found to have a surface score of either 1.5 or 2. All 22 patients with the stage 4 fibrosis were found to have a surface score of 2 or more. The liver surface score and the fibrosis stage showed a statistically significant correlation (rs: 0.9007).

The relationship between liver parenchymal texture and fibrosis (Figure 6)

Eight patients with stage 0 fibrosis were all found to have a fine liver parenchymal texture (parenchymal score 0), and 29 of 34 patients with stage 1 fibrosis were found

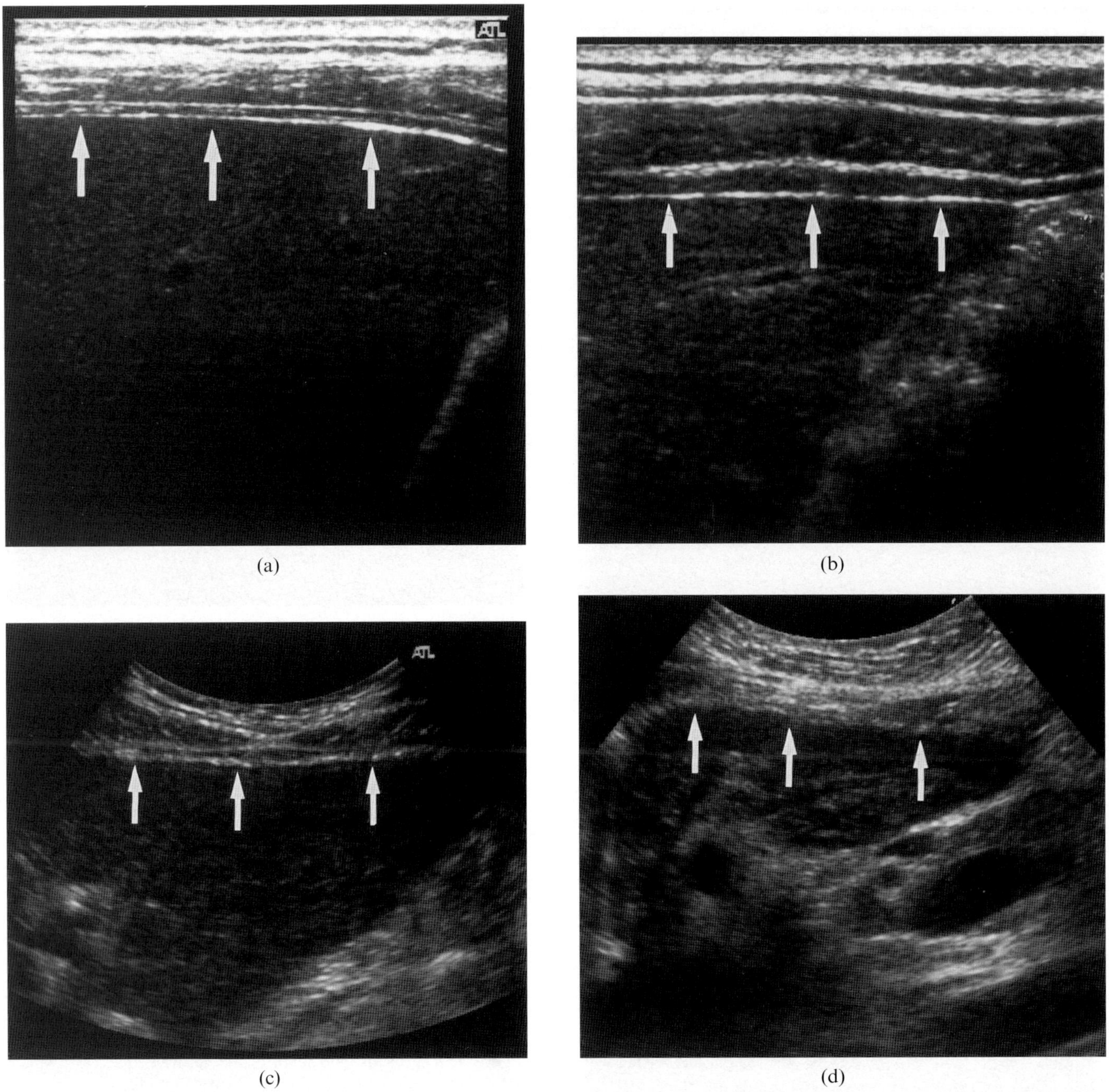

Figure 2. The ultrasound features of the liver surface; (a) a smooth surface with a high frequency probe, (b) a mildly irregular surface with a high frequency probe, (c) an irregular surface with a low frequency probe, and (d) a highly irregular surface with a low frequency probe.

to have a score of 0. Of 26 patients with stage 2 fibrosis, 11 had a score of 0, 14 a score of 1 and 1 a score of 2. Five and 6 patients of the 13 patients with stage 3 fibrosis had a score of 1 and 2, respectively. All 22 patients with stage 4 fibrosis had a parenchymal score of 2 or more. The liver parenchymal score and the fibrosis stage showed a statistically significant correlation (rs: 0.8853).

Relationship between the fibrosis grade and the accumulated scores of the liver edge, surface and parenchymal texture (Figure 7)

The liver edge, surface and parenchymal texture scores were all determined and compared with the histological fibrosis score. Of eight patients with fibrosis stage 0, six patients were found to have a total score of 0 and while two had a total score of 1. 34 patients with stage 1 fibrosis had a total score 1.53 consisting of 2 patients with scores of 0, 11 and a score of 0.5–1, 17 had a score of 1.5–2.0, and 4 had a score of 2.5–3, respectively. 26 patients with stage 2 fibrosis shifted to the progressive fibrosis stage, such as 1 patient with a score of 1.5–2, 10 with a score of 2.5–3, 9 with a score of 3.5–4, and 6 with a score of 4.5–5, respectively. Similarly, 13 patients with stage 3 fibrosis shifted to a progressive fibrosis stage such as 1 patient with a score of 3.5–4, 5 with a score of 4.5–5, and 7 with a score of 5.5–6, respectively. Out of 22 patients with stage 4 fibrosis had a score of 6.5–7.0 and eleven had a score of

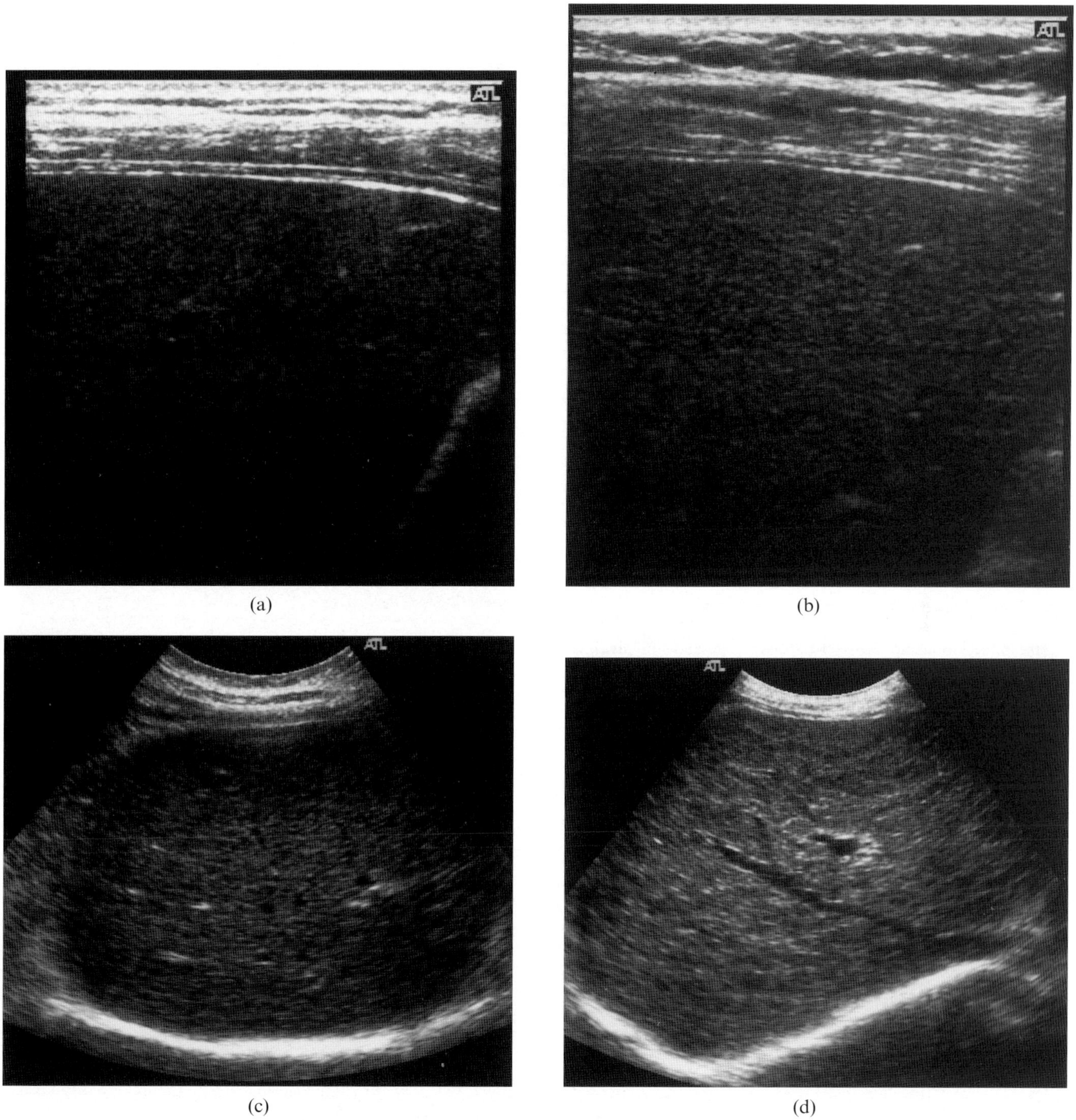

Figure 3. Scores for the ultrasound features of the liver parenchymal texture; (a) fine parenchymal texture with a high frequency probe, (b) a mildly coarse parenchymal texture with a high frequency probe, (c) a coarse parenchymal texture with a low frequency probe, and (d) a highly coarse parenchymal texture with a low frequency probe.

7–7.5, respectively. The fibrosis grade and the accumulated scores of these three parameters were more significantly correlated (positive predictive value, 0.9524) than the correlations of each score alone.

Discussion

Chronic liver diseases with viral infection manifest varying degrees of hepatic fibrosis ranging from no fibrosis to cirrhosis. Yoshida et al revealed that the annual incidence of hepatocellular carcinoma increased from 0.5% among patients with the stage F0 or F1 fibrosis to 7.9% among the patients with stage F4 fibrosis [13]. It has thus become increasingly apparent that the fibrosis stage is a key factor in defining the prognosis and management of chronic liver diseases with a viral infection.

The gold standard in hepatology for the diagnosis of the fibrosis stage has been a histological liver evaluation based on specimens taken either by a needle biopsy or at operation. Recently, non-invasive and reliable assessments for monitoring chronic liver disease using the platelet

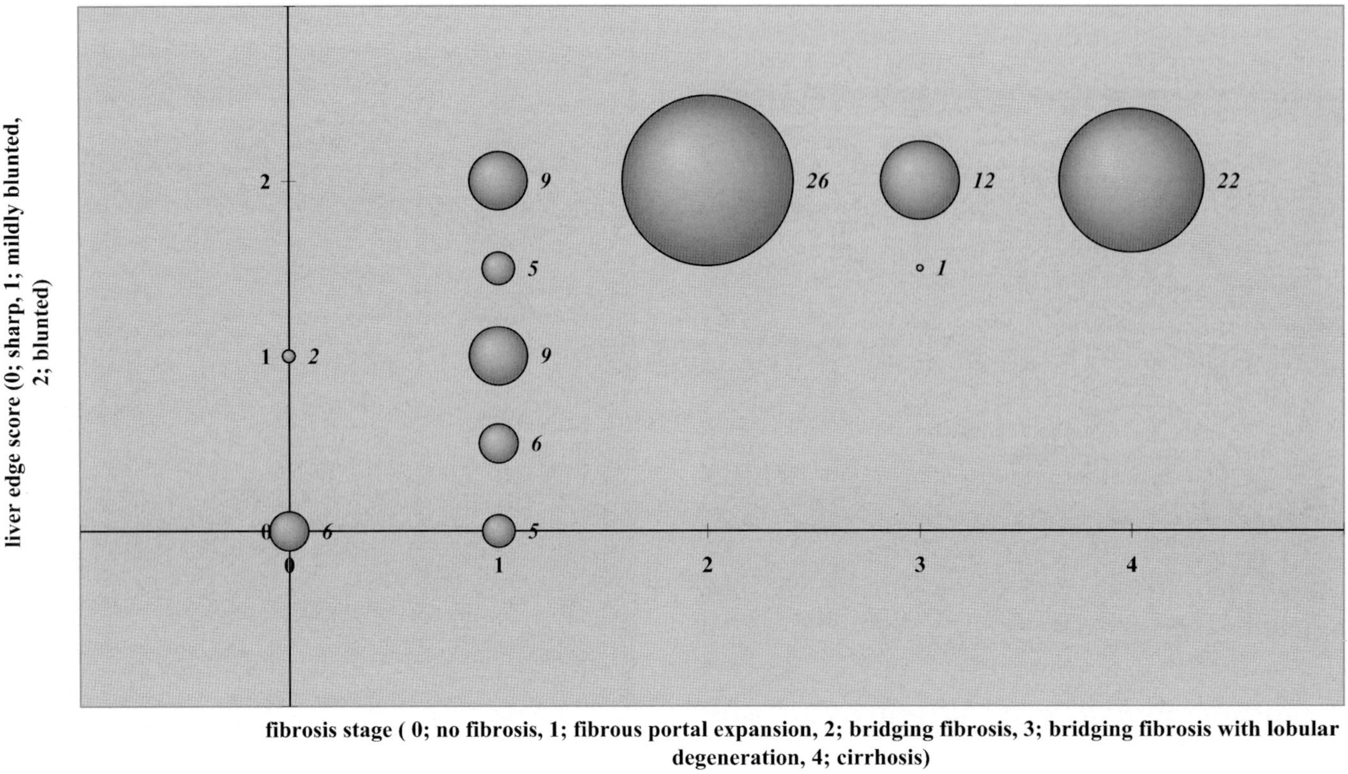

Figure 4. Relationship between the liver edge and fibrosis findings.

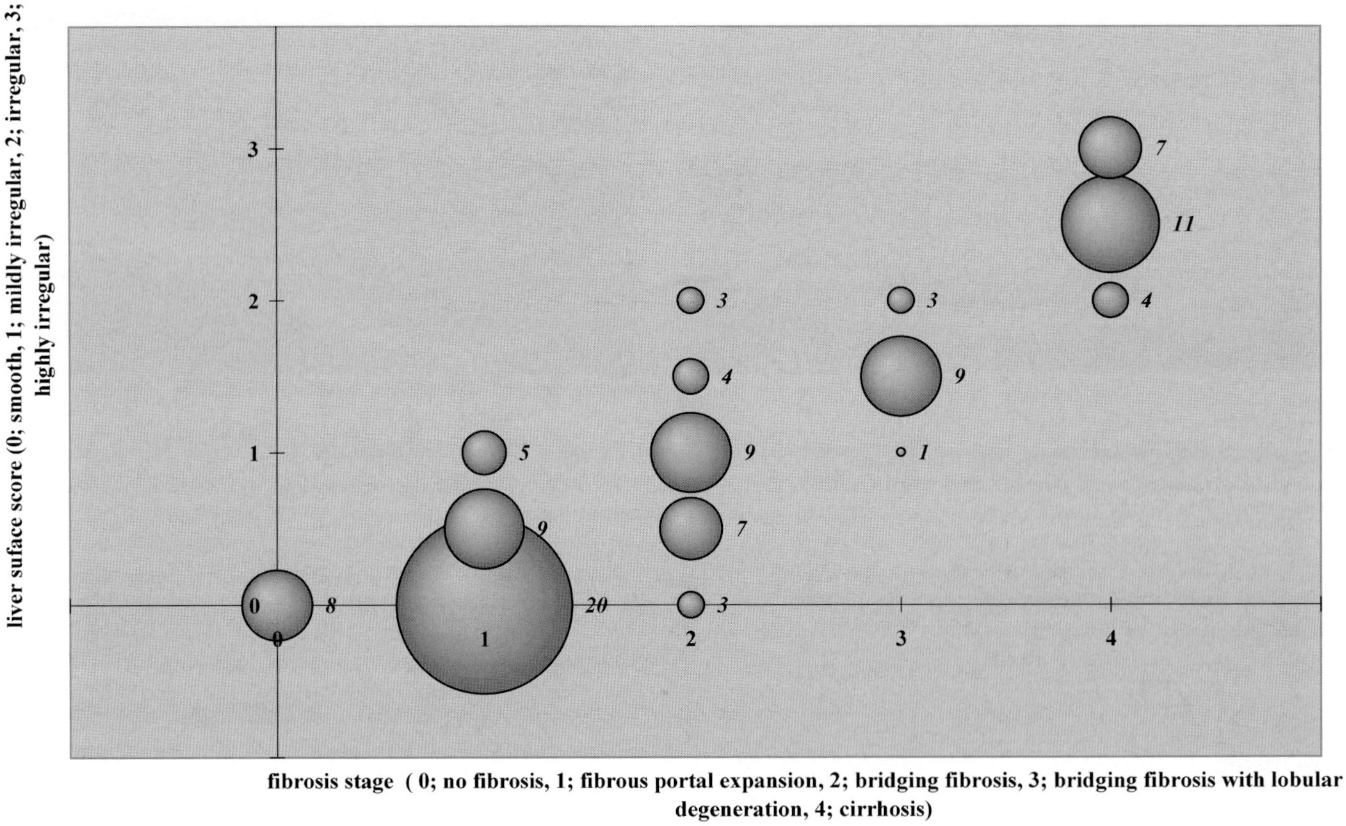

Figure 5. Relationship between the liver surface and fibrosis findings.

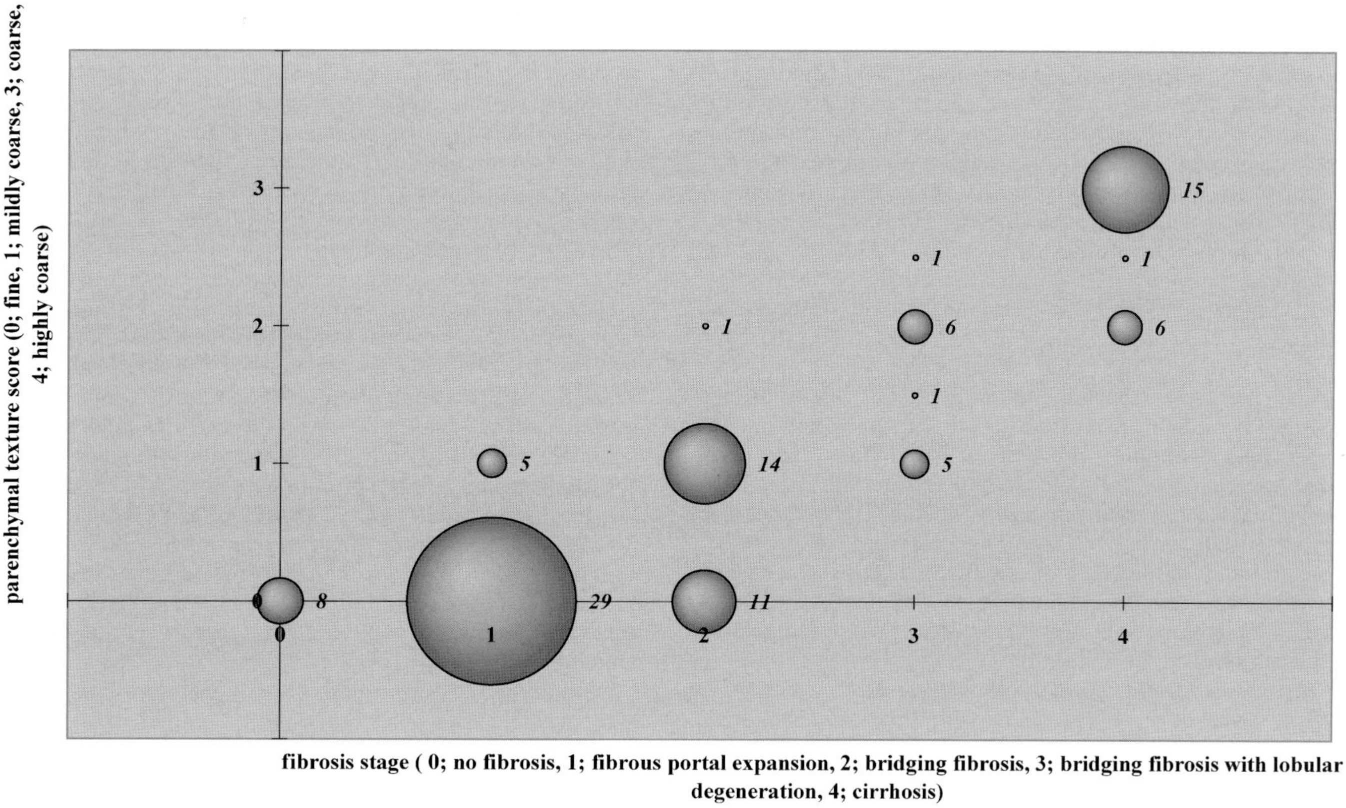

Figure 6. Relationship between the liver parenchymal texture and fibrosis findings.

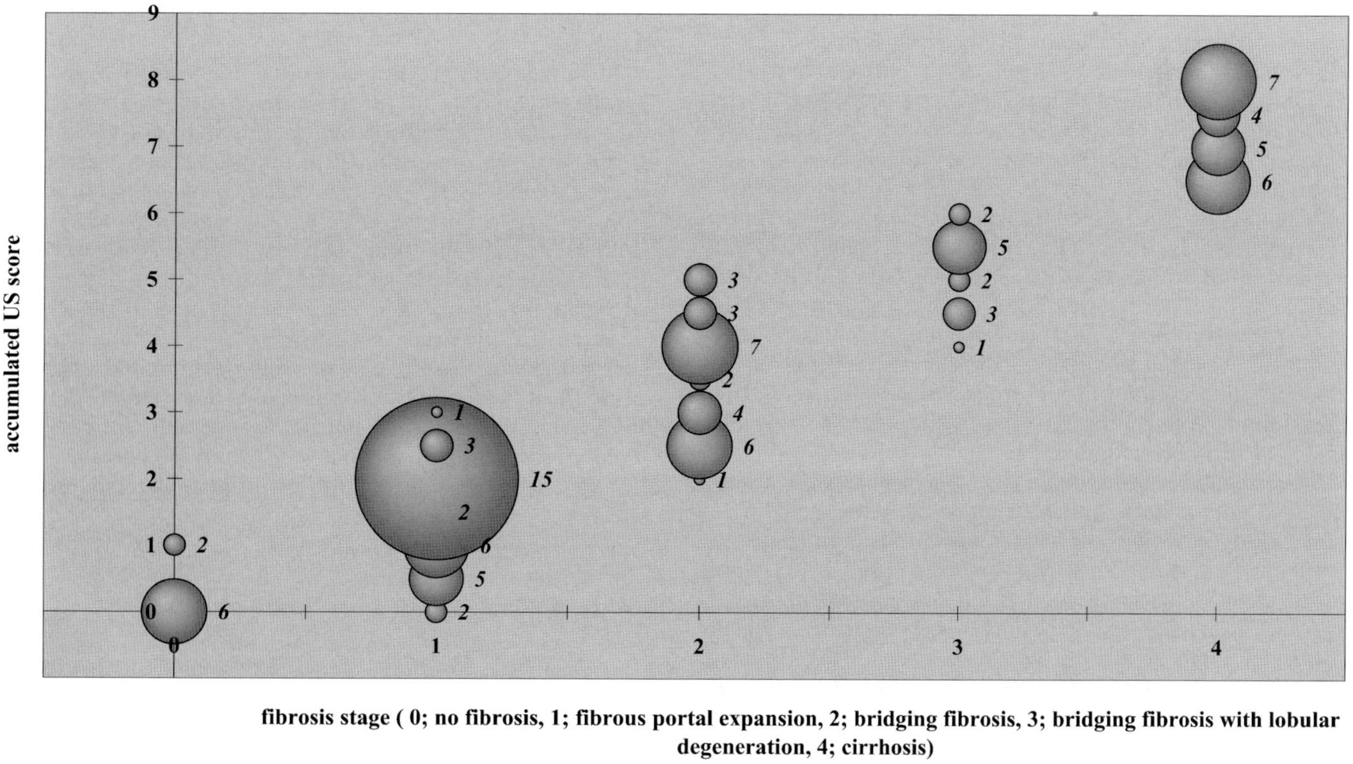

Figure 7. Relationship between the accumulated ultrasound score and fibrosis score findings.

counts [14–16], aspartate aminotransferase (AST)/alanine aminotransferase (ALT) ratio [15, 16], and serum hyaluronan and type III procollagen amino-terminal peptide [17] have been developed. However, none of the currently available tests or modalities can completely replace a histological analysis. Previous studies have assessed several methods for evaluating the fibrosis stage of chronic liver disease using various US parameters. However, there have so far been few studies concerning the accuracy in detecting the signs of compensated cirrhosis by US [5, 18]. Gaiani et al [5] and Hung et al [19] proposed a complex US scoring system using indices of the liver surface, parenchymal echogenecity, the vessel pattern, spleen size etc. to determine the fibrosis stage. In addition, recent advances in ultrasound technology have now made it possible to obtain more precise information about the liver surface, edge and parenchymal texture [8]. Therefore, we conducted this study to clarify whether the US scoring system with a newly developed US equipment based on the conventional parameters of the liver edge, surface and parenchymal texture might obtain sufficiently accurate results in comparison with the histological findings for fibrosis obtained by a liver biopsy.

In this prospective study, among these parameters such as the liver edge, liver surface and liver parenchymal texture, the liver edge was not as specific for evaluating liver fibrosis as the liver surface and parenchymal texture in our study because a mildly blunted (score 1) or blunted edge (score 2) was frequently found in the early fibrosis stage (stage 1) (67.6%). On the other hand, the liver surface and liver parenchymal texture obtained by US showed a better correlation with the histological findings (correlation coefficient of 0.9007 in the liver surface, and 0.8853 in the parenchymal texture).

With conventional US, the liver surface has been most commonly utilized as a sole indicator for the diagnosis of cirrhosis [5, 20–22]. However, numerous papers have reported that the sole factor of the liver surface can not sufficiently distinguish cirrhosis from chronic hepatitis. Gaiani et al confirmed that the stage of cirrhosis may be underestimated when based on a single specimen and clarified that only two US variables, namely liver surface nodularity and the portal vein mean flow velocity, independently contributed to the diagnosis of cirrhosis [5]. In our study, all seven patients with a highly irregular surface were found to have cirrhosis (stage 4 fibrosis) histologically. On the other hand, 15 of 22 patients (68.2%) with cirrhosis were found to have an irregular surface (score 2–2.5), not a highly irregular surface (score 3). Indeed, the results of our study showed a significant correlation between the ultrasound liver surface and the histological fibrosis stage.

An irregular and nodular liver surface may be easily assessed in patients with decompensated liver cirrhosis, particularly in the case of ascites, and it has been observed in 88% of unselected patients with cirrhosis [20]. Gaiani et al reported the findings of a US scoring system, based on the liver, spleen and portal vein features, which identified cirrhosis in 82.2% of the cases [5]. In our study, both the right and the left liver lobes were evaluated for each factor, and the average score for each parameter was calculated. Both the low frequency and the high frequency probes were used to limit the subjective nature of the assessment of the US findings of various degrees. In this prospective study, US was performed with the simultaneous use of low frequency and high frequency probes to determine the sensitivity and probability according to the characteristics of ultrasound. Although our study was limited on account of the relatively small number of patients due to the strict inclusion criteria, 22 patients with an accumulated score of 6.5 or more were all found to have a fibrosis score of 4. Therefore, our scoring system for correctly predicting cirrhosis was found to be 100% sensitive. Furthermore, although the major drawback with US in comparison with the liver histology has been considered to be the failure to detect mild fibrosis or none at all, our scoring system thus provided relatively accurate information about liver fibrosis. When the accumulated US score of 3 was interpreted as mild fibrosis (a fibrosis score of 0 or 1), all 42 patients with stage 0 or 1 fibrosis were categorized into an accumulated US score of 3 or less (a probability of 100%) and 42 of 53 patients with a score of 3 or less were found to have stage 0 or 1 fibrosis (specificity of 79.2%). In addition, the score proposed in our study is easy to obtain and can be applied in every ultrasound laboratory by utilizing regular commercially available US equipment.

Evaluating the ultrasound pattern using either one or two parameters becomes much more complex at the stage of chronic liver disease than that of complete cirrhosis. Our scoring system based on three parameters such as the liver edge, surface and parenchymal texture was able to accurately predict the fibrosis stage (correlation coefficient of 0.9524), especially when distinguishing chronic hepatitis from compensated liver cirrhosis. When an exclusion of liver cirrhosis is requested, then US alone is therefore considered to provide sufficient information based on this scoring system. Furthermore, if a histological analysis can not determine the fibrosis stage correctly due to fragmentation or architectural distortion, then this ultrasound diagnostic modality of fibrosis could replace a histological diagnosis.

In conclusion, we demonstrated that our US scoring system is clinically useful for differentiating patients who have chronic liver disease with minimal or no fibrosis from those with mild to severe fibrosis. These parameters may also be useful for providing prognostic information and also for determining the optimal therapeutic options during the follow-up of patients with chronic liver disease, especially in patients with chronic hepatitis C or B, in order to predict the occurrence of HCC. In addition, further study is called for to determine whether or not the wider use of this scoring system could apply to other forms of hepatic fibrosis such as those suffering from long-term hepatotoxic disease, congenital diseases in children and non-viral infective forms of chronic liver disease in order to obtain an improved response to therapy.

References

1. Fontana RJ, Lok ASF. Noninvasive monitoring of patients with chronic hepatitis C. Hepatology 2002;36:S57–S64.
2. Dohmen K, Shirahama M, Onohara S, Miyamoto Y, Torii Y, Irie K, et al. Differences in survival based on the type of follow-up for the detection of hepatocellular carcinoma: an analysis of 547 patients. Hepatol Res 2000;18:110–21.

3. Dohmen K, Shigematsu H, Irie K, Ishibashi H. Trends in clinical characteristics, treatment and prognosis of hepatocellular carcinoma. Hepato-Gastroenterology 2003;50:1872–7.
4. Celle G, Savarino V, Picciotto A, Magnolia MR, Scalabrini P, Dodero M. Is hepatic ultrasonography a valid alternative tool to liver biopsy? Report on 507 cases studied with both techniques. Dig Dis Sci 1988;33:467–71.
5. Gaiani S, Gramantieri L, Venturoli N, Piscaglia F, Siringo S, D'Errico A, et al. What is the criterion for differentiating chronic hepatitis from compensated cirrhosis? A prospective study comparing ultrasonography and percutaneous liver biopsy. J Hepatol 1997;27:979–85.
6. Tüney D, Aribal ME, Ertem D, Kotiloğlu E, Pehlivanoğlu E. Diagnosis of liver cirrhosis in children based on colour Doppler ultrasonography with histopathological correlation. Pediatr Radiol 1998;28:859–64.
7. Khan KN, Yamasaki M, Yamasaki K, Inoue O, Yatsuhashi H, Koga M, et al. Proposed abdominal sonographic staging to predict severity of liver diseases: analysis with peritoneoscopy and histology. Dig Dis Sci 2000;45:554–64.
8. Nicolau C, Bianchi L, Vilana R. Gray-scale ultrasound in hepatic cirrhosis and chronic hepatitis: diagnosis, screening, and intervention. Seminars in US, CT and MRI 2002;23:3–18.
9. Kutcher R, Smith GS, Sen F, Gelman SF, Mitsudo S, Thung SN, et al. Comparison of sonograms and liver histologic findings in patients with chronic hepatitis C virus infection. J Ultrasound Med 1998;17:321–5.
10. Joseph AEA, Saverymuttu SH, Al-Sam S, Cook MG, Maxwell JD. Comparison of liver histology with ultrasonography in assessing diffuse parenchymal liver disease. Clin Radiol 1991;43:26–31.
11. Ichida F, Omata M, Tsuji T, Ichida T, Inoue K, Uemura A, et al. New Inuyama classification: new criteria for histological assessment of chronic hepatitis. Hepatol Com 1996;6:112–9.
12. Desmet VJ, Gerber M, Hoofnagle JH, Manns M, Scheuer PJ. Classification of chronic hepatitis: diagnosis, grading and staging. Hepatology 1994;19:1513–20.
13. Yoshida H, Shiratori Y, Moriyama M, Arakawa Y, Ide T, Sata M, et al. Interferon therapy reduces the risk for hepatocellular carcinoma: National surveillance program of cirrhosis and noncirrhotic patients with chronic hepatitis C in Japan. Ann Intern Med 1999;131:174–81.
14. Ono E, Shiratori Y, Okudaira T, Imamura M, Teratani T, Kanai F, et al. Platelet count reflects stage of chronic hepatitis C. Hepatol Res 1999;15:192–200.
15. Luo J-C, Hwang S-J, Chang F-Y, Chu C-W, Lai C-R, Wang Y-J, et al. Simple blood tests can predict compensated liver cirrhosis in patients with chronic hepatitis C. Hepato-Gastroenterology 2002;49:478–81.
16. Pohl A, Behling C, Oliver D, Kilani M, Monson P, Hassanein T. Serum aminotransferase levels and platelet counts as predictors of degree of fibrosis in chronic hepatitis C virus infection. Am J Gastroenterol 2001;96:3142–6.
17. Guéchot J, Laudat A, Loria A, Serfaty L, Poupon R, Giboudeau J. Diagnostic accuracy of hyaluronan and type III procollagen amino-terminal peptide serum assays as markers of liver fibrosis in chronic viral hepatitis C evaluated by ROC curve analysis. Clin Chem 1996;42:558–63.
18. Richard P, Bonniaud P, Barthélémy C, Étaix JP, Veyret C, Audigier JC, et al. Valeur de l'ultrasonographie dans le diagnostic des cirrhosis. J Radiol 1985;66:503–6.
19. Hung C-H, Lu S-N, Wang J-H, Lee C-M, Chen T-M, Tung H-D, et al. Correlation between ultrasonographic and pathologic diagnoses of hepatitis B and C virus-related cirrhosis. J Gastroenterol 2003;38:153–7.
20. Di Lelio A, Cestari C, Lomazzi A, Beretta L. Cirrhosis: diagnosis with sonographic study of the liver surface. Radiology 1989;172:389–92.
21. Ferral H, Male R, Cardiel M, Munoz L, Ferrari FQY. Cirrhosis: diagnosis by liver surface analysis with high-frequency ultrasound. Gastrointest Radiol 1992;17:74–8.
22. Śimonovský V. The diagnosis of cirrhosis by high resolution ultrasound of the liver surface. Br J Radiol 1999;72:29–34.

The British Journal of Radiology, *78* (2005), 198–201
DOI: 10.1259/bjr/26977910

A comparative study of evaluation of radiographs, CT and 3D reformatted CT in facial trauma: what is the role of 3D?

[1]A D REUBEN, MRCS, [2]S R WATT-SMITH, MD, [1]D DOBSON and [1]S J GOLDING, FRCR

[1]*Departments of Radiology, University of Oxford and* [2]*Maxillofacial Surgery, John Radcliffe Hospital, Oxford, UK*

Abstract. A panel of 17 trainee maxillofacial surgeons viewed 23 cases of facial trauma, demonstrated on radiographs, axial CT images and three-dimensional (3D) reformatted CT images in a standardized viewing format under standard conditions. Their diagnostic interpretation, extraction of information relevant to surgical management and subjective evaluation of each modality were recorded by standard questionnaire and compared with a gold standard evaluation by a consultant radiologist and surgeon reading based on results of clinical management. There were clear and measurable differences in the viewers' evaluations of radiographs, CT and 3D reformatted images. Overall, surgeons showed more accurate diagnostic reading of radiographs and 3D reformatted images. This was in contrast to their subjective assessment of the clinical value of each modality, which showed a strong preference for 3D over all other techniques and for CT over radiographs. However the perceived benefit of axial CT images over radiographs was not reproduced on objective testing in this group; surgeons appear to perform less well in interpreting CT images than their subjective response to the modality would suggest. This work has supported the view that surgeons value 3D imaging as a front-line tool in the evaluation and management of selected cases of acute facial trauma. We have demonstrated that the perceived benefits of 3D reformatted CT to surgeons appear real.

Facial injuries are clinically significant because they are often complex in nature and may have serious functional and cosmetic sequelae. This makes accurate diagnostic evaluation essential. Modern imaging modalities, especially CT, have been shown to be of value in the assessment and management of acute facial trauma [1–3].

Surgeons frequently need to make their own evaluation of the degree of skeletal disruption revealed by imaging studies when planning initial treatment of facial fractures. 3D images reformatted from CT offer a subjectively attractive medium for displaying skeletal lesions and the technique has attracted interest in the management of patients with facial trauma, among surgeons in particular [4–6]. However to what extent this corresponds to clinicians' objective performance in reading the images has not been studied in detail. This study was undertaken to investigate the objective performance of trainee maxillofacial surgeons in their diagnostic evaluation of facial fractures on different imaging techniques, including 3D reformatted CT, and to determine the degree of correlation with their subjective views of the clinical value of each.

Patients and methods

Preparation of images

Imaging records were selected from 16 patients with acute facial trauma undergoing treatment at the John Radcliffe Hospital, Oxford over a 2 year period. Cases were chosen from radiographs, axial CT studies and 3D images to reflect a representative spectrum of facial trauma, from simple localized fractures to complex transfacial injury. Overall, the study group comprised seven examples of radiographs, nine CT studies and seven cases of 3D reconstruction, treated for the purpose of reading as 23 separate cases (Table 1).

Selected radiographs were occipitomental or occipitofrontal views, as appropriate (Figure 1). All CT studies were obtained using a Pace CT system (General Electric Medical Systems, Slough, UK), using contiguous 1 mm or 3 mm sections through the face, with a 20 cm field of view. Images were reconstructed on a high resolution algorithm using a 512 × 512 matrix, giving a pixel size of 0.39 mm. Representative sections numbering 10 to 15 in each case were selected from each patient to show the important areas of fracture (Figure 2). 3D images were reformatted

Table 1. Sites of fracture in 16 patients, indicating source of images used in the study

Patient	Site(s) of fracture	Radiograph	CT	3D
1	Right maxilla+zygoma	+	+	
2	Transfacial–mid level	+		
3	Left zygoma+maxilla	+		
4	Left maxilla	+		
5	Right zygomatic arch	+		
6	Transfacial–mid level	+		
7	Right maxilla+orbit	+		
8	Transfacial–high level		+	+
9	Transfacial mid level		+	+
10	Right frontal+nasoethmoid		+	+
11	Healed right nasoethmoid		+	+
12	Transfacial–mid and low level		+	+
13	Left maxilla+zygoma		+	
14	Left orbital floor		+	
15	Left and right maxilla		+	+
16	Right maxilla			+

Received 5 January 2004 and in revised form 19 August 2004, accepted 13 October 2004.

Address correspondence to Dr S J Golding.

Current address for Dr Adam D Reuben, Hillcrest, Netherclay, Bishop's Hull, Taunton TA1 5ED, UK.

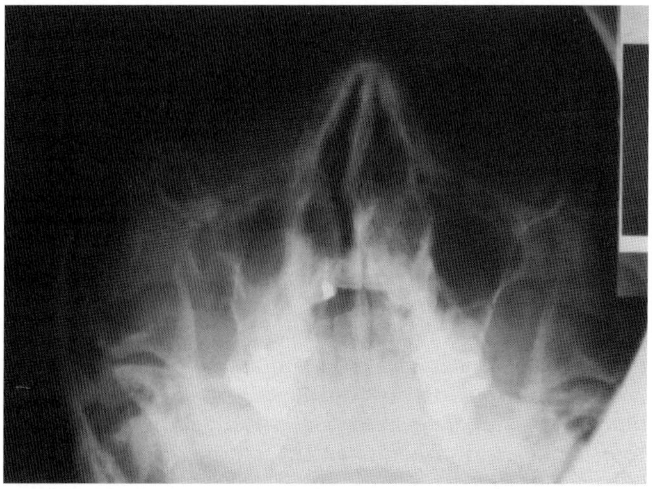

Figure 1. Occipitomental radiograph of the face showing a right zygomaticomaxillary fracture.

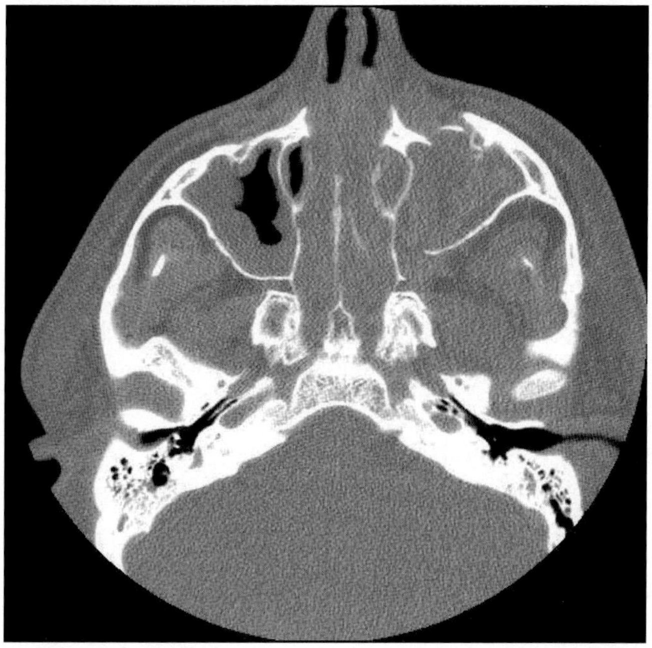

Figure 2. Axial high resolution CT section of a patient showing left zygomaticomaxillary fracture.

from the CT data by surface rendering using a stand-alone processing system and software provided by the Medical Physics Department, University College, London (R Williams, www.medphys.ucl.ac.uk/mgi/workstat.htm). Thresholds were chosen manually in each case to show skeletal details optimally, and to minimize pseudoforamen artefacts (Figure 3).

Evaluation of images

A standard viewing format was created by transferring all images to high resolution VHS video tape. A commercial video camera (Sony Hi 8; Sony, Tokyo, Japan) was used to film radiographs on a light box. The selected CT sections were individually recorded by direct video link from the system computer to the video recorder,

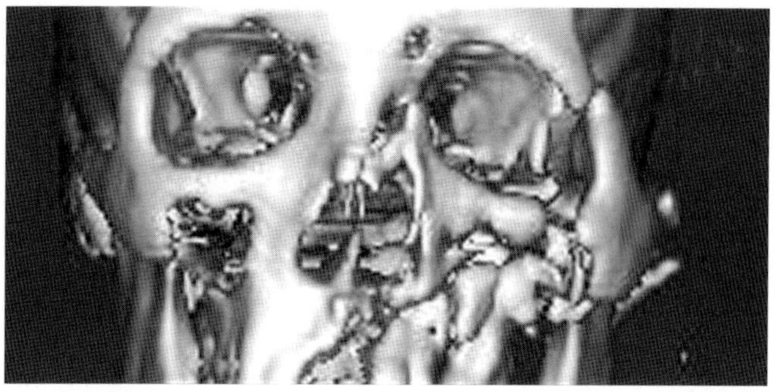

Figure 3. Surface rendered 3D reformatted CT image showing a comminuted fracture of the left zygoma and maxilla.

window width and level display having been set manually for optimal display of bony structures. 3D reformatted CT images were recorded directly from the video output of the processing unit and displayed in frontal view in rotating frame over 180°, in 3° increments, using a light source perspective technique. The video recording was edited on an editing station (Panasonic HD700; Matsushitu Electric Corp. of America, Secaucus, NJ) to create the final viewing format, in which radiographs were displayed for 30 s, each CT section for 10 s and each of the 3D images for 30 s.

A panel of 17 trainee maxillofacial surgeons was recruited from the Eastman Dental Hospital. All viewed the video tape in one session and their diagnostic evaluations and subjective assessments of the cases were collected by means of a standard questionnaire.

The questionnaire began with an introduction explaining what the viewing panel were asked to do. After this the panel viewed each of the 23 cases in turn. They were presented with a list of 19 structures in the face and asked to indicate whether or not they thought each structure was involved by fracture, and if so whether left or right sides, or both. After viewing all cases the panel completed the final section of the questionnaire, which sampled their subjective responses. They graded the ease of interpretation for each three modalities on a five point scale (5 easy, 1 difficult) and were then asked to indicate which of the three types of image they found easiest to view for (a) understanding the pathology and (b) making a diagnosis. Finally they were asked to make a binary decision whether each of the three techniques provided sufficient information for four purposes: diagnosis, assessing the extent of fracture, predicting complications and planning surgery.

Analysis of results

Viewers' responses to part 1 of the questionnaire (objective reading) were evaluated by comparison with a gold standard reading, made by a consultant radiologist and surgeon who had been involved in the clinical care of the patients. This reading was made on both the video presentation and the source images, in order to compensate for possible loss of information in the recording process. However the video reproduction was deemed independently by both expert viewers to represent the original data with acceptable accuracy. The objective reading of the viewing panel of each of the 19 structures potentially involved by fracture were scored against the gold standard reading, giving a mark out of 19 for correctness. The average scores for each imaging modality were calculated from these. To determine the effect of differences between viewers the marks from individual viewers were subject to two-way analysis of variance, and the marks for each modality were compared using Scheffes multiple comparisons. Finally the objective performance of viewers was compared with their subjective response to the questions in the second part of the questionnaire.

Results

Objective responses

Compared against the standard reading, viewers achieved best scores for reading 3D images, followed by their scores for radiographs, with reading of CT performing least well. Mean scores out of 19 from each candidate for 3D images (7 cases) ranged from 12.71 to 15.29 (mean 14.29, standard deviation (SD) 2.31). For radiographs (7 cases) the range was 12.14 to 15 (mean 13.62, SD 2.51) and for CT (9 cases) the range was 10.44 to 13.89 (mean 12.31, SD 3.86). Overall "correct" percentage scores were 75.7% for 3D images, 71.5% for radiographs and 64.7% for CT.

Two-way analysis of variance showed that there was no significant difference between the performances of viewers over the series of scores, indicating that interobserver error could be discounted. It showed additionally that there was significant difference between the scores for each modality ($p<0.0001$), subject to further analysis. This was achieved using Scheffes multiple comparisons, which showed that the differences in results between radiographs and CT and between CT and 3D reformatted CT were significant at the level of testing ($p<0.001$). The difference in results between radiography and 3D images was found to be insignificant ($p<0.001$), there being a 24% probability that this result could have happened by chance.

Overall, analysis of the objective responses indicates that surgical viewers perform better, in terms of recognition of known fracture lines, with both 3D reformatted CT and conventional radiographs, than they do when interpreting conventional CT images.

Subjective responses

All 17 viewers rated the ease of interpretation of each modality, giving an average rating of 5 (excellent) to 3D reformatted CT, 4 to CT and 3 to radiographs. Only 14 viewers indicated which modality they found to provide a better understanding of pathology; 13 (95%) felt that 3D images were best, and 1 thought CT. 12 of the 14 (86%) rated 3D images the best for clarity in making a diagnosis and 2 preferred CT. No viewer preferred radiographs for either purpose. The results showed a more positive subjective response to CT than had been suggested by viewers' objective performance, while reinforcing their overall preference for 3D reformatted CT. Viewers' responses when asked to indicate whether or not each technique provided enough information for diagnosis, assessing extent of injury, predicting potential complications and planning surgery are shown in Table 2.

The results found heavily in favour of 3D reformatted CT, with all 17 viewers reporting that 3D provided enough information on its own in categories 1, 2 and 4. CT was the next preferred modality in general but it was notable that only 50% of viewers felt that radiographs showed enough information for diagnosis, in contrast to their objective scores, and most found radiographs unsatisfactory for assessing fracture extent and planning treatment. All viewers rated each technique less well for predicting potential complications, compared with other clinical uses.

Overall the results show that subjectively viewers show a preference for 3D images over conventional CT and over radiographs, while the objective assessment shows better performance with 3D over conventional CT but also better performance on radiographs over conventional CT.

Discussion

This study demonstrates that surgical viewers find 3D reformatted images to be of the greatest clarity and easiest to interpret of the available imaging modalities in facial trauma. All of those questioned reported that the 3D images presented enough information for diagnosis of the fracture, for assessing the extent of the fracture and for planning surgical treatment in the patient. Statistical analysis confirmed that candidates' objective performance in interpreting 3D reformatted CT was significantly better than when interpreting conventional CT. The results compare favourably with previous studies showing a subjective preference for 3D images among clinicians [7–10] but in addition they documented a significant difference between subjective evaluation and objective performance in this group of surgeons. Objective testing showed that for this group 3D reformatted CT gave the most accurate performance, followed by radiographs and then conventional CT. Statistical analysis revealed the study to be robust and confirmed as significant the differences between 3D and CT and between radiographs and CT. On subjective testing surgeons reported 3D images to be the most easily interpreted, to best provide understanding of the pathology, and to be effective for predicting potential complications and for treatment planning.

A similar study by Alder et al revealed subjective preference for 3D over conventional modalities, which was

Table 2. Viewers' opinions on the clinical role of each technique affirmative responses as a percentage of the total responses for each modality

	Radiograph	Conventional CT	3D images
Does the modality provide enough information for:			
1. Diagnosis of the fracture	50%	88%	100%
2. Assessing the extent of the fracture	25%	87%	100%
3. Predicting potential complications	12%	63%	82%
4. Planning surgical treatment for the patient	37%	81%	100%

reflected in an alteration in surgical approach in 45% of cases [7]. They concluded that 3D images are of greatest benefit for the assessment of mid-face injuries, although they recognized that disparity between those who reported the images to be useful (97%) compared with those who modified their diagnosis (28%) was large. Mayer et al [8] performed subjective and objective analysis of the diagnostic capabilities of 3D reformatted CT as compared with CT and radiographs, finding that 3D provided superior definition of fracture lines (especially horizontal ones) and better appreciation of the extent of comminution. Gillespie et al [1] in their study found 3D to be of greatest value in patients with severe trauma and multiple fractures but less useful in minor trauma where there was no fragment displacement.

A key feature of our results is the lack of correlation between viewers' subjective and objective results with respect to CT. Axial CT images may be held to contain more information than the other techniques but despite their subjective preference for CT over radiographs, surgeons actually performed less well in interpreting CT. These responses may reflect training and familiarity with different imaging modalities, giving a bias to radiographs in particular, which are more likely to be interpreted by surgeons themselves, whereas radiological support is more likely to be available in evaluating CT. If so, our results have implications to the training of junior maxillofacial surgeons, the group used in this study, who are most likely to be engaged in the first-line management of facial trauma. Clinical training and experience may explain the preference for 3D reformatted CT, as these images relate readily to structures with which surgeons are confronted during surgical procedures.

We wished to make an objective comparison of interpretation of different techniques and for this reason chose a standardized viewing method using the medium of videotape and television monitor. This is a familiar method of viewing 3D reformatted CT and may have introduced bias in favour of 3D, to the detriment of the other two techniques. Further study of our own work has also shown rotating frame display to enhance image interpretation. Additionally, the viewing format dictated selectivity of images, which may have introduced limitations in reading CT in particular, although a radiologist and surgeon experienced in this work were satisfied that selected images were a faithful reflection of the fracture in each case. An ideal evaluation would display images in their conventional formats and allow variable time for viewing and assimilation of information, as would be the case in a clinical scenario.

In order to compare techniques we chose to treat each radiograph, CT and 3D reformatted CT as a separate case. However we believe there is a case for a study of the effect of imaging in clinical management, in which all three modalities would be available for each patient and the contribution of each would be evaluated separately. The cases used in this study also varied greatly in their severity and anatomical distribution within the face. It has yet to be established which injuries are more appropriately evaluated with 3D reformation in particular and so for clinically relevant assessment cases could be grouped according to the severity of their injury.

Effective clinical imaging must always be justified by positive influence on clinical management. In facial trauma imaging provides information which is known to contribute to accurate diagnosis and greater understanding of the degree and extent of injury but ideally this should be reflected in reduced operating times, reduction in post-operative complications, shorter hospital stays and improved clinical result. Our study has reinforced the role of 3D reformatted CT in conveying essential information to clinicians dealing with facial injury but we believe that further work is needed to establish precisely where and when each imaging technique should be used for most clinical benefit.

References

1. Gillespie JF, Isherwood I, Barker GR, Quayle AA. 3D reformations of CT in the assessment of facial trauma. Clin Radiol 1987;38:523–6.
2. Johnson DH. CT of maxillofacial trauma. Radiol Clin N Am 1984;112:146–53.
3. Zilka A. CT in facial trauma. Radiol Clin N Am 1984;22:131–44.
4. Gillespie JE, Isherwood I. 3D anatomical images from CT scans. Br J Radiol 1993;59:289–92.
5. Zonneveld FW, Lobregt S, van der Meulen JC, Vaandrager JM. 3D imaging in craniofacial surgery. World J Surg 1989;13:328–42.
6. Zonneveld FW. A decade of clinical 3D imaging, a review. Part 2: clinical applications. Invest Radiol 1994;29:574–89.
7. Alder ME, Deahl ST, Matteson SR. Clinical usefulness of two-dimensional reformatted and three-dimensionally rendered computerised tomographic images. J Oral Maxillofacial Surg 1995;53:375–86.
8. Mayer JS, Wainwright DJ, Yeakley JW, Lee KF. The role of three-dimensional computed tomography in the management of maxillofacial trauma. J Trauma 1988;28:1043–53.
9. Magid D, Michelson JD, Ney D, Fishman EK. Adult ankle fractures: comparison of plain films and interactive 2 and 3D CT scans. Am J Radiol 1990;154:1017–23.
10. DeMarino DP, Steiner E, Poster RB, Katsberg RW, Hengerer AS, Herman GT. 3D CT in maxillofacial trauma. Am J Radiol 1988;138:477–83.

The British Journal of Radiology, *78* (2005), 202–206
DOI: 10.1259/bjr/15237296

MR colonography: baseline appearance of the unprepared rectosigmoid

V L JARDINE, MA, E SALA, MD, PhD, FRCR and D J LOMAS, FRCP, FRCR

Department of Radiology, University of Cambridge & Addenbrooke's Hospital, Cambridge, UK

Abstract. A retrospective review of 100 routine pelvic MR examinations was conducted to evaluate the appearance of the unprepared rectosigmoid colon, with the aim of informing future strategies for minimal preparation MR colonography. All examinations were reviewed by two observers in consensus, and included matched-location axial T_1 weighted and T_2 weighted fat suppressed fast spin echo (FSFSE) images. Analysis revealed that the overall appearance of the faecal material in the colon could simulate tumour in 80% of T_1 weighted and 17% of T_2 weighted images. By matching the images from the two sequences for each patient the faeces had an overall appearance that would mimic tumour in only 7% of cases. However, luminal tumour-mimicking foci of signal occurred frequently, present in 91% of T_1 weighted and 85% of T_2 weighted studies. The results indicate that if bowel-cleansing regimens are to be avoided for MR colonography, effective strategies such as dietary restriction and use of oral contrast agents will be required to reduce luminal signal on T_2 weighting and eliminate polyp-mimicking foci. The results also suggest that T_2 weighted strategies should be further investigated and that combination with T_1 weighted imaging may improve discrimination of lesions from normal faecal material.

Colorectal cancer is the second leading cause of death due to cancer in the UK [1] and USA [2, 3], estimated to cause nearly half a million deaths worldwide each year [4]. The adenoma to carcinoma progression is well understood [5], occurring over several years [6] and providing the opportunity to detect and remove pre-cancerous lesions at a potentially curative stage [4, 7]. As a result several western countries, including the UK, are currently evaluating screening strategies as part of their public health programs.

Population screening ideally requires a sensitive, specific, safe and inexpensive screening test acceptable to the population into which it is introduced. Several methods for detecting colonic polyps and tumours are currently available, including faecal occult blood testing (FOBT) and imaging methods such as colonoscopy, sigmoidoscopy, barium enema and CT colonography.

Current proposed strategies suggest a cheap, simple and relatively insensitive non-imaging method such as FOBT [8] (or in the future faecal deoxyribonucleic acid (DNA) [9] or protein [10] testing) for initial screening. Subsequently, anatomical imaging methods with higher costs and morbidity would be utilized in a selected subpopulation to confirm the presence and location of any lesion. A constraint of current colonic imaging methods is their reliance on cleansing regimens, which are often uncomfortable for patients and associated with their own morbidity [11], especially in a relatively elderly target population. This is a substantial limitation since it may reduce compliance and influence accuracy, in turn undermining the benefit of a population-screening program. However colonic cleansing remains routine since the presence of normal colonic faecal material can compromise diagnostic performance by mimicking or masking tumours and polyps on all imaging techniques [12].

Received 5 January 2004 and in revised form 18 August 2004, accepted 13 October 2004.

Address correspondence to Prof. David J Lomas, University Department of Radiology, Box 219, Level 5, Addenbrooke's Hospital, Cambridge CB2 2QQ, UK.

MRI offers a method for imaging the colon theoretically comparable with CT colonography, but without the burden of ionizing radiation. Initial MR feasibility studies have used air or fluid for colonic distension after cleansing procedures [13–17] to remove faecal material. However a key advantage of MRI is the ability to obtain a wide range of soft tissue contrast and imaging based on different signal characteristics. This has stimulated the investigation of minimal preparation techniques for MR colonography that might avoid colonic cleansing, by utilizing oral agents and/or dietary manipulation to "tag" stool [18–21]. The aim is to consistently change the signal of faeces to prevent it from mimicking or masking tumour, the ideal result being homogeneous material of substantially different signal intensity to the bowel wall and potential lesions. Despite these early attempts to manipulate signal in the colon there has been little work on the "normal" or baseline appearances of the colon at MR, or CT examination.

The aim of this study is to evaluate the appearance of the unprepared rectosigmoid colon and the ability of faeces to mimic tumour in a series of patients undergoing routine pelvic MRI examination. The findings will be used to inform future preparation strategies for an MR colonography technique.

Methods and materials

A retrospective review of consecutive routine pelvic MR examinations obtained between July 2001 and September 2002 (for conditions unrelated to the gastrointestinal tract) was undertaken to obtain 50 male and 50 female studies with faeces within the lumen of the colon. Since the aim of the study was to assess the appearance of the "normal" faecal material within the rectosigmoid colon the following exclusion criteria were used: empty rectosigmoid, previous

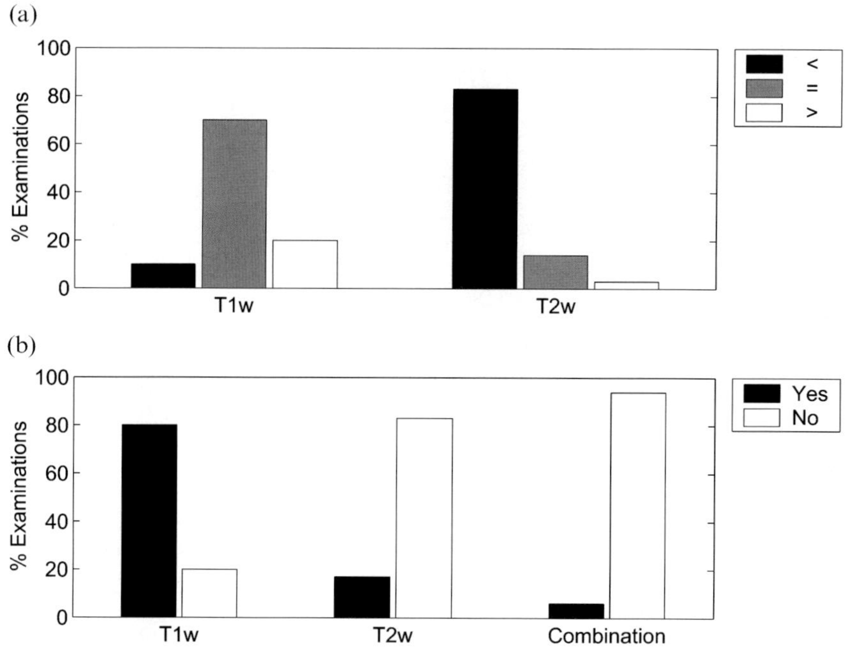

Figure 1. (a) The overall signal intensity of intraluminal material relative to the bowel wall for both T_1 and T_2 weighted studies. (b) The capacity of this luminal signal material to mimic tumour overall for T_1 weighted and T_2 weighted strategies individually, and for the combined analysis of T_1 and T_2 weighting. Wilcoxon signed rank test statistics were used to detect significant differences: intraluminal material of signal intensity similar to that of tumour occurred less frequently on T_2 than T_1 weighted imaging, with combined analysis providing a lower incidence of such tumour-mimicking material than either T_1 weighted or T_2 weighted alone ($p<0.001$ in each case).

rectosigmoid surgery, bowel pathology, pelvic masses distorting the sigmoid colon, previous pelvic radiotherapy or chemotherapy within a year of the examination. Also studies rendered technically inadequate for analysis by motion or prosthesis-related artefacts were excluded.

All examinations were performed using a 1.5 T whole body MR system (GE Medical Systems, Milwaukee, WI) with a pelvic phased array coil. Matched location axial T_1 weighted (echo time (TE) 14 ms, repetition time (TR) 700–750 ms) and fat suppressed T_2 weighted fast spin echo (FSE) (8 echo train length, TE effective 90 ms, TR 3500 ms) images with 256×256 matrix, 5 mm section thickness and a 2.5 mm interslice gap were obtained in each case, covering the pelvis inferior to the aortic bifurcation. The rectum and distal sigmoid colon within the pelvis were evaluated by two observers in consensus for the following features of the intraluminal faecal material: overall contrast relative to the bowel wall, heterogeneity, focal areas of increased or decreased signal that could mimic polypoid lesions, luminal distension of the whole rectosigmoid, and the presence of any free fluid. Statistical analysis was performed using a non-parametric Wilcoxon signed rank test.

Where the colonic wall could not be clearly identified, adjacent gluteal muscle was used as a reference to assess the relative signal intensity of the intraluminal contents since skeletal muscle is of similar signal intensity to the smooth muscle of the colon wall. Focal increases or decreases in signal intensity within the lumen were recorded for areas of bowel containing faeces, not gas. Free fluid was defined as the presence of a gravity dependent fluid level or high T_2 signal collection (comparable with that of the bladder) within the rectosigmoid.

Results

100 examinations of 50 male and 50 female patients aged between 18 years and 87 years (mean age 58 years) were available for assessment. The rectosigmoid colon was fully distended in only 3% of the studies. Free fluid was not present in any of the examinations assessed.

The overall signal intensity of the faecal material relative to the bowel wall for T_1 and T_2 weighted imaging is shown in Figure 1a. The majority of T_1 weighted images showed luminal material of signal intensity similar to that of the bowel wall (70%), whereas most T_2 weighted images demonstrated luminal signal less than that of the wall (83%). The signal intensity of tumour is similar to that of the bowel wall, typically slightly increased in T_2 weighted and decreased in T_1 weighted images [22, 23]. Interpreting the results with this in mind (Figure 1b): in 80% of T_1 weighted studies the overall signal of faeces could mimic tumour, whereas this was the case in significantly fewer T_2 weighted studies (z=6.833, $p<0.0001$): just 17%. Furthermore, matching the T_1 and T_2 weighted images for each examination leaves only 7% with faeces whose overall signal intensity could mimic tumour, significantly less than T_2 weighted alone (z=3.317, $p<0.001$).

Intraluminal faecal material of the rectosigmoid was considered heterogeneous in 97% of T_1 and 89% of T_2 weighted examinations (Figure 2). Foci of signal in the lumen (small areas of different signal intensity to the majority of faeces) occurred in most examinations, with the majority of T_1 weighted images demonstrating luminal foci of decreased signal and most T_2 weighted images foci of increased signal (Figure 3a). On the same basis as above, luminal foci of greater signal intensity than the colon wall on T_1 weighting are unlikely to be tumour, and similarly relatively low signal foci on T_2 weighting are unimportant. However 91% of T_1 weighted studies and 85% of T_2 weighted studies, contained foci whose signal was considered similar to that of tumour (Figure 3b). Even after matching T_1 weighted and T_2 weighted studies 80% of examinations contained luminal foci capable of mimicking polyps (Figure 4).

Discussion

This study was performed to inform which strategies for manipulating intraluminal signal are most likely to succeed

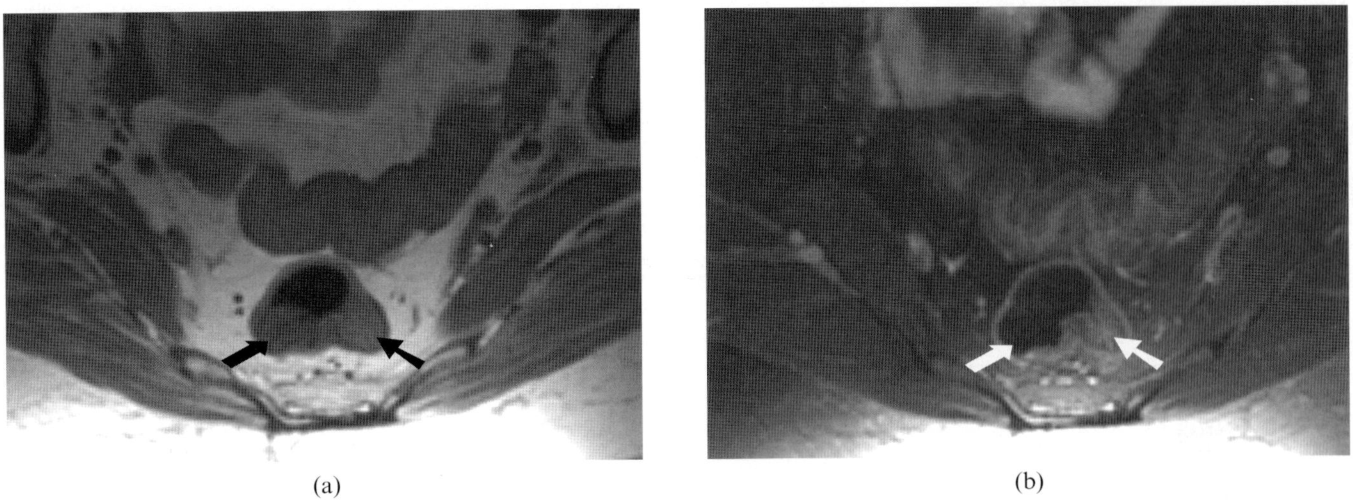

Figure 2. Location matched (a) T_1 weighted and (b) T_2 weighted images of the rectum and pelvic sigmoid colon with heterogeneous faecal material. These images also demonstrate the potential value of comparing multiple sequences to aid differentiation between lesions and intraluminal faeces. On T_1 weighting (a) the area indicated (thick arrow) is of similar signal to the bowel wall and therefore could be tumour. T_2 weighted (b) however demonstrates good negative luminal contrast in this region: no tumour is present. However this strategy is clearly limited: it would be impossible to exclude a lesion in either image at the area indicated by the thin arrow.

in the development of a MR colonography technique that avoids colonic cleansing. Ideally any oral contrast agents and dietary restriction strategies must be safe, cheap, palatable and influence luminal signal consistently and evenly throughout the entire colon, providing maximal contrast between the material and potential lesions. The use of a minimal preparation strategy should also allow easy identification of those who have failed to follow the preparation requirements to reduce the risk of misinterpretation. Furthermore it is clearly fundamental that any preparation strategy must be better tolerated than the standard colonic cleansing methods or there would be little benefit.

Lauenstein et al [18, 20] have investigated the use of barium sulphate as a negative oral contrast agent, utilizing a T_1 weighted three-dimensional (3D) gradient-echo imaging strategy with colonic distension obtained by means of a water enema. This T_1 weighted "dark lumen" technique requires intravenous gadobenate dimeglumine to provide adequate contrast between the lumen and enhancing lesions which would otherwise appear relatively low signal. The same group have also tried oral gadoterate meglumine with a T_1 weighted imaging strategy in conjunction with a dilute gadolinium based water enema [19]. Using this technique tumour appears low signal against a high signal lumen.

Our work indicates that the overall signal of faecal material in the majority of T_1 weighted images is of similar signal intensity to the bowel wall. This is highly problematic since tumour signal is likely to be the same or slightly less than that of the wall on T_1 weighted imaging, so material would commonly mimic lesions. For T_1 weighted imaging without intravenous enhancement the maximum contrast between material and lesions will occur

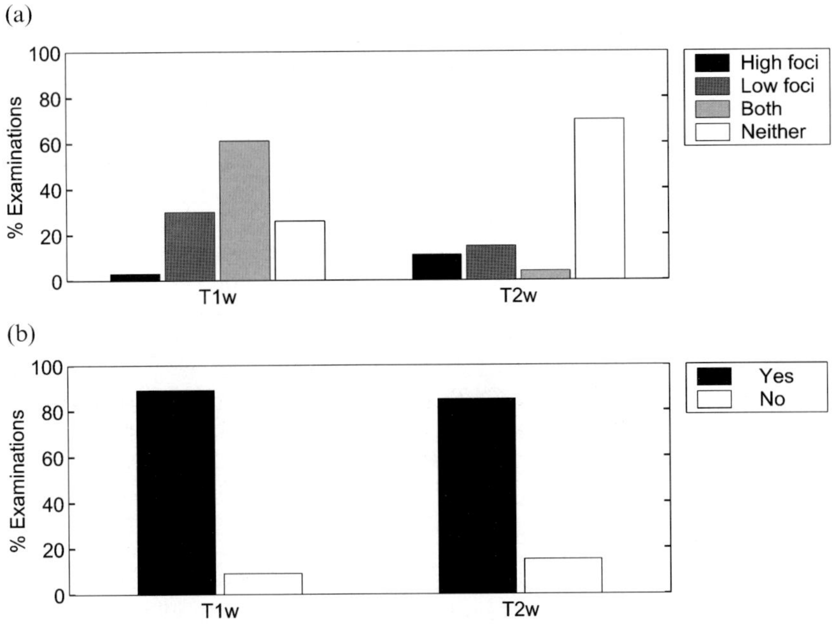

Figure 3. (a) The presence of focal areas of luminal increased or decreased signal intensity compared with the remainder of intraluminal material. The majority of examinations demonstrated heterogeneous material, with foci of increased, decreased, or both increased and decreased signal present in T_1 and T_2 weighted studies. (b) The capacity of luminal foci to mimic colonic lesions in T_1 and T_2 weighted strategies.

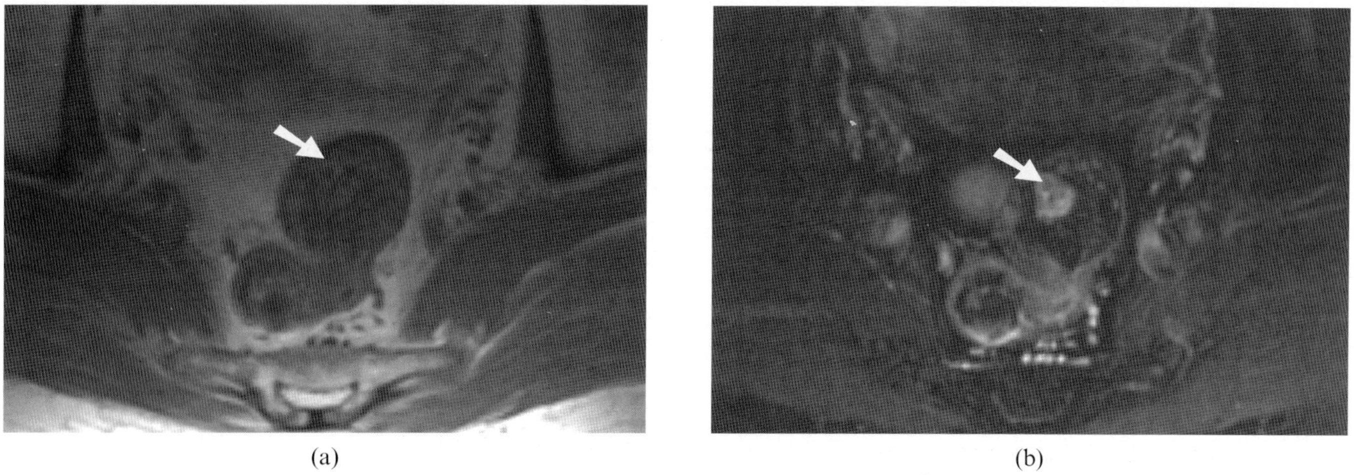

Figure 4. Location matched (a) T_1 and (b) T_2 weighted images of the rectosigmoid colon. A focus of slightly increased signal intensity relative to the bowel wall is demonstrated within the lumen on T_2 weighting, whereas on T_1 weighting this area is of similar signal to the wall. Consequently differentiation between faeces and a lesion is impossible.

when the luminal signal is substantially greater than that of the bowel wall, but does not obscure haustral folds or small polyps. T_1 weighted imaging sequences are currently relatively attractive in terms of their performance, providing good volume coverage within acceptable breath-holding times. This is mainly as a result of the development of angiographic techniques designed to suppress signal from longer T_1 weighted tissues and detect the shortened T_1 in blood resulting from intravenous gadolinium enhancement. Lauenstein et al [18] have pursued the same strategy by enhancing polyps and tumours using intravenous gadolinium media against a dark lumen background with moderate success using barium as an oral contrast agent combined with a low fat, low residue diet. However this strategy requires a pre and post intravenous comparison study typically limiting the examination to one orientation (*i.e.* prone or supine), which may in turn limit evaluation.

In this study the overall signal of faeces on T_2 weighted imaging was lower than that of the bowel wall in the majority of cases, and since the signal of tumour is likely to be the same or slightly greater than the wall a preparation strategy to reduce luminal signal should have the least difficulty in maximizing contrast between material and lesions. Thus a T_2 weighted approach may also prove feasible for minimal preparation MR colonography, provided that the preparation successfully eliminates all the foci of increased signal. These are most likely related to water-retaining high residue fruit and fibrous dietary components that are not fully digested in the proximal intestine. T_2 weighted sequences are generally of lower signal to noise ratio than T_1 weighted sequences and so obtaining adequate coverage within a single breath-hold is likely to be more difficult, although improvements in coil design and system efficiency are gradually overcoming these limitations. Additionally the longer TE employed with T_2 weighted imaging could increase the likelihood of susceptibility artefacts in relation to distension with gases. However, this could be counterbalanced by the use of a T_2 weighted spin echo technique compared with the gradient echo techniques use for T_1 weighting.

A further strategy for MR colonography was implicit from the significant decrease in the incidence of examination in which overall luminal signal was consistent with that of tumour when matched-location T_1 and T_2 weighted images were compared. This suggests that using multiple contrast imaging could be of value, especially if luminal signal manipulation is successful for all the sequences examined. Clearly this raises issues on the effective review of examinations concerning the avoidance of image misregistration and the correlation of two or more sets of images.

This retrospective study does have limitations, primarily that only the rectosigmoid colon was studied. Although the majority of tumours occur in the rectosigmoid it is possible that the appearances in the remainder of the colon may differ. For instance, the hydration of the intraluminal content would be expected to decrease along the length of the colon, which may have biased the results in favour of the T_2 weighted approach described above. This could be enhanced by fasting patients prior to MR colonography and thereby promoting the dehydration of faeces. We did not investigate the diets of those taking part assuming that, as a cross-section of our referral population for pelvic examination, they would reflect a similar range of dietary habits encountered in a population referred for examination of the colon. Similarly patient drug history was not evaluated, although this could also have influenced intraluminal signal. A referred population for screening would inevitably contain individuals taking a range of drugs although this would be likely to be influenced by how the screening population is selected. Finally, although all patients with known colonic pathology were excluded from the study, it is possible that some of the cases reviewed had asymptomatic lesions of the rectosigmoid. Therefore some of the foci of signal noted could have been "false positives", with intraluminal faeces being adequate for image evaluation. The incidence of such lesions would be low, and given the overall results the impact on the findings in this study is likely to be negligible.

The results above suggest that dietary control will be essential as part of any strategy to avoid traditional colonic cleansing. Different food constituents are known to have particular MR characteristics, fats for instance typically giving high signal on T_1 weighting, and water retaining materials such as fruit often producing high signal on T_2 weighting, low on T_1 weighting. Future work will require optimization of suitable diets that can increase the ability to discriminate faeces from tumour and the bowel wall. Ideally the diet will promote homogeneity within the faecal material, avoiding undigested residues that may retain water and produce tumour-mimicking foci. Both diet and oral contrast agents will also be influenced by the individual variation in intestinal transit time and the optimal combinations of diet and oral contrast agent need to be identified.

In conclusion, this study indicates that the unprepared rectosigmoid colon typically contains faeces that is heterogeneous on MRI, potentially mimicking tumour in the majority of cases on T_1 and T_2 weighted imaging either by overall signal intensity or by the presence of foci within intraluminal material. The results suggest that both dietary control and oral contrast agent preparation are essential if colonic cleansing is to be avoided, and that strategies using T_2 weighted and combinations of T_1 weighted and T_2 weighted imaging require further investigation and optimization.

Acknowledgments

The authors would like to acknowledge the assistance of the Fund for Addenbrooke's, Elmore Fund, James Baird Fund and the Radiographers of the MRIS Unit.

References

1. Office for National Statistics. Mortality Statistics 1998. ONS, 1998. Series DH2 no 25.
2. American Cancer Society, Cancer, facts and figures. GA:ACS, 2001. Atlanta GA: American Cancer Society, 2001:5.
3. Reis LAG, Eisner MP, Kosary CL, et al. SEER cancer statistics review. 1973–2000. Bethesda MD: National Cancer Institute, 2000.
4. Boyle P, Leon ME. Epidemiology of colorectal cancer. Br Med Bull 2002;64:1–25.
5. Fearon ER, Vogelstein B. A genetic model for colorectal tumorigenesis. Cell 1990;61:759–67.
6. O'Brein MJ, Winawer SJ, Zauber AG. The National Polyp Study. Patient and polyp characteristics associated with high-grade dysplasia in colorectal adenomas. Gasteroenterology 1990;98:371–9.
7. Winawer SJ, Zauber AG, Ho MN, et al. Prevention of colorectal cancer by colonoscopic polypectomy. New Engl J Med 1993;329:1977–81.
8. Lowenfels AB. Fecal occult blood testing as a screening procedure for colorectal cancer. Ann Oncol 2002;13:40–3.
9. Traverso G, Shuber A, Levin B. Detection of APC mutations in fecal DNA from patients with colorectal tumors. New Engl J Med 2002;346:311–20.
10. Davies RJ, Freeman A, Morris LS, et al. Analysis of minichromosome maintenance protiens as a novel method for detection of colorectal cancer in stool. Lancet 2002;359:1917–9.
11. Toledo TK, Dipalma JA. Review article: colon cleansing preparation for gastrointestinal procedures. Aliment Pharmacol Ther 2001;15:605–11.
12. Lefere PA, Gryspeerdt SS, Dewyspelaere J, et al. Dietary fecal tagging as a cleansing method before CT colonography: initial results - polyp detection and patient acceptance. Radiology 2002;224:393–403.
13. Lomas DJ, Sood RR, Graves MJ, et al. Colon carcinoma: MR imaging with CO2 enema - pilot study. Radiology 2001;219:558–62.
14. Luboldt W, Steiner P, Bauerfeind P, et al. Detection of mass lesions with MR colonography: preliminary report. Radiology 1998;207:59–65.
15. Luboldt W, Bauerfeind P, Wildermuth S, et al. Colonic masses: detection with MR colonography. Radiology 2000;216:383–8.
16. Morrin MM, Hochman MG, Farrell RJ, et al. MR colonography using colonic distension with air as the contrast material: work in progress. AJR Am J Roentgenol 2001;176:144–6.
17. Lauenstein TC, Herborn CU, Vogt FM, et al. Dark lumen MR-colonography: initial experience. Rofo 2001;173:785–9.
18. Lauenstein TC, Goehde SC, Ruehm SG, et al. MR colography with barium-based fecal tagging: initial clinical experience. Radiology 2002;223:248–54.
19. Weishaupt D, Patak MA, Froehlich J, et al. Faecal tagging to avoid colonic cleansing before MRI colography. Lancet 1999;354:835–6.
20. Lauenstein TC, Holtmann G, Schoenfelder D, et al. MR colonography without colonic cleansing: a new strategy to improve patient acceptance. AJR Am J Roentgenol 2001;177:823–7.
21. Ajaj W, Pelster G, Treichel U, et al. Dark lumen magnetic resonance colonography: comparison with conventional colonoscopy for the detection of colorectal pathology. Gut 2003;52:1738–43.
22. Bottomley PA, Hardy CJ, Argersinger RE, et al. A review of 1H nuclear magnetic resonance relaxation in pathology: are T1 and T2 diagnostic? Med Phy 1987;14:1–37.
23. Bottomley PA, Foster TH, Argersinger RE, et al. A review of normal tissue hydrogen NMR relaxation times and relaxation mechanisms from 1-100 MHz: dependence on tissue type, NMR frequency, temperature, species, excision and age. Med Phys 1984;11:425–48.

The British Journal of Radiology, *78* (2005), 207–218
DOI: 10.1259/bjr/41095952

Radiation doses received in the UK Breast Screening Programme in 2001 and 2002

[1]K C YOUNG, PhD, [2]A BURCH, MA MPhil and [1]J M ODUKO, PhD

[1]*National Co-ordinating Centre for the Physics of Mammography, Medical Physics Department, Royal Surrey County Hospital, Guildford GU2 7XX and* [2]*Breast Test Wales, 18 Cathedral Road, Cardiff CF11 9LH, UK*

Abstract. The mean glandular doses (MGD) to samples of women attending for mammographic screening are measured routinely at screening centres in the UK Breast Screening Programme (NHSBSP). This paper reviews a large representative sample of dose measurements collected during screening in the NHSBSP in 2001 and 2002 for 53 218 films, using 290 X-ray sets, for 16 505 women. The average MGD was 2.23 mGy per oblique film and 1.96 mGy per craniocaudal film; similar to those found previously in the NHSBSP for the years 1997 and 1998. Increasing use of sophisticated units with automatic beam quality selection has reduced the radiation dose received by large breasts, with only 2% of oblique mammograms having doses in excess of 5 mGy. The increasing use of large format film has also reduced the doses to this sub-group. However the total dose per woman has increased due to the introduction of two view screening at every visit. The MGD to the standard breast was found to vary from 0.76 mGy to 2.29 mGy, with 97% of units below the recommended upper limit of 2 mGy, illustrating the benefit of strict quality control. A reduction in dose of 3% was observed between the age bands 50–54 years and 60–64 years. This study has confirmed that the proposed national diagnostic reference level (NDRL) of 3.5 mGy for 55 mm thick breasts is an appropriate value to identify systems giving unusually high doses, with just 3.5% of systems exceeding this level. In most cases these higher doses were explained by the design of one particular make of X-ray set and its mode of operation. Average doses for oblique views of average sized breasts were fairly well correlated with the dose to the standard breast, and typically 42% higher. This highlights the need for a revised definition of the standard breast used in the UK to better reflect the exposure factors and doses received in clinical practice.

The National Health Service Breast Screening Programme (NHSBSP) in the UK invites all women aged 50–64 years to attend for X-ray mammography every 3 years. Older women can be screened on request. In 2001–2002 the programme screened 1.5 million women [1]. The programme in England has been extended so that women up to and including the age of 70 years receive routine invitations for screening since the end of 2004. From 2003 all women have two views of the breast taken at every screen instead of just at the first screen. As for all medical X-ray procedures the principles of radiation protection require that the radiation dose be justified and optimized. In order to ensure the justification and optimization of the radiation dose, accurate dose information is required. The two main methods used in the UK for the assessment of patient dose in mammography are described in IPSM Report 59/2 [2]. In the "standard breast method" dose is calculated for a breast model of total thickness 45 mm that comprises a central region with a 50:50 mixture by weight of adipose and glandular tissue and a superficial region of adipose tissue 5 mm thick. The mean glandular dose (MGD) for the standard breast is estimated from measurements with a 40 mm thickness of poly-methyl-methacrylate (PMMA) *i.e.* Perspex or Lucite. The MGD for the standard breast is useful for comparing doses between different mammography systems and for quality control purposes. It is one of the objectives of the NHSBSP that the MGD to the standard breast is 2 mGy or less [3]. This ensures that all the equipment is capable of achieving acceptable doses. The actual doses received by the screened population also depend on other factors, including the breast size and composition, degree of compression, choice of tube voltage, target and filter, and number of films taken. In previous reviews the radiation doses for individual women have been calculated by using the post exposure mAs to estimate incident air kerma and using the conversion factors (g-factors) provided by Dance [4] and reproduced in IPSM Report 59/2 [2]. Recently the method of estimating doses to individual women has been improved with the introduction of additional factors provided by Dance et al [5]. One factor takes account of variations in breast composition with compressed thickness. Another factor adjusts for the use of target/filter combinations such as molybdenum/rhodium and rhodium/rhodium, which were not considered when the original conversion factors were determined.

Measurements of doses to samples of about 50 women attending for screening are recorded routinely at most screening centres and a pilot study collected dose data from screening centres covering the years 1994 and 1995 [6]. A more recent paper used similar methodology to review the doses from screening centres in 1997 and 1998 [7]. This paper reviews new data collected on samples across the NHSBSP during 2001 and 2002 using a similar methodology but with the additional factors in Dance et al [5]. Where dose data are shown (or referred to for comparison) for 1997/8 they have been recalculated using the additional factors described in Dance et al [5]. The aims of this study were:

- To compare doses with previous years;

Received 19 April 2004 and in revised form 6 September 2004, accepted 12 October 2004.

- To investigate the effect of various technical features (*e.g.* model of X-ray set, film–screen speed, film size, method of beam quality selection);
- To investigate the effect of age and breast thickness;
- To verify the suitability of a proposed national diagnostic reference level (NDRL);
- To assess the impact of a change of policy to 2-view screening.

Method

For each unit that participated in the study the following data were collected:

- date of survey
- models of X-ray set, processor, films, screens
- MGD to standard breast and corresponding film density (the "standard optical density")
- availability of 24 cm × 30 cm cassettes
- age of women screened (where available)
- compressed breast thickness and projection for each film in sample
- exposure factors (mAs, kV, target, filter) for each film
- output data for each X-ray set
- method of beam quality selection (automatic or manual)
- mode of automatic beam quality selection (if more than one)

The survey was restricted to the basic screening situation and so more complicated procedures such as magnification mammography were excluded. Data on doses for women attending screening below the age of 50 years as part of a research trial are being collected and have been reported separately [8].

The exposure factors and compressed breast thickness for each mammogram in the sample were recorded by radiographers and supplied to their local medical physics services. These data were entered into a database supplied by the NHSBSP [9]. The physics service added further details including X-ray tube output data and the MGD per mammogram was calculated automatically. All the information was transferred to a central database for subsequent analysis. The view information was coded to distinguish between left and right breasts, mediolateral oblique projection (OB) and craniocaudal projection (CC). In addition, films were categorised as "main" films or "extra" films. The extra films arose where a breast could not be completely covered with a single film. Unless otherwise indicated, the first film was assumed to be the main film. Examinations were categorised as either 1-view (1V) or 2-view (2V). A 2V examination is conducted at the first visit in the NHSBSP and comprises OB and CC films. Until recently the NHSBSP recommendation was to conduct a 1V examination comprising OB films for all subsequent visits. The NHSBSP (in England) has undergone a phased introduction of 2V examinations for all screens by 2003.

The total dose for a screening procedure or "examination" was calculated by summing the doses for all films and averaging over both breasts. This involved summing the doses for both views in a 2V examination, but also adding the doses for any extra films that were taken to cover large breasts.

Where means for MGD or breast thickness have been calculated they are shown in the tables and figures with 95% confidence limits. The distribution of breast thickness was well represented by a normal distribution. As found previously the distribution of MGD was found to be well represented by a lognormal distribution. In practice it was found that the confidence limits for means of MGD were effectively the same whether a normal or a lognormal distribution was assumed. Thus the 95% confidence limits have been reliably estimated by using $\pm$ 2 standard errors of the mean.

The Ionising Radiation (Medical Exposure) Regulations 2000 require employers to establish DRLs for radiodiagnostic examinations [10]. DRLs are defined in the regulations as dose levels for typical medical X-ray examinations for groups of standard-sized patients or standard phantoms and for broadly defined types of equipment. The employer is required to establish DRLs and to ensure that procedures are in place for using them on the understanding that they are not expected to be exceeded for standard procedures when good and normal practice is being followed. The employer is, moreover, obliged to undertake appropriate reviews whenever DRLs are consistently exceeded and to ensure that corrective action is taken when the excessive exposures cannot be clinically justified. The Institute of Physics and Engineering in Medicine (IPEM) along with the National Radiological Protection Board (NRPB), the College of Radiographers (CoR), the Royal College of Radiologists (RCR) and the British Institute of Radiology (BIR) have established a Working Party to provide guidance on the implementation of DRLs for diagnostic X-ray examinations. The Working Party has proposed a dose audit measure for mammography which is the average MGD for mediolateral oblique mammograms for breasts with a compressed thickness of 55 $\pm$ 5 mm [11]. A minimum of 10 women should be included in the dose sample. The proposed National DRL (NDRL) for this dose audit measure is 3.5 mGy. In this study the average MGD for all oblique mammograms (main films only) with a compressed thickness of 55$\pm$5 mm was calculated for each dose survey. For a few surveys the number of OB mammograms in this thickness range was less than 20 (*i.e.* equivalent to less than 10 women) and these were excluded from this analysis.

Results

Data included

20 medical physics departments contributed data to the survey covering 290 X-ray sets used in 75 of the 99 NHS breast screening programmes. The data were collected over the period May 2001 to December 2002 and include doses for 16 505 women. Although most datasets were for a sample of about 50 women on one X-ray set, the sample size varied from 15 to 195.

X-ray technique and systems used

Only 8% of the X-ray sets were used in a mode that selected the beam quality manually. The rest had some form of automatic selection. The tube voltage selected ranged from 23 kV to 34 kV. Where the tube voltage was

Table 1. Proportion of films taken with different target/filter combinations

Target/filter combination used	1997/8	2001/2
Mo/Mo	96%	58.5%
Mo/Rh	3%	40.0%
Rh/Rh	0.4%	1.2%
W/Rh	0.0%	0.2%

Table 2. Breast dose and thickness for main films compared with previous data. (Errors represent 95% confidence limits)

Projection	Mean MGD per film (mGy)		Average thickness (mm)	
	1997/8	2001/2	1997/8	2001/2
Oblique	2.36±0.03	2.23±0.01	54.3±0.2	56.8±0.2
Craniocaudal	1.86±0.02	1.96±0.01	51.5±0.3	54.1±0.2

MGD, mean glandular dose.

selected manually a molybdenum target material was always used, and 97% of films were taken using a molybdenum filter and 3% using a rhodium filter. The average tube voltage selected in manual mode was 28.2 kV. The proportions of films taken with different target/filter combinations are shown in Table 1 and compared with those in 1997/8. All units operated with an anti-scatter grid, which is standard practice within the

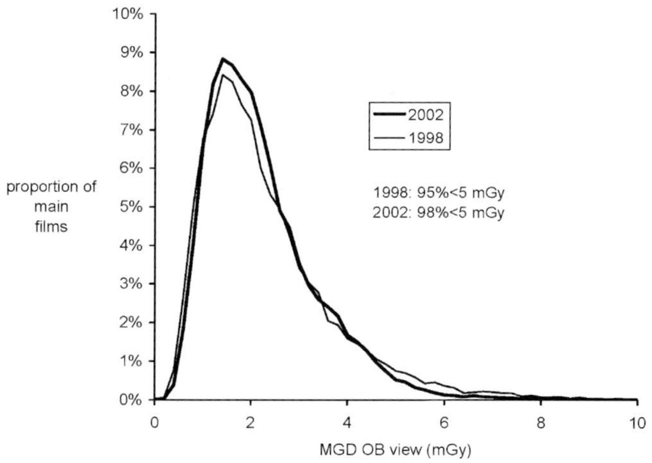

Figure 1. Distribution of mean glandular dose per film for oblique views. Data from the previous dose review in 1997/8 are also shown. Axis represents the mid-point of 0.2 mGy bands.

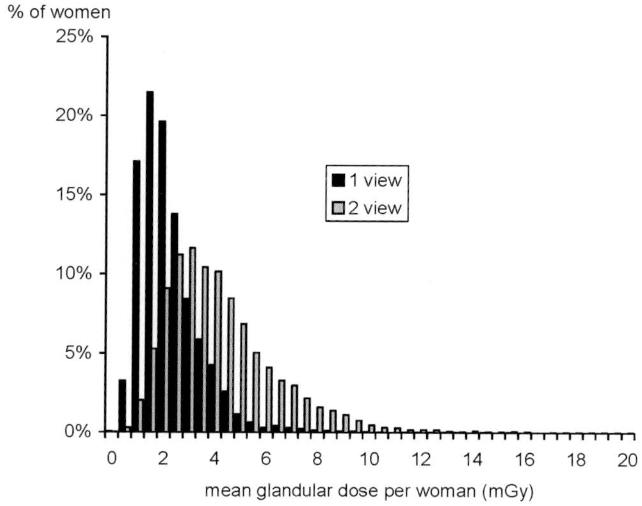

Figure 2. Histogram of mean glandular dose per woman for 1V and 2V examinations. Axis labels represent the mid-point of 0.5 mGy bands.

NHSBSP. Standard optical densities (including base and fog) ranged from 1.11 to 2.11 and averaged 1.71. 89% of the systems had densities that lay within the range 1.50 to 1.90.

Average doses

The average breast doses and thickness recorded for main films are compared with those recorded in 1997/8 in Table 2. The average MGD for OB films decreased from 2.36 mGy to 2.23 mGy, but that for CC films increased from 1.86 mGy to 1.96 mGy. As before the MGD and breast thickness were lower for CC films. Mean thickness increased from 54.3 mm to 56.8 mm for OB and from 51.5 mm to 54.1 mm for CC films. The histograms of doses for OB films are compared in 0.2 mGy bands for 1997/8 and 2001/2 in Figure 1. In 1997/8 5% of films had doses in excess of 5 mGy. In 2001/2 this proportion had fallen to 2%. The average doses for 1V and 2V examinations are compared with the previous data in Table 3. The histograms of the doses for 1V and 2V examinations are shown in Figure 2.

Age

Age was reported for 9839 of the women; of these most were in the usual screening age range of 50–64 years with an average age of 56 years. There were also 8.6% below 50 years and 13% over 65 years. The average dose (main OB films only) and breast thickness for three 5-year age bands

Table 3. Breast dose and thickness for whole examinations compared with previous data. (Errors represent 95% confidence limits)

Examination type	Number of women		Mean MGD per woman (mGy)		Average thickness for OB view (mm)	
	1997/8	2001/2	1997/8	2001/2	1997/8	2001/2
One view	5794	6943	2.48±0.04	2.25±0.03	54.8±0.3	56.3±0.3
Two view	3081	9562	4.19±0.09	4.32±0.05	52.7±0.5	55.6±0.3

MGD, mean glandular dose; OB, oblique projection.

Table 4. Average breast doses and thickness for different age bands. (Errors represent 95% confidence limits)

Age band (years)	Number of films	Average thickness for OB films (mm)	Mean MGD per OB film (mGy)	Ratio of OB dose to the standard breast dose
50–54	5672	56.3±0.4	2.33±0.03	1.60±0.02
55–59	5108	56.4±0.4	2.27±0.03	1.54±0.02
60–64	4564	57.7±0.3	2.25±0.03	1.54±0.02

MGD, mean glandular dose; OB, oblique projection.

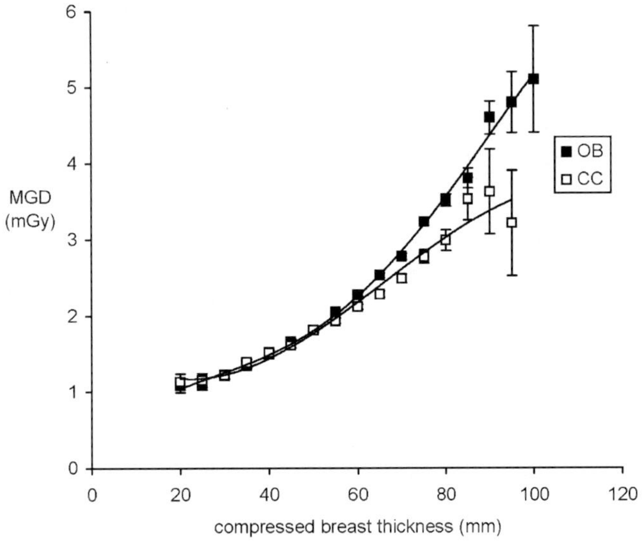

Figure 3. Average mean glandular dose per film (main oblique (OB) and caudocranial (CC) only) as a function of compressed breast thickness. The error bars show 95% confidence limits; for some data points the errors are too small to be seen.

are shown in Table 4. The MGD to the standard breast for the systems that provided age information was 4.2% higher than the average for all the systems and as a result the average doses in Table 4 are higher (by 4.5%) than in Table 2. To minimize the effect of any confounding due to variations in the MGD to the standard breast for the different mammography systems, the average ratio of the dose for the main OB films to the dose to the standard breast was calculated for the three 5 year age bands and is shown in Table 4. This ratio declined by 4% between the age groups 50–54 years and 60–64 years ($p<0.001$, Student's t-test).

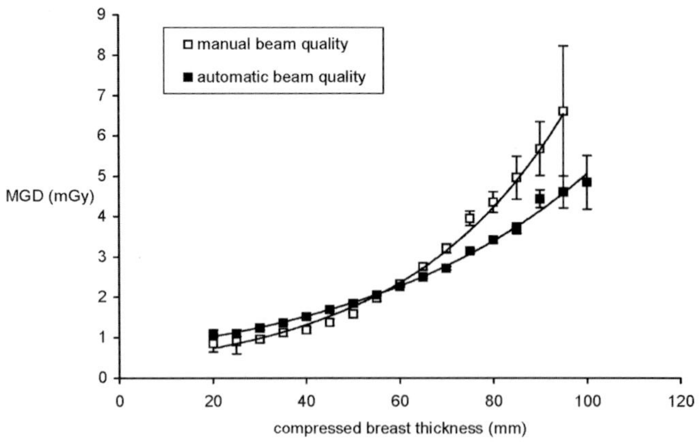

Figure 4. Average mean glandular dose (MGD) per film (main oblique (OB) only) as a function of compressed breast thickness for manual and automatic beam quality selection. The error bars show 95% confidence limits; for some data points the errors are too small to be seen.

Compressed breast thickness and beam quality selection

The average MGDs per OB and CC film are shown as a function of breast thickness in Figure 3. The effect of thickness on MGD where automatic and manual beam quality selection was used is shown in Figure 4. Where manual beam quality selection was employed the MGD increased more rapidly with breast thickness. Average doses per OB film were found to be about 10% lower where X-ray sets were used with automatic rather than manual beam quality selection as shown in Table 5. However, the compressed breast thicknesses are also slightly lower. The average doses per CC film were about the same where X-ray sets were used with automatic rather than manual beam quality selection and the average compressed breast thicknesses slightly lower. The variation in dose with breast thickness for different models of X-ray set is shown in Figure 5. The highest doses were found with the Lorad Mark IV X-ray set (Hologic Inc., Bedford, MA). During the period of the data collection Lorad introduced a new version of their AEC software which was designed to reduce doses. The use of this software is optional and some users may choose to continue with the older version. The data in Figure 5 are shown separately for Lorad systems that use the old and new versions of the software.

Film size

177 of the X-ray sets had the facility to use large format films (24 cm × 30 cm) as well as the standard size (18 cm × 24 cm). For 92 of those units, where the size of

Table 5. Average doses per film for manual and automatic modes of tube potential selection. (Errors represent 95% confidence limits)

kV selection mode	Number of films		Mean MGD per film (mGy)		Average compressed breast thickness (mm)	
	OB	CC	OB	CC	OB	CC
Manual	2768	1608	2.47±0.05	1.93±0.05	58.9±0.5	56.2±0.6
Automatic	29483	17164	2.21±0.01	1.96±0.02	56.6±0.2	53.9±0.2

MGD, mean glandular dose; OB, oblique projection; CC, caudocranial.

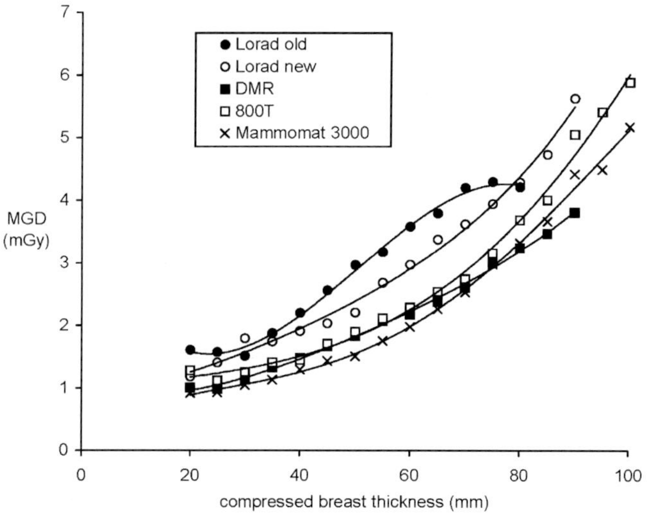

Figure 5. Average mean glandular dose (MGD) per film (main oblique (OB) only) as a function of compressed breast thickness for different models of X-ray set. The Lorad Mark IV is shown for "old" and "new" automatic exposure control software versions. The error bars show 95% confidence limits; for some data points the errors are too small to be seen.

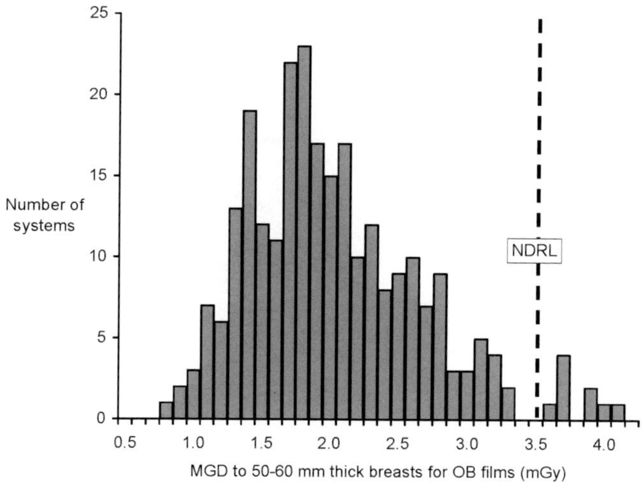

Figure 6. Histogram of the average mean glandular dose (MGD) for main oblique (OB) films for 50–60 mm thick breasts. (Including only those systems where the sample had at least 20 films.)

film was recorded along with the dose data, 8.7% of the films were of the large format. Table 6 shows the number of films per view per breast for those centres with and without the large format film. The average doses per examination for units with and without the facilities for large format film are compared in Table 7.

Standard breast dose

The MGD to the standard breast using 28 kV and a Mo/Mo target filter combination was reported for 285 systems and averaged 1.42±0.04 mGy, and was 6% higher than reported in 1997/8. The minimum was 0.76 and the maximum 2.29 mGy. For nine systems the MGD to the standard breast was above the 2 mGy upper limit required by the NHSBSP. Seven of these nine were Lorad Mark IV X-ray sets, and the other two were a GE DMR (General Electric Medical Systems, Paris, France) and a Siemens Mammomat 3000 (Siemens AG, Erlangen, Germany).

Diagnostic reference level

The average MGD for main OB films for 50–60 mm thick breasts was 2.03±0.08 mGy, with a minimum of 0.85 mGy and a maximum of 4.06 mGy, with a distribution as shown in Figure 6. Nine systems (3.5%) out of the 259 for which data were available exceeded the NDRL of 3.5 mGy. Seven of these systems were Lorad Mark IVs using the old automatic exposure control (AEC) software while the other two were another Lorad Mark IV using the new software, and a GE 800T. Figure 7 shows the MGD for 50–60 mm thick breasts against the MGD

Table 6. Number of films per view per breast

Films per view	Units with only 18 cm × 24 cm films		Units also with 24 cm × 30 cm films	
	OB	CC	OB	CC
1	11289 (93.03%)	7436 (98.18%)	19956 (98.86%)	11235 (99.64%)
2	749 (6.17%)	128 (1.69%)	225 (1.11%)	37 (0.33%)
3	92 (0.76%)	10 (0.13%)	5 (0.02%)	4 (0.04%)
4	5 (0.04%)	0 (0.00%)	1 (0.00%)	0 (0.00%)

OB, oblique projection; CC, caudocranial.

Table 7. Comparison of doses per examination between units having and not having the facility for large format film

Number of views	Large film format available	Number of women	(a) Mean MGD per woman (mGy)	(b) Average MGD to standard breast 28 kV Mo/Mo (mGy)	Ratio of columns (a) to (b)	Dose saved by having large format available
One view	no	2409	2.40±0.06	1.36	1.75	
One view	yes	4594	2.17±0.03	1.47	1.48	16%
Two view	no	3621	4.51±0.08	1.46	3.09	
Two view	yes	5338	4.20±0.06	1.45	2.90	9.4%

MGD, mean glandular dose.

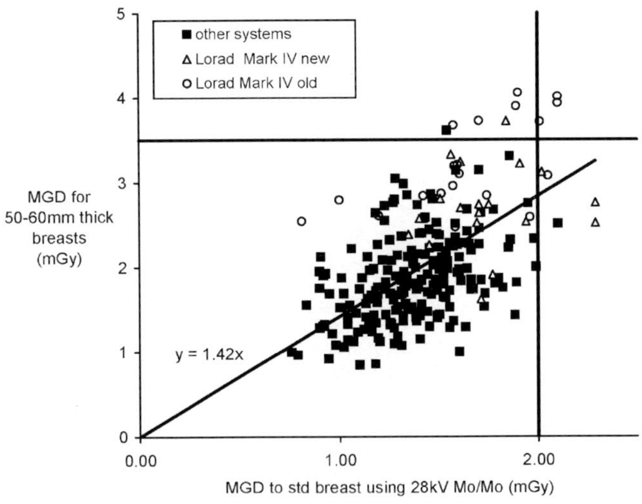

Figure 7. The average mean glandular dose (MGD) for main oblique (OB) films of 50–60 mm thick breasts plotted against the MGD to the standard breast for each unit (using 28 kV and a Mo/Mo target filter combination). Only those systems where the sample had at least 20 films are included. A linear correlation fitted to pass through the origin is shown.

for the standard breast at 28 kV and a Mo/Mo target/filter combination. The Lorad Mark IV X-ray sets are highlighted because they tended to have the highest doses. The regression line shown has a correlation coefficient of 0.54 and a gradient of 1.42. (The regression was set to intercept the origin and has a significance of $p<0.001$.) The systems that exceeded the NDRL were not generally the same systems as those that exceeded the 2 mGy limit to the dose to the standard breast.

Film–screen speed

The average doses to the standard breast for a tube voltage of 28 kV and a Mo/Mo target/filter combination for the most commonly used film–screen combinations are shown in Table 8. From these data a relative speed for each combination has been calculated. The film–screen combination used at a screening centre is one of the main determinants of the average MGD per film as shown in Figure 8. This figure also shows that if one multiplies the average MGD to the standard breast for a given film–screen combination by 1.57 the result approximates the average MGD for OB films. The figure of 1.57 is the

Table 8. Average MGD to the standard breast at 28 kV Mo/Mo for the most commonly used film–screen combinations. Relative speed has been calculated assuming that a speed of 100 results in the average dose to the standard breast 1.42 mGy. (Errors represent 95% confidence limits)

Manufacturer	Film type	Screen	Number of systems	Average MGD to standard breast (mGy)	Relative speed
Agfa	HDR	Detail R	3	0.96±0.10	148
Fuji	UM-MA	AD-M fine	8	1.03±0.24	138
Fuji	UM-MA	UM Medium	6	1.03±0.09	138
Agfa	HDR	Mamoray HD-S	6	1.11±0.15	128
Agfa	HDR	Mamoray Detail S	2	1.18±0.03	121
Kodak	Min-R2000	Min-R2190	26	1.19±0.08	119
Fuji	UM-MA	UM fine	70	1.38±0.06	103
Fuji	AD-M	AD-M fine	53	1.41±0.06	101
Kodak	Min-R2000	Min-R2000	108	1.59±0.05	89

MGD, mean glandular dose.

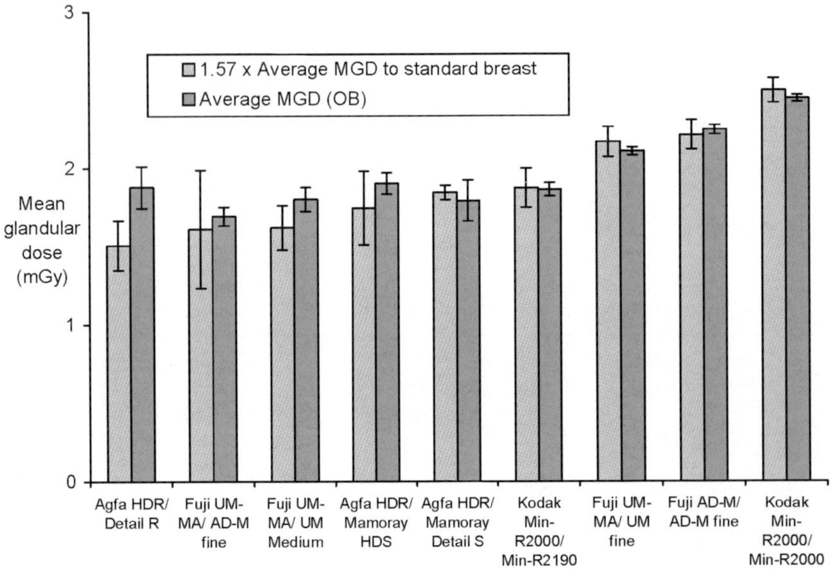

Figure 8. The average mean glandular dose (MGD) for oblique (OB) films and 1.57 times the average MGD to the standard breast at 28 kV Mo/Mo for different film–screen combinations. (Errors represent 95% confidence limits.)

Table 9. Average doses for the most commonly used models of X-ray set. (Where less than four models were included in the survey they were excluded from the analysis)

X-ray set make	X-ray set model	Number of sets	Average MGD for OB films (mGy)	Average MGD to standard breast at 28 kV Mo/Mo (mGy)	Average ratio of OB dose to the standard breast dose at 28 kV Mo/Mo
Lorad	Mark IV (Old AEC)	23	3.05±0.05	1.64±0.14	1.88±0.03
Lorad	Mark IV (New AEC)	19	2.81±0.05	1.74±0.12	1.58±0.03
Planmed	Sophie Classic	4	2.42±0.12	1.50±0.12	1.66±0.09
GE	800T	38	2.36±0.03	1.47±0.09	1.59±0.02
GE	DMR	42	2.10±0.03	1.41±0.09	1.49±0.02
Siemens	Mammomat 300	8	2.32±0.07	1.39±0.18	1.67±0.05
Siemens	Mammomat 3000	119	1.95±0.02	1.35±.04	1.47±0.02
Instrumentarium	Diamond	4	2.42±0.10	1.33±0.12	1.84±0.08
Siemens	Mammomat 2/3	10	2.48±0.09	1.31±0.10	1.90±0.07
Instrumentarium	Alpha RT	12	1.54±0.04	1.17±0.12	1.35±0.04

MGD, mean glandular dose; OB, oblique projection.

average MGD for all main OB films, 2.23 mGy, divided by the average MGD to the standard breast at a tube voltage of 28 kV and a Mo/Mo target/filter combination, 1.42 mGy, for all film–screen combinations.

Model of X-ray set

The average doses for OB films for the more commonly used models of X-ray sets are shown in Table 9. The average doses to the standard breast for each model are also shown for a tube voltage of 28 kV and a Mo/Mo target/filter combination. The highest doses were for the Lorad Mark IV X-ray set used with the old AEC software. The new AEC software resulted in doses that were about 16% lower than with the old software, after allowing for differences due to variations in the dose to the standard breast.

High dose sub-group

A relatively small number of women with the greatest compressed breast thickness received the highest doses. To quantify this, the doses per film for women with a compressed breast thickness in excess of 90 mm are compared in Table 10. A sub-group comprising 0.8% of women screened had a compressed breast thickness greater than or equal to 90 mm for the OB view. A smaller proportion had breasts with a compressed breast thickness greater than or equal to 90 mm in the CC view. The average doses for these women are shown for both automatic and manual beam quality selections. The small proportion (about 9%) of these women who were screened in manual mode had average doses of 6.64 mGy per OB view, which is about 2.7 times the average dose of 2.47 mGy for all women screened in manual mode (Table 5). Those women screened in automatic mode had average OB doses of 4.84 mGy, which is about 2.2 times the average dose of 2.21 mGy for all women screened in automatic mode.

Discussion

Method of dose calculation

In the calculation of the MGD for each film the use of additional factors to compensate for breast composition and the target/filter combination may increase or decrease the dose estimation. However, as discussed previously, the average effect is an increase of about 15% in the doses estimated [8].

Data included

The data analysed here are broadly representative of the NHSBSP and represent the largest study of mammographic doses ever published. The women were almost all in the normal screening age range 50–64 years with an average age of 56 years. About 76% of the NHSBSP programmes participated and data were collected for over half the X-ray sets used by the NHSBSP. The equipment included a wide range of X-ray models and film–screen systems. A few of the datasets submitted were smaller than 50 women. This did not cause a problem for most of the analyses since the data for many different systems were usually averaged. However, the comparison with the

Table 10. Doses for breasts with compressed thickness greater than 90 mm

Method of beam quality selection		All	Manual	Automatic
MGD per film (mGy)	OB	5.07±0.27	6.64±0.86	4.84±0.27
	CC	3.55±0.72	—	3.61±0.74
Number of films (proportion of women)	OB	261 (0.81%)	33 (0.10%)	228 (0.71%)
	CC	28 (0.15%)	1 (0.00%)	27 (0.14%)
Average compressed breast thickness (mm)	OB	95.0±0.5	94.3±1.2	95.1±0.5
	CC	95.8±1.8	96.0	95.8±1.9

MGD, mean glandular dose; OB, oblique projection; CC, caudocranial.

NDRL was not possible in a few cases where less than 20 OB films were included for 50–60 mm thick breasts.

X-ray technique

Modern machines with a choice of filters have replaced most of the X-ray sets used at the time of the dose review of 1997/8 and many have a choice of target material. Some of the changes in X-ray sets have tended to reduce doses (*e.g.* availability of rhodium filters) while others have increased them (*e.g.* selection of lower kV and grid designs that improve contrast but increase dose). In 1997/98 only 15% of the X-ray sets selected the beam quality automatically. In this review 92% of the sets were used in an automatic mode. One consequence of this change is the much greater use of a rhodium filter. Thus the proportion of films taken using a rhodium filter has increased from 3% to 40%. However although many modern machines have an alternative target material such as tungsten or rhodium, these are still relatively rarely used. This is because current guidance in the NHSBSP is that the use of these target materials with film–screen imaging can result in significant loss in contrast as well as a large dose reduction. Standard film densities have increased only slightly from 1.64 to 1.71 since the previous review.

Average doses

The average MGD per OB film has fallen by about 5% since 1997/8. The average MGD for CC films has increased by about 5%. The average thickness for both OB and CC films has increased by about 2.5 mm. This could be due to a real change in the sampled thickness or due to a change in the calibration of thickness displays. It is surprising that average doses have not fallen by more given the widespread use of rhodium filters. However there have been many other changes in the X-ray sets, film processors, films and screens used in the NHSBSP, some of which tend to increase doses. Doses for CC films were about 12% lower than for OB films. Previously CC films had doses that were about 19% lower than OB films. The small difference found in the compressed breast thickness of about 3 mm explains most of this dose difference. The other explanation of the difference is likely to be the effect of pectoral muscle in the oblique views overlying the AEC chamber and causing an increase in the exposure. Changes in AEC design may explain why the difference between the doses for OB and CC films has varied.

The dose for a one view examination was slightly higher than the dose per film because of the additional films per view shown in Table 6. The dose for a two view examination is also much higher because of the additional CC view. The change to two view examinations in every screening round causes by far the greatest change in doses to women attending for screening. Thus the MGD for a full screening examination is now about 4.3 mGy. The decision to change to two view imaging at every screening visit was based on the prediction of an increase in cancer detection [12]. A review of the radiation risks and benefits of such a screening regimen concluded that the benefits greatly exceeded the risks [13]. The dose assumed in that review was an average of 4.5 mGy for a two view screening episode which is consistent with the results reported here.

The average doses found in the UK NHSBSP can be compared with a few similar but smaller studies for other countries. Jamal et al calculated the MGD per film in Malaysia for 300 women examined using three X-ray units [14]. The average MGD was 1.54 mGy and 1.82 mGy for CC and OB films, respectively, which is lower than presented here. However the corresponding average compressed breast thicknesses were also much lower at 37 mm and 44 mm, respectively. Kruger and Schueler reported on patient doses for 6006 women undergoing mammography in the USA using 7 Lorad Mark-IV X-ray sets [15]. They calculated an average MGD per film of 2.6 mGy and a compressed thickness of 5.1 cm for all views combined. Such higher doses can be explained by the use of this particular X-ray set. The use of different conversion factors can also be expected to cause a difference. Bulling and Nicoll have reported on mammographic doses for a screening programme in New Zealand [16]. They reported on doses for 310 women, routinely screened using a GE Senographe 600 operated mainly at 25 kV with Mo/Mo target filter combination. The average MGD per film was about 2.8 mGy with an average thickness of 4.9 cm.

Age

Age information was available for 60% of the women, which allowed the relationship between age and radiation dose to be assessed. Since the system to system variations in dose were quite large it was important to ensure that these differences did not mask or exaggerate any relationship between age and dose. For each X-ray set information on age was usually provided for all the women or for none. The distribution of ages sampled for the different systems was not perfectly uniform, and it was therefore prudent to take the step of normalizing the dose data by dividing by the standard breast dose as in the last column of Table 4. Since it is known that breasts become less glandular with age, one might have expected dose to decline with increasing age. In the previous review a small reduction of about 3% in the normalized dose data between the age bands 50–54 years and 60–64 years was found but was not statistically significant. In this study a 3% reduction is again observed, and is in this case significant because of the larger sample size. A slight increase (3%) in breast thickness over this age range was observed as found previously. In a previous report no effect of age on doses was found when the doses for women in the age range 40–48 years were compared with those in the screening programme [8]. Overall, age appears to have only a very small effect on dose.

Compressed breast thickness and beam quality selection

The compressed breast thickness is a major determinant of the dose per film received by a woman for a given mammography system. Compressed thicknesses were recorded, which ranged from 10 mm to 100 mm with an average thickness of about 57 mm for OB films and 54 mm for CC films. These thicknesses are about 2.5 mm greater than reported in 1997/8 (Table 2). Possible reasons are a real increase in breast size due to increasing obesity in the population, less compression force being applied, or problems with calibration especially with new tilting paddle designs. In the authors' opinion the latter is the most likely.

The difference in thickness largely explains why doses are higher for OB than CC films. However Figure 3 shows that there appears to be an additional factor. For thickness greater than about 60 mm the OB doses were larger even for the same breast thickness. It is likely that the presence of pectoral muscle overlying the AEC chamber is the cause of greater doses for OB films than CC films of the same compressed breast thickness. In general there was a curvilinear relationship between the compressed breast thickness and the dose per film. Where beam quality was manually selected (and usually fixed at a tube voltage of 28 kV with a Mo/Mo target/filter combination) the average dose per film rose from just above 0.9 mGy for a 20 mm thick compressed breast to 5.7 mGy for a 90 mm thick compressed breast. Where X-ray sets were used in an automatic mode the selection of a different tube voltage, target and filter reduced doses for breasts with a compressed thickness greater than about 60 mm. Thus in automatic mode large breasts with a 90 mm thickness received doses which were about 2.2 times that for average sized breasts (55 mm thick). However Figure 5 showed that the change in dose with thickness varied from one model of X-ray set to another. Lorad Mark IV X-ray sets programmed with the old AEC software typically selected 25 kV and a Mo/Mo target filter combination for average sized breasts. As a result the average dose for a 55 mm thick breast was 3.2 mGy. The new AEC software on the Lorad X-ray sets tended to select 28 kV and a Mo/Mo target filter combination for average sized breasts. As a result the average dose for a 55 mm thick breast was 2.7 mGy. For the women with relatively thick breasts on compression, automatic beam quality selection leads to a significant dose reduction. However, the average dose per film for all women screened using automatic beam quality selection shown in Table 5 was not much lower than that of women screened on systems using manual beam quality selection. This is partly explained by higher doses for women with thinner breasts and partly by the increase in dose caused by the use of Lorad X-ray sets. The interpretation of Table 5 is also complicated by the fact that the average compressed breast thicknesses were slightly lower where automatic systems were used. The small differences found may be real leading one to expect lower doses due to thinner breasts or just reflect thickness scale calibration differences between different X-ray sets.

Film size

Many screening centres in the UK do not have the facilities for the larger format 24 cm × 30 cm mammography film. Some women's breasts are too large to fit on the standard sized film and have to be imaged using a mosaic of the standard sized films. This procedure involves a higher dose than if a single large format film were used. The extra dose can be assumed to be approximately proportional to the area of overlap of the films over the breast. In calculating the dose per examination it was assumed here that there was 100% overlap between films and this will have somewhat overestimated the true additional dose. Table 6 shows that some extra films are indeed taken where the larger format film is not available. For OB views about 7% of women required more than one film if the larger format film was not available. Even where the larger format film was available about 1.1% of women still required more than one film per oblique view. Fewer extra films were taken for the CC views, with only about 1.8% of women having extra films if the larger format film was not available. The effect of these differences on doses for examinations was compared in Table 7. It was calculated that there was about a 16% dose saving for single view screening if the larger format film was available. This dose saving fell to 9% for two view screening. Although the potential dose saving achievable by ensuring that all centres had large format film available would not be great for the screened population as a whole, it would be substantial for those women who currently need extra films. Women who had large compressed breast thicknesses were more likely to require extra films. Thus the dose reduction achieved by having the large format available is of most benefit to those women receiving the highest doses. Recent new equipment purchases for the NHSBSP have included funding for equipment to have facilities for both standard and large sizes of cassettes. Funding and radiation dose are not the only issues affecting the use of larger format cassettes. There may be image quality issues (*e.g.* relating to positioning, and effectiveness of compression) and practical ones (*e.g.* space for additional film handling equipment, film viewing arrangements). Nonetheless, more widespread use of large cassettes can be expected in future in the NHSBSP.

Standard breast dose

The MGD to the standard breast may be calculated relatively easily by combining the mAs for correct exposure of a 40 mm thick block of PMMA with values of tube output and beam quality [2]. The advantage of this approach is that the effect of equipment factors can be assessed, while eliminating patient variables. The exposure may be made using standard exposure factors or those selected automatically by the X-ray set. The standard breast doses shown here are for a tube voltage of 28 kV and a Mo/Mo target/filter combination. The limitation of the standard breast method is that it does not indicate the actual doses to individual women. The doses calculated for real breasts are for the beam qualities used clinically which can result in higher or lower doses than expected from the standard breast dose. In general one would expect the standard breast dose to be correlated with average breast doses for any mammography system. In Figure 7 the average MGD for 50–60 mm thick breasts and the MGD to standard breasts were linearly correlated with a coefficient of 0.54. Figure 7 also showed that the dose for an OB film on an average sized breast (*i.e.* 55 mm thick) was about 42% higher than the dose to the standard breast on the same system. This difference is largely explained by the fact that the standard breast is only 45 mm thick. For a few systems a very different relationship between the standard breast dose and the average breast dose was found. This is partly explained by the different beam qualities used. A further consideration is the inhomogeneous nature of breast tissue as compared with PMMA, and what effect that has on the operation of AEC systems.

In a recent review of the performance of mammographic equipment in the NHSBSP, the MGD for the standard breast was found to have gradually risen from 1.28 mGy in 1991 to 1.45 mGy in 2001 where a tube voltage of 28 kV and a Mo/Mo target/filter combination was used [17]. The average MGD to the standard breast was 1.55 mGy in 2001 where the clinically selected factors were used. These data for doses to the standard breast would lead one to expect a similar rise in the dose measurements for women attending screening. In fact this paper shows that such a trend has been counteracted by the changes in beam quality selection (*e.g.* increased use of rhodium filters). Such an apparent contradiction is one reason why a revision of how the MGD is estimated with phantoms is being considered in the UK.

Although the standard breast model has worked well for many years, some problems have become apparent recently and are illustrated by the data presented here. The first issue is that the standard breast model with a 45 mm thickness and 50% glandularity in the central region is not representative of the breasts of women attending for screening. In screening in the UK the average compressed breast has a thickness of approximately 50–60 mm and a glandularity of about 30% [5, 18]. This means that average doses are rather higher than the MGD to the standard breast for a given system. Another issue is the change in the beam quality selection by modern X-ray sets. A few years ago almost all mammography in the NHSBSP was conducted using a tube voltage of 28 kV and a Mo/Mo target/filter combination. Nowadays the beam quality is usually selected automatically depending on breast thickness and composition, and the spectrum used may have significantly higher or lower energies. As a result the use of a phantom comprising 40 mm PMMA results in an atypical spectrum being used to calculate the dose. To fully understand the doses delivered one needs to conduct dose measurements using either exposure data for real breast examinations or simulations with a range of thicknesses of PMMA. These procedures are time consuming and a more appropriate simple single measurement would be useful.

A procedure for measuring dose in mammography with a new standard breast model is being drafted [19]. It is proposed to use published data for the equivalence between PMMA and typical compressed breast to establish a new standard breast simulated with 45 mm PMMA [5]. The entrance air kerma for 45 mm PMMA is equivalent to that for a 53 mm thick breast with a glandularity of 29% in the central region. (Note that this composition was found to be approximately typical for breasts of this compressed thickness for women in the age range 50–64 years). This will bring the UK into line with existing European dose and quality control protocols, which have a standard PMMA phantom with a 45 mm thickness [20, 21]. It is planned to have a new dose recommendation whereby the MGD to the new standard breast model should not exceed 2.5 mGy when exposed using the beam quality selected clinically. In practice this will usually mean as selected automatically by the AEC with the phantom in place. This change in the standard breast model and the applicable dose limit is intended to make the standard dose measurement more relevant to the clinical situation, but have a neutral effect on the proportion of systems meeting the required standard.

Diagnostic reference level

Nine systems (3.5%) exceeded the diagnostic reference level of 3.5 mGy for an OB film of a 55 mm thick breast. Most of these X-ray sets were Lorad models using the old AEC software. The reasons for the high doses were a combination of a high mean glandular dose to the standard breast and a beam quality selection strategy that increased doses for this type of breast. The national DRL appears to be set at the correct level with only 3.5% failing in the NHSBSP where doses are relatively well controlled. It would be undesirable to set a level whereby a substantial proportion of systems failed, leading to dose reductions which might compromise image quality. The national DRL should be kept under review and reduced when this is possible without significantly impacting on image quality. Some screening centres may find that they can set a local DRL that is lower than the national DRL.

Film–screen speed

A major determinant of average breast doses was the type of film–screen combination used. All the film manufacturers offer a choice of screen speeds. Relatively few screening centres choose to use the faster screen options (Agfa Detail R and Detail S; Agfa-Gevaert, Mortsel, Belgium, Fuji UM medium; Fuji Photo Film, Bedford, UK; and Kodak Min-R2190; Eastman Kodak, Rochester, NY) because of the slight loss in image quality involved. The fastest film–screen combination was the Agfa HDR film used with an Agfa Detail R screen, which resulted in an average MGD to the standard breast of 0.96 mGy. The slowest film–screen combination was the Kodak Min-R2000 film used with a Kodak Min-R2000 screen, which resulted in an average MGD to the standard breast of 1.59 mGy. Figure 8 showed that multiplying the standard breast dose by the ratio of the average dose for OB films to the average dose to the standard breast (*i.e.* 1.57) was a very good predictor for the average doses for oblique films for a given film–screen combination. This was possible partly because film–screen speed is such a major determinant of dose. It must be remembered that the choice of film–screen combination affects not only the average doses but also the image quality.

Model of X-ray set

Another determinant of average breast doses is the model of X-ray set used. The average doses for different models of X-ray set varied from 1.54 mGy to 3.05 mGy as shown in Table 9. It was particularly noticeable that the Lorad Mark IV X-ray sets gave the highest doses. This was partly due to the design of the Bucky systems and partly due to the programming of the AEC beam quality selection software. The use of the new AEC software appears to be reducing doses by about 16%. Even with the new software, doses remain higher than for other models. The design factors that cause these differences in dose may or may not also affect image quality, depending on the underlying reasons for the differences.

High dose sub-group

Although the average dose per OB film is 2.2 mGy in the NHSBSP there are subgroups of women for whom the doses are higher. One identifiable sub-group of women who receive larger doses than average comprises those women with relatively thick breasts on compression. It was shown in Table 10 that the small sub-group of women with compressed breasts greater than 90 mm thick had doses for OB films of about 2.7 times the average for a given mammography system operated using manual beam quality selection. Another factor that affects the doses to women is the equipment used. This can be appreciated by examining the doses to the standard breast, which ranged from 0.76 mGy to 2.29 mGy. Although the quality assurance guidelines for the NHSBSP [3] require that the MGD to the standard breast should not exceed 2 mGy nine systems were slightly above this limit. For the mammography system with the highest standard breast dose of 2.29 mGy, breast doses of about 1.6 times the average can be expected. It is assumed here that doses to breasts of all sizes will be greater by approximately this amount. (One can see that this is likely to be true since a major cause of this variation is the variation in the speed of the film–screen system, which can be assumed to be approximately the same for all sizes of breast). Thus using this system one can expect that a few women with large breasts (>90 mm thick) would receive doses of about 10.7 mGy per film (*i.e.* $2.7 \times 1.6 \times 2.47$ mGy) if beam quality were selected manually. In fact only 11 out of 32 250 oblique films (*i.e.* 0.03%) had doses in excess of 10.7 mGy. 99.97% of oblique films had doses of less than 10.7 mGy and this dose per OB film can be regarded as an upper limit to what can normally be expected for a screening mammogram in the NHSBSP. The doses for whole examinations were higher, particularly for 2V examinations. Using the same arguments as above and the data from Table 10 one can estimate the maximum dose for a CC film normally expected. For OB films, doses for the manual mode were used in this calculation as these resulted in higher doses. However there is a lack of data in Table 10 for compressed breasts over 90 mm thick in the CC view, and automatic mode is therefore used to estimate maximum doses. In this case the highest expected dose for a CC film is 5.8 mGy (*i.e.* $1.84 \times 1.6 \times 1.96$ mGy). Thus the maximum dose that may be normally expected for a 2V examination is 16.5 mGy if there is one film per view. In practice only 15 women (0.16%) out of 9562 who had 2V examinations received more than 16.5 mGy even when all extra films were included. Thus one may conclude that a very small proportion of women will receive about 3.8 times (*i.e.* $16.5 \div 4.32$) the average dose in a 2V screening programme, and that this identifiable sub-group should be considered in any risk benefit analysis. A few women will receive doses higher than this, but this is very rare and impossible to predict in advance. Note that some of the highest doses per examination are overestimates because multiple films per view have merely been added together – rather than by taking the amount of overlap into account.

Conclusions

We have reported the results of a very large sample of doses, which give a good representation of the performance of breast screening units in the UK. 97% of units complied with the standard for dose, illustrating the benefit of strict quality control. Increasing use of sophisticated units with automatic beam quality selection has reduced the radiation dose received by large breasts. The increasing use of large format film is also reducing the doses to this sub-group. There has been little change to the average dose per film since the last study in 1997/8 but total dose per woman has increased due to the introduction of two view screening at every visit. A reduction in dose of 3% was observed between the ages 50 years and 64 years. This study has confirmed that the proposed NDRL of 3.5 mGy for 50–60 mm thick breasts is an appropriate value to identify systems giving unusually high doses. Average doses for OB views of average sized breasts were fairly well correlated with the dose to the standard breast, and typically 42% higher. This highlights the need for a revised definition of the standard breast used in the UK to give values that better reflect the doses received in clinical practice. The type of film–screen combination and X-ray set used can explain much of the variation in dose from one system to another. The introduction of a substantial number of Lorad Mark IV X-ray sets has tended to increase doses in the NHSBSP. The use of these X-ray sets needs to be carefully monitored to ensure that national guidelines on doses are followed.

Acknowledgments

The authors would like to acknowledge the work of the many radiographers and physicists throughout the UK who collected the raw data analysed in this paper. We would also like to acknowledge the support of the National Breast Screening Quality Assurance Coordinating Group for Physics. The National Coordinating Office of the NHSBSP funds the work of the National Coordinating Centre for the Physics of Mammography.

References

1. NHS Breast Screening Annual Review 2003: serving women for 15 years. (NHSBSP, Sheffield) 2003.
2. Law J, Dance DR, Faulkner K, Fitzgerald MC, Ramsdale ML, Robinson A. Commissioning and Routine Testing of Mammographic X-ray Systems. (IPSM Report 59/2) York: Institute of Physical Sciences in Medicine, 1994;67–73.
3. Guidelines on Quality Assurance Visits. Sheffield: NHS Breast Screening Programme (NHSBSP Publication No 40). 1998:51–52.
4. Dance DR. Monte Carlo calculation of conversion factors for the estimation of mean glandular breast dose. Phys Med Biol 1990;35:1211–9.
5. Dance DR, Skinner CL, Young KC, Beckett JR, Kotre CJ. Additional factors for the estimation of mean glandular dose using the UK mammography dosimetry protocol. Phys Med Biol 2000;45:3225–40.
6. Burch A, Goodman DA. A pilot survey of radiation doses received in the United Kingdom Breast Screening Programme. Br J Radiol 1998;71:517–27.
7. Young KC, Burch A. Radiation doses in the UK Breast Screening Programme in 1997 and 1998. Br J Radiol 2000;73:278–87.

8. Young KC. Radiation doses in the UK trial of breast screening in women aged 40 to 48 years. Br J Radiol 2002;75:362–70.
9. Young KC. Breast dose surveys in the NHSBSP: Software and instruction manual. (NHSBSP, Sheffield) NHSBSP Report 01/10, October 2001.
10. Ionising Radiation (Medical Exposure) Regulations 2000 (Statutory Instrument No. 1059). London, UK: Her Majesty's Stationary Office, 2000.
11. Guidance on the establishment and use of diagnostic reference levels for medical X-ray examinations. (IPEM Report 88) York: Institute of Physics and Engineering in Medicine, 2004.
12. Blanks RG, Moss SM, Wallis MG. Use of two view mammography compared with one view in the detection of small invasive cancers: further results from the NHSBSP. J Med Screen 1997;4:98–101.
13. Young KC, Faulkner K, Wall B, Muirhead C. Review of radiation risk in breast screening. (NHSBSP, Sheffield) NHSBSP Publication No 54 February 2003.
14. Jamal N, Ng KH, McLean D. A study of mean glandular dose during diagnostic mammography in Malaysia and some of the factors affecting it. Br J Radiol 2003;76:238–45.
15. Kruger RL, Schueler BA. A survey of clinical factors and patient dose in mammography. Med Phys 2001;28:1449–54.
16. Bulling SM, Nicoll JJ. Level and distribution of the radiation dose to the population from a mammography screening programme in New Zealand. Radiat Prot Dosim 1995;57:455–8.
17. Young KC, Ramsdale ML. Performance of mammographic equipment in the UK Breast Screening Programme in 2000/2001. (NHS Cancer Screening Programmes, Sheffield) NHSBSP Publication Number 56, September 2003.
18. Young KC, Ramsdale ML, Bignell F. Review of dosimetric methods for mammography in the UK Breast Screening Programme. Radiat Prot Dosim 1998;80:183–6.
19. Commissioning and Routine Testing of Mammographic X-ray Systems. (IPEM Report 89) York: Institute of Physics and Engineering in Medicine. (Pending publication in 2004)
20. Zoetelief J, Fitzgerald M, Leitz W, Sabel M. European Protocol on dosimetry in mammography. European Commission Report 16263 EN. Luxembourg: European Commission, 1996.
21. Woudenberg S van, Thijssen M, Young K. European protocol for the quality control of the physical and technical aspects of mammography screening. In "European Guidelines for Quality Assurance in Mammography Screening" (Luxembourg, European Commission, 1996).

The British Journal of Radiology, *78* (2005), 219–229
DOI: 10.1259/bjr/12209589

A study of the distribution of dose across the hands of interventional radiologists and cardiologists

M WHITBY, MSc and C J MARTIN, PhD

Health Physics, Department of Clinical Physics and Bio-Engineering, West House, Gartnavel Royal Hospital, Glasgow, UK

Abstract. The magnitude and distribution of doses across the hands of interventional radiologists and cardiologists have been studied. The aims were to determine the region of highest dose, investigate variations in dose distribution, and propose an effective method for dose monitoring. Doses have been measured using sets of up to 18 thermoluminescent dosemeters (TLDs) for 183 single procedures. Important factors influencing the dose to the hand are the type of procedure, particularly the access route, the X-ray equipment used, and the experience of the operator. Radiologists performing percutaneous procedures received the highest doses, because of the proximity of their hands to the X-ray tube. The majority of procedures involve a combination of twisting and prodding actions, and the relative proportions of each determine the parts of the fingers which receive a higher dose. For most interventional radiology and cardiology procedures the bases of the ring and little fingers receive the highest dose. However, during percutaneous procedures the tips of the middle and ring fingers could receive doses which were 20–30% higher than this. For radiologists and cardiologists with a mixed workload, monitoring using TLD rings located at the base of the little or the ring fingers on either hand should provide a reasonable estimate of dose to the most exposed area. Monitoring is recommended for operators who may receive over 50 mSv to their hands per year, and should be considered for operators carrying out therapeutic procedures involving patient dose–area products over 500 Gy cm^2 per month.

There is a potential for staff carrying out interventional procedures in radiology and cardiology departments to receive significant radiation doses to their hands, as they guide and manipulate needles and catheters while viewing with fluoroscopy. The monthly programme of monitoring for finger doses in hospitals in the West of Scotland has recorded doses of tens of mSv for interventional radiologists in some hospitals with annual doses occasionally exceeding 200 mSv. This has required some staff to be designated as classified radiation workers. There is a wide range of doses to the hands of interventional radiologists and cardiologists. Studies at other centres have recorded doses to the hands ranging from less than 0.1 mSv up to 4–5 mSv for individual procedures [1–13] and noted the potential for annual doses to exceed 200 mSv [2, 14–17], so monitoring of the dose to the hands needs to be considered. UK legislation [18] states that the dose limit for the skin of 500 mSv in a calendar year should be applied to the dose averaged over any area of 1 cm^2 regardless of the area exposed. Since the operator's hands may be close to the source of scattered radiation, there can be a large dose gradient across the hands, so a dosemeter worn at an arbitrary location will not necessarily be representative of that to the most exposed area. Thus in order to comply with the requirements of the legislation, the part of the hand likely to receive the highest dose should be identified and information obtained on the dose distribution, in order that the correct location for wearing a dosemeter can be specified. The studies carried out so far that have involved measurements at more than one location on the hand [19], have not contained sufficient data to allow the most exposed part to be identified. Moreover, since there are many types of procedure involving different manipulations which could create different distributions of dose across the hands, a standard monitoring technique may not be appropriate for all operators.

The purpose of this study was to:

- Evaluate the magnitude and distribution of doses to the hands of operators carrying out interventional procedures in radiology and cardiology in a number of centres.
- Determine the regions of the hand receiving the highest doses.
- Investigate whether there are significant variations in dose distribution with different types of procedure.
- Make recommendations about the most effective methods for routine monitoring of dose to the hands.

Routine monitoring of doses to the hands requires a measurement technique which is easy to apply. Thermoluminescent dosemeters (TLDs) are widely used and these can be worn at several different positions on the hands. Standard techniques involve incorporating TLDs into rings that are worn at the bases of fingers, into sheaths which enable dosemeters to be worn near finger tips, or into bands worn around the wrists. However, when a TLD is worn at the finger tip, the touch sensation may be impaired and this can impede the manipulations carried out. The constraints on viable options for the monitoring position have been borne in mind during the study.

Received 3 February 2004 and in final form 4 October 2004, accepted 26 October 2004.

Funding for this work was provided by the UK Health and Safety Executive.

Materials and methods

Calibration and dose distribution measurements

Doses were measured using LiF: Mg, Ti TLD 100 chips, which were read out using a Harshaw 5500 TLD reader (Harshow, Solon, OH). The TLDs were calibrated against air kerma, measured using a Keithley Triad dosimetry system (Keithley, Cleveland, OH) with a 15 cm^3 chamber and a RADCAL 9010 electrometer (Radcal, Monrovia, CA) with a 60 cm^3 chamber. Both systems had calibrations which were traceable to a national standard. The calibration exposures were carried out free in air in a beam of 80 kVp X-rays [20]. A conversion coefficient was applied to derive the soft tissue dose (H_p 0.07) [21]. For each procedure, 12–18 TLDs were used, 6–9 on each hand of the primary operator. No other staff members were monitored. The TLDs were sealed in plastic, wiped with a surgical solution and taped in place after the operator had scrubbed up. A surgical glove was then put on over the top. The positions of the TLDs were chosen to assess the dose gradient across and along the length of the hand, on both the dorsum and palmer aspects (Figure 1).

The principle investigator was present throughout the majority of procedures studied in order to ensure accurate placement of the TLDs on the hand and their removal after each procedure was complete. Observation of practices during the procedures enabled an understanding to be developed of how the exposure of the operators' hands occurred. Factors which could affect the scatter air kerma around the table were recorded. This information included room layout, technique used, views obtained (beam geometry), image intensifier field size (magnification), radiographic runs employed, contrast injection technique, operator position throughout the procedure, dose–area product (DAP) and screening time.

The distribution of scatter air kerma close to the patient, in the positions where the operators' hands might be, was measured using a Radcal 9010 electrometer with a 180 cm^3 chamber. This was achieved by irradiating a RANDO phantom in an X-ray field using typical fluoroscopic settings and positions encountered in practice [23]. A 100 mm grid marked on a polythene sheet, suspended in turn horizontally and vertically at the side of the couch, was used to aid positioning of the ionization chamber.

Procedures monitored

Studies for interventional radiology were carried out at five large teaching hospitals and five district general hospitals, with a range of different equipment, protection and operator experience. Cardiology data were collected at a large teaching hospital, with two different interventional units, which were used by cardiologists from other hospitals with a range of experience. All X-ray units studied were of an undercouch geometry. Only procedures routinely undertaken in most interventional departments were included in the study, since the aim was to establish dose distribution, which would be applicable to the majority of radiologists practising in the UK. Cardiologists were only monitored during percutaneous transluminal coronary angioplasties (PTCA), as these were common procedures which were considered to represent a "worst case scenario", involving lengthy screening times and radiographic runs, for several different views. The manipulations carried out in other cardiology procedures were similar to those in PTCA.

In order to establish the likely dose levels that would be encountered, and gain an impression of the general distribution of dose across the hand, a preliminary study was undertaken for 10 complete interventional radiology sessions. The average dose to the hand per session ranged from 0.07 mSv to 3.5 mSv. Doses from sessions, in which therapeutic procedures were performed, were significantly higher than those involving purely diagnostic angiograms. The preliminary study demonstrated that it would be difficult to establish links between dose distributions across the hand and different procedures from measurements made over complete sessions. Therefore, it was decided that the main study should concentrate on measuring dose distributions for individual procedures. During this study,

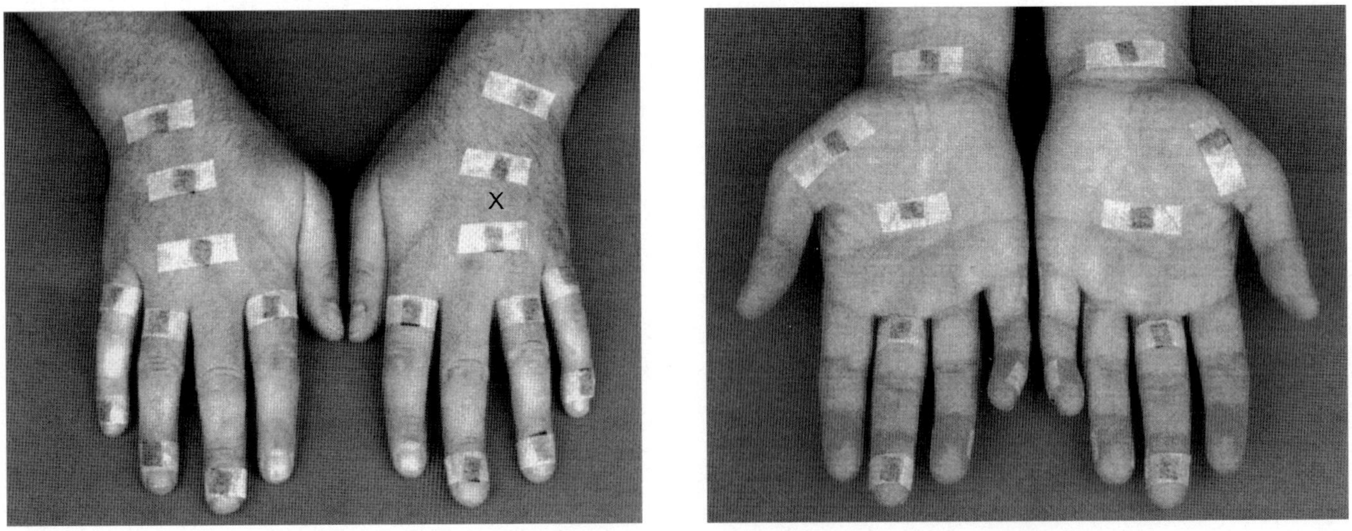

(a) (b)

Figure 1. Positions of thermoluminescent dosemeters (TLDs) used for monitoring (a) the dorsum and (b) the palmer aspects of the hands. The X marks the position of the TLD that was used as the denominator when deriving ratios for doses to different parts of the hands.

Table 1. Procedures for different interventional radiology and cardiology groups studied

Patient access	Procedures studied	Total no. of procedures studied	Data on procedures used to assess dose distribution		
			No. in distribution study	Mean screening time (min)	Mean DAP (Gy cm^2)
Percutaneous	Biliary stent/drainage Percutaneous transhepatic cholangiogram Percutaneous nephrostomy	32	20	10.6	15.4
Internal jugular vein (IJV)	Transjugular intrabepatic portosystemic shunts (TIPS) TIPS Follow-up Transhepatic liver biopsy	27	15	16.3	143.2
Femoral	Angioplasty	28	21	11.8	43.5
	Stents	22	17	12.2	45.5
	Embolisations	19	14	19.1	61.3
	Angiograms	30	13	5.2	76.8
Cardiac Femoral/Radial	Percutaneous transluminal coronary angioplasty (PTCA)	25	25	11.8	61.5

DAP, dose–area product.

measurements were made on 183 individual interventional radiology and cardiology procedures. For the purpose of analysis, these have been split into four groups (Table 1) based on the access route and the resulting position of the operator, as this appeared to have most influence on the doses recorded. The areas in which the operators hands are typically located for the four groups are shown in Figure 2, along with the typical scatter air kerma distributions derived from the ionization chamber measurements. Results from the preliminary study were not included in the final data analysis.

Measurement of dose distribution

In the main study, doses were assessed for single procedures, so that differences in dose distribution relating to the type of procedure could be evaluated. The TLD positions used were based upon results from the preliminary measurements and observations of practices with respect to potential exposure. Those for the early part of the study were chosen to assess doses both to the palmer and dorsum aspects of the hand. In the latter part of the study, doses to the dorsum aspects of the bases and tips of the fingers were assessed as these were found to be the parts receiving the higher doses (Figure 1). The same TLD positions employed during the latter part of the study for interventional radiologists were used for measurements on cardiologists. The doses in the centres of the backs of the hands (TLD X on Figure 1a) were measured for all procedures, and doses to other parts evaluated relative to these. For every procedure studied, the mean doses to either hand were calculated from all the TLDs placed on each of the operator's hands. For the analysis of dose distribution, procedures which did not give a dose to any part of the hand greater than 0.04 mSv were excluded. This left a total of 125 individual procedures in the final analysis of dose distribution for which numbers in the different groups are shown in Table 1, together with the mean screening time and mean patient DAP for each type of procedure. Ratios between the TLD dose to each part of the hand and that for the TLD on the back of the hand were calculated for the hand nearest the X-ray tube.

Results

Magnitude of hand dose

The mean, median and range of all the mean hand doses for every procedure studied within each of the groups are given in Table 2, together with the mean ratio of mean hand dose to DAP. The left hand usually received the highest dose due to the position in which the operator stood, which was linked to the layout of the room. In most cases the dose to the hand furthest from the image intensifier was 40–50% less than to the other hand. The distribution of mean doses for the most exposed hand for all the procedures studied is shown in Figure 3. For a third of the procedures the mean dose was less than 0.02 mSv. The highest doses were recorded during percutaneous procedures and the ratio between the mean dose to the most exposed hand and the DAP for these procedures was significantly higher than for the others. Doses for procedures involving access through the internal jugular vein (IJV) (mainly involving the hepatobiliary region), which were primarily transjugular intrahepatic portosystemic shunt (TIPS), were only slightly lower than for the percutaneous group and indeed the doses to the other hand were only 10–20% less than those to the most exposed hand and the highest for any procedure. Here the DAPs were large, but the ratio between the hand dose and the DAP was almost an order of magnitude less than for the percutaneous procedures. The doses for stents and angioplasties were highest among the group using femoral access. Ratios of hand doses to DAPs for stents and angioplasties were similar to those for IJV, but the ratios for angiograms and embolisations were much lower because a significant proportion of the DAP was due to imaging runs, during which the operator could either keep their hands away from the area under investigation or move away from the couch completely.

Two methods were used by cardiologists for PTCA procedures during the study, one in which vascular access was gained via the radial artery in the hand, and the other via the femoral artery at the groin. Those procedures involving radial access gave significantly higher average doses to the operators' hands, than those using the femoral

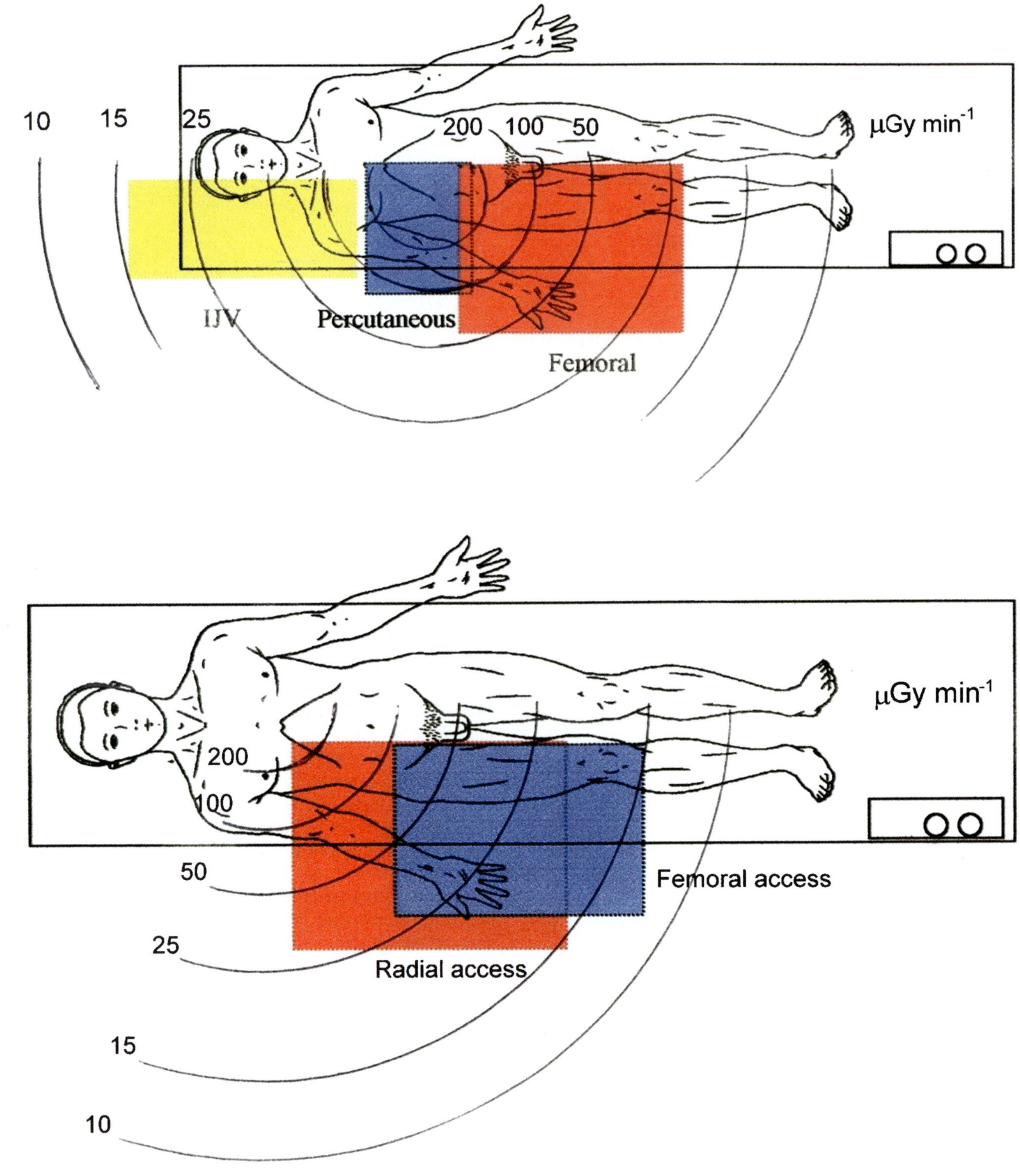

Figure 2. Diagram showing the positions where the hands are located relative to the patient for various points of entry for the different groups of procedures studied, (a) interventional radiology with femoral, internal jugular vein (IJV) and percutaneous access and (b) percutaneous transluminal coronary angiography (PTCA) with radial and femoral access. Contours relate to dose rate distributions measured on one unit and are given in μGy min^{-1}.

artery method (Table 2). This was because of the need for the operators to manipulate the catheter from positions closer to the X-ray field where their hands were exposed on average to a higher level of scattered radiation (Figure 2b). The hands of cardiologists carrying out PTCAs through the radial access route are at a similar distance from the X-ray tube to those of interventional radiologists performing therapeutic procedures via IJV and femoral access routes, and the ratio of the hand dose to the DAP was similar, while the ratio for the femoral access route, where the hand was further from the X-ray tube, was much lower. A lead acrylic screen designed to

Table 2. Mean and median doses to both hands for all the procedures studied

Procedure	Dose (mSv)				Ratio hand dose/DAP ($mSv\ Gy^{-1}\ cm^{-2}$)
	Hand nearest X-ray tube		Hand furthest from X-ray tube		
	Mean	Median (Range)	Mean	Median (Range)	
Percutaneous	0.92	0.46 (0.12–5.37)	0.39	0.22 (0.09–1.98)	0.04
IJV	0.63	0.40 (0.04–2.05)	0.53	0.36 (0.02–1.85)	0.007
Femoral					
Angioplasty	0.21	0.08 (0.02–1.60)	0.10	0.04 (0.02–0.37)	0.007
Stents	0.51	0.27 (0.02–2.72)	0.28	0.14 (0.02–1.61)	0.009
Embolisation	0.14	0.13 (0.04–0.40)	0.07	0.06 (0.02–0.23)	0.002
Angiograms	0.05	0.03 (0.02–0.20)	0.03	0.02 (0.02–0.09)	0.001
Cardiac					
PTCA					
(Femoral)	0.06	0.04 (0.03–0.17)	0.05	0.04 (0.02–0.11)	0.001
(Radial)	0.35	0.29 (0.16–0.76)	0.13	0.12 (0.06–0.26)	0.009

IJV, internal jugular vein; DAP, dose–area product; PTCA, percutaneous transluminal coronary angioplasty.

protect the upper body was used during some procedures. Its use and position varied between individuals and the potential reduction in dose resulting from use of the screen was unclear.

The distribution of dose across the hand

The distributions of dose across the hands of interventional radiologists carrying out procedures via femoral and IJV access routes normalized with respect to the dose to the back of the hand are shown in Figure 4. In all procedures the dorsum and palmer aspects of the body of the hand below the knuckles received similar doses, but the dorsum aspect of the fingers was exposed to a greater dose and the discussion briefly concentrates on this. The doses to the backs of the hands increase from the wrist to the bases of the fingers, and also across the hands rising from the base of the index finger to the base of the little finger. The doses to the tips of the fingers for femoral procedures were either similar to or slightly lower than those to the bases of the fingers. The most exposed parts of the hand for femoral procedures were the ring and little fingers with the base of the little finger receiving the highest dose. During IJV procedures, the dorsum aspect of the hand

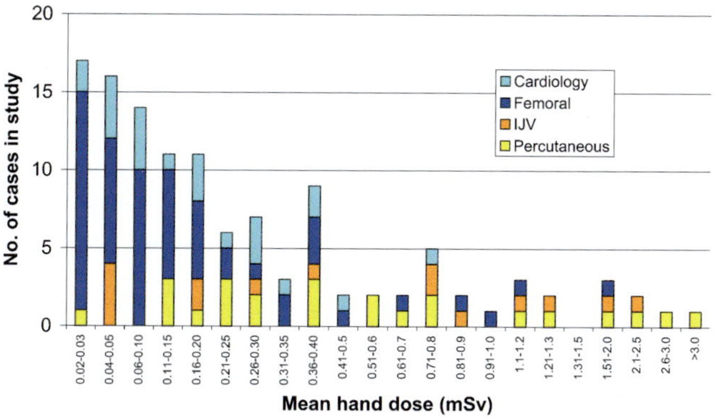

Figure 3. Numbers of procedures where the mean doses to the most exposed hand lay in different dose ranges for each category of procedure. In 62 procedures the mean doses to the hand were below 0.02 mSv and these have been excluded (percutaneous transluminal coronary angiography (PTCA) 2, femoral 36, internal jugular vein (IJV) 12, percutaneous 12).

again received a higher exposure than the palmer side (Figure 4). For IJV procedures, the dose increased all the way from the wrist to the tip of the middle finger for both the palmer and dorsum aspects of the hand. Transversely, the dose across the bases of the fingers again rose from the index finger to the little, while across the tips, doses decreased from the middle finger towards the little finger. The bases of the ring and little fingers and the tip of the middle finger received the highest doses for IJV procedures. The distribution of dose for percutaneous procedures was slightly different (Figure 5). Here the palmer side for the body of the hand received a higher dose than the back, but the dorsum aspect of the fingers received the highest dose. The dose increased continuously from the wrist to the tips of the fingers. There was a small gradient of dose across the base of the fingers rising from the index finger to the little. The tip of the middle (and possibly the index) fingers received the highest dose, which was 20–30% higher than the dose to the base of the ring and little fingers.

Figure 6 shows the distribution of dose across the hands of cardiologists carrying out PTCA procedures. The distributions were similar for all PTCA procedures, independent of radial or femoral access, but were slightly different from those found in radiology in that the doses to the tips of the fingers tended to be lower than those to the rest of the hand. The dose to the bases of the fingers increased from the index finger to the little finger, with again the base of the little finger receiving the highest dose, although not significantly greater than that to the back of the hand. The dose to the wrist could also sometimes be high.

Hand position during interventional procedures

There are a number of factors that influence doses to the hand during any interventional procedure, and these involve the position of the hands, the amount of fluoroscopy/fluorography, the beam geometry and the injection technique. The position and orientation of the hands relative to the scattered radiation field are particularly important in determining the magnitude of the dose and the distribution across the hand, respectively. In order to understand more fully how the dose distributions arise, the movements of the hands during a

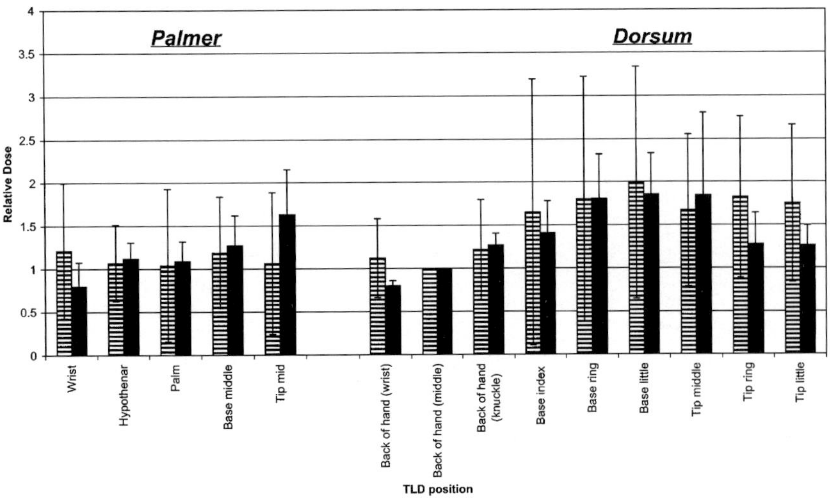

Figure 4. Distribution of dose across the hands for interventional radiology procedures with femoral (cross-hatched) and internal jugular vein (IJV) (black) access. All doses are normalized with respect to that to the centre of the back of the hand (Figure 2). Error bars indicate ±1 standard deviation. TLD, thermoluminescent dosemeter.

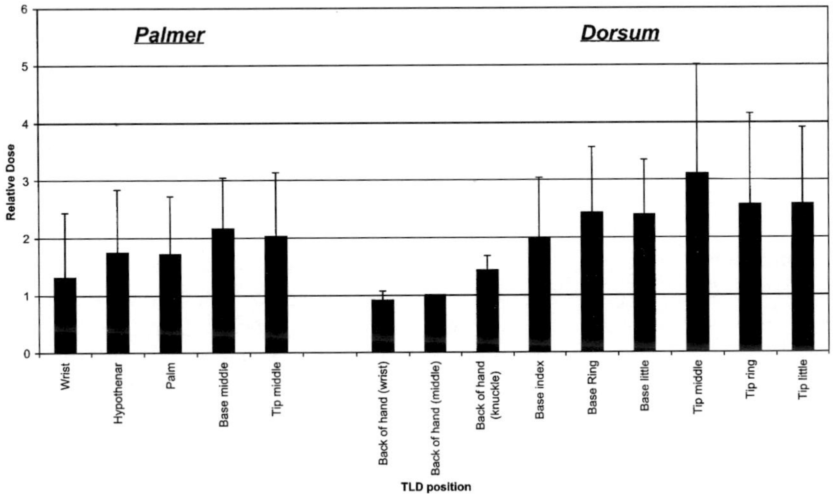

Figure 5. Distribution of dose across the hands for interventional radiology procedures with percutaneous access. All doses are normalized with respect to that to the centre of the back of the hand (Figure 2). Error bars indicate ±1 standard deviation. TLD, thermoluminescent dosemeter.

particular procedure are considered for an operator standing with his/her left hand nearest to the image intensifier. Figure 2a shows the positions of the hands during the three types of interventional procedures and the cardiology procedures studied. Figures 7, 8 and 9 show typical hand configurations used. Most procedures involve a combination of a twisting action in which the hand is more side on to the beam, and a prodding, advancing/retracting motion for which the tips are pointed towards the X-ray source. The proportion of time spent with the hands in each of these configurations is the dominant factor determining whether the side of the hand around the base of the little and ring fingers or the finger tips receive the higher dose.

During femoral access cases where the catheter is introduced into the femoral artery at the groin, the hands can be located anywhere within the shaded box marked femoral (Figure 2a). Once the catheter has been

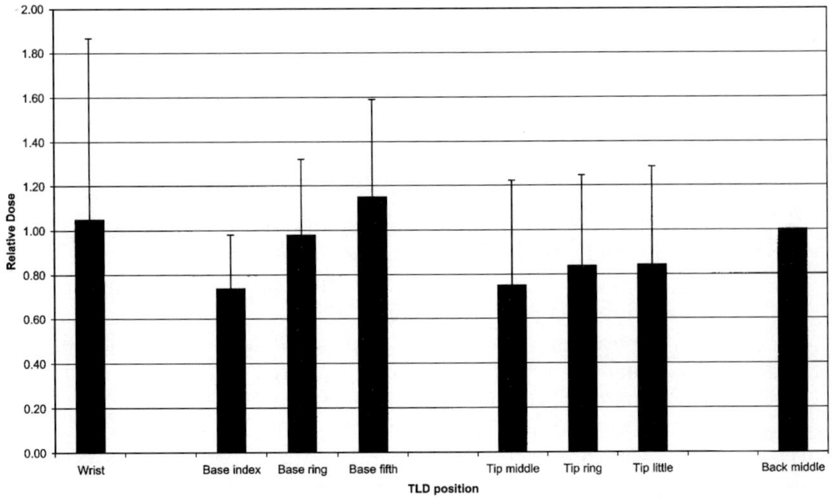

Figure 6. Distribution of dose across the dorsum aspect of the hands for cardiology percutaneous transluminal coronary angiography (PTCA) procedures. All doses are normalized with respect to that to the centre of the back of the hand. Error bars indicate ±1 standard deviation. TLD, thermoluminescent dosemeter.

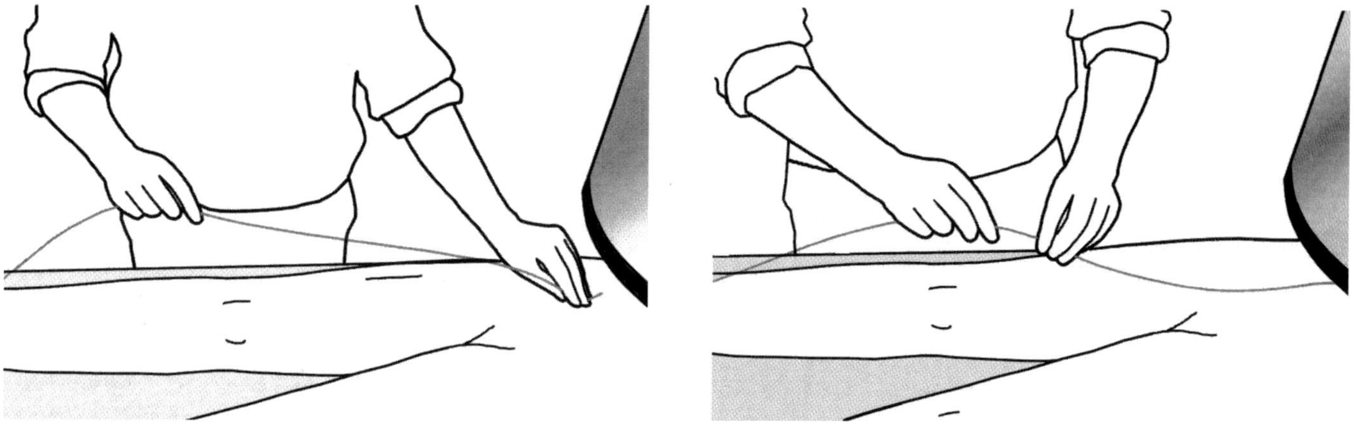

(a) (b)

Figure 7. Hand positions and configurations used for performing (a) the advancing/retracting and prodding actions and (b) the twisting action required for interventional radiology and cardiology procedures with femoral access.

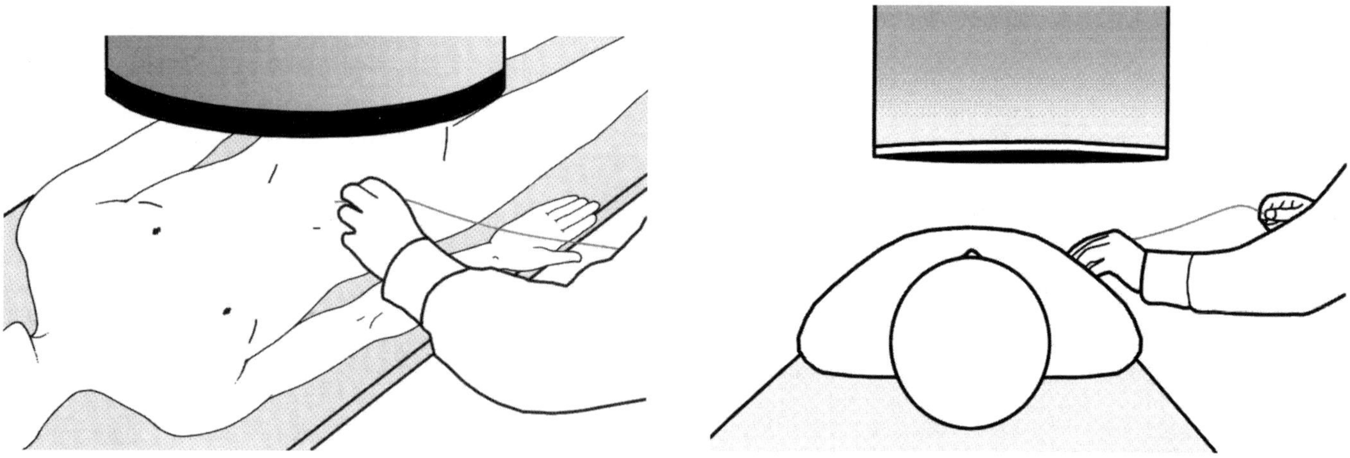

(a) (b)

Figure 8. Hand positions and configurations used for performing percutaneous procedures in which the hand is required to be close to the X-ray beam.

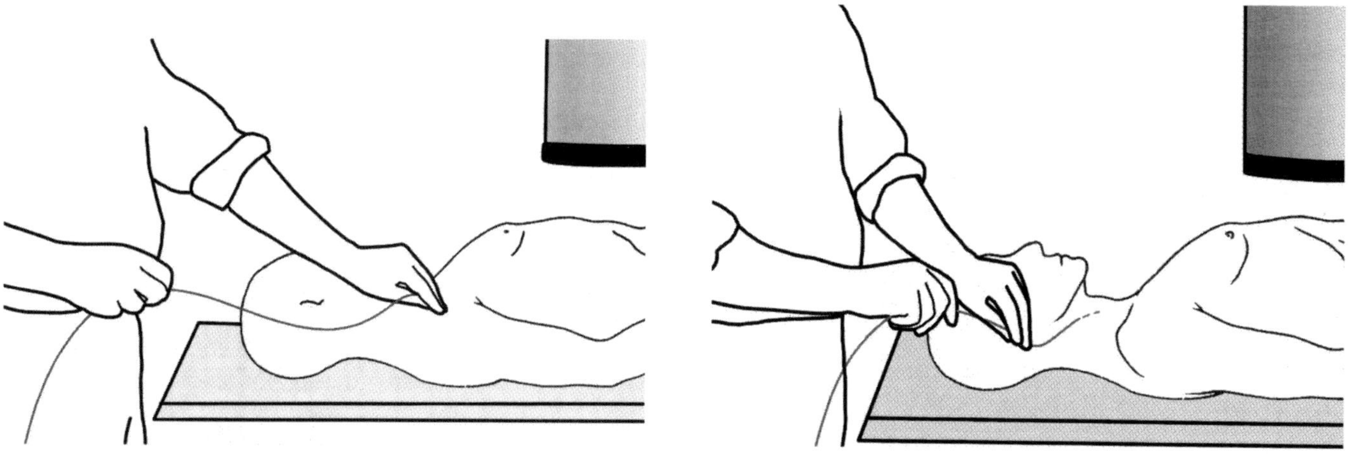

(a) (b)

Figure 9. Hand positions and configurations used for performing (a) the advancing/retracting and (b) the twisting actions required for interventional radiology internal jugular vein (IJV) procedures.

introduced, the left hand is used to advance it under fluoroscopic guidance using a prodding action, while the right hand acts as a guide for the catheter to slip through (Figure 7a). When the catheter has been advanced into the correct area, the left hand may return towards the right to aid in turning and twisting the catheter to manipulate it into the exact location required. The left hand may at times return to the groin to advance or retract the catheter once more. The length of time that the left hand is held at the entry site (groin) and in the prodding position can depend upon the complexity of the individual procedure/ experience of the operator. For the majority of the procedure the hands perform a lateral twisting motion with the hand wrapped around the catheter (Figure 7b). The position of the hands relative to the area under investigation will be dependent upon the type of procedure. During femoral cases, although the area under investigation may vary from the vessels of the upper torso down to the small vessels of the foot, the position adopted by the hands does not stray from the area indicated in Figure 2a. The area of highest dose is in the dorsum aspect of the little finger to the middle finger (Figure 4), because of the orientation of the hands during the predominantly twisting action (Figure 7b).

During percutaneous procedures, the hands take up a position much closer to the area under investigation, and so to the X-ray beam, than during femoral cases in order to manipulate the catheter/needle effectively, hence the higher ratio of hand dose to DAP (Table 2). In the procedures monitored, the area under investigation is centred around the renal and hepatic regions of the body. The movement of the hand is predominantly a prodding action combined with pushing/retracting, resulting in the tips of the fingers being held towards the X-ray field (Figure 8). Hence in these procedures, it is the tip of the middle and probably also the index finger which receive slightly higher doses than the bases of the fingers (Figure 5).

During procedures involving access through the IJV such as TIPS, the hands are located in the shaded box marked IJV (Figure 2a). These procedures involve an equal amount of both the pushing/retracting action (Figure 9a) and remote twisting of the catheter (Figure 9b). In this case the bases of the ring and little fingers and the tip of the middle finger received similar doses (Figure 4).

In cardiology there is considerable overlap between the positions adopted by the hands during procedures via both the femoral and radial access routes (Figure 2b). However, operators using the radial method need to stand closer to the area visualized in the X-ray field for longer periods and so receive higher doses. During cardiology procedures, the predominant movement is a twisting action used in manipulating the catheter (Figure 7b) and injecting contrast, and as a result the base of the little finger receives the highest dose (Figure 6).

Discussion

Interventional radiology

Many factors affect the magnitude and distribution of dose across the hands of interventional radiologists, and this is reflected in the variability of doses measured across all procedures (Figure 3). The following are some of the more important factors.

- The type of procedure will determine the access to the patient, whether by a percutaneous, IJV or femoral approach and this will directly influence the position of the operator in relation to the X-ray field. The hand position and the length of exposure will determine the magnitude of the dose. The type of manipulation required affects the distribution of dose across the hand.
- The equipment used and in particular the dose saving facilities, which will lower the dose to the patient, will reduce the exposure of the operator. Fluoroscopy times can be kept to a minimum, by pulsing the X-ray beam and using equipment software providing facilities such as road mapping [22].
- Operators with lower levels of experience, particularly those undergoing training tend to receive a higher dose to their hands than experienced consultant operators for similar procedures. This can be reflected in increased screening times.
- The room layout will influence the position of the operator and in particular the hand that receives the higher dose.

In addition to the hands, consideration should be given to potential exposure of the eyes, legs [23], and other areas not protected by the lead rubber apron and thyroid collar. In almost all cases the primary operator will receive the highest annual doses. Care should be taken to ensure that nursing and other medical professionals do not receive significant doses to their body or the lens of the eye, particularly when comforting patients, acting as secondary operators or in the role of scrubbed nurse.

Doses to the hands of operators during percutaneous procedures were the highest (Figure 3, Table 2), due to the proximity of the hands to the X-ray field during screening (Figures 2 and 8). Results from this study were in good agreement with results reported elsewhere [2–5, 7–11, 13]. The hands are positioned directly on the patient skin surface in an area of high scattered radiation for lengthy periods. The predominant action that the operator performs is to advance and retract the needle or catheter, and this results in the fingertips of the hand nearest the X-ray tube receiving the highest dose (Figure 5).

The doses for procedures that involved femoral access tended to be less than 0.4 mSv in good agreement with published data [1, 4, 6, 12], although there were a few procedures with doses up to 1.6 mSv (Figure 3, Table 2). The hands are positioned 200–500 mm away from the groin when manipulating the catheter for the majority of the time and therefore in an area of lower scatter. The predominant twisting action used (Figure 7b) is reflected in the distribution of dose across the hand with the most exposed areas being the bases of the little and ring fingers (Figure 4), followed closely by the finger tips, which reflects the need at times to advance/retract the catheter (Figure 7a), particularly during more complex cases or where multiple sites are being investigated.

Those procedures in which the radiologist gains access to the patient via an IJV approach expose the hands to a wide range of doses (Figure 3). Although the hands are located at a distance from the area under investigation, some procedures, in particular TIPS can be technically challenging and are associated with longer screening times giving relatively high doses. The dose distribution is more similar to that during procedures requiring femoral access with the region of highest exposure being around the base of the little and ring fingers. However, the tip of the middle finger also receives a high dose (Figure 4) because prodding and twisting actions are involved to an equal extent (Figure 9). The dose to the other hand is only 10–20% less than that to the primary hand, because the operator is near to the end of the couch and the distance of the two hands from the X-ray beam are more similar.

Cardiology

The factors which affect the magnitude and distribution of doses to the hands during cardiology procedures are similar to those in interventional radiology; namely, the position of the operator, the X-ray equipment used, the experience of the operator and the room layout. Mean doses to the hand for almost all cardiology procedures studied were less than 0.5 mSv (Figure 3). Procedures carried out via a radial access route gave a significantly higher dose to the hands of the operator than those using a femoral puncture technique (Table 2), because of the position of the operator. The advantage of the radial approach is that patient mobility may be achieved more quickly and is therefore the method of choice as it both reduces stress for the patient and increases patient throughput. However, not all patients can be treated in this way and decisions are made on a case by case basis. The increase in exposure to staff from the choice of access route was not considered and did not warrant any re-evaluation of the method.

PTCA investigations require the operator to locate and traverse the coronary artery vessels via the ascending aorta. Once this has been achieved, the operator may carry out an angiogram before progressing towards performing an angioplasty of one or more stenotic sites. The screening required to successfully advance the catheter to the origins of the coronary vessels/stenotic sites, with the operator's hands in the configuration shown in Figure 7a, is minimal relative to the whole procedure. The most time-consuming section of the examination, where most screening and radiographic runs are performed, occurs as the operator attempts to traverse the coronary artery and to visualize and perform the therapeutic part of the procedure, which involves angioplasty of any lesion(s) possibly with the placement of a stent. In this part, the hands will perform the twisting action not dissimilar to that seen in radiology (Figure 7b). The hands are also in this general position during the numerous occasions when any drug therapy or contrast injection is required. As a result, it is the base of the ring and little fingers which receive the higher radiation doses (Figure 6).

Lead screens for shielding the upper body and lens of the eye were used more in cardiology than in radiology in the hospitals studied. A common design is the ceiling suspended leaded window screen, which can also incorporate a lead acrylic skirt at the bottom. This can be placed against the patient in a range of different orientations to provide protection for the operator(s). Although such screens provide good protection to the upper body, particularly during screening or radiographic runs in oblique projections, there was little evidence from the present study to suggest that they provided any significant protection for the hands, nor do manufacturers claim this. The design of the screen must not be too restrictive. It should allow the operator to move their hands in a range of different orientations, while providing them with a clear view of the patient. The operators tend to extend their hands underneath the screen for the majority of procedures, so that although the screens shield the body, little protection is afforded to the hands. Moreover, many operators position the screens poorly, so that the protection they provide is limited.

Extremity monitoring

Implementation of an extremity dose limit relies upon staff using dosemeters on a regular basis. This can be difficult to enforce. Staff are reluctant to use dosemeters in the positions where they might affect their touch sensation and restrict the manipulations they carry out. Therefore, a method of dose monitoring, which is simple, practical and easy to implement is required in order to promote compliance.

Procedures involving femoral access make up around 80% of all interventional radiology procedures undertaken. For femoral access work, the most exposed part of the hand will be the base of the ring and little fingers, and it is recommended that this area on both hands should be monitored using TLD rings. For those procedures in which the radiologist gains access via an IJV approach, such as TIPS, the distribution is similar to that during femoral access, and TLD rings located at the bases of the little or ring fingers on both hands would again be suitable for routine monitoring.

For percutaneous procedures the fingertips of the hand nearest to the X-ray tube, in particular the tips of the middle and probably the index fingers are exposed to the greatest level of scattered radiation. For those operators with a workload that consists mainly of this type of procedure, it could be argued that the most appropriate place to monitor is the tip of the index, middle or ring finger using a TLD finger stall. However, this may be impracticable as these fingers are heavily involved in the manipulation of catheters, and the finger stall would affect the dexterity and tactile ability of the operator. A TLD ring located at the base of the ring or little finger in this situation would still give an accurate estimation of hand dose and since the ratio of the dose to the base and to the tip is approximately 1.2–1.3, an adjustment could be made for radiologists who performed primarily percutaneous procedures. However, for the radiologists performing a typical mix of interventional procedures, ring dosemeters worn on the little/ring fingers of both hands will give the best indication of the dose received by the most exposed areas.

In cardiology, the procedure that had the most potential to expose the hands of the operator to a significant dose was studied. The most exposed area is again at the base of the little finger, because the cardiologist manipulates the catheter laterally for the majority of the procedure during which fluoroscopy is used. Therefore the use of ring dosemeters worn at the bases of the little fingers on either hand are recommended for routine monitoring in cardiology.

If doses for any group exceed 4 mSv per month and 50 mSv per year, then regular monitoring should be considered [24]. Links have been established between neck dose and DAP [17] and leg dose and DAP [23], but the association is more uncertain for hand doses and will depend on both the procedure and the operator. However, the ratios in Table 2 would suggest that staff regularly performing therapeutic interventional radiology procedures, or cardiology procedures via the radial access route, with DAPs totalling over 500 Gy cm^2 per month could receive annual doses to the hands of 50 mSv, as could those regularly performing percutaneous procedures with DAPs over 100 Gy cm^2 per month. Monitoring for a period of 2–3 months is recommended for primary operators falling within these groups in order to establish dose levels and determine whether regular monitoring is required.

Dose reduction

The hands may be protected using shielding devices such as protective screens of various designs or leaded surgical gloves. Anything which could interfere with the manipulations carried out, thereby lengthening the procedure and increasing the dose to the patient, must be avoided. Drop down lead acrylic screens have been employed in radiology, but in the hospitals included in the present study they tended to be confined to use in cardiology, as most radiologists found them too intrusive, as well as raising issues of sterility and space. In cardiology the screens provided good protection for the body and head, but the hands would often be extended under the screen and so receive less protection. The possible dose reduction afforded by surgical gloves incorporating 0.02 mm of lead is debatable, since they only reduce the dose by 15–20% through attenuation [12, 25] and may give the operator a false sense of security. Since the gloves can only be used once, cost is also an issue. Thus in most cases time and distance were the primary methods used to keep hand doses to a minimum.

Feedback from TLD dose monitoring is only available some time after a dose has been received. This does not allow the operator to identify when doses are received and so take action to minimize the dose. Electronic finger dosemeters are available which emit an audible alarm tone if a pre-determined threshold is exceeded (EDD; Unfors Instruments, Billdal, Sweden). This alerts operators when their hands are in a higher dose rate field, so that they can withdraw to a greater distance, if that is appropriate. Electronic finger dosemeters can provide a valuable educational tool for increasing the radiologists' and cardiologists' awareness of when doses are received, and could be applied in training.

Conclusions

Both radiologists and cardiologists are exposed to a wide range of doses to the hand during each procedure they perform. The main factors that affect this dose are the type of procedure, their experience, the X-ray equipment and the layout of the room. Procedures in interventional radiology were divided into three categories (percutaneous, IJV and femoral) relating to the access route which determined the position of the operator. Those radiologists performing cases via percutaneous access routes received the highest doses to their hands, as they required to be closer to the X-ray tube in order to carry out the manipulations.

The distribution of dose across an operator's hands is dependent upon the hand configuration and movement as well as the site of entry. The majority of the procedures involve a twisting action or a prodding, advancing/retracting motion of the hand. The ratio of these two main movements of the hands determines the distribution of dose across the hand for any individual procedure. For a general mix of interventional radiology procedures the most exposed region of the hand is the area from the little finger to the middle finger, with the bases of the fingers often receiving the highest dose. During percutaneous procedures the most exposed parts were the tips of the middle and ring fingers, although the doses were only 20–30% higher than those to the base of the little finger.

For those radiologists whose workload consists of all three types of procedure, monitoring using TLD ring dosemeters worn at the bases of the little or ring fingers on both hands is recommended. In those cases where a radiologist's workload consists mainly of percutaneous procedures, for which the tips of the middle and index fingers may receive higher doses, TLD rings would still provide a reasonable estimate of the dose to the most exposed area. Cardiologists were exposed to doses similar to those for radiologists carrying out femoral access cases and again the most exposed areas of the hand were the bases of the little and middle fingers. Thus use of ring dosemeters on the little finger of either hand is recommended as an effective monitoring method for interventional radiologists and cardiologists.

If hand doses for any group exceed 50 mSv per year, then regular monitoring should be considered. The relationship between hand dose and DAP per procedure performed is variable, but the DAP can be used as an indicator of the likely dose level. If an individual performs a variety of therapeutic interventional procedures or performs cardiology procedures via the radial access route which give DAPs totalling over 500 Gy cm^2 per month, or carries out percutaneous procedures with DAPs over 100 Gy cm^2 per month, monitoring is recommended to establish dose levels.

Acknowledgments

The authors wish to acknowledge the support of the Health and Safety Executive for this project. They also wish to thank the radiologists and cardiologists involved in the study for their forbearance during the extensive dose monitoring performed and the staff of all the radiology and cardiology departments for their support. The hospitals taking part were Gartnavel General Hospital; Southern General Hospital, Glasgow; Glasgow Royal Infirmary; the Western Infirmary, Glasgow; Edinburgh Royal Infirmary; Dumfries and Galloway Royal Infirmary; Stirling Royal Infirmary; Law Hospital; and Ayr Hospital.

References

1. Santen BC, Kan K, Velthuyse JM, Julius HW. Exposure of the radiologist to scattered radiation during angiography. Radiat Phys 1975;115:447–50.
2. Cruikshank JG, Fraser GM, Law J. Finger doses received by radiologists during Chiba needle percutaneous cholangiography. Br J Radiol 1980;53:584–5.
3. Gustafsson M, Lunderquist A. Personnel exposure to radiation at some angiographic procedures. Radiology 1981;140:807–11.
4. Burgess AE, Burhenne HJ. Finger doses in special procedures. Br J Radiol 1984;57:650–1.
5. Lowe FC, Auter M, Beck TJ, Chang R, Marshall FF. Monitoring radiation exposure to medical personnel during percutaneous nephrolithotomy. Urology 1986;XXVIII:221–6.
6. Tryhus M, Mettler FA, Kelsey C. The radiologist and angiographic procedures: absorbed radiation dose. Invest Radiol 1987;22:747–50.
7. Geterud K, Larsson A, Mattsson S. Radiation dose to patients and personnel during fluoroscopy at percutaneous renal stone extraction. Acta Radiologica 1989;30:201–5.
8. Ramsdale ML, Walker WJ, Horton PW. Extremity doses during interventional radiology. Clin Radiol 1990;41:34–6.
9. Felmlee JP, McGouch PF, Morin RL, Classic KL. Hand dose measurements in interventional radiology. Health Physics 1991;60:265–7.
10. Vehmas T, Tikkanen H. Measuring radiation exposure during percutaneous drainages: can should dosemeters be used to estimate finger doses? Br J Radiol 1992;66:1007–10.
11. Vehmas T. What factors influence radiologists' finger doses during percutaneous drainages under fluoroscopic guidance? Health Physics 1993;65:161–3.
12. Damilakis J, Koulourakis M, Hatjidakis S, Karabekios S, Gourtsoyiannis N. Radiation exposure to the hands of operators during angiographic procedures. Br J Radiol 1995;21:72–5.
13. Vehmas T. Radiation exposure during standard and complex interventional procedures. Br J Radiol 1997;70:296–8.
14. Faulkner K. Personal monitoring during fluoroscopy. J Radiol Prot 1992;12:225–31.
15. Law J. Doses to head and arms of radiologists during fluoroscopy. Br J Radiol 1985;58:187–8.
16. Faulkner K, Moores BM. An assessment of the radiation dose received by staff using fluoroscopic equipment. Br J Radiol 1982;55:272–6.
17. Williams JR. The interdependence of staff and patient doses in interventional radiology. Br J Radiol 1997;70:498–503.
18. The Ionising Radiations Regulations. 1999 SI 1999/3232 Stationery Office 1999 ISBN 0 11 0856147.
19. Anderson NE, King SH, Miller KL. Variations in dose to the extremities of vascular/interventional radiologists. Health Physics 1999;76 (Suppl. 2):39–40.
20. Green S, Zamenhof RG. Radiation measurements. Chapter 4. In: Martin CJ, Sutton DG (editors). Practical Radiation Protection in Healthcare. Oxford: Oxford University Press, 2002:58–9.
21. International Commission on Radiological Protection (ICRP). Conversion coefficients for use in radiological protection against external radiation. Publication No. 74. Annals of the ICRP, Vol. 26, 3–4. Oxford: Pergamon Press, 1997.
22. Martin CJ, Sutton DG, Sharp P. Balancing patient dose and image quality. Appl Radiation Isotopes 1999;50:1–19.
23. Whitby M, Martin CJ. Radiation doses to the legs of radiologists performing interventional procedures: are they a cause for concern? Br J Radiol 2003;76:321–7.
24. Martin CJ, Whitby M. Application of ALARP to extremity doses for hospital workers. J Radiol Prot 2003;23:405–21.
25. Marx MV, Ellis JH. Radiation protection of the hand in interventional radiology: Should it fit like a glove? Radiology 1996;200:24–5.

The British Journal of Radiology, *78* (2005), 230–235 © 2005 The British Institute of Radiology
DOI: 10.1259/bjr/28534346

Treatment outcomes and prognostic factors in patients with supratentorial low-grade gliomas

[1]S-A YEH, MD, [2]J-T HO, MD, [3]C-C LUI, MD, [1]Y-J HUANG, MD, [1]C-Y HSIUNG, MD and [1]E-Y HUANG, MD

Department of [1]Radiation Oncology, [2]Neurosurgery and [3]Radiology, Chang Gung Memorial Hospital, Kaohsiung, Taiwan

Abstract. Low-grade gliomas account for 10–15% of all adult primary intracranial tumours. Currently, there is no consensus on the treatment strategy for low-grade gliomas. This study was designed to evaluate the treatment outcomes, prognostic factors and radiation-related late complications, as well as to assess whether or not post-operative radiotherapy has benefit on local control and overall survival in this population. We retrospectively reviewed 93 consecutive adult patients with supratentorial low-grade gliomas diagnosed at our institution from July 1985 to December 1997. All patients underwent surgical intervention and 60 of them received post-operative radiotherapy. With a median follow-up of 110 months for surviving patients, the 5-year overall and progression-free survival rates were 57% and 47%, respectively. 46 patients experienced local progression of disease during the follow-up period. In multivariate analysis, age at diagnosis, extent of surgery and post-operative Karnofsky performance status showed independent prognostic significance for progression-free and overall survival rates. Post-operative radiotherapy had independent prognostic value for progression-free survival. This analysis has changed our practice and we suggest that aggressive surgical resection and post-operative radiotherapy might be considered for patients with low-grade gliomas. Further efforts should be made to optimize radiotherapy techniques and to integrate new therapeutic modalities.

Supratentorial low-grade glioma is a heterogeneous group of brain tumours, accounting for roughly 10–15% of all adult primary intracranial tumours [1]. Because of the relatively slow growth rate of low-grade gliomas, a long expected survival is not unreasonable. Surgical resection or observation alone is the mainstay of treatment. Where the tumours involve critical functional regions of the brain, complete removal would be dangerous and is not feasible. Even with grossly total removal, the infiltrative feature of gliomas often leaves behind some microscopic tumours. The microscopic residual tumours might increase the incidence of local relapse and allow adjuvant therapy to play a role in the management of low-grade gliomas.

This analysis was undertaken to investigate the treatment outcomes of patients with supratentorial low-grade gliomas. Treatment options and potential prognostic factors were evaluated to substantiate their relationship to progression-free survival (PFS) and overall survival. Radiation-related complications were surveyed. These results might contribute to treatment recommendations and exploration of avenues of further research.

Material and methods

From July 1985 to December 1997, 93 consecutive adult patients with supratentorial low-grade gliomas were treated at our hospital. All patients underwent surgical intervention (grossly total resection in 13 patients, subtotal resection (removal of 20~80% of tumour) in 71, biopsy in 9. Tumours were classified according to the World Health Organization grading system [2]. There were grade II astrocytoma in 46 patients, grade II oligodendroglioma in 32 patients and mixed oligoastrocytoma in 15 patients. Only patients who were operated on for the first time were included. The post-operative performance status was assessed using the Karnofsky performance scale (KPS) [3]. Because residual tumours were often found in patients whose operative records mentioned total removal of tumours, the extent of surgery was determined by review of both the operative records and the serial CT scans (pre-operative and post-operative). Data were analysed retrospectively by reviewing the medical records and radiographic images, by telephone or written correspondence and by review of the death certificate. Surveillance for disease status consisted of physical examination and serial radiographic studies. Only patients with definite tumour regrowth on consecutive CT scans were defined as having progression of disease. There were 57 men and 36 women; age range from 18 years to 80 years (median 41 years). The most common locations of tumours was the frontal lobe (69%), followed by the temporal lobe (37%). The most common presenting symptoms were seizure (46%), followed by increased intracranial pressure (headache, nausea, vomiting; 34%). The characteristics of these patients were given in the Table 1.

Received 2 July 2004 and in revised form 11 October 2004, accepted 23 November 2004.

Address correspondence to Dr Shyh-An Yeh, 5F., No.181, Wen-Chuan Road, Zuoying District, Kaohsiung City 81361, Taiwan (R.O.C.).

Radiotherapy

60 patients received post-operative radiotherapy. The median interval between surgical resection and initiation of radiotherapy was 0.9 months (range 0.1–2 months). The prescribed tumour dose ranged from 56 Gy to 70 Gy (median 60 Gy) with daily fractions of 2 Gy, 5 fractions per week. 21 patients received whole brain irradiation (40–46 Gy) followed by focal boost irradiation (total 58–70 Gy). 39 patients received only focal brain irradiation to a total of 56–70 Gy. Radiotherapy was delivered with

Table 1. Clinical characteristics of 93 patients with low-grade gliomas

Characteristics	No. of patients		
	Post-op RT (−)	Post-op RT (+)	Total
Gender			
Male	21	36	57
Female	12	24	36
Age (years)			
⩽40	14	31	45
>40	19	29	48
Extent of surgery			
Total	6	7	13
Subtotal and biopsy	27	53	80
Location			
Frontal lobe	24	40	64
Temporal lobe	12	22	34
Parietal lobe	11	15	26
Corpus callosum	1	18	19
Intraventricle	2	12	14
Others	5	9	14
Histology			
Astrocytoma	17	29	46
Oligodendroglioma	10	22	32
Mixed	6	9	15
KPS			
<70	18	13	31
⩾70	15	47	62

KPS, Karnofsky performance status; Post-op, post-operative; RT, radiotherapy.

10-MV photons through individually shaped, bilateral opposed portals. Focal irradiation fields included the pre-operative tumour volume (contrast-enhanced area or low-attenuation area for non-enhanced tumours) with a 2 cm margin. Evaluation of treatment response was based on the serial changes in neuroradiographic studies. Radiation-related late complications were gauged with SOMA scale [4].

Statistics

The endpoints of this study were overall survival, PFS and radiation-related late complications. Survival was measured from the date of histopathological diagnosis, as was time to tumour progression. Surviving patients were censored at the date of last physician contact. The date of the imaging procedure documenting tumour progression was used to calculate PFS rates. The survival data were analysed using the Kaplan-Meier method [5]. Differences between potentially prognostic subgroups were tested for statistical significance by the log-rank test, with $p<0.05$ indicating significance [6]. All statistically significant prognostic variables in univariate analysis were considered in the multivariate analysis. Multivariate analysis was performed with the Cox regression model to identify independent prognostic factors [7].

Results

The 5-year overall survival and PFS rates were 57% and 47%, respectively. At the time of this retrospective review, 43 patients were alive with a median follow-up of 110 months (range 50–197 months). In terms of overall survival rates, the age at diagnosis, histology, local progression, post-operative radiotherapy, post-operative KPS, extent of surgery and duration of symptoms were identified as significant prognostic factors. Patients undergoing grossly total surgical resection survived longer than those where resection was incomplete (5-year overall survival rate: 92% *vs* 52%, $p=0.0349$). In multivariate analysis, the age at diagnosis, post-operative KPS and extent of surgery continued to show independent prognostic significance for overall survival rates.

When PFS rate was considered, univariate analysis showed that age at diagnosis, histology, post-operative radiotherapy, post-operative KPS, extent of surgery and duration of symptoms had prognostic significance. Patients receiving post-operative radiotherapy had a 5-year PFS rate of 56% as compared with 30% for those with surgery alone ($p=0.0028$, Figure 1). Multivariate analysis confirmed that age at diagnosis, post-operative radiotherapy, post-operative KPS and extent of surgery were independent prognostic factors for PFS rates. The details of univariate and multivariate analysis are listed in Tables 2 and 3.

For patients treated with post-operative radiotherapy, the survival rates of patients receiving 62–70 Gy were not significantly different from the corresponding rates of those receiving 56–60 Gy (5-year overall survival rates: 60% *vs* 70%, $p>0.05$; 5-year PFS rates: 51% *vs* 59%, $p>0.05$). No correlation was found between whole brain irradiation and survival rates. The 5-year overall survival and PFS rates were 70%, 56% for patients without whole brain irradiation and 61%, 57% for those with whole brain irradiation ($p>0.05$).

Local progression

There was local progression in 46 patients. The interval between surgical intervention and the development of local progression ranged from 4 months to 135 months (median 22 months). For patients who had previously undergone gross total surgical resection, all of the tumour recurrences developed in the immediate vicinity of the primary tumours. Salvage treatment included surgery alone in 11 patients, radiotherapy alone in 8 patients and a combination of surgery and radiotherapy in 12 patients. 15 patients did not receive any salvage treatment. Among the 23 patients receiving salvage surgery, malignant dedifferentiation was noted in 9 patients (39%). The 5-year overall survival rate after disease progression was 39% for patients receiving salvage treatment (surgery and/or radiotherapy), and 0% for patients refusing or unable to receive salvage treatment ($p=0.0003$). According to subgroups of different salvage treatment modalities, the 5-year overall survival rates after disease progression were 40%, 37.5% and 42% for patients receiving a combination of surgery and radiotherapy, radiotherapy alone and surgery alone, respectively ($p>0.05$).

Complications

In this article, 23 patients suffered from somnolence during the follow-up period (grade I: 3, grade II: 20) and the 5-year complication-free rate was 74% for all patients. Patients receiving post-operative radiotherapy had a 5-year

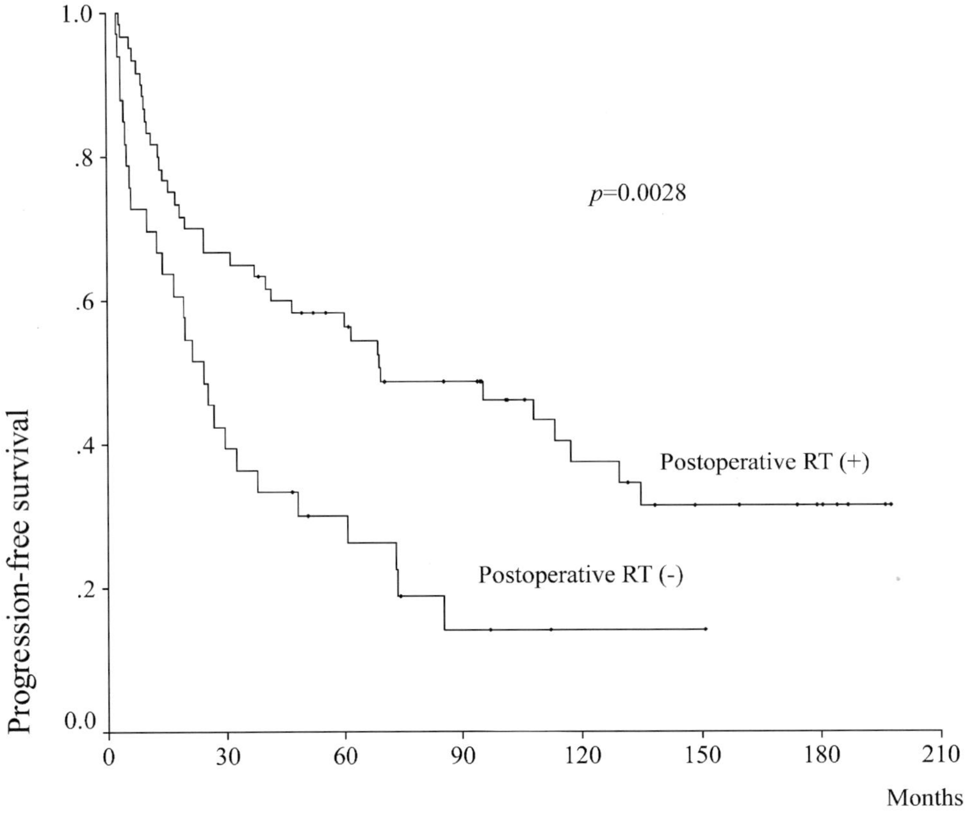

Figure 1. Progression-free survival according to post-operative radiotherapy (RT) status.

complication-free rate (for somnolence) of 72% compared with 77.5% for those who did not have radiotherapy ($p>0.05$). 16 patients had memory impairment (grade I: 5, grade II: 11) and the 5-year complication-free rate was 83% for all patients. Patients treated with post-operative radiotherapy had a higher incidence of memory impairment than those with surgery alone (5-year complication-free rate: 75% *vs* 96%, $p=0.0268$). Among patients receiving post-operative radiotherapy, a radiation dose of 62–70 Gy was not associated with higher incidence of somnolence and memory impairment compared with a radiation dose of 56–60 Gy (5-year complication-free rate, for somnolence: 71% *vs* 73%, $p>0.05$; for memory impairment: 78% *vs* 73%, $p>0.05$). Among those not initially presenting with seizure, seven patients developed seizures (grade II: 7) and the 5-year complication-free rate was 92% for all patients. CT scans of these patients were carefully reviewed to exclude the possible association with tumour progression or recurrence. Patients with post-operative radiotherapy had a 5-year complication-free rate (for seizure) of 95% compared with 86% for patients after surgery alone ($p>0.05$). Among patients receiving post-operative radiotherapy, whole brain irradiation was associated with a higher incidence of somnolence and memory impairment, but the differences did not reach statistical significance (5-year complication-free rate, for somnolence: 64% *vs* 76%, $p>0.05$; for memory impairment: 70% *vs* 78%, $p>0.05$). Two patients had radiation-related low-density white matter changes with irregular enhancement revealed by CT scans. No significant neurological deficits could be attributed to the white matter changes.

Table 2. Prognostic factors for 5-year overall and progression-free survival

Variable	No.	OS	*p*-value	PFS	*p*-value
Age (years)					
≤40	45	80%		71%	
>40	48	37%	<0.0001	25%	<0.0001
Histology					
Astrocytoma	46	37%		28%	
Oligodendroglioma	32	77%		68%	
Mixed	15	79%	0.0001	60%	0.0024
Local progression					
With	46	45%			
Without	47	70%	0.0093		
Post-operative RT					
With	60	66%		56%	
Without	33	42%	0.0189	30%	0.0028
Post-operative KPS					
<70	31	24%		19%	
≥70	62	74%	<0.0001	61%	<0.0001
Total resection					
With	13	92%		84%	
Without	80	52%	0.0349	41%	0.0073
Duration of symptoms					
≤1 months	46	51%		38%	
>1 months	47	64%	0.0288	55%	0.0178

RT, radiotherapy; KPS, Karnofsky performance status; OS, overall survival; PFS, progression-free survival.

Discussion

In this article, the 5-year overall survival and PFS rates were 57% and 47%, respectively. Our treatment results were in agreement with the reported experience [8–12]. The

Table 3. Multivariate analysis data

	Overall survival			Progression-free survival		
	p-value	HR	95%CI	*p*-value	HR	95%CI
Age	0.002	2.736	1.429–5.235	<0.001	3.008	1.707–5.298
Post-operative RT	>0.05			0.016	0.507	0.292–0.881
Post-operative KPS	<0.001	0.227	0.120–0.430	0.001	0.376	0.209–0.676
Total resection	0.016	0.234	0.072–0.764	0.002	0.197	0.070–0.555

HR, hazard ratio; CI, confidence interval; KPS, Karnofsky performance status; RT, radiotherapy.

goal of surgery is to provide a histological diagnosis, relieve symptoms, reduce the tumour burden as much as possible, and guide further treatment. Owing to the infiltrative growth pattern of gliomas, it is difficult to achieve complete removal without producing or exacerbating neurological deficits. Conflicting results regarding the prognostic significance of the extent of surgery have been reported in the literature. There were articles demonstrating that the extent of surgery was an important prognostic factor for survival and local control [8, 13–19]. On the other hand, some investigators reported that the extent of surgery was not correlated with the survival rates of patients with low-grade gliomas [11, 12, 20]. According to our results, the extent of surgery was correlated to PFS and overall survival rates. Therefore, we suggest that a radical surgery should be attempted unless the surgical resection will create significant neurological sequelae.

The influence of histological subtypes on survival was controversial. There were reports that oligodendroglioma was associated with better treatment outcomes [16, 19, 21, 22]. On the other hand, some physicians indicated that if tumours fit the histological criteria of low-grade gliomas, further subdivision might not greatly increase the prognostic value of the histological diagnosis [20, 23]. Our univariate analysis showed that oligodendroglioma was associated with significantly higher overall survival and PFS rates compared with astrocytoma. However, multivariate analysis failed to show an independent prognostic significance of histological subtypes.

The optimal treatment strategy of low-grade gliomas is uncertain. Controversy regarding the indication of post-operative radiotherapy continues to exist. Some investigators suggested that when a complete removal was achieved, no further adjuvant therapy was warranted [24]. On the other hand, Shaw [25] suggested that post-operative radiotherapy should be routinely delivered to all adult patients with histologically verified supratentorial low-grade non-pilocytic gliomas. Several retrospective series demonstrated that post-operative radiotherapy had survival benefit for those who underwent subtotal removal of tumours [15, 21, 24, 26, 27]. Another major uncertainty is the optimal timing of post-operative radiotherapy. Radiotherapy deferred until tumour progression was found to be associated with a longer survival or a trend toward improved survival on univariate analysis, but was not significant in multivariate analysis [16, 23]. Some investigators suggested that radiotherapy could be deferred until tumour progression in young patients despite the extent of surgery [8]. Furthermore, several reports demonstrated that early post-operative radiotherapy had no survival benefit [8, 28–30]. However, there were reports claiming that immediate post-operative radiotherapy could improve overall survival or local control for most patients with low-grade gliomas [11, 15, 25, 27, 31–33]. In our study, patients receiving post-operative radiotherapy had higher overall survival and PFS rates than those with surgery alone regardless of the extent of surgery. Multivariate analysis also showed the independent prognostic significance of post-operative radiotherapy for PFS, but not for overall survival. Our results were in accord with the reported experience [33].

For patients receiving post-operative radiotherapy, the optimal radiation dose has yet to be determined. Some publications indicated the existence of a dose–response relationship for low-grade gliomas [26, 32]. On the other hand, several articles including a large prospective randomized study demonstrated that no clear dose–response relationship could be observed [9, 11, 20, 21]. We also could not demonstrate a dose–response effect of radiotherapy in this study.

The optimal irradiated volume is another important issue that might influence the treatment outcomes. Prior analysis of failure patterns of patients with low-grade gliomas showed that most failures occurred within the irradiated fields [21, 34]. Whole brain irradiation has been reported to have no survival benefit over partial brain irradiation [32]. Furthermore, whole brain irradiation has been considered to be associated with greater morbidity [25]. Our study failed to demonstrate any survival benefit for whole brain irradiation over partial brain irradiation. We also found that there was a trend for patients with whole brain irradiation to have higher incidence of late complications; although this trend did not reach statistical significance. Because prolonged survival could be expected in patients with low-grade gliomas, the irradiated volume should be limited to the pre-operative tumour site (contrast-enhanced area or low-attenuation area for non-enhanced tumours) and multiple conformally shaped treatment fields should be used with the aim of reducing the late complications. Whole brain irradiation is no longer recommended. In general, MRI is more precise and sensitive in brain tumour detection and could offer a greater accuracy in tumour delineation and treatment field determination. MRI or multimodality image fusion (CT and MRI) might be used in the treatment planning process. The advent of intensity-modulated radiotherapy might allow a further reduction in the irradiated volume and radiation dose to normal brain.

Our study revealed that the administration of post-operative radiotherapy was an independent prognostic factor for predicting tumour progression. Patients who had post-operative radiotherapy had a higher incidence of mild memory impairment than those after surgery alone. The radiation-related late complications were limited to grade II of the SOMA scale. These results might further constitute the rationale for the use of adjuvant post-operative radiotherapy. We do not recommend deferring radiotherapy until tumour progression or recurrence. Where tumour progression or recurrence occurs, brain tissue damage due to the tumour itself is unavoidable. Salvage surgery might also remove or damage some normal brain tissue and further compromise the neurological function and quality of life. On the other hand, if the patient undergoes radiotherapy after the first surgical intervention, the incidence of tumour progression or recurrence is significantly decreased at the cost of only a slightly higher incidence of radiation-related neurotoxicities. Based on the above results, we recommend that application of post-operative radiotherapy might be considered for all patients with low-grade gliomas regardless of the extent of surgery and the histological subtypes. The role of radiotherapy should not be only limited to serve as a salvage therapy for local progression or recurrence. For patients who will receive post-operative radiotherapy, we suggest partial brain irradiation to a dose not more than 60 Gy.

The importance of age as a determinant of survival has been demonstrated in the literature; the younger the patients, the better the prognosis [8, 12, 14–20, 23, 29, 30]. In this article, patients younger than 40 years had significantly higher overall survival and PFS rates than those older than 40 years. Multivariate analysis further confirmed the independent prognostic significance of age on overall survival and PFS rates. A long duration of symptoms prior to surgery had been shown to be associated with longer survival in patients with low-grade gliomas [15]. In this study, the median duration of symptoms before histological diagnosis was 1 month and it had significant impact on overall survival and PFS; the longer the duration, the better the prognosis. The possible explanation was that a protracted duration of symptoms was associated with less aggressive tumour behaviour. However, there was no independent prognostic significance in multivariate analysis.

For patients suffering from tumour progression, the optimal management is unclear. In our study, patients undergoing salvage treatment had a significantly better prognosis than those without salvage treatment. In this study, there was a trend for salvage surgery to provide better long-term survival after disease progression. However, the independent prognostic significance of salvage surgery needs to be proved by further studies.

Malignant dedifferentiation has been noted in patients undergoing salvage surgery for progressive or recurrent diseases. In the literature, the reported dedifferentiation rate of low-grade gliomas ranged from 45% to 86% [10, 18, 20, 29]. The gemistocytic variant is known to be particularly prone to malignant progression [35]. It is conceivable that radiotherapy might initiate or accelerate malignant transformation [36]. Among the 23 patients who had salvage surgery in our study, malignant transformation was noted in nine patients. Four of these patients received post-operative radiotherapy. Eight patients had astrocytoma and one had oligodendroglioma. The dedifferentiation rate was 39%. Due to small case numbers, no factors were found to be associated with the occurrence of malignant dedifferentiation.

Conclusions

Based on our results, we recommend that aggressive surgical resection followed by post-operative radiotherapy should be considered for patients with supratentorial low-grade gliomas. The potential survival benefit and dose–response relationship of post-operative radiotherapy for low-grade gliomas need further prospective randomized studies. The treatment strategy for low-grade gliomas is evolving and a multidisciplinary approach is advocated.

References

1. Guthrie BL, Laws ER. Supratentorial low-grade gliomas. Neurosurg Clin N Am 1990;1:37–48.
2. Reifenberger G, Kros JM, Burger PC, Louis DN, Collins VP. Oligodendroglioma. In: Kleihues P, Cavenee WK, editors. Tumours of the nervous system. World Health Organization Classification of Tumours. Lyon: IARC Press, 2000:56–61.
3. Karnofsky DA, Burchenal JH. The clinical evaluation of chemotherapeutic agents in cancer. In: MacLeod CM, editor. Evaluation of chemotherapeutic agents. New York: Columbia University Press, 1949:191–205.
4. Pavy JJ, Denekamp J, Letschert J, et al. Late effects toxicity scoring: the SOMA scale. Int J Radiat Oncol Biol Phys 1995;31:1043–51.
5. Kaplan EL, Meier P. Nonparametric estimation from incomplete observations. J Am Stat Assoc 1958;53:457–81.
6. Peto R, Pike MC, Armitage P, et al. Design and analysis of randomized clinical trials requiring prolonged observation of each patient. Br J Cancer 1977;35:1–39.
7. Cox DR. Regression models and life tables. J Royal Stat Soc 1972;34:187–220.
8. Bahary JP, Villemure JG, Choi S, et al. Low-grade pure and mixed cerebral astrocytomas treated in the CT scan era. J Neurooncol 1996;27:173–7.
9. Karim AB, Maat B, Hatlevoll R, et al. A randomized trial on dose-response in radiation therapy of low-grade cerebral glioma: European Organization for Research and Treatment of Cancer (EORTC) Study 22844. Int J Radiat Oncol Biol Phys 1996;36:549–56.
10. McCormack BM, Miller DC, Budzilovich GN, Voorhees GJ, Ransohoff J. Treatment and survival of low-grade astrocytoma in adults - 1977~1988. Neurosurgery 1992;31: 636–42.
11. Shibamoto Y, Kitakabu Y, Takahashi M, et al. Supratentorial low-grade astrocytoma. Correlation of computed tomography findings with effect of radiation therapy and prognostic variables. Cancer 1993;72:190–5.
12. Vecht CJ. Effect of age on treatment decisions in low-grade glioma. J Neurol Neurosurg Psychiatry 1993;56:1259–64.
13. Berger MS, Deliganis AV, Dobbins J, Keles GE. The effect of extent of resection on recurrence in patients with low-grade cerebral hemisphere gliomas. Cancer 1994;74:1784–91.
14. Jeremic B, Shibamoto Y, Grujicic D, et al. Hyperfractionated radiation therapy for incompletely resected supratentorial low-grade glioma. A phase II study. Radiother Oncol 1998;49:49–54.
15. Laws ER Jr, Taylor WF, Clifton MB, Okazaki H. Neurosurgical management of low-grade astrocytoma of the cerebral hemispheres. J Neurosurg 1984;61:665–73.
16. Leighton C, Fisher B, Bauman G, et al. Supratentorial low-grade glioma in adults: an analysis of prognostic factors and timing of radiation. J Clin Oncol 1997;15:1294–301.
17. Reichenthal E, Feldman Z, Cohen ML, Loven D, Zucker G. Hemispheric supratentorial low-grade astrocytoma. Neurochirurgia 1992;35:18–22.

18. van Veelen ML, Avezaat CJ, Kros JM, van Putten W, Vecht C. Supratentorial low grade astrocytoma: prognostic factors, dedifferentiation, and the issue of early versus late surgery. J Neurol Neurosurg Psychiatry 1998;64:581–7.
19. Whitton AC, Bloom HJ. Low grade glioma of the cerebral hemispheres in adults: a retrospective analysis of 88 cases. Int J Radiat Oncol Biol Phys 1990;18:783–6.
20. Lote K, Egeland T, Hager B, et al. Survival, prognostic factors and the therapeutic efficacy in low-grade glioma: a retrospective study in 379 patients. J Clin Oncol 1997;15: 3129–40.
21. Shaw EG, Scheithauer BW, Gilbertson DT, et al. Post-operative radiotherapy of supratentorial low-grade gliomas. Int J Radiat Oncol Biol Phys 1989;16:663–8.
22. Shaw EG, Scheithauer BW, O'Fallon JR. Supratentorial gliomas: a comparative study by grade and histology. J Neurooncol 1997;31:273–8.
23. Bauman G, Lote K, Larson D, et al. Pretreatment factors predict overall survival for patients with low-grade glioma: a recursive partitioning. Int J Radiat Oncol Biol Phys 1999;45:923–9.
24. Morantz RA. Radiation therapy in the treatment of cerebral astrocytoma. Neurosurgery 1987;20:975–82.
25. Shaw EG. The low-grade glioma debate: evidence defending the position of early radiation therapy. Clin Neurosurg 1995;42:488–94.
26. Fazekas JT. Treatment of grades I and II brain astrocytomas. The role of radiotherapy. Int J Radiat Oncol Biol Phys 1977;2:661–6.
27. Garcia DM, Fulling KH, Marks JE. The value of radiation therapy in addition to surgery for astrocytomas of the adult cerebrum. Cancer 1985;55:919–27.
28. Janny P, Cure H, Mohr M, et al. Low-grade supratentorial astrocytomas. Cancer 1994;73:1937–45.
29. Jubelirer SJ, Rubin M, Shim C. An analysis of 38 cases of low-grade cerebral astrocytoma in adults. W V Med J 1993;89:102–5.
30. Kandil A, Khafaga Y, ElHusseiny G, Allan A, Jamshed A, Schultz H. Low-grade astrocytoma - a retrospective analysis of 102 patients. Acta Oncol 1999;38:1051–6.
31. Shaw EG. Low-grade gliomas: to treat or not to treat? A radiation oncologist's viewpoint. Arch Neurol 1990;47: 1138–40.
32. Shaw EG, Daumas-Duport C, Scheithauer BW, et al. Radiation therapy in the management of low-grade supra-tentorial astrocytomas. J Neurosurg 1989;70:853–61.
33. Karim ABMF, Afra D, Cornu P, et al. Randomized trial on the efficacy of radiotherapy for cerebral low-grade glioma in the adult: European Organization for Research and Treatment of Cancer study 22845 with the medical research council study BRO4: an interim analysis. Int J Radiat Oncol Biol Phys 2002;52:316–24.
34. Pu AT, Sandler HM, Radany EH, et al. Low-grade gliomas: preliminary analysis of failure patterns among patients treated using 3D conformal external beam irradiation. Int J Radiat Oncol Biol Phys 1995;31:461–6.
35. Fuller CE, Perry A. Pathology of low- and intermediate-grade gliomas. Semin Radiat Oncol 2001;11:95–102.
36. Piatt JH, Blue JM, Schold SC, Burger PC. Glioblastoma multiforme after radiotherapy for acromegaly. Neurosurgery 1983;13:85–9.

The British Journal of Radiology, *78* (2005), 236–241 © 2005 The British Institute of Radiology
DOI: 10.1259/bjr/51982166

Daytime pulsed dose rate brachytherapy as a new treatment option for previously irradiated patients with recurrent oesophageal cancer

W HARMS, MD, R KREMPIEN, MD, C GREHN, MD, C BERNS, Phys, F W HENSLEY, PhD and J DEBUS, MD, PhD

Department of Radiooncology, University of Heidelberg, INF 400, 69120 Heidelberg, Germany

Abstract. The aim of this study was to evaluate the feasibility, effects, and toxicity of pulsed dose rate (PDR) brachytherapy for re-irradiation of oesophageal carcinoma. A total of 16 patients (median age 67 years) with inoperable recurrences from oesophageal cancer after primary radio-(chemo)-therapy (median 50 Gy) were re-irradiated using PDR brachytherapy (^{192}Ir, 37 GBq). Treatment was carried out on an outpatient basis applying a weekly 5 Gy daytime schedule (0.5 Gy pulse^{-1} h^{-1}, total dose 15–20 Gy). The dose was prescribed 10 mm from the mid-dwell position and encompassed the clipped tumour extension with 2 cm margins. The use of clips for delineation of tumour extent and catheter movement during irradiations was evaluated. All 61 PDR treatments were applied safely. The median catheter movement was 5 mm, range 2–12 mm. After a median follow-up of 8 months, three patients had a complete and five a partial remission. Body weight increased in 5 of 16 (31%) and was stable in 4 of 16 (25%) patients, respectively. The median grade 2 (RTOG/EORTC) dysphagia-free survival was 17 months. Seven patients experienced grade 1, five grade 2, and one grade 3 late toxicity. Three patients with uncontrolled locoregional disease showed grade 4 complications (oesophago-tracheal fistulae (n=2), fatal arterial bleeding (n=1). Daytime PDR brachytherapy proved to be feasible and provided effective palliation. Toxicity remains a major problem. Thus, total dose should be restricted to <15 Gy in this palliative situation.

Despite the introduction of effective multimodal treatment regimens for oesophageal cancer, locoregional tumour control remains a major problem [1, 2]. The incidence of local recurrence or persistence of cancer as the first site of failure was 45% in the RTOG 85-01 and 39% in the Intergroup 0122 study [3, 4]. The comparable local failure rate with surgery alone was 61% in the Intergroup 0113 study [5]. Additionally, autopsy studies have revealed persistent locoregional disease in more than 75% of patients and visceral metastases in approximately 50% of patients treated either with surgery or radiation [6].

In patients with locoregional recurrences after primary radio-(chemo)-therapy re-irradiation is used only with caution because of the increased probability of normal-tissue complications. In this situation the application of endoluminal brachytherapy may have advantages over external beam radiotherapy (EBRT) since high doses may be applied to the local disease while dose to the spinal cord, lungs and other organs at risk can be spared. In comparison with the commonly used HDR (high dose rate) technique, which represents the gold standard for endoluminal brachytherapy in oesophageal cancer, PDR (pulsed dose rate) brachytherapy with its protracted irradiation schedule offers a potentially wider therapeutic ratio and may therefore reduce toxicity in previously irradiated patients [7–10].

The aim of this study was to introduce daytime PDR brachytherapy in the management of previously irradiated recurrent oesophageal carcinoma and to evaluate its feasibility, effects, and toxicity. Secondly, the routine use of surgical clips for delineating the tumour extent was assessed. Thirdly, catheter movement in the proximal and distal direction during prolonged irradiations was monitored.

Received 1 April 2004 and in revised form 6 September 2004, accepted 15 November 2004.

Materials and methods

Patients

From April 2001 to January 2003, a total of 16 patients (median age 67 years, range 52–79 years) with inoperable recurrences from oesophageal cancer were treated at the Department of Radiooncology of the University of Heidelberg, Germany. Seven patients had previously been treated by definitive external beam radiotherapy and nine by combined radiochemotherapy. The median applied dose was 50 Gy, range 46–60 Gy. Time to recurrence was 15 months, range 4–37 months). All recurrences were proven by histology (n=12 squamous cell carcinoma, n=4 adenocarcinoma). Four patients presented with isolated local recurrences and 12 of 16 with locoregional recurrences. Six of 16 patients had concurrent distant metastasis.

Treatment policy

The staging procedure before the initiation of PDR brachytherapy included abdominal ultrasound, a chest CT, and oesophago-gastroscopy. The chest CT was extended to the upper abdomen to rule out lymph node and liver metastases. All patients were evaluated by an experienced surgeon and deemed inoperable due to the extent of the recurrence or presence of co-morbidities. The indication for re-irradiation was clinically significant dysphagia and a Karnofsky Index >60%. Only patients with good performance status were eligible since each weekly outpatient treatment lasted 10 h per 5 Gy fraction. Patients with lower clinical performance status, involvement of the tracheo-bronchial tree, or reduced life-expectancy were referred for palliative stent placement or chemotherapy. All patients were treated solely with endoluminal PDR brachytherapy. The standard treatment schedule consisted of four fractions of PDR brachytherapy 1 week apart with 5 Gy per fraction. Since reasonable clinical data on re-irradiation for oesophageal cancer is scarce and little is known about toxicity we used lower doses for smaller tumours. Thus, in three patients with small recurrences the total dose was limited to 15 Gy (Table 1).

Brachytherapy

In all patients an oesophageal endoscopy was performed before starting brachytherapy in order to mark the upper and lower extension of the visible tumour with surgical clips. This approach was chosen to delineate precisely the tumour extent at the time of brachytherapy. The intention was to keep the brachytherapy volumes as small as possible so as to reduce toxicity. A chest X-ray was performed immediately after clip placement to document the position of the radiopaque markers (Figure 1). For subsequent insertions bony landmarks defined after the first treatment were used for definition of the planning target volume.

The catheter was placed via the oral (catheter diameter >8 mm) or nasal route (diameter ≤8 mm) by the radiation oncologist. The procedure was performed after simple local anaesthesia with xylocaine spray and mild sedation with 1–2 mg midazolam intravenously. A self-made catheter consisting of two single hollow tubes (outer tube: oesophageal tube, Rüsch GmbH, Kernen-Rommelshausen, Germany; inner tube: duodenal tube, B. Braun Melsungen AG, Melsungen, Germany), which were placed within each other, was used for endoluminal irradiation. This approach ensured the central positioning of the 6 Fr brachytherapy catheter (Nucletron, Veenendaal, The Netherlands) within the oesophageal applicator (Figure 2). The applicators had an outer diameter ranging from 6 mm to 10 mm. The final position of the catheter loaded with a ribbon of dummy seeds was controlled by fluoroscopy.

A PDR afterloading machine (microSelectron; Nucletron, Veenendaal, The Netherlands) with a single stepping source (^{192}Iridium, 37 GBq) was used for brachytherapy. Centre-to-centre separations of the dwell positions were 5 mm. A standard dose of 5 Gy was applied weekly with 0.5 Gy per pulse per hour. The brachytherapy dose was prescribed to 10 mm off axis at mid-dwell position without computerized optimization [9]. The active length encompassed the clipped tumour extension with a 2 cm proximal and distal margin. This schedule resulted in total treatment times of approximately 10 h and was administered on an outpatient basis. A single PDR pulse given every hour lasted only a couple of minutes. In between the hourly pulses the patients were disconnected from the afterloading device. All patients had intravenous access for hydration and needed continuous suction of saliva since, owing to the inserted catheter, swallowing was impossible. After initial sedation with midazolam no further sedation was required during treatment.

Evaluation of catheter movement

Since the PDR schedule resulted in prolonged irradiation times catheter movement was assessed during irradiations in all patients. For this purpose the location of the catheter was documented twice during pulsed brachytherapy by repeated simulations. The variation of catheter localization was expressed as movement of the

Table 1. Treatment parameters and results. Brachytherapy (BT) treatment schedule and clinical outcome (CR complete remission, PR partial remission, SD stable disease, PD progressive disease) on last day of follow-up (FU). Body weight was monitored during follow-up and classified as gain + (>+2 kg), no change ± (±2 kg), and loss − (>−2 kg)

Patient number	BT total dose (Gy)	Extent recurrence (cm)	Response last FU	Body weight	RTOG/EORTC [11] grade 3/4 late toxicity	FU (months)	Status
1	20	6×3	SD	−	No	4	Alive
2	15	3×1	CR	±	No	12	Alive
3	20	5×3	PD	−	Oesophago-tracheal fistula	6	Dead
4	20	4×1	PD	−	Oesophago-tracheal fistula	9	Dead
5	15	2×1	PR	+	No	8	Alive
6	20	4×2	PR	±	No	10	Alive
7	20	3×3	PR	±	No	8	Alive
8	20	7×2	SD	−	No	4	Dead
9	20	3×1	CR	+	No	19	Alive
10	20	3×2	PD	−	Severe fibrosis	17	Dead
11	20	3×2	SD	±	No	8	Alive
12	20	4×2	PR	+	No	12	Alive
13	20	6×2	PD	−	Fatal bleeding	6	Dead
14	20	5×2	PD	−	No	5	Dead
15	20	4×1	PR	+	No	7	Alive
16	15	3×1	CR	+	No	14	Alive

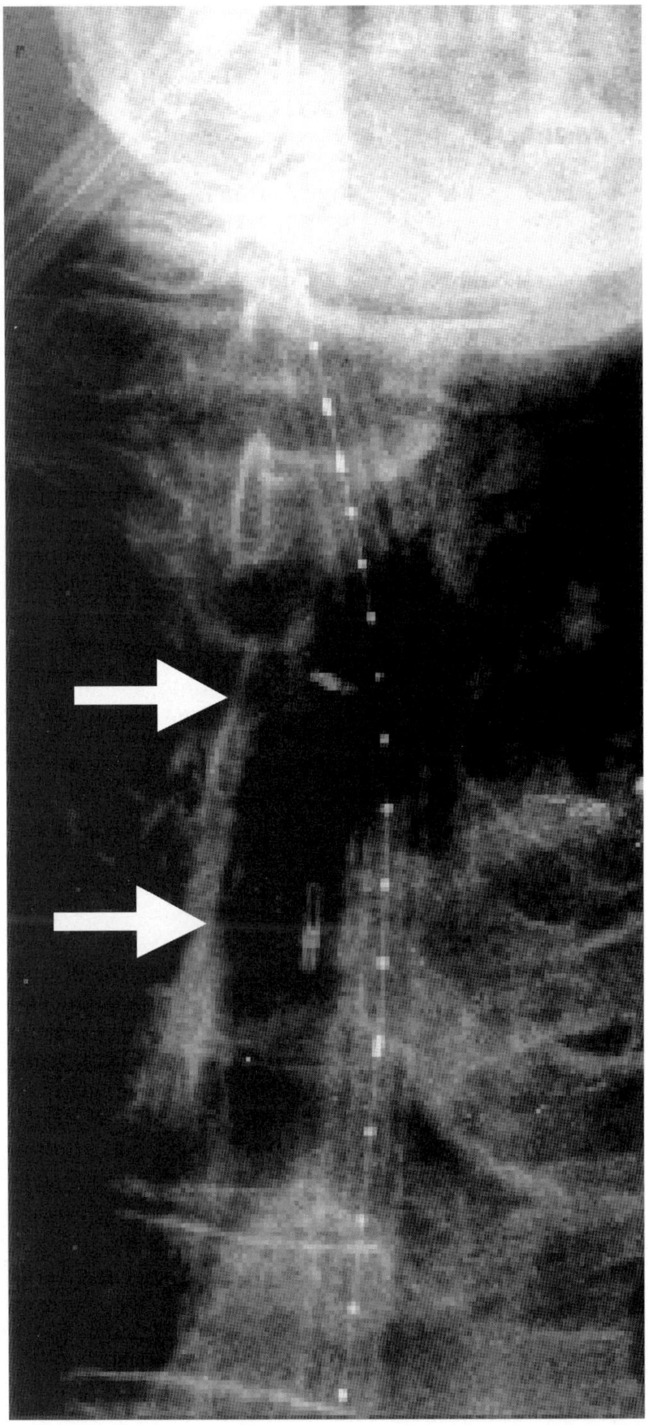

Figure 1. This image shows the oesophageal brachytherapy catheter containing a ribbon of dummy seeds. Two surgical clips (arrows) delineate the cranial and caudal extent of the oesophageal recurrence.

mid-dwell position in cranial or caudal direction in millimetres when compared with the initial simulation film. The bony structures of the thoracic vertebrae served as a reference.

Follow-up program

All patients were followed up at 6 weekly intervals up to 3 months, and 3 monthly thereafter. At the time of presentation physical examination, barium swallow, and chest CT (including the upper abdomen) were performed. Routine endoscopy was performed 6 weeks after completing of brachytherapy. Thereafter, we performed endoscopy every 3 months. Acute and late effects on the oesophagus and the mucosa were assessed according to the RTOG/EORTC toxicity criteria [11]. Changes in body weight were observed during follow-up and classified as gain (>+2 kg), no change ($\pm$2 kg), and loss (<-2 kg). The median follow-up for all patients was 8 months (range 4–19 months).

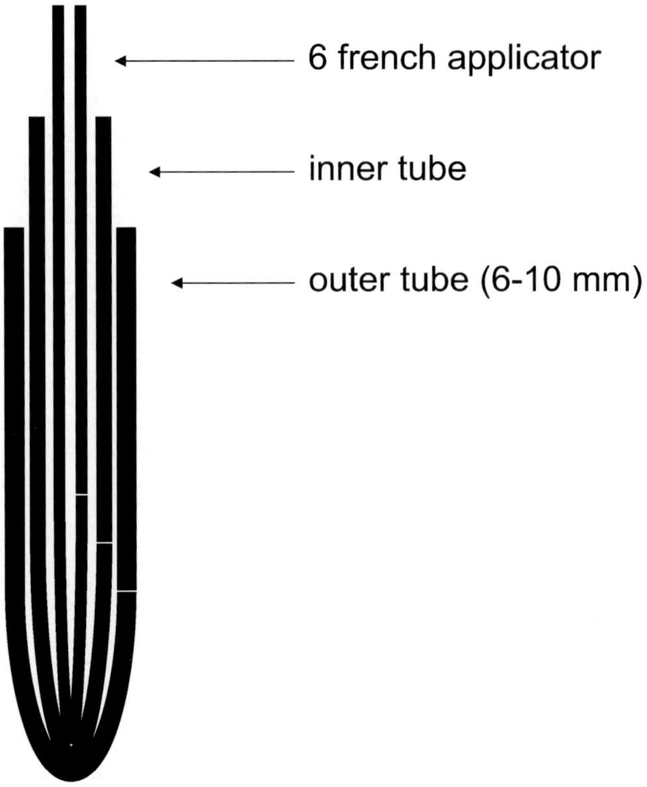

Figure 2. Schematic drawing of the oesophageal applicator: a self-made catheter consisting of two single hollow tubes (outer tube: oesophageal tube, Rüsch GmbH, Kernen-Rommelshausen, Germany; inner tube: duodenal tube, B. Braun Melsungen AG, Melsungen, Germany), which were stuck into each other, was used for endoluminal irradiation. This approach ensured central positioning of the 6 Fr brachytherapy catheter (Nucletron, Veenendaal, The Netherlands) within the oesophageal applicator. The applicators had outer diameters ranging from 6 mm to 10 mm.

Statistical evaluation

Overall survival time was defined as the time from the beginning of PDR brachytherapy to the death of the patient [12]. Partial remission (PR) was defined as a $\geqslant$50% reduction of tumour extent evaluated by endoscopy, barium oesophagography and CT during follow-up. Complete remission (CR) and progressive disease (PD) were respectively defined as: no evidence of local tumour; and further tumour growth of more than 25%. No change (NC) was defined either as a $<$ 50% reduction of tumour extent or progression $\leqslant$25%.

Results

Clip placement, catheter movement

We observed no complications related to the placement of either the clips or the brachytherapy catheters. Marking the extent of the tumour with clips improved definition of the planning target volume. The clips are loosely adherent to the oesophageal mucosa. Therefore an X-ray should be taken immediately after endoscopy or at least before any oral intake to document the localization of the surgical clips. The median catheter movement in the proximal or distal direction, when compared with the initial simulation films was 5 mm and ranged from 2 mm to 12 mm.

Feasibility of PDR brachytherapy

All 61 PDR brachytherapy treatments were feasible. The treatment courses were applied safely and no complications occurred during protracted irradiations. The daytime PDR brachytherapy schedule was tolerated well by 12 of 16 patients, while the remaining 4 patients complained about the prolonged irradiation time.

Clinical outcome

The median overall survival was 8 months, range 4–19 months. At final analysis 10 of 16 patients were alive. One patient died 5 months after the initiation of brachytherapy from a cardiac arrest. The other five patients died from systemic progression (n=2) or locoregional progression with oesophago-tracheal fistulae (n=2). One patient suffered a fatal arterial bleed.

The response rate on the last day of follow-up was 50% (see Table 1). Persisting local control with a follow up ranging from 12 months to 19 months was observed in three patients who presented with relatively small local recurrences. The median actuarial grade 2 dysphagia-free survival was 17 months (Figure 3). Body weight was improved in 5 of 16 (31%) and stable in 4 of 16 (25%) patients, respectively.

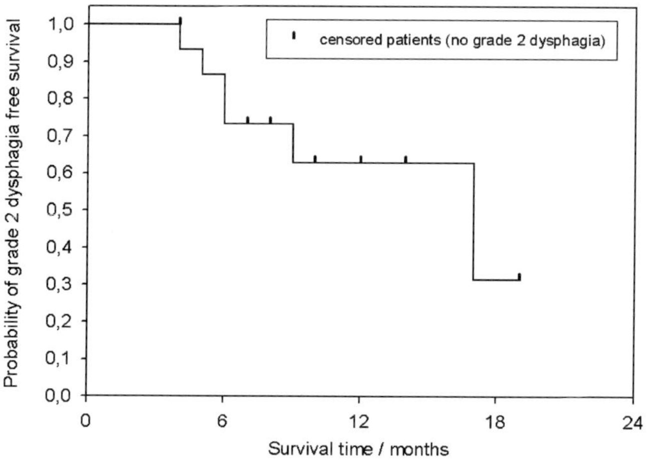

Figure 3. Grade 2 (RTOG/EORTC) dysphagia-free survival after daytime pulsed dose rate (PDR) brachytherapy for re-irradiation of patients with recurrent oesophageal cancer. The endpoint of this analysis was the occurrence of grade 2 dysphagia (unable to take solid food normally, swallowing semi-solid food, dilatation may be indicated) during follow-up.

Toxicity (RTOG/EORTC)

In terms of acute toxicity, the majority of patients (12 of 16) experienced mild dysphagia (grade 1) while 3 patients showed grade 2 (moderate dysphagia) and 1 grade 3 (severe dysphagia) dysphagia. We evaluated oesophageal late effects since 13 of 16 patients were followed $\geqslant$6 months. On the last day of follow-up seven patients had slight difficulties in swallowing solids (grade 1), five patients were unable to take solid food normally (grade 2), and one patient was able to swallow only liquids (grade 3). Three patients suffering from uncontrolled locoregional disease presented with grade 4 complications. One patient died due to a fatal arterial bleed 6 months after the initiation of brachytherapy while two patients presented with oesophago-tracheal fistulae 4 and 7 months after treatment, respectively. All patients suffering from grade 3/4 toxicity (EORTC/RTOG [11]) were treated with a total dose of 20 Gy (Table 1).

Discussion

Treatment of recurrent oesophageal cancer after primary radio-(chemo)-therapy is difficult and no general therapeutic rules are available. Possible treatment options include stent placement, feeding gastrostomy, photodynamic therapy, chemotherapy, radiotherapy and palliative resection [13–17]. Brachytherapy, in comparison with EBRT, offers rapid decrease in the extent of endoluminal tumour thus rapidly improving swallowing whilst delivering relatively low doses to the surrounding normal tissues, particularly spinal cord, lung and adjacent normal oesophageal mucosa [18]. Several studies have shown that HDR brachytherapy is effective in the curative or palliative treatment of oesophageal cancer [19].

For the following reasons, we introduced a daytime PDR brachytherapy treatment schedule for endoluminal re-irradiation of recurrent oesophageal cancer. PDR brachytherapy combines the technical advantages of HDR (single stepping source, dose optimization) with the radiobiological advantages of continuous low dose rate (CLDR) brachytherapy. Thus, PDR offers, owing to its protracted irradiation schedule, a potentially wider therapeutic ratio than HDR and this may reduce toxicity [7, 8]. This applies especially to patients presenting with recurrences after full courses of previous radio-(chemo)-therapy. In comparison with CLDR brachytherapy, PDR offers flexible fractionation, and a more straightforward technical approach: a single stepping source replaces multiple line sources and advanced treatment planning (optimization, 3D treatment planning) is possible [20]. The 10 h daytime treatment schedule we used was feasible and acceptable to most of our patients. We are aware that the prolonged treatment time is a major disadvantage of the proposed method, but protracted irradiation was the only way to improve the therapeutic index of re-irradiation.

If we are using a prolonged treatment time and tailoring the treated length exactly to the endoscopical findings we need to know the extent of catheter movement during the treatment course. The comparison of repeated simulations revealed a relatively small median catheter movement of 5 mm (range 2–12 mm) during irradiations. Thus, applying 2 cm margins in each direction seems to be a reasonable compromise between the intended small treatment volumes and catheter movement. Since it is necessary to pass a scope through the tumour this technique is restricted to patients presenting with recurrences that do not completely obstruct the oesophageal lumen. In our experience this is true for most patients presenting with oesophageal recurrences after primary radiochemotherapy. In this study we encountered no problems in placing clips on the endoscopically visible tumour.

Since a theoretical basis for estimating equivalence of CLDR to PDR brachytherapy [7, 8] was not described until 1991, relevant clinical data on PDR brachytherapy is scarce. So far no studies have been published applying PDR brachytherapy in patients with recurrent oesophageal cancer. In the current study the median overall survival was 8 months. Treatment response was 50% and body weight was improved in 31% and stable in 25% of the patients, respectively. The median actuarial grade 2 (RTOG/EORTC) dysphagia-free survival was 17 months. These data are comparable with the published series applying HDR brachytherapy for palliation [14, 18, 19]. Small recurrences treated with a total dose of 15 Gy had reasonable survival rates indicating that this dosage may be a good compromise between treatment response and toxicity.

Sharma et al [18] retreated 15 patients with recurrent oesophageal cancer after a previous course of radiotherapy with two 6 Gy fractions of HDR brachytherapy. The authors observed strictures in 4 of 15 patients and ulcerations in 3 of 15 patients and concluded that toxicity remains a major concern in previously irradiated patients. Yu et al [14] published the largest re-irradiation series in the literature and reported on 81 patients with recurrent oesophageal carcinoma after primary radiotherapy. 21 patients failed to complete re-irradiation due to deterioration in general health (n=9) or major complications (oesophageal perforation n=8, fatal haemorrhage n=4). These findings are supported by our data. Three patients (19%) presented with grade 4 complications (oesophago-tracheal fistulae (n=2) or fatal arterial bleed (n=1). All these patients suffered from uncontrolled locoregional disease. Thus, it remains unclear whether grade 4 toxicity is truly treatment-related or due to progressive disease. We are aware that with the limited follow-up the true late toxicity rate may not be completely assessed. Conversely, the median overall survival of our patients is consistent with that reported in the literature: 6–8 months [14, 19]. Our data, with a median follow-up of 8 months, may give a reasonable estimate of the potential late effects of oesophageal re-irradiation using PDR brachytherapy in this particular selected group. Nevertheless, toxicity remains a major problem in previously irradiated patients and reduction of toxicity needs to be addressed in further studies. All patients who experienced grade III/IV toxicity had been treated with a total dose of 20 Gy. Thus, total dose should be restricted to 15 Gy in this palliative situation. Although we have reported on only small patient numbers this is supported by the fact that in the 15 Gy group no major toxicity occurred and reasonable survival times have been achieved.

In conclusion, daytime PDR brachytherapy proved feasible and provided effective palliation in previously irradiated patients with recurrent oesophageal cancer. Since toxicity remains a major problem the applied dose should be restricted to 15 Gy in this context. Taking into account the heterogeneity in this patient population it is important to offer each patient individualized treatment options.

References

1. Fietkau R, Grabenbauer GG, Sauer R. Radiotherapy of esophageal cancer. Results following radiotherapy alone and simultaneous radiochemotherapy and intracavitary irradiation. Strahlenther Onkol 1994;170:69–78.
2. Fritz P, Wannenmacher M. Radiotherapy in the multimodal treatment of esophageal carcinoma. A review. Strahlenther Onkol 1997;173:295–308.
3. Cooper JS, Guo MD, Herskovic A, et al. Chemoradiotherapy of locally advanced esophageal cancer: long-term follow-up of a prospective randomized trial (RTOG 85-01). Radiation Therapy Oncology Group. JAMA 1999;281:1623–7.
4. Minsky BD, Neuberg D, Kelsen DP, et al. Final report of Intergroup Trial 0122 (ECOG PE-289, RTOG 90-12): Phase II trial of neoadjuvant chemotherapy plus concurrent chemotherapy and high-dose radiation for squamous cell carcinoma of the esophagus. Int J Radiat Oncol Biol Phys 1999;43:517–23.
5. Kelsen DP, Ginsberg R, Pajak TF, et al. Chemotherapy followed by surgery compared with surgery alone for localized esophageal cancer. N Engl J Med 1998;339: 1979–84.
6. Mandard AM, Chasle J, Marney J. Autopsy findings in 111 cases of esophageal cancer. Cancer 1981;48:329–35.
7. Brenner DJ, Hall EJ. Conditions for the equivalence of continuous to pulsed low dose rate brachytherapy. Int J Radiat Oncol Biol Phys 1991;20:181–90.
8. Fowler J, Mount M. Pulsed brachytherapy: the conditions for no significant loss of therapeutic ratio compared with traditional low dose rate brachytherapy. Int J Radiat Oncol Biol Phys 1992;23:661–9.
9. Gaspar LE, Nag S, Herskovic A, Mantravadi R, Speiser B, the Clinical Research Committee, American Brachytherapy Society, Philadelphia, PA. American Brachytherapy Society (ABS) consensus guidelines for brachytherapy of esophageal cancer. Int J Radiat Oncol Biol Phys 1997;38:127–32.
10. Harms W, Krempien R, Hensley FW, Berns C, Wannenmacher M, Fritz P. Results of chest wall reirradiation using pulsed-dose-rate (PDR) brachytherapy molds for breast cancer local recurrences. Int J Radiat Oncol Biol Phys 2001;49:205–10.
11. Seegenschmiedt MH, Sauer R. Systematik der akuten und chronischen Strahlenfolgen. Strahlenther Onkol 1993;169:83–95.
12. Kaplan EL, Meier P. Nonparametric estimation from incomplete observation. J Am Stat Ass 1958;53:457–82.
13. Carlini S, Grauso F, Perri P, et al. Role of surgery in the treatment of recurrent esophageal cancer. Hepatogastroenterology 1997;44:187–91.
14. Yu ZH, Miao YJ, Yin WB, Gu XZ. Irradiation of recurrent esophageal carcinoma. Zhonghua Zhong Liu Za Zhi 1986;8:294–6.
15. Seitz JF, Renou C, Perrier H, et al. Recurrence after surgical treatment of epidermoid cancers of the esophagus. Therapeutic approach in 19 patients. Gastroenterol Clin Biol 1997;21:287–92.
16. Wannenmacher M. Strahlentherapie bei Tumorrezidiven im Gastrointestinaltrakt. Chirurg 1985;56:499–502.
17. Christie NA, Buenaventura PO, Fernando HC, et al. Results of expandable metal stents for malignant esophageal obstruction in 100 patients: short-term and long-term follow-up. Ann Thorac Surg 2001;71:1797–801.

18. Sharma V, Mahantshetty U, Dinshaw KA, Deshpande R, Sharma S. Palliation of advanced/recurrent esophageal carcinoma with high-dose-rate brachytherapy. Int J Radiat Oncol Biol Phys 2002;52:310–5.
19. Sasha D, Harrison LB. The role of brachytherapy for palliation. Semin Radiat Oncol 2000;10:222–39.
20. Martin T, Kolotas C, Dannenberg T. New interstitial HDR brachytherapy technique for prostate cancer: CT based 3D planning after transrectal implantation. Radiother Oncol 1999;52:257–60.

The British Journal of Radiology, 78 (2005), 242–244
DOI: 10.1259/bjr/15227254

Short communication

Abnormal hepatic vein Doppler waveform in patients without liver disease

[1]J F PEDERSEN, MD, PhD, [1]A Z DAKHIL, MD, [1]D B JENSEN, MD, [2]B SØNDERGAARD, MD and [2]P BYTZER, MD, PhD

Departments of [1]Radiology and [2]Medical Gastroenterology, Glostrup University Hospital, Denmark

Abstract. In patients with liver cirrhosis Doppler ultrasound often detects absence of the retrograde (hepatopetal) flow phase in the hepatic vein, suggestive of an increased stiffness of the liver parenchyma around the vein. This is rarely or never reported in healthy control persons. We examined the frequency of absent retrograde flow in a consecutive series of 139 patients referred for abdominal ultrasound. We used state-of-the-art ultrasound scanners, and placed the Doppler gate so that in non-forced end-expiration it would sample the right hepatic vein 4–6 cm from the vena cava. There was no association between the hepatic vein flow pattern and age, sex or body mass index. 43 of 139 studied patients showed absent retrograde flow. Review of the case records revealed liver disease in 26 patients and no sign of liver disease in 17 patients. We suggest that absent retrograde flow in the hepatic veins may be seen not only in patients with overt liver disease but also in apparently liver-healthy patients.

The hepatic vein Doppler waveform normally shows a triphasic pattern with two hepatofugal phases related to atrial and ventricular diastole, and a short phase of retrograde (hepatopetal) flow caused by the pressure increase in the right atrium at atrial systole [1]. Absence of this retrograde flow phase is seen in about half of patients with cirrhosis, and is believed to reflect an increased stiffness of the liver parenchyma around the liver veins [1, 2]. This pattern may also be seen in fibrosis, elevated aminotransferases, fatty liver, chronic hepatitis C and in metastatic liver disease [2–6]. However, we have seen an abnormal curve on occasion in patients without known liver disease and without any other ultrasound indication of liver disease.

It is not clear what action should be taken when an "abnormal" hepatic vein flow curve is unexpectedly revealed. In this study we therefore examine the frequency of abnormal Doppler curves in a sample of our patient population, and explore the possible explanations of the abnormal curves in apparently liver-healthy individuals.

Material and methods

During a 2 month period we registered all patients >18 years old without cardiac arrhythmia who had an abdominal ultrasound study, including the liver, performed by one of the authors (JFP, DBJ, AD). Only patients referred from a department in our hospital were included, to ensure that a case record would be available. Whenever the Doppler waveform showed absence of the retrograde flow phase the two remaining authors were informed (PB, BS). They would evaluate the case notes and decide whether there was evidence of liver disease.

The ultrasound examinations were performed with state-of-the art ultrasound units with convex abdominal probes (Elegra and Antares; Siemens, Issaquah, WA; HDI 5000 sonoCT; Philips Medical Systems, Bothell, WA). The Doppler gate was placed so that in non-forced end-expiration it would sample the right hepatic vein 4–6 cm from the vena cava. The Doppler tracing was documented on video print. The curve pattern was categorized into: triphasic; biphasic, without a retrograde flow phase; flat, monophasic (<10% fluctuation) [1] (Figure 1). Triphasic curves were considered normal, biphasic and monophasic curves were considered abnormal. The patients body mass index (BMI) was calculated according to the formula BMI=weight/height^2 (kg m^{-2}).

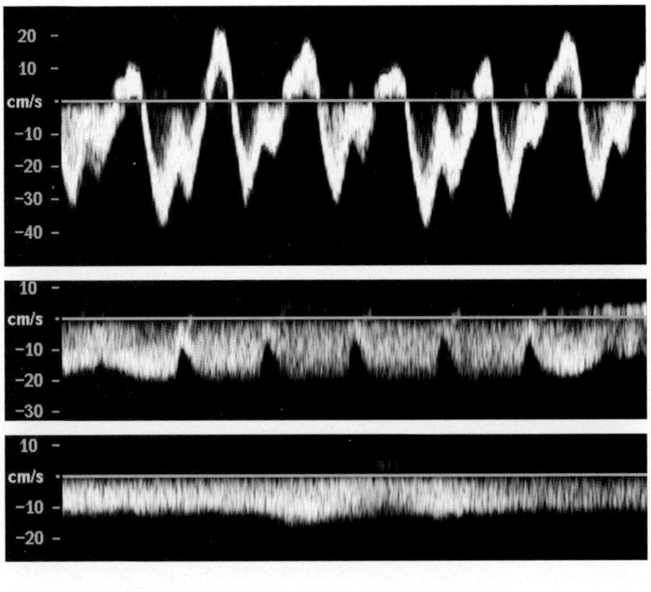

Figure 1. Hepatic vein Doppler waveforms. From top to bottom: normal triphasic waveform with two hepatofugal and one hepatopetal (retrograde) velocity peaks; biphasic waveform without retrograde flow phase; flat (monophasic) waveform.

Received 23 July 2004 and in revised form 1 October 2004, accepted 15 November 2004.

Table 1. Comparison of 96 patients with a normal (triphasic) hepatic vein Doppler curve and 43 patients with abnormal (biphasic and monophasic) curves. Patients with abnormal curves are divided according to evidence of liver disease

	No. of patients	Sex ratio (F/M)	Mean age (years)	Mean BMI (kg m^{-2})
Normal Doppler curve	96	49/47	55.6	25.3
Abnormal Doppler curve	43	18/25	56.9	26.4
No liver disease	17	10/7	56.6	25.2
Proven liver disease	26	8/18	57.1	27.2

BMI, body mass index.

For the statistical analysis of quantitative data we used the two-sample rank sum test (Mann-Whitney) and for qualitative data we used Fisher's exact test. $p<0.05$ was considered significant.

Results

A total of 139 patients entered the study, 67 females and 72 males, mean age 56 years (range 19–91 years). The majority (84%) were referred from the surgical and medical gastroenterology departments. 96 patients (69%) had normal triphasic Doppler waveforms of the hepatic veins. There was no significant difference between patients with normal and with abnormal Doppler tracings concerning mean age, sex ratio and BMI (Table 1), and the fraction of abnormal curves was not higher in patients from the gastroenterology departments than in the remainder, 31% *vs* 32%.

Among the 43 patients with abnormal tracings the ultrasound study suggested liver disease in 23. Review of the case notes revealed liver disease in 20 patients, whereas three patients with ultrasound signs of steatosis and one with MR-verified hepatic haemangiomata lacked biochemical signs of liver disease. Furthermore, two patients without ultrasound signs of liver disease were diagnosed with alcohol related liver disease and CMV hepatitis, respectively. Thus, hepatic disease was diagnosed in 26 patients with abnormal liver vein tracings (cirrhosis, 3; alcohol related liver disease, 14; non-alcoholic steatohepatitis, 3; hepatitis, 1; metastases, 4; haemangiomata, 1). No liver disease could be suggested in 17 patients – ultrasound showed gall bladder calculi in three of them, 1–3 1 cm hepatic cysts in two (considered trivial), and normal liver and gallbladder in 12 patients. Among the patients with abnormal Doppler curves there was no statistical difference between patients with and without liver disease concerning age, sex ratio and BMI (Table 1).

Discussion

Assessment of the hepatic vein Doppler waveform extends the examination time only marginally. Furthermore, application of colour Doppler imaging will make it extremely fast and simple to ensure that there is a retrograde flow phase in the hepatic veins. A short flash of colour shift in the hepatic veins will prove flow reversal, so that recording of a spectral curve can be reserved for examinations with no colour shift.

We found no association between the hepatic vein flow pattern and age, sex or BMI, leaving the relation between waveform and hepatic pathology to be examined. In their first report on Doppler waveforms of the hepatic veins Bolondi and co-workers observed no abnormal curves in 65 healthy volunteers [1]. Similarly, in subsequent studies no abnormal tracings were obtained from 50 [3], 36 [6], 30 [7] and 25 [8] healthy volunteers, and a recent study reported normal liver vein Doppler curves in 48 of 49 healthy volunteers [5]. Taken together these studies suggest that healthy individuals almost always have normal triphasic liver vein Doppler curves. It therefore appears likely that an abnormal Doppler tracing detected in an apparently liver-healthy patient may still indicate some degree of liver abnormality.

Our study deals with a group of 139 adult patients referred for an abdominal ultrasound examination. The patients were unselected, but predominantly referred from the gastroenterology departments. In 43 patients we found an abnormal hepatic vein Doppler curve, which in 26 of them could be explained by liver disease. In the remaining 17 patients (12% of the examinations) the case records gave no indication of liver disease.

The study thus confirms both that abnormal hepatic vein flow curves may be seen in a spectrum of hepatic disorders, and also, more interestingly, that an abnormal hepatic vein waveform is quite common in apparently liver healthy patients, which to our knowledge has not been reported by others. We suggest that an abnormal hepatic vein Doppler curve, believed to reflect an increased stiffness of the liver parenchyma around the hepatic veins, may be a non-specific indicator of liver abnormality, also in individuals with normal liver biochemistry.

Our study was not designed to answer the natural next question, if and to which extent further diagnostic work-up should be considered, but with the present knowledge we find it justified to ignore an abnormal hepatic vein Doppler curve in a patient with no clinical sign of liver disease. We plan further studies to reveal whether an abnormal hepatic vein waveform may be transient, or whether in some patients it may mark a step towards future development of overt liver disease.

References

1. Bolondi L, Bassi SL, Gaiani S, et al. Liver cirrhosis: changes of Doppler waveform of hepatic veins. Radiology 1991;178:513–6.
2. Colli A, Fraquelli M, Andreoletti M, Marino B, Zuccoli E, Conte D. Severe liver fibrosis or cirrhosis: Accuracy of US for detection - analysis of 300 cases. Radiology 2003;227:89–94.
3. Colli A, Cocciolo M, Riva C, et al. Abnormalities of Doppler waveform of the hepatic veins in patients with chronic liver disease: correlation with histologic findings. AJR Am J Roentgenol 1994;162:833–7.

4. Dietrich C, Lee J-H, Gottschalk R, et al. Hepatic and portal vein flow pattern in correlation with intrahepatic fat deposition and liver histology in patients with chronic hepatitis C. AJR Am J Roentgenol 1998;171:437–43.
5. O'Donohue J, Ng C, Catnach S, Farrant P, Williams R. Diagnostic value of Doppler assessment of the hepatic and portal vessels and ultrasound of the spleen in liver disease. Eur J Gastroenterol Hepatol 2004;16:147–55.
6. Herbay A, Frieling T, Haussinger D. Association between duplex Doppler sonographic flow pattern in right hepatic vein and various liver diseases. J Clin Ultrasound 2001;29:25–30.
7. Arda K, Ofelli M, Calikoglu U, Olcer T, Cumhur T. Hepatic vein Doppler waveform changes in early stage (Child-Pugh A) chronic parenchymal liver disease. J Clin Ultrasound 1997;25:15–9.
8. Teichgräber UKM, Gebel M, Benter T, Manns MP. Characterisation of hepatic venous flow via duplex Doppler sonography. Ultraschall Med 1997;18:267–71.

The British Journal of Radiology, 78 (2005), 245–251
DOI: 10.1259/bjr/33540239

Short communication

Techniques and trouble-shooting in high spatial resolution thin slice MRI for rectal cancer

[1]G BROWN, MD, MRCP, FRCR, [2]I R DANIELS, FRCS, [1]C RICHARDSON, DCRD, [3]P REVELL, DCR, [2]D PEPPERCORN, FRCR and [4]M BOURNE, DMRD, FRCR

[1]*Department of Radiology, Royal Marsden Hospital, Fulham Road, London SW3 6JJ,* [2]*Pelican Cancer Foundation, Pelican Centre, North Hampshire Hospital, Aldermaston Road, Basingstoke, Hants RG24 9NA,* [3]*Siemens Medical, Siemens House, Oldbury, Bracknell, Berkshire RG12 8FZ and* [4]*Department of Radiology, University Hospital of Wales, Heath Park, Cardiff CF14 4XW, UK*

Abstract. MRI is increasingly advocated as an optimal method of staging rectal cancer. The technique enables depiction of the relationship of tumour to the mesorectal fascia and may thus identify tumours at risk of positive circumferential margin involvement at surgery. Depth of extramural spread may also be accurately measured and tumour deposits within the mesorectum are shown. It is important that a high spatial resolution technique is used in order to accurately depict these features and care should be taken in ensuring that images acquired cover the entire rectal tumour and mesorectum. This paper describes the technique of high spatial resolution rectal cancer imaging and the potential technical pitfalls in acquiring good quality images. Important factors to consider include: adequate scan duration to achieve high spatial resolution images with sufficient signal to noise ratio, careful positioning of the pelvic phased array coil, use of T_2 weighted turbo spin-echo rather than T_1 weighted imaging and careful planning of scans to ensure that images are obtained perpendicular to the rectal wall.

Colorectal carcinoma is the second most common cause of cancer death in the UK. Rectal cancer comprises up to 50% of all cases and accurate pre-operative staging is assuming increasing importance with the availability of effective pre-operative neoadjuvant therapies. The international TNM classification [1] is the most widely used staging system based on the depth of tumour into and beyond the bowel wall, the number of nodal metastases and the presence or absence of distant metastases. In addition, pre-operative assessment of the relationship of tumour or tumour deposits in relation to the potential circumferential resection margin (the mesorectal fascia) is of importance as tumour involvement of this margin in the resection specimen predicts for local recurrence [2] and poor survival [3]. Demonstration of these features pre-operatively is of importance in selecting patients for neoadjuvant therapy prior to surgery.

Three principal imaging techniques, endoluminal ultrasound, endorectal and pelvic phased array MRI, have been studied in the staging of rectal cancer. All of these modalities have been subject to attention because of their ability to distinguish tumour from rectal wall. However, unlike endoluminal ultrasound and endorectal MRI, high spatial resolution MRI consistently depicts the mesorectal fascia [4] and anatomical structures that relate to total mesorectal excision surgery for rectal cancer [5]. The technique enables accurate measurement of depth of extramural spread [4], identification of tumour deposits within the mesorectum [6] and prediction of tumours with positive circumferential margin involvement [7]. It is important that a high spatial resolution technique is used in order to accurately stage tumours and measure depth of extramural spread. Care should be taken in ensuring that images acquired adequately cover the rectal tumour and mesorectum and that overstaging is prevented by ensuring that images are obtained perpendicular to the rectal wall. The aim of this paper is to describe the technique of high spatial resolution rectal cancer imaging and the potential technical pitfalls in acquiring good quality images.

Received 29 March 2004 and in revised form 6 October 2004, accepted 25 November 2004.

Address correspondence to Dr Gina Brown, Consultant Radiologist and Honorary Senior Lecturer, Department of Radiology, The Royal Marsden Hospital NHS Trust, Downs Road, Sutton, Surrey SM2 5PT, UK.

Method

Indications and patient preparation

The examination should be performed for all patients with histologically proven rectal carcinoma who present for disease staging. The referring surgeon should indicate the tumour position (in terms of height above the anal verge) and any history of past pelvic pathology and surgery. Ideally the imaging should be performed before the multidisciplinary meeting to aid in the pre-operative decision making process. Ensuring that the patient is comfortable and pain free will ensure a good quality examination free from unwanted motion artefact. Patients need to be fully informed about the length of time of the scans and be positioned comfortably in the supine position within the scanner. There is no role for purgative bowel preparation or enemas. Small bowel movement is not a problem in our experience and therefore anti-peristaltic agents are not indicated. The patient is placed supine on the table and the flexible multi-element phased array body/pelvic coil is placed firmly around the pelvis to ensure good compression and to minimize the possibility of motion. A full bladder is unnecessary and is uncomfortable with the compression from the body coil.

Hardware

Magnet

A 1.0 T/1.5 T system can be used. All of the images presented here have been produced with a 1.5 T machine. The main consequence of using a 1.0 T magnet is the longer image acquisition times. Equally good images can be produced on these machines.

Coil choice

Surface coils: Surface coils, such as the endorectal coil, are designed to maximize signal return from the small area being imaged [8–12]. These coils comprise an oval receive only loop coil mounted on the inner surface of an inflatable balloon and have the advantage of placement against the surface of the tissue being imaged such as the rectal wall. These coils can produce images of very high signal with little unwanted signal from tissues around but their principal limitation is their small volume of sensitivity. The area that can be imaged using such coils amounts to a total distance of one coil diameter away from the coil with a very rapid drop in signal intensity beyond the immediate vicinity of the coil (Figure 1). A gap of several millimetres is present between the surface of the coil and the surface of the lesion and the balloon needs to be distended in order to maintain the position of the loop coil close to the primary tumour. Although the coil design permits improved signal to noise ratio, allowing image acquisition using a smaller field of view and thinner slices it is of limited value in the routine staging of rectal cancer. This relates to the use of any endoluminal technique wherein stenosis, stricturing, pain and discomfort, bowel wall motion, difficulty placing the probe in the upper rectum and coil migration all hamper image acquisition. These are significant limitations of using an endoluminal technique and therefore such devices are not recommended in the routine staging of rectal cancer.

Phased array coils: These coils gain the advantages of the surface coil by obtaining higher signal but with greater coverage than a single surface coil and improved homogeneity.

Sequences recommended in the local staging of rectal cancer

Initial localization images, in the coronal and sagittal planes are needed to plan the high resolution images of the pelvis and rectum as follows:

Sequence 1

- The first series is the sagittal T_2 weighted fast spin echo (T2W-FSE), which enables identification of the primary tumour (Table 1).

Sequence 2

- The second series is the large field of view axial sections of the whole pelvis from the iliac crest to the symphysis pubis (Table 1).

These first two sequences give a crude visualization of the primary tumour, possible sites of nodal involvement and direction of the rectal wall to enable the crucial high spatial resolution sequences 3 and 4 to be planned to enable characterization of nodes and detailed staing of the extent of the primary tumour.

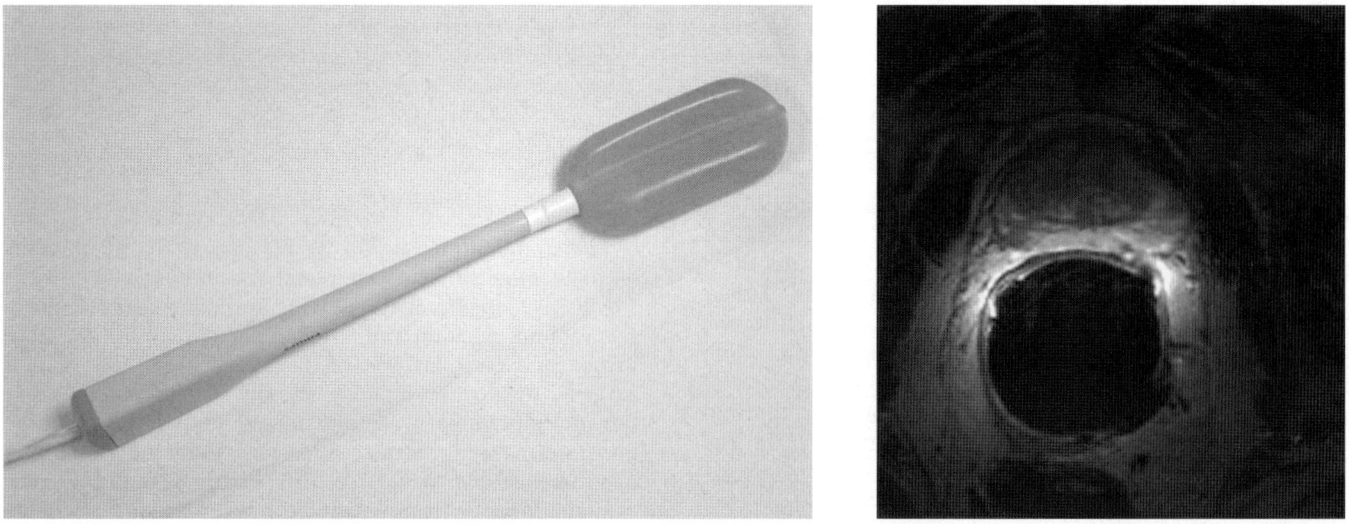

(a) (b)

Figure 1. (a) Endorectal coil and (b) T_2 weighted image using the endorectal coil. The bowel wall layers are shown but there is insufficient detail from the surrounding mesorectum to adequately stage rectal tumours.

Table 1. Sequence 1 and 2: standard 5 mm sagittal and axial scans

Scanner	Philips TSE	Siemens TSE	GE FSE
TR (ms)	5080 (sagittal) 4018 (axial)	3000–6000	4000
TE (ms)	132 (sagittal) 80 (axial)	100	110
No. of slices	23 (20 axial)	24	24
Thickness/gap	3 (sagittal) 5/1 (axial)	5/0	5/0
Interleaved	No	Yes	No
ETL	23	8	8
Matrix in phase direction	512	512	512
Matrix in frequency direction	370/70% for sagittal 256/100% (axial)	256	288
Phase encoding direction	AP	AP	AP
Field of view (mm)	250	240	250
Phase	250	240	250
Frequency	250	240	250
No. of acquisitions	3 (sagittal) 2 (axial)	2	2
Flow compensation	Yes	Yes	Yes
Sat Bands	Anterior/superior	Anterior	Anterior

TR, repetition time; TE, echo time; TSE, turbo spin echo; FSE, fast spin echo; AP, anteroposterior; ETL, echo train length.
GE, Milwaukee, W; Siemens, Erlangen, Germany; Philips, Best, The Netherlands.

Sequence 3

While the second sequence is being acquired, the high-resolution images can be planned (Table 2). The sagittal T_2 weighted images obtained are used to plan T_2 weighted thin-section axial images through the rectal cancer and adjacent perirectal tissues. It is critical that these images are performed perpendicular to the long-axis of the rectum (Figure 2). The images are obtained by using a 16 cm field of view and 3 mm section thickness.

Table 2. Sequence 3 and 4: high resolution oblique axial and coronal scans (for low tumours)

Scanner	Philips TSE	Siemens TSE	GE FSE-XL
TR (ms)	5362	6590	5100
TE (ms)	100	136	85
No. of slices	16	24	28
Thickness/gap	3/0.3	3	3
Interleaved	Yes	Yes	No
ETL	16	8	8
Matrix in phase encoding	256	256	256
Matrix in frequency – encoding	256/90%	256	256
Phase encoding direction	FH	FH	SI
Field of view (mm)	160	160	160
RFOV	100%	100%	160
Foldover	RL	RL	No phase wrap
No. of acquisitions	6	4	4
Sat Bands	None	SI	SI
Scan duration (min:s)	7:35	7:36	8:40
Other	No DRIVE Prep phase auto		Phase correct: on Flow comp on Tailored RF fast

TR, repetition time; TE, echo time; TSE, turbo spin echo; FSE, fast spin echo; ETL, echo train length; FH, foot to head; SI, superior inferior; RL, right to left; RFOV, rectangular field of view; RF, radiofrequency.
Philips, Best, The Netherlands; Siemans, Erlangen, Germany; GE, Milwaukee, WI.

Sequence 4

The rapid change in calibre of the rectal lumen at the level of the anorectal junction limits the usefulness of oblique axial imaging alone. At this level axial images may not show the rectal wall in its entirety and clear delineation between the outer edge of the rectal wall and the levator

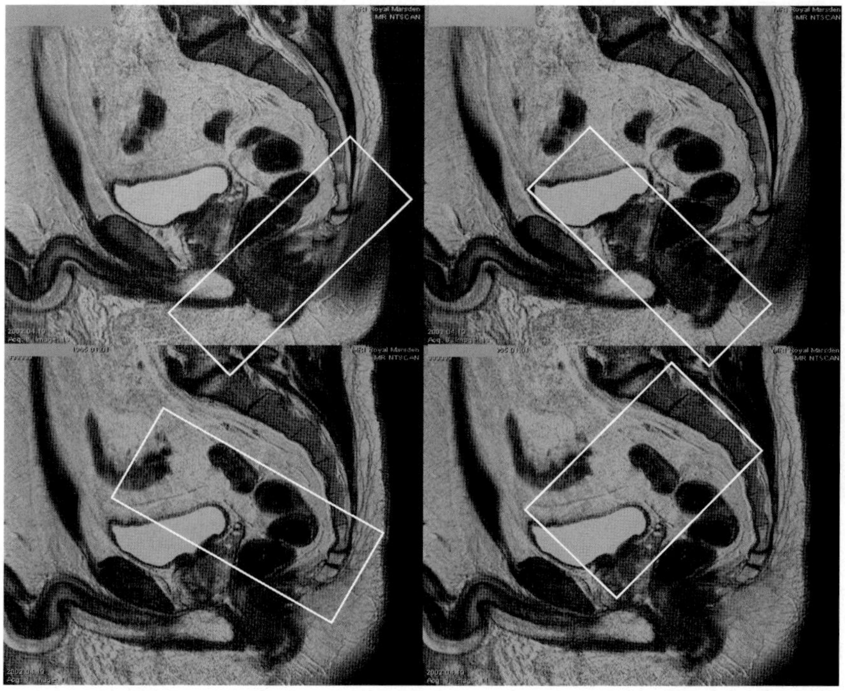

Figure 2. Planning the high resolution images. Images are acquired orthogonal to the long axis of the rectum. Note that for a low tumour, an additional oblique coronal scan (top right image) is also acquired, which is planned along the long axis of the anal canal.

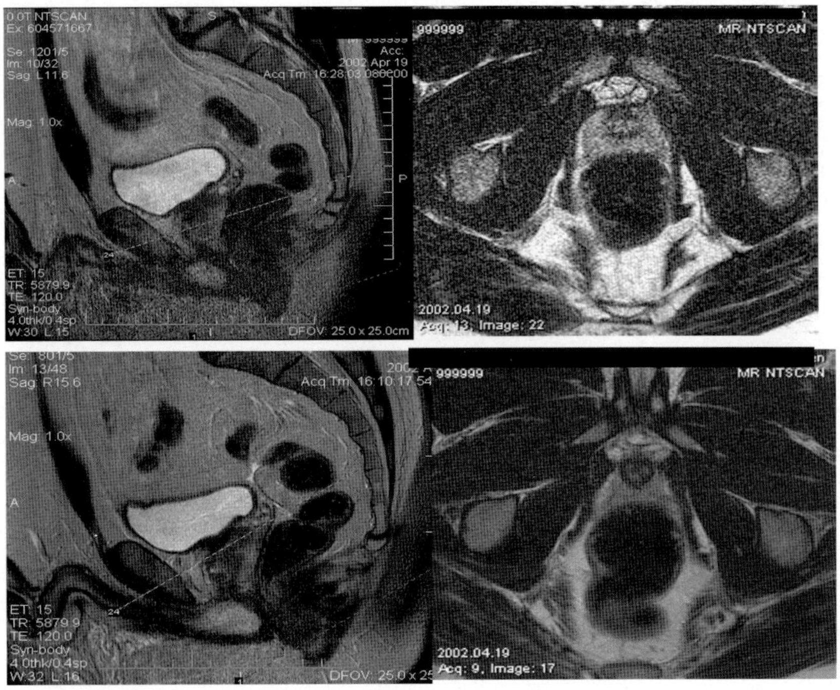

Figure 3. Poor coil positioning. The images shown (top left and right) have been obtained with the lower edge of the pelvic coil placed at the level of the symphysis pubis. Consequently there is poor signal to noise ratio from the lower rectum and anal sphincter region. Repositioning the coil restores adequate signal to noise ratio.

muscle may not be possible. This can potentially lead to overstaging. It is therefore useful to utilize a high spatial resolution coronal imaging sequence, for lower third rectal tumours, which will show the levator, the sphincter complex, the intersphincteric plane and the relationship to the rectal wall most optimally (Figure 2).

Potential factors that may impair the quality of images

Coil positioning

In order to prevent poor signal to noise from the anorectal junction (Figure 3), it is important that the phased array coil is centred optimally to ensure adequate coverage of the rectum, mesorectum and anal sphincter complex. Thus there should be adequate coverage from the level of the sacral promontory to below the symphysis pubis (Figure 4).

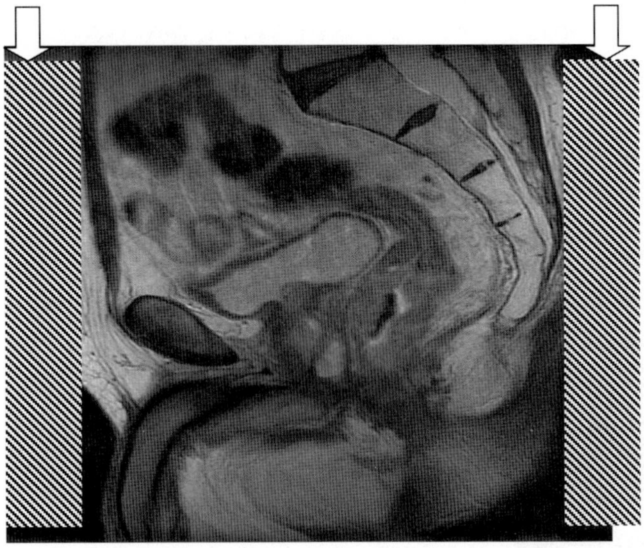

Figure 4. It is important to centre the coil correctly to the whole rectum. Thus the lower edge of the coil needs to be placed so that it lies at least 10 cm below the symphysis pubis in order to ensure adequate signal is obtained from the lower rectum and anorectal junction. The upper most limit for coil placement is the sacral promontory.

Choice of sequences

T_1 weighted imaging: Although the availability of short repetition time/echo time (TR/TE) volume imaging can provide images of high spatial resolution, images obtained fail to depict either tumour or the layers of the bowel wall due to similar relaxation rates of tumour and bowel wall (Figure 5).

Fat saturation and contrast enhancement: Contrast enhancement has not been shown to be an effective method for the local staging of rectal cancer [9, 13]. A contrast enhanced technique requires the high signal

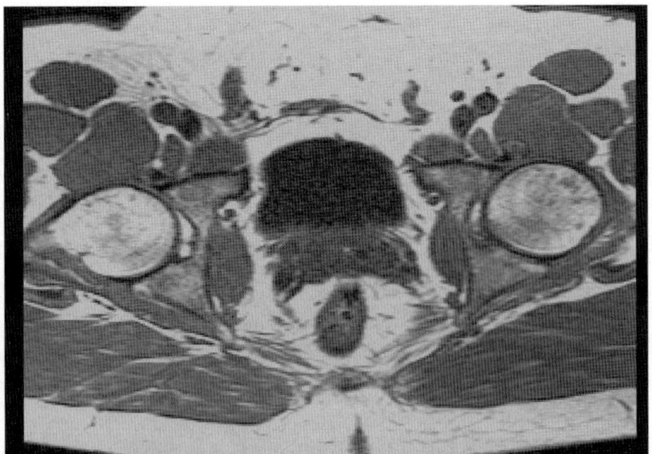

Figure 5. A T_1 weighted image (repetition time (TR) 500 ms, echo time (TE) 10 ms) has been obtained with a high spatial resolution 1 mm^3 voxel but the bowel wall layers cannot be distinguished.

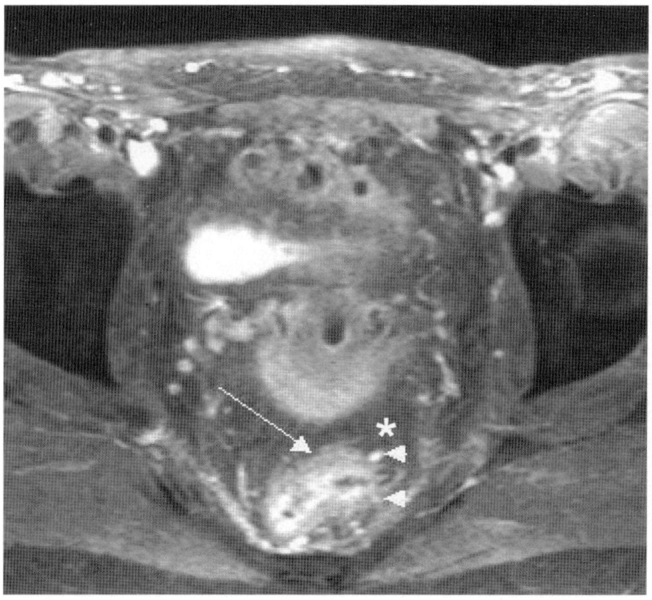

Figure 6. T_1 fat saturated image with contrast enhancement. The bright fat signal intensity from perirectal fat (asterisk) has been suppressed and is of low signal intensity, there is florid enhancement of the entire bowel wall (arrow) and perirectal vessels (arrowheads) which would not be readily distinguishable from tumour if it were present.

from surrounding perirectal fat on T_1 weighted images to be suppressed to permit visualization of high signal enhancement of tumour. This results in a further reduction in signal to noise ratio and potential overstaging of tumours due to enhancement of adjacent non-tumour tissue namely vessels, desmoplastic reaction and normal nodes (Figure 6).

T_2 weighted fast spin-echo (T_2 FSE): T_2 weighted images of the rectal wall and pararectal tissues result in visualization of individual bowel wall layers and tumour returns a brighter signal than the muscle coat but lower signal intensity than perirectal fat and thus superior depiction of tumour when compared with T_1 weighted images (Figure 7).

Thus T_1 fat saturated or short tau inversion recovery (STIR) imaging of the rectum and perirectal tissues offers no additional staging information and should not be used.

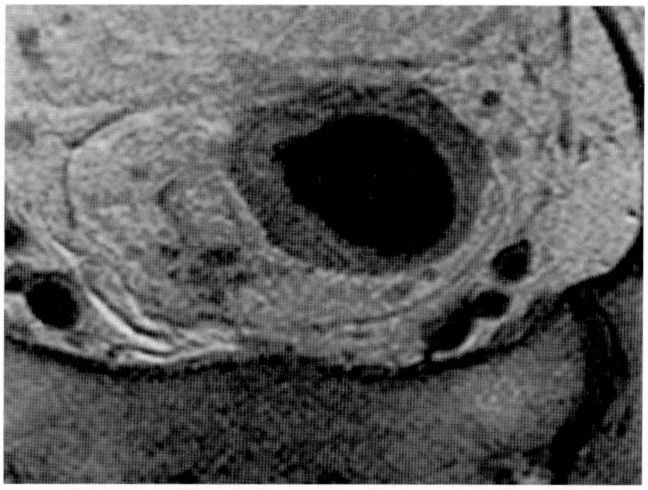

Figure 8. Cross-talk. The image has been degraded by noise resulting from cross-talk. This varies with machines and manifests as loss of signal. This is overcome by interleaving slices during the high resolution acquisition.

Cross-talk: This varies with machines and patients and is manifested on the images obtained as loss of signal and unexpected loss of detail (Figure 8). This is overcome by interleaving slices during the high resolution acquisition or increasing the slice gap.

Tumour not seen on initial sagittal sequences: On occasion, lack of clinical detail or the presence of a

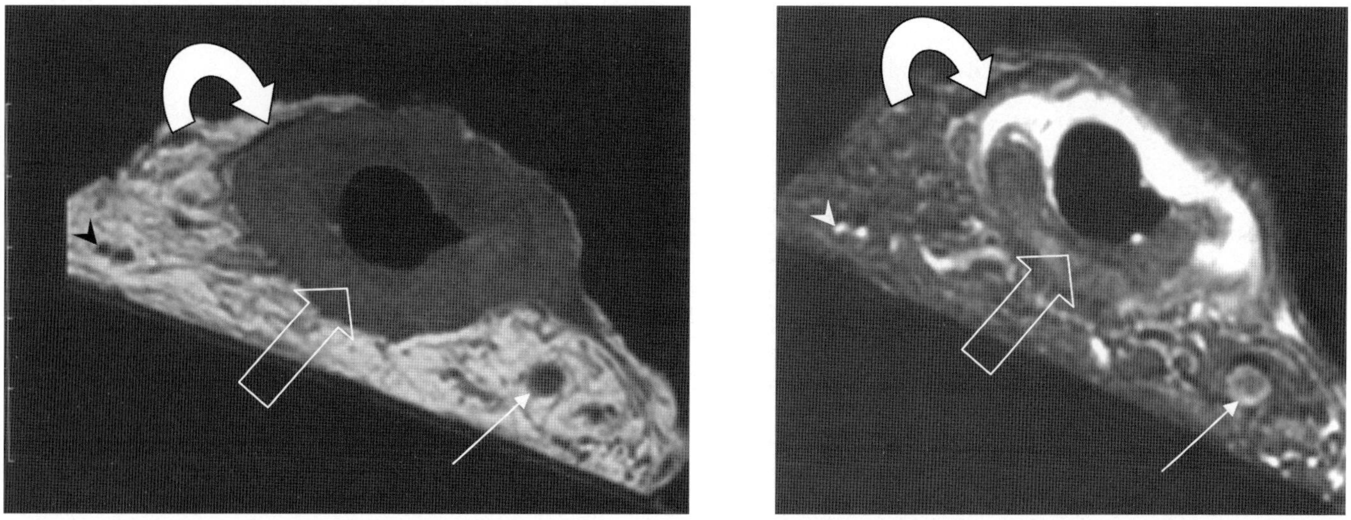

(a) (b)

Figure 7. (a) T_1 weighted (repetition time (TR)=500 ms, echo time (TE) 10 ms) and (b) T_2 fast spin echo (FSE) (TR>3000 ms, TE 105 ms) axial images of rectal tumour. The bowel wall layers cannot be seen on the T_1 weighted images. Vessels (arrowhead), lymph node (arrow), tumour (open arrow) and muscle coat (curved arrow) all return very similar signal intensities making distinction between structures difficult on the T_1 weighted image. This compares with the T_2 weighted image, which shows clear separation of tumour and bowel wall layers due to high inherent tissue contrast.

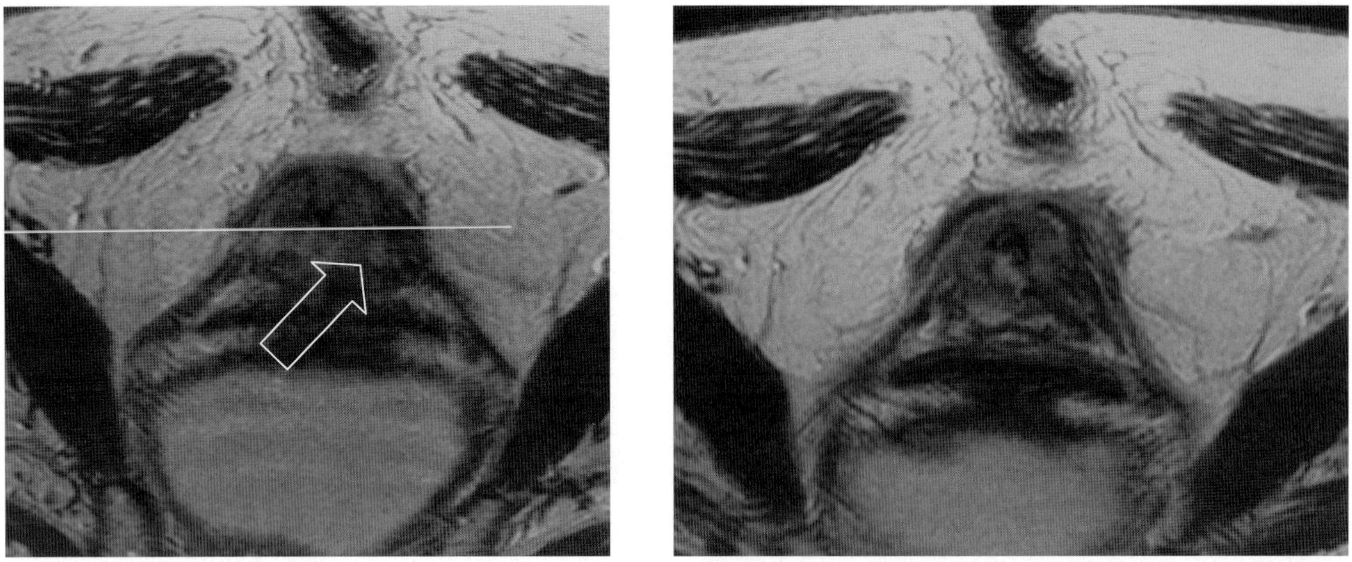

(a) (b)

Figure 9. Motion artefact. (a) This characteristically produces a series of bands that degrade the image. (b) This can often be overcome by ensuring the patient is not in discomfort, by repositioning the patient and ensuring adequate abdominal compression and repeating the sequence again after swapping phase and frequency directions.

small tumour prevents the tumour being seen on the sagittal images. In these instances, tumour may only be visible on the high resolution images. In order to ensure that the tumour has not been missed it will be necessary to perform high resolution scans along the entire length of the rectum (as shown in Figure 2).

Patient unable to tolerate long scan: Some patients (<5%), either due to co-existing medical conditions or claustrophobia, find the scan impossible to tolerate; a combination of patient discomfort, excessive motion of the anterior abdominal wall may result in motion artefact. This is seen as horizontal bands across the image (Figure 9). Of all of the sequences the oblique high resolution scans are the most important. The sagittal views can be shortened by altering the parameters; the large field of view axials are performed last and may even be omitted if the patient is in considerable discomfort.

Discussion

High spatial resolution MRI is gaining acceptance as a method of determining the local stage of rectal cancer [4, 7, 10, 14, 15]. In comparison with endoluminal techniques such as endorectal ultrasound, MRI offers inherent advantages [16], namely the ability to assess all tumours including bulky obstructing or stricturing tumours. The large field of view afforded by high spatial resolution MRI using the surface coil permits assessment of the entire mesorectum as well as the relationship of tumour to the mesorectal fascia which forms the radial margins in rectal cancer surgery using total mesorectal excision. High contrast resolution using T_2 weighted fast spin-echo sequences enables perirectal fibrosis to be readily distinguished from tumour by virtue of signal intensity characteristics and its ability to depict the outer muscle coat as a distinct layer on MR images permits accurate assessment of the depth of extramural spread from the outer muscle coat [4, 7]. However, as yet there is no role for MRI in the assessment of early tumours (T1), adenomatous polyps, or resolving the staging of T1 and T2 tumours in patients being considered for local excision of their tumour. Endorectal techniques are likely to be more useful in such patients and high frequency probes have the potential to identify superficially invasive T1 tumours suitable for cure by local excision [17].

The introduction of the pelvic phased array coil has enabled a major advance in the detail and reproducibility of rectal cancer imaging. It has now been shown to be of high accuracy in assessing the depth of extramural spread and predicting the relationship of tumour close to the mesorectal fascia and is thus a clinically effective method of locally staging all patients with the disease.

References

1. Sobin L, Wittekind C, editors. TNM classification of malignant tumours (5th edn). New York: John Wiley & Sons, 1997.
2. Adam IJ, Mohamdee MO, Martin IG, Scott N, Finan PJ, Johnston D, et al. Role of circumferential margin involvement in the local recurrence of rectal cancer. Lancet 1994;344:707–11.
3. Hall NR, Finan PJ, al-Jaberi T, Tsang CS, Brown SR, Dixon MF, et al. Circumferential margin involvement after mesorectal excision of rectal cancer with curative intent. Predictor of survival but not local recurrence? Dis Colon Rectum 1998;41:979–83.
4. Brown G, Richards CJ, Newcombe RG, Dallimore NS, Radcliffe AG, Carey DP, et al. Rectal carcinoma: thin-section MR imaging for staging in 28 patients. Radiology 1999;211:215–22.
5. Brown G, Kirkham A, Williams GT, Bourne M, Radcliffe AG, Sayman J, et al. High-resolution MRI of the anatomy important in total mesorectal excision of the rectum. AJR Am J Roentgenol 2004;182:431–9.
6. Bartram CI, Brown G. Endorectal ultrasound and magnetic resonance imaging in rectal cancer staging. Gastroenterol Clin North Am 2002;31:827–39.

7. Brown G, Radcliffe AG, Newcombe RG, Dallimore NS, Bourne MW, Williams GT. Preoperative assessment of prognostic factors in rectal cancer using high-resolution magnetic resonance imaging. Br J Surg 2003;90:355–64.
8. Schnall MD, Furth EE, Rosato EF, Kressel HY. Rectal tumor stage: correlation of endorectal MR imaging and pathologic findings [see comments]. Radiology 1994;190:709–14.
9. Indinnimeo M, Grasso RF, Cicchini C, Pavone P, Stazi A, Catalano C, et al. Endorectal magnetic resonance imaging in the preoperative staging of rectal tumors. Int Surg 1996;81:419–22.
10. Blomqvist L, Machado M, Rubio C, Gabrielsson N, Granqvist S, Goldman S, et al. Rectal tumour staging: MR imaging using pelvic phased-array and endorectal coils vs endoscopic ultrasonography. Eur Radiol 2000;10:653–60.
11. Drew PJ, Farouk R, Turnbull LW, Ward SC, Hartley JE, Monson JR. Preoperative magnetic resonance staging of rectal cancer with an endorectal coil and dynamic gadolinium enhancement. Br J Surg 1999;86:250–4.
12. Joosten FB, Jansen JB, Joosten HJ, Rosenbusch G. Staging of rectal carcinoma using MR double surface coil, MR endorectal coil, and intrarectal ultrasound: correlation with histopathologic findings. J Comput Assist Tomogr 1995;19:752–8.
13. Okizuka H, Sugimura K, Yoshizako T, Kaji Y, Wada A. Rectal carcinoma: prospective comparison of conventional and gadopentetate dimeglumine enhanced fat-suppressed MR imaging. J Magn Reson Imaging 1996;6:465–71.
14. Beets-Tan RG, Beets GL, Vliegen RF, Kessels AG, Van Boven H, De Bruine A, et al. Accuracy of magnetic resonance imaging in prediction of tumour-free resection margin in rectal cancer surgery. Lancet 2001;357:497–504.
15. Radcliffe A, Brown G. Will MRI provide maps of lines of excision for rectal cancer? Lancet 2001;357:495–6.
16. Brown G, Davies S, Williams GT, Bourne MW, Newcombe RG, Radcliffe AG, et al. Effectiveness of preoperative staging in rectal cancer: digital rectal examination, endoluminal ultrasound or magnetic resonance imaging? Br J Cancer 2004;91:23–9.
17. Brown G, Richards CJ, Bourne MW, Newcombe RG, Radcliffe AG, Dallimore NS, et al. Morphologic predictors of lymph node status in rectal cancer with use of high-spatial-resolution MR imaging with histopathologic comparison. Radiology 2003;227:371–7.

The British Journal of Radiology, *78* (2005), 252–254
DOI: 10.1259/bjr/50653404

Case report

Selective conformal radiotherapy for arteriovenous malformation involving the spinal cord

[1]K KISHI, MD, PhD, [1]S SHIRAI, MD, [2]T SONOMURA, MD and [1]M SATO, MD

[1]*Department of Radiology, Wakayama Medical University (WMU), Kimiidera 811-1, Wakayama City, 641-0012 and* [2]*Department of Radiology, Kishiwada Tokushukai Hospital, Japan*

Abstract. Radiotherapy has seldom been used in the treatment of arteriovenous malformations (AVM) involving the spinal cord because of the cord's limited radiation tolerance. A 57-year-old woman with progressive myelopathy due to AVM was treated with a selective conformal radiation therapy (55.6 Gy/20 days) on the nidus region preserving the spinal cord, drainer veins and involved bones. The drainers and symptoms were minimized at the end of treatment and disappeared over 2 years. This case illustrates the usefulness of selective conformal radiation therapy.

Radiotherapy has been rarely used for arteriovenous malformations (AVMs) involving the spinal cord because of the low radiation tolerance of the spinal cord [1]. Radiotherapy using a selective three-dimensional plan to focus on the nidus region while preserving the spinal cord, drainer veins, and involved bones has been used successfully in one patient.

Case report

A 57-year-old woman was first referred to an orthopaedic surgeon, complaining of a growing mass on her right back. A blue and flat birthmark had been asymptomatic since her neonatal period, and had been neglected for decades. After accidentally bruising her back 2 months earlier, she began suffering back pain, shoulder stiffness, and gradual swelling of a mass. On admission, the mass measured 13 cm × 20 cm. During pre-operative assessment, she developed a progressive myelopathy, with intolerable pain, abnormal sensation below the thorax, unsteadiness in the upright position, and impaired micturition. She was referred to the radiotherapy department and was dependent on a wheel chair.

A colour Doppler ultrasound study found turbulent high-velocity flow signals [2] in the mass. CT myelograpy revealed compression of the dural sac and spinal cord from the 7th cervical vertebra to 2nd thoracic vertebra (Figure 1a). Abnormal enhancement was found in the right erector spinae muscles (Figure 1b) and mass. Numerous cystic lesions in these vertebral bodies indicated a risk of fracture. MRI revealed distended epidural veins compressing the spinal cord (Figure 2a). T_2 enhancement in the spinal cord was observed from C3 to C6, suggesting the presence of congestive myelopathy [3]. The abnormally enhanced region in the erector spinae muscles was due to the nidus for the epidural veins, and also for signal change in the vertebral bones [4]. The angiogram showed a typical AVM pattern with a number of feeding arteries. Early venous filling coincided with the abnormal enhancement (Figure 1c). Embolisation, surgery and combination therapy were not possible because of the large number of feeders with possible anastomoses, and of the large size of the mass.

Three-dimensional conformal radiation therapy targeted to a volume including the nidus region was planned on CT images (Figure 1d) using eight beams. This was equivalent to the gross tumour volume (GTV) defined in ICRU report 50. A total dose of 55.6 Gy in 20 fractions in 4 weeks was given, which was equivalent to 64 Gy in 32 fractions in 6 and a half weeks using the linear quadratic model with an alpha/beta ratio of 3 Gy. The mean dose of the planning target volume (PTV) that completely included the nidus region was 49 Gy. The mean dose for the spinal cord was 20 Gy, the maximum dose 34.9 Gy and normal tissue complication probability between the C5 and the T2 level was 0%. The estimated probability for myelopathy within 5 years (TD1/5) [5] was 1%. The dose to the distended epidural veins and affected vertebral body was no higher than the spinal cord dose.

The patient complained of a transient slight increase in her lower leg pain for a few days during the first week. The difficulty passing urine diminished in the second week. She became able to walk independently and a rehabilitation program was started. MRI on the 21st day of radiotherapy showed no compression of the spinal cord, and a shrunken epidural vein (Figure 2b). MRI 1 year later showed complete disappearance of the epidural venous distension and the spinal compression (Figure 2c). No T_2 enhancement of the cord was found. CT scans showed a reduction in the lytic areas. There has been no sign of myelopathy and no recurrence of symptoms for 3 years.

Received 12 November 2003 and in revised form 26 October 2004, accepted 23 November 2004.

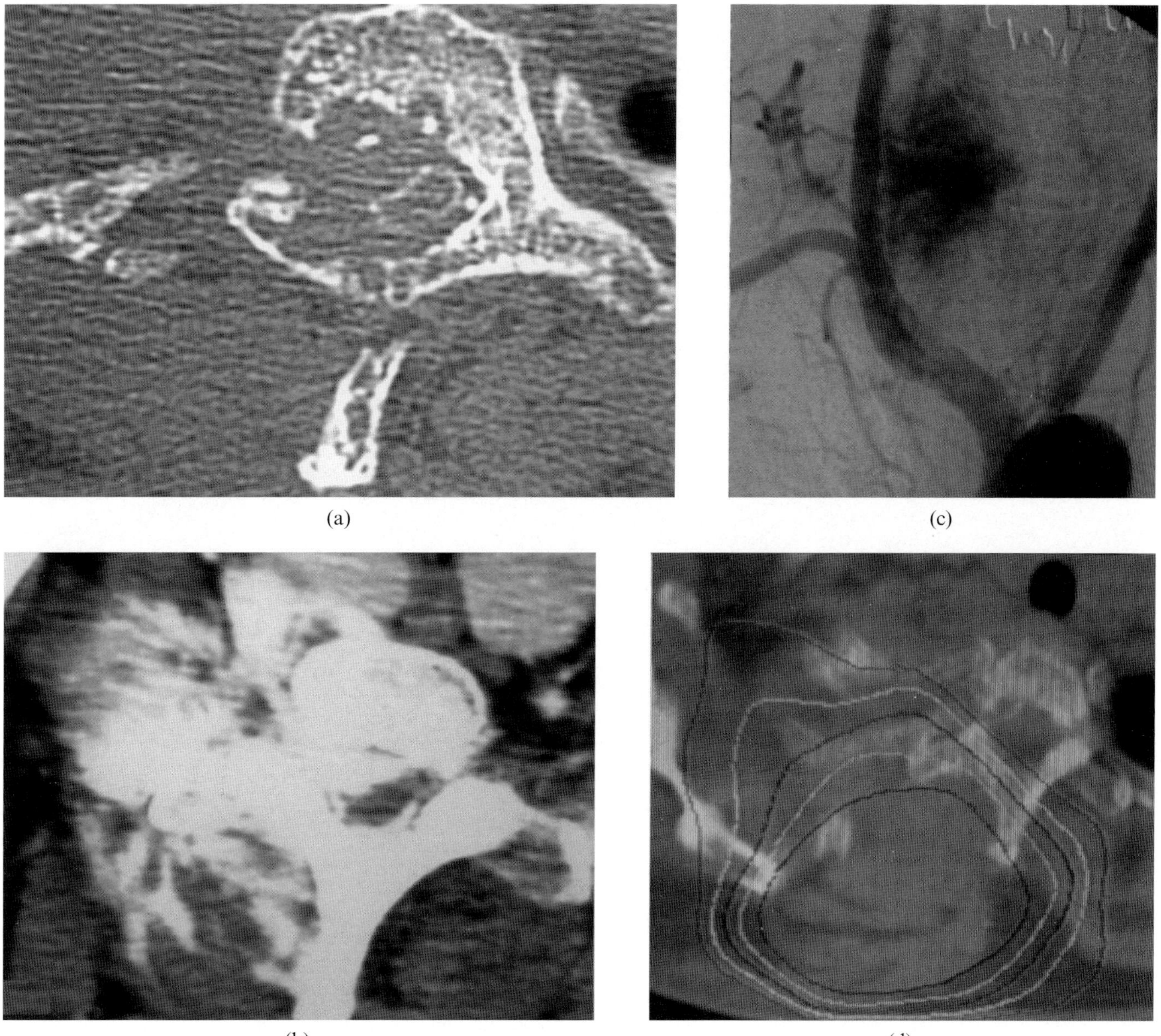

Figure 1. Before radiotherapy. (a) CT image during myelograpy. Compression of dural sac and spinal cord. Porous change of vertebral body. (b) Enhanced CT image. Abnormal enhancement in the right spinal erector muscles. (c) Early venous filling. (d) Dose distribution curves in radiation planning. From inside to outside, each line indicates 100%, 90%, 70%, 50%, and 30% of the prescribed dose.

Discussion

The radiation was selectively targeted on the nidus, to decrease the transnidal flow that was responsible for the cord compression, congestion [3], and artery steal [6].

On the other hand, doses to the spinal cord, affected vertebral bones and draining veins were intentionally reduced. The lower tolerance dose of the spinal cord has long been the major constraint in giving radiotherapy [5, 7, 8]. The dose used here is associated with a 5% risk of myelopathy or necrosis within 5 years from treatment (TD5/5) (47 Gy on 20 cm of spinal cord [5]). A compressed, or haemodynamically abnormal spinal cord [6] might have an even lower tolerance dose. Thus the radiation dose given was below tolerance. The dose to the lytic vertebral body was intentionally decreased to avoid further demineralization. The dose given to the distended drainage veins was also restricted because venous impairment could be an explanation for frequent post-radiosurgery haemorrhage (7–10%) in less selective treatment [9], and because the distended veins were not an essential target. High dose radiotherapy causes a loss of tissue elasticity.

Recent developments in radiation therapy systems have enabled planning of sophisticated dose distributions, overcoming the problems of sparing organs at risk, and focusing an effective dose on the nidus. The only previous report on treatment planning for spinal AVM was a technical report on the Cyberknife system [10]. In this case a good clinical outcome was achieved through technical progress, based on a knowledge of physiology and radiotherapy physics.

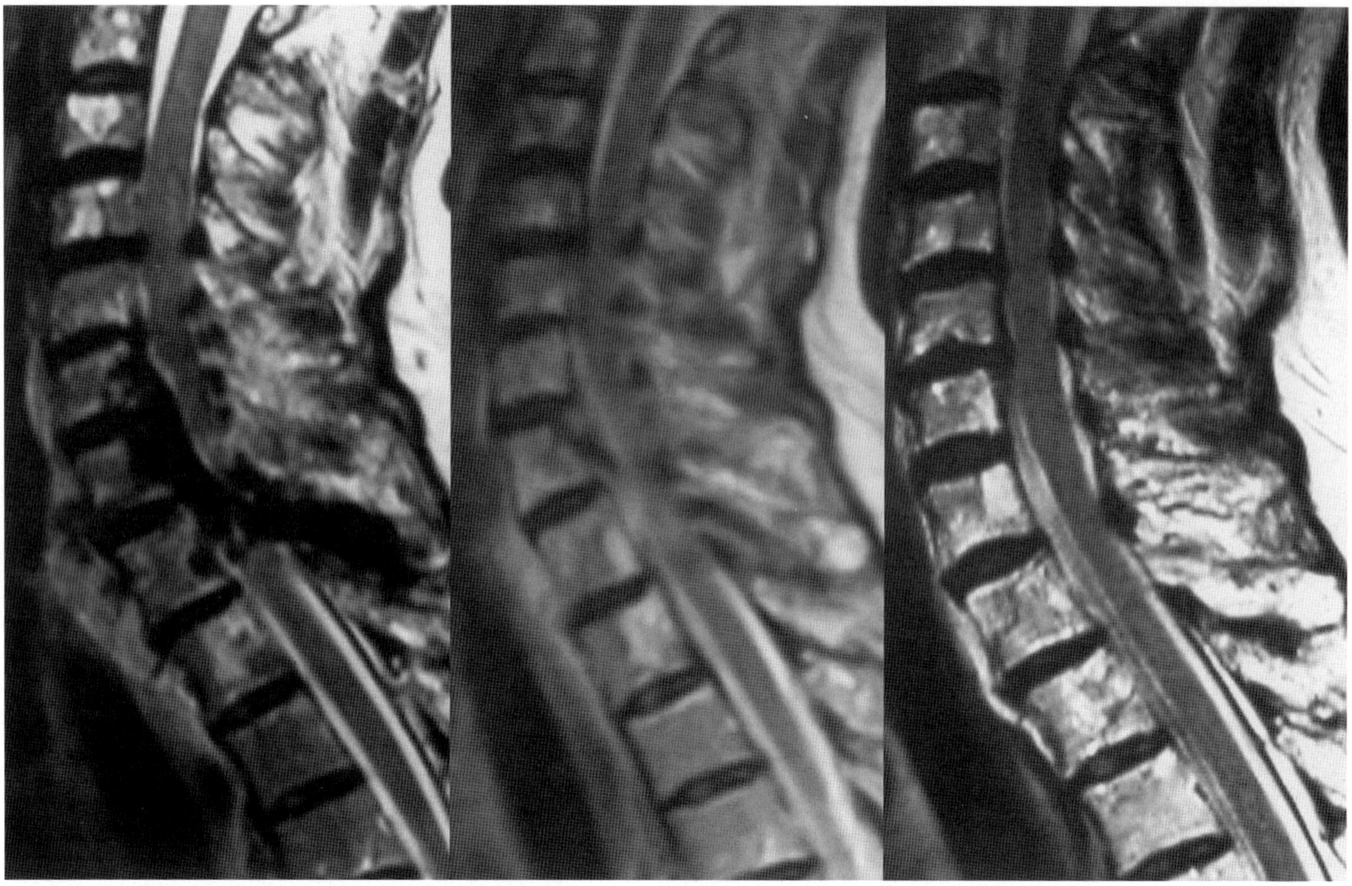

(a) (b) (c)

Figure 2. During and after radiotherapy. (a) T_2 weighted MRI. Distended epidural veins. Note T_2 hyperintensity in the spinal cord. (b) MRI image on the 21st day. The spinal cord was not compressed. The epidural vein was shrunk. (c) MRI image 1 year later. Complete disappearance of the epidural venous. No T_2 enhancement in the spinal cord.

References

1. Schulz U, Bamberg M. Relationship between curative radiation therapy of paravertebral tumors and the incidence of radiation myelitis. Tumori 1978;64:305–12.
2. Li JC, Cai S, Jiang YX, Dai Q, Zhang JX, Wang YQ. Diagnostic criteria for locating acquired arteriovenous fistulas with color Doppler sonography. J Clin Ultrasound 2002;30:336–42.
3. Kataoka H, Miyamoto S, Nagata I, Ueba T, Hashimoto N. Venous congestion is a major cause of neurological deterioration in spinal arteriovenous malformations. Neurosurgery 2001;48:1224–9; discussion 1229–30.
4. Modic MT, Hardy RW Jr, Weinstein MA, Duchesneau PM, Paushter DM, Boumphrey F. Nuclear magnetic resonance of the spine: clinical potential and limitation. Neurosurgery 1984;15:583–92.
5. Emami B, Lyman J, Brown A, Coia L, Goitein M, Munzenrider JE, et al. Tolerance of normal tissue to therapeutic irradiation. Int J Radiat Oncol Biol Phys 1991;21:109–22.
6. Taylor CL, Selman WR, Ratcheson RA. Steal affecting the central nervous system. Neurosurgery 2002;50:679–88; discussion 688–9.
7. Schultheiss TE. Spinal cord radiation tolerance. Int J Radiat Oncol Biol Phys 1994;30:735–6.
8. Yamada S, Hoshi A, Takai Y, Hoshino F, Mochizuki Y, Kanehira C, et al. [Radiation tolerance dose of the spinal cord following conventionally fractionated irradiation]. Gan No Rinsho 1987;33:1189–92.
9. Friedman WA, Bova FJ, Bollampally S, Bradshaw P. Analysis of factors predictive of success or complications in arteriovenous malformation radiosurgery. Neurosurgery 2003;52:296–307; discussion 307–8.
10. Ryu SI, Chang SD, Kim DH, Murphy MJ, Le QT, Martin DP, et al. Image-guided hypo-fractionated stereotactic radiosurgery to spinal lesions. Neurosurgery 2001;49:838–46.

The British Journal of Radiology, *78* (2005), 255–256
DOI: 10.1259/bjr/36083619

Case report

Small cell carcinoma of the colon: barium study and CT findings

[1]H C KIM, MD, [1]S I PARK, MD, [2]S J PARK, MD, [1]H C SHIN, MD, [3]M-H OH, MD, [1]H H KIM, MD, [1]W K BAE, MD and [1]I Y KIM, MD

Department of [1]Diagnostic Radiology and [3]Pathology, Soonchunhyang University, Cheonan Hospital, 23–20 Bongmyung-dong, Cheonan, Chungcheongnam-do, 330-721 and [2]Department of Diagnostic Radiology, College of Medicine, Soonchunhyang University, Bucheon Hospital, 1174 Jung-dong, Wonmi-gu, Bucheon, Gyeonggi-do, 420-021, Republic of Korea

Abstract. Extrapulmonary small cell carcinoma is a rare neoplasm. It is an aggressive malignant tumour characterized by rapid local progression and early metastasis. We report a case of small cell carcinoma arising in the transverse colon in a 34-year-old man who presented with epigastric pain. On CT, a poorly enhancing bulky mass encircling the transverse colon with extensive regional lymph node metastases was observed. A segmental annular narrowing with thick interhaustral folds of the transverse colon was found by barium enema examination. This is the first report of barium study and CT findings of extrapulmonary small cell carcinoma of the colon.

Extrapulmonary small cell carcinoma is a rare malignant condition that can arise from various organs, such as the salivary gland, pharynx, oesophagus, stomach, small bowel, colorectum, gallbladder, uterus, kidney and skin [1, 2]. This neoplasm manifests highly aggressive behaviour and the prognosis is generally poor, especially when involving the gastrointestinal tract [1–3]. Small cell carcinoma of the colon is rare, and constitutes about 1.5% of all colon cancers [4]. To our knowledge, the radiological findings regarding small cell carcinoma of the colon have not been previously described in the English literature. We present the barium enema and CT findings of a case of small cell carcinoma of the colon.

Received 5 August 2004 and in revised form 20 October 2004, accepted 25 November 2004.

Case report

A 34-year-old man was hospitalized due to epigastric pain. Physical examination revealed a palpable mass in left upper abdomen. Chest radiography showed no pathological findings. An abdominal CT scan was performed on an eight-channel multislice helical CT scanner (LightSpeed Ultra; General Electric, Milwaukee, WI). It revealed a poorly enhancing mass encircling the transverse colon (Figure 1a) and extensive adjacent lymph node metastasis (Figure 1b). Barium enema examination showed mild annular narrowing with thickening of interhaustral folds in the transverse colon (Figure 2). The proximal and distal margins of the lesion showed gradual tapering without shouldering. Colonoscopy showed a semicircular ulcerating and fungating mass in the transverse colon.

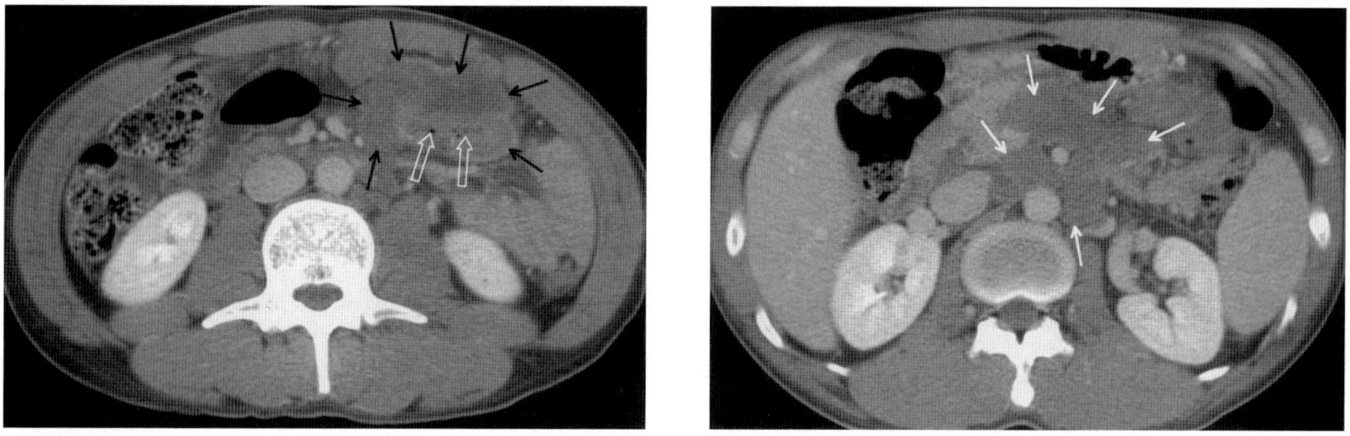

(a) (b)

Figure 1. Post contrast enhanced CT images of the small cell carcinoma of the colon. (a) Axial CT image shows bulky poorly enhancing mass (black arrows) encircling the transverse colon (open arrows). (b) Axial CT image obtained 55 mm above the mass shows extensive metastatic lymph node enlargement (white arrows) in the both para-aortic areas and along the mesenteric root.

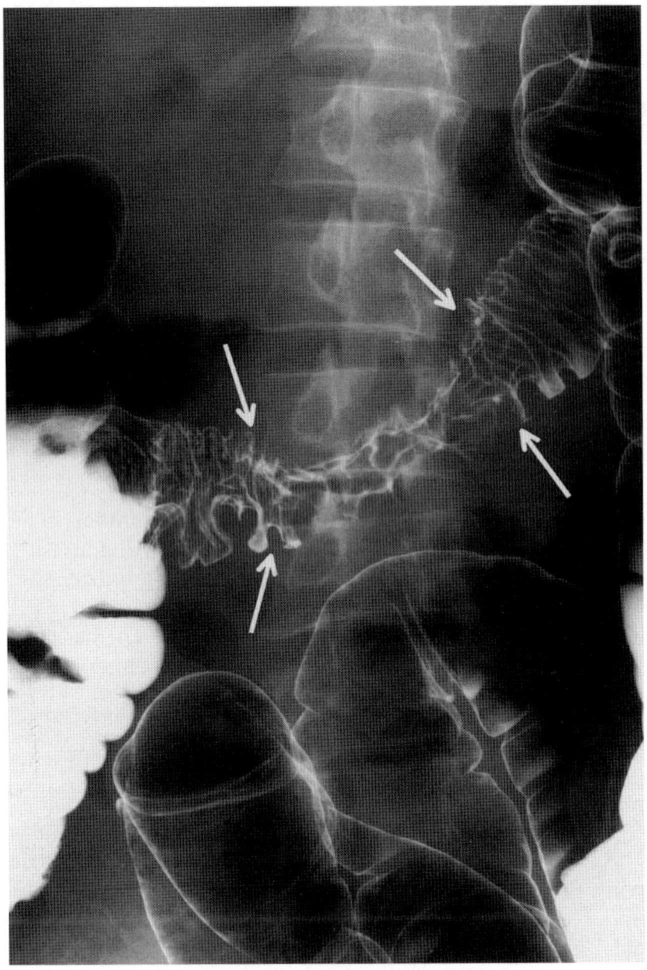

Figure 2. Barium enema examination shows mild annular narrowing of the transverse colon with thick interhaustral folds due to circumferential invasion by the small cell carcinoma. The proximal and distal margins of the lesion (arrows) are gradually tapered.

Microscopic examination obtained from colonoscopic biopsy showed that the mass is composed of small cells with hyperchromatic nuclei, coarse chromatin, inconspicuous nucleoli and little cytoplasm. Immunohistochemical examination revealed diffuse positivity for CD56, synaptophysin, and neuron-specific enolase, and negativity for cytokeratin, leukocyte common antigen, CD3 and CD20, which was consistent with small cell carcinoma. The patient is being treated by systemic chemotherapy.

Discussion

Extrapulmonary small cell carcinoma has been understood as a distinct disease entity with biological behaviour and prognosis different from those of other carcinomas of a given site [1, 2]. The pathological features of extrapulmonary small cell carcinoma are similar to those of pulmonary small cell carcinoma [5]. They have small neoplastic cells with a markedly hyperchromatic nucleus and scanty cytoplasm. They frequently showed neuroendocrine differentiation by immunohistochemical staining for neuron-specific enolase, chromogranin and synaptophysin [3].

The diagnosis of extrapulmonary small cell carcinoma of the colon should be made only when the possibility of metastasis from a tumour arising in the lung has been excluded. Although a chest CT scan was not performed in our case, chest radiographs were normal at presentation and remained normal over a 6 month follow up period.

Small cell carcinoma is rare in the colon or rectum, accounting for about 1.5% of all colorectal carcinomas [4]. In a review of previous reports on small cell carcinoma of the colon, radiological findings have not been described in the English literature. Our case showed a poorly enhancing bulky exophytic mass encircling the transverse colon on CT. The barium enema showed mild annular narrowing and thick interhaustral folds without overhanging edges, which were different from typical findings seen in ordinary annular colonic adenocarcinomas. Small cell carcinoma of the colon is a neuroendocrine tumour that can originate from the mucosa as well as the submucosa, and the barium enema appearances of our case were more suggestive of a submucosal lesion invading the mucosa than a mucosal lesion. However, the precise site of origin of the tumour could not be identified histologically because the pathological specimen was only obtained from colonoscopic biopsy, and not from a gross specimen obtained at operation. Additionally, our case could not easily be differentiated from circumferential involvement of the transverse colon by lymphoma from the CT and barium enema findings. Because colonic lymphomas are relatively less common and show diverse imaging features [7], specific differential imaging features between colonic lymphoma involvement and our case could not be found.

In conclusion, we present the barium study and CT findings of a very rare case of extrapulmonary small cell carcinoma of the colon.

References

1. Remick SC, Hafez GR, Carbone PP. Extrapulmonary small-cell carcinoma. A review of the literature with emphasis on therapy and outcome. Medicine 1987;66:457–71.
2. Galanis E, Frytak S, Lloyd RV. Extrapulmonary small cell carcinoma. Cancer 1997;79:1729–36.
3. Matsui K, Kitagawa M, Miwa A, Kuroda Y, Tsuji M. Small cell carcinoma of the stomach: a clinicopathologic study of 17 cases. Am J Gastroenterol 1991;86:1167–75.
4. Saclarides TJ, Szeluga D, Staren ED. Neuroendocrine cancers of the colon and rectum. Results of a ten-year experience. Dis Colon Rectum 1994;37:635–42.
5. Oesterling JE, Hauzeur CG, Farrow GM. Small cell anaplastic carcinoma of the prostate: a clinical, pathological and immunohistological study of 27 patients. J Urol 1992; 147:804–7.
6. Rubesin SE, Laufer I. Tumors of the colon. In: Levine MS, Rubesin SE, Laufer I, editors. Double contrast gastrointestinal radiology, Philadelphia, USA: Saunders, 2000:357–416.
7. Lee HJ, Han JK, Kim TK, Kim YH, Kim AY, Kim KW, et al. Primary colorectal lymphoma: spectrum of imaging findings with pathologic correlation. Eur Radiol 2002;12:2242–9.

The British Journal of Radiology, 78 (2005), 257–260
DOI: 10.1259/bjr/54676183

Case report
Pilomatrix carcinoma of the axilla: CT and MRI features

[1]T NIWA, MD, [1]T YOSHIDA, MD, [1]T DOIUCHI, MD, [2]T HIRUMA, MD, [2]K KUSHIDA, MD, [3]A MITSUDA, MD, [3]Y KAMEDA, MD, ^{3}H HAYASHI, MD, [4]K FUJII, MD and [5]T INOUE, MD

Departments of [1]Radiology, [2]Orthopaedic Surgery, [3]Pathology, Kanagawa Cancer Centre, 1-1-2 Nakao, Asahi-ku, Yokohama, 241-0815, [4]Depatment of Radiology, Yamato Tokusyukai Hospital, 4-4-12, Chuou, Yamato, 242-0021 and [5]Department of Radiology, Yokohama City University School of Medicine, 3-9 Fukuura, Kanazawa-ku, Yokohama, 236-0004, Japan

Abstract. Pilomatrix carcinoma, a rare malignant soft tissue tumour, is the malignant variant of pilomatricoma. We report a case of pilomatrix carcinoma of the axilla. CT demonstrated a well-circumscribed, sand-like calcified mass. MRI showed diffusely inhomogeneous, mixed signal intensities with inhomogeneous enhancements. The MRI findings were different from those previously reported for pilomatricoma.

Pilomatricoma is a rare benign dermal or subcutaneous tumour originating in the hair matrix, usually located in the head or neck [1, 2]. The malignant variant of pilomatricoma, called "pilomatrix carcinoma" or "calcified epithelial carcinoma of Malherbe" is extremely rare. To our knowledge, the imaging features of primary pilomatrix carcinoma of the axilla have not been previously reported. We report the radiological findings, including CT and MRI, in a case of pilomatrix carcinoma of the axilla.

Case report

A 54-year-old man was referred to our institution for left shoulder pain. Plain radiograph showed soft tissue lesion with calcifications in the left axilla (Figure 1a). The patient had not previously noticed this mass.

CT was performed after intravenous administration of contrast material and showed a well-defined, axillary soft tissue mass, 3 cm × 3.5 cm × 6 cm in size. The mass contained sand-like mottled calcifications and cystic components (Figure 1b). To further characterize the mass, MRI examination was performed with a 0.3 T unit (MRP-7000AD; Hitachi, Tokyo, Japan). MR sequences included spin-echo T_1 weighted images (repetition time (TR)= 600 ms, echo time (TE)=25 ms) before and after intravenous administration of gadolinium contrast agent (gadopentetate dimeglumine (0.5 mmol ml^{-1}), Magnevist; Nihon Schering, Osaka, Japan), and fast spin-echo T_2 weighted (TR=4000 ms, TE=117 ms, echo train length=8) images in axial and coronal planes. MRI demonstrated a well-circumscribed subcutaneous mass. Both T_1 and T_2 weighted images showed a diffusely inhomogeneous mass containing a mixture of low and high signal intensity areas (Figure 1c, d). Inhomogeneous enhancement was observed after intravenous administration of contrast agent (Figure 1e). No enhancement was observed in several portions of the mass. No neurovascular involvement was identified. Chest CT did not identify any metastases.

Surgical excision was performed. The excised specimen consisted of a multinodular mass in subcutaneous fat. The cut surface of the lesion showed multiple white nodules along with small calcifications and a cystic component (Figure 2a). Histological examination demonstrated nests of proliferating basaloid cells transitioning to shadow cells (Figure 2b). The tumour cells showed atypia and mitoses (Figure 2c). The cystic area contained necrotic debris. This histological pattern in association with the presence of shadow cells and increased mitotic activity led to the diagnosis of pilomatrix carcinoma.

Received 29 June 2004 and in revised form 22 September 2004, accepted 25 November 2004.

Discussion

Pilomatrix carcinoma is a rare malignant variant of pilomatricoma. Pilomatrix carcinomas occur more often in middle-aged to older individuals, more commonly in men, and show a predilection for the posterior neck, upper back and pre-auricular areas. The size of pilomatrix carcinoma has been reported ranging from 0.5 cm to 20 cm, with a mean of 3.95 cm, whereas that of pilomatricoma ranged from 0.5 cm to 3.0 cm [3]. The average size of these tumours is slightly larger than the size of benign pilomatrixomas [1].

To our knowledge only a few reports have described the imaging findings associated with pilomatrix carcinoma, and precise CT and MRI features of primary pilomatrix carcinoma have not been described. Venexan et al [4] reported a recurrent pilomatrix carcinoma invading the temporal bone in the post-auricular region and described the MRI findings of the tumour as containing a mixture of areas of mildly decreased signal intensity, thought to be due to the extensive calcification and scattered areas of high signal in T_2 weighted images. Campoy et al [2] reported MRI findings of a recurrent pilomatrix carcinoma of soft tissue in the back invading the spinal canal at the level of the mid thoracic spine. They described the lesion as having a long T_2 and intermediate signal intensity on T_1 weighted images [2]. However, the report did not describe precise MRI characteristics of the tumour.

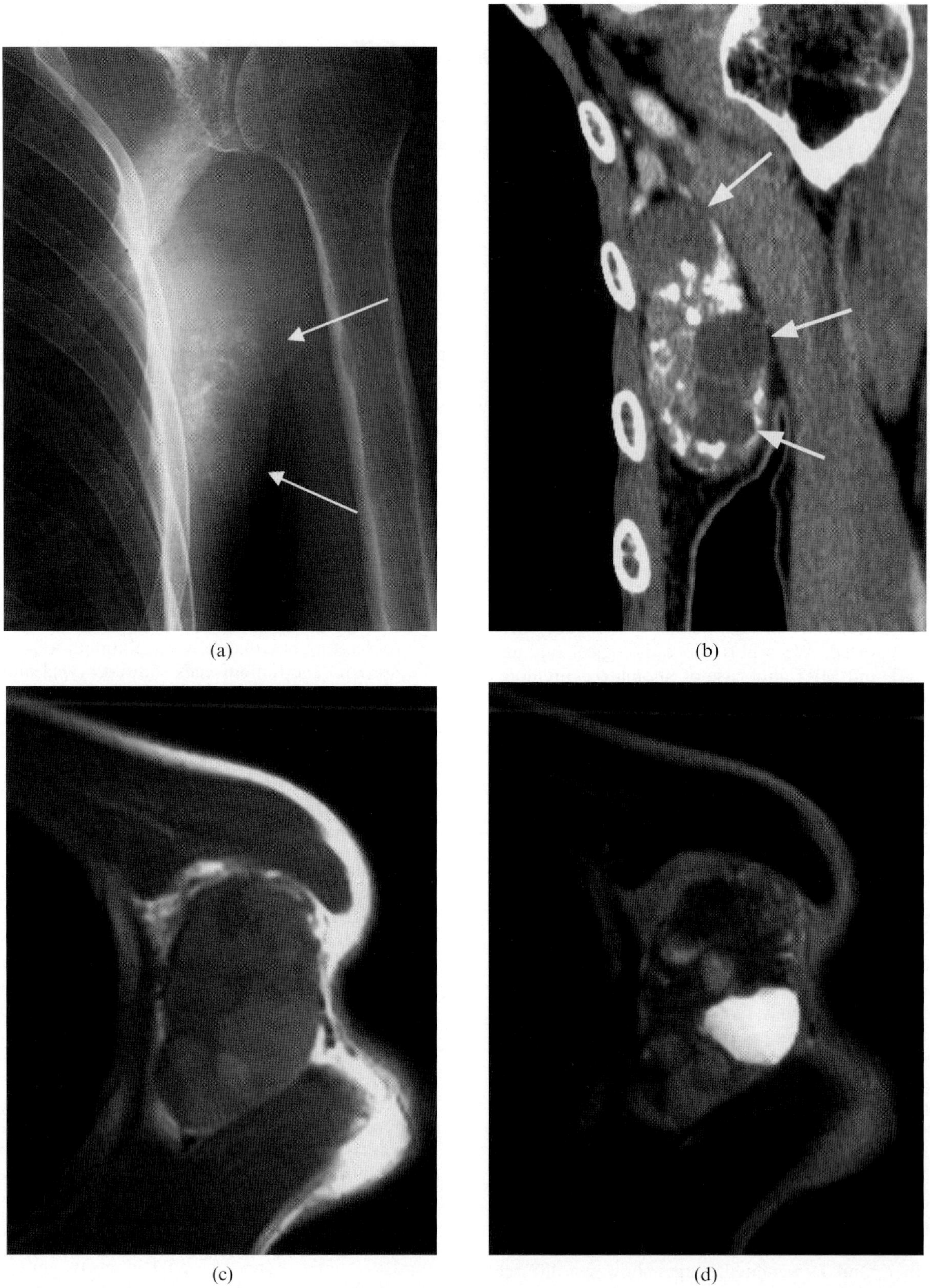

Figure 1. 54-year-old man with left axillar mass. (a) Plain radiograph shows a soft tissue mass with amorphous dotted calcifications in the left axilla (arrows). (b) Coronal multiplanar reformated CT image (window width=250 HU, window level=50 HU) after administration of intravenous contrast material shows a well-circumscribed mass with multiple small calcifications and cystic components (arrows). (c) Axial T_1 weighted MR image shows a diffusely inhomogeneous mass with a mixture of low signal intensity and slightly high signal intensity areas. (d) Axial T_2 weighted MR images shows a mixture of high signal intensity and low signal intensity areas. (*Continued.*)

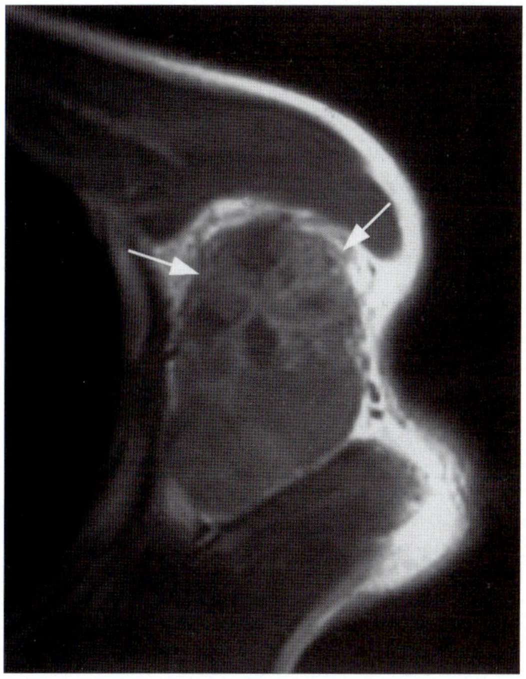

(e)

Figure 1. (*cont.*) (e) Axial T_1 weighted image after intravenous administration of gadolinium contrast agent (gadopentetate dimeglumine) shows diffusely inhomogeneous enhancement (arrows).

The radiological findings of a pilomatricoma typically demonstrate a well-circumscribed lesion with homogeneous or sand-like calcifications on plain radiograph and CT studies, and a homogeneous or slightly inhomogeneous mass on unenhanced and gadolinium containing contrast medium-enhanced MRI studies [5–7].

In the present case, plain radiographs and CT revealed a well-circumscribed, sand-like mottled calcified lesion, an appearance characteristic of pilomatricoma. However, MRI showed diffusely inhomogeneous areas, a finding not characteristic of pilomatricoma. Areas of low signal intensity in the T_2 weighted images may correspond to calcifications, and the diffusely inhomogeneous signal intensities observed with contrast medium enhancement may relate to varying degrees of proliferating tumour. The high signal intensity areas seen in the unenhanced T_1 and T_2 weighted images may represent cystic spaces forming in an area of tumour necrosis.

The histological appearance of a pilomatricoma typically shows small basophilic cells with large basophilic nuclei, scant cytoplasm, and poorly demarcated cell boundaries at the tumour periphery. Transition occurs toward the centre of the mass as cells lose basophilic nuclear material and transform into shadow (ghost) cells with a central pale area and a tendency to calcify [5, 8]. Common malignant features of pilomatrix carcinoma include proliferation of hyperchromatic and vesicular basaloid cells containing numerous mitoses, necrosis in

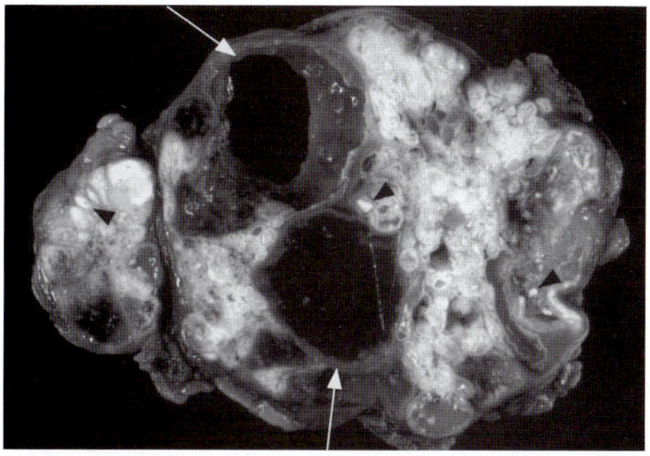

(a)

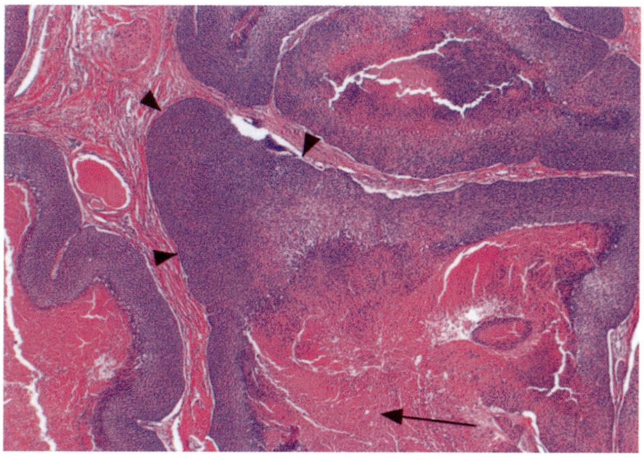

(b)

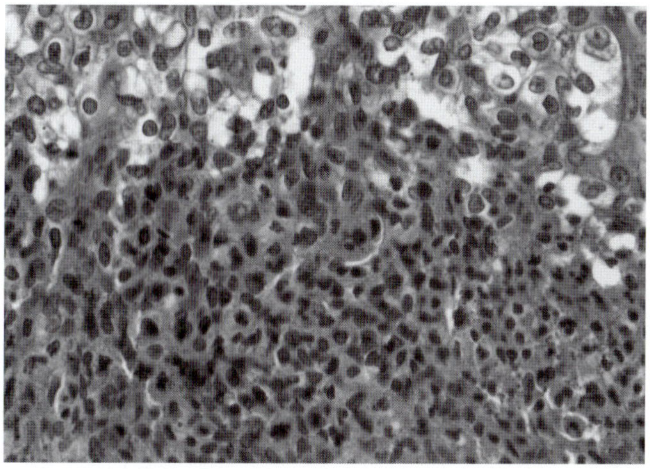

(c)

Figure 2. Pathological findings. (a) Cut surface of the excised specimen shows a multinodular mass with calcifications (arrowheads) and cystic components (arrows). (b) Microscopic examination shows a proliferation of basophilic cells (arrowheads) and shadow cells (arrow) (haematoxylin and eosin (H&E) $\times$ 40). (c) The tumour cells show pleomorphism, vesicular nucleus, mitoses, and prominent nucleoli (H&E $\times$ 400).

the centre of the lesion, and infiltration into fat or underlying structures [1, 8]. In the present case, the lesion contained mitoses and an area of necrosis, which are signs of malignancy. However, the tumour margin was well-circumscribed and no infiltrative changes were identified on both radiological and histological examination.

With regard to the biological behaviour of pilomatrix carcinoma, recurrence is a frequent event [8]. Wide excision should be a basic principle of treatment of pilomatrix carcinoma, which is associated with a low rate of tumour recurrence, whereas pilomatrix carcinoma recurred in more than 50% of cases in which a simple excision was performed [3]. Distant metastases are rare but have been reported in several cases. In the present case, the tumour was an incidental finding and there was no evidence of infiltration or metastasis.

In summary, we report a rare case of pilomatrix carcinoma in the axilla. Although the findings of a well-circumscribed mass and sand-like calcification are typical of pilomatricoma, the diffusely inhomogeneous MR findings with cystic changes are more suggestive of pilomatrix carcinoma.

References

1. Sau P, Lupton GP, Graham JH. Pilomatrix carcinoma. Cancer 1993;71:2491–8.
2. Campoy F Jr, Stiefel P, Stiefel E, Loizaga JM, Arduan J, Campoy F. Pilomatrix carcinoma: role played by MR imaging. Neuroradiology 1989;31:196–8.
3. Hardisson D, Linares MD, Cuevas-Santos J, Coutreas F. Pilomatrix carcinoma: a clinicopathologic study of six cases and review of the literature. Am J Dermatopathol 2001;23:394–401.
4. Vanexan KS, el Gammal T, Soong VY. Scalp pilomatrix carcinoma as an extra-axial mass. South Med J 1991;84:371–3.
5. De Beuckeleer LH, De Schepper AM, Neetens I. Magnetic resonance imaging of pilomatricoma. Eur Radiol 1996;6:72–5.
6. Ichikawa T, Nakajima Y, Fujimoto H, Koyama A, Honma M, Yatsuzuka M, et al. Giant calcifying epithelioma of Malherbe (pilomatrixoma): imaging features. Skeletal Radiol 1997;26: 602–5.
7. Haller JO, Kassner G, Ostrowitz A, Kottmeler K, Perfschuk LP. Pilomatrixoma (calcifying epithelioma of Malherbe): radiographic features. Radiology 1977;123:151–3.
8. Niedermeyer HP, Peris K, Hofler H. Pilomatrix carcinoma with multiple visceral metastases. Report of a case. Cancer 1996;77:1311–4.

The British Journal of Radiology, *78* (2005), 261–264
DOI: 10.1259/bjr/55389916

Case report

Successful treatment of a chronic post-traumatic 5-year-old osteoporotic vertebral compression fracture by percutaneous vertebroplasty

[1]F G IRANI, MBBS, MD, [1]J P MORALES, MD, [1]T SABHARWAL, MBBCH, FRCSI, FRCR, [1]R DOURADO, DCR, [1,2]A GANGI, MD, PhD and [1]A ADAM, FRCP, FRCS, FRCR

[1]*Department of Radiology, Guy's and St Thomas' Hospital, London, UK and* [2]*University Louis Pasteur, Strasbourg, France*

Abstract. Osteoporotic vertebral compression fracture (VCF) is a frequently encountered clinical problem associated with chronic pain and disability. Conservative treatment in the form of bed rest, pain control and bracing may create a vicious circle, in which reduced activity leads to further reduction in bone density and fracture risk. Percutaneous vertebroplasty (PVP) is an accepted treatment modality for osteoporotic vertebral body collapse present for less than 1 year, vertebral myeloma, haemangioma, metastasis and recent traumatic fractures (between 3 and 12 months). We describe an osteoporotic patient in whom successful PVP was performed, under general anaesthesia using CT and fluoroscopic guidance, in a post-traumatic 5-year-old VCF with complete alleviation of debilitating pain. In the light of our experience, we suggest that PVP should be carried out in a series of similar patients to asses its value as a treatment option in patients with chronic osteoporotic vertebral fractures for pain relief and improvement in mobility, independent of fracture age.

Osteoporosis is a chronic debilitating disease, which has reached epidemic proportions in Western societies and which has substantial social and economic consequences. Each year more than 700 000 vertebral compression fractures (VCFs) secondary to osteoporosis are diagnosed in the USA, resulting in 115 000 hospital admissions, 161 000 physician office visits and 5 million restricted activity days annually [1]. In the European Union there are said to be almost 435 000 VCF per year. Osteoporotic VCFs are a leading cause of disability and morbidity in the elderly, adversely affecting quality of life, physical function, psychosocial performance, mental health and survival [2, 3]. Treatment of VCFs is largely conservative, in the form of bed rest, pain control, and occasionally bracing. Hormone replacement therapy (HRT), calcitonin and biphosphonates are effective in maintaining or increasing bone mass and reducing the risk of compression fractures, but are often not prescribed until the disease is diagnosed by the presence of a fracture [4, 5]. Percutaneous vertebroplasty (PVP) with acrylic cement (polymethylmethacrylate, PMMA) is a minimally invasive procedure aimed at preventing further vertebral collapse and producing pain relief in patients with pathological vertebral bodies. It was first described by Galibert et al in 1984 for treatment of an aggressive vertebral haemangioma [6].

The procedure alleviates pain in 75–90% of patients with osteoporotic VCFs [3] and is now an established modality of treatment. Several studies have documented the effectiveness of PVP for pain relief in VCFs that are 1–4 months old [7]. This report describes a patient in whom PVP was performed in a chronic 5-year-old VCF with complete alleviation of debilitating pain.

Received 26 March 2004 and in final form 13 October 2004, accepted 25 November 2004.

Address correspondence to Dr Tarun Sabharwal, Consultant Radiologist, Department of Radiology, 1st Floor Lambeth Wing, St Thomas' Hospital, Lambeth Palace Road, London SE1 7EH, UK.

Case report

We were asked to consider a 58-year-old female patient with a chronic anterior wedge compression fracture of T12 vebebral body for PVP. The patient was a known asthmatic with reduced lung function and shortness of breath on exertion. She had been on long-term beclometasone therapy. In June 1997, following a horse-riding accident, she developed severe pain in the back. The plain thoracic radiographs revealed an anterior wedge compression fracture of the body of T12. She was treated conservatively with analgesics and bed rest. However her pain persisted.

In 2000–2001 she was referred to her local pain specialist and treated with several epidural injections of morphine but these did not relieve her pain. Therefore, an epidural catheter was introduced for patient controlled analgesia, which proved very effective. However, on three subsequent occasions, the procedure failed owing to entry site infection. The patient was then referred to our pain clinic. As further treatment with intrathecal opiates was considered inappropriate, we were asked to assess the feasibility of PVP.

Plain radiographs of the thoracolumbar spine showed an anterior wedge compression fracture of the T12 vertebral body with 25–40% reduction in height. A limited CT study with sagittal reconstruction showed no obvious disruption of the anterior and posterior vertebral walls and intact superior and inferior endplates. The bones showed evidence of reduced mineral content suggestive of osteoporosis, which was confirmed by a dual energy X-ray absorptiometry (DXA) scan.

We explained to the patient that published studies have shown vertebroplasty to be successful in the treatment of recent traumatic vertebral fractures (3–12 months) and that the likelihood of pain relief was uncertain in relation to chronic fractures. On examination, there was severe localized tenderness at the T12 vertebral spinous process without kyphotic deformity.

A pre-procedure MRI scan revealed anterior wedging of the T12 vertebral body, with minimal posterior retropulsion causing indentation on the thecal sac. However the involved vertebral body was isointense on T_1 weighted scan and showed minimal signal increase on T_2 weighting (Figure 1a) and short tau inversion recovery (STIR) sequences (Figure 1b). The scan showed no evidence of facet arthropathy, spinal canal stenosis or disc herniation. Full informed written consent was obtained. The procedure was performed in the CT suite under general anaesthesia, as the patient was not able to tolerate sedoanalgesia. Blood pressure, ECG and oxygen saturation were monitored continuously. She was placed prone on the CT table and the procedure performed under combined CT and fluoroscopic guidance.

Using a posterior lateral approach, the overlying skin, subcutaneous tissue and periosteum of T12 vertebra were infiltrated with local anaesthetic. An 11 G bone biopsy needle (OptiMed Cemento set, High Wycombe, UK), was introduced into the centre of the T12 vertebral body via a

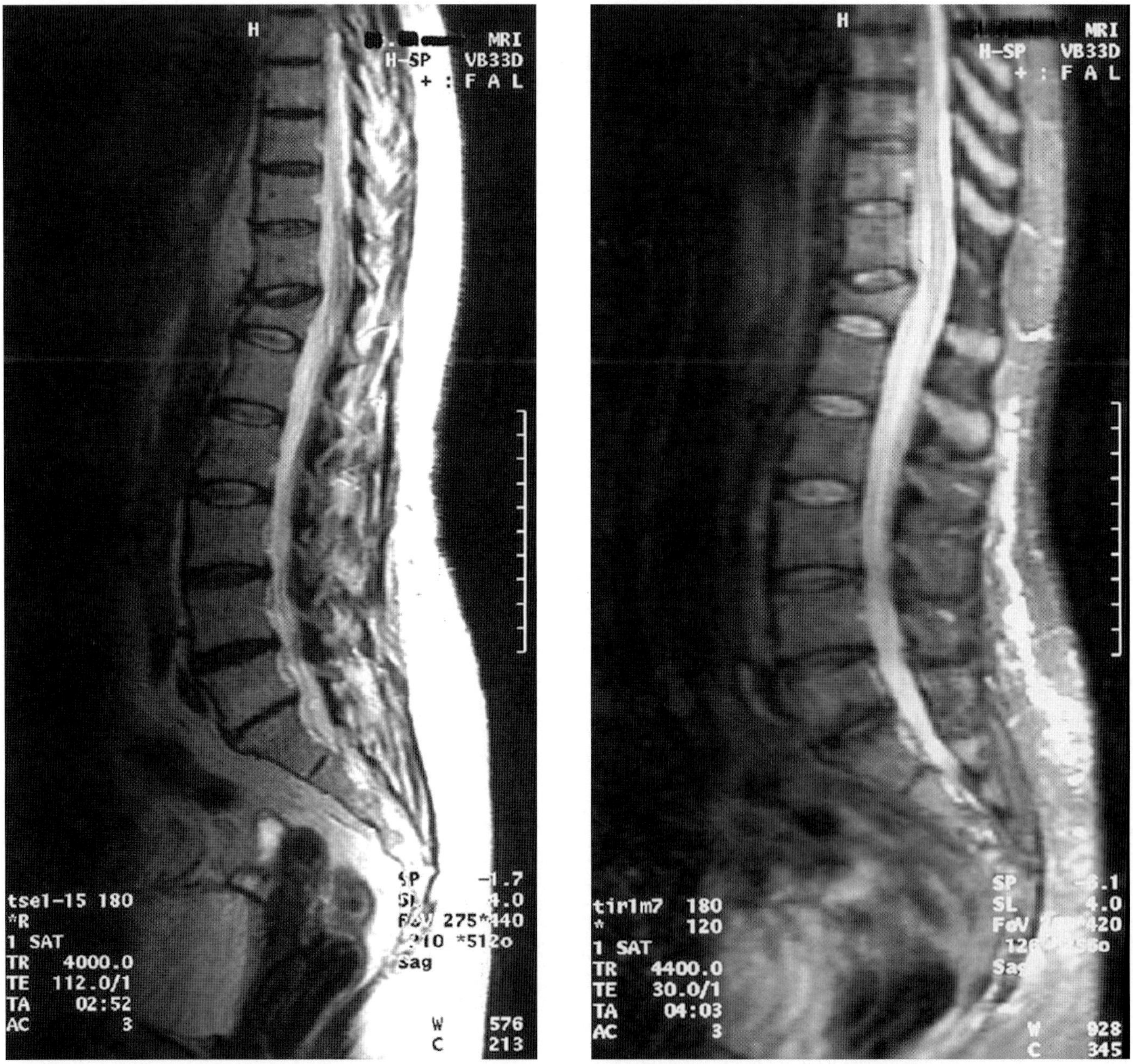

(a) (b)

Figure 1. (a) T_2 weighted and (b) short tau inversion recovery (STIR) images showing anterior wedge compression of T12 vertebra with minimal increase in signal intensity of the vertebral body.

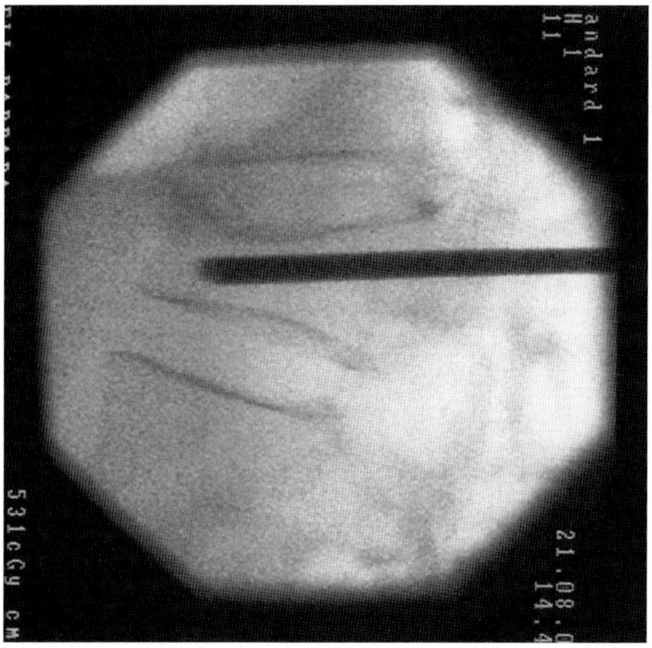

Figure 2. Lateral radiograph showing final placement of needle in the anterior portion of the T12 vertebral body.

unilateral left intercostovertebral route. Once satisfactory placement of the needle was confirmed on fluoroscopy and CT (Figure 2), 4 ml of cement (PMMA) (Osteopal® V Vertebroplasty; Biomet Merck, Altdorf, Switzerland) was injected into the vertebral body, under continuous lateral fluoroscopic control. Fluoroscopy and CT images showed adequate filling of the cement in the anterior two-thirds of the vertebral body (Figure 3). No epidural, paravertebral, discal or venous leakage of cement was noted.

At 24 h follow up, the patient reported significant pain relief and decreased need for analgesics. On 3, 6 and 12 monthly follow up the patient has had complete pain relief

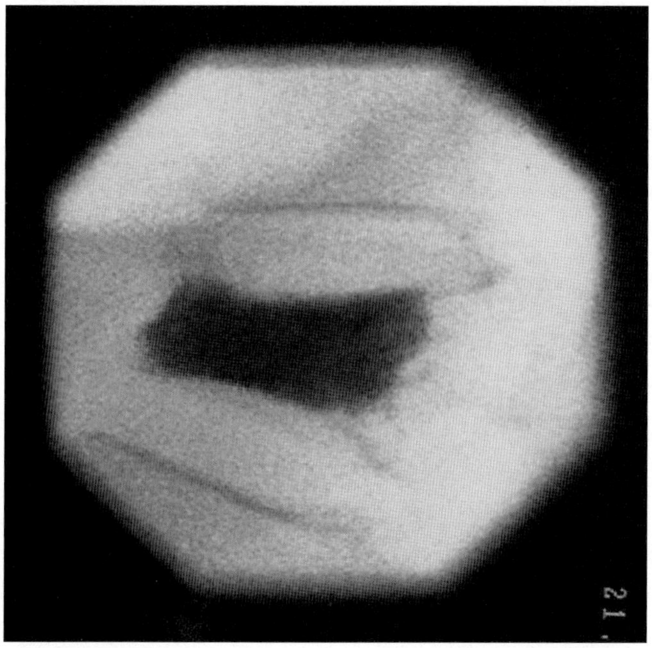

Figure 3. Lateral radiograph demonstrating adequate filling of the anterior two-thirds vertebral body with cement (PMMA).

from the T12 compression fracture site, with no use for narcotic analgesics.

Discussion

Osteoporosis, as a result of bone mineral loss may be primary (age related) or secondary (commonly due to steroid use) [3, 8]. Chronic steroid use for asthma, chronic obstructive airways disease, rheumatoid arthritis, lymphoma, multiple myeloma and transplantation predispose to the development of secondary osteoporosis and insufficiency fractures due to accelerated bone resorption by osteoclasts [3]. Cumulative prednisolone doses are strongly associated with the risk of development of vertebral fractures [9]. Our patient was a post-menopausal woman on long term steroid therapy for asthma, both of which are high risk factors for the development of osteoporosis and VCF. PVP is the injection of radio-opaque bone cement (*e.g.* PMMA) into the painful osteoporotic compression fracture or painful pathological vertebral body (*e.g.* multiple myeloma, metastatic disease and haemangioma), with use of imaging guidance [10]. It is an established therapeutic alternative for treatment of painful VCFs in patients refractory to medical and conservative treatment, where surgery is poorly tolerated and frequently unsuccessful due to the poor quality of osteoporotic bone. Surgery is usually employed in patients with neurogenic complications [11]. PVP has been shown to be effective in acute and subacute fractures, 1 to 4 months old [7]. A recent study suggests treatment within a few weeks of a painful VCF, as a lengthy period of non-operative treatment may lead to continued collapse of the fractured vertebra [8]. Indications for intervention within days of a painful VCF include post-fracture complications such as pneumonia and thrombophebitis, and intolerance to narcotic analgesics [8]. However, it is safest to perform the procedure 3–4 weeks after the fracture, to allow time for consolidation of the fractured posterior elements and clotting of the venous plexus, both of which help to decrease the risk of leakage of cement [11].

According to Gangi et al [12] the ideal candidate for PVP is one who presents within 4 months of the fracture, has midline non-radiating back pain that increases with weight bearing and which is exacerbated by manual palpation of the spinous process of the involved vertebra.

Treatment after 6 months was thought to be less successful in relieving pain [3]. However, there is increasing evidence of the usefulness of PVP in the treatment of chronic osteoporotic VCFs. Kaufmann et al [7] found PVP to provide very effective pain relief and improvement in mobility in chronic VCFs (duration of pain before PVP ranging from 1 week to 104 weeks, mean 19 weeks) with a reduction in the requirement of analgesia. They concluded that patient selection for PVP should not be based on the age of the VCF but on evidence of non-healing of the fracture on the isotope bone scans or MRI images. Brown et al [13] in a retrospective review of 41 patients with symptomatic VCF with mean and median fracture ages of 40.4 months and 28 months, respectively, reported pain relief in 80% patients and improved mobility in 49% patients following PVP. Our case suggests that PVP may be beneficial in the treatment of 5-year-old chronic fractures. Bone scans are helpful in differentiating acute from chronic fractures. Acute fractures show increased uptake of tracer and are highly predictive of positive clinical response after PVP [3]. However, increased tracer uptake may be seen as long as 12 months after fracture [3, 7]. MRI is very useful in patient selection as it provides both functional and anatomical information. Marrow signal changes help determine the age of the fracture. Acute and subacute fractures are hypointense on T_1 weighted images and hyperintense on T_2 weighted and STIR sequences suggestive of marrow oedema [3, 8]. Fully healed compression fractures become isointense to normal bone marrow on T_1 and T_2 weighted sequences. Hypointense signal on both T_1 and T_2 weighted images is suggestive of healing with sclerosis. If suspected a confirmatory CT scan should be performed, as needle placement and injection of PMMA in such cases will be difficult and yield suboptimal radiological and clinical results [3].

In our patient, the MR was equivocal and showed the involved vertebra to be isointense to bone marrow on T_1 weighting, with only minimal increased signal on T_2 weighted and STIR images. There is anecdotal evidence that equivocal non-contrast MRI scans in patients with severe pain would benefit from gadolinium enhancement as the involved vertebrae show contrast enhancement and they do well with PVP.

Pain in VCFs is thought to be caused by compressive forces acting on the nociceptor endings within the bone matrix. Increasing the rigidity and strength of the bone through the injection and subsequent hardening of PMMA cement reduces bone deformation and painful micromotion at the fracture site. This is the consolidation effect. In addition, pain relief is thought to be affected by the destruction of sensitive nerve endings in the matrix by the PMMA cement, which is directly toxic because of enhanced production of free oxygen radicals and heating during cement polymerization [8, 12, 14].

Immediate and long-term outcomes of PVP are very encouraging. Immediate pain relief within 24–48 h after PVP has been seen in 75–90% of patients [10, 12, 13, 15, 16]. In our patient both immediate and long term (14 months) pain relief was noted with significant improvement in her mobility. In view of our experience in this case, we suggest that a study of the effectiveness of PVP in VCFs over 1 year old is indicated.

References

1. Riggs BL, Melton LJ III. The world wide problem of osteoporosis: insights afforded by epidemiology. Bone 1995;17(s):505–11.
2. Phillips FM. Minimal invasive treatment of osteoporotic vertebral compression fractures. Spine 2003;28(s):45–53.
3. Bernadette Stallemeyer MJ, Zoarski GH, Obuchowski AM. Optimising patient selection in percutaneous vertebroplasty. JVIR 2003;14:683–96.
4. Kim DH, Silber JS, Albert TJ. Osteoporotic vertebral compression fracture. Instr Course Lect 2003;52:541–50.
5. McGraw JK, Lippert JA, Minkus KD, Rami PM, Davis TM, Budzik RF. Prospective evaluation of pain relief in 100 patients undergoing percutaneous vertebroplasty: results and follow up. JVIR 2002;13:883–6.
6. Galibert P, Deramond H, Rosat P, Le Gars D. Preliminary note on the treatment of vertebral angioma by percutaneous acrylic vertebroplasty. Neurochirugie 1987;33:166–8.
7. Kaufmann TJ, Jensen ME, Schweickert PA, Marks WF, Kallmes DF. Age of fracture and clinical outcome of percutaneous vertebroplasty. AJNR Am J Neuroradiol 2001;22:1860–3.
8. Mathis JM, Barr JD, Belkoff SM, Barr MS, Jensen ME, Deramond H. Percutaneous vertebroplasty: a developing standard of care for vertebral compression fractures. AJNR Am J Neuroradiol 2001;22:373–81.
9. Walsh LJ, Lewis SA, Wong CA, et al. The impact of oral corticosteriod use on bone mineral density and vertebral fractures. Am J Respir Crit Care Med 2002;166:691–5.
10. McGraw K, Cardella J, Barr JD, et al. Society of interventional radiology quality improvement guidelines for percutaneous vertebroplasty. JVIR 2003;14(s):311–5.
11. Garfin SR, Reilley MA. Minimally invasive treatment of osteoporotic vertebral body compression fracture. Spine J 2002;2:76–80.
12. Gangi A, Guth S, Imbert JP, Marin H, Dietemann JL. Percutaneous vertebroplasty: Indications, technique, and results. RadioGraphics 2003;23:e10; published online as 10.1148/rg.e10.
13. Brown DB, Gilula LA, Sehgal M, Shimony JS. Treatment of chronic symptomatic vertebral compression fractures with percutaneous vertebroplasty. AJR Am J Roentgenol 2004;182:319–22.
14. Niv D, Gofeld M, Devor M. Causes of pain in degenerative bone and joint disease: a lesson from vertebroplasty. Pain 2003;105:387–92.
15. Grados F, Depriester C, Cayrolle G, Hardy N, Deramond H, Fardellone P. Long term observations of vertrebal osteoporotic fractures treated by percutaneous vertebroplasty. Rheumatology 2000;39:1410–4.
16. Cortet B, Cotten A, Boutry N, Flipo RM, et al. Percutaneous vertebroplasty in the treatment of osteoporotic vertebral compression fractures: an open prospective study. J Rheumatol 1999;10:2222–8.

The British Journal of Radiology, 78 (2005), 265–268
DOI: 10.1259/bjr/30325507

Case report

Pseudocyst rupture into the portal vein diagnosed with MRI

A RIDDELL, MB BS, FRCS, FRCR, K JHAVERI, MD and M HAIDER, MD, FRCP(C)

Department of Medical Imaging, University Health Network, Princess Margaret Hospital, 610 University Avenue, Toronto, M5G 2M9, Canada

Abstract. We report on the first documented case of rupture of a pancreatic pseudocyst into the portal vein diagnosed with MRI.

The development of a pseudocyst is a common complication of pancreatitis. Complications related to pseudocysts include rupture into adjacent viscera [1, 2], haemorrhage [3], disseminated fat necrosis [4, 5], arthritis [6], and vascular complications – pseudoaneurysm formation [7] and portal vein thrombosis [8, 9]. Pseudocyst rupture into either the portal or splenic vein is a rare complication. The diagnosis is usually made at endoscopic retrograde cholangiopancreatography (ERCP) or surgery. We report a case where this diagnosis was made with MRI and describe the MRI features. After an extensive literature search we believe this is the first documented case where the diagnosis was made using this technique.

Case report

A 42-year-old female was transferred to our institution for management of the complications of chronic pancreatitis. She had no history of gallstones or alcohol abuse. At the time of transfer she was haemodynamically stable, afebrile with no signs of sepsis. An ultrasound on admission showed large volume ascites and a pseudocyst in the region of the neck of the pancreas. Analysis of the ascitic fluid showed a high amylase content 272 U l^{-1} (normal <1). A CT scan confirmed the presence of a 3 cm pseudocyst posterior to the neck of the pancreas. No contrast was present within the portal vein and there was cavernous transformation at the porta hepatis indicating this to be chronic (Figure 1). Sludge was present within the gallbladder, but no calculi.

The patient was discharged but re-admitted a month later. In the interim she had suffered a pulmonary embolism and was treated with warfarin sodium (Coumadin; Bristol-Myers Squibb Pharma Company, New York, NY). Her international normalized ratio (INR) was difficult to stabilize and anticoagulation was complicated by a retroperitoneal bleed. She was re-admitted for the insertion of an inferior vena cava (IVC) filter and for anticoagulation stabilization. On admission her INR was 1.1 and her activated partial thromboplastin time (aPPT) 45.5 s (range 28–40 s). CT was performed confirming a large retroperitoneal haematoma within the left psoas muscle. The pancreatic pseudocyst was still present and remained stable in size. An ultrasound confirmed lack of flow within the portal vein and also showed similar echogenic debris within the portal vein and pseudocyst (Figures 2a, b). MRI was performed during the same admission, which confirmed the presence of a large left psoas muscle haematoma. The signal intensity of the portal vein was that of fluid (low on T_1 and high on T_2 weighted images with no enhancement following gadolinium administration) rather than blood products, as would be expected in portal vein thrombosis. The T_2 weighted breath-hold fast recovery sequence (Figure 3a) showed similar high signal intensity within the portal vein as seen in the intrahepatic bile ducts, rather than the signal void expected from a patent portal vein. The T_1 weighted coronal images (Figure 3b, c) demonstrate homogeneous low signal within the pseudocyst and portal vein confirming the presence of fluid, rather than thrombus within these structures. The T_2 weighted radial slab (Figure 4) showed similar signal intensity returned from the biliary tree, pseudocyst and portal vein. Direct

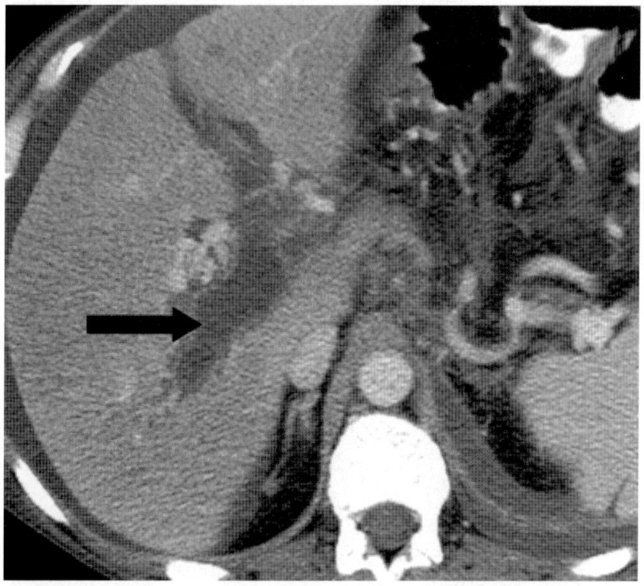

Figure 1. This contrast enhanced CT shows low attenuation thrombus within the portal vein (black arrow) and small serpiginous contrast filled collaterals indicative of cavernous transformation.

Received 12 March 2004 and in revised form 19 October 2004, accepted 25 November 2004.

Current address for Dr Angela Riddell, Department of Radiology, The Royal Marsden Trust, Downs Road, Sutton, Surrey SM2 5PT, UK.

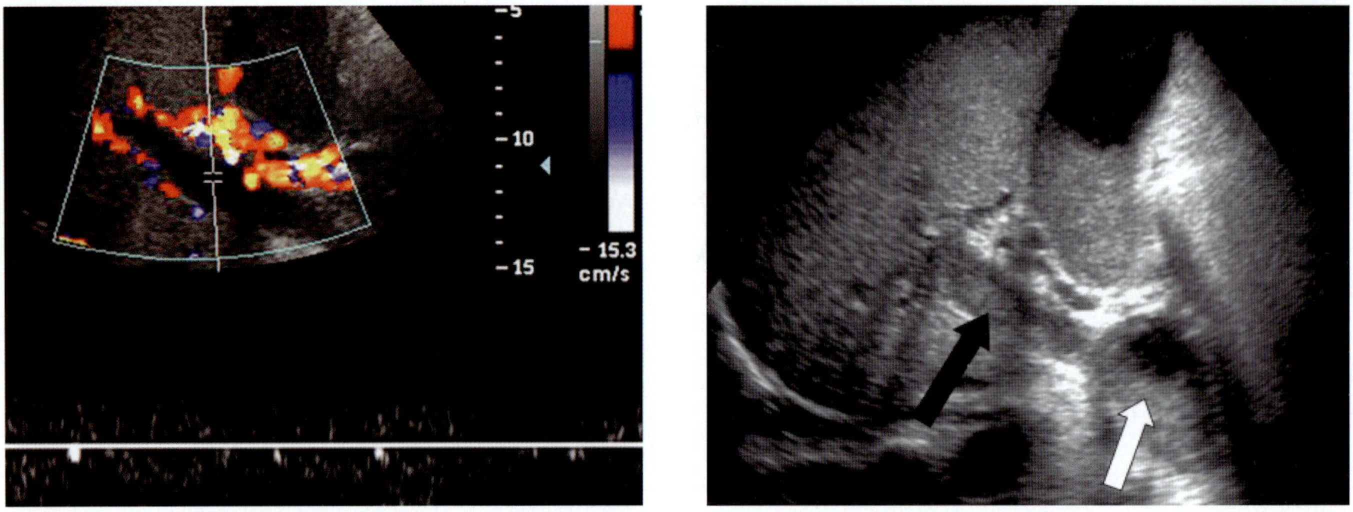

(a) (b)

Figure 2. (a) Lack of flow within the portal vein is confirmed on ultrasound, with no flow on the spectral Doppler trace. Colour Doppler signal is seen in the portal collaterals. (b) This grey scale image shows echogenic material within the portal vein (black arrow), which is similar in appearance to that seen in the pseudocyst (white arrow). Sludge is seen layering in the gallbladder.

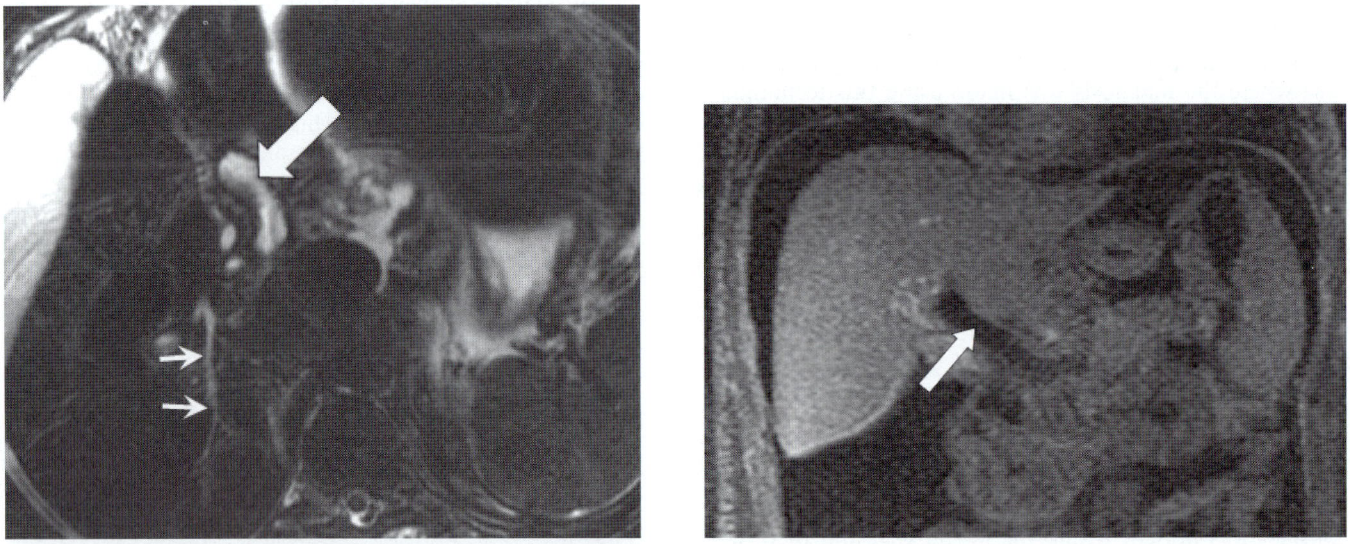

(a) (b)

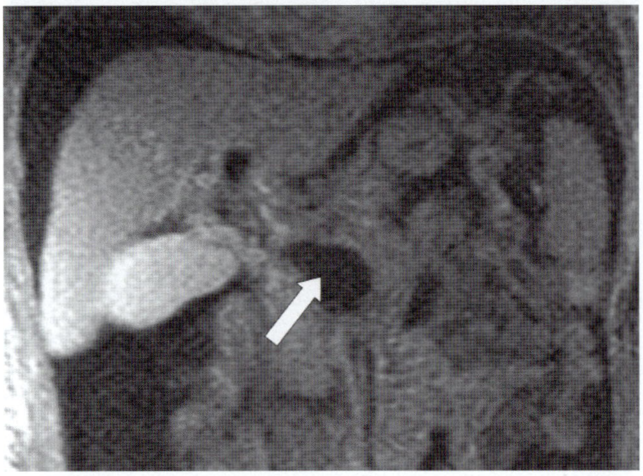

(c)

Figure 3. (a) Axial breath hold fast recovery (BHFR) T_2 weighted image shows high signal fluid within the left portal vein (white arrow) and also within biliary radicals (white arrow heads). On this sequence flowing blood within a normal portal vein would be of low signal intensity, and thrombus of heterogeneous intermediate signal intensity. The pseudocyst, which is caudal to this image, had the same signal intensity as the portal vein. The patient also has ascites, predominantly surrounding the anterolateral margin of the liver. (b, c) Coronal T_1 weighted images show homogeneous low signal intensity within (b) the portal vein (white arrow) and (c) anterior pseudocyst (white arrow), consistent with fluid rather than thrombus.

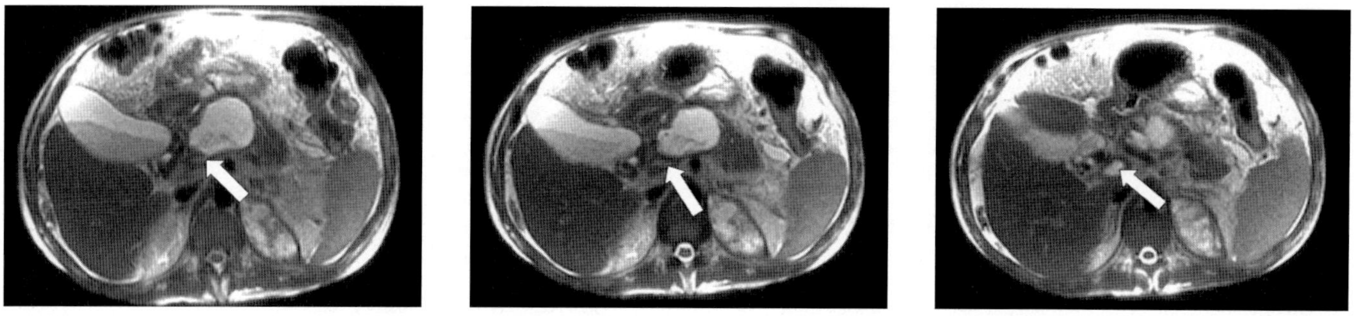

(a) (b) (c)

Figure 5. A series of three axial single shot fast spin echo (SSFSE) T_2 weighted images show a tract passing from (a) the posterior aspect of the pseudocyst to (c) the main portal vein.

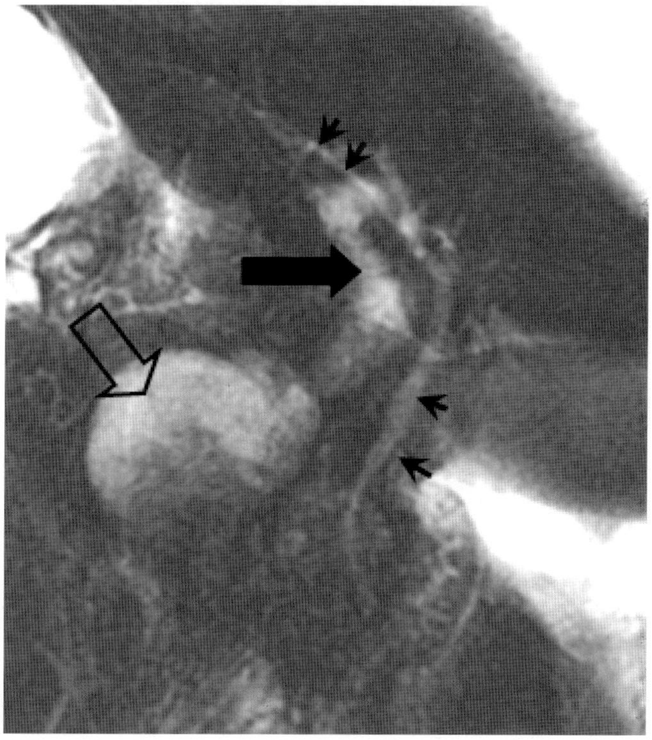

Figure 4. This T_2 weighted radial slab image shows high signal fluid within the common bile duct and biliary tree (black arrowheads), the pseudocyst (open black arrow) and the portal vein (black arrow). Signal would not normally be returned from flowing blood within the portal vein.

communication between the portal vein and the pseudocyst was demonstrated on axial single shot fast spin echo (SSFSE) T_2 images (Figure 5). No communication was seen between the pancreatic duct and the pseudocyst. The patient remains asymptomatic from the pancreatic-portal vein fistula and she has been treated conservatively but is under close clinical surveillance.

Discussion

The mechanism of the fistula formation is controversial, but it has been hypothesized that it occurs soon after thrombosis of the portal vein, when the portal system is cut off from the systemic circulation. The pancreatic enzymes then cause erosion of the wall of the vein and breakdown the fresh thrombus, substituting the vein contents with material from the pseudocyst [10].

There have been 11 cases of a fistulous communication between a pancreatic pseudocyst and either the portal or splenic vein reported to date. All these patients had a history of chronic pancreatitis secondary to alcohol abuse [4, 6, 9–17]. The majority of patients presented with abdominal pain, some with acute-on-chronic pancreatitis. Several showed signs of disseminated fat necrosis and arthritis [6, 11, 13, 15]. In the cases described to date, the diagnosis has been made by invasive imaging techniques such as ERCP (five cases) or surgically (three cases). Two cases were diagnosed by percutaneous splenoportography [16].

In our case the diagnosis was made with MRI, which confirmed the presence of the fistulous tract and the presence of static fluid within the portal venous system giving supportive evidence of the pseudocyst-portal vein communication. This provided a definitive diagnosis in a non-invasive manner. Although ERCP does provide a dynamic view of the ductal and portal systems it is invasive, with a 6.7% risk of inducing pancreatitis [18]. Also, if there is no communication between the main pancreatic duct and the pseudocyst, the pseudocyst-portal fistula will not be demonstrated at ERCP. The treatment depends on the patient's clinical symptoms. Asymptomatic patients, such as in our case, have been treated conservatively. Patients with signs of sepsis or disseminated fat necrosis are usually treated surgically by a pancreaticoenterostomy. We feel this case report illustrates the great strength of MRI, with its ability to characterize different soft tissue elements and highlights its use in the diagnosis of this rare complication of pancreatitis. Thus obviating the need for an invasive means of diagnosis.

References

1. Shah P, Pamakan R. Spontaneous rupture of a pseudocyst of the pancreas into the stomach. Am J Gastroenterol 1989;84:1466–7.
2. Sbrocehi RD, Anderson MC. Erosion of adjacent organs by pancreatic pseudocysts. Am Surg 1984;50:191–6.
3. Kelly SB, Gauhar T, Pollard R. Massive haemorrhage from a pancreatic pseudocyst. Am J Gastroenterol 1999;94:3638–41.
4. Zeller M, Hetz HH. Rupture of a pancreatic cyst into the portal vein. Report of a case and generalized fat necrosis. JAMA 1966;195:181–5.

5. Sorensen EV. Subcutaneous fat necrosis. A review and two case reports. J Clin Gastroenterol 1988;10:71–5.
6. Hammar A, Sand J, Lumio J, Hirn M, Honkonen S, Tuominen L, et al. Pancreatic pseudocystportal vein fistula manifests as residivating oligoarthritis, subcutaneous, bursal and osseal necrosis: a case report and review of literature. Hepato-Gastroenterology 2002;49:273–8.
7. White AF, Baum S, Buranasiri. Aneurysms secondary to pancreatitis. AJR Am J Roentgenol 1976;127:393–6.
8. Warshaw AL, Jin G, Ottinger LW. Recognition and clinical implications of mesenteric and portal vein obstruction in chronic pancreatitis. Arch Surg 1987;122:410–5.
9. McCormick PA, Chronos N, Burroughs AK, McIntyre N, McLaughline JE. Pancreatic pseudocyst causing portal vein thrombosis and pancreatico-pleural fistula. Gut 1990;31: 561–3.
10. Procacci C, Mansueto GC, Graziani R, Bicego E, Pederzoli P, Mainardi P, et al. Spontaneous rupture of a pancreatic pseudocyst into the portal vein. Cardiovasc Interv Radiol 1995;18:399–402.
11. Skarsgard ED, Ellison E, Quenville N. Spontaneous rupture of a pancreatic pseudocyst into the portal vein. Can J Surg 1995;38:459–63.
12. Yamamoto T, Hayakawa K, Kawakami S, Nishimura K, Katsuma Y, Hayashi N, et al. Rupture of a pancreatic pseudocyst into the portal venous system. Abdom Imaging 1999;24:494–6.
13. Potts JR. Pancreatic-portal vein fistula with disseminated fat necrosis treated by pancreaticoduodenectomy. Southern Med J 1991;84:632–5.
14. Steenberg WV, Ponette E. Pancreaticoportal fistula: a rare complication of chronic pancreatitis. Gastrointest Radiol 1990;15:299–300.
15. Willis SM, Brewer T. Pancreatic duct-portal vein fistula. Gastroenterology 1989;97:1025–7.
16. Takayama T, Kato K, Sano H, Katada N, Takeichi M. Spontaneous rupture of a pancreatic pseudocyst into the portal venous system. AJR Am J Roentgenol 1986;147:935–6.
17. Takayma T, Kato K, Katada N, Nishimura D, Shibata T, Kato K, et al. Radiological demonstration of spontaneous rupture of a pancreatic pseudocyst into the portal system. Am J Gastroenterol 1982;76:55–8.
18. Freeman ML, DiSario JA, Nelson DB, Fennerty MB, Lee JG, Bjorkman DJ, et al. Risk factors for post-ERCP pancreatitis: a prospective, multicenter study. Gastrointest Endosc 2001;54:425–34.

The British Journal of Radiology, 78 (2005), 269–271
DOI: 10.1259/bjr/28214940

Case report

Erythropoietin-producing renal cell carcinoma arising from autosomal dominant polycystic kidney disease

[1]Y HAMA, MD, [1]T KAJI, MD, [2]K ITO, MD, [2]M HAYAKAWA, MD, [1]M TOBE, MD and [1]S KOSUDA, MD

Departments of [1]Radiology and [2]Urology, National Defense Medical College, 3-2 Namiki, Tokorozawa, Saitama, Japan

Abstract. Erythropoietin (EPO)-producing renal cell carcinomas (RCC) in patients with chronic renal failure secondary to autosomal dominant polycystic kidney disease (ADPKD) has not previously been reported. We report a case of EPO-producing RCC associated with ADPKD in a 66-year-old woman, and discuss the clinical and radiological findings.

Erythropoietin (EPO)-producing renal cell carcinomas (RCC) in patients with chronic renal failure is uncommon [1]. The occurrence of EPO-producing RCC in a patient with autosomal dominant polycystic kidney disease (ADPKD) has not previously been reported [2–4]. Here, we report a case of EPO-producing RCC in a patient with ADPKD and discuss the clinical and radiological findings.

Case report

A 66-year-old woman, receiving maintenance haemodialysis for 8 years owing to chronic renal failure secondary to ADPKD, was referred to our institution for evaluation of polycythaemia. She had manifested no anaemia for more than 4 months without using recombinant human EPO. Her red blood cell count was 606×10^6 cells mm^{-3}, the haemoglobin concentration was 16.4 g dl^{-1}, and the haematocrit was 53.3%. The serum EPO level was 893 mU ml^{-1} (normal: 9.1–32.8 mU ml^{-1}). Ultrasound (US) scan showed a homogeneous, round, echogenic area medial to the middle of the left kidney (Figure 1a). Contrast-enhanced CT scan obtained during the nephrographic phase showed a homogeneously enhancing mass arising from the medial aspect of the left kidney (Figure 1b). On digital subtraction angiography, the lesion was shown to be highly vascularized and supplied mainly by direct branches of the left renal artery (Figure 1c). Pre-operative selective embolisation of the left renal artery was performed using gelatin sponge particles. She underwent radical nephrectomy with curative intent. Pathological examination revealed clear cell RCC. Immunohistochemical staining of the resected specimens showed production of erythropoietin in the tumour cells. Although an elevated serum EPO level decreased to 61 mU ml^{-1} 2 weeks after the nephrectomy. Based on the immunohistochemical and clinical findings, EPO was considered to be produced by RCC arising from ADPKD.

Discussion

Serum erythropoietin may be increased in patients on chronic haemodialysis secondary to acquired polycystic disease of the kidneys. The development of RCC in ADPKD is rare and the association of RCC and ADPKD is controversial [2, 3, 5]. The majority of reported cases have been shown to be an incidental finding either on surgical exploration or at autopsy [6]. The serum EPO level is usually low in long-term haemodialysis patients with anaemia [7]. However, increased levels of serum EPO and haemoglobin have been observed in haemodialysis patients because the renal proximal tubule cells produce EPO into the fluid of cysts [4, 8, 9]. Thus, the diagnosis of EPO-producing RCC in such cases is difficult due to overlapping clinical features and marked distortion of architecture [10].

US often fails to reliably differentiate benign haemorrhagic cysts from other complications in patients with ADPKD [11]. CT remains the most widely used modality for assessment and has helped refine the diagnostic work-up of renal masses by allowing image acquisition in various phases of renal enhancement after intravenous administration of a single bolus of contrast material. The nephrographic phase is the most sensitive for tumour detection [12], because the renal parenchyma enhances homogeneously in this phase, allowing a better opportunity for discrimination between the normal renal medulla and masses [13]. In end-stage ADPKD, most of the renal parenchyma is replaced by cysts and fibrotic tissues, and detection of RCC becomes much easier because of the intense enhancement of RCC.

MRI has certain advantages in evaluating patients with ADPKD. The high soft tissue contrast resolution to evaluate the kidneys, cysts, and the possible development of cancer, have shown MRI to be of particular importance in assessing ADPKD patients and defining the possible development of RCC [14]. However, in the present case, clinical signs, US and CT findings were sufficient to reach a pre-operative diagnosis of RCC, and further investigation by MRI was not necessary. Selective angiography, performed for pre-operative embolisation of the tumour vessels, strongly suggested the diagnosis of RCC, although the availability of reliable non-invasive investigations, routine diagnostic angiography is no longer recommended [15].

In conclusion, although a single case cannot be generalized to other ADPKD cases, a continuous increase

Received 1 September 2004 and in revised form 8 October 2004, accepted 6 December 2004.

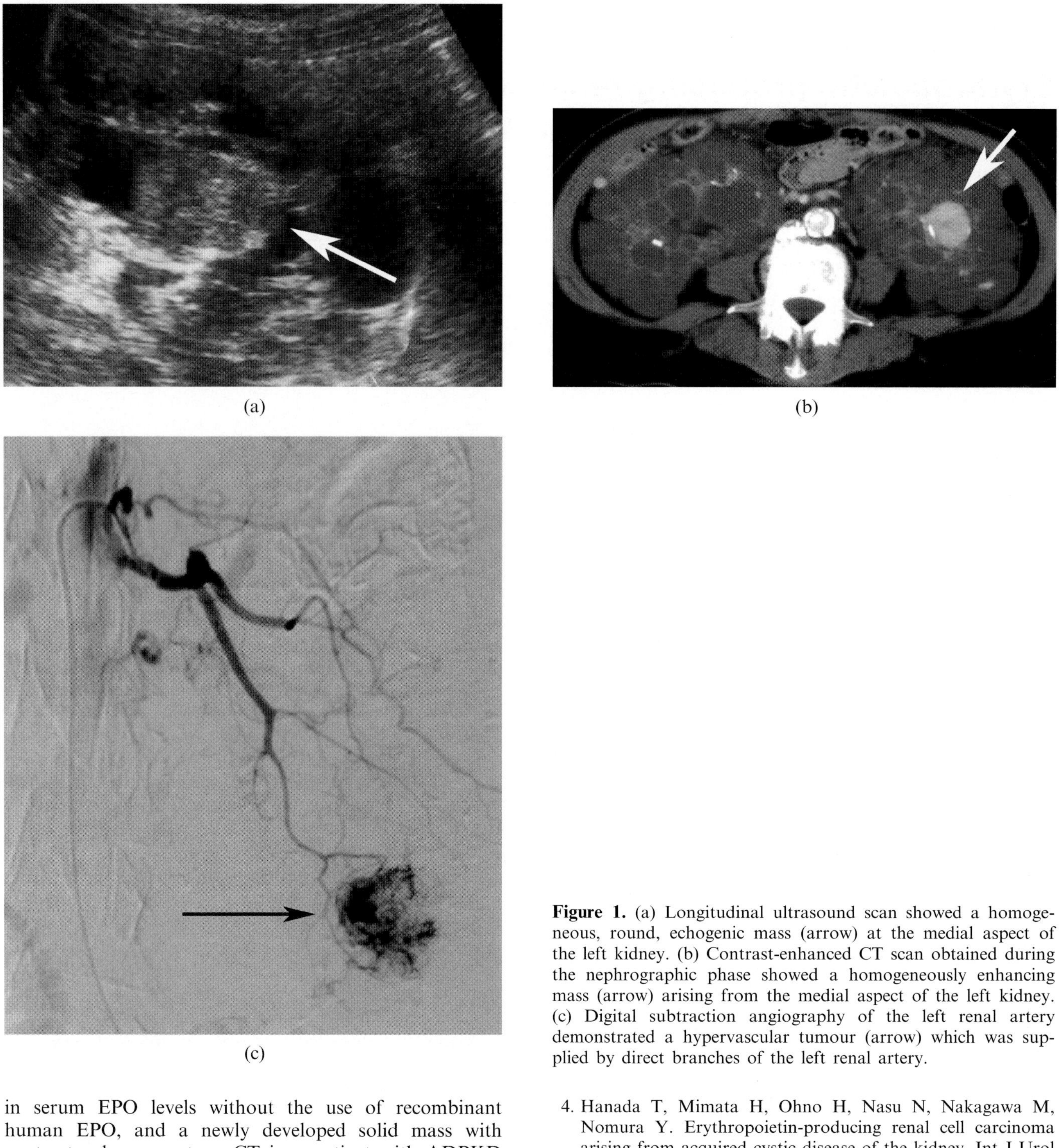

Figure 1. (a) Longitudinal ultrasound scan showed a homogeneous, round, echogenic mass (arrow) at the medial aspect of the left kidney. (b) Contrast-enhanced CT scan obtained during the nephrographic phase showed a homogeneously enhancing mass (arrow) arising from the medial aspect of the left kidney. (c) Digital subtraction angiography of the left renal artery demonstrated a hypervascular tumour (arrow) which was supplied by direct branches of the left renal artery.

in serum EPO levels without the use of recombinant human EPO, and a newly developed solid mass with contrast enhancement on CT in a patient with ADPKD may suggest the diagnoses of an EPO-producing RCC.

References

1. Sakamoto S, Igarashi T, Osumi N, Imamoto T, Tobe T, Kamiya M, et al. Erythropoietin-producing renal cell carcinoma in chronic hemodialysis patients: a report of two cases. Int J Urol 2003;10:49–51.
2. Walters W, Braasch WC. Surgical aspects of polycystic kidneys. Surg Gynecol Obstet 1934;58:649–53.
3. Keith DS, Torres VE, King BF, Zincki H, Farrow GM. Renal cell carcinoma in autosomal dominant polycystic kidney disease. J Am Soc Nephrol 1994;4:1661–9.
4. Hanada T, Mimata H, Ohno H, Nasu N, Nakagawa M, Nomura Y. Erythropoietin-producing renal cell carcinoma arising from acquired cystic disease of the kidney. Int J Urol 1998;5:493–5.
5. Jurgensen JS, Muller V, Kettritz U, Woywodt A, Gobel U, Luft FC. A malignant 'incidentaloma' in a patient with autosomal dominant polycystic kidney disease. Nephrol Dial Transplant 1999;14:490–2.
6. Hemal AK, Khaitan A, Singh I, Kumar M. Renal cell carcinoma in cases of adult polycystic kidney disease: changing diagnostic and therapeutic implications. Urol Int 2000;64:9–12.
7. Erslev AJ, Caro J, Miller O, Silver R. Plasma erythropoietin in health and disease. Ann Clin Lab Sci 1980;10:250–7.
8. Edmunds ME, Devoy M, Tomson CR, Krishna U, Clayworth A, Durrant ST, et al. Plasma erythropoietin levels and acquired cystic disease of the kidney in patients receiving regular haemodialysis treatment. Br J Haematol 1991;78:275–7.

9. Eckardt KU, Mollmann M, Neumann R, Brunkhorst R, Burger HU, Lonnemann G, et al. Erythropoietin in polycystic kidneys. J Clin Invest 1989;84:1160–6.
10. Kumar S, Cederbaum AI, Pletka PG. Renal cell carcinoma in polycystic kidneys: case report and review of literature. J Urol 1980;124:708–9.
11. Gupta S, Seith A, Sud K, Kohli HS, Singh SK, Sakhuja V, et al. CT in the evaluation of complicated autosomal dominant polycystic kidney disease. Acta Radiol 2000;41:280–4.
12. Sheth S, Scatarige JC, Horton KM, Corl FM, Fishman EK. Current concepts in the diagnosis and management of renal cell carcinoma: role of multidetector CT and three-dimensional CT. Radiographics 2001;21:S237–54.
13. Yuh BI, Cohan RH. Different phases of renal enhancement: role in detecting and characterizing renal masses during helical CT. AJR Am J Roentgenol 1999;173:747–55.
14. Mosetti MA, Leonardou P, Motohara T, Kanematsu M, Armao D, Semelka RC. Autosomal dominant polycystic kidney disease: MR imaging evaluation using current techniques. J Magn Reson Imaging 2003;18:210–5.
15. Hemal AK, Khaitan A, Singh I, Kumar M. Renal cell carcinoma in cases of adult polycystic kidney disease: changing diagnostic and therapeutic implications. Urol Int 2000;64:9–12.

The British Journal of Radiology, 78 (2005), 272–281
DOI: 10.1259/bjr/55402388

Pictorial review

Non-infectious manifestations of stem cell transplantation

D BECKETT, MBBS and J OLLIFF, MBBS, FRCR

Queen Elizabeth Hospital, Edgbaston, Birmingham B15 2TH, UK

Abstract. Stem cell transplantation (SCT) is now commonplace within medical practice. With growth in transplant activities, outcomes are likely to continue to improve. Increasing numbers of the population now face life after transplantation. The aetiology of post transplant complications is multifactorial. Background knowledge of SCT and common, radiographically detectable, non-infective complications are important in everyday clinical practice. A review of these complications using a variety of imaging modalities is presented and the process of SCT briefly described. Tumour recurrence is outside the remit of this review.

Stem cell transplantation (SCT) is now commonplace within medical practice [1, 2]. Estimates suggest 30 000–40 000 SCT are performed annually worldwide [3]. The role of SCT is restoration of immunohaemopoietic function in the recipient after elimination of the underlying disease. Autologous transplantation involves high dose chemotherapy with stem cell rescue, the stem cells having been collected from the patient during periods of low tumour load. Allogeneic transplantation is when another individual, a sibling, haplo-identical parent or unrelated individual, is used as the donor. In order to maximize graft viability a full or near human leukocyte antigen (HLA) match is required. Varying conditioning regimens aim to ablate the existing recipient marrow and tumour load and to suppress graft rejection. While true in myelo-ablative regimens, mini-allogeneic or non-myelo-ablative transplantation seeks to facilitate engraftment and augment the "graft versus tumour" effect. Early transplant related morbidity and mortality is reduced through the use of less toxic conditioning. Still in its infancy, this form of transplantation is largely experimental.

Following suitable pre-conditioning, donor cells harvested from marrow or peripheral blood are infused into the recipient. These have usually been accumulated by extracorporeal separation of peripheral stem cells following cellular mobilization of the donor using granulocyte colony stimulating factor. A varying degree of engraftment ensues, but for up to approximately 21 days the patient is haematologically and immunologically incompetent. This period of engraftment has been shown to be reduced by the use of peripheral blood stem cell infusion. Full immunological restitution may take up to 1 year following transplant. In addition regimens using cyclosporin are used in the prophylaxis of graft-versus host disease (GVHD).

Conventional SCT has established roles within the management of lymphohaemopoietic, immunological, metabolic and other conditions, as well as non-haematological malignancies (Table 1).

With growth in transplant activities, outcomes are likely to continue to improve. Increasing numbers of the population now face life after transplantation. Cure, however, comes with a price. Transplant morbidity is high.

A multifactorial aetiology for post transplantation complications was given by Wingard et al, in which total body irradiation, chemotherapy, GVHD and immunodeficiency act alone or in combination [3]. While non-infective manifestations account for a significant proportion of transplant related morbidity and may affect all organ systems, infection within the setting of SCT, is common and remains the most significant cause of morbidity and mortality.

Received 5 January 2004 and in revised form 4 October 2004, accepted 13 October 2004.

Imaging

Imaging has a central role in the initial diagnosis and staging of SCT complications. Both during SCT and thereafter, clinicoradiological collaboration allows prompt management of complications. Plain radiography is used initially in suspected abdominal and pulmonary pathology, as well as in the investigation of musculoskeletal disease in the post transplant period. CT and high resolution computed tomography (HRCT) are useful in the classification of pulmonary pathology [4]. Interpretation of imaging findings should be related to the time elapsed since SCT. Furthermore CT guides the physician with regard to subsequent diagnostic procedures. CT and MRI form the mainstay of investigation of cerebral pathology. The widespread availability of MRI has seen an increase in the use of this modality.

Ultrasound, CT and MRI all have a role in the investigation of abdominal pathology, including veno-occlusive disease. Conventional contrast studies have a limited role. The role of the radiologist is pivotal during every step of the patient management.

Musculoskeletal complications

Long term musculoskeletal complications are not uncommon (Table 2), and these include benign and malignant conditions [5–11]. Psoriatic arthropathy is reported in the literature but not commonly seen [11]. More commonly, reduction in bone mineral density

Table 1. Indications for stem cell transplantation

Haematological malignancy	• Acute leukaemia (AML/ALL) • Chronic leukaemia (CLL/CML) • Lymphoma • Myelodysplasia and myelofibrosis
Non-haematological malignancy	• Testicular cancer
Haematological disorders	• Aplastic anaemia • Fanconi's anaemia • Thalassemia • Sickle cell anaemia
Miscellaneous conditions	• Primary immunodeficiency states (severe combined immunodeficiency disorder) • Hereditary genetic disorders (*e.g.* Hurler's syndrome)

AMC, acute myeloid leukaemia; ALL, acute lymphocytic leukaemia; CLL, chronic lymphocytic leukaemia; CML, chronic myeloid leukaemia.

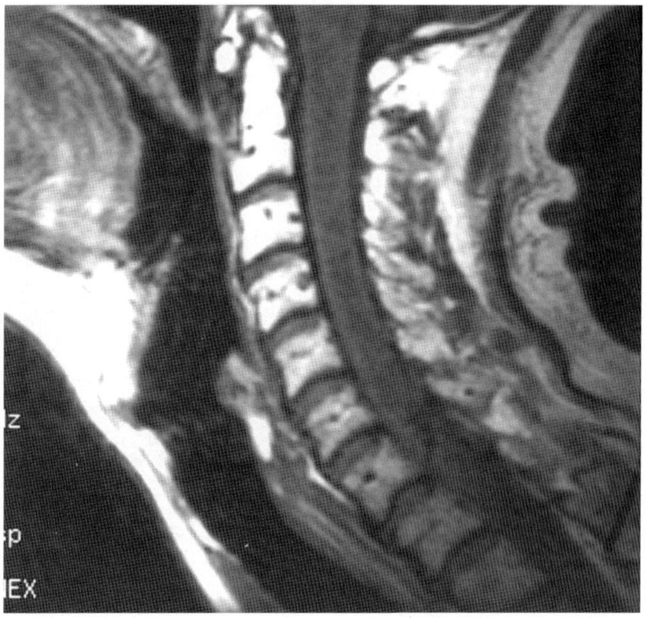

Figure 1. Marrow signal change following stem cell transplantation. T_1 weighted MRI sequence of the cervical spine demonstrates diffuse increase in the marrow signal reflecting the increase in yellow marrow seen following high dose irradiation therapy.

occurs, peaking at 6 months following SCT and is associated with chemoradiotherapy, steroid usage and malnutrition [10].

Skeletal abnormalities previously associated with external beam irradiation are now being seen in long term survivors of SCT (enchondromas, slipped femoral epiphysis, metaphyseal abnormalities, osteochondromas) who have received total body irradiation (TBI) [7].

Signal changes within the marrow have been observed on MRI following high doses of irradiation during pre-conditioning (Figure 1). Red marrow within the axial skeleton is replaced by fat containing yellow marrow. The subsequent signal change is best appreciated on T_1 weighted MRI sequences. The bone marrow shows a steady and marked increase in the pre-contrast signal intensity. The converse, *i.e.* increased volume of low signal red marrow, may be seen in patients receiving granulocyte colony stimulating factor. Stem cell harvesting using repeated trephine aspiration from the ileum causes focal abnormalities which may be seen on plain radiography and CT (Figure 2).

Avascular necrosis has an incidence of 4.3% at 5 years [6]. Symptoms develop between 2 months and 132 months with the femoral head being the most commonly affected site (Figure 3). Significant morbidity is seen with up to half of these patients requiring joint replacement. Patient age, a diagnosis of aplastic anaemia or acute leukaemia, GVHD and prophylactic treatment with steroids have all been associated with an increased risk of avascular necrosis [6].

Neuropathological complications

Neurological complications are frequent, particularly during the first 3 months following SCT and affect patient survival [12]. The peak occurrence for neurological complications is quoted to be at week 3–4 following SCT. Central nervous system (CNS) related mortality accounts for approximately 15–20% of overall early transplant related mortality [13]. With the development of metabolic encephalopathy (seen in up to a third of patients with CNS complications) patient survival within 100 days falls from 87% to 27%.

There is a complex interplay between pre-conditioning with chemoradiotherapy, the immunohaematological incompetence within the transplant period, GVHD and GVHD prophylaxis in causation of neuropathological

Table 2. Musculoskeletal manifestations of stem cell transplantation

Pathological process	Pathology	Predisposing factors
Benign	Osteoporosis	Conditioning, malnutrition, GVHD prophylaxis
	Osteochondromas	Conditioning
	Metaphyseal growth abnormalities	Conditioning
	Slipped femoral epiphysis	Conditioning
	Avascular necrosis (AVN)	Conditioning, AL, AA, GVHD, GVHD prophylaxis, Age >16 years
	Enchondromas	Conditioning
Malignant	Osteosarcoma	Conditioning regimens
	Malignant fibrous histiocytoma	
Unusual	Transmitted psoriatic arthritis	Immunologically mediated through donor cells

GVHD, graft versus host disease; AL, acute leukaemia; AA, aplastic anaemia.

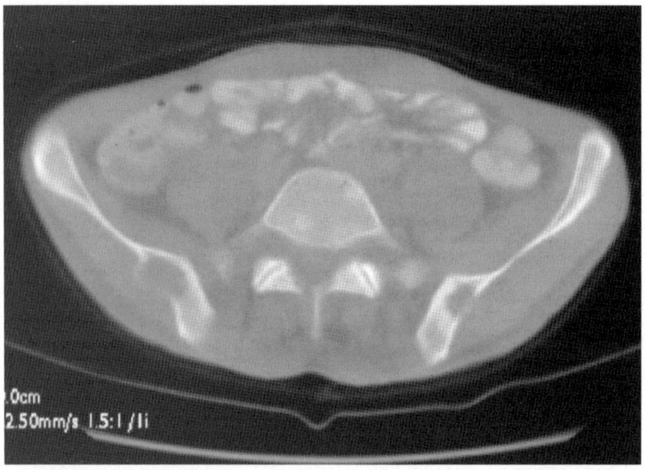

Figure 2. Routine follow up CT in a 29-year-old male following autologous stem cell transplant taken at the level of sacro-iliac joints. Bilateral lucencies with a narrow zone of transition are demonstrated within both posterior iliac wings from trephine marrow aspiration.

complications [12, 14]. Complications may be broadly classified into treatment induced, cerebrovascular and GVHD. Anecdotal reports of inflammatory demyelinating polyneuropathy and immune-mediated myelopathy have been described [15]. Multifocal cerebral demyelination with fulminant, widespread white matter lesions on MRI is documented [16].

Cerebrovascular

Cerebrovascular events may complicate SCT [12–17] (Figure 4). Contributing factors include TBI, haemopoietic incompetence and platelet refractoriness. Cerebral infarction is more common than haemorrhage. TBI is associated with an increased risk of cerebrovascular events. Subdural haematoma (SDH) is common within the haemorrhagic group. The main risk factor for development of SDH is platelet refractory disease [17]. SDH is more common within autologous transplantation [17]. Resolution with conservative management is expected. Anecdotal reports of subarachnoid haemorrhage as a sequlae to Cyclosporin neurotoxicity and GVHD cerebral angiitis have been described [18–20].

Treatment induced

Total body irradiation

Standard autologous and allogeneic SCT involves pre-conditioning with TBI. A standard regimen would consist of eight fractions over 4 days (approximately 14.4 Gy). Cerebral infarction, diffuse white matter disease, and cortical atrophy have been reported with this form of conditioning.

Cyclosporin neurotoxicity

Regimens incorporating Cyclosporin are used in the prophylaxis of GVHD following allogeneic SCT. Patients

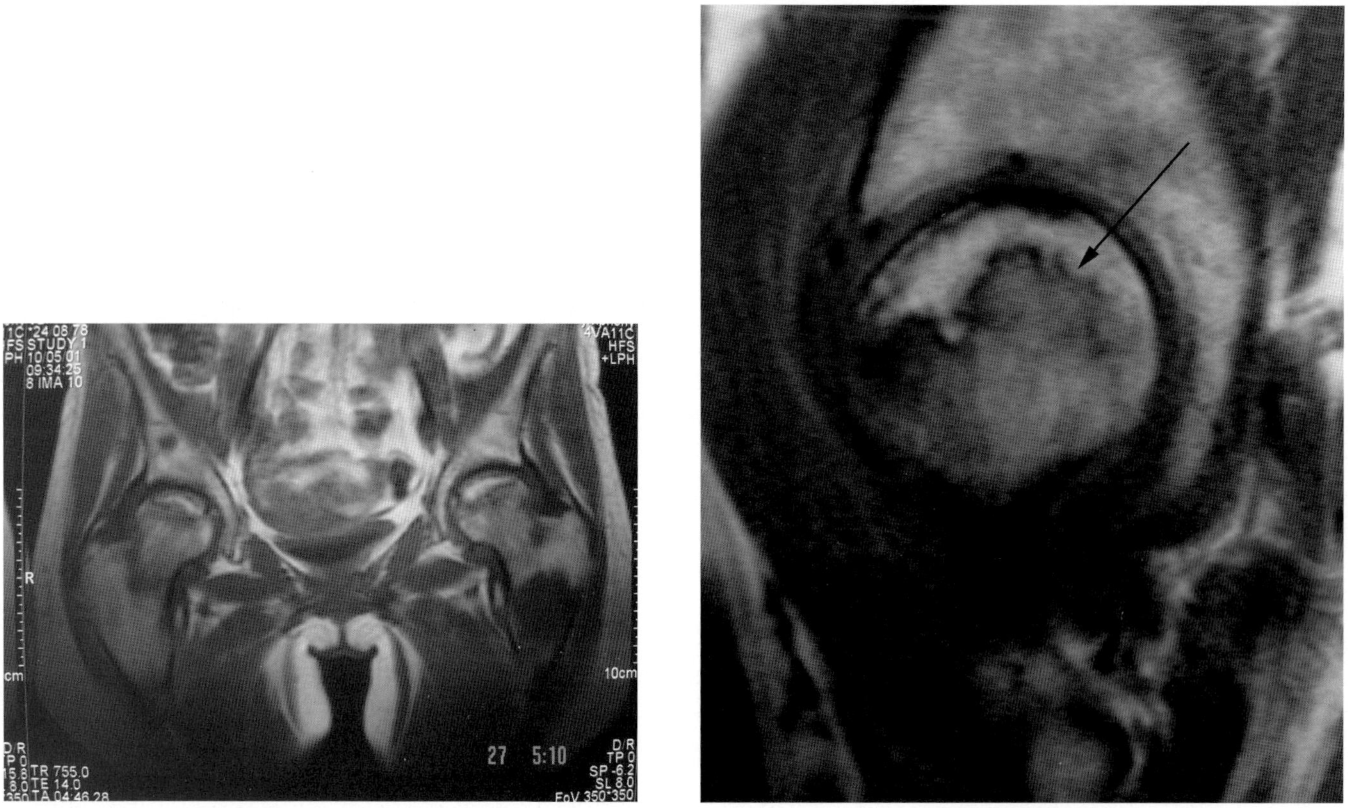

(a) (b)

Figure 3. Avascular necrosis. 35-year-old female with bilateral hip pain at 1 year following a matched unrelated transplant. The patient had recently completed a course of steroids for an episode of GVHD. (a) Coronal T_1 weighted MRI image of the hips and (b) sagittal T_1 weighted MRI of the left hip showing a serpiginous zone of low signal around the avascular area (arrow).

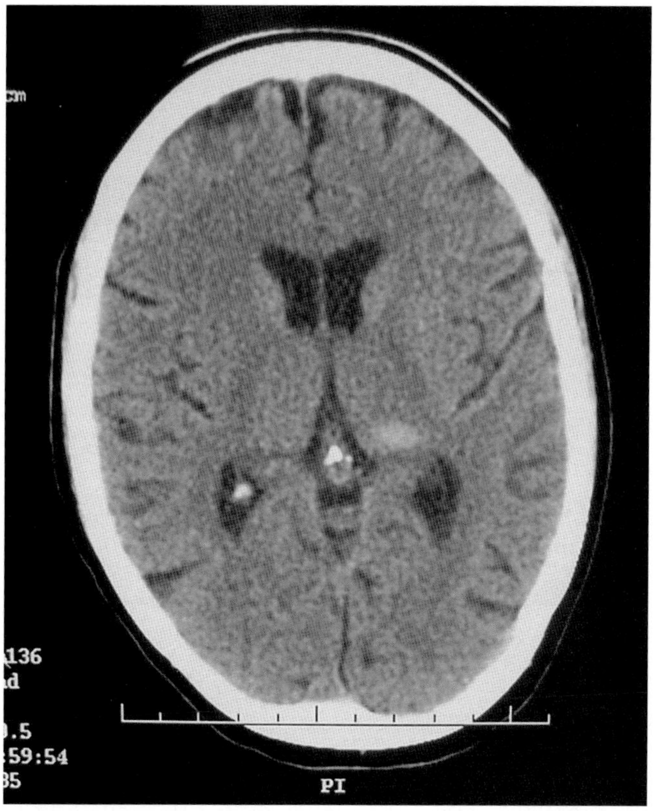

Figure 4. Axial CT of the head through the level of the lateral ventricles. An area of high attenuation is seen within the left thalamus demonstrating a thalamic haemorrhage. A minor degree of cortical atrophy within the frontal lobes is shown.

may continue with Cyclosporin prophylaxis for a variable time period dependant on initial transplant (myelo-ablative *vs* non-myelo-ablative), and ongoing GVHD. It is not uncommon for patients to remain on Cyclosporin for up to 2 years and beyond. Cyclosporin neurotoxicity has been characterized by hypertension, seizures and reversible posterior leukoencephalopathy [21–23]. Low attenuation on CT and increased signal on T_2 MR which characteristically does not enhance are typical radiographic findings.

Specific conditioning prior to SCT may alter the pattern of toxicity [24]. TBI has been associated with white matter lesions while those conditioned with chemotherapy develop mixed cortical and white matter lesions.

Secondary malignancy

Chromosomal instability, immunosuppression, conditioning with TBI and viral pathogens have been linked to the development of malignant disease within the post-transplant period [25]. The risk of developing a solid tumour at 15 years post SCT is in the order of 7–8% [25]. Head and neck squamous cell carcinoma, melanoma, and solid tumours of brain and thyroid are seen (Figure 5). Reported neoplasms of bone following total body irradiation include osteosarcoma, fibrosarcoma, malignant fibrous histiocytoma and chondrosarcoma.

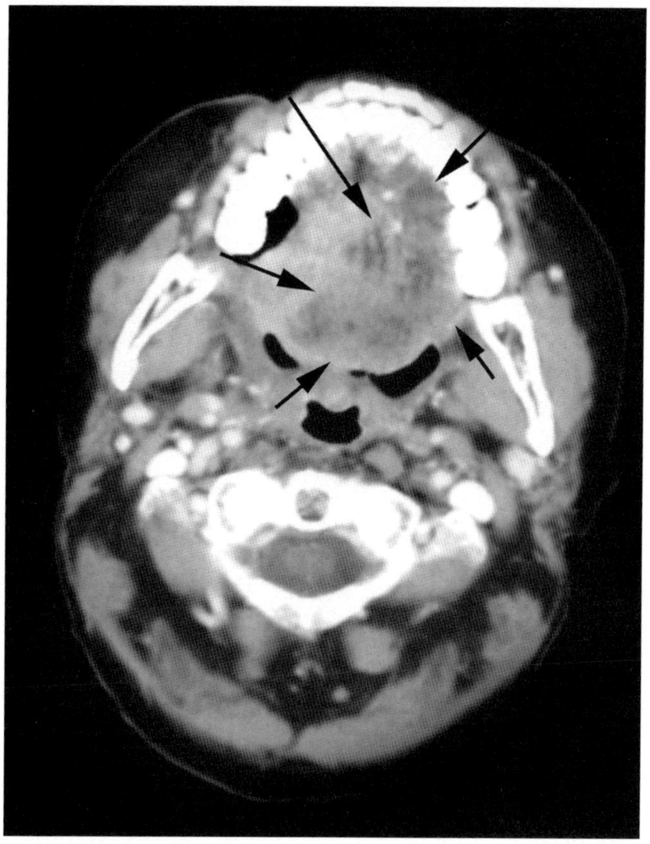

Figure 5. Biopsy proven squamous cell carcinoma of the roof of the mouth in a 39-year-old female, 8 years following stem cell transplantation. Contrast enhanced axial CT through the roof of the oral cavity. A heterogeneous mass involving the roof of the mouth adherent to the alveolar aspects of the maxilla is demonstrated (arrows). There was no evidence of bony destruction.

Cardiothoracic pathology

Pulmonary system

Pulmonary complications in the setting of SCT are a common cause of morbidity and mortality [26].

Three discrete phases which reflect the immunological state of the patient have been identified [26]. The neutropenic phase, lasting up to 30 days is characterized by alveolar haemorrhage, drug toxicity and capillary leak syndrome. The second phase, 30–100 days, consists of radiation/drug induced damage. The third, or late phase, is strongly associated with chronic GVHD (cGVHD). Accordingly, bronchiolitis obliterans, bronchiolitis obliterans with organizing pneumonia (BOOP), and lymphocytic interstitial pneumonitis (LIP) are seen within this phase.

0–30 days

Non-cardiogenic pulmonary oedema occurs frequently within SCT [27]. There is a strong correlation with the time of engraftment. Circulating lymphocytes are thought to be involved. Up to 25% of patients may develop this form of capillary leak syndrome (CLS) [27]. Pulmonary features tend to be accompanied by hepatic and renal dysfunction. CLS is seen in both allogeneic and autologous transplantation. With engraftment occurring earlier in allogeneic transplantation, CLS will be seen earlier

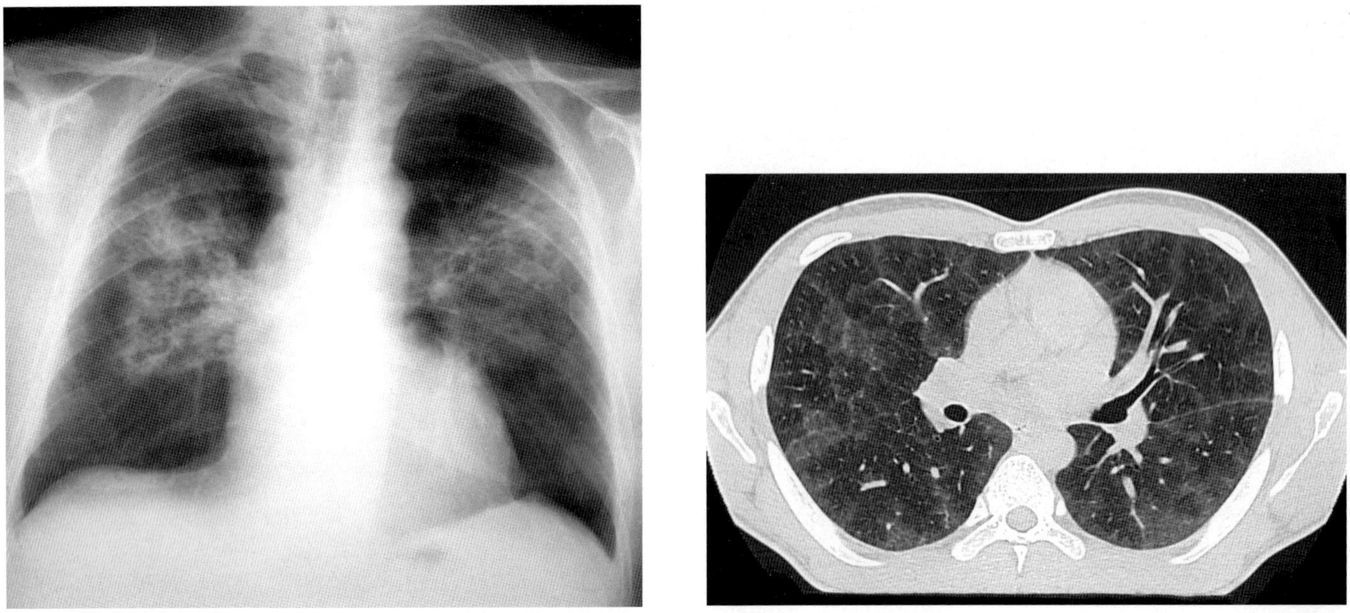

(a) (b)

Figure 6. Diffuse alveolar haemorrhage. (a) Chest radiograph taken 22 days following allogeneic SCT shows bilateral alveolar opacification. (b) CT from a different patient with dyspnoea taken at 29 days following transplantation demonstrates patchy ground glass attenuation within the mid zones.

within this group. Classical septal lines, alveolar oedema and pleural effusions are seen. Capillary leak syndrome may also develop in response to granulocyte stimulating factor treatment or chemotherapy.

Diffuse alveolar haemorrhage (DAH) may occur early or late within the transplant period, although DAH tends to be associated with granulocyte recovery (first 30 days) [28, 29]. DAH is linked to the conditioning regimen, infections and inflammatory pneumonitis. DAH has been reported in up to 20% of patients. Patients may present with dyspnoea (96%), fever (67%) and cough (56%) [29]. Haemoptysis is rare. Up to 90% require ventilation and high dose methlyprednisolone (1.5 g day^{-1}) for about 4 days. Mortality is significantly higher within allogeneic transplantation and those presenting with late haemorrhage [29]. Radiographic findings include bilateral reticular or patchy alveolar opacities, usually in the mid to lower lung zones (Figure 6a). Rapid progression to a severe diffuse alveolar pattern is characteristic. On CT small areas of ground glass attenuation confined to the secondary lobules can be seen. The pattern is non-specific and has a variety of causes (infectious, neoplastic, idiopathic and inhalational disorders) (Figure 6b).

Drug toxicity changes are non-specific and include ground glass opacification, nodules, consolidation and later fibrosis [30]. These tend to occur within phases 1 or 2.

Late onset pulmonary complications

Chronic pulmonary complications affect approximately 10% of patients [28]. Abnormal pulmonary function is associated with higher non-relapse mortality [21, 32].

Obliterative bronchiolitis and obliterative bronchiolitis with organizing pneumonia

Obliterative bronchiolitis is seen in up to 15% of patients with cGVHD [33–35]. Typical presentation is at 6–12 months. Little or no treatment exists apart from treating the underlying GVHD. Mortality is up to 40%.

Histologically there is inflammation and lymphocytic infiltration with progressive destruction of the small airways.

Hyperinflation of the lungs, flattening of the diaphragm, and recurrent pneumothoraces are seen on the chest radiograph. HRCT may show decreased pulmonary vasculature, peribronchial thickening, and areas of air trapping, seen best on expiratory HRCT (Figure 7). Ventilation scans show reduced tracer activity in areas of obliteration of bronchiolar walls, along with atelectatic areas.

Organizing pneumonia may be associated with or without obliterative bronchiolitis. Typically, a meandering pattern of multifocal consolidation may be seen on the chest radiograph or CT (Figure 8). CT is of use in targeting for open lung biopsy. Biopsy confirms an organizing pneumonia in the absence of micro-organisms.

Lymphocytic interstitial pneumonitis

LIP is seen more frequently within the setting of allogeneic transplantation. There is a strong association with cGVHD and patients frequently show other manifestations of cGVHD [36]. Histology shows lymphocyte infiltrate of the interstitium with alveolar sparing. The chest radiograph and cross sectional imaging show diffuse micronodular opacification. Consolidation is not typical early on in the disease process. HRCT findings include diffuse bilateral ground glass opacification and poorly defined centrilobular nodules, subpleural nodules, thickening of the bronchovascular bundles, cystic airspaces and patchy ground glass (Figure 9). Interstitial damage may progress to fibrosis with impaired gas exchange and respiratory dynamics. A definitive diagnosis may be made by open lung biopsy. Treatment primarily consists of steroids and immunosuppression to arrest cGVHD.

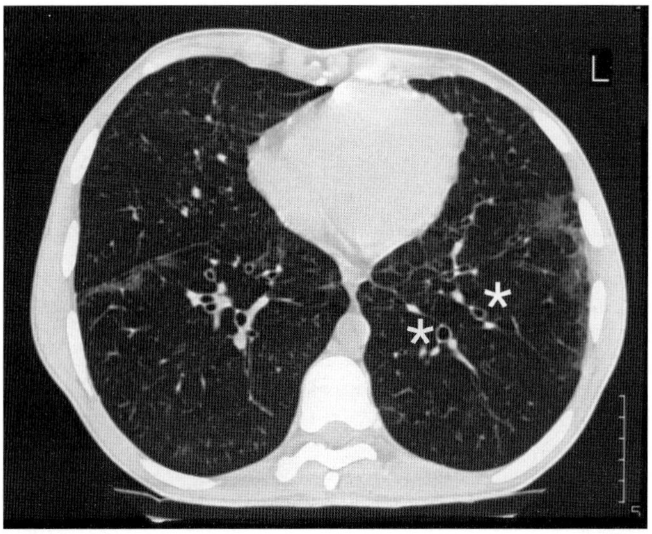

Figure 7. Bronchiolitis obliterans. High resolution CT shows decreased pulmonary vasculature and subsegmental bronchial dilatation (asterisk). Obvious areas of air trapping giving the "mosaic perfusion" appearance are not readily apparent. (Image courtesy of Dr J Reynolds. Consultant Radiologist at Heartlands and Solihul Hospital, Birmingham.)

Cardiovascular pathology

Cardiotoxic events result from intensive conditioning during SCT [37–41]. Cardiotoxicity may be associated with septic shock, pneumonitis or multiorgan failure. Although infrequent, cardiomyopathy has been observed [39–41]. Overall, major cardiotoxic events are infrequent (<1%) [37]. Various subclinical events have been reported and include impaired systolic and diastolic function [38]. Complications related to catheter placement are seen within interventional radiology [42] (Figure 10). Occlusion caused by thrombus, and/or fibrin sheath formation are common (Figure 11). Catheter migration and malfunction have been reported.

Gastrointestinal/hepatobilary manifestations

Acute abdominal complications in SCT may be broadly categorised as those arising from intensive conditioning through chemoradiotherapy, acute or chronic GVHD, or miscellaneous conditions.

Chemoradiotherapy

Chemotherapy and TBI may cause ileocolitis, pancreatitis, cholangitis, appendicitis, gastric perforation and hepatic veno-occlusive disease (VOD) [43]. VOD has a reported incidence of 0–70% [44]. 30% of patients are affected within the first 2 weeks. The aetiology of VOD is complex and not fully understood. It is thought that chemoradiotherapy leads to endothelial injury of small hepatic veins and sinusoids [45]. Concentrated antineoplastic agents within the centrilobular zone leads to necrotic oedematous hepatocytes obstructing sinusoidal flow. Tumour necrosis factor alpha is released leading to cytotoxicity and coagulation. Histopathology shows

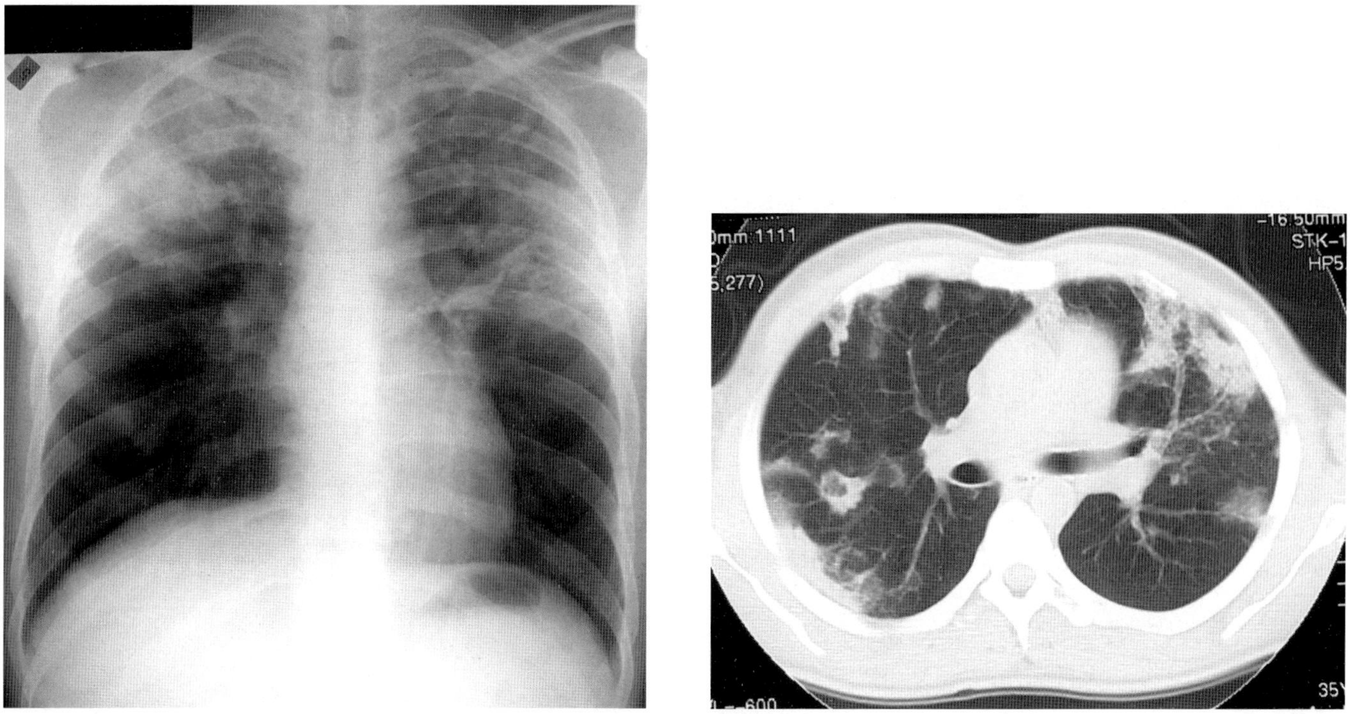

(a) (b)

Figure 8. Organizing pneumonia. 32-year-old male with increasing breathlessness at 5 months following stem cell transplantation. (a) Chest radiograph demonstrates upper zone, peripheral areas of consolidation and interstitial shadowing. (b) CT demonstrates areas of ill defined ground glass attenuation in association with more focal areas of consolidation in a predominantly subpleural distribution. (Images courtesy of Dr J Reynolds. Consultant Radiologist at Heartlands and Solihul Hospital, Birmingham.)

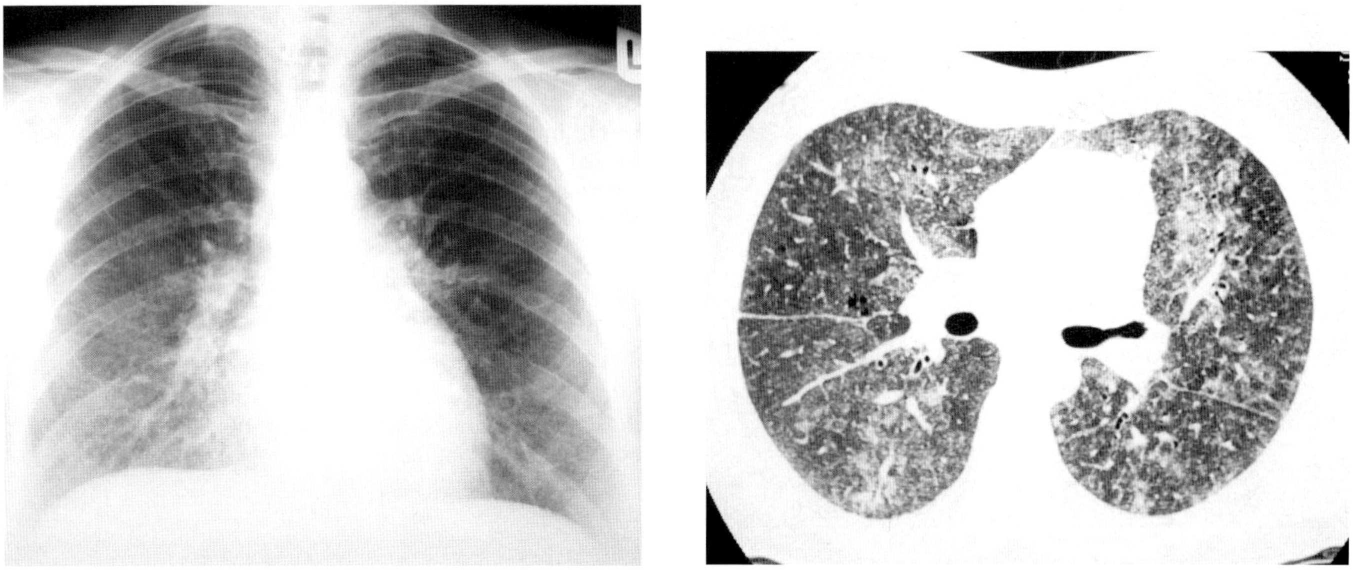

(a) (b)

Figure 9. Lymphocytic interstitial pneumonitis. 33-year-old male with increasing breathlessness 3 months following stem cell transplantation. (a) Chest radiograph demonstrates bilateral mid and lower zone pulmonary nodules measuring 1–5 mm in the absence of clinical infection. (b) High resolution CT through the lower lobes demonstrates widespread nodules throughout the lungs and patchy ground glass opacification. (Images courtesy of Dr J Reynolds. Consultant Radiologist at Heartlands and Solihul Hospital, Birmingham.)

centrilobular congestion, oedema, venular occlusion, atrophy of pericentral hepatocytes, recanalization of venules and centrilobular cholestasis. Diagnosis is non-specific. Clinical presentation is that of jaundice, weight gain and ascites. Radiographically detectable findings include hepatomegaly with or without major hepatic vein collapse, gallbladder thickening, ascites and bidirectional or reversed portal flow on Doppler [45]. Liver biopsy is used to differentiate VOD from other causes of hepatic dysfunction (infective, GVHD, drug induced toxicity) [46].

Neutropenic colitis (NC) is an acute necrotizing inflammatory condition predominantly affecting the caecum and right colon. NC is rare within the setting of SCT [47]. Ischaemia, secondary bacterial invasion and sepsis are seen. If untreated patients may develop transmural necrosis and perforation. CT findings include

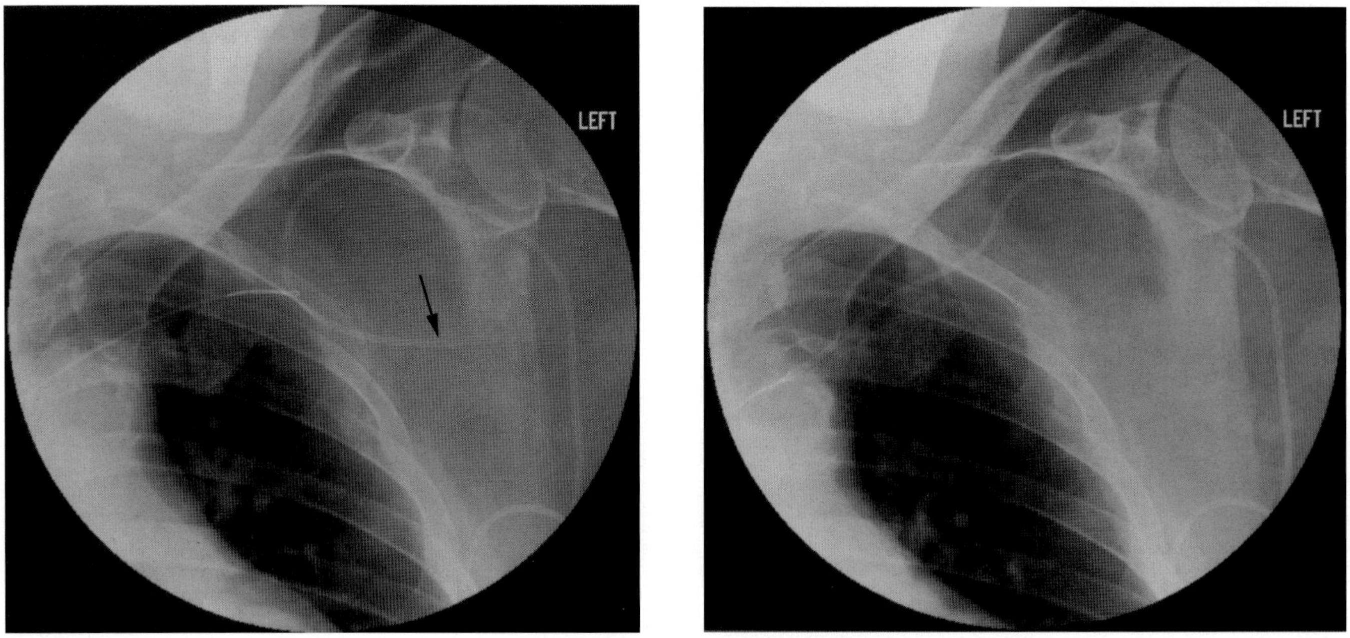

(a) (b)

Figure 10. A misplaced single lumen central venous catheter. (a) The tip is seen to lie within the left axillary vein (arrow). (b) Using a common femoral vein approach the tip is snared and manipulated into the correct position. (Images courtesy of Dr P Crowe. Consultant Radiologist at Heartlands and Solihul Hospital, Birmingham.)

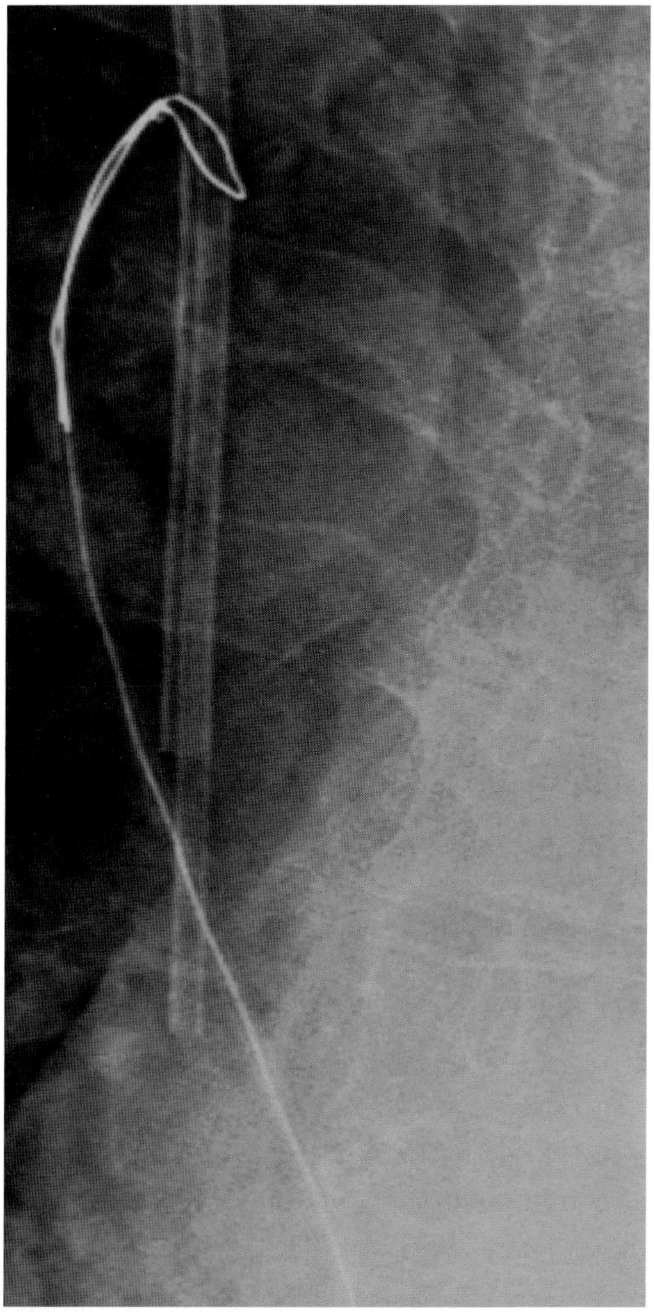

Figure 11. A snare catheter via a femoral vein approach may be used to strip the tip of a central venous catheter when a fibrin sheath is seen to overlie the tip. (Image courtesy of Dr P Crowe. Consultant Radiologist at Heartlands and Solihul Hospital, Birmingham.)

bowel wall thickening, pericolic inflammatory changes and pneumoperitoneum (Figure 12).

GVHD

GVHD refers to the process by which donor T-cells may elicit disease within recipient tissue. 60% of patients may be affected. GVHD is characterized as acute or chronic depending whether presentation is before or after 100 days from SCT. Any organ system may be involved.

Chronic involvement of the oesophagus and stomach is occasionally seen. If untreated cGVHD may lead

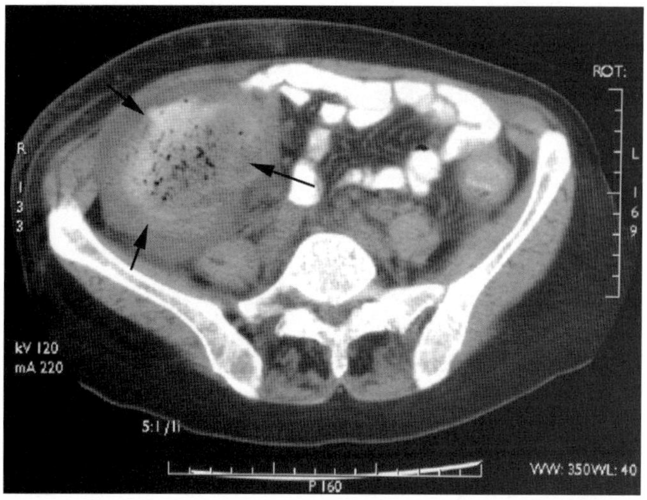

Figure 12. Neutropenic colitis. 28-year-old male with abdominal pain. CT with oral contrast through the level of the caecum in a neutropenic patient. There is marked thickening of the caecum (arrows) and descending colon. The caecal pole is dilated and there is streaking of the mesenteric and retroperitoneal fat planes.

to stricture and web formation of the oesophagus requiring endoluminal dilatation. Isolated cases of oesophageal and bowel carcinoma have been reported in the literature.

Diffusely affected abnormal, dilated, fluid filled loops of small bowel with or without bowel wall thickening are seen [48]. Granulation tissue replaces destroyed bowel mucosa. The characteristic target sign of mucosa oedema with abnormal contrast enhancement of the bowel wall is a feature on contrast enhanced CT [49].

Miscellaneous

An increased incidence of cholelithiasis is seen in patients following SCT [43]. Splenic and renal infarction has been described [43]. Pneumatosis intestinalis is a rare yet important phenomenon within SCT [50, 51]. The aetiology is multifactorial. Chemoradiotherapy, GVHD and corticosteroids have been implicated [50]. Presentation is with diarrhoea, abdominal pain and bleeding per rectum. The right colon is predominantly affected [50]. Pneumatosis intestinalis is predominantly linear on plain radiography.

Post-transplant lymphoproliferative disorder

The cumulative probability of developing post-transplant lymphoproliferative disorder (PTLD) has been estimated at 1.6% at 4 years [52]. The pathology involves uncontrolled, B-cell derived donor lymphocyte proliferation. PTLD is strongly associated with Epstein-Barr virus in the setting of stem cell transplantation. Risk factors include T-cell depletion, HLA mismatch, conditioning, and a diagnosis of primary immunodeficiency. Clinical presentation is with fever and associated lymphadenopathy of the bowel, spleen, liver and other organs.

Conclusion

Specificity of diagnosis is achieved with clinicoradiological collaboration. Knowledge of the transplant process and multifactorial nature of the ensuing complications is required for the successful management of this patient subgroup.

References

1. Molina A, Popplewell L, Kashyap A, Nademance A. Stem cell transplantation in the new millennium: report from city of Hope National Medical Centre. Clin Transplant 2000: 317–42.
2. Evans A, Steward CG, Lyburn ID, Grier DJ. Imaging in haematopoietic stem cell transplantation. Clin Radiol 2003;58:201–14.
3. Wingard JR, Georgia B, Vogelsang H, Deeg J. Stem cell transplantation: supportive care and long term complications. Haematology 2002;422:1–31.
4. Graham NJ, Muller NL, Miller RR, Shepherd JD. Intrathoracic complications following allogeneic bone marrow transplantation: CT findings. Radiology 1991;181:153–6.
5. Torii Y, Hasegawa Y, Kubo T, Kodera Y, Minami S, Morishita Y, et al. Osteonecrosis of the femoral head after allogeneic bone marrow transplantation. Clin Orthop 2001;382:124–32.
6. Socie G, Cahn JY, Carmelo J, Vernant JP, Jouet JP, Ifrah N, et al. Avascular necrosis of bone after allogeneic bone marrow transplantation: analysis of risk factors for 4388 patients by SFGM. Br J Haematol 1997;97:865–70.
7. Fletcher BD, Crom DB, Krance RA, Kun LE. Radiation induced bone abnormalities after bone marrow transplantation for childhood leukaemia. Radiology 1994;191: 231–5.
8. Vela-Ojeda J, Diaz de Leon L, Tripp-Villanueva F, Sanchez-Cortes E, Ayala-Sanchez M, Garcia-Ruiz Esparza MA, et al. Malignant fibrous histiocytoma after allogeneic bone marrow transplantation. Bone Marrow Transplant 1999;24: 1029–31.
9. Asai T, Myoui A, Fujimoto T, Hara J, Aozasa K, Yoshikawa H. Osteosarcoma after bone marrow transplantation for ALL. Int J Clin Oncol 2002;7:318–21.
10. Buchs N, Helg C, Collao C, Chapuis B, Slosman D, Bonjour JP, et al. Allogeneic bone marrow transplantation is associated with a preferential femoral neck bone loss. Osteoporosis Int 2001;12:880–6.
11. Daikeler T, Gunaydin I, Einsele H, Kanz L, Kotter I. Transmission of psoriatic arthritis by allogeneic bone marrow transplantation for CML from an HLA identical donor. Rheumatology 1999;38:89–90.
12. Antonini G, Ceschin V, Morino S, Fiorelli M, Grangnani F, Mengarelli A, et al. Early neurological complications following allogeneic bone marrow transplant for leukaemia: a prospective study. Neurology 1998;50:1441–5.
13. Bleggi-Torres LF, de Medeiros BC, Werner B, Neto JZ, Loddo G, Pasquini R, et al. Neuropathological findings after bone marrow transplantation: an autopsy study of 180 cases. Bone Marrow Transplant 2000;25:301–7.
14. De Brabander C, Cornelissen J, Smitt PA, Vecht CJ, van den Bent MJ. Increased incidence of neurological complications in patients receiving an allogeneic bone marrow transplantation from alternative donors. J Neurol Neurosurg Psychiatry 2000;68:36–40.
15. Openshaw H, Slalkin NE, Parker PM, Forman SJ. Immune mediated myelopathy after allogeneic marrow transplantation. Bone Marrow Transplant 1995;15:633–6.
16. Kelly P, Staunton H, Lawler M, Brennan P, Jennings S, Unger ER, et al. Cerebral demyelination twenty years following allogeneic bone marrow transplant. J Neuropathol Exp Neurol 1996;55:992–8.
17. Graus F, Siaz A, Sierra J, Arbaiza D, Rovira M, Carreras E, et al. Neurological complications of autologous and allogeneic bone marrow transplantation in patients with leukaemia: a comparative study. Neurology 1996;46:1004–9.
18. Teksam M, Casey SO, Michel E, Truwit CL. Subarachnoid hemorrhage associated with cyclosporin A neurotoxicity in a bone marrow recipient. Neuroradiology 2001;43:242–5.
19. Ma M, Barnes G, Pulliam J, Jezek D, Baumann RJ, Berger JR. CNS angiitis in GvHD. Neurology 2002;59:1994–7.
20. Padovan CS, Bise K, Hahn J, Sostak P, Holler E, Kolb HJ, et al. Angiitis of the central nervous system after allogeneic bone marrow transplantation. Stroke 1999;30: 1651–6.
21. Teive HA, Brandi IV, Camargo CH, Bittencourt MA, Bonfim CM, Friedrich ML, et al. Reversible posterior leukoencephalopathy syndrome associated with bone marrow transplantation. Arquivos de Neuro-Psiquiatria 2001;59:784–9.
22. Shbarou RM, Chao NJ, Morgenlander JC. Cyclosporin A-related cerebral vasculopathy. Bone Marrow Transplant 2000;26:801–4.
23. Bartynski WS, Grabb BC, Zeigler Z, Lin L, Andrews DF. Watershed imaging features and clinical vascular injury in cyclosporin A neurotoxicity. J Comput Assist Tomogr 1997;21:872–80.
24. Bartynski WS, Zeigler Z, Spearman MP, Lin L, Shadduck RK. Etiology of cortical and white matter lesions in cyclosporin-A FK-506 neourotoxicity. AJNR Am J Neuroradiol 2001;22:1901–14.
25. The Committee for the Compilation of Materials on Damage Caused by the Atomic Bombs in Hiroshima and Nagasaki. Iijima S, Gushima K, Imahori S. Hiroshima and Nagasaki: the physical, medical, and social effects of the atomic bombings. New York: Basic Books, Inc., 1981:1–706.
26. Worthy SA, Flint JD, Muller NL. Pulmonary complications after bone marrow transplantation. HRCT and pathologic findings. Radiographics 1997;17:1359–71.
27. Cahill RA, Spitzer TR, Mazumder A. Marrow engraftment and clinical manifestations of capillary leak syndrome. Bone Marrow Transplant 1996;18:177–84.
28. Palmas A, Tefferi A, Myers JL, Scott JP, Swensen SJ, Chen MG, et al. Late onset pulmonary complications after allogeneic bone marrow transplantation. Br J Haematol 1998;100:680–7.
29. Afessa B, Tefferi A, Litzow MR, Peters SG. Outcome of diffuse alveolar haemorrhage in haematopoietic stem cell recipients. Am J Respir Crit Care Med 2002;166:1364–8.
30. Patz EF Jr, Peters WP, Goodman PC. Pulmonary drug toxicity following high-dose chemotherapy with autologous bone marrow transplantation. J Thorac Imaging 1994;9: 129–34.
31. Crawford SW, Pepe M, Lin D, Benedetti F, Deeg HJ. Abnormalities of pulmonary function tests after marrow transplantation predict nonrelapse mortality. Am J Respir Crit Care Med 1995;152:690–5.
32. Springmeyer SC, Flournoy N, Sullivan KM, Storb R, Thomas ED. Pulmonary function changes in long-term survivors of allogeneic marrow transplantation. In: Gale RP, editor. Recent advances in bone marrow transplantation. NY: Alan R. Liss Inc. 1983:343–53.
33. Sullivan KM, Mori M, Sanders J, et al. Late complications of allogeneic and autologous marrow transplantation (Review). Bone Marrow Transplant 1992;10:127–34.
34. Philit F, Wiesendanger T, Archimbaud E, et al. Post-transplant obstructive lung disease ("bronchiolitis obliterans"): a clinical comparative study of bone marrow and lung transplant patients. Eur Resp J 1995;8:551–8.

35. Sharples LD, Tamm M, McNeil K, et al. Development of bronchiolitis obliterans syndrome in recipients of heart-lung transplantation, early risk factors. Transplantation 1996;61:560–6.
36. Boeckh M, Riddell SR, Cunningham T, et al. Increased risk of late CMV infection and disease in allogeneic marrow transplant recipients after ganciclovir prophylaxis is due to a lack of CMV-specific T cell responses. Blood 1996;88:302a, 1195, (Abstract).
37. Murdych T, Weisdorf DJ. Serious cardiac complications during bone marrow transplantation at the University of Minnesota, 1977–1997. Bone Marrow Transplant 2001;28:283–7.
38. Kupari M, Volin L, Suokas A, Hekali P, Ruutu T. Cardiac involvement in bone marrow transplantation: serial changes in left ventricular size, mass and performance. J Intern Med 1990;227:259–66.
39. Gottdiener JS, Appelbaum FR, Ferrans VJ, Deisseroth A, Ziegler J. Cardiotoxicity associated with high-dose cyclophosphamide therapy. Arch Intern Med 1981;141: 758–63.
40. Braverman AC, Antin JH, Plappert MT, Cook EF, Lee RT. Cyclophosphamide cardiotoxicity in bone marrow transplantation: a prospective evaluation of new dosing regimens. J Clin Oncol 1991;9:1215–23.
41. Ramrakha PS, Marks DI, O'Brien SG, et al. Orthotopic cardiac transplantation for dilated cardiomyopathy after allogeneic bone marrow transplantation. Clin Transplant 1994;8:23–6.
42. Moosa HH, Julian TB, Rosenfeld CS, Shadduck RK. Complications of indwelling central venous catheters in bone marrow transplant recipients. Surg Gynaecol Obstetrics 1991;172:275–9.
43. Day DL, Carpenter BL. Abdominal complications in pediatric bone marrow transplant recipients. Radiographics 1993;13:1101–12.
44. Carreras E, Granena A, Rozman C. Hepatic veno-occlusive disease after bone marrow transplant. Blood Reviews 1993;1:43–51.
45. Van den Bosch MA, Van Hoe L. MR imaging findings in two patients with hepatic veno-occlusive disease following bone marrow transplantation. Eur Radiol 2000;8:1290–3.
46. Storek J. Liver dysfunction in the early post bone marrow transplant period. Casopis Lekaru Ceskych 1996;135:295–8.
47. Avigan D, Richardson P, Elias A, Demetri G, Shapiro M, Wheeler C. Neutropenic enterocolitis as a complication of high dose chemotherapy with stem cell rescue in patients with solid tumours. A case series with a review of the literature. Cancer 1998;83:409–14.
48. Belli AM, Williams MP. Graft versus host disease: findings on plain abdominal radiography. Clin Radiol 1988;39:262–4.
49. Jones B, Fishman EK, Kramer SS, Siegelman SS, Saral R, Yeager AM, et al. Computer tomography of gastrointestinal inflammation after marrow transplantation. AJR Am J Roentgenol 1986;146:691–5.
50. Day DL, Ramsay NK, Letourneau JG. Pneumatosis intestinalis after bone marrow transplantation. AJR Am J Roentgenol 1988;151:85–7.
51. Bates FT, Gurney JW, Goodman LR, Santamaria JJ, Hansen RM, Ash RC. Pneumatosis intestinalis in bone marrow transplantation patients: diagnosis on routine chest radiographs. AJR Am J Roentgenol 1989;152:991–4.
52. Fischer A, Blanche S, Le Bidois J, et al. Anti-B-cell monoclonal antibodies in the treatment of severe B-cell lymphoproliferative syndrome following bone marrow and organ transplantation. N Engl J Med 1991;324:1451–6.

Book reviews

Cranial neuroimaging and clinical neuroanatomy. Atlas of MR imaging and computed tomography. Edited by H-J Kretschmann and W Weinrich, pp viii + 451, 2004 (Georg Thieme-Verlag, Stuttgart), €199.00
ISBN 3-13-672603-0

This book is ostensibly an atlas of cerebral anatomy, which will be well known to the large number of Radiologists since it has been in press in previous editions since 1986. The book has progressively grown since then and is now extremely comprehensive. The main value of this book is the lavish and beautifully prepared illustrations that appear throughout it. The first section of the book is basically an overview and introduction. The second starts with a basic description of imaging techniques and of global neuroanatomy but the main portion of it is a series of comparative cross-sectional anatomical diagrams paired with appropriate T_1 and T_2 magnetic resonance images. The images are of good quality and the diagrams are beautiful in quality and appear to be extremely anatomically accurate. Coronal, axial and sagittal images are presented and appropriate CT sections are also presented through the base of skull and upper cervical spine. These include sagittal CT as well as magnetic resonance. The CTs are derived from post mortem cadaver samples and therefore show bony anatomy exquisitely. This main atlas section is followed by a specialist series of anatomical illustrations of brainstem anatomy again sumptuously illustrated and compared with matching MR-based images. Section 3 deals with the topography of the facial skeleton using illustrations to identify anatomical areas and relationships. Section 4 describes the topography of the pharynx and craniocervical junction and section 5 describes the anatomy of the bony skull and the cerebrospinal fluid (CSF) spaces. This chapter is again beautifully illustrated although many of the illustrations are clearly very similar to those in other sections, the areas of interest are highlighted and this does make for clear demonstration of the anatomy. Section 4 also includes illustrations of the cerebral vasculature and the vascular territories within the brain and descriptive anatomy of the cranial nerves as well as descriptive anatomy of the prosencephalic lobes and of major gyri and sulci. This chapter along with several others are illustrated by the 3D renderings from TM's Computer-based Atlas Of Cerebral Anatomy which will be familiar to many Neuroradiologists. Chapter 6 starts to deal with neurofunctional systems showing the anatomical distribution of fibres and nuclei in the major functional systems such as the trigeminal, medial lemniscus, gustatory system, auditory system and others. Chapter 7 provides an overview of the current status and knowledge about neuro transmitters in the brain and chapter 8 describes the imaging techniques that have been applied throughout the atlas.

This is basically a bench reference book for people who are reporting cerebral scans and wish to be certain that the relational anatomy of the systems involved in patient symptoms agrees with the imaging findings. It is also a nice book for people starting to learn neuroantomy at a fairly higher level such as specialist trainees in neuroradiology. If I have one complaint about this book it is that the layout is a little confusing and it is actually quite difficult to find things that you might want to specifically look at except by flicking through and spotting the appropriate illustration. This is not helped by the fact that the illustrated atlas components of the book which are in many ways its most valuable component, are not actually included in the Table of Contents or separately identified in a Table of Illustrations which would have made it far easier to find the areas that you want. Despite this it is an excellent book and it certainly has a place on my bookshelf and I will also be recommending it to trainees who are at the stage of needing to learn neuroanatomy to any level of complexity.

A JACKSON

MRI manual of pelvic cancer. By P A Hulse and B M Carrington, pp 251, 2004 (Martin Dunitz Ltd, London, UK), £75.00
ISBN 1-85996-069-3

This new multi-author British text that has been compiled to provide radiologists with a working knowledge of MRI in the various pelvic cancers. Its publication occurs at a time when cancer imaging generally is assuming increasing importance.

The first chapter outlines the role of MRI in tumour staging and the second describes the techniques used in pelvic cancer. The third is longer and gives an overview of pelvic anatomy both in clear text and with the use of high quality images. In all of these early chapters there is a refreshing absence of MRI physics, which one often has to wade through in some other texts.

The rest of the book is dedicated to individual chapters on the various pelvic cancers. As with the anatomy chapter, the images are of excellent quality and well annotated. The last two chapters describe the appearances of pelvic metastases and that of residual or recurrent disease, which can be very difficult to evaluate.

For those on the learning curve for this type of work, the book should be close at hand when reporting examinations. It combines clear and concise text along with many excellent images of each cancer type. I would not hesitate to recommend that it should be available in all MRI departments carrying out pelvic cancer evaluation.

J ROBERTS

The British Journal of Radiology, 78 (2005), 283–284
DOI: 10.1259/bjr/17730869

Case of the month

Whispering enigma

[1]H ANSARI, MRCP, [1]T PATANKAR, FRCR and [2]A JACKSON, PhD, FRCR, FRCP

[1]*Department of Radiology, Hope Hospital, Manchester M6 8HD and* [2]*Imaging Science and Biomedical Engineering, Department of Medicine, Stopford Building, Oxford Road, Manchester M13 9PT, UK*

A 73-year-old lady presented with headaches, dizzy spells and left sided subjective tinnitus. Headaches had been long lasting, intermittent, in the frontal and temporal regions, and dizzy spells were occasional with light-headedness, with no episodes of falls or loss of consciousness. Significant previous medical history included hiatus hernia, irritable bowel disease, trigeminal neuralgia, and spondylosis. Clinical examination was normal with no cerebellar signs. Rinnes and Webers tests were normal. An MR scan (3 Tesla, Achieva; Philips Medical System, Best, Netherlands) was performed to rule out an acoustic neuroma.

What is the radiological abnormality demonstrated in Figure 1? What are the radiological findings in Figure 2? What is the diagnosis? How would you explain tinnitus on the basis of the imaging findings?

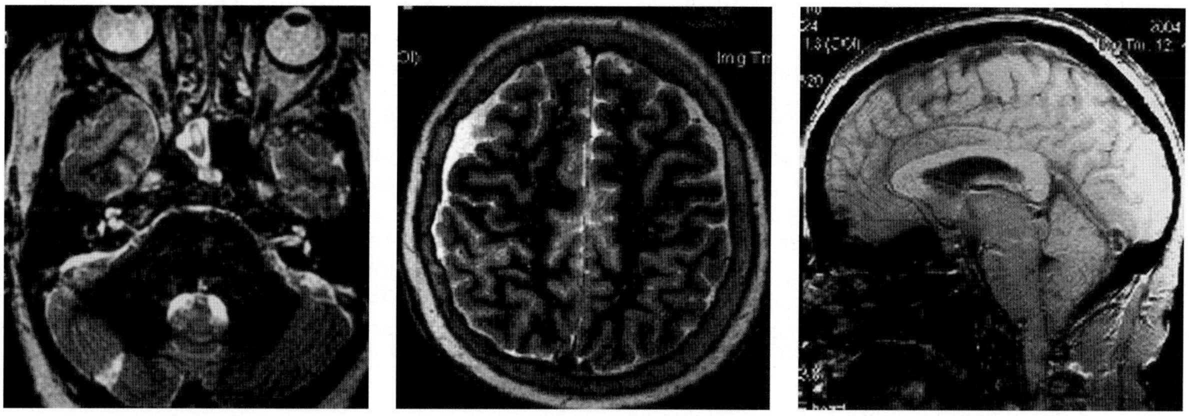

(a) (b) (c)

Figure 1. (a,b) Axial T_1 weighted inversion recovery sequence. (c) Sagittal T_1 weighted fast field echo.

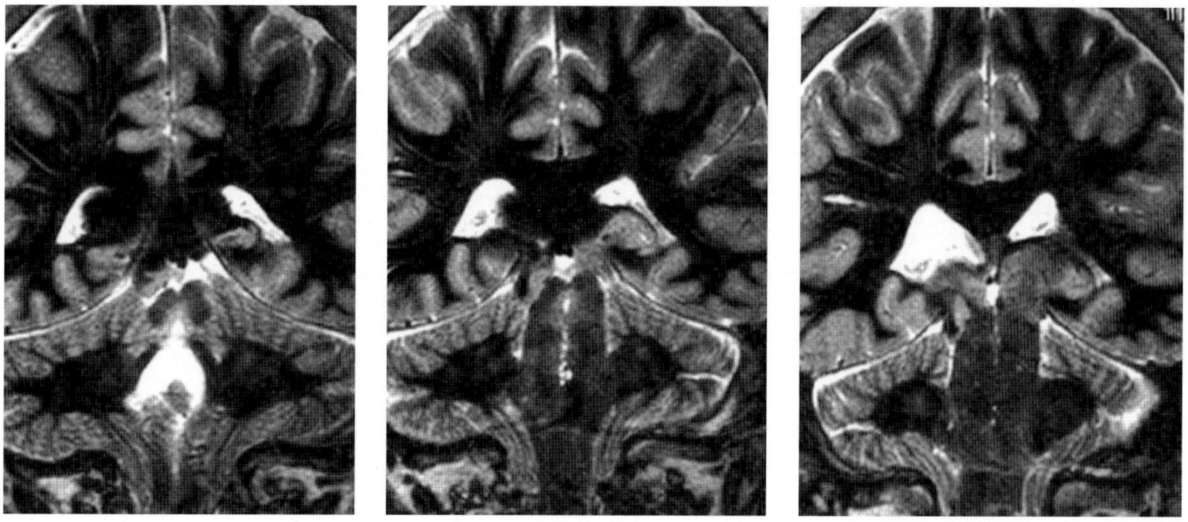

(a) (b) (c)

Figure 2. (a,b,c) Coronal T_2 weighted inversion recovery sequence.

Received 27 July 2004 and in revised form 3 December 2004, accepted 5 January 2005.

The radiological abnormality in Figure 1 is a marked thickening of the diploic spaces, with marked skull softening and descent of the vertex. There is also downward descent of the cerebellar tonsils in the foramen magnum.

The radiological finding in Figure 2 is herniation of the parahippocampal gyrus around the tentorial hiatus, which is causing direct compression of the superior and inferior colliculus on the right side. There is also a smaller herniation on the left causing compression of the superior colliculus.

The diagnosis is Paget's disease.

Compression of the inferior colliculus as a result of the herniation of the parahippocampal gyrus in Paget's disease leads to tinnitus.

Discussion

Sound travels from the cochlear hair cells, along the eighth nerve to reach the cochlear nucleus located on the lateral–ventral side of the brain stem under the cerebellum. From the cochlear nucleus, axons stream out mainly along the trapezoid body to join superior olivary nuclei. Axons arising from the superior olivary nuclei join the crossed and uncrossed axons from the cochlear nucleus to form the lateral lemniscus, and eventually synapse in the inferior colliculus on the ventral side of mid-brain just below the thalamus. Most of the cells in the inferior colliculus send their axons to the medial geniculate body of the thalamus in the ipsilateral side of the brain. The cells in the medial geniculate body then send their axons to the ipsilateral primary auditory cortex in the superior temporal gyrus.

Tinnitus is the perception of sound in one or both ears or in the head in the absence of external stimuli. Although the exact physiological causes of tinnitus are not known, a wide variety of ear diseases and disorders including impacted cerumen, acoustic neuroma, Meniere's disease, acoustic over stimulation, open eustachian tube and otosclerosis have been implicated. Medications, most notably aspirin-containing compounds, aminoglycosides and non-steroidal anti-inflammatory drugs may also produce tinnitus.

Tinnitus can be classified in two categories: objective tinnitus, that produced by para-auditory structures, and subjective tinnitus generated by the sensorineural auditory system, subjective tinnitus being much more prevalent than objective tinnitus [1].

Objective tinnitus may be pulsatile or non-pulsatile. Pulsatile tinnitus is attributed to increased turbulence of blood flow, and majority of these cases are attributed to benign intracranial hypertension, atherosclerotic coronary artery disease and glomus tumours.

Subjective tinnitus originates within the auditory system and can be caused by abnormal conditions in the cochlea, the cochlear nerve, the ascending auditory pathway, or the auditory cortex. Functional MRI studies have shown abnormal inferior colliculus activation in lateralized tinnitus patients [2].

Paget's disease of bone, is a disease of unknown aetiology, characterized by excessive and abnormal remodelling of bone. The skull is involved in about two thirds of cases and radiological changes being often advanced by the time of diagnosis. It typically causes enlargement of bone, generalized thickening of vault, middle and outer tables with accentuated trabecular pattern.

Paget's disease complicates the skull in form of basilar invagination owing to softening of bone, malignancy (osteosarcoma and fibrosarcoma) and narrowing of basal foramina, which in turn causes cranial nerve lesion, especially deafness, and occasional compression of medulla oblongata or upper spinal cord. Encroachment on the labyrinthine capsule, distortion of cochlea with osseous fractures between basal and middle turns, and cochlear capsule demineralization have been reported [3].

Tinnitus, vertigo, or both have been reported in about 20% of patients with Paget's disease. Patients with Paget's disease of the temporal bone, are known to have pulsatile tinnitus [4]. In a case review of 165 patients with skull involvement in Paget's disease 31 had tinnitus, 20 of whom had pulsatile tinnitus [5] which some authors attributed to increase in the size and number of the blood vessels and extensive arteriovenous shunting, which is frequently encountered in these cases [6]. The unique feature in our case was the patients clinical presentation with subjective tinnitus, which is unusual and in our opinion is due to inferior collicular compression secondary to her Paget's disease.

References

1. Schleuning AJ. Tinnitus. In: Bailey BJ, editor. Head and neck surgery – otolaryngology (2nd edn). Philadelphia, PA: Lippincott – Raven, 1998.
2. Melcher JR, Sigalovsky IS, Guinan JJ Jr, Levine RA. Lateralized tinnitus studied with functional magnetic resonance imaging: abnormal inferior colliculus activation. J Neurophysiol 2000;83:1058–72.
3. Phelps PD, Lloyd GA. Diagnostic imaging of the ear (2nd edn). London, UK: Springer-Verlag, 1983:209.
4. Sismanis A. Pulsatile tinnitus. A 15-years experience. Am J Otol 1998;19:472–7.
5. Davies DG. Pagets disease of the temporal bone. Acta Otolaryngol 1968;65(Suppl. 242):1–47.
6. Nager GT. Pagets disease of the temporal bone. Ann Otorhinolaryngology 1984;84 Suppl (22):2.

Correspondence

(The Editors do not hold themselves responsible for opinions expressed by correspondents)

Posterior fossa treatment

The Editor—Sir,

The interesting and commendable comparisons of conventional, conformal and intensity-modulated coplanar radiotherapy plans for posterior fossa treatment of medulloblastoma patients [1] confirm the widely held doubts about application of intensity-modulated radiotherapy (IMRT) techniques in children. The associated "dose bath" effect obtained with IMRT could be deleterious not only to growing tissues in terms of deleterious functional effects but also there is the potential enhanced increased risk of stochastic effects such as induction of second malignancy [2].

This treatment planning exercise will be informative to British radiotherapy centres that possess the techniques used in the study, although there is a risk of complacency because of our characteristic insular approach to radiotherapy. The availability of more sophisticated proton beams abroad allows for better dose distributions than those demonstrated. The French group (Paris/Orsay) are developing a cochlear sparing technique [3] and at the Northeast Proton Therapy Centre (Boston), sparing of spinal exit dose to include only 0.7 cm of the vertebral body has now been achieved, with good *in vivo* verification in terms of the delineation of bone marrow changes on MRI [4].

We British are accustomed to shortages and severe economic constraints in healthcare, but the time has arrived to consider offering the best available treatment based on improvements in physical dose distributions, particularly to our children. I would encourage our most highly specialist centres to obtain proton therapy planning software so that the appropriate isodose comparisons can be made in individual cases. This will allow clinicians and parents of children to be better informed of the potential advantages. It can only be a matter of time before Government will decide to invest in high energy particle therapy within the UK, but in the meantime we should strive to educate ourselves and prepare for such necessary developments.

Yours etc.,

B JONES

Department of Clinical Oncology
Queen Elizabeth University Hospital
Birmingham B15 2TH

(Received 28 October 2004 and accepted 3 November 2004)
DOI: 10.1259/bjr/25200453

References

1. Breen SL, Kehagioglou P, Usher C, Plowman PN. A comparison of conventional, conformal and intensity-modulated coplanar radiotherapy plans for posterior fossa treatment. Br J Radiology 2004;77:768–74.
2. Miralbell R, Lomax A, Cella L, Schneider U. Potential reduction of the incidence of radiation-induced second cancers by using proton beams in the treatment of pediatric tumors. Int J Radiat Oncol Biol Phys 2002;54:824–9.
3. Jones B, Rosenberg I. Particle Therapy Co-operative Oncology Group (PTCOG 40) Meeting, Institute Curie 2004. Br J Radiol 2005;78:99–102.
4. Adams J, Liebsch NJ (personal communication, October 2004).

Author's reply

The Editor—Sir,

Professor Jones and I both share a concern over an IMRT low dose "bath" in the exit tissues through which the multiple beams exit – and the growing facial bones of the child is a prime example for that concern when planning the posterior fossa boost in medulloblastoma therapy – both from the growth/development and oncogenesis view points.

That proton beam therapy may improve the dosimetry of posterior fossa radiotherapy is of interest and the cochlear dose advantage is potentially important in a disease where the co-morbid agent Cisplatin is also prescribed.

That paediatric medulloblastoma is the topic under discussion here is pertinent in that the first phase of treatment involves whole neuraxis radiotherapy. The Boston proton technique, cited by Jones, manages whole craniospinal radiotherapy with very little dose to the vertebral bodies and other anterior exit structures. However, late reverse spinal lordosis, commonly observed in the 250 KV era and due to a dose gradient across the vertebral body of a young child, is a likely late event. High skin and bone canthal entry doses were a disadvantage when proton beam therapy was compared with radioisotope plaque therapy for retinoblastoma. New techniques bring new considerations.

That proton facilities are becoming more user friendly is a practical advance.

With the foregoing in mind, we agree with Jones that modern proton radiotherapy needs a home in the UK and the "absent" exit dose advantage is a potential bonus in paediatric work (as exemplified here) in addition to its focal and conformal advantages.

[1]P N PLOWMAN
[2]C USHER

[1]Department of Radiotherapy
St. Bartholomew's Hospital
The Hospital for Sick Children
Great Ormond Street
London
[2]Physics Department
Radiotherapy
St. Bartholomew's Hospital
London

(Received 2 December 2004 and accepted 2 December 2004)
DOI: 10.1259/bjr/71080454

BIR CORPORATE MEMBER SCHEME

The BIR Corporate Member Scheme is aimed at all companies with an interest in radiology and allied sciences. For an annual subscription member companies are offered an attractive benefits package. To find out why your company should join the leading edge companies listed below, please contact Mr Adrian C Laws, Marketing Manager, British Institute of Radiology, 36 Portland Place, London W1B 1AT. Tel: +44 (0) 20 7307 1404.

Agfa-Gevaert Ltd
Tel: 020 82314900
Contact Mr M Hill, Business Manager Medical Imaging and PACS Systems
Product Code: 1, 2, 3, 4, 6, 9, 10, 12, 13, 14, 15, 20, 22 and 23

Alliance Medical Ltd
Tel: 01295 671223
Contact Mr Charles Fox, Marketing Executive
Product Code: 1, 4, 5, 16, 20 and 21

Amersham Health
Tel: 01494 798666
Contact Mr D G Rothery, Marketing Manager
Product Codes: 1, 2, 3, 4, 5 and 6

Bard Limited
Tel: 01293 606864
Contact Ms T Empson, Product Manager
Product Code: 2

B.M.V.A.
Tel: 01483 689838
Contact Dr R Bowden, Meetings Officer
Product Codes: 1, 3, 4, 9, 10 and 21

Bracco UK Ltd
Tel: 01628 851500
Contact Mr A Quinn, Product Manager
Product Codes: 1, 2 and 5

BVM Medical Ltd
Tel: 01455 614555
Contact Jay Tailor, Managing Director
Product Codes: 2 and 18

Cerner Corporation (UK)
Tel: 01452 831533
Contact Mr C Harrison, Client Executive
Product Codes: 9, 10, 13 and 20

Clinical Press Ltd
Tel: 0117 9420256
Contact Professor Paul Goddard, Chairman
Product Codes: 17 and 21

Cook (UK) Ltd
Tel: 01462 482884
Contact Mr Iain Mackintosh, regional Manager - Diagnostic and Interventional Products
Product Code: 2

Department of Radiography & Imaging Sciences (St Martin's College, Lancaster)
Tel: 01524 384640
Contact Mr Philip Harris, Acting Head of Department
Product Code: 21

Dictaphone International
Tel:020 78785000
Contact Dr F Brabant, Director of Product Management
Product Codes: 9 and 13

E-Z-EM Ltd
Tel: 01869 366900
Contact Mr Martin Suggitt, Product Manager
Product Codes: 1, 2 and 8

Ferrania UK Ltd
Tel: 01344 312100
Contact Mr Alan Budge, General Marketing Manager
Product Codes: 1, 3, 4, 9, 10, 13, 14, 15 and 18

Fuji Photo Film (UK) Ltd
Tel: 01234 326780
Contact Mr R G Brown, Strategic Business Manager
Product Codes: 1, 3, 4, 6, 9, 10, 12, 13, 14, 15, 18 and 22

GE Medical Systems
Tel: 01753 874000
Contact Mr A Trivett, Managing Director
Product Codes: 1, 2, 3, 4, 6, 8, 9, 10, 15, 18 and 22

Guerbet Laboratories Ltd
Tel: 01908 522888
Contact Mr Trevor Furniss, General Manager
Product Code: 1 and 2

Insignia Medical Systems Ltd
Tel: 01420 540206
Contact Mr Richard Dormer, Managing Director
Product Code: 9

Kimal plc
Tel: 01895 270951
Contact Mr S Clarke, Technical Director
Product Code: 2

Kingsmoor Publications Ltd
Tel: 01371 812960
Contact Mr David Roberts, Managing Director
Product Code: 17

Kodak Ltd
Tel: 01442 844473
Contact Mr Chris Wright, Marketing Manager UK and Ireland
Product Codes: 1, 3, 4, 6, 8, 9, 10, 12, 13, 14, 15, 18, 21, 22 and 23

Landauer, Inc.
Tel: 01865 373008
Contact Dr T Finnigan, Director, European Operations
Product Code: 8

Lanmark
Tel: 01494 675535
Contact Mrs Liz Beckmann, Director
Product Codes: 6, 9, 10, 13, 17 and 20

Lodestone Patient Care Limited
Tel: 020 89449630
Contact Mrs J Hill, Director of Operations
Product Code: 1, 3 and 21

Medical Imaging Systems Limited
Tel: 020 82059500
Contact Mr P W Sykes, Director
Product Code: 1

Mirada Solutions Ltd
Tel: 01865 265500
Contact Dr Clare Jones, VP Marketing
Product Codes: 1, 4, 6, 9, 10, 13, 21 and 22

Nucletron UK Ltd
Tel: 018297 71111
Contact Mr J Banks, Managing Director
Product Codes: 6 and 8

Pantak Medical Systems Agfa NDT
Tel: 0118 9310310
Contact Mr R Howton, Managing Director
Product Codes: 1, 6, 7 and 8

Philips Medical Systems
Tel:01737 230400
Contact Ms Anita Littlechild, Marketing Communications Manager
Product Codes: 1, 2, 9, 10, 22 and 23

Samsung SDS Europe Ltd
Tel:020 83807000
Contact Mr G Wheeler, Sales Manager (Medical)
Product Codes: 1, 9, 10, 13, 15, 16 and 20

Schering Health Care Ltd
Tel: 01444 232323
Contact Mr Chris Matthews, Product Manager
Product Codes: 1, 2 and 3

Sectra Ltd
Tel: 020 86106033
Contact Jan Wolfram, Managing Director
Product Codes: 9 and 10

Siemens Medical Solutions
Tel: 01344 396317
Contact Mr Mike Bell, Manager, Advertising and Exhibitions
Product Codes: 1, 2, 3, 4, 6, 9, 15 and 22

Sony Scientific and Medical
Tel: 01932 816267
Contact R Holt, Marketing Manager
Product Code: 14

Sonosite Ltd
Tel: 01767 313117
Contact Ms Gillian Duffy, European Marketing Director
Product Codes: 3

Southern Scientific Ltd
Tel: 01903 604000
Contact Mr Stephen Adams, Sales Manager
Product Codes: 1, 3, 4, 8, 10, 12 and 22

Toshiba Medical Systems UK
Tel: 01293 653700
Contact Mr S M Weeden, Manager X-ray Products
Product Codes: 1, 2, 3, 4, 9, 10 and 15

Varian Oncology Systems
Tel: 01293 531244 (UK)
Contact Mr Rolf Stähelin (Switzerland - tel. 00 41 417498844), Marketing Manager, Europe
Product Code: 6

Vertec Scientific Ltd
Tel: 01734 817431
Contact Mr B Hipgrave, Managing Director
Product Codes: 1, 4, 6, 8 and 12

Wardray Premise Ltd
Tel: 020 83989911
Contact Mr R Beach, Sales Manager
Product Codes: 8, 18 and 20

Wolverson X-Ray
Tel: 01902 637333
Contact Mr N Bacon, Sales Director
Product Codes: 1, 8, 15, 18 and 23

Xograph Imaging Systems
Tel: 01666 501501 or 07000 for X-ray
Contact Mr N Staff, Technical Director
Product Codes: 1, 8, 12, 14, 15, 18, 22 and 23

PRODUCT CODES

1. Diagnostic X-ray including NMR and CT
2. Interventional radiology
3. Ultrasound
4. Nuclear medicine
5. Radiopharmaceuticals
6. Radiotherapy and oncology
7. Radiobiology
8. Radiation protection
9. PACS
10. Image processing
11. Nuclear fuel cycle service
12. Quality assurance
13. Radiology data management computer systems
14. Video printing
15. Equipment leasing
16. Hospital-shared services
17. Medical publishing
18. X-ray consumables distribution
19. Electricity generation
20. Medical reporting systems
21. Education
22. Mammography
23. Dental X-ray

Meetings & Courses

Nuclear medicine in oncology
17 March 2005
London, UK
Further details: The British Institute of Radiology, 36 Portland Place, London W1B 1AT.
Tel: 0207 307 1406. Fax: 0207 307 1414.
Email: registrations@bir.org.uk. Visit: www.bir.org.uk

Image display workstations
12 April 2005
London, UK
Further details: The British Institute of Radiology, 36 Portland Place, London W1B 1AT.
Tel: 0207 307 1406. Fax: 0207 307 1414.
Email: registrations@bir.org.uk. Visit: www.bir.org.uk

MR angiography
15 April 2005
London, UK
Further details: The British Institute of Radiology, 36 Portland Place, London W1B 1AT.
Tel: 0207 307 1406. Fax: 0207 307 1414.
Email: registrations@bir.org.uk. Visit: www.bir.org.uk

Prepare yourself for PACS
6 May 2005
London, UK
Further details: The British Institute of Radiology, 36 Portland Place, London W1B 1AT.
Tel: 0207 307 1406. Fax: 0207 307 1414.
Email: registrations@bir.org.uk. Visit: www.bir.org.uk

President's Conference 2005
25–26 May 2005
London, UK
Further details: The British Institute of Radiology, 36 Portland Place, London W1B 1AT.
Tel: 0207 307 1406. Fax: 0207 307 1414.
Email: registrations@bir.org.uk. Visit: www.bir.org.uk

IMRT
8 July 2005
Manchester, UK
Further details: The British Institute of Radiology, 36 Portland Place, London W1B 1AT.
Tel: 0207 307 1406. Fax: 0207 307 1414.
Email: registrations@bir.org.uk. Visit: www.bir.org.uk

International Cancer Imaging Society Meeting and 5th Annual Teaching Course
3–5 October 2005
Beurs van Berlage, Amsterdam, The Netherlands
Further details: The British Institute of Radiology, 36 Portland Place, London W1B 1AT.
Tel: 0207 307 1406. Fax: 0207 307 1414.
Email: icis@bir.org.uk. Visit: www.icimagingsociety.org.uk

Achieva 3.0T research and clinical benefits readily apparent at University of Manchester

Clinicians at first Achieva 3.0T site exploit high SNR and multi-channel RF architecture in many applications.

Within just two weeks of arriving at the University of Manchester in April 2004, the world's first Achieva 3.0T system was up and running. During the ensuing eight weeks, clinicians affirmed the Achieva's capabilities in clinical and research examinations ranging from BOLD imaging, MR spectroscopy, and diffusion-weighted imaging to angiographic, musculoskeletal and abdominal scanning. In addition, the high field strength, combined with the FreeWave spectrometer scalable up to 32 RF channels, convinced Manchester radiologists Prof. Alan Jackson, Dr. Charles Hutchinson, and scientist Prof Steve Williams, that Achieva 3.0T will contribute significantly to a multitude of emerging applications.

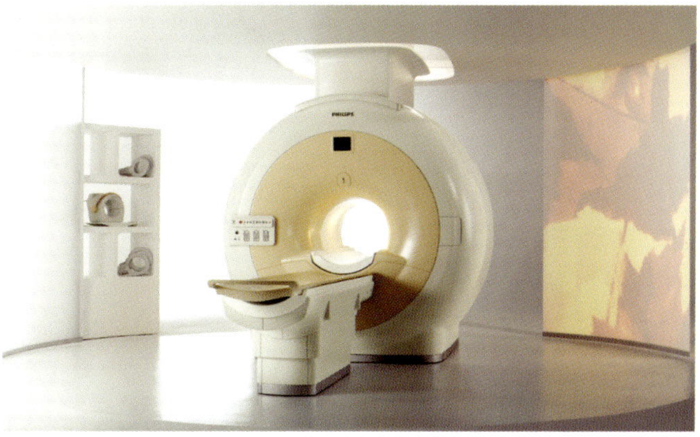

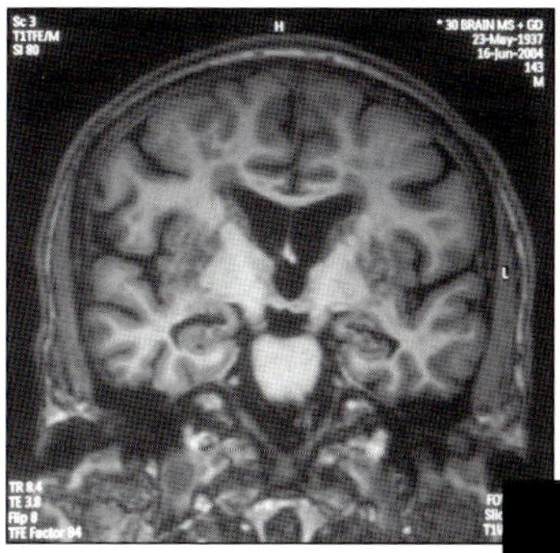

High-resolution T1w 3D volume. Voxels are 0.9mm in all three planes, allowing the data to be reformatted into any plane without loss of image quality. In the coronal plane the layers of grey and white matter in the hippocampus can be distinguished.

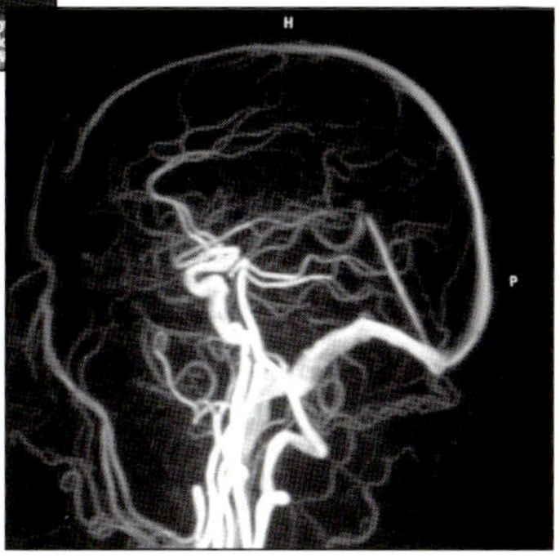

Sagittal MIP, time-of-flight MRA of cranial vessels. Using SENSE with the 8-channel head coil gives a scan time of less than 6 mins for this high resolution acquisition.

"Because we received the world's first scanner of its type we weren't expecting to start out at a very great rate", says Prof. Alan Jackson, Chair in Neuroradiology at Manchester. "In fact, what we got was a high performance well-designed machine that we were able to use clinically immediately and effectively. Many of the problems we anticipated we might encounter at 3.0T haven't surfaced. The image quality is excellent and we are very favourably impressed."

Achieva 3.0T performance leaves no doubt about 3.0T clinical potential

Appreciating that 3.0T offers twice the signal-to-noise as 1.5T is one thing – actually witnessing the benefits is another, says Prof. Jackson. "We've been doing quite a lot of very high resolution imaging of the brain in very reasonable times by virtue of Achieva's gradient performance. You can see individual third branch arteries going out on to the cortex, which would be unexpected at 1.5T or lower fields."

Achieva revolutionises DWI

In addition to routine phase contrast angiography with SENSE, diffusion-weighted imaging clinical studies have been exceptional, adds Prof. Jackson. "We've been doing diffusion research here for years, and Achieva 3.0T has revolutionised DWI. A colleague has already written a paper based on two or three image sets acquired with Achieva after just one week of sequence optimisation. Furthermore, the diffusion tensor tractography, using 32 and 64 diffusion directions, has superb spatial resolution – we're able to produce beautiful, isotropic, multi-directional data sets, something we really couldn't do before. This will be invaluable in white matter fibre tract research."

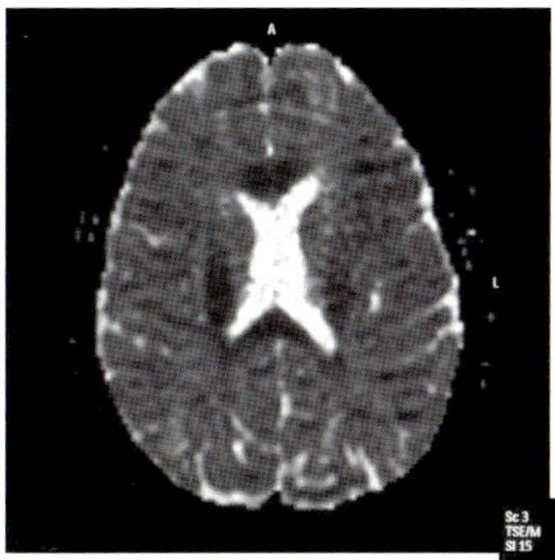

Calculated ADC map from DWI-EPI, normal brain. A relatively large matrix is used with SENSE factor 2.0 to reduce the echo time, which minimises the distortions normally associated with EPI.

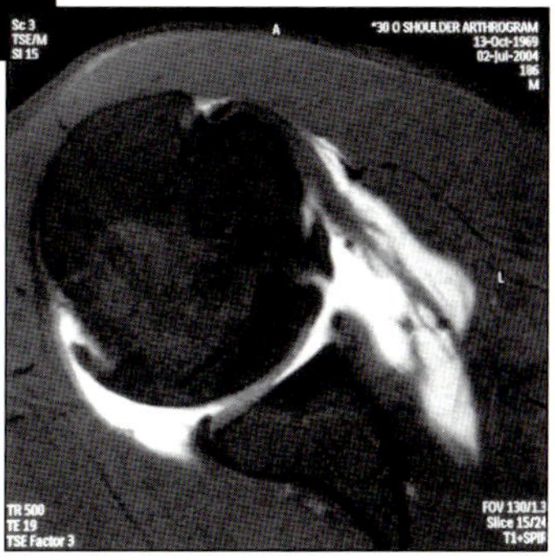

Axial view, shoulder arthrogram, in a patient with a history of traumatic injury to the joint. The cartilage can be clearly visualised and there is irregular thickening of the periosteum on the anterior aspect of the glenoid.

Volume 78| **April 2005**

BJR British Journal of Radiology

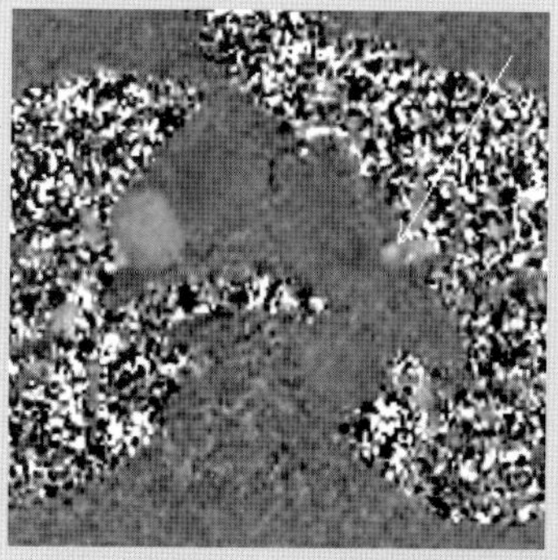

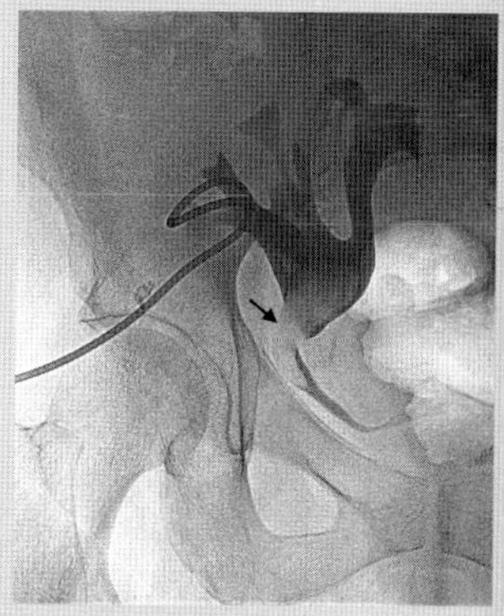

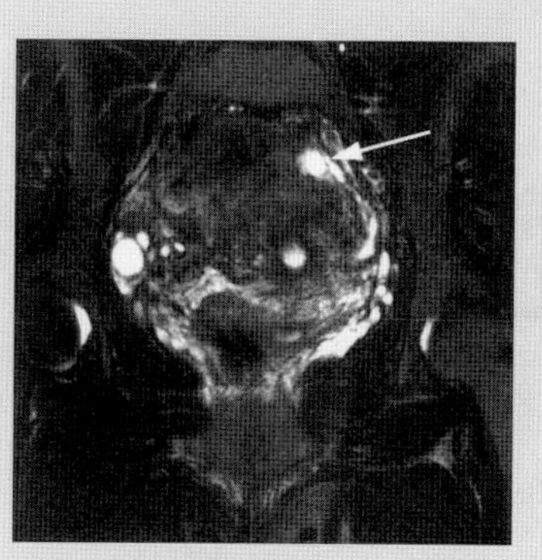

Full papers

Perioperative monitoring of flow and patency in native and grafted internal mammary arteries using a combined MR protocol

A comparison of fast MRI of hips with and without parallel imaging using SENSE

Colour Doppler ultrasound mapping of chest wall lesions

Three-dimensional anal endosonography may improve diagnostic confidence of detecting damage to the anal sphincter complex

Comparison of full-field digital mammography and film–screen mammography: image quality and lesion detection

Automatic selection of non-coplanar beam directions for three-dimensional conformal radiotherapy

In vivo absorbed dose measurements in mammography using a new real-time luminescence technique

Editorial
Short communications
Case reports
Pictorial review
Case of the month
Correspondence
Book reviews

Published by

BIR The British Institute of **Radiology**

http://bjr.birjournals.org

ISSN 0007-1285

BJR

ISSN 0007 1285

THE BRITISH JOURNAL OF RADIOLOGY

Aims and Coverage

The *British Journal of Radiology* is the official peer-reviewed monthly research journal of the British Institute of Radiology. It is a multidisciplinary journal covering all clinical and technical aspects of diagnostic imaging, radiotherapy and oncology, medical physics and radiobiology. BJR is an international journal containing papers both from the UK and overseas, and is circulated to Full Members of the BIR and to libraries worldwide.

Authors are strongly advised to submit manuscripts online using Editorial Manager^{TM}, at http://bjr.edmgr.com. Online submission will expedite the peer-review process. Instructions to Authors are available on request from the Refereeing Administrator at the address given below, and are also available on the BIR's website at www.bir.org.uk

Editorial Board

Overseas Advisory Panel

BRITISH INSTITUTE OF RADIOLOGY & RÖNTGEN SOCIETY

Published by the British Institute of Radiology, 36 Portland Place, London W1B 1AT, UK.
Editorial enquiries: Tel: +44 (0)20 7307 1424; Fax: +44 (0)20 7307 1414
Email: publications@bir.org.uk
Advertising sales and enquiries: please contact Gareth Liddiatt at McMillan Scott: Tel: +44 (0)20 7878 2313
Email: gareth@mcmslondon.co.uk
www.bir.org.uk www.birjournals.org bjr.edmgr.com

Subscriptions

Subscriptions fulfilment is carried out by PSP Subscriptions, BMA House, Tavistock Square, London WC1H 9JR, UK (Telephone +44 (0)20 7383 6270; Fax +44 (0)20 7383 6402; email subscriptions@bmjgroup.com). The 2005 annual subscription rate for the printed version of BJR is £524 (includes 12 issues plus two Special Issue). Subscriptions are on a calendar basis only.

Institutional BJR subscribers have free access to both BJR Online and Imaging Online, and are offered a 33% discount on a print subscription to the BJR's quarterly review journal Imaging (see http://imaging.birjournals.org).

US Mailing Agent

The British Journal of Radiology (ISSN 0007 1285) is published monthly by the British Institute of Radiology, c/o Mercury Airfreight Int. Ltd, 365 Blair Road, Avenel, NJ 07001. The Dollar price for US direct subscribers is $786. Periodicals Postage Paid at Rahway NJ. Postmaster: send address corrections to the British Journal of Radiology, c/o Mercury Airfreight Int. Ltd, 365 Blair Road, Avenel, NJ 07001.

Back Issues

Back issues can be ordered from Vine House Distribution, Waldenbury, North Common, Chailey, East Sussex BN8 4DR, UK (Telephone +44 (0)1825 723398; Fax +44 (0)1825 724188). Price is £40 per issue.

BJR Online

BJR Online, produced in association with HighWire Press, is available free of charge to BIR members and Institutional print subscribers: http://bjr.birjournals.org. Enquiries to publications@bir.org.uk

Typeset, printed and bound by The Charlesworth Group, Wakefield, UK. Telephone +44 (0)1924 204830.

BJR

VOLUME 78

Number 928

Contents

April 2005

Front cover: *The illustrations used on the front cover of this issue of BJR can be found on pages 296, 344, and 346. We thank the authors for granting us permission to use their figures.*

Editorial

Page

- Ultrasound exposure measurement: a hidden science? — 289
  F A Duck

Full papers

- Perioperative monitoring of flow and patency in native and grafted internal mammary arteries using a combined MR protocol — 292
  N I Stauder, A M Scheule, U Hahn, M Fenchel, F S Eckstein, U Kramer, C D Claussen and S Miller
- A comparison of fast MRI of hips with and without parallel imaging using SENSE — 299
  M Ryan, P Cunningham, C Cantwell, D Brennan and S Eustace
- Colour Doppler ultrasound mapping of chest wall lesions — 303
  C Görg, T Bert, K Görg and M Heinzel-Gutenbrunner
- Three-dimensional anal endosonography may improve diagnostic confidence of detecting damage to the anal sphincter complex — 308
  A F Christensen, B Nyhuus, M B Nielsen and H Christensen
- Comparison of full-field digital mammography and film–screen mammography: image quality and lesion detection — 312
  A Fischmann, K C Siegmann, A Wersebe, C D Claussen and M Müller-Schimpfle
- Automatic selection of non-coplanar beam directions for three-dimensional conformal radiotherapy — 316
  J Meyer, S M Hummel, P S Cho, M M Austin-Seymour and M H Phillips
- *In vivo* absorbed dose measurements in mammography using a new real-time luminescence technique — 328
  M C Aznar, B Hemdal, J Medin, C J Marckmann, C E Andersen, L Bøtter-Jensen, I Andersson and S Mattsson

Short communications

- Further evidence for biological effects resulting from ionizing radiation doses in the diagnostic X-ray range — 335
  S Anoopkumar-Dukie, A McMahon, A Allshire and T J Conere
- Comparison between 1 T MRI and non-MRI based volumetry in inoculated tumours in mice — 338
  B Cornelissen, V Kersemans, L Jans, L Staelens, R Oltenfreiter, T Thonissen, E Achten and G Slegers

Case reports

■ An ovary in luteal phase mimicking common iliac lymph node metastasis from a primary cutaneous peripheral primitive neuroectodermal tumour as revealed by 18-fluoro-2-deoxyglucose positron emission tomography 343
K-C Ho, K-K Ng, T-C Yen and H-H Chou

■ Papillary necrosis causing hydronephrosis in renal allograft treated by percutaneous retrieval of sloughed papilla 346
S Kamath, M P Moody, J C Hammonds and I P Wells

■ The absent kidney in $^{99}Tc^{m}$-MAG3 renogram: a dramatic reversible consequence of contrast nephrotoxicity superimposed on renal obstruction 349
I Kayani, A M Groves, R Syed, N Nagabushan, F Pakzad, E M Prvulovich and J B Bomanji

■ MRI and CT findings of cryptococcal vaginitis 353
S Ranganathan, F Moosa, A Kamarulzaman and L M Looi

■ The reverse target sign in liver disease: a potential ultrasound feature in cirrhotic liver nodules characterization 355
G J Kraus, P Schedlbauer, S Lax, D Zebedin and F Flueckiger

■ Re-treatment of a lung tumour using a simple intensity-modulated radiotherapy approach 358
A W Beavis, A Abdel-Hamid and S Upadhyay

Pictorial review

■ Diseases of the submandibular gland as demonstrated using high resolution ultrasound 362
F Alyas, K Lewis, M Williams, A B Moody, K T Wong, A T Ahuja and D C Howlett

Correspondence

■ EBM and the diagnosis of hepatocellular carcinoma 370
P J A Robinson

■ Authors' reply 371
A K Burroughs, K T T Fung, F T W Li, M L Raimondo, D Maudgil, A Mancuso, J M Tibballs, A A Watkinson and D Patch

Case of the month

■ An unusual cause of rectal bleeding 373
A M Kaiser and C Spanos

Book reviews 376

Meetings and courses 377

BIR Company Subscribers 378

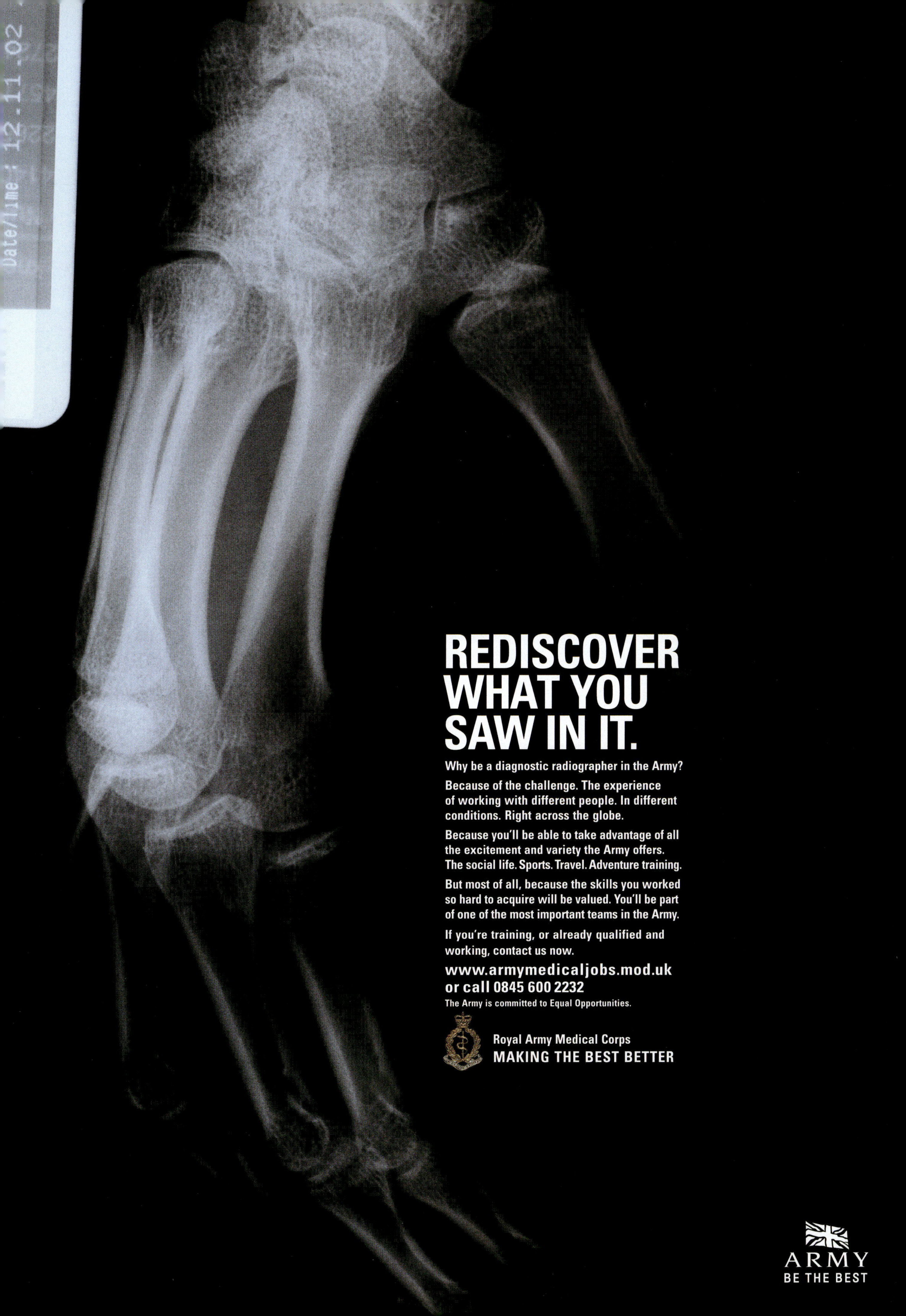
Date/Time : 12.11.02
REDISCOVER WHAT YOU SAW IN IT.
Why be a diagnostic radiographer in the Army?
Because of the challenge. The experience of working with different people. In different conditions. Right across the globe.
Because you'll be able to take advantage of all the excitement and variety the Army offers. The social life. Sports. Travel. Adventure training.
But most of all, because the skills you worked so hard to acquire will be valued. You'll be part of one of the most important teams in the Army.
If you're training, or already qualified and working, contact us now.
www.armymedicaljobs.mod.uk
or call 0845 600 2232
The Army is committed to Equal Opportunities.
Royal Army Medical Corps
MAKING THE BEST BETTER
ARMY
BE THE BEST

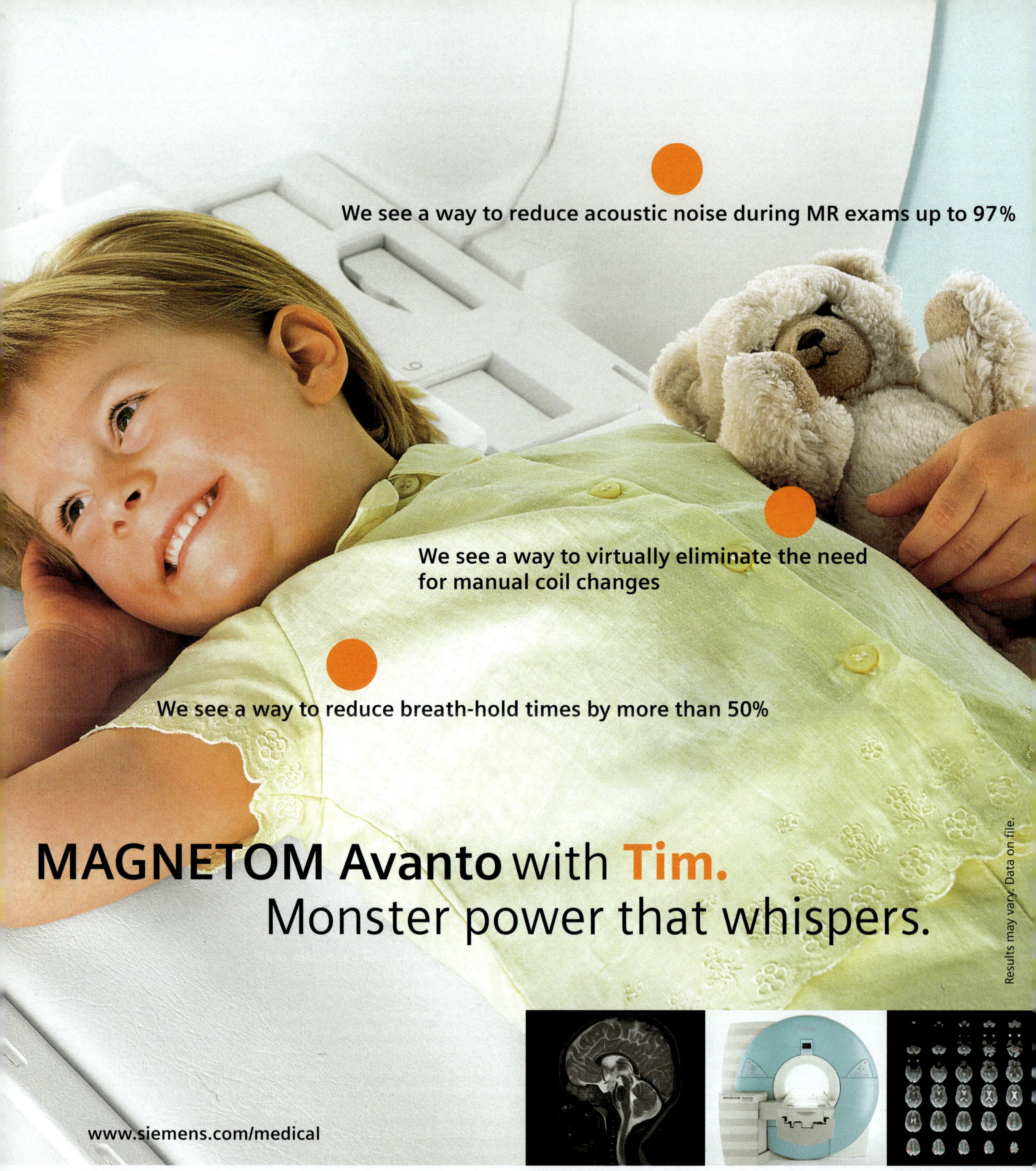

M-Z848-2-7600

Proven Outcomes in Magnetic Resonance.

MAGNETOM® Avanto, the world's first Tim™ system, takes sound to a new, and very low level. While still delivering powerful gradient performance unmatched by anything else – and essential for today's most demanding applications. MAGNETOM Avanto's AudioComfort enables an acoustic noise reduction of up to 30 dB(A).

MAGNETOM Avanto. It looks different. It sounds different. It works differently, too. To learn more, visit us at www.siemens.com/Tim.

Siemens **Medical Solutions** that help

SIEMENS
medical

The British Journal of Radiology, *78* (2005), 289–291
DOI: 10.1259/bjr/30873859

Guest editorial
Ultrasound exposure measurement: a hidden science?

F A DUCK, PhD, DSc

Medical Physics Department, Royal United Hospital NHS Trust, Bath BA1 3NG, UK

The measurement of radiation is central to the safe and effective management of radiological imaging. Diagnostic ultrasound now constitutes a substantial percentage of imaging practice. At present, however, there is very little equivalent investment in the measurement of exposure to ultrasound. This editorial explores how this has come about and what may be done to respond to the present situation.

The data for use of ultrasound in diagnostic imaging speak for themselves. During the year 2003/2004, 5 937 383 ultrasound scans were reported to the Department of Health as being carried out in NHS Trusts in England [1]. This is 19.4% of all reported imaging tests. The total was about 300 000 scans more than the previous year, slightly greater than the combined growth reported for CT and MRI. In addition, much ultrasound activity probably remains unreported, being carried out in hospital departments other than radiology or within the expanding sector of primary care. Some years ago it was estimated that 25% of all imaging worldwide was due to ultrasound, and one may speculate that this is still an underestimate of the true activity.

Exact estimates for the numbers of scanners installed are less easy to determine. In my own Trust and local health community there are approximately 40 ultrasound scanners in current use. 27 of these have been installed since January 2000. This may be compared with a current complement of approximately 50 X-ray rooms, one CT scanner and one MR scanner. So, broadly, there are similar numbers of X-ray installations as ultrasound scanners. However, the comparison alters considerably when comparing ultrasound transducers with X-ray tubes, where clearly the former considerably outnumber the latter. This Trust serves a population of about 400 000 and these figures may well mirror the experience of similar acute trusts over the rest of the country.

One cause of the extensive use and continuing growth in diagnostic ultrasound has been its enviable reputation as a safe modality for imaging. About 35% of reported scans are still carried out in obstetrics and gynaecology, where safety of the unborn child takes absolute priority. Although now only one of many uses, obstetrics established ultrasound as a preferred safe modality, substantially replacing the use of X-ray imaging with its known hazard. Nevertheless, ultrasound examinations do expose the patient to external radiation, albeit associated with different hazards than those from ionizing radiation. As a result, the science of ultrasound exposure measurement has grown in partnership with its clinical use, creating knowledge of ultrasound fields and exposure on which to base estimates of hazard and to limit risk.

Rules can be great generators of activity. The Ionising Radiation (Medical Exposure) Regulations (IR(ME)R) have resulted in many more measurements being performed to quantify patient exposure to diagnostic radiological procedures. The Regulations and the resultant dose-related measurements have helped to maintain and reinforce the balance between clinically effective use of ionizing radiation, and the risks associated with its use. For ultrasound imaging, the regulation which has had the greatest impact on exposure differs from IR(ME)R in several respects. It operates, not in the UK but in the USA, through its Food and Drug Administration (FDA) [2]. It sets a control on the design of ultrasound scanners, placing limits on the allowed ultrasound output for medical use. And its emphasis has resulted in a substantial investment in acoustic measurement by manufacturers, so that they can declare to the FDA the values of specific acoustic quantities and place their scanners "on the market" in the USA. The most important overall limit, established over 20 years ago, is still applied: estimated *in situ* spatial peak temporal-average intensity must not exceed 720 mW cm^{-2}. These FDA regulations strictly only have force in the USA; however, several other countries have also adopted these FDA regulations. Thus a US law has served to constrain ultrasound exposure in an international market. Acoustic measurement became embedded in the industrial scanner design process.

At the same time and on a much smaller scale, a few independent laboratories equipped themselves to carry out measurements of acoustic output. Calibration facilities such as those at the UK National Physical Laboratory, led by Dr Roy Preston, established robust calibration services, and themselves made measurements on commercial scanners. Ultrasound laboratories were established by NHS medical physics departments such as that in Newcastle under Dr Tony Whittingham and our own in Bath. Evidence emerged of occasional errors by manufacturers: these were largely corrected. But of greater general importance was the evidence from long-term studies of a general trend towards increased acoustic output. Clinical users were asking for improved performance and manufacturers competed to gain commercial edge; Doppler techniques evolved and limits to acoustic imaging were pushed. Independent surveys demonstrated an increasing availability of equipment capable of approaching the exposure limits set by the FDA. Nevertheless, such independent acoustic output measurements remain limited to very few active departments. The cost to set up an effective ultrasound measurement system, including appropriate hydrophones and acquisition and

Received 11 January 2005 and accepted 11 February 2005.

computing systems, often proved too great a challenge to a cash-strapped service when judged against more robust arguments for equipment for ionizing radiation measurement. Furthermore, even the basic measurement of total acoustic power required sensitive radiation force balances, which at that time were available only to those laboratories capable of designing and building them in-house.

Life moved on. Earlier FDA limits prevented the use of Doppler systems in the USA, leaving pioneers in Europe to demonstrate the value of Doppler in obstetric imaging. The US reaction was to remove the specific intensity limit placed on obstetric exposure, allowing manufacturers to make available, for obstetric applications, intensities which had previously been reserved for peripheral vascular applications only. Agreement to relax the regulation occurred, however, only with an additional agreement to introduce so-called "safety indices": the Thermal Index (TI) and the Mechanical Index (MI) [3–5]. These safety indices are now displayed on most new scanners, and are intended to guide users in the safe use of the scanner. For those involved in ultrasound exposure, however, this represented a considerable escalation in the challenge of acoustic measurement. Acoustic power must be measured to calculate TI, with special arrangements to measure "power per centimetre" from imaging arrays. MI requires measurement of hydrophone position and acoustic frequency, as well as peak rarefaction pressure, where acoustic pressure alone previously had been sufficient. Much more significantly, however, the measurement strategy changed from an investigation of conditions giving rise to maximum exposure, to a measurement regimen applied to all conditions for which a safety index value might be displayed. Users were now expected to note and act upon the displayed value whereas, before, the user had almost no information on which to control output for safety reasons. This resulted, for example, in general caution against the use of Doppler in early pregnancy. The introduction of a safety index display has, at least in principle, enabled users to determine Doppler conditions with low TI and to use these conditions preferentially.

Comparison between exposure measurements for diagnostic radiology and for diagnostic ultrasound is, perhaps, illuminating. Output of X-ray equipment is evaluated using an ionization chamber to measure exposure and a tube potential divider to estimate tube potential. More recent emphasis on patient exposure and dose has resulted in the widespread installation and use of dose–area product (DAP) meters, and the introduction of surveys with thermoluminescent dosemeters to establish and use diagnostic reference levels. Risk assessment depends on well-established Monte Carlo modelling and comparison with an established body of scientific bio-effects evidence. By comparison, ultrasound measurement uses a hydrophone to measure the acoustic pressure wave and a radiation force balance for total acoustic power. *In situ* estimation of acoustic exposure may be modelled, and temperature rise can be estimated. Whilst detailed differences exist, there is close equivalence in principle between ultrasound and X-rays. Both have established methods for measuring key parameters of the radiation. Both have models to predict radiation exposure *in situ*. Both have means to convert measured exposure to dose, although this is, at present, more highly developed for ionizing radiation than for ultrasound, for which the concept of dose has still to be properly developed. Most notably, ultrasound lacks robust means to predict risk.

But the measurement challenge for ultrasound and the costs are significant. Manufacturers are now obliged to measure the acoustic conditions relating to the full range of scanner settings, and to calculate all the safety indices according to the defining formulae. They must also take account of equipment variability, most notably that resulting from the variability of transducer manufacture. For those involved with independent measurement, full evaluation of the correctness of the displayed index values is generally impossible except for very simple scanners, within any reasonable time scale. The calculation of TI in pulsed Doppler mode, for example, requires axial intensity profiles to be measured, which demands automated hydrophone scanning to be practical. Indeed, such are the financial implications for industry that feasibility studies are in place to compute rather than measure acoustic quantities, based on validated computer models.

Although a full evaluation is beyond the scope of any independent laboratory, it is possible for an experienced laboratory to carry out spot checks of equipment for selected, critical output conditions. This is happening in a small number of hospitals and laboratories and not surprisingly, evidence is now emerging of discrepancies between displayed safety index values and those measured independently. For the larger part, the differences are small, and often the measured value is lower than that displayed, so erring on the side of caution. Nevertheless, some large errors have been found and reported. Clearly, a means designed to inform users about safety must have their confidence, and there remains work to be done both by industry and independent laboratories to ensure that the indices can always be relied upon to give valid guidance. For hospitals this requires, necessarily, investment in appropriate measurement equipment and allocation of scientists' and technologists' time to the task.

The safety indices were developed to advise the user of possible thermal and mechanical hazard. For the measurement scientist, an alternative sensible approach is to avoid the limitations of calculation inherent in the TI and to measure temperature rise directly. This approach carries the added advantages for hospital-based laboratories of relative simplicity, low cost, and speedy measurement. The development of the Thermal Test Object by the National Physical Laboratory is one approach which has provided valuable results reported in two projects funded by the Department of Health [4]; this approach deserves more extensive evaluation than it has experienced so far. However, the highest temperature rises are at the transducer surface, and measurement and management of surface temperature remains a central issue for both manufacturers and users. Many clinical scanners may cause the transducer surface to heat by 20°C in air, and can cause temperatures very close to the limit allowed by the International Electrotechnical Commission (IEC), 43°C, when in contact with the skin [5]. Of particular concern is the behaviour of interstitial transducers, especially transvaginal. A recent study from the Medical Physics Department at St George's Hospital has demonstrated that some scanner conditions may cause unacceptably high surface temperatures for some transvaginal transducers [6].

Many challenges remain. High-fidelity acoustic measurements require appropriate measurement devices, suitable for laboratory-based and for field measurements. It is commonly inconvenient or impossible to take a scanner away from its clinical setting for measurement. There is a pressing need for a well-engineered, portable commercial acoustic power meter capable of measuring acoustic power down to 10 mW or less. This would make available a direct and simple means to confirm the accuracy of displayed TI for imaging, and for identifying critical conditions for transducer heating. Hydrophone technology is well developed, and the challenges of phase calibration and spatial and temporal resolution associated with higher-frequency beams are being met. Modern ultrasound imaging systems now operate with complex sequences of ultrasound pulses of a variety of waveforms, where current hydrophone-based measurement systems may sometimes be inadequate. Non-linear propagation effects must be managed properly, and there will be measurement challenges in carrying out all measurements under low-amplitude, quasi-linear conditions. Whilst hydrophone technology is well developed, the practical use still remains clumsy even now. Hydrophones in buckets worked well as the measurement need developed, but it is time to have available an integrated easy-to-use portable package including hydrophone, positioning, data acquisition and output. Such a system would enable on-line measurement of pressure waveform, acoustic frequency, MI and temporal-average intensity, all key quantities for exposure measurement. Partnership between hospitals, standards laboratories, academics and industry is essential to progress. The UK is particularly fortunate in having local scientific and technical skills of both the National Physical Laboratory (Teddington, UK) and Precision Acoustics (Dorchester, UK) to support this area.

The availability of measurement equipment is only part of the story. Ultrasound measurement must become part of the scientific ethos of all NHS Trusts, mediated through their medical physics and bioengineering services. Commitment to a regimen of measurement support should be integrated within the risk management policies of Trusts, so ensuring accountability and the ability to respond robustly to the question "What evidence to you have that your ultrasound scanners are safe to use on patients?" Training in ultrasound measurement is already integrated within the IPEM training scheme for Medical Physicists and Clinical Engineers, and skill development for these scientists will become part of their continued professional development, supported by the national occupational standards for Healthcare Scientists. As a result, NHS Trusts will have available local skills to support and advise on ultrasound output and safety of ultrasound scanning in all disciplines.

I have heard it suggested that ultrasound measurements should lie with a central Government-funded laboratory, and that manufacturers should submit all new equipment to such a laboratory for measurement, prior to offering it for sale in the UK. This suggestion has some merit and the establishment of this type of specialist laboratory would provide a valuable resource, making available specialist skills, measurement equipment and ultrasound beam data of importance to all users of ultrasound. It seems unlikely, however, that users would tolerate significant delays between the introduction of a new scanner, transducer or mode, and the output being confirmed as appropriate for use. The task itself is substantial, with new systems, modes, and transducers being introduced monthly, and beam complexity challenging the current measurement technology. With the advent of fully computer-managed scanners, software upgrades are often distributed direct to users. Furthermore, the precedents are not good for the longevity of such a laboratory, given the recent decision to close the Medical Devices Agency "Ultrasound Equipment Evaluation Project". Such centrally-funded schemes always ultimately close because funding is linked to political expediency. Consequently, the clear priority is to establish a desire at a local level to engage with this task, and by so doing to embed scientific understanding at the point of service delivery.

The measurement of radiation is central to the tradition of radiology. The success of diagnostic ultrasound has resulted in the introduction into healthcare of very large numbers of ultrasound scanners, now approaching in number that of X-ray installations. Current hospital practice makes little or no attempt to evaluate the ultrasound radiation generated by this equipment and there is little investment in measurement tools, personnel or commitment of time to this role. Given the capital investment in ultrasound scanners, perhaps approaching £2 million per Trust, it is difficult indeed to find an argument against the purchase of a hydrophone and power balance for a few thousand pounds, or the investment in skills to understand their use and interpret the findings. Ultrasound exposure measurement still remains a sparsely-practiced science. It would be greatly to the benefit of the health service, for the users of ultrasound scanners and for the patients who are exposed to ultrasound waves, to have a visible and recognised ultrasound measurement service as an integral part of the radiation protection service within each hospital.

References

1. Department of Health, Hospital Activity Statistics: Imaging and radiodiagnostics: NHS organisations in England 2003–04. www.performance.doh.gov.uk
2. Food and Drug Administration - Centre for Devices and Radiological Health. Information for manufacturers seeking marketing clearance of diagnostic ultrasound systems and transducers. Sept 30,1997. US Department of Health and Human Services. www.fda.gov/cdrh/ode/ulstran.pdf
3. American Institute of Ultrasound in Medicine/National Electrical Manufacturers Association (AIUM/NEMA), UD 3-1992, Standard for Real-Time Display of Thermal and Mechanical Acoustic Output Indices on Diagnostic Ultrasound Equipment. Rockville, Maryland: AIUM, 1992.
4. Shaw A, Pay NM, Preston RC. Assessment of the likely thermal index values for pulsed Doppler ultrasonic equipment – Stages II and III: Experimental assessment of scanner/transducer combinations. NPL Report CMAM 12, April 1998. National Physical Laboratory, Teddington.
5. IEC Standard 60601-2-37: Medical electrical equipment – Particular requirements for the safety of ultrasonic medical diagnostic and monitoring equipment. Geneva: International Electrotechnical Commission, 2002.
6. Killingbeck ALT, Newey VR, Chan J, Buland CM, Nassiri DK. A survey of probe self-heating in diagnostic inter-cavitary probes. Ultrasound 2004;12:248.

The British Journal of Radiology, 78 (2005), 292–298
DOI: 10.1259/bjr/16043862

Perioperative monitoring of flow and patency in native and grafted internal mammary arteries using a combined MR protocol

[1]N I STAUDER, MD, [2]A M SCHEULE, MD, [1]U HAHN, MD, [1]M FENCHEL, MD, [2]F S ECKSTEIN, MD, [1]U KRAMER, MD, [1]C D CLAUSSEN, MD and [1]S MILLER, MD

[1]*Department of Diagnostic Radiology and* [2]*Department of Thoracic, Cardiac and Vascular Surgery, Eberhard-Karls-University, Tübingen, Hoppe Seyler-Str. 3, 72076 Tübingen, Germany*

Abstract. The objective of this study was to evaluate graft flow (f) and patency (p) in patients with internal mammary artery (f,p) and venous (p only) grafts using a combined MR protocol with phase-contrast technique and MR angiography. 42 patients with 42 left internal mammary artery (LIMA) and 63 venous grafts were examined pre and 6 months post coronary artery bypass graft (CABG) surgery. Phase-contrast flow measurements were applied to the IMA. Post-operatively, a contrast enhanced MR angiogram was performed to assess bypass patency. LIMA/venous grafts were occluded in 3/42 and 13/63, respectively. Flow in LIMA decreased from 19.4 ± 10.4 ml min^{-1} m^{-2} pre-operatively to 13.4 ± 9.7 ml min^{-1} m^{-2} post-operatively ($p<0.002$). In contrast, flow in the native right IMA increased from 17.6 ± 8.7 ml min^{-1} m^{-2} pre-operatively to 24.8 ± 9.0 ml min^{-1} m^{-2} post-operatively ($p<0.001$). MRI allows a combined assessment of bypass patency and flow. This study protocol may be applicable to perioperative follow-up studies in patients after CABG surgery.

In patients with coronary artery disease (CAD) surgical re-vascularization is performed to treat angina and/or heart failure. Treatment is either by internal mammary artery (IMA) coronary artery bypass graft (CABG) or homologous venous CABG. Patients usually have a reduction of clinical symptoms and an increase in quality of life after re-vascularization [1]. However thoracic discomfort can persist in a subgroup of patients after surgical therapy. These symptoms are often difficult to distinguish from angina pectoris and the question of bypass occlusion or bypass stenosis may be raised. At present, the diagnostic method of choice in this situation is invasive catheter angiography to investigate coronary artery and bypass status. Here, previous studies revealed an incidence of bypass occlusion during the first year of up to 5% for IMA grafts and up to 20% for venous grafts [2, 3]. MRI has been tested as an early non-invasive alternative diagnostic tool [4, 5]. It was found, that information about patency of bypass grafts could be obtained by quantitative flow measurements [6, 7]. Furthermore, several authors demonstrated the feasibility of assessing the morphology of bypass grafts by MRI [8–10]. However, visualization of IMA bypass grafts was found to be difficult with two-dimensional (2D) spin echo and 2D gradient echo sequences. This was mainly due to the smaller diameter of IMA bypass grafts compared with venous bypass grafts [4, 7]. Even though the morphological delineation of the bypass grafts could be improved by contrast enhanced 3D MR angiography (ceMRA), the visualization of the vascular mediastinal course was still hampered by metallic clip artefacts and the depiction of the distal anastomosis remained problematic [9, 10]. A combination of flow measurements and ceMRA could be beneficial to improve the diagnostic evaluation of IMA grafts.

The purpose of this study was to evaluate a combined protocol for assessment of patency and flow quantification of LIMA bypass grafts, and patency alone for venous grafts. Also mean flow in the IMA vessels was followed before and after surgical re-vascularization.

Material and methods

Patient study

42 patients (39 males, 3 females; mean age of 61.4 ± 8.5 years old) were studied with MRI before and 7.3 ± 2.3 months after CABG surgery. A total of 105 grafts (42 LIMA and 63 venous grafts) were placed. The LIMA grafts were exclusively solitary grafts attached to the left anterior descending artery (LAD). Concerning the venous grafts, 31 were anastomosed to an area supplied by the LAD, 46 to an area supplied by the Ramus circumflexus (RCX) and 36 to an area supplied by the right coronary artery (RCA). The total number of distal anastomoses was $n=155$ (42 LIMA and 113 venous).

Medical history was obtained from patients pre- and post-operatively concerning chest discomfort and amount of tolerable exercise. Participation in the study was voluntary and patients were enrolled after giving written informed consent. The study was approved by the review board of our hospital.

MRI

MR examinations were performed with a 1.5 T whole-body system Magnetom Vision (Siemens Medical Systems,

Received 15 October 2003 and in final form 16 September 2004, accepted 26 September 2004.

Erlangen, Germany) using a phased-array surface coil and prospective ECG-triggering. Pre-operatively, all patients had flow quantification (FQ) through the ascending aorta and both the IMA. Post-operatively besides the FQ, ceMRA was also performed. At first, a transverse T_1 weighted fast spin echo sequence (repetition time (TR)=RR interval (cardiac cycle between two R waves on electrocardiogram), echo time (TE) 12 ms, field of view (FOV) 320 mm × 320 mm, matrix 256 × 256, slice thickness 5 mm, length of echo-train n=3 echos) was applied for the examination of mediastinal anatomy and location of the bypass grafts. After that the aortic arch was localized, flow measurement was performed perpendicular to the ascending aorta, 1 cm proximal to the branching of the brachiocephalic trunk. A phase contrast FLASH 2D sequence (TR 24 ms, TE 5 ms, flip angle 20°, FOV 250 mm × 250 mm, matrix 256 × 256, slice thickness 5 mm, velocity encoding 250 cm s^{-1}, spatial resolution 0.98 mm × 0.98 mm, two signal averaging measurements) was applied. The number of phases over the cardiac cycle was adapted to the heart rate of the patient and calculated as follows:

$$\text{number of phases} = (\text{RR interval} - 10\%)/\text{TR} \quad (1)$$

with TR=24 ms.

Furthermore, flow measurements of the IMA were performed at the level of the bifurcation of the pulmonary trunk perpendicular to the course of the vessel. Velocity encoding was 75 cm s^{-1}. Flow was determined for the left (LIMA) as well as for the right IMA (RIMA). Identical protocols were used for pre- and post-operative examinations.

Post-operatively for the ceMRA a 3D FLASH sequence (TR 3.8 ms, TE 1.4 ms, flip angle 30°, FOV 300 mm × 300 mm, matrix 160 × 256, slab thickness 132 mm, 44 partitions, interpolated to 88 partitions and a resulting voxel size of 1.5 mm × 1.9 mm × 1.2 mm, no ECG-triggering) was used. The determination of transit time was done with a Turbo FLASH 2D sequence. A power injector (Medrad Spectris, Volkach) was used to inject 3 ml Gd-DTPA (Magnevist®) for the evaluation of transit time and 25 ml Magnevist® for the ceMRA, respectively, both followed by 30 ml 0.9% NaCl into an antecubital vein at a flow rate of 2.5 ml s^{-1}. Calculation of the delay time between injection of contrast agent and start of image acquisition was done according to the formula:

$$\text{delay[s]} = \text{transit time[s]} - \text{acquisition time}/4\text{[s]} \quad (2)$$

Data analysis of ceMRA

Two experienced investigators reading localization and patency of bypass grafts by source images as well as maximal intensity projections (MIP) in a consensus mode. Information about the type of the bypass graft and the supplied areas of the bypass grafts was present at the time of reading.

For data analysis the IMA graft was subdivided into five segments: branching from the subclavian artery, proximal third, middle segment, distal third and anastomosis to LAD. An IMA graft was considered "open" if the full course of the vessel including the distal anastomosis was visible or if blood flow with a biphasic flow curve could be measured in the IMA graft although the vessel was not be continuously depicted at ceMRA (*e.g.* anastomosis of the vessel to the LAD). The vessel was rated "occluded", if there was a visualization stop in the graft course without contrasted areas in the more distal parts of the graft and no measurable flow in the graft.

Venous bypasses were evaluated and subdivided in segments as follows: branching from the ascending aorta, proximal segment, distal segment, anastomosis. The vessel was considered "open", if the graft was continuously visible distal to the aortic anastomosis. The venous graft was rated "occluded", if only the proximal anastomosis and/or a short proximal stub was seen, or if the vessel was not visible at all.

The subjective quality of bypass delineation (visibility) was ranked with a five-step scale: excellent=4, good=3, fair=2, poor=1 and not visible=0.

Flow measurement by MRI

The standard software of the MR system (Numaris, Siemens, Version 3B 31A) was used for image post-processing and flow quantification analysis. The lumens of the native IMA vessels and grafted LIMA were identified on magnitude images of the flow quantification sequence. A region of interest (ROI) was drawn manually around the lumen, and a reference ROI to correct flow measurements against cephalocaudal respiratory motion was placed into adjacent mediastinal fat. Both ROIs were automatically transferred to phase images by the software.

The IMA flow values were determined as absolute values in millilitres per minute, as index values corrected for body surface area, and as a percentage of aortic flow ($F_{IMA/Aorta}$).

Statistical analysis

Mean and standard deviation of functional parameters were calculated from pre- and post-operative measurements. The significance regarding changes of functional parameters was determined by a student's t-test. The level of significance was set to $p<0.05$. Interobserver and intra-observer variability of flow measurements before and after re-vascularization were determined by two independent investigators using the Bland and Altman approach [11].

Results

Complete pre-operative and follow up data could be obtained in all patients. Duration of the examination was 40–50 min pre-operatively, and 45–55 min post-operatively, and was well tolerated by all patients.

In five cases selective visualization of the bypass grafts by coronary artery angiography and in three cases a spiral multidetector CT of the thorax (Volume Zoom, Siemens, 4 × 1 mm, 120 ml Imeron 400®) was performed due to chest pain (*i.e.* angina, atypical chest pain, intermittent thoracic discomfort).

MR angiography

At ceMRA, 38 of 42 (93%) LIMA grafts were rated open and 4 of 42 occluded. 13 of 42 (31%) distal LIMA

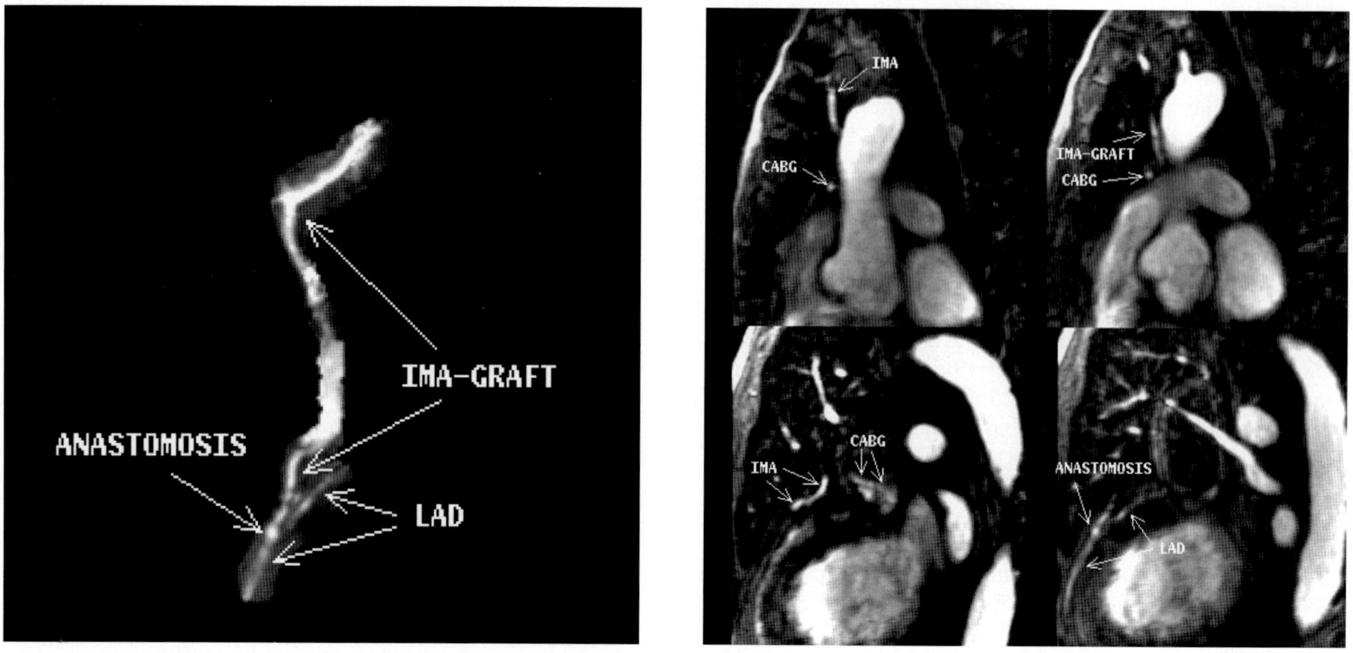

(a) (b)

Figure 1. (a) Maximum intensity projection (MIP) reconstruction of an internal mammary artery (IMA) graft including the distal anstomosis to the left anterior descending artery. Discontinuity through clip artefacts. (b) Single slice images of the MR angiography of the same patient.

anastomosis could be detected (visualization=0.7 ± 1.3). In Figure 1a MIP reconstruction of an IMA graft including the distal anastomosis to the LAD is given. Figure 1b demonstrate single slice images of the MRA in the same patient.

50 of 63 (80%) venous grafts were rated open and 13 of 63 (20%) for occluded. 12 of 34 (35%) sequentially bypasses and 7 of 113 (6%) distal anastomosis of venous grafts could be detected. Detailed results of the ceMRA are summarized in Table 1. One of four LIMA vessels which were rated occluded by ceMRA demonstrated sudden disruption in the middle segment. However, flow measurement revealed a residual flow of 5 ml min^{-1} m^{-2} suggesting that the vessel was highly stenosed but patent. Owing to clinical symptoms, a selective catheter examination was performed confirming a pronounced stenosis of the LIMA graft and occlusion of the sequential venous graft. The solitary venous CABG had a small diameter but was patent as seen in the ceMRA. A biphasic flow pattern with a flow of 26 ml min^{-1} m^{-2} was present in the LIMA graft of another patient with poor contrast enhancement and disrupted LIMA bypass by ceMRA (Figure 2). Due to the flow measurement the LIMA graft was rated open. Selective bypass catheterization proved the patency of the LIMA bypass (Figure 3).

The assessment of the visual quality of LIMA and venous bypass grafts in the various segments of the vessels is demonstrated in Table 2.

Table 1. Graft patency of 63 (with 113 distal anastomoses) venous and 42 LIMA grafts by MRA versus MRI (MRA combined with IMA graft flow measurements)

	Venous	Venous	Venous	LIMA	LIMA
	LAD	RCX	RCA	LAD	Distal anastomosis
MRA: patent	25/31	44/46	32/36	38/42	13
MRA+FQ patent	—	—	—	40/42	13

LIMA, left internal mammary artery; LAD, left anterior descending artery; RCX, ramus circumflexus; RCA, right coronary artery; MRA, magnetic resonance angiography; FQ, flow quantification.

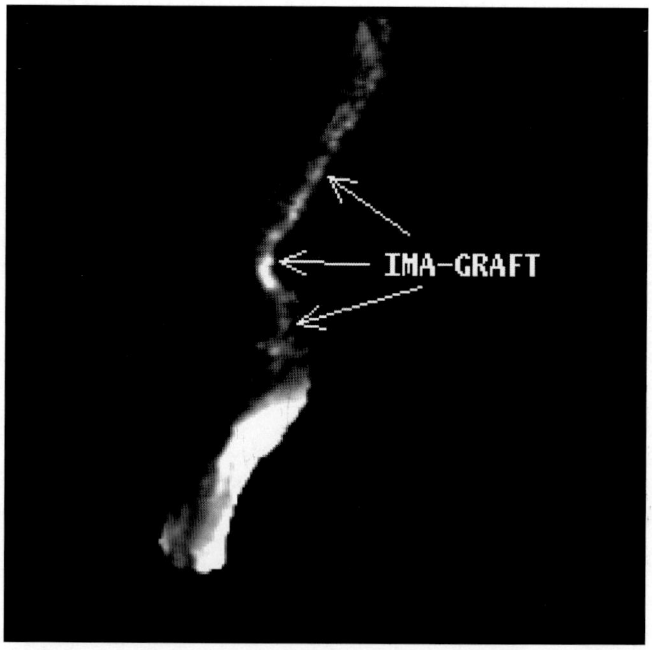

Figure 2. MR angiography maximum intensity projection poorly demarcated left internal mammary artery graft with disruption.

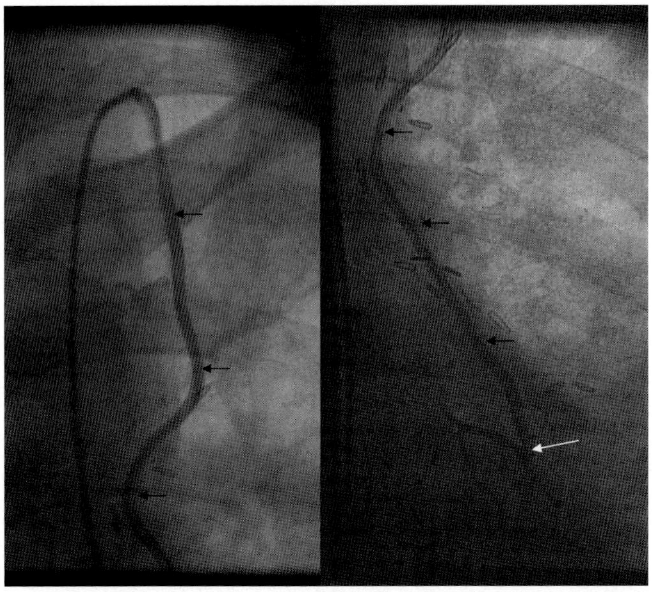

Figure 3. Selective bypass catheterization of the same patient: left internal mammary artery (LIMA) graft well contrasted. Short black arrows: LIMA graft. Long white arrow: anastomosis to left anterior descending artery.

Comparison of pre- and post-operative flow measurements in LIMA and RIMA

Pre-operatively the flow pattern of the IMA vessels had a systolic maximum (Figure 4a). Quantitative assessment of pre-operative flow in LIMA grafts revealed a range of 15–92 ml (19.4 ± 10.4 ml min^{-1} m^{-2}). Characteristic changes of flow patterns were observed, when comparing pre- and post-operative IMA flow curves, with a post-operative biphasic flow pattern having a lower systolic and a maximum diastolic peak (Figure 4b). Post-operatively there was a significant decrease in quantitative flow values, with a range of 5–90 ml (13.4 ± 9.7 ml min^{-1} m^{-2}, $p<0.002$). A significant decrease ($p<0.02$) in $F_{LIMA/Aorta}$ was present pre-operatively (0.76 ± 0.38) compared with post-operatively (0.54 ± 0.37). In contrast, there was a significant increase in mean flow in the native RIMA from 17.6 ± 8.7 ml min^{-1} m^{-2} pre-operatively to 24.8 ± 9.0 ml min^{-1} m^{-2} post-operatively ($p<0.001$). Similarly there was a significant increase ($p<0.005$) of $F_{RIMA/Aorta}$ from 0.76 ± 0.38 pre-operatively to 1.1 ± 0.59 post-operatively. An identical flow pattern in the RIMA was observed pre- and post-operatively, with a monophasic early systolic flow maximum. Representative flow measurement in a LIMA graft is shown in Figure 5.

Table 2. Visibility of the left internal mammary artery (LIMA) and venous grafts by magnetic resonance angiography

	Proximal	First part	Second part	Distal part	Anastomosis
LIMA	1.6 ± 1.6	2.8 ± 1.2	2.5 ± 1.1	1.5 ± 1.4	0.7 ± 1.3
CABG	3.7 ± 0.6	3.2 ± 0.9	2.0 ± 1.3	—	0.1 ± 0.3

CABG, coronary artery bypass graft.

The intraobserver variability of flow measurements was $5.6 \pm 3.7\%$ in the native IMA vessels (pre-operative LIMA/RIMA, post-operative RIMA) and $17.2 \pm 9.4\%$ in the LIMA graft. The interobserver variability was $10.5 \pm 5.7\%$ for the evaluation of the native IMA vessels and $22.4 \pm 12.1\%$ for the LIMA grafts.

Discussion

In the present study MRI was used to non-invasively follow up patients after surgical myocardial re-vascularization. The imaging protocol comprised several important determinants of the patients cardiovascular condition, such as bypass patency as well as the flow in the IMA at several time points. As a key finding we observed a significant decrease of mean flow in the LIMA graft post-operatively, whereas mean flow in the native RIMA increased after surgery. 93% of LIMA grafts and 80% of venous grafts were considered patent and 31% of distal

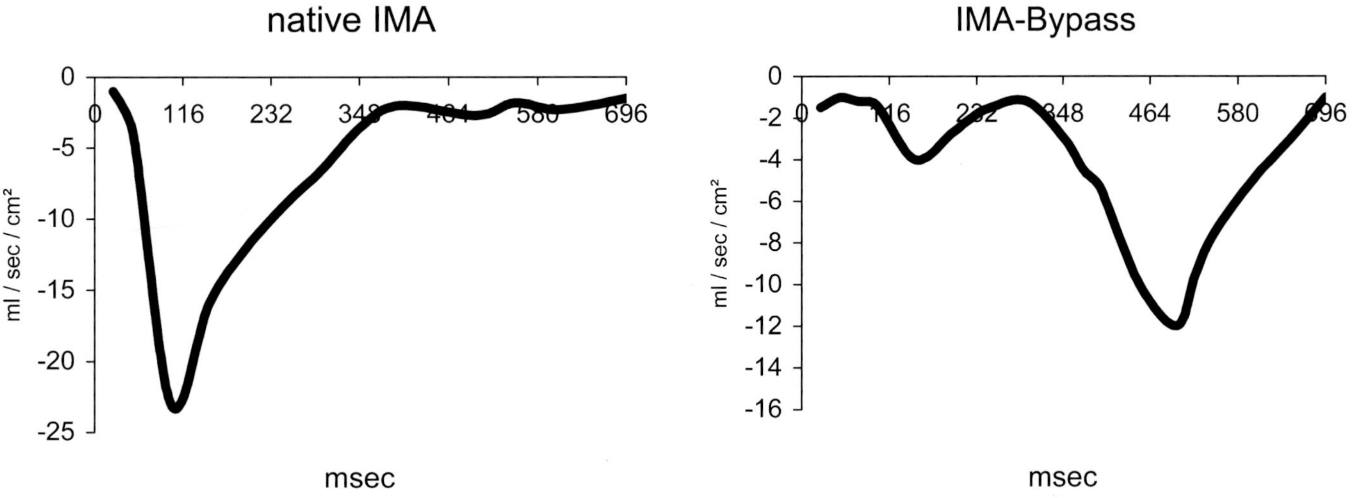

(a) (b)

Figure 4. Representative left internal mammary artery (LIMA) flow quantification pre- and post-operatively of the same patient. (a) Pre-operatively monophasic flow pattern with systolic maximum. (b) Post-operatively biphasic flow pattern in LIMA graft with maximum diastolic peak.

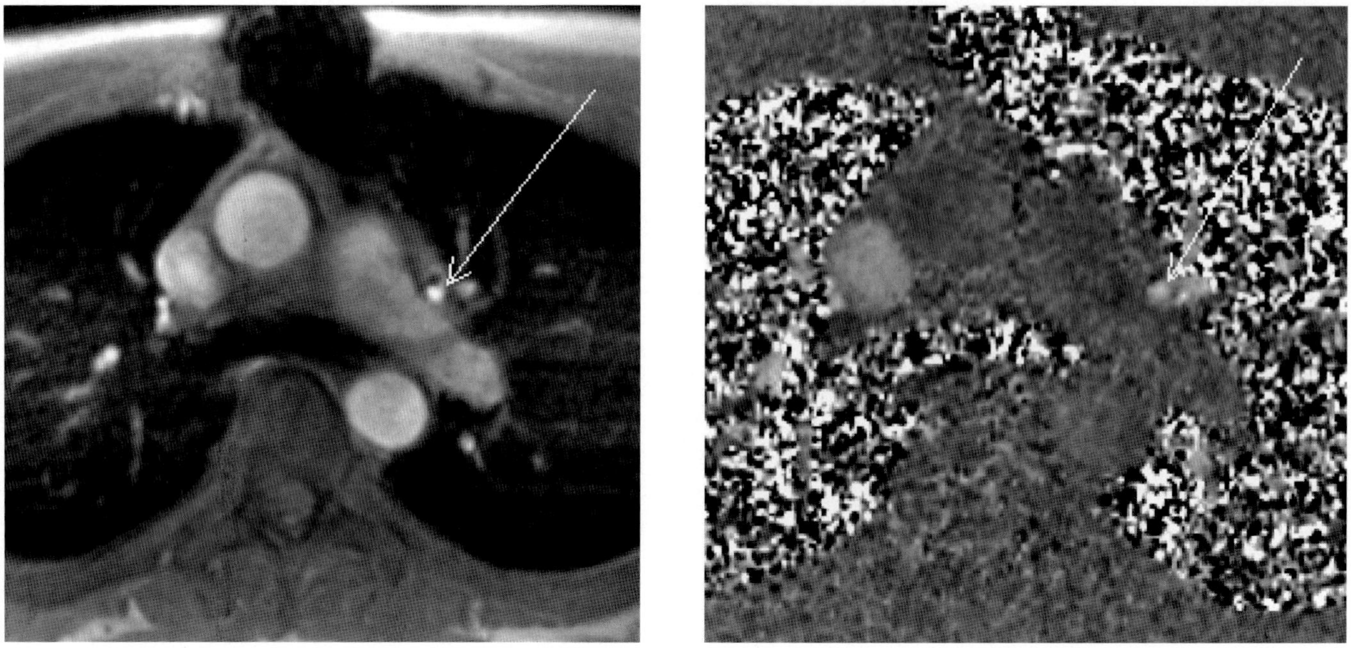

(a) (b)

Figure 5. (a) Magnitude- and (b) Phase-Image of the post-operative flow quantification sequence. The arrows show the left internal mammary artery graft.

LIMA anastomosis could be demonstrated. There was a decrease in visibility of graft segments near the heart.

MR angiography

Since the beginning of the 1990s various MRI methods have been investigated in the assessment of CABG. MRI studies of CABG have been performed comparing the role of spin-echo and gradient-echo techniques. Here spin-echo techniques revealed a sensitivity ranging between 79% and 98% and a specificity between 72% and 85% [4, 13]. Using gradient-echo techniques sensitivities between 88% and 98% and specificities between 86% and 91% were found [5, 13]. Kalden et al [8] recently reported on the use of HASTE imaging in the assessment graft patency with a sensitivity of 95% and a specificity of 93%. A major limitation was the reduced spatial resolution and difficulty in the assessment of the small diameter IMA grafts (sensitivity 80–93%, specificity 50–100%). The authors proposed that this method might be used as a localizer for subsequent ceMRA.

Contrast enhanced 3D MR angiographic methods have been available since the middle of the 1990s. Studies employing ceMRA yielded sensitivities for bypass patency of between 93% and 95% and specificities of between 67% and 97% [9, 10, 14].

Several studies have reported difficulties in the evaluation of IMA grafts because of the small vessel diameter and numerous surgical clips [4, 7]. Clips in the region of the LIMA also proved to be the limiting factor in the evaluation of our data, especially when MIP reconstructions were evaluated (Figure 1a). In patent vessels, the proximal segment of the bypass was clearly visible (2.8 ± 1.2). The distal anastomosis of the LIMA could be detected in 31% of all cases, whereas in previous studies this region could not be assessed [5, 10]. The individuals' breath holding capability was a limiting factor considering the duration of ceMRA-sequence (21 s). ECG-triggering would probably improve the assessment of bypass segments adjacent to the heart owing to the reduction of pulsation artefacts, however this would further prolong the data acquisition and scan times.

Another alternative used in the morphological examination of bypass grafts by MRI is the navigator technique [15]. However, such sequences require long period of data acquisition.

True fast imaging with steady-state precession (true FISP) is another promising new technique for cardiac MRI. True FISP images have a higher contrast to noise ratio (CNR) than images acquired with FLASH sequences [16]. Bunce et al [17] recently reported that the accuracy for detection of coronary artery bypass graft patency was similar with gadolinium-enhanced MRA and true FISP angiography, with a trend toward more false-positive findings for occlusion and reduced visualization of arterial grafts with true FISP angiography.

Flow measurements

Beyond the morphological delineation of bypass grafts flow measurements were found to be accurate in quantifying blood flow in CABG [6, 7]. In contrast to its application for assessment of major thoracic vessels, such as the aorta or the pulmonary arteries, partial volume effects are of major relevance in the determination of flow volumes in small vessels such as coronary arteries and bypass grafts. At the vessel boundary, voxels may contain both signal from vessel and from surrounding tissue. Partial volume effects can degrade the results of this technique and may lead to an overestimation of flow volumes [18]. Nevertheless, phase contrast flow measurements in small diameter phantom models, as well as in the coronary arteries of animals, were proven to be feasible and provided accurate reproducibility [19]. While Tang et al [18] first proposed that 9–16 pixels would be necessary in order to acquire exact flow measurement results, Hofmann et al [20] proposed that 4 pixels covering the vessel diameter would produce acceptable accuracy. These conditions were used in the present study, and the IMA flow values and flow patterns observed confirm in this. Kreitner et al [21] also found absolute flow values in IMA grafts of 53.3 ± 51.2 ml min^{-1}.

In our patients, LIMA flow was significantly higher pre-operatively compared with post-operative flow values. This may be due to the dissection of peripheral LIMA branches post-operatively. Other groups reported higher flow values post-operatively in the native RIMA compared with the LIMA bypass graft [6, 22]. The significant increase of native RIMA blood flow post-operatively may be due to a compensatory blood flow to territories supplied by the dissected LIMA branches beforehand. This finding has never previously been reported. Ishida et al [12] recently noted, that velocity encoded cine MR blood flow measurement at baseline is highly useful in predicting significant stenosis in IMA grafts. Severe stenoses were detected with a sensitivity of 86% and a specificity of 88% [12]. A clinical application could be the serial assessment of graft function, which is useful in detecting gradual increases in graft stenosis before the onset of total occlusion. Even more information can be obtained by measurement of the flow reserve. Langerak et al [23] recently reported, that a newly developed turbo field echo planar imaging (TFEPI)-technique allowed accurate assessment of flow reserve in bypass grafts without breath holding [23].

A major limitation of our study is the absence of a gold standard for comparison, as for ethical reasons, cardiac catheterization or CT was only performed in symptomatic patients. As such we may be under-reporting false negative results. This emphasizes the fact that the results of patency and flow on both MRA and flow quantification may not reflect the true graft status in all patients. The lower values of flow volume in the post-operative LIMA grafts may represent stenosis [12] even in the absence of symptoms.

In the present study the combination of MRA and 2D-phase contrast flow quantification was beneficial in clinical practice and their individual limitations reduced.

In summary the present study demonstrates the feasibility of MRI in following up patency and flow in LIMA grafts with an acceptable examination time. Patients with persisting ischaemic symptoms after surgical myocardial re-vascularization, could be offered a non-invasive method to evaluate their bypass graft patency and this would used to help identify those patients who need re-intervention.

Acknowledgments

The study was promoted by the Dr Karl-Kuhn foundation in Tübingen, Germany.

References

1. Coronary Artery Surgery Study (CASS). A randomized trial of coronary artery bypass surgery. Circulation 1983;5:951–60.
2. Lytle BW, Loop FD, Cosgrove DM, Ratliff NB, Easley K, Taylor PC. Long-term (5 to 12 years) serial studies of internal mammary artery and saphenous vein coronary bypass grafts. J Thorac Cardiovasc Surg 1985;9:248–58.
3. Cameron A, Davis KB, Green G, Schaff HV. Coronary bypass surgery with internal-thoracic-artery grafts – effects on survival over a 15-year period. N Engl J Med 1996;334: 216–9.
4. Rubinstein RI, Askenase AD, Thickman D, Feldman MS, Agarwal JB, Helfant RH. Magnetic resonance imaging to evaluate patency of aortocoronary bypass grafts. Circulation 1987;76:786–91.
5. Aurigemma GP, Reichek L, Axel L, Schiebler M, Harris C, Kressel HY. Noninvasive determination of coronary artery bypass graft patency by cine magnetic resonance imaging. Circulation 1989;80:1595–602.
6. Debatin JF, Strong JA, Sostman HD, Negro-Vilar R, Paine SS, Douglas JM, et al. MR characterization of blood flow in native and grafted internal mammary arteries. J Magn Reson Imaging 1993;3:443–50.
7. Galjee MA, van Rossum AC, Doesburg T, Hofman MBM, Falke THM, Visser CA. Quantification of coronary artery bypass graft flow by magnetic resonance phase velocity mapping. Magn Reson Imag 1996;14:485–93.
8. Kalden P, Kreitner KF, Wittlinger T, Voigtlander T, Krummenauer F, Kestel J, et al. Assessment of coronary artery bypass grafts: value of different breath-hold MR imaging techniques. AJR Am J Roentgenol 1999;172:1359–64.
9. Vrachliotis TG, Bis KG, Alibadi DA, Shetty AN, Safian R, Simonetti O. Contrast-enhanced breath-hold MR angiography for evaluating patency of coronary artery bypass grafts. AJR Am J Roentgenol 1997;168:1073–80.
10. Wintersperger BJ, Engelmann MG, von-Smekal A, Knez A, Penzkofer HV, Hofling B, et al. Patency of coronary bypass grafts: assessment with breath-hold contrast-enhanced MR angiography: value of a non-electrocardio-graphically triggered technique. Radiology 1998;208:345–51.
11. Bland JM, Altman DG. Statistical methods for assessing agreement between two methods of clinical measurement. Lancet 1986;1:307–10.
12. Ishida N, Sakuma H, Cruz BP, Shimono T, Tokui T, Yada I, et al. MR flow measurement in the internal mammary artery-to-coronary artery bypass graft: comparison with graft stenosis at radiographic angiography. Radiology 2001;220: 441–7.
13. Galjee MA, van Rossum AC, Doesburg T, van Eenige MJ, Visser CA. Value of magnetic resonance imaging in assessing patency and function of coronary artery bypass grafts. Circulation 1996;93:660–6.
14. Brenner P, Wintersperger B, von Smekal A, Agirov V, Böhm D, Kreuzer E, et al. Detection of coronary artery graft patency by contrast enhanced magnetic resonance angiography. Eur J Cardio-thoracic Surg 1999;15:389–93.
15. Langerak SE, Vliegen HW, de Roos A, Zwinderman AH, Jukema JW, Kunz P, et al. Detection of vein graft disease using high-resolution magnetic resonance angiography. Circulation 2002;105:328–33.
16. Carr JC, Simonetti O, Bundy J, Li D, Pereles S, Finn JP. Cine MR angiography of the heart with segmented true fast imaging with steady-state precession. Radiology 2001;219: 828–34.
17. Bunce NH, Lorenz CH, John AS, Lesser JR, Mohiaddin RH, Pennel DJ. Coronary artery bypass graft patency: assessment with true FISP imaging with steady-state precession versus gadolinium-enhanced MR angiography. Radiology 2003;227: 440–6.
18. Tang C, Blatter DD, Parker DL. Accuracy of phase-contrast flow measurements in the presence of partial-volume effects. J Magn Reson Imaging 1993;3:377–85.

19. Li HF, Clarke GD, Peshock RP, Lui H, NessAiver M. MRI k-space segmentation using phase encode groupings: the accuracy of quantitative measurements of pulsatile flow. Med Phys 1995;22:391–9.
20. Hofman MBM, Visser FC, van Rossum AC, Vink GQM, Sprenger M, Wetserhof N. In vivo validation of magnetic resonance blood flow measurements with limited spatial resolution in small vessels. Magn Reson Med 1995;33:778–84.
21. Kreitner KF, Voigtländer T, Witllinger T, Dahm M, Kalden P, Meyer J, et al. Flow quantification in coronary and bypass vessels with MR phase contrast technique. Radiologe 2000;40:143–9.
22. Walpoth BH, Müller MF, Genyk I, Aeschbacher B, Kipfer B, Althaus U, et al. Evaluation of coronary bypass flow with color-Doppler and magnetic resonance imaging techniques: comparison with intraoperative flow measurements. Eur J Cardio-thoracic Surg 1999;15:795–802.
23. Langerak SE, Vliegen HW, Jukema JW, Kunz P, Zwinderman AH, Lamb HJ, et al. Value of magnetic resonance imaging for the noninvasive detection of stenosis in coronary artery bypass grafts and recipient coronary arteries. Circulation 2003;107:1502–8.

The British Journal of Radiology, *78* (2005), 299–302
DOI: 10.1259/bjr/23825228

A comparison of fast MRI of hips with and without parallel imaging using SENSE

[1]M RYAN, FFR RCSI, [1]P CUNNINGHAM, FFR RCSI, [1]C CANTWELL, AFRCSI, [1]D BRENNAN, FRCR and [2]S EUSTACE, FRCR

[1]*Cappagh National Orthopaedic Hospital, Finglas, Dublin 11, Ireland and* [2]*Mater Misericordiae Hospital, Eccles Street, Dublin 7, Ireland*

Abstract. This study was undertaken to qualitatively and quantitatively compare fast MRI of hips with and without parallel imaging using SENSE (sensitivity encoding). 27 patients underwent MRI of the hips with coronal T_1 turbo spin echo (TSE) (repetition time (TR) 500 ms, effective echo time (TEeff) 15 ms, Turbo Factor 4), coronal IR-TSE (TR 2000 ms, TEeff 30 ms, inversion time (TI) 160 ms, Turbo Factor 20) and axial T_2 TSE (TR 3000 ms, TEeff 80 ms, Turbo Factor 20) weighted images acquired with and without SENSE with a reduction factor of 2. Conventional imaging was performed in 8 min and 36 s. Images acquired with SENSE were acquired in 5 min and 31 s without a discernible reduction in image quality or a significant quantitative reduction in image signal to noise ratio, contrast to noise ratio or edge enhancement.

Previous authors have described the use of parallel imaging techniques, SENSE (Sensitivity Encoding MRI) and SMASH (Simultaneous Acquisition of Spatial Harmonics) to accelerate MR image acquisition. In this role, parallel imaging techniques have been employed to facilitate breath hold techniques in the abdomen, cine imaging of the heart and bolus tracking at MR angiography [1–4]. To date its application to facilitate rapid imaging of the extremities has been employed in a single study evaluating the role of SMASH to allow fast imaging of the shoulder [5]. To date, no publication has qualitatively and quantitatively assessed the use of SENSE in allowing fast imaging of the extremities [6, 7].

This study was undertaken to compare the quality and diagnostic accuracy of images of the hips acquired by fast MRI sequences with and without SENSE (parallel imaging).

Subjects and methods

Patients

27 consecutive patients referred for MRI of the hips were included in the study.

Imaging

All patients underwent imaging on a 1.5 T Philips Intera system (Philips Medical Systems, Best, The Netherlands) using a Synergy body coil and a 40 cm field of view (FOV). Each patient was imaged with coronal T_1 weighted turbo spin echo (TSE) (repetition time (TR) 500 ms, effective echo time (TEeff) 15 ms, Turbo Factor 4), coronal inversion recovery (IR)-TSE (TR 2000 ms, TEeff 30 ms, inversion time (TI) 160 ms, Turbo Factor 20) and axial T_2 weighted TSE (TR 3000 ms, TEeff 80 ms, Turbo Factor 20) sequences with and without SENSE employed with a reduction factor of two. The same contrast parameters and number of excitations were used for both sets of sequences. A 256×256 matrix was used to generate both sets of images. Slice number and thickness (3 mm) was identical in both image sets.

Received 12 February 2004 and in revised form 6 July 2004, accepted 9 November 2004.

Address correspondence to Dr Stephen Eustace, Department of Radiology, Cappagh National Orthopaedic Hospital, Finglas, Dublin 11, Ireland.

Image interpretation

Qualitative

In each case images were read independently blinded to the imaging technique, with discrepancies when present resolved by consensus. In each case, evaluation was made of the acetabular labrum, articular cartilage and bone marrow of the femoral head. Image quality was scored as poor=1, satisfactory=2, good=3 in each case.

Quantitative

Subsequently each image was evaluated on an EasyVision workstation (Philips Medical Systems) using region of interest mapping to determine image signal to noise ratio, contrast to noise ratio (the difference between signal to noise ratios at two sites), and edge enhancement of bone marrow, fat and muscle (based on the rate of change in signal intensity through a straight line on acquired images).

In each case regions of interest were selected by two reviewers who used side by side monitor evaluation of conventional images and SENSE images to ensure that identical regions of interest were selected on both sets of images.

Results

Acquisition time

Coronal IR TSE, coronal T_1 weighted TSE and axial T_2 weighted TSE images of the hips were acquired in 8 min 36 s in total. When SENSE was added with a reduction

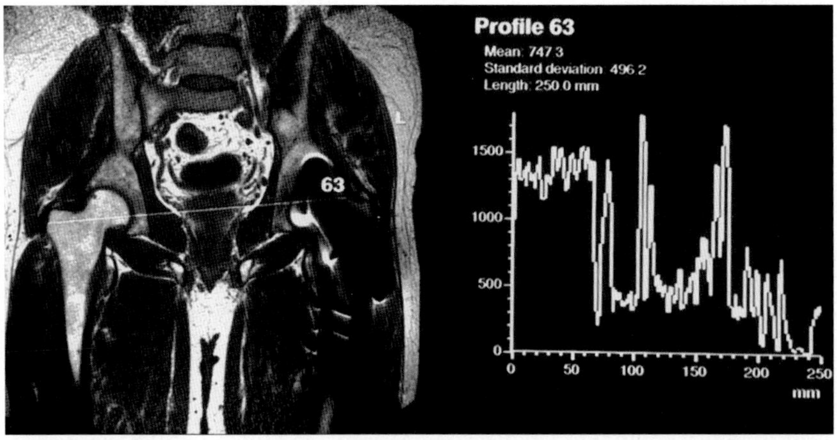

(a)

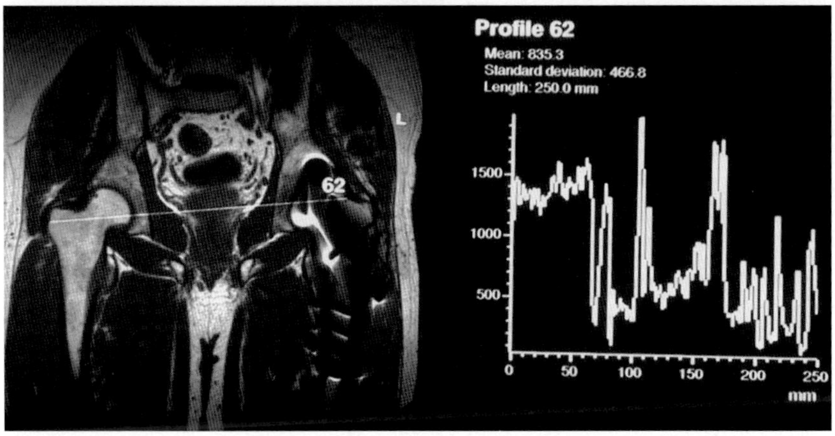

(b)

Figure 1. 50-year-old male with right hip pain. (a) Coronal turbo spin echo (TSE) T_1 weighted image without sensitivity encoding (SENSE), (repetition time (TR) 500 ms, effective echo time (TEeff) 15 ms, turbo factor (TF) 4, low high filling of K space) showing pattern of signal change through a line drawn through both hips (left prosthesis) with associated graph depicting signal intensity change per millimetre. (b) Coronal TSE T_1 weighted image with SENSE, (TR 500 ms, TEeff 15 ms, TF 4, low high filling of K space) showing almost identical pattern of signal change through a line drawn through both hips (left prosthesis) with associated graph depicting almost identical signal intensity change per millimetre.

factor of 2, the total imaging time was reduced to 5 min 31 s.

Side by side image interpretation

Recorded image quality of conventional images and of those with SENSE was identical in 27 of 27 patients.

Findings included eight normal studies, nine patients had osteoarthritis of the hips, three patients had femoral head avascular necrosis, six patients had acetabular dysplasia, and one patient had a fracture of the femoral neck. No perceived difference in image quality of images acquired with and without sense was documented using a 3 point scoring system.

Assessment of marrow was recorded as good (3) by both readers in all cases. Assessment of the acetabular labrum was recorded as good (3) in all cases with the exception of two patients with osteoarthritis and two patients with acetabular dysplasia where the labrum evaluation was considered satisfactory (2) on both sets of images by both readers. Assessment of acetabular cartilage was considered good (3) in nine patients (eight normals, one patient post fracture), and satisfactory (2) in remaining cases by both readers.

Workstation image evaluation

Quantitative evaluation of images was on the basis of review of T_1 weighted images with and without SENSE. Quantitative assessment of coronal IR TSE and axial TSE T_2 weighted images was not undertaken as the effect of SENSE on image quality and acquisition time is the same for all sequences if all other parameters (matrix, slice thickness and field of view) remain unchanged.

In 27 patients, the recorded mean signal to noise of fat was 1080/88 without sense compared with a mean of 984/81 when imaged with SENSE ($p<0.5$).

In 27 patients, the recorded mean signal to noise of muscle was 366/88 without sense, compared with 290/81 when imaged with SENSE ($p<0.5$).

The contrast to noise yielded by comparing the mean signal of fat and muscle relative to the mean signal of noise was 740/88 without sense, compared with 632/81 when imaged with SENSE ($p<0.5$).

No significant difference in edge enhancement was documented on the images with and without SENSE.

Discussion

The last decade has seen the widespread introduction of fast imaging sequences supported by the tandem development of flexible localizing gradients. Such developments have allowed dramatic reduction in acquisition times paving the way for innumerable new clinical applications previously vulnerable to motion, including diffusion imaging in the brain, gated cardiac techniques and abdominal applications such as magnetic resonance cholangiopanceatography (MRCP) [6]. Although not primarily benefiting from motion reduction, fast techniques have allowed

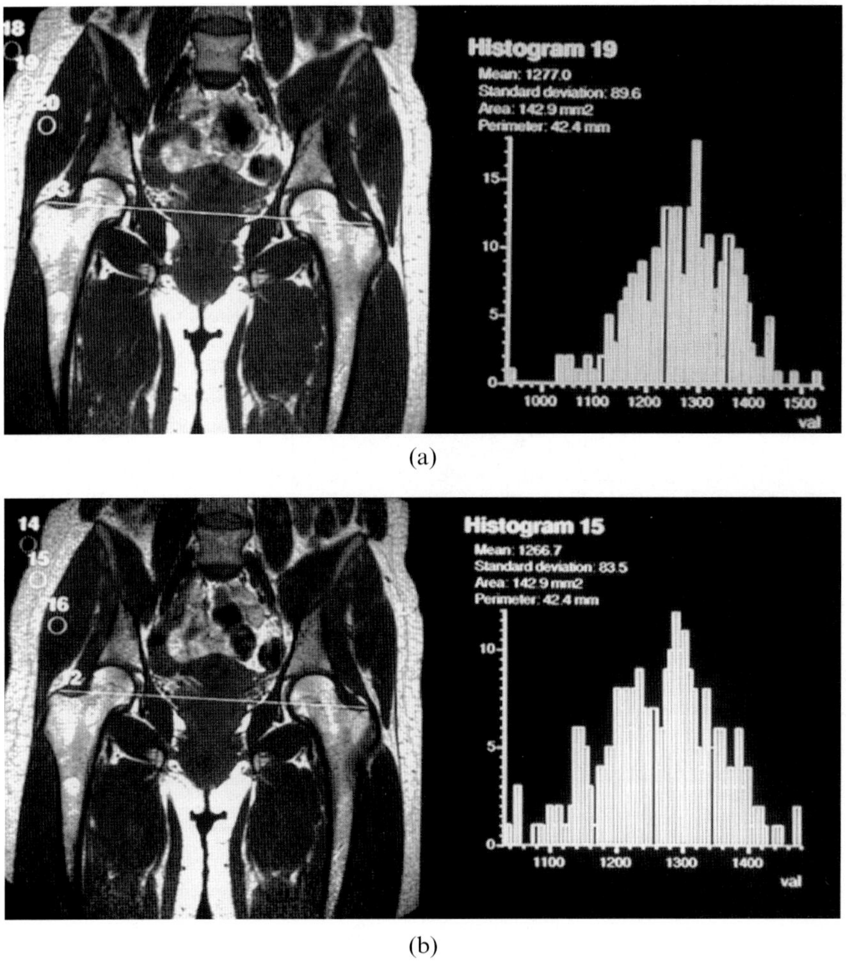

Figure 2. 32-year-old female with bilateral hip pain. (a) Coronal turbo spin echo (TSE) T_1 weighted image without sensitivity encoding (SENSE), (repetition time (TR) 500 ms, effective echo time (TEeff) 15 ms, turbo factor (TF) 4, low high filling of K space) showing 250 pixel regions of interest yielding noise (14), muscle signal (15), and fat signal (16) with associated histogram indicating range and mean signal intensity in fat (1277). (b) Coronal TSE T_1 weighted image with SENSE, (TR 500 ms, TEeff 15 ms, TF 4, low high filling of K space) showing 250 pixel regions of interest yielding noise (18), muscle signal (19), and fat signal (20) with associated histogram indicating range and mean signal intensity in fat (1266).

dramatic increases in patient throughput in the extremities without a reduction in image quality. Recognizing that there is a limit to potential reduction in acquisition times afforded by fast sequences and optimized gradients alone, this report reviews the potential of parallel imaging techniques to produce further acquisition time reductions without significant impact on the diagnostic quality of the acquired images. The paper specifically reviews the impact of image reduction times on contrast, edge enhancement, image signal and diagnostic effectiveness of acquired images.

Parallel imaging techniques employ phased array surface coils and allow reconstruction algorithms to unwrap or unalias useful information and signal acquired in neighbouring coils outside the field of view of individual coil elements [6, 7]. In such a way fewer phase encode steps are required to fill image K space within each coil element, as potential deficiencies are filled by unwrapped information to generate a high spatial resolution image. Intuitively this process should result in both a reduction in image acquisition time and also a reduction in image signal. However, the relative reduction in image signal versus acquisition time and relative impact of SENSE acquired images on diagnostic accuracy when employed to image the extremities has not been previously assessed.

In this report, we employed optimized turbo spin echo sequences to allow imaging of both hips with a total acquisition time of 8 min 36 s compared with 5 min 30 s when the same parameters were employed with SENSE. Although one might predict that the application of SENSE with a reduction factor of 2 would result in a direct halving of acquisition time, in practice, the implementation of SENSE requires the acquisition of a sensitivity map prior to image acquisition at a cost of 50 s. Further reductions in acquisition time are likely to be generated by the development of more complex phased array surface coils with a further increase in the number of individual coil elements. The necessity to acquire a sensitivity map to localize signal prior to imaging also increases the possibility of misregistration if there is motion between mapping and signal acquisition. Since the SENSE technique involves a reduction in phase encoding steps, which is compensated by the addition of unwrapped information, one would anticipate a significant reduction in image signal. This reduction is determined as a factor of the reduction factor. Therefore a reduction factor of two as employed in this study should theoretically lead to a drop off in signal to noise of 1.4 and so on. Such an expected reduction in image signal was not encountered in this study. Such a result may reflect the reduction in scan acquisition time. The increased acquisition speed using SENSE results in less time for proton dephasing resulting in preservation of image signal. The SNR also depends on slice setup and individual coil design. The under sampling of K space by increasing the distance of sampling positions while maintaining the maximum K values will allow spatial resolution to be maintained. In this study no significant reduction in image signal, contrast or edge enhancement was recorded. Owing to the entirely independent physics of the encoding effect, SENSE does not interfere with any of the numerous known contrast mechanisms or acquisition schemes. The SENSE approach can therefore be applied to practically all known MRI techniques [6].

In summary, the results of this study suggest that parallel imaging techniques particularly SENSE can be successfully employed to image the extremities. The use of SENSE allows a reduction in acquisition times without a significant reduction in subjective image quality or objective workstation assessment of image signal, contrast or edge enhancement.

References

1. Sodickson DK, Griswold MA, Jacob PM. SMASH imaging. Magn Reson Imaging Clin N Am 1999;7:237–54.
2. Sodickson DK, McKenzie CA, Ohlinger MA, et al. Recent advances in image reconstruction, coil sensitivity, calibration, and coil array design for SMASH and generalized parallel MRI. MAGMA 2002;13:158–63.
3. Sodickson DK, McKenzie CA. A generalized approach to parallel magnetic resonance imaging. Med Phys 2001;28: 1629–43.
4. Bydder M, Larkman DJ, Hajnal JV. Generalised SMASH imaging. Magn Res Med 2002;47:160–70.
5. Magee T, Shapiro M, Williams D, Richard Ramnath R, Simon J. Usefulness of the simultaneous acquisition of spatial harmonics technique during MRI of the shoulder. AJR Am J Roentgenol 2003;181:961–4.
6. Van den Brink JS, Watanabe Y, Kuhl CK, et al. Implications of SENSE MR in routine clinical practice. Eur J Radiol 2003;46:3–27.
7. Willinek WA, Gieseke J, von Falkenhausen M, Neuen B, Schild HH, Kuhl CK. Sensitivity encoding for fast MR imaging of the brain in patients with stroke. Radiology 2003;228:669–75.

The British Journal of Radiology, 78 (2005), 303–307 © 2005 The British Institute of Radiology
DOI: 10.1259/bjr/28232950

Colour Doppler ultrasound mapping of chest wall lesions

[1]C GÖRG, MD, [1]T BERT, MD, [1]K GÖRG, MD and [2]M HEINZEL-GUTENBRUNNER, MD

[1]*Department of Internal Medicine, Philipps-University, Baldingerstraße, Marburg and* [2]*Institute of Medical Biometry and Epidemiology, Philipps-University, Bunsenstraße 3, Marburg, Germany*

Abstract. Spectral curve-analysis of arterial flow signals (FS) in patients with pulmonary lesions is able to discriminate FS of bronchial arteries (BA) from FS of pulmonary arteries (PA). In patients with chest wall lesions a different FS from that of the BA/PA can be obtained. The aim of the study was to evaluate and characterize arterial supply of chest wall lesions using quantitative colour Doppler ultrasound (CDS). Between September 2002 and June 2003, 29 consecutive patients with chest wall lesions were examined by CDS. 16 lesions were located strictly to the chest wall (group I). 13 lesions had a chest wall lesion with pulmonary extension (group II). The following parameters were prospectively determined: (1) qualitative CDS (absence or evidence of vascularity); (2) quantitative CDS of intercostal or non-intercostal located arterial FS (resistive index (RI) and pulsatility index (PI)); (3) number of different arterial FS in one lesion using CDS-mapping. In a control group of 17 healthy volunteers quantitative measurement of RI and PI of the intercostal artery (ICA) was performed. 4 of 29 patients (14%) had no FS by CDS mapping. Quantitative CDS parameters of the control group were mean RI of ICA 0.88 ($\pm$0.056); mean PI of ICA 2.88 ($\pm$0.643); of group I mean RI of ICA 0.79 ($\pm$0.127) mean PI of ICA 1.93 ($\pm$0.641), and of group II mean RI of ICA 0.79 ($\pm$0.144), mean PI of ICA 2.1 ($\pm$1.015), mean RI of non-ICA 0.68 ($\pm$0.675) mean PI of non-ICA 2.5 ($\pm$2.506). Median RI as well as PI-value obtained within the chest wall (ICA) do not differ between group I, group II, and the control group. Within group II impedance measurements discriminates intercostal from non-intercostal arterial supply. In 29 patients 37 different arterial FS were obtained. None of the 16 patients in group I and 8 of the 13 patients in group II had 2 or more different FS. Lesions strictly located to the chest wall had an arterial supply characteristic for ICA by quantitative CDS. Chest wall lesions with pulmonary extension demonstrate a complex arterial supply by quantitative CDS.

Colour Doppler ultrasound (CDS) can be used as a qualitative or a quantitative method to describe flow patterns in pleurally based pulmonary lesions. Qualitative CDS pattern show characteristic findings in various pulmonary lesions [1–6]. Quantitative CDS of arterial flow signals (FS) enables discrimination of FS of bronchial arteries (BA) characterized by a monophasic low impedance flow pattern from FS of pulmonary arteries (PA) characterized by a triphasic high impedance flow pattern [4–8]. In a recent study [9] of chest wall based pulmonary lesions a variable impedance, monophasic flow pattern could discrimate from FS of PA and FS of central BA by spectral analysis. The aim of the present study is to evaluate and characterize arterial supply of chest wall lesions with quantitative CDS.

Patients and methods

Between September 2002 and June 2003, 29 consecutive patients with chest wall lesion were referred to our ultrasound laboratory and prospectively examined by B-mode ultrasound as well as quantitative and qualitative CDS. Diagnosis was histologically confirmed in all patients (Table 1). 16 lesions were strictly located in the chest wall and demarcated by pleural effusion from pulmonary tissue in eight cases. 13 lesions were predominantly located in the chest wall with pulmonary extension. 14 patients had a small size lesion with a largest diameter less than 4 cm, in 15 patients the lesion largest diameter was $\geqslant$4 cm. The range of lesion size was 2 cm to 14 cm. The age ranged from 18 years to 81 years.

The following quantitative and qualitative CDS parameters were determined:

(1) Qualitative CDS of lesions was classified as absence of FS in all parts or evidence of FS in the lesion;
(2) Quantitative measurement of resistive index (RI) and pulsatility index (PI) were performed in all FS studied;
(3) Number of different arterial FS in a lesion were counted and classified as follows:

Arterial vessels were assumed to be from the intercostal artery (ICA) by the following parameters:

Table 1. Diagnosis in 29 patients with chest wall lesions (group I) and chest wall lesions with pulmonary extension (group II)

	Benign diseases	Malignant diseases
Group I	2 lipoma	6 metastases
	1 abscess	3 plasmocytoma
	1 pleural scar	3 malignant lymphoma
Group II	2 abscesses	4 metastases
		4 lung cancer
		2 PNET
		1 malignant lymphoma

PNET, primitive neuroectodermal tumour.

Received 26 November 2003 and in final form 6 October 2004, accepted 15 November 2004.

(1) a strictly intercostal location;
(2) a nearly horizontal flow direction, and;
(3) a high impedance monophasic flow.

Arterial vessels were assumed to be from the bronchial artery (BA) by

(1) a pulmonary location;
(2) a variable flow direction; and
(3) a low impedance monophasic flow.

Arterial vessels were assumed to be from the pulmonary artery (PA) by

(1) a pulmonary location;
(2) a centrifugal flow direction from the hilum towards the surface of the lung; and
(3) a high impedance predominantly triphasic flow.

Arterial vessels were assumed for tumour neoangiogenesis (TN) by a nearby constant flow that lacked systolic–diastolic variation [7].

In a control group of 17 healthy volunteers quantitative measurement of RI and PI of the intercostal artery was performed.

Ultrasound was performed with a real time scanner with 3.5–8 MHz curved and linear array transducers (Acuson, Sequoia, Mountain View, CA) using tissue harmonic imaging. Ultrasound studies were performed by two authors experienced in CDS (CG and KG). Colour Doppler settings were optimized to achieve the greatest sensitivity to allow the detection of low flow. For evaluation of qualitative vascularity of pleural-based lesions power Doppler imaging was primarily used. For classification of flow direction colour Doppler imaging was performed. Colour gain setting was adjusted to a level just below the level creating artefacts. The colour box was designed as small as possible and the wall filter and pulse repetition frequency (PRF) were lowered. At least three similar, sequential Doppler waveforms were obtained while the subject suspended respiration. The single tracing obtained was selected for analysis.

For statistical analysis the Kruskal-Wallis test was applied.

Results

Qualitative CDS of lesions

Four of 29 patients (14%) had no FS by CDS mapping: The underlying diseases were abscesses (n=2) and lipoma (n=2). The remaining 25 patients had FS which includes 13 patients with strictly chest wall lesion, and 12 patients with pulmonary extension.

Quantitative CDS of lesions

Mean values of impedance indices of the ICA in the control group are shown in Figure 1. Impedance values were: control group mean RI 0.876 (±0.056), mean PI 2.877 (±0.643) (Figure 2); group I mean RI 0.793 (±0.127), mean PI 1.929 (±0.641) (Figure 3); group II mean ICA-RI 0.788 (±0.144), mean non-ICA-RI 0.675 (±0.446), mean ICA-PI 2.088 (±1.015), mean non-ICA-PI 2.520 (±2.506) (Figure 4). In all 25 patients values of impedance indices of FS obtained within the chest wall did not differ from FS obtained in intercostal arteries of healthy volunteers (Figure 1). Within group II 12 non ICA-FS located within pulmonary tissue were obtained in 8 patients and could be discriminated from intercostal arterial supply by spectral curve analysis. Mean values of impedance indices of the ICA and non ICA in group II are shown in Figure 1.

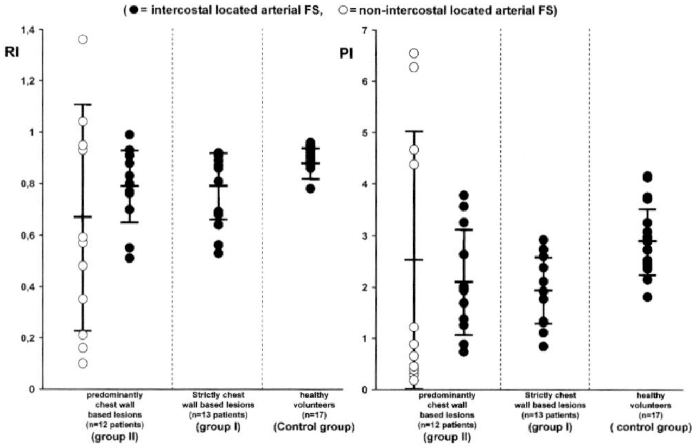

Figure 1. Values of resistive-index (RI) and pulsatility-index (PI) (mean ± sd) of 37 spectral curves in 25 patients with chest wall lesions.

Number of different FS in a lesion

Four patients had no FS, 17 patients had one FS, 5 patients had two different FS, 2 patients had three different FS, 1 patient had four different FS (Figures 5–7). In total 37 different FS were seen in 25 patients. 25 patients had ICA-FS, 12 patients had non-ICA-FS which included PA-FS (n=5), BA-FS (n=4) and TN-FS (n=3).

Statistical analysis

RI values with alpha correcture do not differ between the three groups (p=0.037). The PI values do differ between the three groups (p=0.002). The p-values for comparison of impedance measurements within group II were not significant (p=0.55 for RI, p=0.63 for PI).

Discussion

Thoracic ultrasound is limited by complete sound reflection of the aerated lung. Nevertheless B-mode-ultrasound and qualitative CDS can provide additional information about the aetiology of based lesions diagnosed by chest radiography [1–6]. In the last decade several studies have shown a sensitivity and specificity of up to 95% for the differentiation of benign lesions from malignant lesions by impedance measurement of spectral curves [2, 4–6]. In these studies benign lesions such as pneumonia and atelectasis were characterized by a high impedance triphasic FS derived from PA. In malignant pulmonary lesions a low impedance monophasic FS was seen [2, 4–6]. Whereas some authors interpreted this FS as vessels of tumour neoangiogenesis (TN), a recent study identified the low impedant monophasic FS as BA by histological analysis [7]. Central BA form a vascular ring

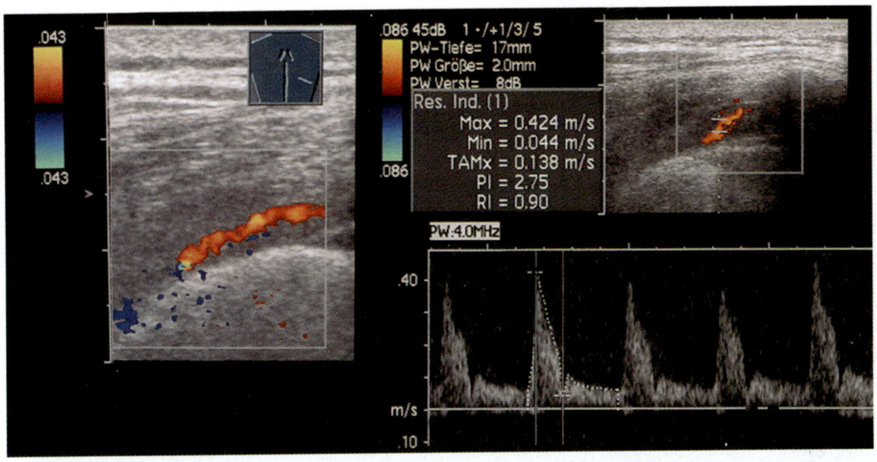

(a) (b)

Figure 2. (a) Visualization of an intercostal artery in a healthy volunteer by power Doppler ultrasound. (b) A monophasic high impedant arterial flow pattern was seen suggesting an intercostal artery (ICA).

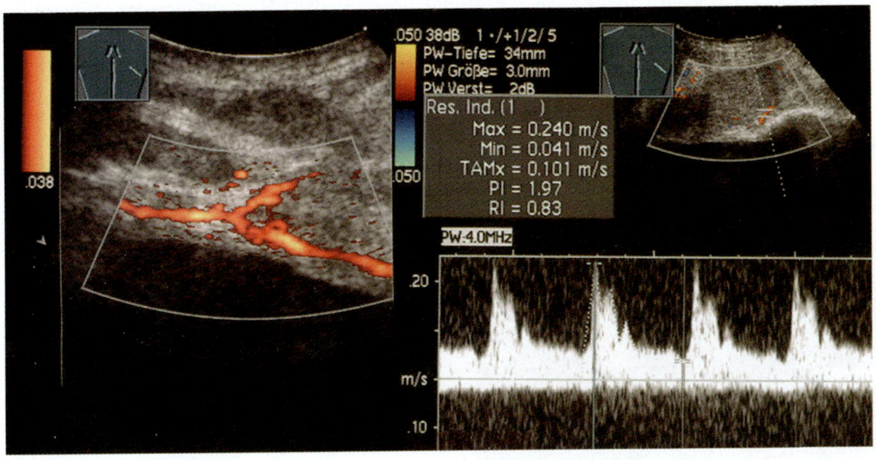

(a) (b)

Figure 3. 56-year-old patient with lung cancer and metastases within the chest wall. (a) On power Doppler ultrasound a large vessel was seen in the tumour which infiltrates the chest wall. The tumour involvement is bordered by a pleural effusion. (b) A monophasic high impedant arterial flow pattern was seen suggesting an intercostal artery (ICA).

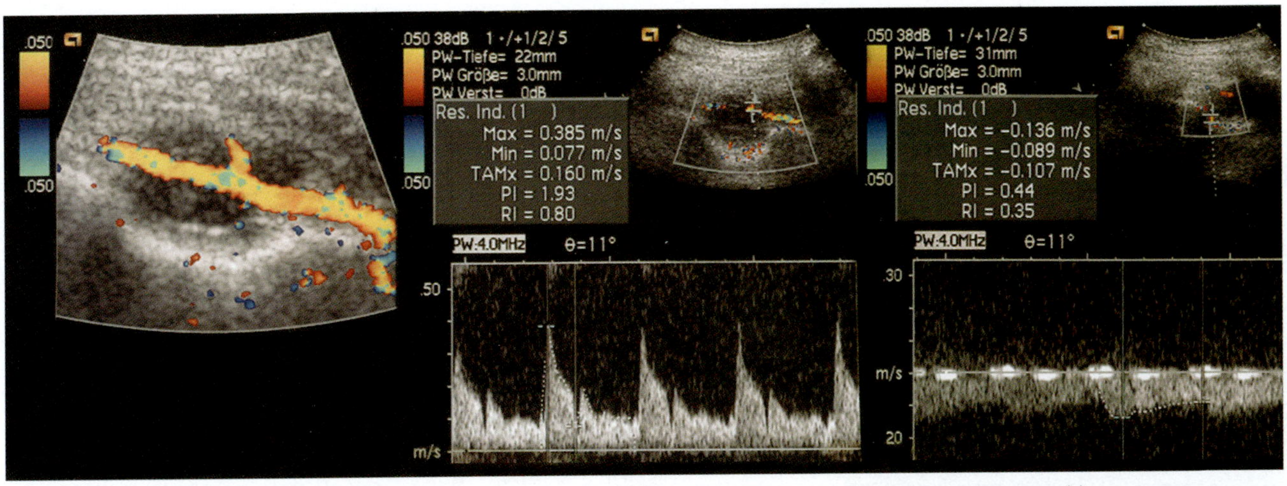

(a) (b) (c)

Figure 4. 33-year-old patient with a primitive neuroectodermal tumour (PNET) of the chest wall with infiltration of pulmonary tissue. (a) On colour Doppler ultrasound a vessel was seen centrally in the tumour. (b) A monophasic high impedant arterial flow pattern was seen suggesting an intercostal artery (ICA). (c) In the periphery of the lesion a monophasic low impedant arterial flow pattern was seen suggesting a peripheral bronchial artery (BA) origin.

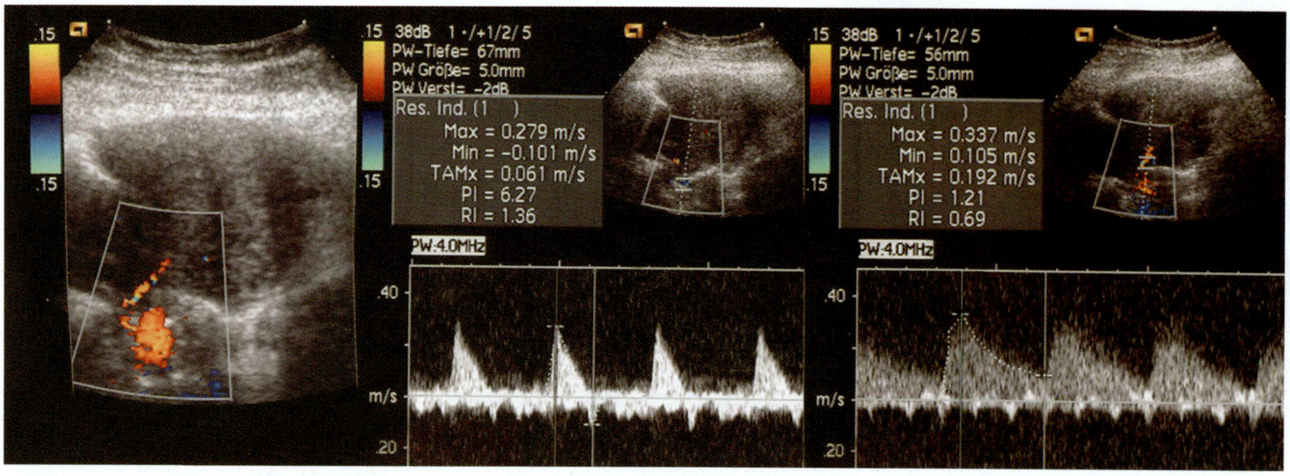

(a) (b) (c)

Figure 5. 34-year-old patient with testicular cancer and pleuropulmonary metastases, which infiltrate the chest wall. (a) On colour Doppler ultrasound mapping vessels were seen in the central region of the tumour. (b) A triphasic high impedant arterial flow pattern was seen suggesting a pulmonary artery (PA) origin. (c) Beneath the PA an additional flow signal (FS) characterized as a monophasic low impedant arterial flow pattern was seen suggesting a central bronchial artery (BA) origin.

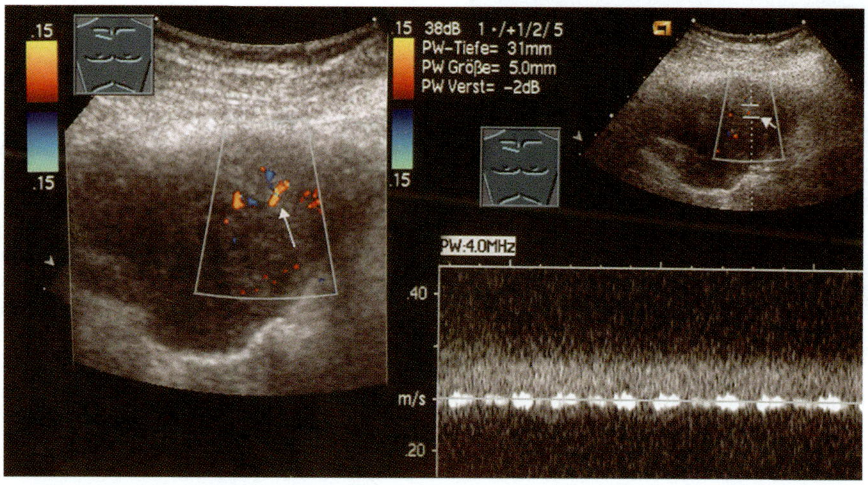

(a) (b)

Figure 6. (a) On colour Doppler ultrasound mapping small vessels were seen in the central region of the tumour (arrow). (b) A monophasic nearby constant flow pattern that lacks systolic–diastolic variation was seen suggesting tumour neoangiogenesis (TN).

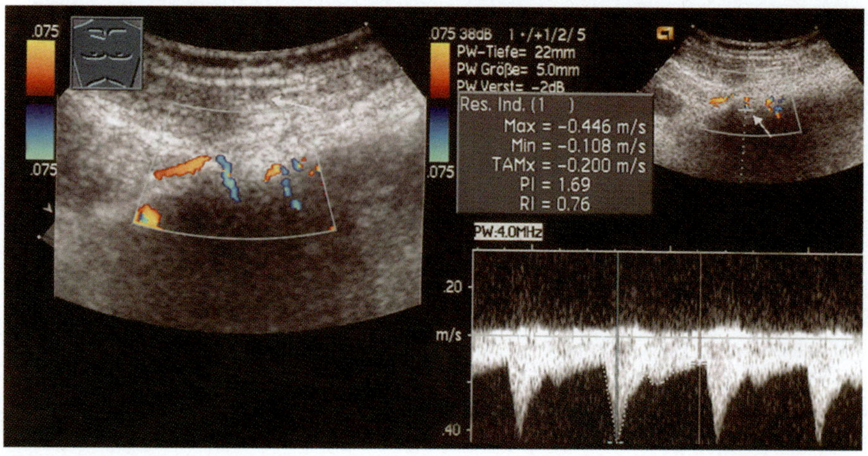

(a) (b)

Figure 7. (a) On colour Doppler ultrasound mapping small vessels originated in the chest wall were seen in the peripheral region of the tumour. (b) A monophasic high impedant arterial flow pattern was seen suggesting an intercostal artery (ICA) origin.

around the lung hilum from which branches centrifugally course along the bronchial tree. Peripheral BA lies within the interlobar and interlobular septa and supply the visceral pleura. In contrast to BA true vessels of TN are rarely found by CDS because of its slow flow [10]. They are characterized by a nearly constant flow that lacks systolic–diastolic variation [8]. In chest wall lesions this study characterized an additional arterial supply identified as ICA derived which could discriminate from PA, BA, and TN by spectral curve analysis. It should be emphasized that in almost 50% of pulmonary lesions various arterial FS can be identified [9]. Therefore a variable nutritional supply of the tumour is suspected corresponding to the complex arterial supply of the lung.

In conclusion, quantitative CDS indicates a variable arterial supply of chest wall lesions which strongly depends on location of lesions. A single spectral analysis is not helpful for tissue characterization. Lesions strictly located to the chest wall had an ICA supply. Chest wall lesions with pulmonary extension demonstrated a complex arterial supply.

References

1. Gehmacher O, Mathis G, Kopf A, Scheier M. Ultrasound imaging of pneumonia. Ultrasound Med Biol 1995;21: 1119–22.
2. Yuan A, Chang DB, Yu CJ, Kuo SM, Luh KT, Yang PC. Color Doppler sonography of benign and malignant pulmonary masses. AJR Am J Roentgenol 1994;163:545–9.
3. Mathis G, Dirschmid K. Pulmonary infarction: sonographic appearance with pathologic correlation. Eur J Radiol 1993;17:170–4.
4. Yuan A, Yang PC, Lee L, Wu HD, Kuo SH, et al. Reactive pulmonary artery vasoconstriction in pulmonary consolidation by color Doppler ultrasonography. Ultrasound Med Biol 2000;26;49–56.
5. Civardi G, Fornari F, Cavanna L, Di Stasi M, Sbolli G, et al. Vascular signals from pleural-based lung lesions. Studied with pulsed Doppler ultrasonography. J Clin Ultrasound 1993; 21:617–22.
6. Hsu WH, Ikezoe J, Chen CY, Kean PC, Hsu CP, et al. Color Doppler ultrasound pulsatile flow signals of thoracic lesions: Comparison of lung cancer and benign lesions. Ultrasound Med Biol 1998;24:1087–95.
7. Hsu WH, Ikezoe J, Chen CY, Kean PC, Hsu CP, et al. Color Doppler ultrasound signals of thoracic lesions: Correlation with resected histologic specimens. Am J Respir Crit Care Med 1996;153:1938–51.
8. Babo VM, Müller KMG, Huzky A, et al. Die Bronchialarteriographie bei Erkrankungen der Lunge. Radiologie 1979; 19:506–13.
9. Görg C, Seifart U, Görg K, Zugmaier G. Color Doppler mapping of pulmonary lesions: evidence of dual arterial supply by spectralanalysis. J Ultrasound Med 2003;22:1033–9.
10. Harvey CJ, Albrecht T. Ultrasound of focal liver lesions. Eur Radiol 2001;11:1578–93.

The British Journal of Radiology, *78* (2005), 308–311
DOI: 10.1259/bjr/72038963

Three-dimensional anal endosonography may improve diagnostic confidence of detecting damage to the anal sphincter complex

A F CHRISTENSEN, MD, B NYHUUS, MD, M B NIELSEN, MD, DMSc and H CHRISTENSEN, MD, PhD

Department of Radiology, Section of Ultrasound, Rigshospitalet and Department of Neurology, Bispebjerg Hospital, University of Copenhagen, Denmark

Abstract. The aim of study was to investigate the differences between three-dimensional (3D) endosonography and two-dimensional (2D) endosonography in visualizing damage to the anal sphincter complex. 33 patients with a history of damage to the anal sphincters were examined with a 10 MHz rotating endoprobe. Cross-sectional images of the anal sphincters were stored on a 3D system during retraction of the endoprobe through the anal canal. Cross-sectional images (2D) were compared with reconstructed projections (3D) according to five parameters relating to damage of different parts of the sphincter muscles as well as scar-tissue formation in the rectovaginal septum. Depending on whether the investigator felt confident in diagnosis of scar tissue being present or not a numerical value of 1 or 0 was assigned. In this way a scale from 0 to 5 points was achieved, which ideally should be identical in 3D and 2D. Overall both observers felt diagnostic confidence in a median of five parameters (range 4–5) using 3D, compared with a median of four parameters (range 3–5) using 2D (p=0.001). When only assessing the four parameters relating to damage of different parts of the sphincter-muscles the observers felt diagnostic confidence in eight more cases using 3D than 2D. This difference did not reach statistical significance. The overall agreement between the two observers comparing all five parameters was 98.2% using 3D and 87.9% using 2D. 3D anal endosonography improves diagnostic confidence in detecting damage to the anal sphincter complex. The agreement between the two observers was acceptable using 2D but better when using 3D. The 3D method may improve the selection of patients for surgical repair of the anal sphincter complex.

Anal incontinence following damage to the anal sphincter muscles during vaginal delivery occurs in up to 7% of cases [1, 2]. The treatment in severe cases is surgery. This is preceded by anal endosonography [3], which has been shown to provide highly accurate imaging of anal sphincter morphology with a high spatial resolution, and has become the gold standard for demonstration of sphincteric defects [4, 5]. However, the technique is limited to a two-dimensional (2D) visualization of the structures. With a new technique, three-dimensional (3D) endosonography, any projection (*e.g.* coronal and sagittal) can be reconstructed [6, 7]. The aim of this study was to investigate the differences between the two endosonographic techniques in visualization of damage to the anal sphincter complex.

Materials and methods

33 consecutive female patients, median age 33 years (range 24–58 years), with suspected damage to the anal sphincter muscles were examined with anal endosonography in the period from July 2001 to September 2002. Endosonography was performed using a B-K Medical (Herlev, Denmark) type 2102 ultrasound apparatus with a rotating endoprobe type 1850 and a 10 MHz transducer type 6004 (focus 1.5–4 cm), which produces 360° axial images of the anal sphincter muscles. The transducer was covered with a water-filled hard sonolucent plastic cone (diameter 1.7 cm) [5]. The ultrasound apparatus had a built-in 3D module (B-K Medical, Herlev, Denmark), with which the axial images of the anal sphincters were stored on a hard disc during retraction of the endoprobe through the anal canal using a mechanical retractor with a constant retraction rate. Afterwards, by means of the 3D module, any projection (*e.g.* coronal or sagittal) could be reconstructed.

All examinations were retrospectively reviewed by two observers and the axial (2D) projections (Figure 1a), *i.e.* the true scanning plane, reviewed from the 3D dataset, were compared with reconstructed projections (3D: coronal, sagittal as well as the original axial projections) (Figure 1b) for the following five parts of the anal sphincter apparatus: (1) internal anal sphincter; (2) puborectalis muscle; (3) external anal sphincter in the middle third of the anal canal; (4) external anal sphincter in the distal third of the anal canal; (5) distal part of the rectovaginal septum. Depending on whether the investigator felt diagnostic confidence about damage/scar tissue being present or not (Figure 2) a numerical value of 1 or 0 was assigned for each of the five locations. In this way a scale from 0 to 5 points were achieved, that ideally should be identical in 3D and 2D.

Received 22 March 2004 and in revised form 23 August 2004, accepted 15 November 2004.

Address correspondence to Anders Fogh Christensen, Department of Radiology, Section of Ultrasound x4123, Rigshospitalet, Blegdamsvej 9, 2100 Copenhagen, Denmark.

This study was supported by grants from: Mogens Andreasen fonden and Ragnhild Ibsens Legat for Medicinsk forskning.

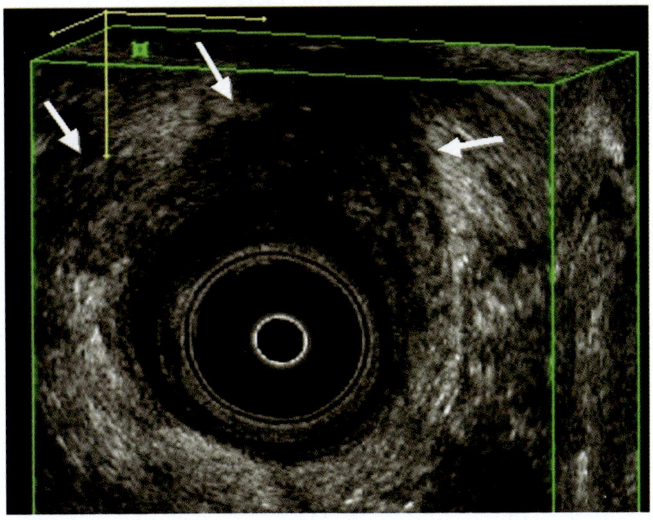

(a)

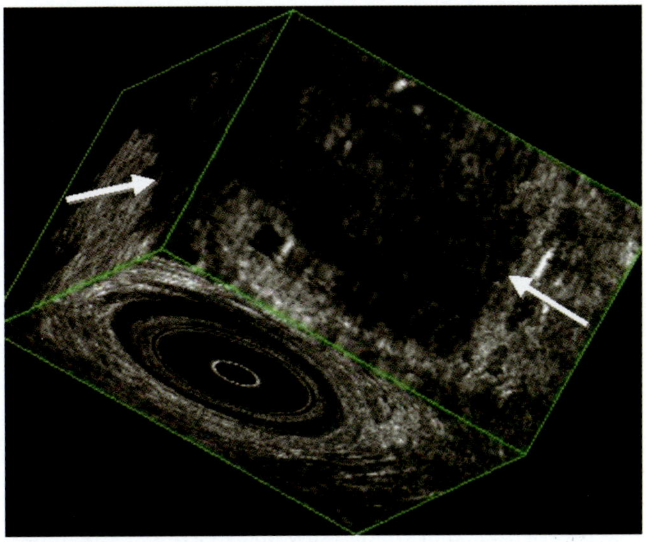

(b)

Figure 1. (a) Transverse anal endosonogram (2D), corresponding to the original axial image, shows large hypoechoic defect in the external anal sphincter (arrows). (b) 3D projection of the same patient (right) shows the sphincteric defect (arrows) extending cranially (upper right) towards the rectovaginal septum.

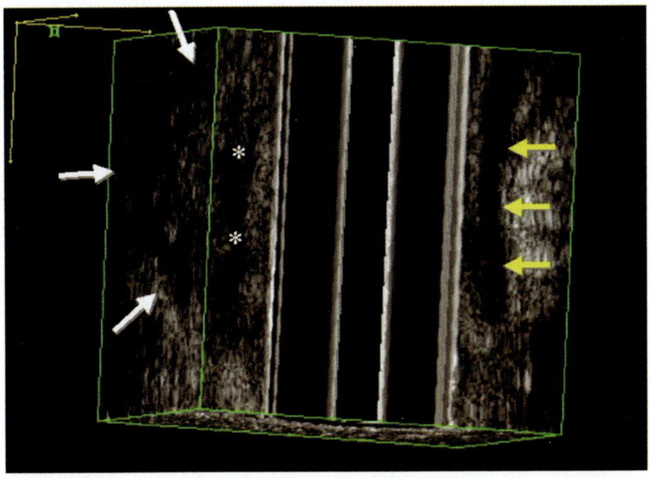

Figure 2. 3D coronal projection of the anal sphincter muscles. To the right the hypoechoic internal sphincter is clearly seen (yellow arrows), to the left hypoechoic scar tissue in the external sphincter (arrows) involves the internal anal sphincter as well (*).

Data analysis was performed by SPSS for Windows version 9.0 (SPSS Inc., Chicago, IL). Non-continuous related variables were compared by the Wilcoxon signed rank-test. Interobserver agreement was calculated as $(N-\text{agreement} \times 100)/N-\text{total}$, where N is number of patients.

Results

Data are presented in Table 1. Both observers felt diagnostic confidence in median five parameters (range 4–5) using 3D, compared with median four parameters (range 3–5) using 2D ($p=0.001$). The lowest number of cases in which both observers shared diagnostic confidence was 31 in 3D and 1 in 2D, both concerning presence of scar tissue in the rectovaginal septum.

When isolating the four parameters relating to damage to different parts of the sphincter muscles the observers felt diagnostic confidence in eight more cases using 3D than 2D. This difference did not reach statistical significance when the parameters were compared separately, but only when they were compared together.

The overall agreement between the two observers comparing all five parameters were 98.2% using 3D and 87.9% using 2D. The agreement ranged from 63.6% to 100% with the parameters on 2D and from 93.9% to 100% with the parameters in 3D.

Table 1. Number of cases in which the two observers A and B were in agreement of whether 2D or 3D anal endosonography were able or unable to determine possible damage to the anal sphincter complex

Part of anal sphincter complex	2D			3D			
	able	unable	disagree	able	unable	disagree	Prevalence of scar/defects on 3D
Internal anal sphincter	27	1	5	33	0	0	1 (3%)
Puborectalis muscle	32	0	1	32	0	1	0 (0%)
External anal sphincter, midlevel	33	0	0	33	0	0	33 (100%)
External anal sphincter, distal part	31	0	2	33	0	0	5 (16%)
Rectovaginal septum	1	20	12	31	0	2	9 (28%)

Discussion

Anal endosonography using a single scanning plane (2D) has been validated histologically [8], intraoperatively [9] and physiologically [10] as the primary tool in the assessment of sphincteric defects and has replaced the previously used needle electromyography mapping of the external anal sphincter [3, 11, 12]. In detail endosonography has been reported to be reproducibly better than MRI with endocoil at visualizing the internal anal sphincter [13] and possibly for differentiating scar tissue from the external anal sphincter whereas MRI is considered the most accurate in evaluation of the external anal sphincter itself [14]. 2D endosonography has not previously been compared with the new technique of 3D endosonography. In this retrospective study, based on the diagnostic confidence concerning possible damage to the anal sphincter complex in five well demarcated areas, the use of 3D endosonography increased the diagnostic confidence and offered an improved agreement between two observers.

A detailed assessment of the possible damage to the anal sphincter complex is important for selection of patients for surgical repair of the anal sphincters [3, 12, 15, 16]. The results of the present study indicate that 3D endosonography is better at providing these data than 2D endosonography for the anal sphincter muscles and especially in detecting scar tissue in the distal rectovaginal septum. The rectovaginal septum, named by some the rectovaginal fascia, has been defined as a sheet of strong connective-type tissue between the rectum and the vagina [17]. The septum fuses with the vaginal wall anteriorly, the fascia over the levator muscles laterally and the anterior rectal wall posteriorly. Obstetric trauma is associated with damage/defects primarily to the distal part of the rectovaginal septum [18] as well as elongation of the length of the septum [19] and defects in the septum have been associated with rectocele formation [17]. Surgical repair involving repair of the rectovaginal septum has been shown to be an effective treatment of rectocele and symptoms of obstructed defecation/incontinence caused by the rectocele [20, 21]. However surgical repair in combination with sphincteric repair does not seem to give any clear benefits [21, 22]. Perhaps the lack of a way to visualize the extent of the scar tissue can explain these results. A recent study [23] has reported a sensitivity and positive predictive value for standard pre-operative evaluation of rectovaginal septum support that was less than 40%, and the authors emphasize the need for new methods to evaluate the area.

With 2D endosonography and transverse images the anal sphincter muscles are usually described at three levels only (the upper, middle or lower third of the anal canal) and the radial extent of scar tissue in hours of the clock. An additional advantage of 3D anal endosonography is the possibility to measure the size of a sphincter tear in any projection as well as the length of the remaining intact sphincter muscle. We did not include measurements of maximum size of tear in this study because 2D and 3D are not comparable in this respect.

The interobserver agreement for diagnosing sphincter disruption using 2D endosonography has previously been shown to be high with values exceeding 80% and complete agreement between observers in cases of large tears involving both the internal and the external anal sphincter [24]. This correlates well with an overall agreement between observers in this study of 88% using 2D. In comparison values below 50% have been described for endoanal MRI [13]. To our knowledge no comparison of interobserver agreement for diagnosing sphincteric damage using 3D endosonography has been performed. In this study the values for interobserver agreement using 3D reached 98% clearly exceeding the values found using 2D.

The ability of 3D endosonography to review images in all projections resembles MRI, but the resolution appears to be better. For endosonography, slice thickness for reconstruction is 0.2 mm, which corresponds to the obtained resolution in a voxel size of 0.2 mm^3 in longitudinal projections. In comparison the best resolution by MRI will have a voxel size of at least 0.6 mm^3 [25, 26]. The high resolution in the reconstructed projections facilitates differentiation of damage to the thin structures of the anal sphincter complex.

In conclusion, 3D may improve the diagnostic confidence in detecting damage to the anal sphincter complex and especially the presence of scar tissue in the distal rectovaginal septum. The interobserver agreement is improved using 3D endosonography. This may result in a better selection of patients for surgical sphincter repair.

References

1. Macarthur C, Bick DE, Keighley MR. Faecal incontinence after childbirth. Br J Obstet Gynaecol 1997;104:46–50.
2. Groutz A, Fait G, Lessing JB, et al. Incidence and obstetric risk factors of postpartum anal incontinence. Scand J Gastroenterol 1999;34:315–8.
3. de Leeuw JW, Vierhout ME, Struijk PC, Auwerda HJ, Bac DJ, Wallenburg HC. Anal sphincter damage after vaginal delivery: relationship of anal endosonography and manometry to anorectal complaints. Dis Colon Rectum 2002;45: 1004–10.
4. Frudinger A, Halligan S, Bartram CI, Price AB, Kamm MA, Winter R. Female anal sphincter: age-related differences in asymptomatic volunteers with high-frequency endoanal US. Radiology 2002;224:417–23.
5. Nielsen MB. Endosonography of the anal sphincter muscles in healthy volunteers and in patients with defecation disorders. Acta Radiol Suppl 1998;416:1–21.
6. Williams AB, Bartram CI, Halligan S, et al. Alteration of anal sphincter morphology following vaginal delivery revealed by multiplanar anal endosonography. Br J Obstet Gynaecol 2002;109:942–6.
7. Gold DM, Bartram CI, Halligan S, Humphries KN, Kamm MA, Kmiot WA. Three-dimensional endoanal sonography in assessing anal canal injury. Br J Surg 1999;86:365–70.
8. Sultan AH, Kamm MA, Talbot IC, Nicholls RJ, Bartram CI. Anal endosonography for identifying external sphincter defects confirmed histologically. Br J Surg 1994;81:463–5.
9. Sultan AH, Nicholls RJ, Kamm MA, Hudson CN, Beynon J, Bartram CI. Anal endosonography and correlation with in vitro and in vivo anatomy. Br J Surg 1993;80:508–11.
10. Sultan AH, Kamm MA, Hudson CN, Thomas JM, Bartram CI. Anal-sphincter disruption during vaginal delivery. N Engl J Med 1993;329:1905–11.
11. Willis S, Faridi A, Schelzig S, et al. Childbirth and incontinence: a prospective study on anal sphincter morphology and function before and early after vaginal delivery. Langenbecks Arch Surg 2002;387:101–7.

12. Buhr HJ, Kroesen AJ. Rolle der bildgebung bei analinkontinenz [The importance of diagnostics in faecal incontinence. Endosonography]. Chirurg 2003;74:4–14.
13. Malouf AJ, Williams AB, Halligan S, Bartram CI, Dhillon S, Kamm MA. Prospective assessment of accuracy of endoanal MR imaging and endosonography in patients with fecal incontinence. AJR Am J Roentgenol 2000;175:741–5.
14. Rociu E, Stoker J, Eijkemans, et al. Fecal incontinence: endoanal US versus endoanal MR imaging. Radiology 1999;212:453–8.
15. Bartram C. Anal endosonography after sphincter repair. Abdom Imaging 1999;24:574–5.
16. Williams AB, Spencer JA, Bartram CI. Assessment of third degree tears using three-dimensional anal endosonography with combined anal manometry: a novel technique. Br J Obstet Gynaecol 2002;109:833–5.
17. Richardson AC. The rectovaginal septum revisited: its relationship to rectocele and its importance in rectocele repair. Clin Obstet Gynecol 1993;36:976–83.
18. Briel JW, de Boer LM, Hop WC, Schouten WR. Clinical outcome of anterior overlapping external anal schincter repair with internal anal schincter imbrication. Dis Colon Rectum 1998;42:688–9.
19. Kuhn RJ, Hollyock VE. Observations on the anatomy of the rectovaginal pouch and septum. Obstet Gynecol 1982;59: 445–7.
20. Zbar AP, Lienemann A, Fritsch H, Beer-Gabel M, Pescatori M. Rectocele: pathogenesis and surgical management. Int J Colorectal Dis 2003;18:369–84.
21. Singh K, Cortes E, Reid WM. Evaluation of the fascial technique for surgical repair of isolated posterior vaginal wall prolapse. Obstet Gynecol 2003;101:320–4.
22. Lechaux JP, Lechaut D, Bataille P, Bars I. Traitement de la rectocele par voie perinale avec prothese-Transperineal repair of rectocele with prostetic mesh. A prospective study. Ann Chir 2004;129:211–7.
23. Burrows LJ, Sewell C, Leffler KS, Cundiff GW. The accuracy of clinical evaluation of posterior vaginal wall defects. Intern Urogynecol J 2003;14:160–3.
24. Gold DM, Halligan S, Kmiot WA, Bartram CI. Intraobserver and interobserver agreement in anal endosonography. Br J Surg 1999;86:371–5.
25. Rociu E, Stoker J, Eijkemans MJ, Lameris JS. Normal anal sphincter anatomy and age- and sex-related variations at high-spatial-resolution endoanal MR imaging. Radiology 2000;217:395–401.
26. Beets-Tan RG, Beets GL, van der Hoop AG, et al. High-resolution magnetic resonance imaging of the anorectal region without an endocoil. Abdom Imaging 1999;24:576–81.

The British Journal of Radiology, *78* (2005), 312–315
DOI: 10.1259/bjr/33317317

Comparison of full-field digital mammography and film–screen mammography: image quality and lesion detection

[1]A FISCHMANN, MD, [1]K C SIEGMANN, MD, [1]A WERSEBE, MD, [1]C D CLAUSSEN, MD and [1,2]M MÜLLER-SCHIMPFLE, MD

[1]*Department of Diagnostic Radiology, University Hospital Tübingen, Hoppe-Seyler-Str. 3, 72076 Tübingen and* [2]*Städtische Kliniken Frankfurt/Main, Central Institute of Radiology, Germany*

Abstract. The objective of this study is to compare image quality and lesion detection for full field digital mammography (FFDM) and film–screen mammography (FSM). In 200 women we performed digital mammography of one breast and film–screen mammography of the other breast. Imaging parameters were set automatically. Image quality, visualization of calcifications and masses were rated by three readers independently. Mean glandular dose was calculated for both systems. We found no significant difference in mean glandular dose. Image quality was rated by reader A/B/C as excellent for FFDM in 153/155/167 cases and for FSM in 139/116/114 cases ($p<0.03/0.001/0.001$). Microcalcifications were detected by FFDM in 103/89/98 and by FSM in 76/76/76 cases ($p<0.01/0.06/0.01$). Detection of masses did not differ significantly. FFDM provided significantly better visibility of skin and nipple-areola region ($p<0.01$). FFDM demonstrated improved image quality compared with film–screen mammography. Microcalcification detection was also significantly better with the digital mammography system for two of the three readers.

Digital technology is replacing conventional film–screen systems in all aspects of clinical radiology. Several digital mammography systems based on different physical concepts have been introduced and approved by the Food and Drug Administration in the last few years [1]. The first system introduced was the full field digital mammography (FFDM) system based on amorphous silicon (General Electric Medical Systems, Milwaukee, WI), followed by the charge coupled device (CCD)-based slot-scan-system (Fischer Imaging, Denver, CO) and the FFDM based on amorphous selenium (LoRad, Danbury, CT).

Since November 2000 we have used a GE FFDM unit with a soft copy review workstation. The spatial resolution of the unit for high contrast objects is 5 line pairs mm^{-1} (lp mm^{-1}). This is below the minimum requirements for film–screen mammography (FSM) in Europe, which require a spatial resolution of at least 10 lp mm^{-1} (>10 lp mm^{-1} acceptable, >13 lp mm^{-1} desirable) [2]. The system has, however, a higher detective quantum efficiency (DQE) and contrast resolution [3, 4]. This allows for better contrast resolution of structures at a spatial resolution of 1–4 lp mm^{-1}, where the human eye performs best. Therefore the European guidelines for screening mammography exclude digital mammography from the higher requirements in spatial resolution [2]. A study using FFDM with screening patients showed a better detection of calcifications and better visualization of dense breast parenchyma compared with FSM [5]. However, few prospective clinical studies comparing image quality have been published [6–8].

The aim of this study was to compare image quality and lesion detection of FFDM and FSM in a prospective randomized study on the same woman without double radiation exposure of the breasts, a method already used in other studies [9].

Received 5 May 2004 and in revised form 20 October 2004, accepted 23 November 2004.

Materials and methods

This study included 200 consecutive women without visible or palpable breast lesions, who were referred for mammography after individual counselling by a physician. Criteria for exclusion were visible breast asymmetry, previous breast surgery and/or known breast lesions and inflammation. Women below the age of 40 years were excluded to reduce radiation risk. The detector size of the Senographe 2000D is 19 cm × 23 cm, therefore women with breasts too large to be imaged with one exposure were excluded as well. All participants gave informed consent. The study was approved by the local ethics committee. In one patient breast cancer was detected during the course of the study. The mammograms of this patient were not available during this study owing to further external therapy, therefore the remaining 199 patients formed the study population.

All participants received an FFDM of one breast and a FSM of the other, with random allocation of the modalities to the breasts. All images of one patient were taken by one radiographer compressing the breasts with identical force to identical thickness with both modalities. Using this method, comparison between an individual's breasts could be performed without additional radiation dose. Image parameters were set by both systems automatically in standard mode. FSM was performed using a GE Senographe DMR+ with Kodak MinR 2000 film–screen system (Kodak, Rochester, NY), and developed using a Kodak Xomat M35 developer with RP Xomat chemicals at 33.5℃. Imaging parameters were recorded for each exposure. Entrance skin dose was measured on a phantom for every set of patient parameters. These parameters were used to calculate mean glandular dose according to the method by Sobol and Wu [10]. FFDM was performed using the GE Senographe 2000D. Comparison was made on hardcopies, printed on a Kodak DryView 8610 laser-printer. Printout parameters were set in standard mode.

Table 1. Classification of parenchymal density

Class	Size of a lesion that could be missed
1	<0.5 cm
2	0.5 to 1 cm
3	1 to 2 cm
4	>2 cm

To measure breast density, we used a classification modified from the one used in the BI-RADS®-Lexicon by the American College of Radiology [18]. The tissue density is classified into four groups according to the size of lesions that cannot be excluded (Table 1). In this way we provide a measurement for exclusion of opacities especially for inhomogeneous breast parenchyma.

Comparison was performed independently by three radiologists with 2, 4 and 10 years experience in mammography. FFDM and FSM were rated separately according to multiple criteria (Table 2), with both modalities rated in each session. To reduce reader bias, the evaluation of digital and conventional images of each patient were separated by at least 1 month. Images from 50 patients were rated twice to estimate intrareader-variability. Significance was tested with the sign-test and McNemar test. Statistical evaluation was performed on the statistic software JMP 4.0 for Windows NT (SAS Institute Inc. Cary, NC).

Results

FFDM used significantly more Rh/Rh (rhodium/rhodium) as anode-filter-combination compared with FSM: in craniocaudal view (CC) in 102 cases with FFDM compared with 8 times with FSM, in mediolateral-oblique view (MLO) in 110 cases with FFDM compared with 7 cases with FSM. Mean glandular dose was slightly higher with FFDM with 1.63 mGy (0.85–3.36 mGy) in CC-view compared with 1.45 mGy (0.35–3.60 mGy) for FSM. In MLO-view the corresponding values were 1.70 mGy (1.00–3.16 mGy) for FFDM and 1.52 mGy (0.46–3.49 mGy) with FSM (Table 3). These differences were not significant.

Table 2. Criteria of classification

Criteria	Classification
Detection of the pectoral muscle	Visible/not visible
Visibility of the nipple	Excellent/good/mediocre/not visible with and without bright light
Visibility of the skin	Excellent/good/mediocre/not visible with and without bright light
Breast density	Highly dense/dense/mostly fatty/fatty see Table 1
Sharpness	Sharp/slightly unsharp/unsharp
Contrast in parenchymal tissue	Excellent/good/mediocre/inadequate
Contrast in fatty tissue	Excellent/good/mediocre/inadequate
Detection of microcalcifications	No calcs/probably no calcs/probably calcs/calcs
Diagnostic quality for microcalcifications	Excellent/good/mediocre/inadequate
Detection of masses	No/probably no masses/probably masses present/masses
Diagnostic quality for masses	Excellent/good/mediocre/inadequate
Overall image quality	Excellent to inadequate (school marks)

Table 3. Mean glandular dose calculations in mediolateral oblique (MLO) and craniocaudal (CC)-view

	Parameter	FSM	FFDM
MLO	Average dose [mGy]	1.52	1.70
	Standard deviation	0.58	0.40
	Minimum–maximum	0.46–3.49	1.00–3.16
	Average tube voltage [kV]	27.24	28.81
	Standard deviation	1.01	1.43
	Minimum–maximum	24–29	25–32
	Average tube-current-time product [mAs]	87.42	73.71
	Standard deviation	40.63	19.53
	Minimum–maximum	21–223	25–115
CC	Average dose [mGy]	1.45	1.63
	Standard deviation	0.55	0.38
	Minimum–maximum	0.35–3.60	0.85–3.36
	Average tube voltage [kV]	27.0	28.81
	Standard deviation	1.21	1.35
	Minimum–maximum	22–31	25–32
	Average tube current [mAs]	83.31	70.74
	Standard deviation	37.81	18.22
	Minimum–maximum	21–236	27–120

FSM, film–screen mammography; FFDM, full field digital mammography.

FFDM significantly facilitated mammographic positioning. The pectoral muscle was depicted on the CC-view by Reader A/B/C with FFDM in 96/111/110 cases compared with 76/84/88 cases with FSM ($p<0.02/0.001/0.01$). This difference is demonstrated in Figure 1.

The largest difference was in the depiction of the nipple (Figure 1) which was rated as excellent for FFDM even without bright light in 161/141/189 cases, for FSM in 6/7/103 cases ($p<0.0001/0.0001/0.02$). With the use of a bright light FFDM improved to 192/161/192 excellent cases, FSM to 52/55/177 cases ($p<0.0001/0.0001/0.01$). The depiction of the skin was rated excellent in 195/173/193 cases for FFDM and in 32/10/172 cases for FSM ($p<0.0001/0.0001/0.01$), which improved with the use of a bright light to 197/168/194 cases for FFMD and 158/104/191 cases with FSM (n.s. for reader C). Inter-reader concordance was low for skin and nipple detection with kappa-values ranging from −0.06 to 0.47.

Image quality was rated as excellent for FFDM in 153/155/167 cases and for FSM in 139/116/114 cases ($p<0.03/0.001/0.001$). Contrast in parenchymal and fatty tissue was rated heterogeneously: while reader A and B found better contrast with FFDM in parenchymal tissue ($p<0.05$), reader C found a better contrast in fatty tissue ($p<0.01$). All three readers classified the breast parenchyma on digital mammograms to be less dense than the film–screen images ($p<0.01/0.0001/0.01$), with good inter-reader and intrareader agreement (kappa-values of 0.47–0.77).

Another difference was in the detection of microcalcifications, which were detected with FFDM in 103/89/98 cases (kappa-values from 0.57 to 0.84) and with FSM in

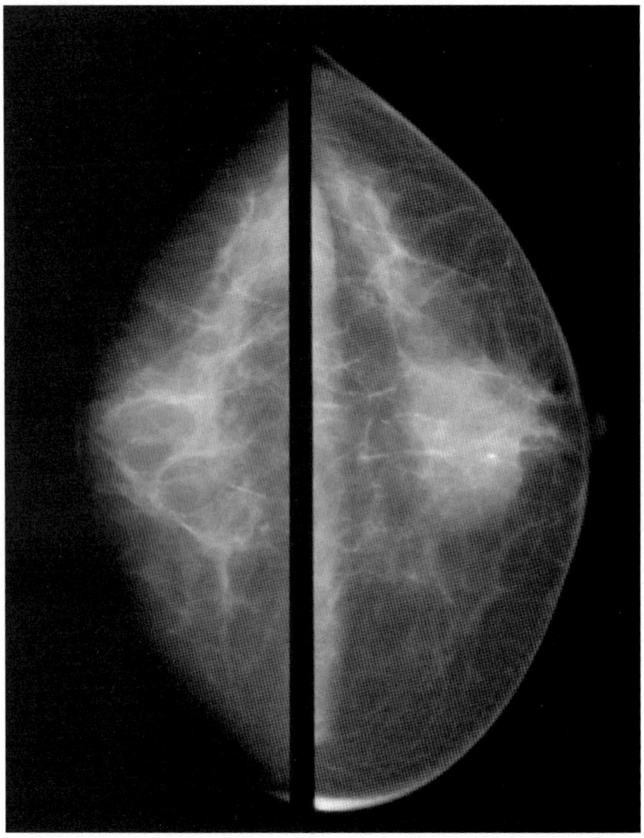

Figure 1. Caudocranial-exposures, left film–screen mammography, right full-field digital mammography. Better depiction of m. pectoralis right and nipple.

76/76/76 cases (kappa-values from 0.51 to 0.62). This difference was significant for two readers and showed a strong tendency for the third one ($p<0.02/0.07/0.02$), while no differences were found in the diagnostic classification of these microcalcifications. No significant differences were found in the detection of masses although all readers were significantly more certain in the exclusion of masses ($p<0.02/0.04/0.01$).

Discussion

This study compared both image quality and detection on FFDM and FSM using three experienced readers. The FFDM images were printed and compared under the same viewing conditions as the FSM. The readers were more experienced in FSM, however, all of the readers had read at least 100 digital mammograms prior to reading this study. Soft copy review may have allowed more manipulation of the images and possibly higher image quality scores for the digital images [11, 12]. Despite this and the readers being more used to FSM for diagnostic mammography, FFDM was at least equal to FSM in all examined parameters.

Breast composition, size, compression force and thickness of each patient were identical with both modalities. In contrast to early studies on phantoms that showed possible dose reduction of up to 50% [13] we found a tendency for a higher mean glandular dose with FFDM that was not significant. While the dose used by FFDM was in the range reported in other studies, the mean glandular dose used by the FSM was exceptionally low compared with data published by other workgroups [14].

In agreement with studies on phantoms [13, 15] and on patients [5, 6], we found a better detection of microcalcifications which was statistically significant for two out of three readers, considering the fact that two different breasts were examined. Even with FSM, which provides a spatial resolution of more than 15 lp mm^{-1}, the minimal size of detectable calcification is 130 μm [16]. In a phantom study FFDM proved to be superior to FSM especially in the detection of small calcifications in the 125–140 μm size range [17]. This indicates that the predominant limiting factor is the signal-to-noise ratio of the microcalcifications compared with the surrounding tissue rather than the theoretical maximal resolution for high contrast objects. For small calcifications, the contrast decreases rapidly with the size of the calcifications. In a clinical setting, the higher contrast resolution of FFDM seems to be more important than the detail resolution of FSM. Concerns that the lower spatial resolution could limit the characterization of calcifications have not been proven in clinical studies. Fischer et al [5] have shown that the FFDM system has a higher reliability in characterizing calcifications than FSM. Because of the ongoing discussion about soft-copy reading, we decided to perform this study with laser print-outs of the FFDM images, realising that this would limit the possibilities of digital mammography, especially concerning contrast resolution. Nevertheless we found no parameter which was rated to be superior in FSM.

In contrast to phantom studies [13] we found no improvement in the detection of masses with FFDM. The reason for this seems to be that the detection appears to be limited by inhomogeneous parenchymal background and irregular structures rather than by small contrast differences. The advantages in contrast resolution in parenchymal and fatty tissue, however, made the diagnostic classification or exclusion of masses significantly easier with FFDM. This was also seen in the classification of parenchymal density. With FFDM the readers rated the breast parenchyma to be less dense and they were able to exclude smaller lesions because of the higher contrast resolution.

A clear advantage of FFDM was the better depiction of skin and nipple without the use of a bright light. This can reduce reading time (Figure 2). The inter-reader variability for these parameters, especially for reader C, can be explained by a different threshold for excellent images. While A and B rated most of the images to be either good or mediocre, with few excellent images, reader C distributed the images between excellent and good, involuntarily reducing the original four-step-scale to three steps.

Another advantage is the better depiction of the pectoral muscle in CC-view (Figure 2), which is an important factor for perfect positioning according to the image quality assurance criteria [2]. As FFDM does not require a film-cassette and cassette-holder, the detector reaches approximately 2 mm closer to the chest wall. The pectoral muscle, as well as parenchymal tissue or carcinomas situated close to the chest wall can be better visualized this way.

The major limitation of this study is that owing to the differences between digital and conventional images it is not possible to blind the readers to the modalities. To reduce possible reader bias, we decided to read the

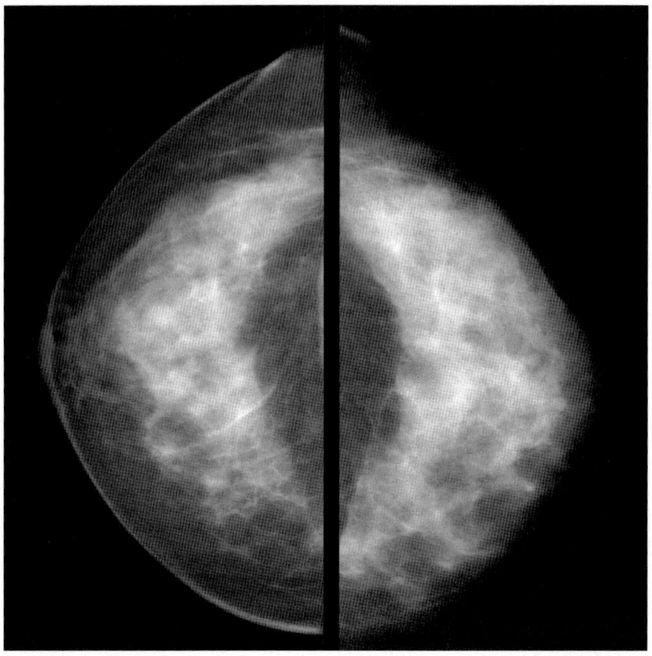

Figure 2. Caudocranial-exposures, left full-field digital mammography (FFDM), right film–screen mammography (FSM). Clearly recognizably better depiction of skin and nipple-areola region FFDM. Breast parenchyma was rated to be less dense with FFDM.

different studies of each patient in separate sessions. Another limitation is the method to compare two different techniques by comparing differences between one individuals breasts. This could bias the results, as there might have been differences in the number of calcifications in the breasts. To reduce this bias, breasts were randomized to the modalities and possible differences were considered in the calculations.

A further limitation is the subjective character of the parameters examined. As the radiologist is one of the major limiting factors in breast imaging, the non-objective parameters play an important role in the diagnostic process. For the acceptance of a new imaging modality, it is important that the radiologists "like" the pictures. Therefore we consider the measurement of subjective factors to be an important part in the evaluation of FFDM.

Overall the full field digital mammography system (FFDM) was equal or superior to film–screen mammography (FSM) for all of the image quality and detection parameters studied. The FFDM was also judged superior in the following image quality comparisons: (1) overall image quality; (2) skin and nipple depiction; and (3) pectoralis muscle depiction. The FFDM was superior to FSM in detecting microcalcifications for two out of the three readers. No difference was found in the detection of masses. The full field digital mammography system provided high quality diagnostic mammograms that were equal or superior to film–screen mammograms.

Acknowledgments

This study was supported by grant No. 2-0-0 by the AKF of the University of Tübingen.

References

1. Bick U. Full-field digital mammography. Fortschr Röntgenstr 2000;12:957–64.
2. (EUREF) European Protocol for the Quality Control of the Physical and Technical Aspects of Mammography Screening. "European Guidelines for Quality Assurance in Mammography Screening" Appendix 5: Digital mammography, 1999.
3. Muller S. Full-field digital mammography designed as a complete system. Eur J Radiol 1999;1:25–34.
4. Vedantham S, Karellas A, Suryanarayanan S, Albagli D, Han S, Tkaczyk EJ, et al. Full breast digital mammography with an amorphous silicon-based flat panel detector: physical characteristics of a clinical prototype. Med Phys 2000;3: 558–67.
5. Fischer U, Baum F, Obenauer S, Luftner-Nagel S, Von Heyden D, Vosshenrich R, et al. Comparative study in patients with microcalcifications: full-field digital mammography vs screen-film mammography. Eur Radiol 2002;11: 2679–83.
6. Obenauer S, Luftner-Nagel S, von Heyden D, Munzel U, Baum F, Grabbe E. Screen film vs full-field digital mammography: image quality, detectability and characterization of lesions. Eur Radiol 2002;7:1697–702.
7. Lewin JM, Hendrick RE, D'Orsi CJ, Isaacs PK, Moss LJ, Karellas A, et al. Comparison of full-field digital mammography with screen-film mammography for cancer detection: results of 4,945 paired examinations. Radiology 2001;3: 873–80.
8. Lewin JM, D'Orsi CJ, Hendrick RE, Moss LJ, Isaacs PK, Karellas A, et al. Clinical comparison of full-field digital mammography and screen-film mammography for detection of breast cancer. AJR Am J Roentgenol 2002;3:671–7.
9. Thilander-Klang AC, Ackerholm PH, Berlin IC, Bjurstam NG, Mattsson SL, Mansson LG, et al. Influence of anode-filter combinations on image quality and radiation dose in 965 women undergoing mammography. Radiology 1997;2:348–54.
10. Sobol WT, Wu X. Parametrization of mammography normalized average glandular dose tables. Med Phys 1997;4:547–54.
11. Pisano ED, Cole EB, Major S, Zong S, Hemminger BM, Muller KE, et al. Radiologists' preferences for digital mammographic display. The International Digital Mammography Development Group. Radiology 2000;3:820–30.
12. Funke M, Obenauer S, Hermann KP, Fischer U, Grabbe E. Soft copy versus hard copy findings in digital mammography. Radiologe 2002;4:265–9.
13. Obenauer S, Hermann KP, Schorn C, Fischer U, Grabbe E. Full-field digital mammography: dose-dependent detectability of breast lesions and microcalcinosis. Fortschr Röntgenstr 2000;12:1052–6.
14. Hermann KP, Obenauer S, Marten K, Kehbel S, Fischer U, Grabbe E. Average glandular dose with amorphous silicon full-field digital mammography - clinical results. Fortschr Röntgenstr 2002;6:696–9.
15. Obenauer S, Hermann KP, Schorn C, Funke M, Fischer U, Grabbe E. [Full-field digital mammography: a phantom study for detection of microcalcification]. Fortschr Röntgenstr 2000;7:646–50.
16. Karssemeijer N, Frieling JT, Hendriks JH. Spatial resolution in digital mammography. Invest Radiol 1993;5:413–9.
17. Rong XJ, Shaw CC, Johnston DA, Lemacks MR, Liu X, Whitman GJ, et al. Microcalcification detectability for four mammographic detectors: flat-panel, CCD, CR, and screen/film). Med Phys 2002;9:2052–61.
18. Breast Imaging Reporting and Data System (BI-RADS) 4th Edition, American College of Radiology, Reston VA, 2004.

The British Journal of Radiology, *78* (2005), 316–327 © 2005 The British Institute of Radiology
DOI: 10.1259/bjr/13015047

Automatic selection of non-coplanar beam directions for three-dimensional conformal radiotherapy

[1,2]J MEYER, PhD, [1]S M HUMMEL, RT(T), CMD, [1]P S CHO, PhD, [1]M M AUSTIN-SEYMOUR, MD and [1]M H PHILLIPS, PhD

[1]*University of Washington Medical Center, Department of Radiation Oncology, Box 356043, Seattle, WA 98195, USA and* [2]*Universität Würzburg, Klinik für Strahlentherapie, Josef-Schneider-Str. 11, D-97080 Würzburg, Germany*

Abstract. An algorithm is described, based on ray-tracing and the beam's-eye-view, that exhaustively searches all permitted beam directions. The evaluation of the search is based on a general cost function that can be adapted to the clinical objectives by means of parameters and weighting factors. The approach takes into account the constraints of the linear accelerator by discarding beam directions that are not permitted. A sensitivity analysis was carried out to determine appropriate parameters for different sized organs, and a prostate case was used to benchmark the approach. The algorithm was also applied to two clinical cases (brain and sinus) to test the benefits of the approach compared with manual angle selection. The time to perform a beam direction search was approximately 2 min for the coplanar and 12 min for the non-coplanar beam space. The angles obtained for the prostate case compared well with reports in the literature. For the brain case, the mean dose to the right and left optic nerves was reduced by 12% and 50%, respectively, whilst the target dose uniformity was improved. For the sinus case, the mean doses to the right and left parotid glands were reduced by 54% and 46%, respectively, to the right and left optic nerves by 37% and 62%, respectively, and to the optic chiasm by 39%, whilst the target dose uniformity was also improved. For the clinical cases the plans based on optimized beam directions were simpler and resulted in better sparing of critical structures compared with plans based on manual angle selection. The approach provides a practical alternative to elaborate and time consuming beam angle optimization schemes and is suitable for routine clinical usage.

The maximum radiation dose that can be deposited in a tumour is limited by the tolerance dose of the surrounding vital organs and critical structures [1]. Inherent objectives for a three-dimensional conformal radiation therapy (3D-CRT) treatment plan are to use beam directions such that the irradiation of the organs at risk (OAR) is minimized so as to reduce normal tissue complications, and to ensure an adequate dose coverage of the planning target volume (PTV).

This work concentrates on conventional 3D-CRT since it still constitutes most clinical treatments despite the increasingly widespread availability of intensity-modulated radiation therapy (IMRT). It was suggested by Webb [2] that only about 30% of clinical problems require the use of IMRT. The impetus of this work is to bridge the gap between 2D treatment planning and computer optimization of IMRT, since the efficacious use of 3D-CRT relies strongly on the judicious selection of non-coplanar beam angles. Rosen estimated in an industrial report in 1999 that only about one-third of facilities performed 3D-CRT regularly [3], but this number has probably increased significantly since then.

The use of non-coplanar 3D-CRT beams, as opposed to coplanar arrangements, has the potential to produce superior plans due to its increased ability to avoid critical structures [4–6]. The beam angle orientation problem has been the subject of a number of studies. The different approaches are based on geometric/volumetric methods [7–13], dose-based objectives [13–16], radiobiological objectives [5, 13] or IMRT specific objectives [17–19].

The geometric and volumetric methods for 3D-CRT are based on the assumption that the avoidance of the OAR is fundamental to the planning process. Further steps, such as optimization of beam weights [20, 21], beam portals [22, 23] or beam intensity modulation [2, 24], can be carried out independently during the next planning stage to achieve target dose homogeneity and to satisfy the dose constraints on the OAR. The work presented in this paper is also based on this principle.

The approaches based on dose and radiobiological objectives as well as IMRT-specific algorithms, are more complex and some of them integrate the beam angle search into the actual plan optimization process [18, 19]. While these approaches have the most potential to find the optimal plan, they are computationally expensive since it is necessary to perform dose calculations during the optimization process. Furthermore, the standard deterministic optimization algorithms are not sufficient to prevent the algorithm becoming trapped in local minima [14, 25–27]. The computational effort required to obtain optimal solutions, *e.g.* ranging from hours [18] up to days [6], makes some of these approaches prohibitive for routine clinical use, even when sophisticated methods are applied that reduce the computation time by an order of magnitude [28].

For coplanar plans, and only one or two OARs, it is fairly straightforward for an experienced dosimetrist to judge which beam directions are preferable. However, it is not feasible for a human planner to exploit the entire beam

Received 16 April 2004 and in revised form 9 September 2004, accepted 29 November 2004.

This work was partially supported by a grant from Elekta Oncology Systems.

space when multiple OARs of different size and radiosensitivity are present. Another difficulty stems from the inability to deliver isocentric beams from any direction owing to limitations relating to the dimensions of the treatment couch, linac design, patient dimensions and the location and size of the tumour. To represent accurately the permitted directions for each individual treatment requires precise modelling of the linac, the couch and the patient. This task is complex since the permitted beam space is a function of the relative location of the tumour [29–31].

Several attempts to automate the process of selecting beam directions have been described in the literature. Chen et al [8] and Myrianthopoulos et al [9] used the beam's-eye-view (BEV) to obtain 2D plots of the percentage volume of OAR irradiated versus the gantry angle as an aid to select beam directions. Rowbottom et al [13] went a step further by combining the BEV volumetric approach with a simple dose model and biological considerations to obtain a single objective score for each beam direction. Pugachev and Xing [17] formulated an IMRT specific score function that was based on the maximum dose deliverable through a portal by means of an intensity modulated beam. The current work is similar to the work of the above authors. The BEV was used as a means to search for beam directions [8, 9], the cost function was introduced to obtain a score for each beam direction [13] and an exhaustive search was conducted to explore the non-coplanar beam space [17]. An exhaustive search circumvents the local minima problem and ensures that the results are reproducible independently of the starting conditions. In addition, the current work takes into account the couch-gantry-patient dimensions, evaluates the optimization by means of logical rules and uses a unique cost function for which optimal parameters were derived.

Methods and materials

A beam direction search tool (BDST) was developed and implemented on the University of Washington treatment planning system (TPS) PRISM [32]. This tool evaluates a cost function, C_i for each beam direction, $\Phi_i(\xi,\psi)$, in the domain $i=1...t$, where t is the total number of beam directions considered, and where each beam direction is defined by the gantry angle, ξ, and the couch angle, ψ. The BDST starts with both the gantry angle and couch angle set to zero, and then systematically works through all other permitted directions by increasing first the gantry angle and then the couch angle by multiples of a chosen angular increment, ϖ. Beam directions that would cause the gantry to collide, either with the couch or with the patient, are excluded from the search. The beam space for the Elekta SL20 series linac (Elekta, Crawley, UK) was modelled for different treatment sites in combination with the Elekta Precise™ couch and the female Rando™ phantom (The Phantom Laboratory, Salem, NY), by assuming a constant isocentre distance of 100 cm. An example of the beam space for tumours in the head is shown in Figure 1, where $\Phi^P(\xi,\psi)$ denotes the permitted directions. Note that PRISM uses different angle conventions to the Elekta accelerator and therefore two axes are plotted in Figure 1.

Each beam portal is shaped to match the projection of the PTV into the BEV and so only the rays represented by the solid circles in Figure 2a are considered. For each

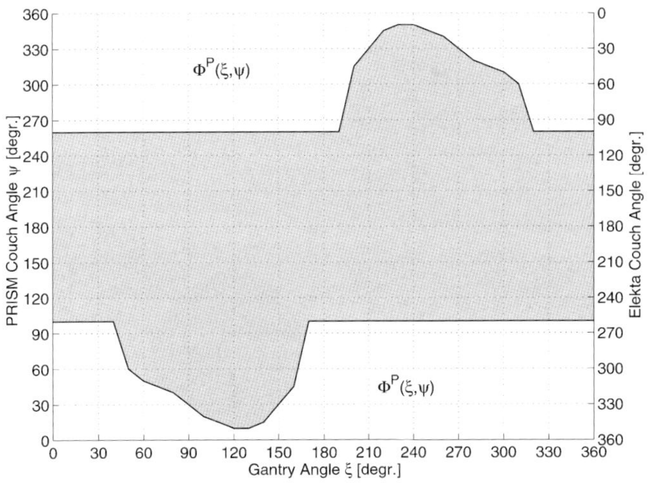

Figure 1. The area that is unshaded denotes the permitted beam space $\Phi^P(\xi,\psi)$. The shaded region represents angles that result in a gantry collision and are, therefore, excluded from the beam search.

beam direction the BDST first computes distances along ray paths as illustrated in Figure 2b. For ray, j, these distances are the depth from the patient entry surface to the PTV, $d_j(\text{PTV})$, the depth from the patient entry surface to each OAR in the beam, $d_j(\text{OAR}_k)$, where k is an index for the OAR in question, and the path length through the OAR, $l_j(\text{OAR}_k)$. By definition the central ray is the one that passes through the isocentre. The rays are projected onto a Cartesian grid located at a distance of 120 cm from the source (Figure 2) such that they are separated by equal increments, s, at the isocentre plane.

The BDST uses the $d_j(\text{PTV})$ values to determine the mean depth to the PTV entry surface for the ith beam direction, $d_i(\text{PTV})$, and similarly calculates a mean depth to each OAR_k entry surface, $d_i(\text{OAR}_k)$. It also estimates the fractional volume of each OAR_k irradiated, $v_i(\text{OAR}_k)$, using the ray path lengths, ray separations s and a pre-calculation of the total OAR_k volume.

The cost function was designed such that the lower its value the more preferable is the beam direction and it has two components that are added together. The first component, $C_i(\text{PTV})$, is based on the mean depth of the PTV, and the second, $C_i(\text{OAR})$, is a penalty term, which depends on the amount of OAR irradiation, thus

$$C_i = C_i(\text{PTV}) + C_i(\text{OAR}) \quad (1)$$

The first component term is computed using the equation

$$C_i(\text{PTV}) = 1 - \exp(-\mu d_i(\text{PTV})) \quad (2)$$

where μ is the linear attenuation coefficient in water for the proposed beam energy. The exponential term, with μ set to a value of $0.0495\ \text{cm}^{-1}$ throughout this paper, corresponds to the attenuation of a 6 MV photon beam in water. Thus, the value of $C_i(\text{PTV})$ approaches zero when the PTV is at shallow depths and approaches unity for very large depths, so favouring those beam directions where the PTV is close to the beam entry surface.

As several different OARs may be included in any particular beam direction, the second component is a weighted average of individual costs computed for each OAR in turn, where different weighting factors, w_k, may

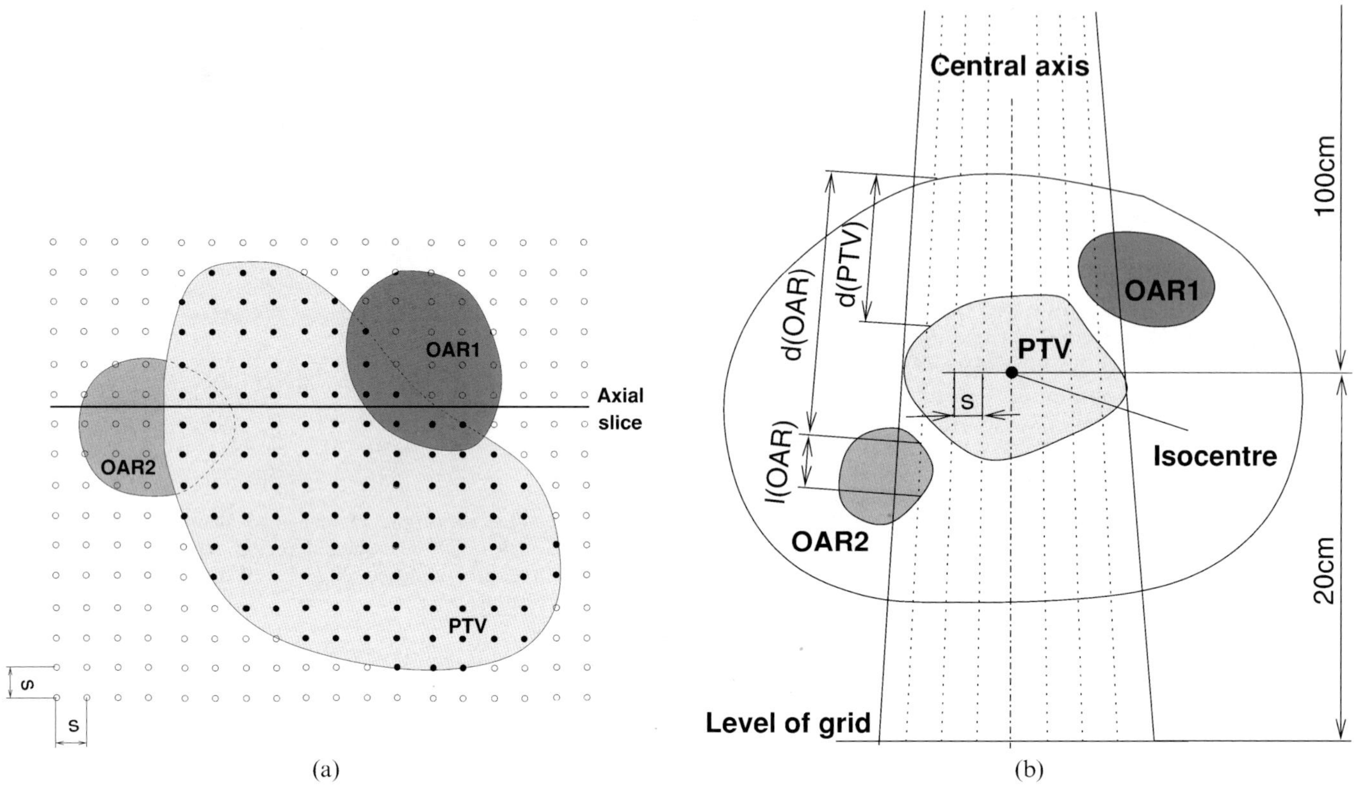

Figure 2. Ray-tracing geometry: (a) beam's-eye-view (BEV) illustrating the grid with uniform spacing s and (b) axial slice with planning target volume (PTV) and two organs at risk (OAR).

be assigned to give each different OAR a different relative importance.

Each OAR has both a "depth cost" and a "volume cost". The depth cost for the kth OAR is calculated using the equation:

$$C_i(d_i(\mathrm{OAR}_k)=\exp(-\mu d_i(\mathrm{OAR}_k)) \quad (3)$$

The same value of μ is used as in Equation 1, but, unlike Equation 1, this gives higher costs (approaching unity) for the shallower depths where the relative dose to the OAR will be greater. If the OAR is completely outside the beam edge in the BEV the depth cost is set to zero.

The volume cost for each OAR is set equal to the fractional volume irradiated, $v_i(\mathrm{OAR}_k)$, which is already conveniently in the range zero to one. In combining the volume and depth costs a factor λ (where $0<\lambda<1$) was introduced so as to control the relative importance of depth and volume, and to ensure that the total cost remains within the range 0 to 1; thus the cost associated with irradiating the kth OAR in the ith beam direction is quantified by:

$$C_i(\mathrm{OAR}_k)=\lambda v_i(\mathrm{OAR}_k)+(1-\lambda)C_i(d_i(\mathrm{OAR}_k)) \quad (4)$$

The angle optimization tool was designed so that the user specified the number of beam directions, nb, required for a plan and the minimum angle separation, φ, between selected angles. To further ensure beam diversity at least one of all nb beams had to be separated by an angle δ, with $90^\circ \leqslant \delta \leqslant 120^\circ$ from the other beams that were selected. An empirical value of $\delta=90^\circ$ was assumed throughout the work presented in this paper to ensure some dose uniformity in the PTV.

The optimization started by discarding all the beam directions that were not permitted within the specified gantry and couch ranges. The algorithm then iterated through the remaining angle combinations of ξ and ψ and created a rank list with the beam directions sorted according to the lowest cost. The direction that topped the list was selected as the first beam. The second direction was selected subject to the criterion that the absolute angle between the first and the second direction was greater or equal to φ. The value of φ depends on the total number of beams and the location of the tumour. However, experience has shown that a minimum separation of 40–45° usually results in satisfactory plans. If the angle was not large enough, the algorithm proceeded to the next position in the rank list until it found an appropriate direction. After the second direction was selected, the algorithm searched for the third direction in the rank list that was separated by a minimum angle φ from any of the previously selected beam directions. The same procedure was carried out for all nb beam directions. For the selection of the last beam direction, the algorithm also examined whether any of the previously selected beam directions and the current candidate direction were separated by at least δ, otherwise the angle was discarded and the algorithm proceeded to the next best direction until one meeting the criterion was found.

Parameter value selection

Ray-tracing resolution

The trade-off between computation time and a fine spatial resolution was explored by varying the value of

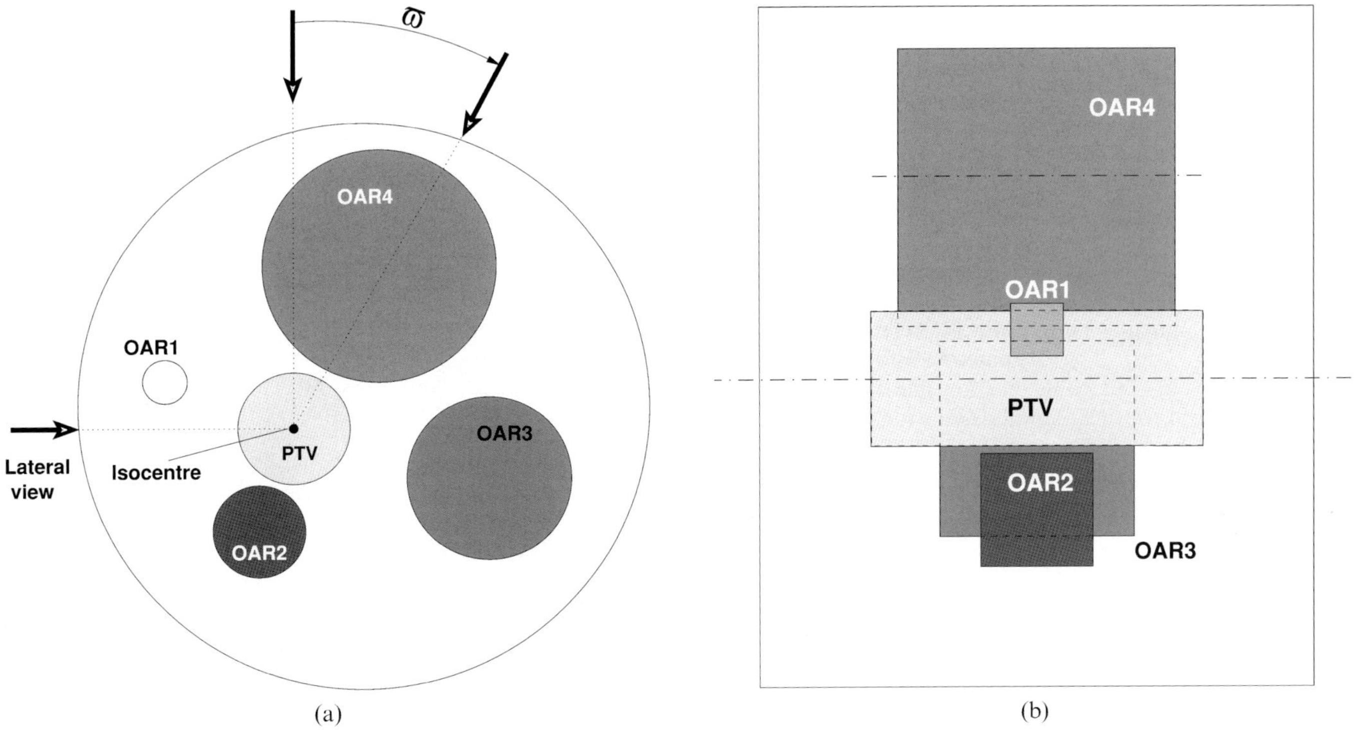

Figure 3. Test plan. (a) Axial slice and (b) lateral view (from left side).

s. Since the selection of *s* depends on the size of the organ, a simple test plan, shown in Figure 3, was produced with OAR of different realistic sizes, *i.e.* Ø(OAR1)=10 mm, Ø(OAR2)=20 mm, Ø(OAR3)=35 mm and Ø(OAR4)=50 mm. The axial length of each OAR was equal to its diameter, as illustrated in Figure 3b, and the diameter of the PTV was 25 mm. The diameter of the external contour was 120 mm. For the purpose of this sensitivity analysis, ψ was set to zero (reducing the search space to coplanar beam arrangements) the gantry range was set to $\xi \in \{0°-360°\}$, the angle resolution $\varpi=10°$, $\lambda=0.2$, $nb=5$, $\varphi=45°$ and the weighting factors were set to unity. The values of *s* investigated were 1 mm, 2 mm, 3.3 mm, 5 mm and 10 mm. The variation of the total cost (Equation 1) as a function of the ray-trace resolution was analysed. All the computation for this work was carried out on a PC running Linux with a CPU speed of 2.4 GHz.

Angle resolution

Beam directions were sampled at uniform angle intervals ϖ, as illustrated in Figure 3. For the search to be effective it is essential to keep ϖ as small as possible. If the resolution is too coarse, potentially good beam directions could be missed. To determine an appropriate value for ϖ, the beam space for the test plan in Figure 3 was searched for different values of ϖ, namely 2°, 5°, 10°, 15° and 30°. The grid increment, *s*, was set to 3.3 mm and the other parameters remained as described in the previous paragraph.

Clinical examples

The BDST was first applied to a prostate case and the resulting beam arrangement compared with clinically approved beam directions from the literature. The tool was then tested on two clinical cases with tumours in the head.

Prostate comparison

The prostate is well suited for an initial comparison since the anatomy is comparable from patient to patient and coplanar beam arrangements are standard. In our institution, the gantry angles for standard 3D conformal prostate treatments are based on the recommendations by Pickett et al [33]. It is a coplanar 6-field conformal technique with opposing lateral beams and opposed oblique beams angled between 30° and 45° off the lateral beam position. The lateral beams penetrate through the femoral heads and the lateral oblique beams are placed such that they minimize the irradiation of the bladder, the rectum and the femoral heads. The dose to the femoral heads can be controlled by the relative beam weights of the opposed lateral beams.

For the first run, the BDST was applied to an arbitrarily selected prostate case with the parameters for the search set to $\xi \in \{0°-360°\}$, $\psi \in \{0°\}$, $s=3.3$ mm, $\varpi=1°$, $\varphi=40°$, $\lambda=0.2$ and $nb=6$. Only the rectum and the bladder were considered OAR and the corresponding weighting factors, w_k, were set to 10 and 5, respectively.

For the second run $nb=5$ and ϖ was increased to 5°. In addition, the femoral heads were considered critical organs. The weighting factors applied were 10 for the rectum, 1 for the bladder and 2 for both femoral heads. These parameters were chosen following the findings by Rowbottom et al [13] who utilized a cost function with volumetric and biological elements to optimize the beam directions for prostate treatment with similar weighting factors.

Clinical case studies

Tumours in the head are especially suited for non-coplanar beam arrangements since numerous critical structures of different importance are to be spared and the permitted beam space is much larger since beams directed through the top of the head are an option. Two cases were studied to test the algorithm. Case I was a patient with a brain tumour and Case II was a patient with a sinus tumour. For each, an experienced senior dosimetrist had produced a 3D-CRT plan, which was used to treat the patient. These will be referred to as the conventional plans. The dosimetrist was confined to non-IMRT beams but could use any means available for 3D-CRT clinical routine planning. This included the use of non-coplanar beams, different energies, optimization of the MLC aperture, customized blocks, electron beams and wedges. These plans were compared, retrospectively, with plans based on beam directions obtained from the beam direction search, and these will be referred to as the optimized plans. The same dosimetrist produced the optimized plans using the same treatment planning tools as previously. Uniform margins of 5 mm for the brain case and 7 mm for the sinus case were applied, to the clinical target volume (CTV) in order to obtain the PTVs and a voxel size of 3.3 mm was used to calculate the final dose distribution. An additional margin of 5 mm was applied to the PTV for the purpose of the beam direction search. This was done to account for the fact that lateral electron transport takes place when the beams are delivered, and without this additional margin, beam directions for which the projection of an OAR is very close to the PTV, but does not overlap with it, might appear to be good. However, when the radiation is delivered the electron transport would result in a high dose to the OAR. The optimized plans were required to use an equal number of beams as the conventional plans. The beam weights and wedge angles were optimized manually for the first case study (brain) and re-optimized with simulated annealing for the second case study (sinus). The plans were compared by means of dose–volume histograms (DVH) and statistical evaluation based on the recommendations for reporting target volume and dose specifications for IMRT plans [34], which is based on ICRU50 [1]. Further evaluation makes use of the Webb and Nahum model [35] for tumour control probability (TCP), the Lyman-Kutcher-Burman model [36, 37] for normal tissue complications probability (NTCP) and the radiation conformity index [38] to the 95% isodose surface (RCI_{95}). The parameters for the NTCP model were based on data published by Emami et al [39].

Case study I: brain

A 12-year-old paediatric patient with a cavernous meningioma was selected. The PTV was located in-between the temporal lobes and overlapped approximately 25% of the right optic nerve (Figure 4). The patient had an acute onset of blindness in his right eye before radiotherapy. The left optic nerve was in close proximity to the PTV. The total dose prescribed to the PTV was 50.4 Gy. Since the tumour was impinging on the optic nerves it was important to reduce the dose to these structures, despite a tolerance dose of approximately 50 Gy, so as to further minimize the impact on the patient's eyesight. This was considered important given the young age of the patient.

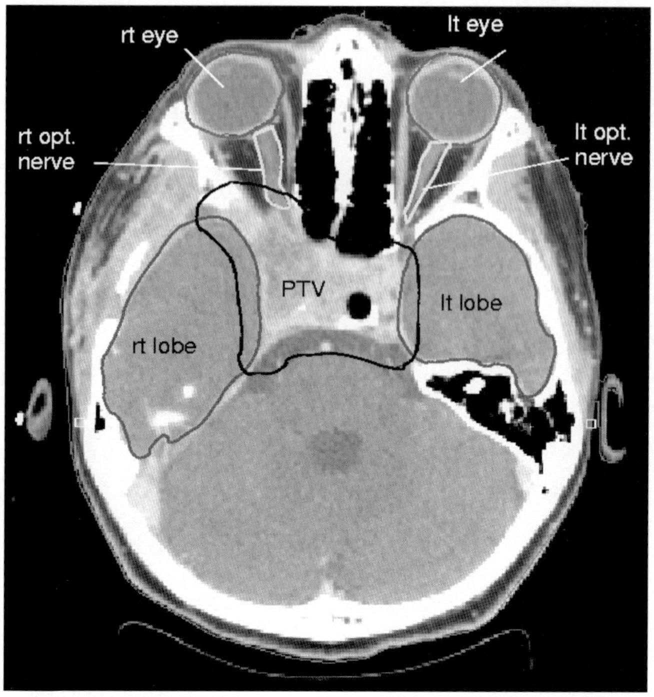

Figure 4. Brain case: axial CT slice through a paediatric meningioma.

The conventional plan consisted of three wedged beams. Two of the beams were opposed lateral coplanar 6 MV beams ($\Phi_1(90°,0°)$ and $\Phi_2(270°,0°)$) and the third was a left superior oblique 18 MV beam ($\Phi_3(100°,300°)$). For the optimized plan the following parameters were applied for the beam direction search: $\xi \in \{0°-360°\}$, $\psi \in \{0°-100°,260°-360°\}$, $s=0.33$, $\varpi=10°$, $\varphi=45°$, $\lambda=0.2$, $nb=3$ and the weighting factors w_k for the OAR were set to 7, 5, 10 and 8, corresponding to the right and left eye, and the right and left optic nerve, respectively. A higher weighting was given to the OAR on the right lateral side compared with the corresponding counterparts on the left because of the overall location of the tumour and the proximity to the right optic nerve. The optic nerves were considered the most important structures, followed by the eyeballs. To allow a fair comparison, both plans were scaled to D_{95} so that the 95% isodose surface covered the entire PTV.

Case study II: sinus

The second clinical case investigated was a large T4N0M0 sinus adenocarcinoma. A coronal slice through the centre of the tumour is shown in Figure 5. The volume of the PTV was approximately 128 cm^3 and was close to the brain stem and the parotid glands. Superiorly, the PTV protruded between the eyeballs, which made it difficult to spare the optic nerves and the optic chiasm while at the same time delivering the prescribed dose of 70 Gy to the PTV. It was aimed for tolerance doses of 50 Gy for the optic nerves and the optic chiasm, 52 Gy for the brain stem and 10 Gy to the lens to minimize the risk of cataracts. A secondary priority was to prevent xerostomia by reducing the dose to the parotid glands.

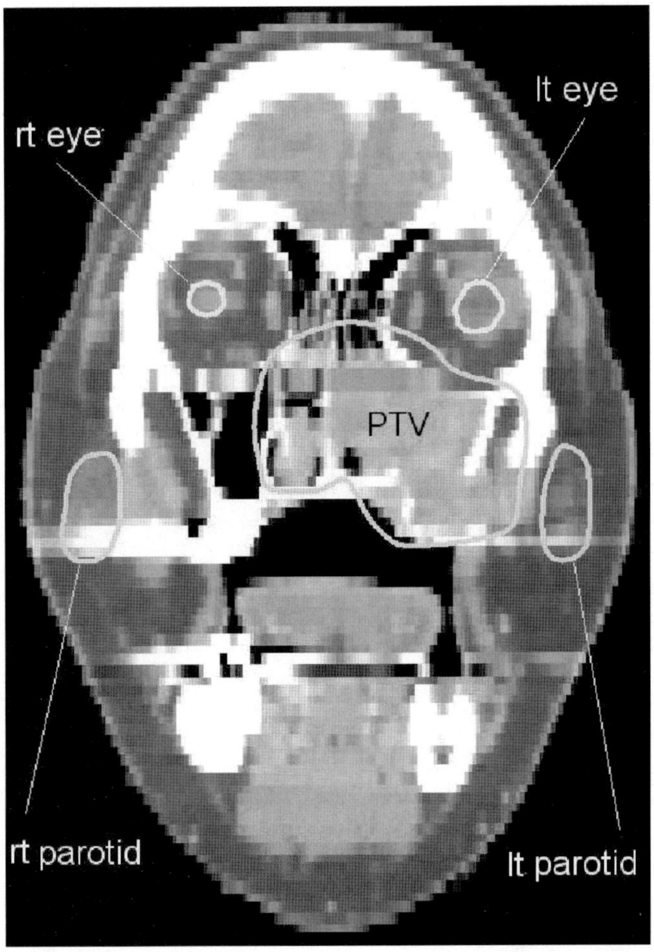

Figure 5. Sinus case: coronal CT slice through tumour.

The conventional plan made use of six beams consisting of two anterior oblique 6 MV beams ($\Phi_1(335°,0°)$ and $\Phi_2(20°,0°)$), a superior oblique 18 MV beam ($\Phi_3(90°,310°)$), a left lateral 6 MV beam ($\Phi_4(90°,0°)$), a right lateral 10 MV beam ($\Phi_5(270°,0°)$) and an anterior 6 MV beam ($\Phi_6(0°,0°)$). All but the anterior beam made use of a wedge and utilized customized beam blocks.

The following parameters were used for the beam direction search for the optimized plan: $\xi \in \{0°-360°\}$, $\psi \in \{0°–100°,260°–360°\}$, s=3.3 mm, ϖ=10°, φ=45°, nb=6 and the weighting factors w_k for the OAR were set to 7, 7, 5, 8, 9, 9, 10, 10, 10, 1 and 1 corresponding to the right and left eye, the spinal cord, the brain stem, the right and left optic nerve, the optic chiasm, the right and left lens and the right and left parotid gland, respectively.

Results

Parameter value selection

The results of the beam direction search for the test plan in Figure 3 are given as a function of the ray-trace resolution in Table 1 and as a function of the angular resolution in Table 2. With respect to both tables, the time to perform the search is given in column two and the top five angles in the rank list, and the selected angles are given in the third and fourth columns, respectively. Each individual cost term in Equation 1 was analysed for all of the test cases. Only the total cost is plotted as a function of the ray-trace resolution, s, in Figure 6a and as a function of the angle resolution, ϖ, in Figure 6b.

Prostate comparison

The time to perform the first run, for which the femoral heads were not considered OAR, was 112 s. The optimal gantry angles were found to be: 273°, 96°, 56°, 313°, 233° and 136° corresponding to the ranks #1, #3, #149, #158, #163 and #173. The first two angles were virtually opposed lateral fields rotated marginally, mainly to minimize the irradiation of the rectum, but also to reduce irradiation of the bladder. The rest of the beams were angled off the lateral beams by $\pm$40°, which corresponds to the minimum angle separation φ.

The second run lasted 24 s and included the femoral heads as critical structures. The following gantry angles were selected by the BDST: 300°, 65°, 115°, 255° and 340° corresponding to ranks #1, #6, #7, #10 and #45, respectively. Figure 7 shows a comparison with the cost

Table 1. The results of the beam direction search as a function of the ray-trace resolution s

Ray-trace resolution, s (cm)	Computation time (s)	Top 5 ranked angles, ξ (degrees)	Selected angles, ξ (degrees)
0.1	67	330, 240, 150, 250, 340	330, 240, 150, 60, 180
0.25	11	320, 140, 330, 150, 340	320, 140, 240, 170, 350
0.33	7	320, 260, 140, 330, 240	320, 260, 140, 230, 350
0.5	3	320, 260, 140, 330, 240	320, 260, 140, 230, 350
1.0	1	320, 260, 140, 330, 340	320, 260, 140, 350, 230

Table 2. The results of the beam direction search as a function of the angle resolution ϖ

Angle resolution, ϖ (degrees)	Computation time (s)	Top 5 ranked angles, ξ (degrees)	Selected angles, ξ (degrees)
2	34	320, 318, 252, 254, 256	320, 252, 140, 72, 350
5	14	320, 255, 260, 245, 140	320, 255, 140, 350, 65
10	7	320, 260, 140, 330, 240	320, 260, 140, 230, 350
15	5	255, 330, 240, 150, 315	255, 330, 150, 225, 75
30	2	330, 240, 150, 60, 180	330, 240, 150, 60, 180

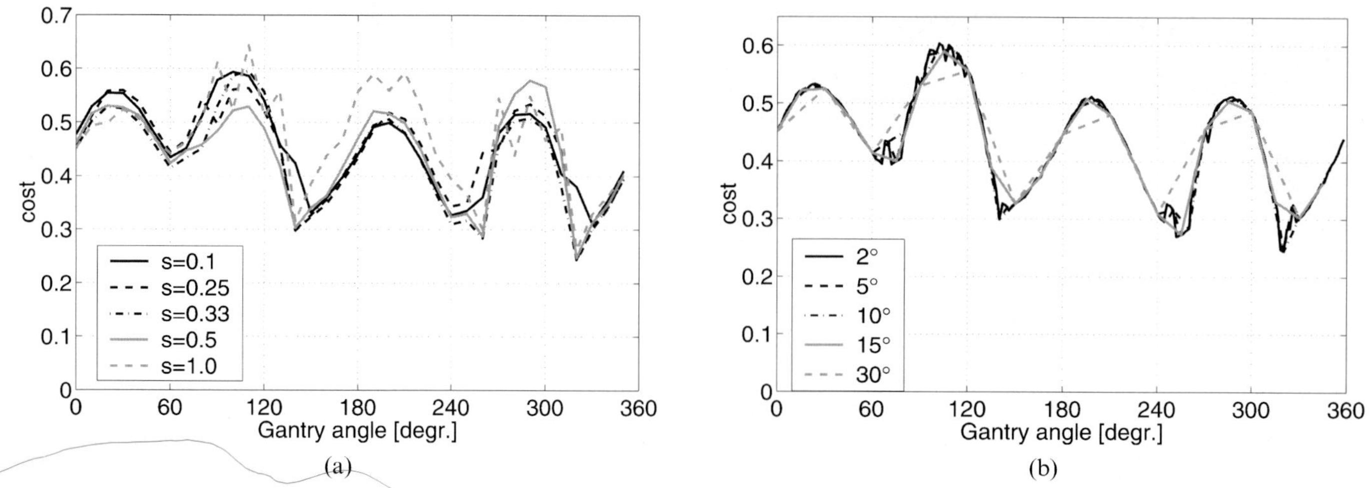

Figure 6. Cost as a function of (a) the ray-tracing resolution, *s*, and (b) as a function of the angle resolution, ϖ, for the test case in Figure 3.

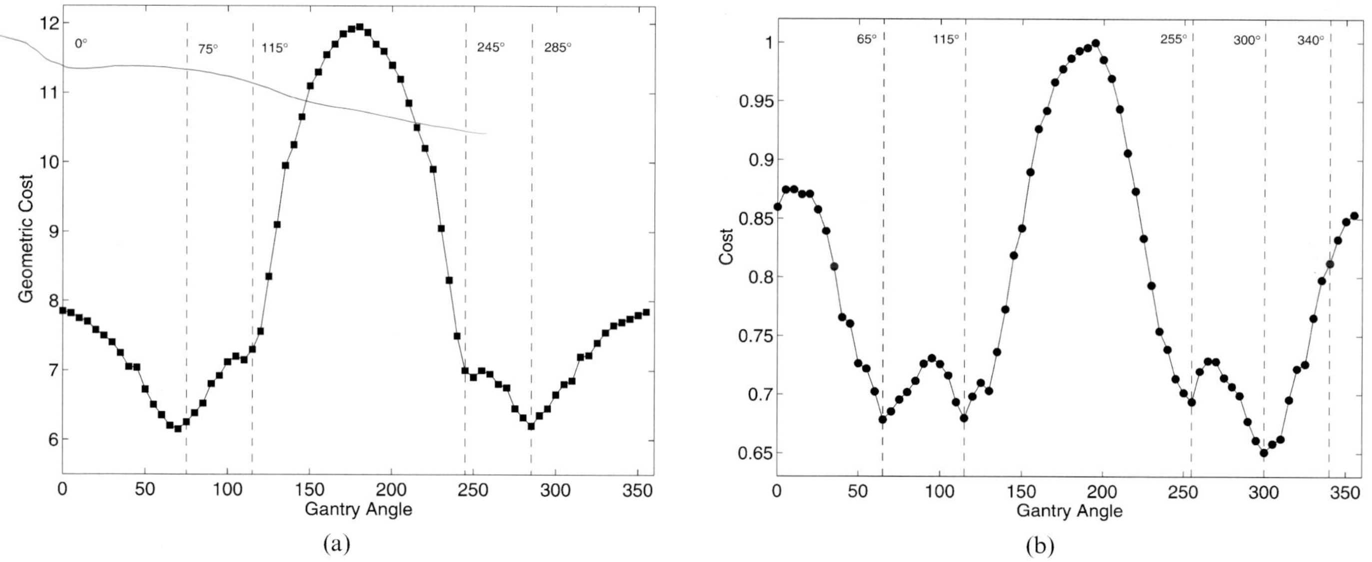

Figure 7. Cost function *vs* gantry-angle plot for prostate: (a) Graph reproduced from Rowbottom et al [13]. (b) Normalized cost corresponding to prostate case. The vertical lines indicate the selected gantry angles. Note that different cost functions were used and therefore the overall magnitude of the graphs is not comparable.

function *vs* gantry angle plot obtained by Rowbottom et al [13] (Figure 7a) and our results (Figure 7b).

Clinical case studies

The times to perform the beam direction searches were 11 min for the brain case and 12 min for the sinus case. The normalized cost distributions over the permitted beam space are depicted in Figure 8a for the brain case and in Figure 8b for the sinus case. The beam space that was not permitted is depicted with a cost of unity (white). The numbers next to the diamonds denote the overall rankings. For the optimized treatment plan wedges were applied to all three beams for the brain case but no wedges were necessary for the sinus case. The beam energy for all optimized beams was 6 MV.

DVHs for the brain case are shown in Figure 9, and the corresponding statistical evaluation is given in Table 3. The graphs corresponding to the critical structures on the left side of the patient are depicted in black and those corresponding to the right side are in grey, and the conventional plan is plotted with dashed lines; whereas the optimized plan is plotted with solid lines. Both plans are within the dose specifications and do not violate the constraints.

For the sinus case, DVHs are shown in Figure 10 for the PTV, the brain stem, the parotid glands, the optic nerves and the optic chiasm. The dose to the spinal cord was negligibly low for both the conventional and optimal plans. As the plans could not be normalized to the D_{95} of 70 Gy, due to the high dose to the optic chiasm for the conventional plan, they were scaled such that the maximum doses in the PTV were comparable. The statistical evaluation, including additional statistical information for the lenses, is given in Table 4.

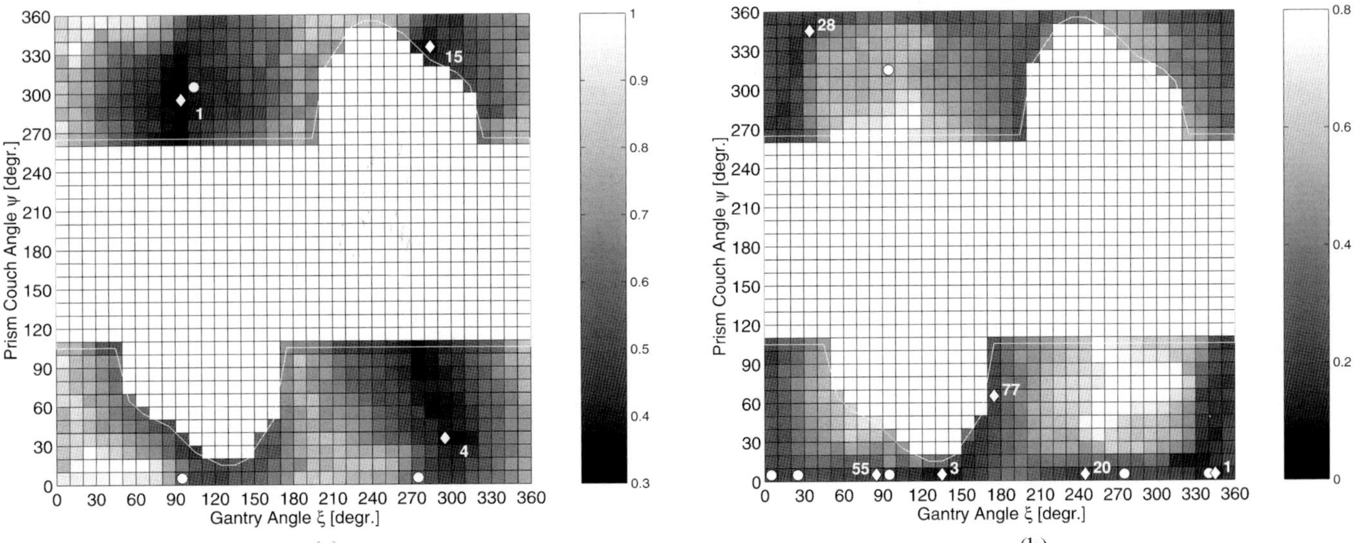

Figure 8. Normalized cost distribution over the beam space $\Phi^P(\xi,\psi)$. A circle corresponds to the conventional and a diamond to the optimized plan. The grey-scale bar represents the cost values. (a) Brain case and (b) sinus case.

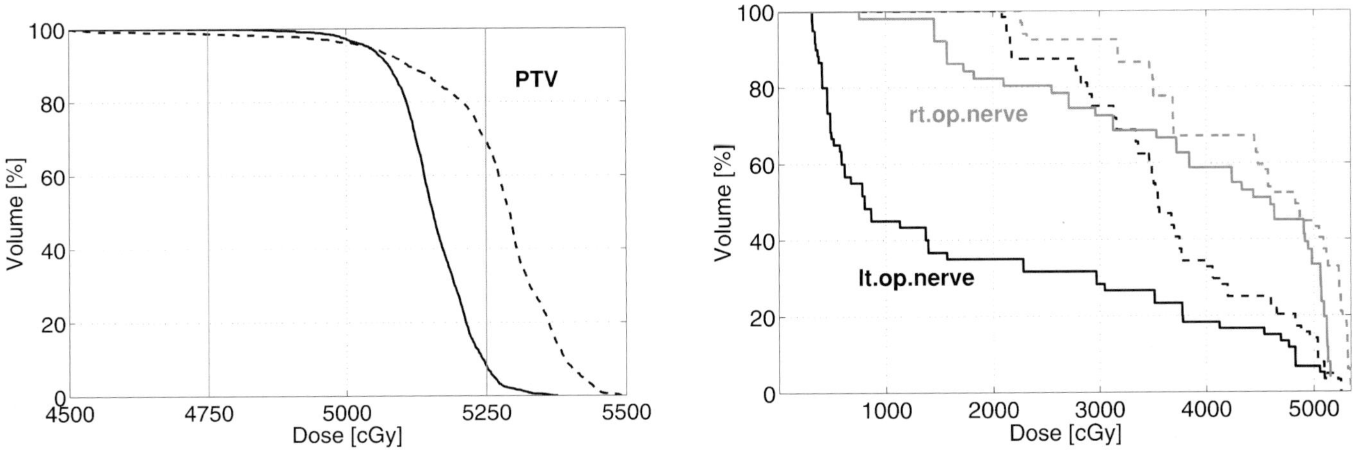

Figure 9. Brain case: dose–volume histograms for the conventional plan (dashed) and the optimized plan (solid): (a) planning target volume (PTV) and (b) optic nerves. The vertical lines in (a) denote the ±5% dose range.

Table 3. Case I. Brain: statistical evaluation

Structure	Plan	Dose [Gy]				in [%]		
		Min.	Mean	Max.	D_{95}	V100	NTCP	RCI
PTV	Conv.	45.0	52.5	55.0	50.4	95	n.a.	0.27
	Optim.	47.1	51.4	53.8	50.4	95	n.a.	0.23
Right optic nerve	Conv.	22.5	44.4	53.4	n.a.	n.a.	0.26	n.a.
	Optim.	7.5	39.0	51.6	n.a.	n.a.	0.07	n.a.
Left optic nerve	Conv.	20.8	36.7	52.5	n.a.	n.a.	0.01	n.a.
	Optim.	3.1	18.3	51.2	n.a.	n.a.	<0.01	n.a.

PTV, planning target volume; Conv., conventional; Optim., optimized; D_{95}, dose that covers 95% of the PTV; V100, percentage of the PTV receiving the prescribed dose; NTCP, normal tissue complication probability; RCI, radiation conformity index; n.a., not applicable.

Discussion

Parameter value selection

The weighting factors for this set-up were all set to unity so there was no preference for one OAR over another, and hence the cost for the OAR only reflects the relative penalty for its location and the partial volume irradiated. Owing to the normalization, the cost terms are also independent of the size of the OAR. Assuming that the finest ray-trace resolution and the smallest value of ϖ result in the most accurate results, the anticipated tendency can be seen. The higher the value of s, the more deviation can be observed. This was most marked for the smallest OAR with a diameter of 10 mm. In Table 1 it can be seen that

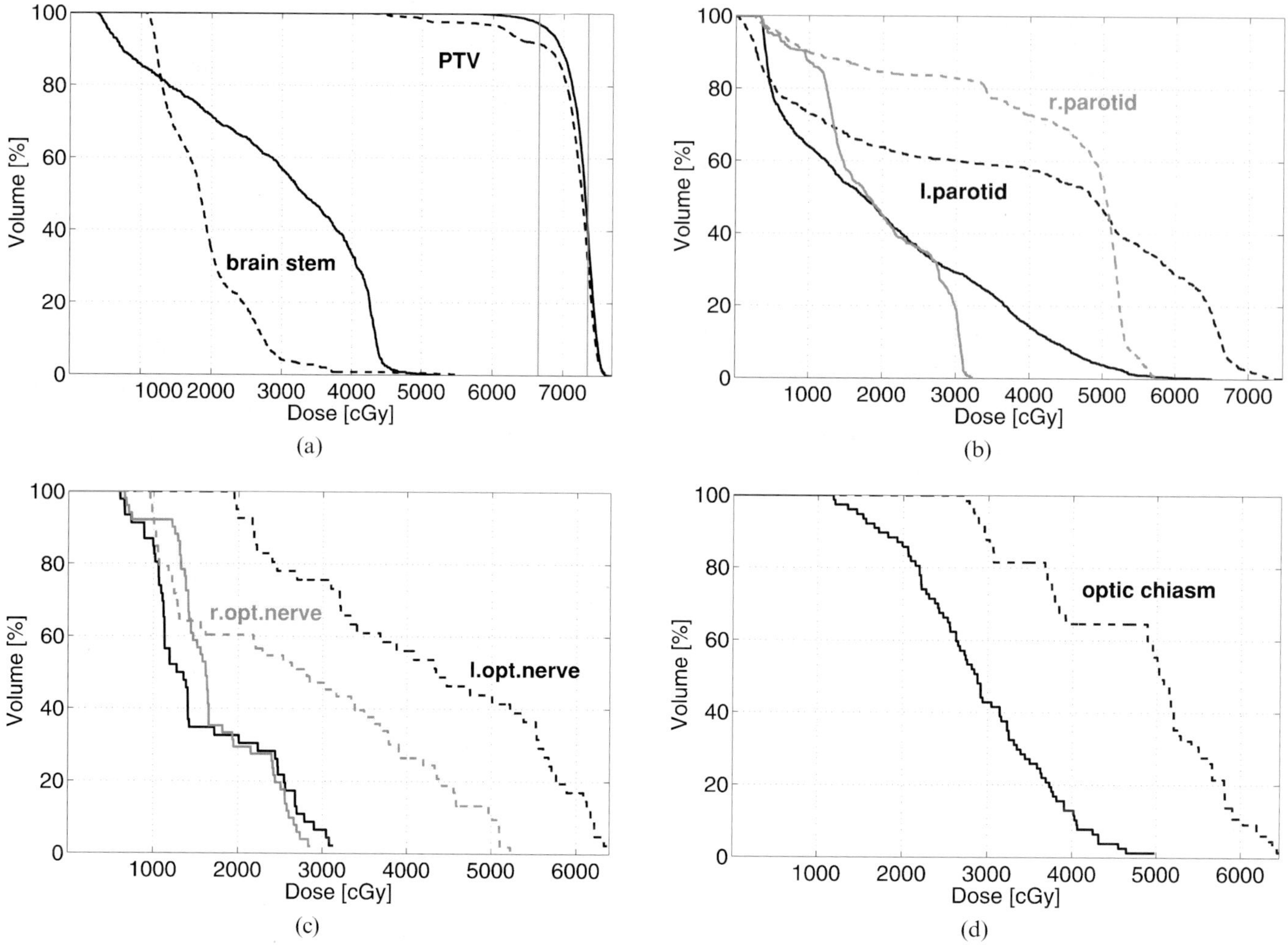

Figure 10. Sinus case: dose–volume histogram for the conventional plan (dashed) and the optimized plan (solid): (a) planning target volume (PTV) and brain stem, (b) parotid glands, (c) optic nerves and (d) optic chiasm. The vertical lines in (a) denote the $\pm5\%$ dose range.

Table 4. Case II. Sinus: statistical evaluation

Structure	Plan	Dose [Gy]				in [%]		
		Min.	Mean	Max.	D95	V100	TCP	NTCP
PTV	Conv.	42.7	71.5	76.6	62.2	83	73	n.a.
	Optim.	58.0	72.9	77.0	68.0	89	94	n.a.
Brain stem	Conv.	10.7	18.7	55.7	n.a.	n.a.	n.a.	0.5
	Optim.	3.7	29.5	52.2	n.a.	n.a.	n.a.	0.5
Right parotid	Conv.	2.5	42.4	57.7	n.a.	n.a.	n.a.	40
	Optim.	3.5	19.7	32.4	n.a.	n.a.	n.a.	<0.1
Left parotid	Conv.	0.1	37.9	74.6	n.a.	n.a.	n.a.	31
	Optim.	3.4	20.5	65.0	n.a.	n.a.	n.a.	0.3
Right optic nerve	Conv.	9.6	27.8	52.3	n.a.	n.a.	n.a.	1.5
	Optim.	6.6	17.5	25.6	n.a.	n.a.	n.a.	<0.1
Left optic nerve	Conv.	19.5	42.8	63.9	n.a.	n.a.	n.a.	12
	Optim.	6.0	16.2	31.3	n.a.	n.a.	n.a.	<0.1
Optic chiasm	Conv.	27.0	47.2	64.6	n.a.	n.a.	n.a.	1.4
	Optim.	11.8	29.0	49.8	n.a.	n.a.	n.a.	<0.1
Right lens	Conv.	7.6	8.3	9.1	n.a.	n.a.	n.a.	–
	Optim.	4.4	6.6	10.3	n.a.	n.a.	n.a.	–
Left lens	Conv.	13.4	16.5	19.0	n.a.	n.a.	n.a.	–
	Optim.	4.5	9.8	15.7	n.a.	n.a.	n.a.	–

PTV, planning target volume; Conv., Conventional; Optim., optimized; D_{95}, dose that covers 95% of the PTV; V100, percentage of the PTV receiving the prescribed dose; NTCP, normal tissue complication probability; RCI, radiation conformity index; n.a., not applicable.

the resolution 3.3 mm, 5 mm and 10 mm resulted in the same four beam directions to top the rank list with the first three of the selected beams being the same. However, reducing the resolution to 1 mm and 2.5 mm, the algorithm found beam directions with a lower cost.

The selection of the value for the angle resolution ϖ for the exhaustive search determines how efficiently the beam space is scanned. A value of 10° for ϖ was acceptable; larger intervals could be used for larger OAR (>20 mm). Based on these results, values of s=3.3 mm and ϖ=10° were selected for the clinical case studies due to the small size of the optic nerves. A value of φ=45° was chosen for the minimum angle separation for the clinical cases with non-coplanar beam arrangements. A minimum angle separation is required to avoid overlapping beams within the body, and so prevents an unnecessarily high dose to the tissue located between the beam entrance surface and the tumour. In terms of dose homogeneity it is also desirable to have the beams maximally separated in space [11, 40]. The accumulation of all of the beams from one general direction makes it difficult to achieve target dose uniformity and difficult to conform the high dose region to the shape of the tumour.

Prostate comparison

To validate the approach a comparison was drawn with our own prostate technique (first run) and with the extensive work that has been carried out on prostate planning at the Institute of Cancer Research and Royal Marsden Hospital [13] (second run). For the latter, Figure 7 illustrates that in both cases the gantry angles were selected in the valleys of the graph such that irradiation of the femoral heads was minimized. Based on clinical experience, *e.g.* symmetry of the beams leading to dose uniformity, Rowbottom et al [13] decided also to select an anterior beam (0°) although the cost was higher than for other candidate gantry angles. The comparison of the cost *vs* gantry-angle plot revealed that the current methodology can reproduce both a standard 6-field beam arrangement as well as individualized beam angles that correspond well to the findings by other researchers.

Clinical case studies

For each of the clinical test cases, the non-coplanar beam directions were checked by placing the treatment mask on the treatment couch, setting up the isocentre and positioning the couch and the gantry in the acquired positions. None of the beam directions violated any geometrical constraints imposed by the linac.

Case study I: brain

In Figure 8a the locations of the angles that were selected manually for the conventional plan are superimposed (circles) on the cost distribution of the beam direction search. The existence of multiple local minima can be observed in the cost distribution, indicated by the low cost regions (dark). The non-coplanar beam with gantry angle 100° and couch angle 300° lies within the low cost area and shows that the dosimetrist was successful in approaching the best non-coplanar beam direction. The dosimetrist might have chosen a slightly different angle for reasons not directly considered in the beam direction search such as dose uniformity in the PTV. The two standard lateral coplanar beams with gantry angles 90° and 270° are not optimal with respect to the cost function used for the beam direction search.

Comparing the DVH for the brain case in Figure 9 shows that the optimized plan is superior to the conventional plan for both the critical structures and the PTV. The PTV is more uniformly irradiated and the cold volume considerably reduced. This is also reflected in the statistical evaluation in Table 3. The NTCP values indicate that both plans do not overdose any critical structures and that the probability of complications is very low. However, any improvements are worthwhile, especially for a paediatric patient. In addition, the improved sparing of OAR without compromising the dose to the PTV is an important foundation for dose escalation, which can only be achieved safely if the OARs are not exposed to toxic dose levels.

Case study II: sinus

The cost distribution in Figure 8b shows that the BDST finds two non-coplanar beam directions (ranks #28, #77) of which #77 is located on the edge of the permitted beam space. It is a posterior beam that penetrates through the brain stem. In fact, it is this beam that enables better coverage of the PTV since it complements the other beams. It is also most likely that this beam direction would have not been explored during manual angle selection.

The fact that the best beam with rank #1 is almost identical with one beam selected manually at gantry angle 335° highlights that the dosimetrist again made a good selection. One might wonder why there is no beam positioned in the low cost region on the bottom right and the top left of Figure 8b. After the first beam with rank #1 was selected all the beams in close proximity with a low rank were discarded if they were within a certain minimum angle φ. Furthermore, some of the beam angles are redundant. A simple example would be a vertex field that can be delivered using either $\Phi_i(90°,270°)$ or $\Phi_i(270°,90°)$.

The DVH in Figure 10 shows that dose uniformity in the PTV was improved in the optimized plan. More importantly, the cold spot was greatly reduced which is reflected in the increase in the TCP value from 73% to 94%. The mean dose to the brainstem is higher for the optimized plan, which is due to the posterior beam. However, the maximum dose is lower, which is reflected in the similar NTCP values for both plans. All the other statistical values in Table 4 are clearly in favour of the optimized plan with greatly reduced mean and maximum doses for the parotid glands, the optic nerves and the optic chiasm. The most important difference between the two plans is the much improved sparing of both parotid glands. It has been reported that a mean parotid dose of more than 26 Gy slows salivary flow [41] and doses over 40 Gy may result in total dysfunction of salivary production [42]. The mean dose for the right parotid gland was reduced from 42 Gy to 20 Gy (improvement of 54%) for the optimized plan, which resulted in a reduction of the NTCP from 40% to <0.1%. For the left parotid gland, the improvement in the NTCP was approximately 46%. This indicates that both parotid glands would be virtually complication free. The sixth beam selected (rank #77) went straight through the brain stem but avoided all the other critical structures. This selection was due to the design of the cost function and the choice of the weighting factors, which all had a similar magnitude. The weighting factors were based on common sense, but were chosen somewhat arbitrarily insofar as the magnitudes, as well as the relative difference could have been selected differently. Selecting weighting factors that are similar in magnitude can be considered as a soft constraint, and this is necessary if multiple objectives, in this case multiple OAR, are present. If one weighting factor is much higher than all the others, then this could result in a solution where only the one particular OAR would be spared. It should also be remembered that the individual cost terms are normalized to the volume of the respective organ, requiring the entire organ volume to be contoured. The beam weight for the beam that went straight through the brain stem was set relatively low by the beam weight optimization procedure. This is an interesting observation as it paves the way for the application of the BDST for IMRT planning [43]. If this particular beam were replaced by an IMRT beam it would have probably received a much higher overall weighting since IMRT has the ability to spare critical structures by modulating the intensity across the field.

The main advantage of the BDST is its ability to search the permitted beam space within a time frame that is acceptable for clinical practice and to select beam directions in a rule-based manner. The approach is inferior to beam angle optimization techniques that integrate dose calculations, optimize wedge angles, etc. Nevertheless the results of this work have shown that the BDST is able to suggest beam directions that result in plans with greatly improved sparing of critical structures and is, therefore, a good compromise to more elaborate techniques. In this work, all the suggestions in terms of selected beam directions by the BDST were accepted. In clinical routine, however, the dosimetrist might only select some of the beam directions suggested by the BDST and combine them with standard beam directions or beam directions that have a high cost but when the portal is split into two subfields (*e.g.* one on the left and one on the right side of the spinal cord), or if the intensity is modulated, result in preferable beam directions.

The BDST has shown that small changes in the beam directions (see clinical case I) can already result in considerable improvements in the reduction of dose to the normal tissues. It is noteworthy that none of the beams for the clinical case II made use of wedges or different energies, which highlights that the conventional plan was more complex and simpler plans might be possible.

It would be of further interest to evaluate the trade-offs between the speed and the quality of a plan based on the current approach and more sophisticated techniques that include dose calculations during the optimization procedure. The cost maps obtained could be used to predetermine and separate the "good" beam directions from the "bad" ones. This could then be used as an input for more complex stochastic optimization procedures similar to the approach described by Pugachev et al [28] who used prior knowledge to reduce the optimization time.

Conclusion

A general algorithm has been presented that explores the entire permitted beam space to determine beam directions that minimize the irradiation of healthy tissues and critical structures. The algorithm can be adjusted to different clinical goals and is a valuable tool for 3D-CRT treatment planning. The beam directions obtained for the prostate case compared well with standard beam directions and other work described in the literature. For the brain and the sinus cases the optimized plans were simpler and better than conventional plans. It is anticipated that the plans could be further improved if the intensity of the conformal beams could be modulated. Indeed, the fact that one beam penetrated through the brain stem in order to spare the other OAR makes it an interesting starting point for further research on the use of the BDST for IMRT, especially with regard to forward planned IMRT [44].

Acknowledgments

The author would also like to thank Dr Homayon Parsai for his assistance with LaTeX during the preparation of this manuscript.

References

1. ICRU50. Prescribing, Recording and Reporting Photon Beam Therapy. Bethesda, MD: International Commission on Radiation Units and Measurements, 1993.
2. Webb S. Intensity-modulated radiation therapy. Bristol and Philadelphia, USA: Institute of Physics Publishing, 2001.
3. Rosen LR, quote in 'Software and hardware advances bring greater accuracy, reduced toxicity to radiation therapy', Technology Trends, May 1999.
4. Derycke S, Van Duyse B, De Gersem W, De Wagter C, De Neve W. Non-coplanar beam intensity modulation allows large dose escalation in stage III lung cancer. Radiother Oncol 1997;45:253–61.
5. Söderström S, Brahme A. Which is the most suitable number of photon beam portals in coplanar radiation therapy? Int J Radiat Oncol Biol Phys 1995;33:151–9.
6. Pugachev A, Li JG, Boyer AL, Hancock SL, Le QT, Donaldson SS, et al. Role of beam orientation optimisation in intensity-modulated radiation therapy. Int J Radiat Oncol Biol Phys 2001;50:551–60.
7. Haas OC, Burnham KJ, Mills JA. Optimisation of beam orientation in radiotherapy using planar geometry. Phys Med Biol 1998;43:2179–93.
8. Chen GT, Spelbring DR, Pelizzari CA, Balter JM, Myrianthopoulos LC, Vijayakumar S, et al. The use of beam's eye view volumetrics in the selection of non-coplanar radiation portals. Int J Radiat Oncol Biol Phys 1992;23:153–63.
9. Myrianthopoulos LC, Chen G, Vijayakumar S, Halpern H, Spelbring R, Pelizzari CA. Beam's eye view volumetrics: an aid in rapid treatment plan development and evaluation. Int J Radiat Oncol Biol Phys 1992;23:367–75.
10. Ezzell GA. Genetic and geometric optimisation of three-dimensional radiation therapy treatment planning. Med Phys 1996;23:293–305.
11. Das SK, Marks LB. Selection of coplanar or noncoplanar beams using three-dimensional optimisation based on maximum beam separation and minimized nontarget irradiation. Int J Radiat Oncol Biol Phys 1997;38:643–55.
12. Rowbottom CG, Webb S, Oldham M. Beam-orientation customisation using an artificial neural network. Phys Med Biol 1999;44:383–99.
13. Rowbottom CG, Webb S, Oldham M. Improvements in prostate radiotherapy from the customization of beam directions. Med Phys 1998;25:1171–9.
14. Bortfeld T, Schlegel W. Optimisation of beam orientations in radiation therapy: some theoretical considerations. Phys Med Biol 1993;38:291–304.
15. Rowbottom CG, Oldham M, Webb S. Constrained customization of non-coplanar beam orientations in radiotherapy of brain tumours. Phys Med Biol 1999;44:2251–62.
16. Pugachev AB, Boyer AL, Xing L. Beam orientation optimisation in intensity-modulated radiation treatment planning. Med Phys 2000;27:1238–45.
17. Pugachev AB, Xing L. Pseudo beam's-eye-view as applied to beam orientation selection in intensity-modulated radiation therapy. Int J Radiat Oncol Biol Phys 2001;51:1361–70.
18. Djajaputra D, Wu Q, Wu Y, Mohan R. Algorithm and performance of a clinical IMRT beam-angle optimisation system. Phys Med Biol 2003;48:3191–212.
19. Li Y, Yao J, Yao D. Automatic beam angle selection in IMRT planning using genetic algorithm. Phys Med Biol 2004;49:1915–32.
20. Mohan R, Mageras GS, Baldwin B, Brewster LJ, Kutcher GJ, Leibel S, et al. Clinically relevant optimisation of 3-D conformal treatments. Med Phys 1992;19:933–44.
21. Wu X, Zhu Y. An optimisation method for importance factors and beam weights based on genetic algorithms for radiotherapy treatment planning. Phys Med Biol 2001;46: 1085–99.

22. van Dalen S, Keijzer M, Huizenga H, Storchi PR. Optimisation of multileaf collimator settings for radiotherapy treatment planning. Phys Med Biol 2000;45:3615–25.
23. De Gersem W, Claus F, De Wagter C, Van Duyse B, De Neve W. Leaf position optimisation for step-and-shoot IMRT. Int J Radiat Oncol Biol Phys 2001;51:1371–88.
24. Bednarz G, Michalski D, Houser C, Huq MS, Xiao Y, Anne PR, et al. The use of mixed-integer programming for inverse treatment planning with pre-defined field segments. Phys Med Biol 2002;47:2235–45.
25. Söderström S, Gustafsson A, Brahme A. The clinical value of different treatment objectives and degrees of freedom in radiation therapy optimisation. Radiother Oncol 1993;29: 148–63.
26. Stein J, Mohan R, Wang XH, Bortfeld T, Wu Q, Preiser K, et al. Number and orientations of beams in intensity-modulated radiation treatments. Med Phys 1997;24:149–60.
27. Alber M, Nuesslin F. An objective function for radiation treatment optimisation based on local biological measures. Phys Med Biol 1999;44:479–93.
28. Pugachev A, Xing L. Incorporating prior knowledge into beam orientation optimisation in IMRT. Int J Radiat Oncol Biol Phys 2002;54:1565–74.
29. Kessler ML, McShan DL, Fraass BA. A computer-controlled conformal radiotherapy system. III: graphical simulation and monitoring of treatment delivery. Int J Radiat Oncol Biol Phys 1995;33:1173–80.
30. Meyer J, Mills JA, Haas OC, Burnham KJ, Parvin EM. Accommodation of couch constraints for coplanar intensity modulated radiation therapy. Radiother Oncol 2001;61: 23–32.
31. Furhang EE, Hanley J, Chiu-Tsao ST, Toner S, Fan P, Gliedman P, et al. Clearance assurance for stereotactic radiosurgery and radiotherapy. Med Phys 2002;29:45–50.
32. Kalet IJ, Jacky JP, Austin-Seymour MM, Unger JM. Prism: a new approach to radiotherapy planning software. Int J Radiat Oncol Biol Phys 1996;36:451–61.
33. Pickett B, Roach 3rd M, Horine P, Verhey L, Phillips TL. Optimisation of the oblique angles in the treatment of prostate cancer during six-field conformal radiotherapy. Med Dosim 1994;19:237–54.
34. Intensity Modulated Radiation Therapy Collaborative Working Group. Intensity-modulated radiotherapy: current status and issues of interest. Int J Radiat Oncol Biol Phys 2001;51:880–914.
35. Webb S, Nahum AE. A model for calculating tumour control probability in radiotherapy including the effects of inhomogeneous distributions of dose and clonogenic cell density. Phys Med Biol 1993;38:653–66.
36. Lyman JT. Complication probability as assessed from dose-volume histograms. Radiat Res 1985;Suppl 8:S13–9.
37. Kutcher GJ, Burman C. Calculation of complication probability factors for non-uniform normal tissue irradiation: the effective volume method. Int J Radiat Oncol Biol Phys 1989;16:1623–30.
38. Knöös T, Kristensen I, Nilsson P. Volumetric and dosimetric evaluation of radiation treatment plans: radiation conformity index. Int J Radiat Oncol Biol Phys 1998;42:1169–76.
39. Emami B, Brown JLA, Coia L, Goitein M, Munzenrider JE, Shank B, et al. Tolerance of normal tissue to therapeutic irradiation. Int J Radiat Oncol Biol Phys 1991;21:109–22.
40. Sailer SL, Rosenman JG, Symon JR, Cullip TJ, Chaney EL. The tetrad and hexad: maximum beam separation as a starting point for noncoplanar 3D treatment planning: prostate cancer as a test case. Int J Radiat Oncol Biol Phys 1994;30:439–46.
41. Eisbruch A, Ten Haken RK, Kim HM, Marsh LH, Ship JA. Dose, volume, and function relationships in parotid salivary glands following conformal and intensity-modulated irradiation of head and neck cancer. Int J Radiat Oncol Biol Phys 1999;47:1458–60.
42. Makkonen TA, Nordman E. Estimation of long-term salivary gland damage induced by radiotherapy. Acta Oncol 1987;26:307–12.
43. Meyer J, Phillips MH. Beam direction optimisation for anatomy-based IMRT using beam's-eye-view metric, Poster presentation at the UK Radiation Oncology Conference 2003, University of Bath, Bath, UK, 7–9 April 2003.
44. Xiao Y, Galvin L, Hossain M, Valicenti R. An optimised forward-planning technique for intensity modulated radiation therapy. Med Phys 2000;27:2093–9.

The British Journal of Radiology, *78* (2005), 328–334
DOI: 10.1259/bjr/22554286

In vivo absorbed dose measurements in mammography using a new real-time luminescence technique

[1]M C AZNAR, MSc, [2]B HEMDAL, BSc, [2]J MEDIN, PhD, [1]C J MARCKMANN, PhD, [1]C E ANDERSEN, PhD, [1]L BØTTER-JENSEN, DSc, [3]I ANDERSSON, MD, PhD and [2]S MATTSSON, PhD

[1]*Radiation Research Department, Risø National Laboratory, DK-4000 Roskilde, Denmark,* [2]*Department of Medical Radiation Physics, Lund University, Malmö University Hospital, SE 205 02 Malmö, Sweden and* [3]*Department of Diagnostic Radiology, Lund University, Malmö University Hospital, SE 205 02 Malmö, Sweden*

Abstract. A dosimetry system based on radioluminescence (RL) and optically stimulated luminescence (OSL) from carbon doped aluminium oxide (Al_2O_3:C) crystals was developed for *in vivo* absorbed dose measurements in mammography. A small cylindrical crystal of Al_2O_3:C (diameter 0.48 mm and length 2 mm) was coupled to the end of a 1 mm diameter optical fibre cable. Owing to their small size and characteristic shape, these probes can be placed on the body surface in the field of view during the examination, without compromising the reading of the mammogram. Our new technique was tested with a mammography unit (Siemens Mammomat 3000) and screen–film technique over a range of clinically relevant X-ray energies. The results were compared with those obtained from an ionization chamber usually used for the determination of absorbed dose in mammography. The reproducibility of measurements was around 3% (1 standard deviation) at 4.5 mGy for both RL and OSL data. The dose response was found to be linear between 4.5 mGy and 30 mGy. The energy dependence of the system is around 18% between 23 kV and 35 kV. *In vivo* measurements were performed during three patient examinations. It was shown that entrance and exit doses could be measured. The presence of the small probes did not significantly interfere with the diagnostic quality of the images. Entrance doses estimated by RL/OSL results agreed within 3% with entrance surface dose values calculated from the ionization chamber measurements. These results indicate a considerable potential for use in routine control and *in vivo* dose measurements in mammography.

Mammography is the most effective method to screen asymptomatic women in selected age groups in order to detect early stages of breast cancer. It is however estimated that when saving 20 women (age 40–50 years) through regular mammography screening, one lethal cancer may be induced by the radiation [1]. It is therefore necessary to monitor the radiation dose in mammography. The risk from radiation is currently described by the average absorbed dose to the glandular tissue. This quantity is called the average glandular dose (AGD) and is normally derived from measurement of the entrance surface air kerma (ESAK), the half-value layer (HVL) and the compressed breast thickness. Published conversion factors [2, 3] are used to calculate the AGD for different breast thicknesses from the ESAK value with the assumption that the breast composition is 50% fat and 50% glandular tissue. In recent years, these conversion factors have been extended [4, 5] to a larger interval of breast thicknesses and also to account for other breast compositions and X-ray spectra.

Accordingly, there are special demands on quality control in mammography, both internationally [3, 6, 7] and nationally [8]. In Sweden, there is a legal need [9] to make direct patient measurements in mammography screening for at least 20 patients each year using the European protocol on dosimetry in mammography [3].

Usually an ionization chamber is used to measure ESAK and HVL without any patient present. The tube output, *i.e.* the air kerma (mGy) relative to the tube loading (mAs) is measured behind the compression plate and should be specified at a reference point 45 mm above the breast support (cassette table) and laterally centred 60 mm from the chest wall side of the table edge. For each patient exposure, the mAs-value and compressed breast thickness are recorded (as well as the anode/filter combination and tube potential, if those parameters could be changed). Then the ESAK value can be calculated for that particular exposure. As an alternative, thermoluminescence dosemeters (TLDs) on the breast can be used as a simple method of determining ESAK [3]. In this case the measured entrance surface dose (ESD), defined in terms of absorbed dose in air at the skin surface including the contribution from backscatter, has to be divided by an appropriate backscatter factor (BSF), which is tabulated as a function of HVL (BSF is 1.07 for HVL=0.25 mm Al and 1.13 for 0.65 mm Al).

The aim of this work was to develop a small size, high-sensitivity optical fibre dosemeter capable of measuring real-time entrance as well as exit absorbed doses and dose rates in mammography, and to test the dosemeter with respect to reproducibility, linearity of the signal with absorbed dose, energy dependence, backscatter and breast thickness simulated with a phantom. Finally we wanted to use the dosemeter for *in vivo* entrance and exit measurements in real mammography examinations in order to see whether the disturbances from the dosemeters on the image are acceptable in routine mammography screening and whether this technique has a potential for use in a quality control programme for mammography.

Received 19 April 2004 and in revised form 12 November 2004, accepted 20 December 2004.

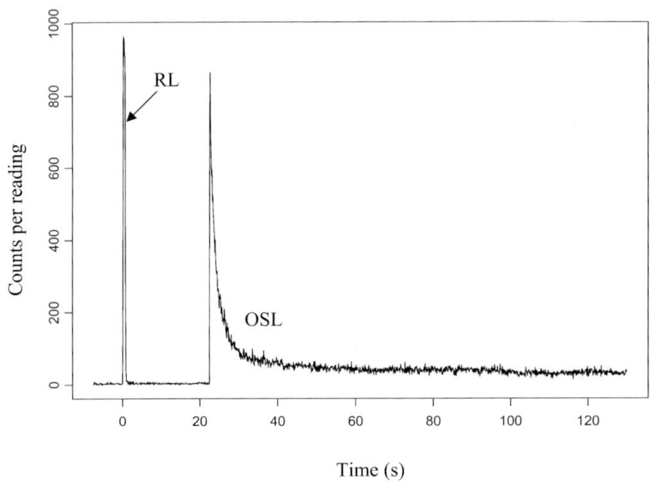

Figure 1. Schematic representation of radioluminescence (RL) and optically stimulated luminescence (OSL) signals from a typical exposure (the absorbed dose is approximately 10 mGy). The exposure starts at time zero and the RL is collected during the exposure. The OSL is shown collected during a time which starts approximately 20 s after the end of the exposures.

Materials and methods

The RL/OSL dosemeter system

Most crystalline materials produce luminescence when exposed to ionizing radiation owing to the presence of impurities or defects in the lattice. One has to distinguish between two different signals: radioluminescence (RL), which is emitted promptly during irradiation; and luminescence that is emitted when the crystal is stimulated either by heat, referred to as thermoluminescence (TL) or, as in our case, by laser light referred to as optically stimulated luminescence (OSL). The instantaneous RL signal is proportional to the dose rate while the OSL is proportional to the absorbed dose in the crystalline detector. Figure 1 shows an example of RL and OSL signals obtained for a single exposure from the mammography unit corresponding to an air kerma of approximately 10 mGy, which can be considered equal to the absorbed dose in air for the photon beam qualities included in the study.

The RL/OSL dosimetry system presented in this study uses carbon-doped aluminium oxide (Al_2O_3:C) as a sensor crystal. Al_2O_3:C was chosen among various potential luminescent materials in view of its excellent OSL properties [10, 11]. The effective atomic number of Al_2O_3:C is 10.2 and its density is 3.97 g.cm^{-3}. Al_2O_3:C emits both RL and OSL in the blue region (~420 nm). The Al_2O_3:C detector (2 mm long, 0.48 mm in diameter; provided by Landauer Inc., Stillwater Crystal Growth Division, USA) is connected to the optical system via a 10 m long optical fibre cable made of a 0.48 mm polymethylmethacrylate (PMMA) core (Super Eska GK-20, Mitsubishi Rayon Co., Ltd., Japan). The total diameter of the fibre cable, including cladding and jacket, is 1 mm. To produce OSL, a green laser beam (532 nm, 20 mW) is focused through a dichroic colour beamsplitter and transported via the optical fibre into the Al_2O_3:C crystal. The stimulated OSL signal is carried back from the crystal in the same fibre and reflected by the beamsplitter into a photomuliplier (PM) tube. A set of filters in front of the PM tube minimizes the scattered green light from the laser. The dosemeter system used in this study consists of two optical units, which are controlled using a standard laptop computer, equipped with a data acquisition card and a Labview interface (both products of National Instruments, Austin, USA). This configuration enables the system to be compact and uses only one optical fibre per dosemeter. A schematic drawing of the RL/OSL dosimetry system is provided in Figure 2.

Two probes were used, and are referred to as "fibre #48" and "fibre #49". The sensitivity of the probes is dependent on the manufacturing process of Al_2O_3:C, the size of the crystal and the optical coupling. As a consequence, fibre #48 is more sensitive than fibre #49, and was therefore used for exit dose measurements. Apart from the difference in sensitivity, the two probes exhibit the same behaviour. Hence, unless otherwise specified, only results from fibre #49 are presented in the following sections.

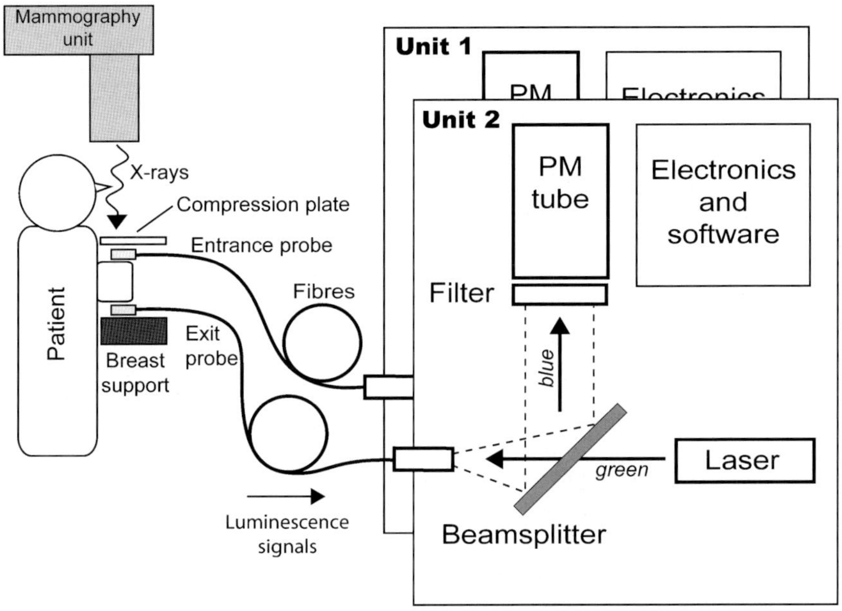

Figure 2. Schematic diagram of the radioluminescence/optically stimulated luminescence (RL/OSL) dosimetry system.

Protocol and data analysis

In all experiments performed in the present work except for the *in vivo* measurements (see below), the RL and OSL signals were acquired according to the schematic arrangement shown in Figure 1, *i.e.* the RL is collected during the exposure, and the laser light is switched on shortly after the end of the exposure to collect the OSL signal. Because the RL signal is collected during irradiation, it is potentially affected by the signal arising from fluorescence generated in the optical fibre (referred to as "stem effect"). However, for photon beam qualities used in mammography the signal generated in the light guide was found to be insignificant compared with the signal coming from the crystal (<1%). The stem effect is not present when the OSL signal is acquired, since it is not read out during the irradiation. Independent absorbed dose estimates were obtained by integrating either the complete RL signal, or the OSL signal for a fixed duration. For both signals (RL and OSL), a background correction is performed, and the raw signal from each probe is corrected to account for sensitivity differences. It was sufficient to integrate the OSL signal for about 100 s to provide a reliable estimate of the relatively small absorbed doses in mammography. However, in the following results, the RL signal generates a higher number of counts per reading for a given absorbed dose than the OSL signal and is consequently considered more accurate.

As mentioned in a previous work [12], the RL signal is subject to sensitivity changes with accumulated absorbed dose. As a consequence, for an irradiation at a constant dose rate, the RL signal will increase. In the case of mammography however, the resulting absorbed doses are too small for any significant changes in RL sensitivity to occur (about 0.2% for an absorbed dose of 10 mGy).

Description of the mammography system and the conventional test equipment

All experiments were performed with a mammography unit (Siemens Mammomat 3000; Siemens, Erlangen, Germany) using a Mo/Mo anode/filter combination. The tube potential ranged from 23 kV to 35 kV. A screen–film system (Kodak Min-R 2190/Min-R 2000, 36℃, 90 s; Eastman Kodak, Rochester, NY) was used. Whenever relevant, the signals from the RL/OSL dosemeter were compared with the reading of a flat ionization chamber (type TB23344 from PTW Freiburg, Germany) connected to an electrometer (Solidos 300, RTI, Mölndal, Sweden).

A PMMA phantom (area 240 mm × 150 mm) was combined to various thicknesses and was used to simulate the presence of breast tissue. The HVL measurements were performed using aluminium foils with a purity of at least 99.99% and varying thicknesses of 0.208 mm, 0.094 mm, 0.091 mm, 0.046 mm and 0.026 mm (Goodfellow, Cambridge, UK) as well as a lead diaphragm (1 mm thickness, 16 mm × 15 mm).

In vivo measurements

Before any *in vivo* measurements were performed, images of the probes positioned on a PMMA phantom, a common quality control phantom for mammography (RMI 156, Gammex RMI, Middleton, WI) and a phantom with human breast tissue in formalin surrounded by polyethylene [13] were acquired. Three experienced radiologists evaluated those images, and gave their approval for the use of the probes during patient examination. *In vivo* measurements were scheduled on three women coming to an ordinary screening examination (selected to have different breast sizes and densities).

Fibre #49 was attached to the compression paddle in such a way that it was compressed between the compression paddle and the upper part of the breast during the examination. Fibre #48 was positioned on the table of the mammography unit, and was then in contact with the inferior surface of the breast (see Figure 2). The fibres were positioned with each crystal laterally centred 60 mm from the chest wall side of the breast support so that they would not be superimposed on the mammograms. Craniocaudal (CC) and mediolateral oblique (MLO) projections were used. Lead markers were attached to the compression paddle on its upper side in order to obtain a more precise estimate of the compressed breast thickness [14] 60 mm from the chest wall side of the breast support for each patient image. Except for these preparations, the standard procedure for mammography screening was followed, including the use of a tube potential of 29 kV.

Each patient received four exposures (two for each breast). RL data were acquired for each individual exposure. However, OSL readings were only performed after each patient's examination was completed. Hence, for each patient, four RL measurements and one OSL measurement (representing the sum of four exposures) were acquired. This protocol was chosen in order to avoid delays due to the longer OSL reading procedure.

Finally, the radiologists evaluated the images from all three examinations to assess the interference of the probes with the diagnostic quality of the image. One expert radiologist also evaluated the screening images in order to quantify the glandularity of the breast parenchyma according to a modified Wolfe classification [15].

HVL, ESAK and AGD were evaluated according to the European protocol on dosimetry in mammography [3]. ESD was evaluated from ESAK using a backscatter factor of 1.084 corresponding to a measured HVL of 0.369 mm Al for the anode/filter combination Mo/Mo and the tube potential of 29 kV. The backscatter factor was interpolated from tabulated values of 1.08 and 1.09 at HVL 0.35 and 0.40 mm Al, respectively [3]. The same values were tabulated for breast tissue and PMMA as the scattering material.

Results and discussion

Reproducibility and linearity

The RL/OSL fibres and the ionization chamber were positioned underneath the compression plate of the mammography unit. No extra build-up or backscatter material was used. 13 exposures were made at 29 kV and 40 mAs corresponding to an air kerma of 4.5 mGy. RL and OSL data were evaluated for both fibres, and normalized to ionization chamber readings. The results are presented in Table 1 and indicate that the overall reproducibility of the system is approximately 3% at 4.5 mGy. The uncertainty in the RL data is dominated by counting statistics, while additional factors (such as laser

Table 1. Reproducibility of the radioluminescence/optically stimulated luminescence (RL/OSL) system (expressed as the relative standard deviation of 13 measurements at 29 kV for an air kerma of 4.5 mGy)

Signal	RL (counts/pC)	OSL (counts/pC)
Fibre #48	1.9% (1 SD)	2.7% (1 SD)
Fibre #49	2.5% (1 SD)	2.8% (1 SD)

SD, standard deviation.

instability) seem to increase the uncertainty in the OSL results. The dose–response of the RL/OSL system was also investigated at 29 kV, and Figure 3 shows that the output is linear with dose between 40 mAs and 250 mAs (4.5–30 mGy). The minimum detectable absorbed dose, calculated as 3 times the standard deviation of the background, is below 50 µGy for both fibres for the RL signal, and approximately about 200 µGy for the OSL signal.

Energy dependence

The variation in response of Al_2O_3:C as a function of tube potential was investigated using the same experimental set-up as described above, keeping the tube loading constant at 40 mAs during all measurements. The RL and OSL data were normalized to the simultaneous reading of the ionization chamber. The energy dependence of this ionization chamber is of the order of 1% for the range of energies used in the study (PTW Calibration Certificate, calibration traceable to national standards of the German National Laboratory, PTB, Braunschweig).

Figure 4 shows the obtained results as a function of HVL. The response of the Al_2O_3:C crystal was found to increase by 18% when the tube potential is increased from 23 kV to 35 kV, corresponding to an HVL range of 0.3–0.41 mm Al.

For the range of energies studied, the Al_2O_3:C crystal can be considered as a "photon detector", *i.e.* the energy deposition in the detector volume can be directly related to the incident photons and not to the secondary electrons

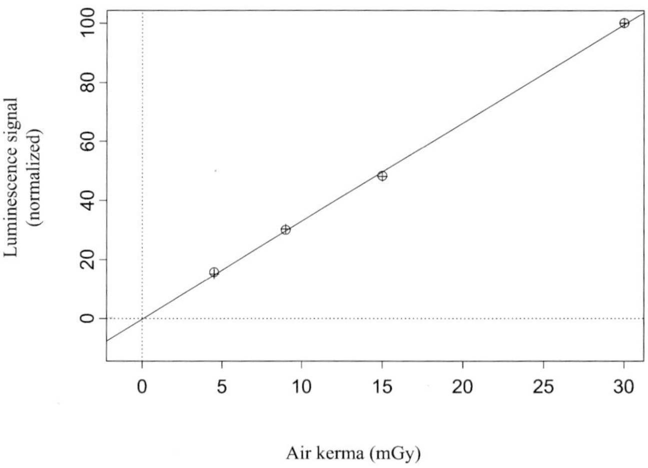

Figure 3. Linearity of dose–response at 29 kV (R-squared >0.999). Data are normalized to their value at a 250 mAs exposure, corresponding to an air kerma of 30 mGy (radioluminescence (RL): crosses, optically stimulated luminescence (OSL): circles).

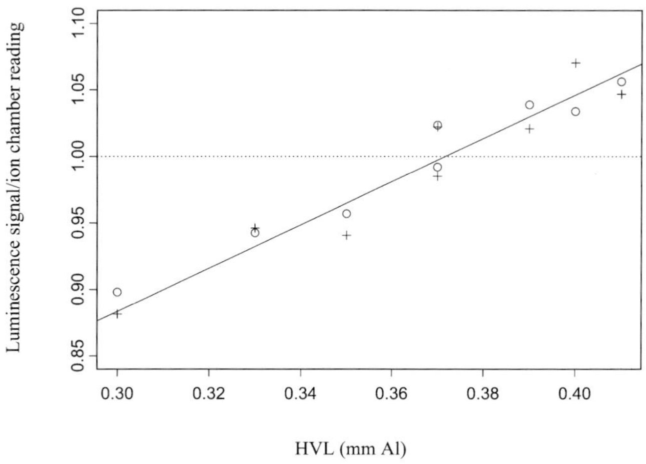

Figure 4. Energy dependence of the luminescence signals compared with the ionization chamber (radioluminescence (RL): crosses, optically stimulated luminescence (OSL): circles). RL and OSL readings are divided by the simultaneous ionization chamber readings. Data are normalized to read unity at 29 kV.

emitted in the material surrounding the detector. This is a reasonable approximation considering the size of the detector and the short range of the emitted electrons, which is less than 8 µm even for the highest maximum energy [16].

Backscatter

Backscatter factors for the RL/OSL probes were defined as:

$$BSF = \frac{S_{phantom}}{S_{air}}$$

where $S_{phantom}$ is the signal at a point on the surface of the PMMA phantom and S_{air} is the signal free in air at the same point without the phantom.

The phantoms used ranged from 1 cm to 6 cm in thickness. The tube potential was kept at 29 kV. Three exposures were performed in each setting, leading to one RL measurement per exposure, and one OSL measurement after each set of three exposures. The results are presented in Table 2.

The data in Table 2 suggest that full backscatter is achieved with 1 cm of PMMA. The average backscatter

Table 2. Measurements of backscatter from a polymethylmethacrylate (PMMA) phantom. Three exposures were performed in each set up

Thickness (x) of PMMA (cm)	Tube loading per exposure (mAs)	RL BSF (x cm/0 cm) of PMMA	OSL BSF (x cm/0 cm) of PMMA
1	40	1.071	1.084
2	80	1.067	1.046
3	140	1.058	1.047
4	200	1.060	1.065
4.5	200	1.057	1.081
6	200	1.075	1.083
Mean $\pm$1 SD (n=6)		1.064$\pm$0.003	1.068$\pm$0.008

RL, radioluminescence; OSL, optically stimulated luminescence; BSF, back scatter factor.

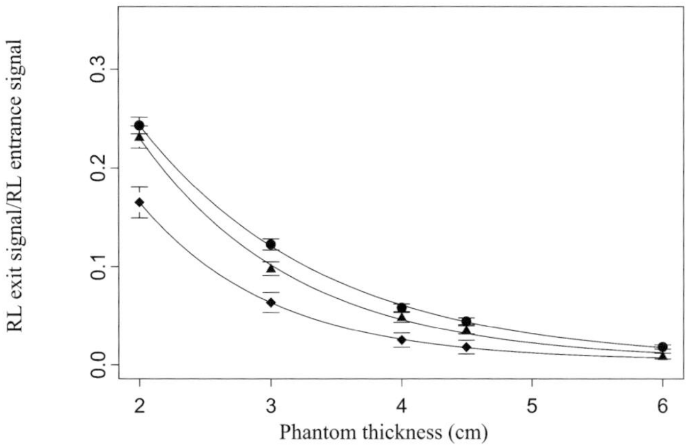

Figure 5. Measurements with one probe (fibre #49) at the entrance surface, the other (fibre #48) at the exit surface of a polymethylmethacrylate (PMMA) phantom. (radioluminescence (RL) exit)/(RL entrance) signals are presented for 23 kV (diamonds), 29 kV (triangles) and 35 kV (circles).

factor is 1.066 ± 0.004 ($n=12$) for the pooled RL and OSL data (ignoring differences in uncertainties and assuming that the measurements are independent) where the indicated uncertainty (expressed as one standard deviation) only includes the observed random variation from measurement to measurement. The observed backscatter factor is slightly lower than the value of 1.084 for TLDs with PMMA or breast tissue as the scattering material [3]. This discrepancy may reflect differences in geometry or in energy response of the different materials [17].

Influence of phantom thickness (exit/entrance measurements)

The sensitivity of the RL/OSL probes is sufficient to measure exit doses in typical exposures. In the following experiment, the thickness of the PMMA phantom was varied between 2 cm and 6 cm, while the tube potential ranged from 23 kV to 35 kV. Fibre #49 was positioned at the entrance surface of the phantom, while fibre #48 was placed on the exit surface. The ratio "exit RL signal/ entrance RL signal" was calculated in each case and corrected for the difference in sensitivity. As illustrated in Figure 5, the exit/entrance RL signal ratio decreases with increasing phantom thickness, and with decreasing tube potential. Uncertainty bars were determined by counting statistics. Only in the most extreme case (6 cm PMMA and 23 kV) was the sensitivity of the exit probe too low to provide a reliable RL signal. The OSL data provide similar results, but with considerably higher uncertainties for the low dose points.

In vivo measurements

Except for the first patient, the fibres were positioned in such a way that their shadows did not superimpose on the mammograms. The compression paddle was not fixed in the lateral direction, which accidentally led to superposition of the fibres in one image of the first screening examination in spite of apparent separation before the breast compression. After further separation of the fibres to about 20 mm, they were not superimposed for the next two patients. Three radiologists viewed the images and stated that neither the fibre dosemeters nor the lead markers disturbed the reading of the mammograms due to their small sizes and characteristic shapes that could not be confused with structures in the breast, either benign or malignant (see Figure 6). Single calcifications could have been obscured, but this was not considered to impair significantly early breast cancer detection.

The estimated compressed breast thickness, ESAK and AGD are presented in Table 3 together with estimated glandularity and breast parenchymal category, which was found to be the same for each breast of the same woman. Table 4 summarizes the results from RL/OSL measurements, compared with the calculated ESD from the ionization chamber measurements. RL and OSL results are expressed as counts, and are corrected for the difference in sensitivity of the two probes. For

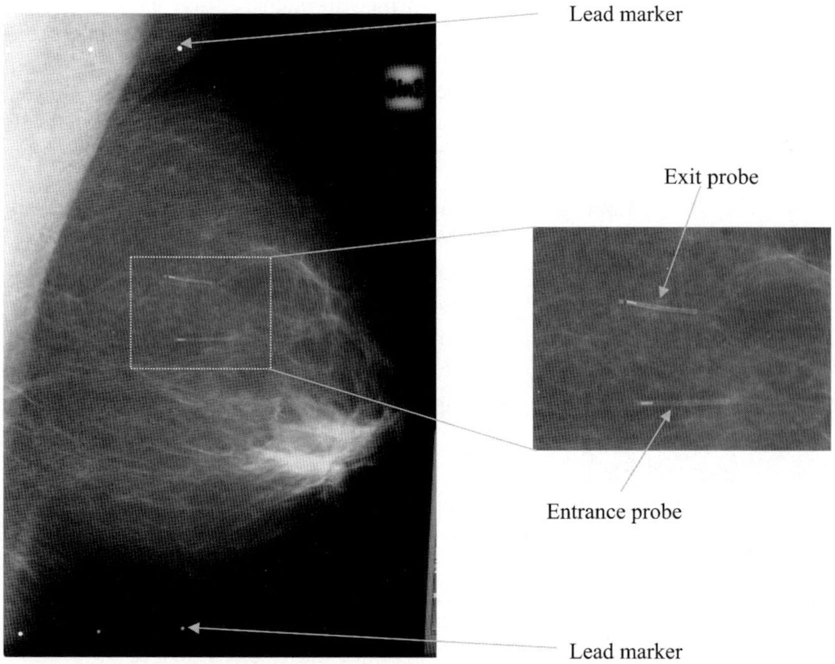

Figure 6. Impact of the radioluminescence/ optically stimulated luminescence (RL/OSL) fibres on a mediolateral oblique (MLO) mammogram. Lead markers 60 mm from the chest wall side of the breast support are indicated by arrows.

Table 3. Patient image data and entrance surface air kerma (ESAK) and average glandular dose (AGD) values determined from the ionization chamber measurements. CC, cranio-caudal; MLO, mediolateral oblique

Patient-image number	Parenchymal Category (0–3)	Glandularity (%)	Breast	Projection	Thickness indicator (mm)	Compressed breast thickness (mm)	Tube loading (mAs)	ESAK (mGy)	AGD (mGy)
1-1	3	85	Left	CC	50	55.9	93	11.1	1.94
1-2			Right	CC	44	52.3	72.1	8.5	1.59
1-3			Left	MLO	53	56.8	83.5	10.0	1.71
1-4			Right	MLO	54	60.5	80.8	9.8	1.56
2-1	2	75	Left	CC	28	34.8	29.4	3.2	0.91
2-2			Right	CC	26	33.0	28.9	3.1	0.93
2-3			Left	MLO	26	34.2	27.5	3.0	0.86
2-4			Right	MLO	25	34.2	29.1	3.1	0.91
3-1	1	25	Left	CC	65	72.5	99.5	12.6	1.65
3-2			Right	CC	66	76.4	126	16.1	2.00
3-3			Left	MLO	68	78.5	133	17.2	2.06
3-4			Right	MLO	62	70.7	102	12.8	1.72

Table 4. Entrance surface dose (ESD) determined for each breast image from the ionization chamber measurements and radioluminescence/optically stimulated luminescence (RL/OSL) *in vivo* data. RL and OSL counts have been corrected for sensitivity differences between fibre #48 and fibre #49

Patient-image number	ESD (mGy)	RL entrance (counts)	RL exit (counts)	OSL entrance (counts)	OSL exit (counts)	RL entrance/ (ESD per image) (counts/mGy)	OSLentrance/ (ESD per patient) (counts/mGy)	RL exit/ entrance	OSL exit/ entrance
1-1	12.0	10532	281			487		0.027	
1-2	9.2	8084	207	10683	281	489	1143	0.026	0.026
1-3	10.8	9779	266			503		0.027	
1-4	10.6	9354	173			491		0.018	
2-1	3.5	2945	187			473		0.063	
2-2	3.4	2952	205	3353	239	486	1090	0.069	0.071
2-3	3.2	2955	181			510		0.061	
2-4	3.4	3155	209			514		0.066	
3-1	13.6	12107	286			494		0.024	
3-2	17.5	15410	283	15875	322	489	1099	0.018	0.020
3-3	18.6	17037	307			509		0.018	
3-4	13.9	12571	271			504		0.022	

measurements at a fixed tube potential (here, 29 kV), the sum of the entrance RL signal seems to be a reliable estimator of the entrance surface dose, as the ratio "RL entrance/ESD" has a standard deviation of 3% (*i.e.* within the uncertainty associated with the system). The exit doses could also be measured *in vivo* during all 12 exposures, as seen from the "RL exit" signal (this signal was at least 4 times higher than the background signal in all cases). The ratio of exit to entrance doses can be obtained for each individual image via RL analysis, or for each patient via OSL analysis. These estimates agree within ±10%.

Conclusions

A new small size, high-sensitivity optical fibre dosemeter capable of measuring real-time entrance as well as exit absorbed doses and dose rates in mammography, was developed. The system has been tested in clinical mammography and it was found that the reproducibility is of the order of 3% (1 standard deviation) at an air kerma of 4.5 mGy. The response is linear with absorbed dose between at least 4.5 mGy and 30 mGy. The energy dependence for the range of beam qualities tested (23–35 kV) is around 18%. The BSF is approximately 1.07.

In vivo entrance and exit dose measurements of three women undergoing a standard mammography screening examination showed that the technique can be used for estimation of ESD and that the disturbances from the dosemeters on the image are acceptable. It is concluded that this technique has considerable potential for use in a quality control programme for mammography.

Acknowledgments

The authors are much obliged to all the staff at the Mammography section, Department of Diagnostic Radiology, Malmö University Hospital, Sweden for providing the opportunity to perform this study and especially for their help when the *in vivo* measurements were performed. We would also like to thank Jan B Olsen in Oslo, Norway, for providing the breast tissue phantom. The group at Risø National Laboratory gratefully acknowledges financial support from Landauer Inc., Chicago, IL, USA.

References

1. Andersson I, Janzon L. Reduced breast cancer mortality in women under age 50: updated results from the Malmo Mammographic Screening Program. J Natl Cancer Inst Monogr 1997;(22):63–7.
2. Dance DR. Monte Carlo calculation of conversion factors for the estimation of mean glandular breast dose. Phys Med Biol 1990;35:1211–9.
3. Zoetelief J, Fitzgerald M, Leitz W, Säbel M. European protocol on dosimetry in mammography. EUR 16263, 1996.
4. Dance DR, Skinner CL, Young KC, Beckett JR, Kotre CJ. Additional factors for the estimation of mean glandular breast dose using the UK mammography dosimetry protocol. Phys Med Biol 2000;45:3225–40.
5. van Engen R, Young K, Bosmans H, Thijssen M. Addendum on digital mammography, European Guidelines for Quality Assurance in Mammography Screening 2003 EUREF.
6. EURATOM. The European medical exposure directive 97/43. Council Directive 97/43/Euratom of 30 June 1997 on health protection of individuals against the dangers of ionizing radiation in relation to medical exposure, 1997.
7. Perry N, Broeders M, de Wolf C, Törnberg S, editors. European Guidelines for Quality Assurance in Mammography Screening (3rd edn). 2001 European Commission, EUREF.
8. Socialstyrelsen. National Board of Health and Welfare. Screening with Mammography for early Detection of Breast Cancer 1998. SoS-report 1998:17 (Stockholm, in Swedish).
9. SSI, Swedish Radiation Protection Authority, Regulations and general advice on diagnostic standard doses and reference levels within medical X-ray diagnostics, SSI FS 2002:2 (Stockholm, in Swedish, non-authorised translation to English is available at www.ssi.se), 2002.
10. Bøtter-Jensen L, McKeever SWS. Optically stimulated luminescence dosimetry using natural and synthetic materials. Radiat Prot Dosim 1996;65:273–80.
11. Bøtter-Jensen L, Agersnap Larsen N, Markey BG, McKeever SWS. Al_2O_3:C as a sensitive OSL dosemeter for rapid assessment of environmental photon dose rates. Radiat Meas 1997;27:295–8.
12. Aznar MC, Andersen CE, Bøtter-Jensen L, Bäck SÅJ, Mattsson S, Kjær-Kristoffersen F, et al. Real-time optical-fibre luminescence dosimetry for radiotherapy: physical characteristics and applications in photon beams. Phys Med Biol 2004;49:1655–69.
13. Olsen JB, Sager EM. Subjective evaluation of image quality based on images obtained with a breast tissue phantom: comparison with a conventional image quality phantom. Br J Radiol 1995;68:160–4.
14. Burch A, Law J. A method for estimating compressed breast thickness during mammography. Br J Radiol 1995;68:394–9.
15. Wolfe JN. Breast parenchymal patterns and their changes with age. Radiology 1976;121:545–52.
16. ICRU Stopping powers for electrons and positrons, ICRU Report 37, 1984.
17. Chan HP, Doi K. Monte Carlo simulation studies of backscatter factors in mammography. Radiology 1981;139: 195–9.

The British Journal of Radiology, *78* (2005), 335–337
DOI: 10.1259/bjr/24426084

Short communication

Further evidence for biological effects resulting from ionizing radiation doses in the diagnostic X-ray range

[1]S ANOOPKUMAR-DUKIE, MSc, [2]A McMAHON, BSc, HND, [1]A ALLSHIRE, PhD and [2]T J CONERE, MSc, PhD

[1]*Department of Pharmacology and Therapeutics, University College Cork, Wilton, Cork, Ireland and* [2]*Medical Physics Department, Cork University Hospital, Wilton, Cork, Ireland*

Abstract. In this study we assessed cell response to ionizing radiation doses in the diagnostic X-ray range, using metabolic performance as the biological end point. HeLa cells were irradiated between 3.5 mGy (standard deviation (SD=2.5%) and 55.1 mGy (SD=0.9%) with 110 kV X-rays, and after 7 days metabolic capacity of cultures was measured spectrophotometrically with resazurin. Cells receiving 7.5 mGy or greater showed impaired proliferation. At 7.5 mGy this effect was prevented by nitric oxide synthase inhibitor N G-monomethyl-L-arginine but not by ascorbic acid or p38 MAPK inhibitor SB203580. We conclude that HeLa cell proliferation is adversely affected by doses within the range of some radiological examinations, through a mechanism involving nitric oxide.

There is currently much debate concerning the biological effects of low dose ionizing radiation [1–3] and whether a threshold dose exists for such effects. The International Commission on Radiological Protection (ICRP) [4] has adopted the so-called "linear-no threshold" hypothesis to estimate the risks for the stochastic effects of ionizing radiation. Under this hypothesis, the biological effect is assumed to be proportional to the radiation dose received, with no dose threshold for such effects. Hence the ICRP adopted a cautious approach in the light of scientific knowledge at that time and subsequently many national regulatory bodies have based their radiation exposure dose limits for occupationally exposed workers and members of the public on risk estimates derived using this model. However, there have been relatively few data obtained at low doses to support such an important concept. In this pilot study we have used enzymatic reduction of resazurin (Alamar Blue) to resorufin [5] as a sensitive indicator of cell response to the lower dose levels found in diagnostic radiology. We also assessed the effects of some potentially protective agents on radiation response.

Methods

The HeLa cell line purchased from American Type Culture Collection through LGC Promochem (Middlesex, UK) was routinely cultured in Minimal Essential Medium with Eagle's salts (Hepes modification) supplemented with 10% fetal bovine serum, gentamycin (20 μg ml^{-1}), L-glutamine (2 mM), sodium bicarbonate (1.5 g l^{-1}) and sodium pyruvate (1 mM). HeLa cells in exponential growth phase were irradiated to a range of doses from 3.5 mGy (standard deviation (SD)=2.5%) to 55.1 mGy (SD=0.9%) in 25 cm^2 culture flasks, using an Argostat Plus TS-5 X-ray unit (Picker, Dublin, Ireland) operating at 110 kV. For irradiation, the flasks were inverted so that the surface to which the cells were attached was uppermost, to minimize dose variations due to meniscus effects etc. These acute radiation doses were delivered over 100 ms (3.5 mGy), 200 ms (7.5 mGy) and increasing to 250 ms for the higher dose points. Radiation output was measured prior to every exposure using a calibrated Unfors Mult-O-Meter radiation dose detector (Billdal, Sweden) inserted into a suitably modified culture flask similar to those used for irradiation of cells. These dose measurements were confirmed by thermoluminescent dosimetry, and total dose uncertainty was estimated at $\pm$5%.

Following irradiation the cells were washed with phosphate buffered saline, trypsinised (0.25% w/v) and centrifuged at 400 $\times$ g. Upon resuspension in fresh culture medium, cells were counted using the trypan blue method and 5×10^3 trypan blue-excluding cells ml^{-1} were seeded in 96 well micro-titre plates. Culture medium over the cells was replaced at day 4 and again at day 7, in the latter case supplemented with resazurin (44 μM). Seven hours later resazurin reduction to resorufin was still within the linear range (<50%), and was measured spectrophotometrically at 570 nm and 600 nm using a Tecan Sunrise plate reader and X-read software (Salzburg, Austria).

Additional experiments were performed at 7.5 mGy, in which the antioxidant ascorbic acid (AA, 200 μM), nitric oxide synthase (NOS) inhibitor N G-monomethyl-L-arginine (LNMMA, 1 mM) or p38 mitogen-activated protein kinase (MAPK) inhibitor SB203580 (10 μM) were added separately to cell cultures 40 min prior to irradiation, and remained until 10 min after irradiation, for a total period of 1 h. Data were analysed using *t*-test and Graphpad Instat software (California, USA). Significance levels were defined as $p<0.05$ (*), $p<0.01$ (**) and $p<0.001$ (***).

Received 19 July 2004 and in revised form 24 September 2004, accepted 7 December 2004.

Address correspondence to Dr Tom Conere, Medical Physics Department, Cork University Hospital, Wilton, Cork, Ireland.

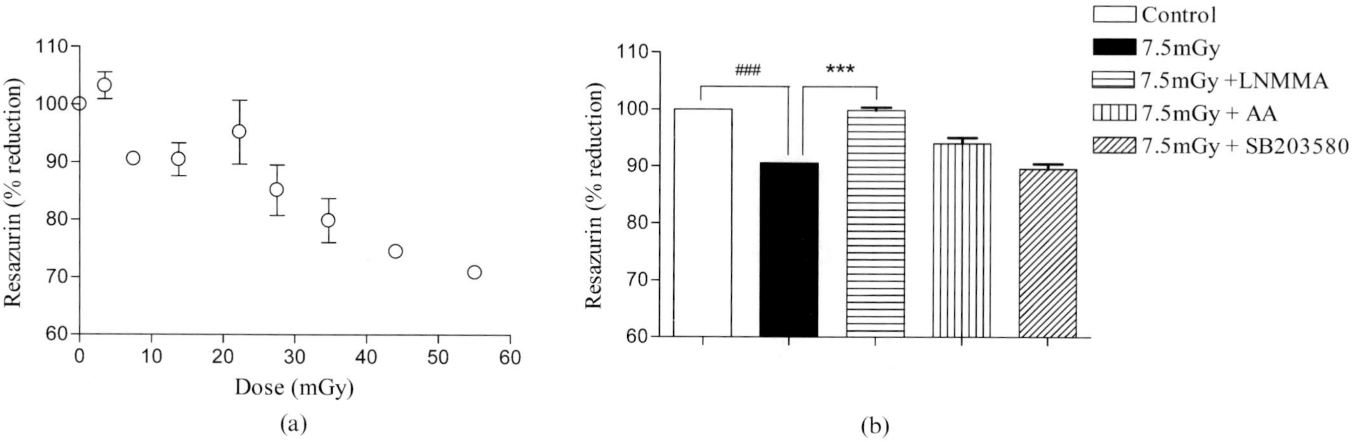

Figure 1. (a) Response of HeLa cells to low-dose X-ray irradiation, measured 7 days post irradiation as capacity for resazurin reduction. Data are means and standard deviation (SD) for three independent experiments, except for control (zero dose) and 7.5 mGy where n=6. (b) Protection against the irradiation effect at 7.5 mGy by LNMMA (1 mM) but not by ascorbic acid (AA, 200 μM) or p38 MAPK inhibitor SB203580 (10 μM). Data are means and (SD) for three independent experiments.

Results

Figure 1a shows that irradiation over the range 7.5–55.1 mGy significantly impaired subsequent cell proliferation, as indicated by resazurin reduction capacity of cultures, whereas response of cells irradiated at 3.5 mGy was not distinguishable from controls. More detailed examination of the effect at 7.5 mGy (Figure 1b) showed that inhibition of NO production with the NOS inhibitor LNMMA abolished this irradiation effect. By contrast, presence of the antioxidant ascorbic acid during cell irradiation did not confer protection. Nor did the p38 MAPK inhibitor SB203580, which had been found in separate experiments to protect HeLa cells irradiated at 5 Gy.

Discussion

The results presented in Figure 1 demonstrate adverse effects on HeLa cells of doses as low as 7.5 mGy, consistent with observations in other cell types and using different endpoints [2, 6]. Furthermore this present work implicates NO as a mediator of the effect at 7.5 mGy, on the basis of the protection afforded cells by the NOS inhibitor LNMMA. NO modulates cell radiosensitivity [7], and ionizing radiation increases NO production by inducing NOS expression [8] and stimulating constitutive NOS [9]. The cytotoxic effects of ionizing radiation (at higher doses than used here) have been attributed to mitochondria-dependent generation of both reactive oxygen and nitrogen species via an amplification mechanism involving mitochondrial permeability transition [10]. Other authors have described inhibition of mitochondrial respiratory complex I by NO [11] and the role of calcium signalling in activating NOS [12]. Thus changes in cellular calcium concentrations following radiation insult could lead to metabolic inhibition via increased production of NO. At present we are investigating these mechanisms further.

Since ascorbic acid is a good scavenger of both hydroxyl and peroxynitrite radicals, its failure to attenuate the effect of cell irradiation at 7.5 mGy suggests that neither species plays a critical role. Furthermore, at this low dose p38 MAPK is not implicated on the basis that p38 inhibitor SB203580 conferred no protection. By contrast, p38 inhibition fully protects HeLa cells irradiated at 5 Gy against metabolic impairment (unpublished observations).

The highly significant (p<0.001) 9.2% decrease in resazurin reduction at 7.5 mGy would imply a corresponding decrease of 4.3% at 3.5 mGy if a "linear-no-threshold" model applied. However we observed that resazurin reduction by cells irradiated at 3.5 mGy was marginally though not significantly stimulated. Thus these data leave open for now the question regarding the existence of a dose threshold.

In conclusion, this pilot study provides evidence of adverse effects to HeLa cells at 7.5 mGy, as measured by an assay of cellular proliferation. NO is a critical mediator of this injury but hydroxyl radical or peroxynitrite are probably not. Although we could not establish the existence of a dose threshold, if it exists then it must be below 7.5 mGy. In this context, other authors have reported cellular damage at 1.2 mGy [6]. Therefore further work is required to elucidate this point, given its importance for radiation protection and the whole concept of risk estimates based on the "linear no-threshold" model of radiation effects.

Acknowledgments

We acknowledge the assistance of Eugene O'Sullivan, Senior Physicist, Department of Medical Physics, Cork University Hospital and the financial support of the Cork based charity Aid Cancer Treatment.

References

1. Dendy PP, Brugmans MJP. Low dose radiation risks. Br J Radiol 2003;76:674–7.
2. Goldberg Z, Schwietert CW, Lehnert B, Stern R, Nami I. Effects of low-dose ionizing radiation on gene expression in human skin biopsies. Int J Radiat Oncol Biol Phys 2004;58:567–74.

3. Prasad KN, Cole WC, Haase, GM. Radiation protection in humans: extending the concept of as low as reasonably achievable (ALARA) from dose to biological damage. Br J Radiol 2004;77:97–9.
4. International Commission on Radiological Protection (ICRP). 1990 Recommendations of the International Commission on Radiological Protection. Ann ICRP 1991;60:1–3.
5. O'Brien J, Wilson I, Orton T, Pognan F. Investigation of the Alamar Blue (resazurin) fluorescent dye for the assessment of mammalian cell cytotoxicity. Eur J Biochem 2000;267: 5421–6.
6. Rothkamm K, Löbrich M. Evidence for a lack of DNA double-strand break repair in human cells exposed to very low x-ray doses. Proc Natl Acad Sci USA 2003;100:5057–62.
7. Verovski VN, Van den Berge DL, Soete GA, Bols BL, Storm GA. Intrinsic radiosensitivity of human pancreatic tumour cells and the radiosensitising potency of the nitric oxide donor sodium nitroprusside. Br J Cancer 1996;74:1734–42.
8. MacNaughton WK, Aurora AR, Bhamra J, Sharkey KA, Miller MJ. Expression, activity and cellular localization of inducible nitric oxide synthase in rat ileum and colon post-irradiation. Int J Radiat Biol 1998;74:255–64.
9. Leach JK, Black SM, Schmidt-Ullrich RK, Mikkelsen RB. Activation of constitutive nitric-oxide synthase is an early signalling event induced by ionizing radiation. J Biol Chem 2002;277:15400–6.
10. Leach JK, Van Tuyle G, Lin PS, Schmidt-Ullrich R, Mikkelsen RB. Ionizing radiation-induced, mitochondria-dependent generation of reactive oxygen/nitrogen. Cancer Res 2001;61:3894–901.
11. Brown GC, Borutaite V. Inhibition of mitochondrial respiratory complex I by nitric oxide, peroxynitrite and S-nitrosothiols. Biochim Biophys Acta 2004;1658:44–9.
12. Traaseth N, Elfering S, Solien J, Haynes V, Giulivi C. Role of calcium signaling in the activation of mitochondrial nitric oxide synthase and citric acid cycle. Biochim Biophys Acta 2004;1658:64–71.

The British Journal of Radiology, *78* (2005), 338–342
DOI: 10.1259/bjr/20260420

Short communication

Comparison between 1 T MRI and non-MRI based volumetry in inoculated tumours in mice

[1]B CORNELISSEN, PhD, [1]V KERSEMANS, MSc, [2]L JANS, MD, [1]L STAELENS, PhD, [1]R OLTENFREITER, Pharm, [1]T THONISSEN, MSc, [2]E ACHTEN, MD, PhD and [1]G SLEGERS, PhD

[1]*Laboratory of Radiopharmacy, Ghent University, Harelbekestraat 72, B-9000 Gent and* [2]*Department of Radiology and Magnetic Resonance Imaging, Ghent University Hospital, De Pintelaan 185, B-9000 Gent, Belgium*

Abstract. Tumour volume is an important therapeutic endpoint for mouse tumour models in the evaluation of new chemotherapeutic drugs and in pre-clinical evaluation of new radioimmunotherapy pharmaceuticals. In this study, two 1 T MRI-based methods both using T_1–T_2 hybrid weighting, a manual method (determination of the area per slice) and a semi-automated method (using thresholding), are compared with two classical methods, the abovementioned calliper method and volumetry by water displacement after dissection of the tumour. Interoperator and intraoperator differences for both MRI-based methods were good (no differences $p<0.05$ using a repeated measures analysis of variance (ANOVA) test). Correlation between the different methods was excellent. No significant differences were obtained ($p<0.05$), except for the semi-automated method, because it automatically excludes necrotic regions from the tumour. Therefore, we conclude that both manual and semi-automated tumour volumetry in subcutaneous tumour bearing athymic mice by low-field MRI are accurate and reliable methods. The semi-automated method is especially useful for larger tumour volumes, since it accounts for necrotic areas within the tumour.

Tumour volume is an important therapy endpoint in cancers treated with chemotherapy and radiotherapy. Tumour volume measurements are widely used in the staging and evaluation of therapy of various types of tumours in humans, such as brain, prostate, cervical and many other tumours. Regarding MR-based volumetry, manual measurements, semi-automated systems (based on region growing) and automated systems (based on segmentation) have been reported [1–7]. In this study, we report the comparison of MR-based volumetry methods with conventional methods (sliding calliper measurement) in tumour inoculated mice.

In an analogy with the human situation, tumour volume is an important therapeutic endpoint for mouse tumour models in the evaluation of new chemotherapeutic drugs [8] and in pre-clinical evaluation of new radioimmunotherapy pharmaceuticals [9, 10]. The most commonly used method for determination of tumour volume of subcutaneously inoculated tumours in mice is calliper measurement, because of its simplicity. However, due to the approximation of the (ellipsoid) shape of the tumour, this method is prone to error [11]. Volume measurement with MRI-based methods is needed to avoid the propagation of these errors when using the tumour volume for normalization of other parameters, *e.g.* uptake of a radiopharmaceutical compound. Waterton et al [12] performed a comparison between ultrasound, MR and calliper measurements in mice bearing a subcutaneous tumour. However, they did not report comparisons with a gold standard. In this study, two MRI-based methods, a manual method (determination of the area per slice) and a semi-automated method (using thresholding), are compared with two classical methods, the abovementioned calliper method and volumetry by water displacement after dissection of the tumour (gold standard).

Received 4 June 2004 and in revised form 4 November 2004, accepted 13 December 2004.

Materials and methods

Tumour inoculation

Male Swiss athymic mice (20–25 g) were obtained from Bioservices (Schaijk, The Netherlands). All animals were treated according to the regulations of the Belgian law and animal experiments were approved by the local ethical committee. Athymic mice were inoculated subcutaneously in the right flank with 5.10^6 cells of HT29, a colon adenocarcinoma, as previously described [8]. Tumours were allowed to grow for 2 to 6 weeks. The *in vivo* tumour genesis was 100%. If tumour size approximately reached the desired size (from 0.196 cm^3 to 2.352 cm^3, as determined by water volumetry), the mice were included in the MRI study. Mean tumour size was 1.048 ± 0.687 cm^3.

MR image acquisition

The animals were anaesthetised with an intraperitoneal injection of 100 µl of a medetomidin/ketamin – mixture (Domitor, Orion, Espoo, Finland; Ketalar, Parke-Davis, Zaventem, Belgium), 0.1 mg ml^{-1} and 5 mg ml^{-1} in water, respectively. After sedation, the animals were placed in a home-built mouse holder in which sterile conditions could be maintained. Two of these holders were fixed into a small surface flex coil.

MRI was performed on a clinical 1 T whole body system (Magnetom SP; Siemens, Erlangen, Germany). The position of the tumour was localized by coronal and sagittal scout images. Imaging was centred on this position.

Prior to the imaging of the series of mice described below, a comparison was made between three-dimensional (3D) dual echo steady state (DESS), T_1 and T_2 weighted images (axial 3D DESS, repetition time/echo time (TR/TE)=25.7 ms/9.0 ms, 128×256 matrix, slice thickness 1.0 mm, field of view (FOV) 124 mm × 124 mm × 42 mm, taking 21 min 05 s; axial T_1 weighted spin echo, a TR/TE=500 ms/15.0 ms, 128×256 matrix, slice thickness 3.0 mm, taking 4 min 19 s; and axial T_2 weighted spin echo, a TR/TE=3204 ms/119.0 ms, 90×256 matrix, slice thickness 3.0 mm, taking 10 min 18 s. We selected the 3D DESS sequence for further analyses. The DESS sequence (dual-echo in the steady state) acquires two gradient-echo signals in one repetition time, a fast imaging with steady state precession (FISP) and a reversed FISP (PSIF) signal. During image reconstruction, the strong T_2 weighted PSIF signal is added to the FISP signal. This yields images with improved signal-to-noise (two raw data sets added) and has stronger T_2 contrast all within a measurement time comparable with a FISP sequence [13]. The 3D DESS sequence not only yielded better signal-to-noise ratios but also significantly better delineation of the tumour, as compared with the T_1 and T_2 weighted sequences. Moreover, 3D DESS yielded better tumour to muscle and tumour to fatty tissue ratios. 3D techniques offer superior spatial resolution, and they do not suffer from interslice saturation and they do not yield interslice gaps (contiguous slices were acquired throughout the tumour without intersectional space). Additionally, they are much faster comparing the same image quality obtained by 2D sequences. For all these reasons, we decided in favour of the 3D DESS sequence.

Manual volume measurements

Manual volumetry was performed on a MagicView 1000 workstation (Siemens AG, Erlangen, Germany). The tumour was delineated in each slice. Summing the obtained areas and multiplication with the slice thickness resulted in the tumour volume. Three operators (BC, VK and RO) independently performed the manual volumetry three times on different days. The rationale to use non-radiologists to perform the repetitive measurements of the manual method was that tumour volume measurements are typically performed by MR-technologists, and not by the local radiologists. Interoperator and intraoperator reliability was assessed from these data.

Semi-automated region growing measurements

The semi-automatic measurement is based on region growing [3]. A seed point was manually selected in the most intensely coloured part of the tumour. All non-diagonal adjacent voxels that have signal intensities above a certain threshold were included in the volume. For every newly included voxel, this algorithm was repeated until no voxels were added. An advantage of this method is that non-enhanced (necrotic) areas are automatically detected and not included (Figure 1). The measurements were performed twice on two different days by BC and TT, who have experience in radiology, but are not radiologists, for the abovementioned reasons. Interoperator and intraoperator reliability was assessed from these data.

Calliper measurements

Volumetry by calliper measurement is performed by measuring (a) the short and (b) the long axis of the tumour by calliper. The volume of the tumour is calculated from the estimation of an ellipsoid: $V=0.5 \times a^2 \times b$ [11].

Water displacement measurements

To measure the volume of the tumour by water displacement volumetry, the tumour was resected. Subcutaneously inoculated tumours, which do not have adjacent tissue infiltration, are easy to resect by an experienced technologist. Additionally, the lining of the tumour is very well defined by 3D DESS MRI. The tissues measured by MRI-based methods and water displacement are therefore the same. After dissection of the tumour, water displacement volumetry is performed immediately to prevent shrinking of the tumour due to dehydration. A scheme of the home-built system is shown in Figure 2. The system consists of three connected recipients, A, B (reading error 0.005 ml) and C (reading error 0.005 ml), filled with water. The water levels in B and C are marked on the recipients. The tumour is placed in recipient A, which is large, and thus not suited for exact volume readings. By placing the tumour in recipient A, the liquid level in

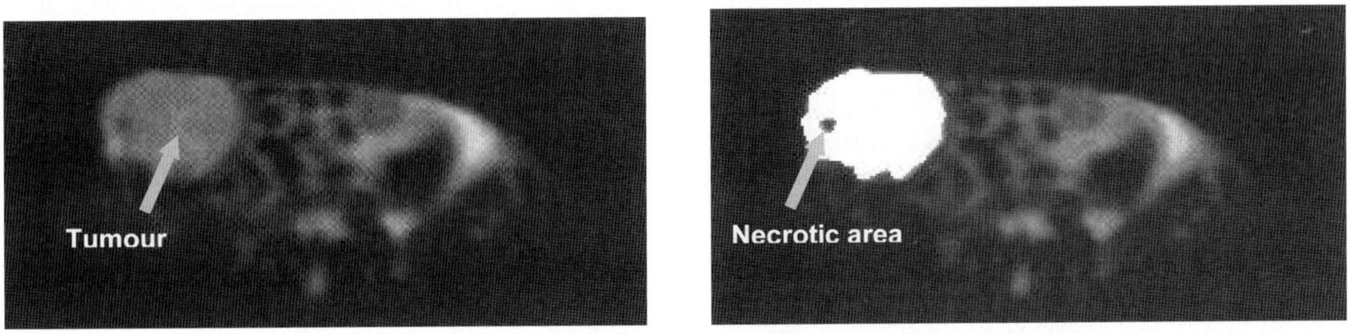

(a) (b)

Figure 1. Region growing tumour volumetry on 1 T MR images. (a) Axial slice through the tumour. (b) The same slice with a section of the "grown" tumour volume. As shown, non-enhanced parts of the tumour are not included in the volume.

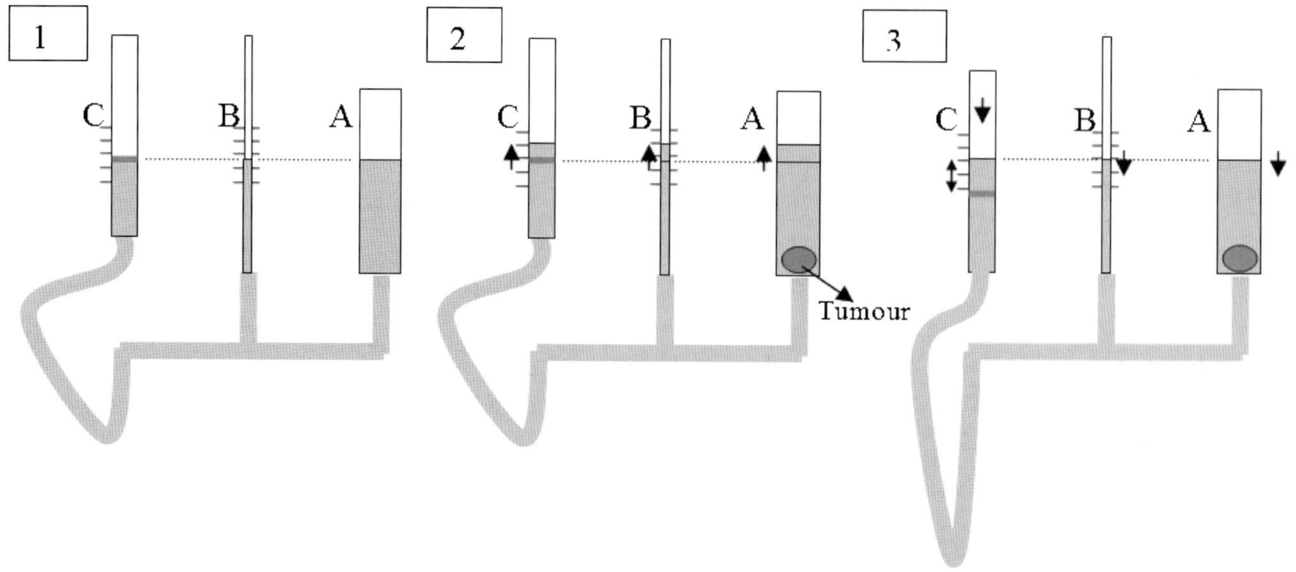

Figure 2. Schematic representation of the home-built water-displacement volumetry system.

pipette B and C also rises. B is used as calibration for the initial water level. Pipette C is now moved downwards until the water level in B has reached its original level. The difference in C corresponds with the volume of the tumour.

Statistics

In order to assess intraoperator differences and interoperator differences, a repeated measures analysis of variance (ANOVA) was performed on the data set of manual volume measurements after confirming that the data were normally distributed by means of the Shapiro-Wilks test. Furthermore, the data from the manual volume measurements were compared with those obtained from water displacement measurements. This was done by performing a paired samples *t*-test, comparing the mean of the three observations from the manual volume measurements and the values obtained from the water displacement measurements. Semi-automated and calliper measurements were also compared with the water displacement values by means of a paired samples *t*-test.

Results

Shapiro-Wilks analysis showed normally distributed results for all manual volume measurements. Repeated measurement ANOVA results for interoperator and intraoperator differences for the manual volumetry on MR images revealed no significant ($p<0.05$) interoperator differences between the measurements performed by any of the three operators on different days. Furthermore, no significant differences were found between the values obtained by the three operators.

A matrix regression analysis of all four methods showed good correlation between all four methods ($r^2>0.95$, $p<0.0001$). Bland-Altman plots of all measurements *vs* gold standard are shown in Figure 3.

Comparison between the calliper method and the water displacement method yielded no significant difference ($p=0.7064$). Correlation was good ($r^2=0.9583$). Bland-Altman analysis showed a mean overestimation of the tumour volume of 0.056 cm^3 (2.81%) compared with the gold standard. The Bland-Altman plot also shows a larger deviation for larger tumour volumes.

The manual method took approximately 5 min per mouse per operator. Linear regression analysis showed good correlation between operators and between repeated measurements of the same operator ($r^2>0.95$; $p<0.003$). Comparison of the manual volume and water displacement methods also showed no significant difference between the gold standard and the values obtained by any of the three operators ($p=0.1945$ (RO); $p=0.1281$ (BC); $p=0.1221$ (VK)). Correlation was good ($r^2>0.9738$). Bland-Altman analysis showed a mean underestimation of the tumour volume of 0.102 cm^3 (5.13%) compared with the gold standard.

The region growing method took approximately 1 min per mouse per operator. However, comparison between the region growing method and the water displacement method did yield a significant difference ($p=0.0155$). Also here, correlation was good ($r^2=0.9907$). Bland-Altman analysis showed a mean underestimation of the tumour volume of 0.076 cm^3 (3.77%) compared with the gold standard. Interoperator and intraoperator reliability for the region growing method was good: Shapiro-Wilks coefficients for all repeated measurement sets were >0.95. No significant ($p<0.05$) interoperator differences were found between the measurements performed by any of the two operators on different days. Furthermore, no significant differences were found between the values obtained by the two operators.

Discussion

In this paper, we evaluated the use of four different techniques for measurement of the volume of subcutaneous tumours in mice. Calliper measurement, and two MRI-based methods (a manual method and a region growing method) are compared with water displacement.

Calliper measurement is mostly used when assessing tumour volume in therapy evaluation studies on large

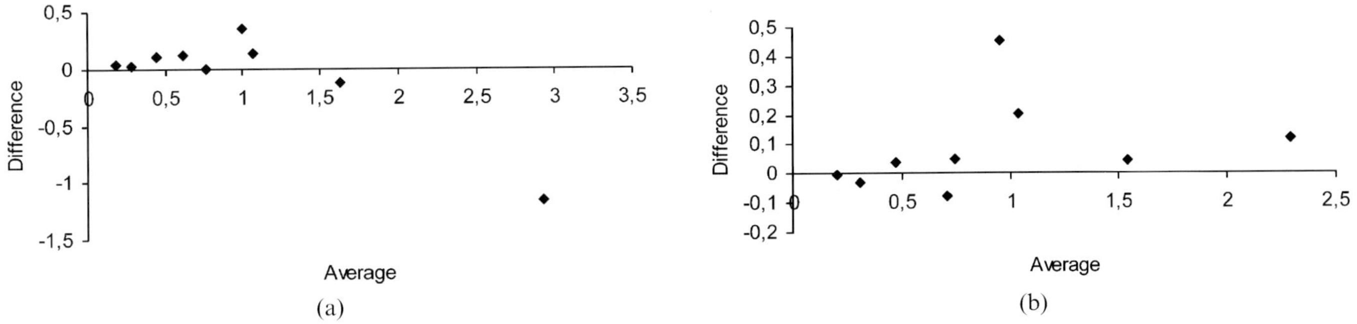

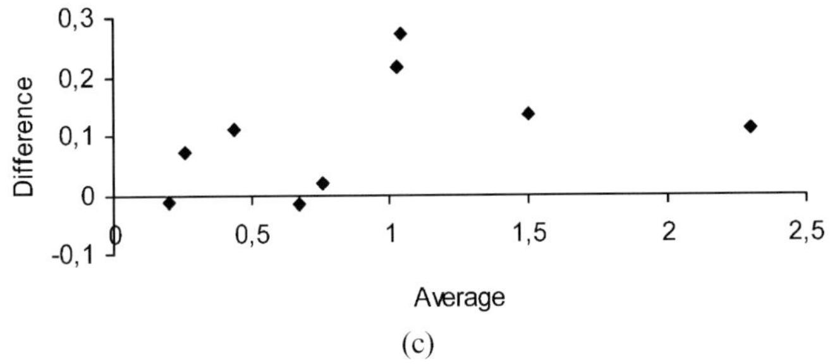

Figure 3. Bland-Altman plots for all methods compared with water volumetry. (a) Water *vs* calliper. (b) Water *vs* manual (region of interest (ROI)-drawing). (c) Water *vs* semi-automated (region growing).

numbers of mice. However, the accuracy of the method is doubtful, especially when larger tumour volumes are included. This is also shown by our results. Therefore, we wanted to examine the use of classical non-dedicated 1 T MRI for tumour volume measurements of subcutaneous tumours.

The large deviations from the gold standard as measured with the calliper method imply that calliper measurement is not suited for pre-clinical studies using large tumours. One possible way to overcome this issue is to use many mice and thus levelling out the mistakes made by calliper measurement. By using MRI-based methods the number of animals can be reduced drastically.

Despite the fact that dedicated small animal strong field MRI systems are available, we used a simple clinical 1 T machine, which is routinely used in clinical practice. The main advantage of this approach is the more abundant availability of clinical 1 T systems, and their reduced cost compared with dedicated systems. However, a disadvantage is the poorer image quality compared with dedicated systems. Nevertheless, our results show that 1 T systems are suitable for application in volumetry of inoculated mouse tumours. Owing to its large cost, the use of MRI-based volumetry is not justified in the case of small tumours. However, when using sliding calliper measurements, huge errors are encountered when trying to measure large tumours (*i.e.* larger than 1.5 cm^3). Moreover, when using tumour models which present large necrotic areas (or a large number of smaller necrotic areas), sliding calliper measurements cannot account for these necrotic parts, thus causing errors in the measurement of the tumour tissue. MRI-based methods can account for these necrotic areas (see below). A third, less important reason why MRI-based volume measurements should be considered, is its superior spatial resolution. Especially in subcutaneously inoculated tumours, the volume of the tumour can be measured very accurately and reproducibly.

The fact that semi-automated volume measurements yielded significantly different values compared with the gold standard is explained by the exclusion of necrotic tissue areas by the semi-automated method. Necrosis is primarily seen in larger tumours. Indeed, when excluding tumours bigger than 1.5 cm^3 as measured by water volumetry, the Wilcoxon signed-rank test does not show any significant difference between both groups (assymptomatic significance=0.063). The paired samples *t*-test could not been used anymore because the data for region growing volumetry were not normally distributed anymore (Shapiro-Wilks coefficient=0.87). Interoperator and intraoperator reliability for the region growing method was however good. Therefore, it is recommended to use the semi-automated method for the measurement of tumour volumes in mice, because it is both reliable and accurate for smaller tumour volumes ($<$1.5 cm^3). In the case of larger tumours, the method is reliable and it accounts for necrotic areas within the tumour.

Conclusion

Both manual and semi-automated tumour volumetry in subcutaneous tumour bearing athymic mice by low-field MRI are accurate and reliable methods. The semi-automated method is especially useful for larger tumour volumes, since it accounts for necrotic areas within the tumour.

References

1. Coakley FV, Kurhanewicz J, Lu Y, Jones KD, Swanson MG, Chang SD, et al. Prostate cancer tumor volume: measurement with endorectal MR and MR spectroscopic imaging. Radiology 2002;223:91–7.
2. Gibbs P, Buckley DL, Blackband SJ, Horsman A. Tumour volume determination from MR images by morphological segmentation. Phys Med Biol 1996;41:2437–46.
3. Joe BN, Fukui MB, Meltzer CC, Huang Q-S, Day RS, Greer PJ, et al. Brain tumor volume measurement: comparison of manual and semiautomated methods. Radiology 1999;212: 811–6.

4. Kaus MR, Warfield SK, Nabavi A, Black PM, Jolsz FA, Kikinis R. Automated segmentation of MR images of brain tumors. Radiology 2001;218:586–91.
5. Lundin P, Engström BE, Karlsson FA, Burman P. Long-term octreotide therapy in growth hormone-secreting pituitary adenomas: evaluation with serial MR. Am J Neuroradiol 1997;18:765–72.
6. Mayr NA, Taoka T, Yuh WT, Denning LM, Zhen WK, Paulino AC, et al. Method and timing of tumor volume measurement for outcome prediction in cervical cancer using magnetic resonance imaging. Int J Radiat Oncol Biol Phys 2002;52:14–22.
7. Stamey TA, McNeal JE, Yemoto CM, Sigal BM, Johnstone IM. Biological determinants of cancer progression in men with prostate cancer. JAMA 1999;281:1395–400.
8. End DW, Smets G, Todd AV, Applegate TL, Fuery CJ, Angibaud P, et al. Characterisation of the antitumour effects of the selective farnesyl protein transferase inhibitor R115777 in vivo and in vitro. Cancer Res 2001;6: 131–7.
9. Orlova A, Bruskin A, Sjöström A, Lundqvist H, Gedda L, Tolmachev V. Cellular processing of 125I- and 111In-labelled epidermal growth factor (EGF) bound to cultured A431 tumor cells. Nucl Med Biol 2000;27:827–35.
10. Sundberg AL, Almqvist Y, Orlova A, Blomquist E, Jensen HJ, Gedda L, et al. Combined effect of gefitinib ('Iressa', ZD1839) and targeted radiotherapy with 211At-EGF. Eur J Nucl Med Mol Imaging 2003;30:1348–56.
11. Van den Berg AP. Enkele kernpunten bij onderzoekskunst en bewerking van resultaten. Personal communication.
12. Waterton JC, Alott CP, Pickford R, Hamilton EA, Valcaccia B. Assessment of mouse tumour xenograft volumes in vivo by ultrasound imaging, MRI and calliper measurement. Proceedings of the 19th LH Gray Conference: Quantitative Imaging in Oncology 146–149; Eds Faulkner K, Carey B, Crellin A, Harisson RM. BIR, London 1997.
13. Hardy PA, Recht MP, Piraino D, Thomasson D. Optimization of a dual echo in the steady state (DESS) free-precession sequence for imaging cartilage. J Magn Reson Imaging 1996;6:329–35.

The British Journal of Radiology, *78* (2005), 343–345
DOI: 10.1259/bjr/95232584

Case report

An ovary in luteal phase mimicking common iliac lymph node metastasis from a primary cutaneous peripheral primitive neuroectodermal tumour as revealed by 18-fluoro-2-deoxyglucose positron emission tomography

[1]K-C HO, [2]K-K NG, [1]T-C YEN and ^{3}H-H CHOU, MD

[1]*Department of Nuclear Medicine,* [2]*Department of Radiology and* [3]*Division of Gynecologic Oncology, Department of Obstetrics and Gynecology, Chang Gung Memorial Hospital and University, Taoyuan, Taiwan*

Abstract. A 30-year-old female underwent surgical removal of a primary cutaneous peripheral primitive neuroectodermal tumour (PNET) of the left thigh. A subsequent 18-fluoro-2-deoxyglucose (FDG) positron emission tomography (PET) scan showed abnormal accumulation of FDG in the left upper pelvic region, consistent with metastasis to a left common iliac node. A series of follow-up imaging studies revealed that a cyst of the corpus luteum of ovary was responsible for the abnormal FDG accumulation.

Primary cutaneous peripheral primitive neuroectodermal tumours constitute a rare presentation of peripheral neuroectodermal tumours (PNETs), which are mainly observed in deep soft tissue. Although primary cutaneous peripheral PNET has a more favourable outcome than other forms of PNET, distant metastasis is still a major concern [1–3]. 18-fluoro-2-deoxyglucose (FDG) positron emission tomography (PET) has proven valuable in detecting primary and local recurrent soft tissue sarcomas [4, 5]. FDG PET is therefore potentially useful for the initial staging and follow-up studies of PNET. Since lymph nodes are possible sites for distant metastases in primary cutaneous PNET [2, 3], any abnormal FDG uptake in the region of the lymph nodes should be carefully examined. We report here a false-positive FDG PET finding for a metastatic common iliac lymph node. Uptake of FDG was later found to be attributable to the luteal phase of left ovary, which was located in the left upper pelvic region. The pattern of uptake in a corpus luteum cyst using FDG PET scanning and possible causes of increased ovarian FDG uptake are discussed.

Case report

A 30-year-old female had a superficial, soft tissue lump in the posterior left thigh for 1 year. The raised mass was freely movable and painless. She conceived 1 month after a small mass was noted, and the mass grew slowly throughout pregnancy. An epidermal cyst was the initial diagnosis. 1 month after delivery, local excision of the mass was performed. Histopathology revealed PNET of the skin, confirmed by immunohistochemical studies. Thereafter, she underwent whole body CT, a bone scan, an MRI for the abdomen and lower limbs, and a whole body PET scan. All were negative for a malignant lesion. Owing to negative section margins and negative images results, she did not receive adjuvant chemotherapy or radiotherapy. 5 months after the initial operation, she had a whole body FDG PET scan for regular follow-up. A focal area of increased FDG uptake (maximum standard uptake value was 4.68) in the left common iliac lymph node region was revealed (Figure 1A). A CT scan, which was performed for further confirmation, revealed an enlarged (3.7 cm) complex cystic lesion in the left external iliac region (Figure 1B). A metastatic lesion to the left common iliac lymph node could not be ruled out. Subsequent ultrasound demonstrated rich flow in the left ovary with a resistive index value lower than 0.4, indicating a hypervascular lesion, and consistent with either a tumour or a corpus luteum cyst. MRI findings were compatible with a left adnexal lesion with no evidence of intra-abdominal lymphadenopathy (Figure 1C), but an intraovary metastatic lesion could not be differentiated from a corpus luteum cyst. After reviewing the patient's menstrual history, another MRI and ultrasound were performed 2 weeks later to rule out the possibility of a false-positive finding. In the follow-up MRI, a corpus luteum cyst was found in a normal-sized left ovary (Figure 2). This dynamic change was also observed with colour Doppler flow. This patient has been followed up regularly and has remained disease-free for 18 months.

Discussion

Peripheral PNET is a highly malignant neoplasm usually involving bone and/or the deeper soft tissues [6]. Rarely it occurs as a primary, superficially-based neoplasm in children and young adults [1]. Deeply located PNETs are aggressive neoplasms with a capability for widespread metastasis. Because reports concerning

Received 16 August 2004 and accepted 25 November 2004.

Address correspondence to Dr Hung-Hsueh Chou, Division of Gynecologic Oncology, Department of Obstetrics and Gynecology, Chang Gung Memorial Hospital & Chang Gung University, 5 Fu-Shin Street, Kueishan, Taoyuan 333, Taiwan.

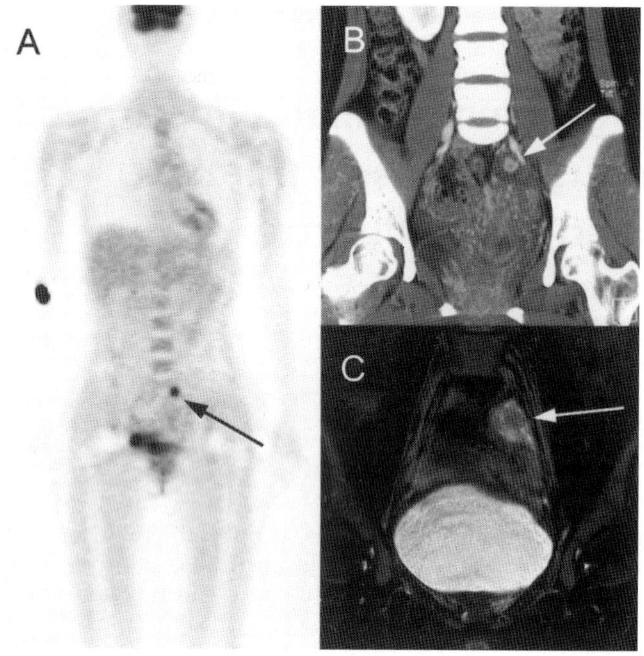

Figure 1. (A) FDG PET scan revealed an FDG avid lesion in the left common iliac lymph node region. (B) CT scan showed a 3.7 cm complex cystic lesion in the left adnexa. (C) T_2 weighted coronal MR image with fat suppression (repetition time (TR)=4000 ms, echo time (TE)=99 ms) demonstrated a comparable left adnexa lesion near the common iliac lymph node region.

primitive cutaneous peripheral PNET are limited, predictions regarding the behaviour of these tumours are not easy [3]. Although cutaneous presentations of peripheral PNET may represent a clinically favourable subset of PNETs [1], distant metastases to lung, bone and lymph node have been reported [2, 3]. PNET, a soft tissue sarcoma variance, is a possible candidate for FDG PET scans [4, 5]. We used PET for initial staging and for locating possible recurrence in a patient presenting initially with a primary cutaneous peripheral primitive neuroectodermal tumour.

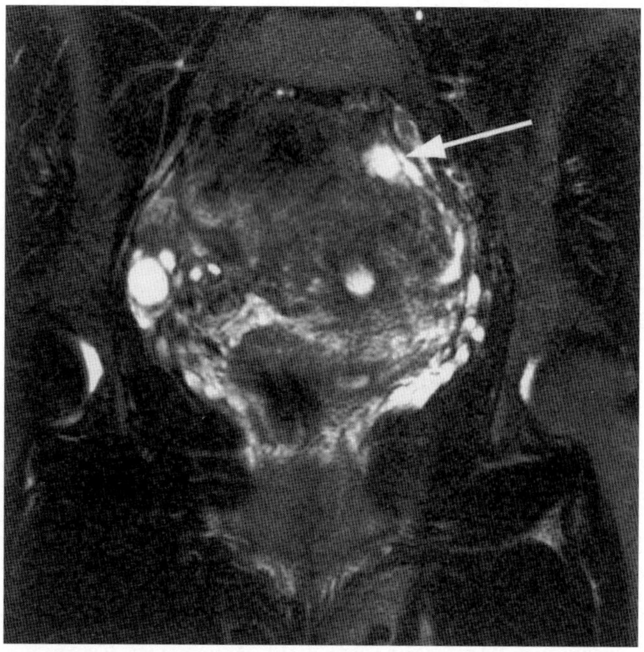

Figure 2. Follow-up T_2 weighted coronal MR image with fat suppression (repetition time (TR)=5269 ms, echo time (TE)=132 ms) showed multiple small cystic changes in rosette form in the left ovary, compatible with lutein cysts.

In this study, the follow-up FDG PET scan (5 months after wide excision treatment) demonstrated a focal increased FDG uptake near the left common iliac lymph node region, possibly located at the lymphatic drainage route of the primary tumour at the posterior aspect of the left thigh. As lymph nodes were possible metastatic sites for primary cutaneous PNET, left common iliac lymph node metastasis was suspected initially. A false-positive PET scan owing to a corpus luteum cyst was confirmed by a series of follow-up image studies.

False-positive FDG PET findings in corpus luteum cysts of the ovary have been reported previously. In a study to correlate FDG PET and histopathological findings of asymptomatic adnexal masses, one of five corpus luteum cysts (20%) showed a false-positive result [7]. False-positive FDG uptake was found in two corpus luteum cysts in another study for pre-operative assessment of asymptomatic adnexal tumours [8]. In a recent study using PET/CT to assess normal ovarian FDG uptake, increased uptake into functional ovarian cysts was observed in 15 of 21 pre-menopausal patients without known gynaecological malignancy [9]. Corpus luteum development is a complex process involving mechanisms that are similar to wound healing and tumour formation. An essential component of corpus luteum development is the recruitment of a blood supply [10]. The mechanisms associated with such development may explain how the ovary in luteal phase was considered to be a "tumour-like" mass with higher FDG uptake in PET imaging and revealed a low resistive index of ultrasound in our case.

In summary, both malignant and functional ovarian lesions can exhibit abnormal FDG uptake. Detection of a dominant functional ovarian cyst on CT and discussion of the menstrual cycle phase with patient in question should assist in differentiating physiological from malignant FDG ovarian uptake [9].

References

1. Hasegawa SL, Davison JM, Rutten A, Fletcher JA, Fletcher CD. Primary cutaneous Ewing's sarcoma: immunophenotypic and molecular cytogenetic evaluation of five cases. Am J Surg Pathol 1998;22:310–8.
2. Chow E, Merchant TE, Pappo A, Jenkins JJ, Shah AB, Kun LE. Cutaneous and subcutaneous Ewing's sarcoma: an indolent disease. Int J Radiat Oncol Biol Phys 2000;46:433–8.
3. Banerjee SS, Agbamu DA, Eyden BP, Harris M. Clinicopathological characteristics of peripheral primitive neuroectodermal tumour of skin and subcutaneous tissue. Histopathology 1997;31:355–66.
4. Schwarzbach MH, Dimitrakopoulou-Strauss A, Willeke F, Hinz U, Strauss LG, Zhang YM, et al. Clinical value of [18-F] fluorodeoxyglucose positron emission tomography imaging in soft tissue sarcomas. Ann Surg 2000;231:380–6.
5. Lucas JD, O'Doherty MJ, Cronin BF, Marsden PK, Lodge MA, McKee PH, et al. Prospective evaluation of soft tissue masses and sarcomas using fluorodeoxyglucose positron emission tomography. Br J Surg 1999;86:550–6.

6. Lee CS, Southey MC, Slater H, Auldist AW, Chow CW, Venter DJ. Primary cutaneous Ewing's sarcoma/peripheral primitive neuroectodermal tumors in childhood. A molecular, cytogenetic, and immunohistochemical study. Diagn Mol Pathol 1995;4:174–81.
7. Fenchel S, Grab D, Nuessle K, Kotzerke J, Rieber A, Kreienberg R, et al. Asymptomatic adnexal masses: correlation of FDG PET and histopathologic findings. Radiology 2002;223:780–8.
8. Fenchel S, Kotzerke J, Stohr I, Grab D, Nussle K, Rieber A, et al. Preoperative assessment of asymptomatic adnexal tumors by positron emission tomography and F-18 fluorodeoxyglucose. Nuklearmedizin 1999;38:101–7.
9. Lerman H, Metser U, Grisaru D, Fishman A, Lievshitz G, Even-Sapir E. Normal and abnormal 18F-FDG endometrial and ovarian uptake in pre- and postmenopausal patients: assessment by PET/CT. J Nucl Med 2004;45:266–71.
10. Smith MF, McIntush EW, Smith GW. Mechanisms associated with corpus luteum development. J Anim Sci 1994;72:1857–72.

The British Journal of Radiology, *78* (2005), 346–348
DOI: 10.1259/bjr/12933217

Case report

Papillary necrosis causing hydronephrosis in renal allograft treated by percutaneous retrieval of sloughed papilla

[1]S KAMATH, MD, MRCP, [2]M P MOODY, FRCS, [2]J C HAMMONDS, FRCS and [1]I P WELLS, MRCS, LRCP, FRCR

Departments of [1]Radiology and [2]Urology, Derriford Hospital, Plymouth PL6 8DH, UK

Abstract. Obstructive uropathy is the second most common urological complication in a transplanted kidney. The usual causes of obstruction are ureteral stenosis and calculi. Papillary necrosis as a cause of obstruction in a transplant kidney is extremely rare with only one prior report published. Moreover, percutaneous removal of sloughed papilla in a transplant kidney has not previously been reported. We report an unusual case of a sloughed papilla causing hydronephrosis of a transplant kidney and its successful percutaneous removal. The recognition of renal papillary necrosis is important, not only because it can be a sign of acute rejection but also it because it can lead to obstruction, infection and potentially the loss of the transplant as exemplified by our case. Rapid diagnosis and meticulous retrieval technique are the crucial factors in minimizing the complications due to obstruction of a transplanted kidney by sloughed papilla.

Obstruction to a transplant kidney can result from a variety of causes including ureteral anastomotic stenosis, urolithiasis, blood clot and fungal ball. However, a sloughed papilla resulting from papillary necrosis as a cause of obstruction in a transplant kidney is extremely rare and has only been reported once to date [1]. Moreover, the percutaneous removal of the sloughed papilla in a transplant kidney has not previously been reported. We report the successful percutaneous removal of a sloughed papilla, causing hydronephrosis of a transplant kidney.

Case report

A 57-year-old diabetic woman presented with a 1-week history of fever, dysuria and decreasing urine output leading to anuria for 2 days. She had received a cadaveric renal transplant 4 years previously for adult polycystic kidney disease.

Examination revealed pyrexia of 38.4℃, tachycardia of 98 beats per minute (bpm) and tenderness over the transplant in the right iliac fossa. Her biochemistry revealed a urea of 31.5 mmol l^{-1} and a creatinine of 559 μmol l^{-1}. Blood cultures revealed proteus bacteraemia. The previous renal function tests performed 2 months before admission had revealed the following: urea 15 mmol l^{-1} and creatinine 210 μmol l^{-1}.

Ultrasound demonstrated a moderate hydronephrosis of the transplant kidney with an obstructing lesion at the pelviureteric junction. A provisional diagnosis of pyonephrosis of the transplant kidney leading to bacteraemia was made. Percutaneous nephrostomy was performed, which drained cloudy urine. A nephrostogram confirmed a smooth filling defect in the renal pelvis, which extended into the proximal ureter (Figure 1).

The obstructing lesion was thought to be amenable to percutaneous removal, which was performed 2 weeks later. A nephrostogram immediately prior to the attempted removal demonstrated a large defect (papillary ulcer) in the lower pole calyces with extensive loss of papillary tissue (Figure 2). The obstructing lesion was therefore thought to be a sloughed renal papilla. The nephrostomy tract into the transplant kidney was dilated up to 30 Fr and using a nephroscope the soft white tissue obstructing the pelviureteric junction of the transplant ureter was

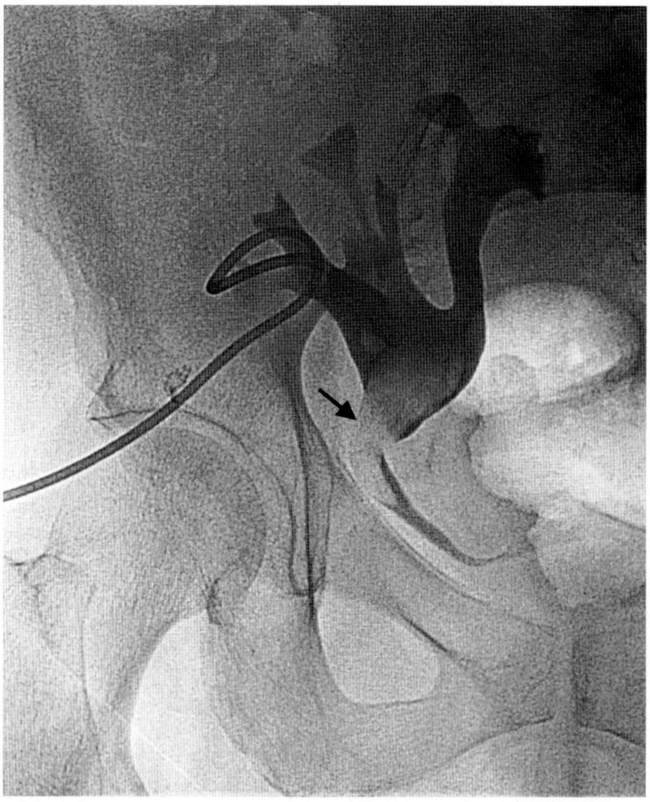

Figure 1. Nephrostogram of the transplant kidney demonstrates a large filling defect (arrow) in the renal pelvis extending into the proximal ureter causing partial obstruction.

Received 18 August 2004 and in revised form 27 October 2004, accepted 25 November 2004.

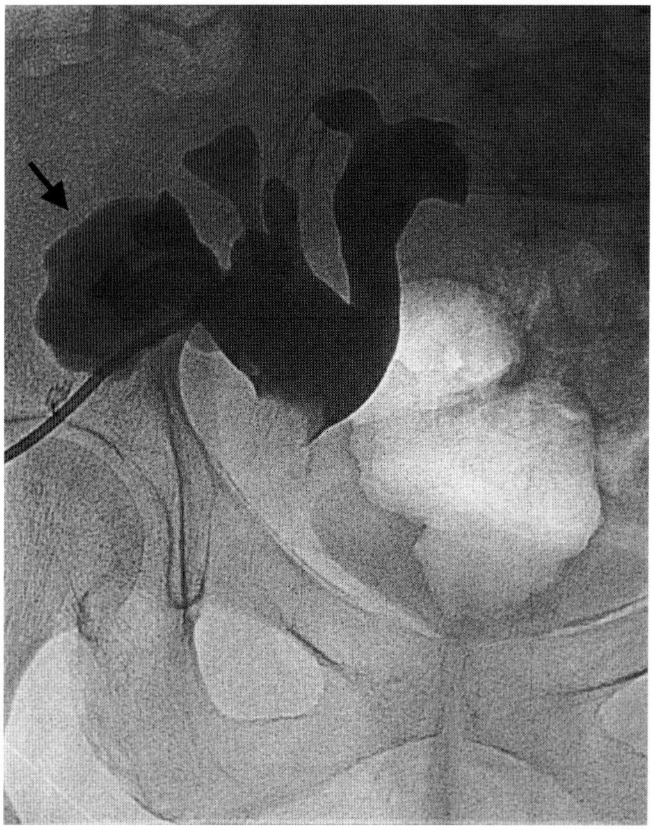

Figure 2. A large sloughed papilla in the renal pelvis extending into the proximal ureter has resulted in complete obstruction to the kidney. A large papillary ulcer (arrow), which is the donor site for the sloughed papilla is demonstrated.

removed in pieces. Subsequently, there was free flow of contrast down the ureter into the bladder (Figure 3) and the specimen was sent for histology. The histology revealed tissue consistent with necrotic sloughed papilla.

The patient continued to improve on antibiotics. Following removal of her nephrostomy drainage catheter, the patient was discharged home 6 days later.

Discussion

The urological complications following renal transplantation vary from 2.9% to 13.4% [2–4]. These include obstructive uropathy, urinary leaks, distal ureteric fistulas (necrosis), vesicoureteral reflux and renal calculi.

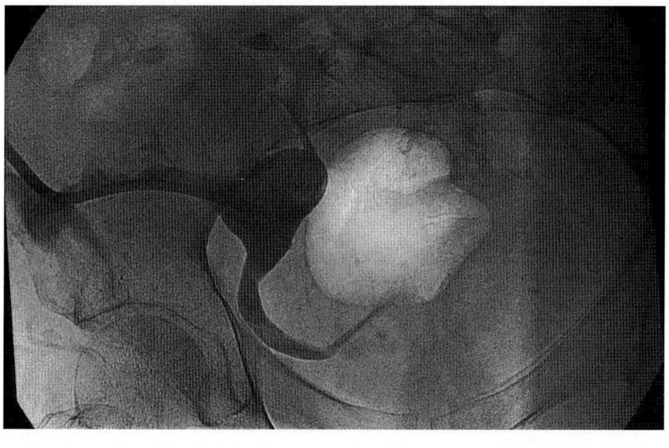

Figure 3. Following percutaneous retrieval of sloughed papilla, there is relief of obstruction.

Obstructive uropathy is second only to urinary leaks as the most frequent urological complication in a transplanted kidney [5] and usually occurs after 1 year following transplantation [6]. While the usual causes of obstruction are ureteral stenosis and calculi, unusual causes include granulomatous disease [7] and fungal bezoars [8]. In the past, a significant proportion of patients with renal transplant underwent open surgical procedures for the treatment of obstruction [9]. However with advances in technology these complications are now treated more often by percutaneous and/or endoscopic techniques.

Obstruction to a native kidney from a sloughed papilla resulting from renal papillary necrosis is a well-recognized entity [10]. Similarly, renal papillary necrosis in a transplant kidney is not unusual. However, hydronephrosis resulting from obstruction to a transplant kidney from a sloughed renal papilla is extremely unusual and only one such case has been reported to date [1].

Papillary necrosis in renal transplant patients is most commonly associated with acute or chronic rejection [11] causing ischaemia due to decreased perfusion of the renal medulla. However, it can also be found in acute tubular necrosis, diabetes, acute bacterial or fungal infection and analgesic usage [11–18]. Renal papillary necrosis, though thought to be a rather late complication in patients with a renal allograft, (an average of 28.1 months after transplantation) can occur as early as 2 months after transplantation [11].

The abnormality in transplant renal morphology following papillary necrosis varies from dilatation and clubbing of calyces in milder form to severe deformity with papillary ulcers and extensive loss of papillary tissue as in our case [11, 13]. Recognition of renal papillary necrosis is important not only because it can be a sign of acute rejection but also because it can lead to various complications such as obstruction, infection and potentially the loss of the transplant. In the only previously reported case of obstructed transplanted kidney due to sloughed papilla, the patient underwent nephrectomy. However, we demonstrate that percutaneous/endoscopic removal of the sloughed papilla is possible resulting in relief of obstruction and improvement in the renal function. To our knowledge, this is the first reported case of percutaneous retrieval of a sloughed papilla from a transplant renal pelvis with subsequent relief of obstruction.

References

1. Shapeero LG, Vordermark JS. Papillary necrosis causing hydronephrosis in the renal allograft. Sonographic findings. J Ultrasound Med 1989;8:579–81.
2. Sert S, Gulay H, Hamaloglu E, Haberal M. Urological complications in 350 consecutive renal transplants. Br J Urol 1990;66:568–71.
3. Shoskes DA, Hanbury D, Cranston D, Morris PJ. Urological complications in 1,000 consecutive renal transplant recipients. J Urol 1995;153:18–21.
4. Mehta SN, Kennedy JA, Loughridge WG, Douglas JF, Donaldson RA, McGeown MG. Urological complications in 119 consecutive renal transplants. Br J Urol 1979;51:184–7.

5. Pappas P, Giannopoulos A, Stravodimos KG, Zavos G, Alexopoulos T, Boletis J, et al. Obstructive uropathy in the transplanted kidney: definitive management with percutaneous nephrostomy and prolonged ureteral stenting. J Endourol 2001;15:719–23.
6. Benoit G, Thiounn N, Opsal C, Hiesse C, Moukarzel M, Neyrat N, et al. Urologic complications in kidney transplantations. Indication for endo-urologic techniques. Presse Med 1991;20:2050–1.
7. Rich LM, Piering WF. Ureteral stenosis due to recurrent Wegener's granulomatosis after kidney transplantation. J Am Soc Nephrol 1994;4:1516–21.
8. Kamel G, Stephan A, Barbari A, Kilani H, Karam A, Zeineh S, et al. Obstructive anuria due to fungal bezoars in a renal graft recipient. Transplant Proc 2003;35:2692–3.
9. Oosterhof GO, Hoitsma AJ, Witjes JA, Debruyne FM. Diagnosis and treatment of urological complications in kidney transplantation. Urol Int 1992;49:99–103.
10. Vijayaraghavan SB, Kandasamy SV, Mylsamy A, Prabhakar M. Sonographic features of necrosed renal papillae causing hydronephrosis. J Ultrasound Med 2003;22:951–6.
11. Kaude JV, Stone M, Fuller TJ, Cade R, Tarrant DG, Juncos LI. Papillary necrosis in kidney transplant patients. Radiology 1976;120:69–74.
12. Edmondson RP, Fawcett IW, Jones NF, Thompson AE, Wing AJ. Papillary necrosis in a transplanted kidney. Br Med J 1972;1:547.
13. Knepshield JH, Feller HA, Leb DE. Papillary necrosis due to Candida albicans in a renal allograft. Arch Intern Med 1968;122:441–4.
14. Whitworth JA, Leroux-Robert C, Meyrier A, Morel-Maroger L, Scetbon V, Sraer JD. Papillary necrosis in renal allografts-report of 2 cases. Aust N Z J Med 1975;5:69–71.
15. Tuma S, Chaimowitz C, Erlik D, Gellei B, Rosenberger A, Better OS. Fatal papillary necrosis in a kidney graft. JAMA 1976;235:754–5.
16. Hoffman JC, Schnur MJ, Koenigsberg M. Demonstration of renal papillary necrosis by sonography. Radiology 1982;145:785–7.
17. Kincaid-Smith P. Histological diagnosis of rejection of renal homografts in man. Lancet 1967;2:849–52.
18. Eknoyan G, Qunibi WY, Grissom RT, Tuma SN, Ayus JC. Renal papillary necrosis: an update. Medicine 1982;61:55–73.

The British Journal of Radiology, 78 (2005), 349–352 © 2005 The British Institute of Radiology
DOI: 10.1259/bjr/30076658

Case report

The absent kidney in ^{99}Tc^{m}-MAG3 renogram: a dramatic reversible consequence of contrast nephrotoxicity superimposed on renal obstruction

I KAYANI, FRCR, A M GROVES, FRCR, R SYED, FRCS, N NAGABUSHAN, MRCP, F PAKZAD, MRCS, E M PRVULOVICH, MSc, MD and J B BOMANJI, MB BS, MSc, PhD

Institute of Nuclear Medicine, Middlesex Hospital, Mortimer Street, London W1T 3AA, UK

Abstract. ^{99}Tc^{m}-mercaptoacetyltriglycine (MAG3) renogram is a robust imaging technique used to delineate upper urinary tract obstruction. The changes observed on the renogram are often reversible on relief of obstruction. We present two cases illustrating the extreme consequence of contrast nephrotoxicity on pre-existing obstructed kidneys. In one case, this led to severe impairment of perfusion and uptake observed on ^{99}Tc^{m}-MAG3 renogram and in the second case virtual non-visualization of the obstructed kidney. Subsequent treatment of obstruction, led to dramatic improvement in renal function. It is important for clinicians, nuclear medicine physicians and radiologists to be aware of the potential of contrast nephrotoxicity in obstructed kidneys.

^{99}Tc^{m}-mercaptoacetyltriglycine (MAG3) is an integral part of investigation in patients with suspected upper urinary tract obstruction [1–3]. The ^{99}Tc^{m}-MAG3 renogram helps confirm obstruction, estimate differential renal function and monitor the success of interventional procedures to relieve obstruction. As part of pre-intervention assessment, patients may receive intravenous (IV) contrast, usually for intravenous urogram (IVU) examination or less commonly during CT angiogram for the assessment of pelviureteric junction (PUJ) obstruction. There is a well-documented risk of nephrotoxicity following administration of IV contrast media [4–6]. This is rare (less than 2%) in patients with normal renal function but occurs in up to 25% of patients with predisposing conditions [5, 6]. Contrast nephrotoxicity may be superimposed on changes owing to urinary obstruction in the ^{99}Tc^{m}-MAG3 renogram.

We present two cases where severe but reversible unilateral renal impairment occurred following intravenous contrast administration.

Case one

A 73-year-old female was admitted for further investigation and treatment of right pelviureteric obstruction. There was a history of intermittent right loin pain and urinary tract infection but during the course of admission she remained clinically well and asymptomatic. A ^{99}Tc^{m}-MAG3 renogram performed at her referring hospital 1 month prior to admission had demonstrated reduced perfusion of the right kidney compared with the left kidney, with right cortical tracer retention and 37% of total function in right kidney.

Further assessment with a CT angiogram (Siemens Somatom Plus 4 Volume Zoom, Forcheim, Germany) with 130 ml of Iohexol (300 mg Iodine ml^{-1}) was performed. This showed normal cortical thickness but reduced perfusion of the right kidney with the right renal artery stretched over a dilated right renal pelvis (Figure 1). A ^{99}Tc^{m}-MAG3 scan 4 days later (Figure 2a) showed virtually no tracer activity in the right kidney and a normal left kidney. 2 days later a Doppler ultrasound confirmed perfusion of the right kidney but with an elevated resistive index (RI) of 0.88. A repeat ^{99}Tc^{m}-MAG3 scan (Figure 2b), performed the following day (8 days post CT angiogram) showed tracer uptake in the right kidney with a prolonged nephrogenic phase of activity and a differential function of 17%. A week later, a retrograde ureterogram confirmed a right PUJ obstruction and a ureteric stent was placed. Ureteric brushings were negative for malignancy on cytological examination.

A ^{99}Tc^{m}-MAG3 scan performed 7 weeks after ureteric stent placement (Figure 2c) showed significant recovery of right-sided renal perfusion and function with good excretion of tracer. The right kidney now contributed 30% of total renal function. Further ^{99}Tc^{m}-MAG3 follow-up studies have shown no change in differential function or outflow pattern of tracer from the right kidney.

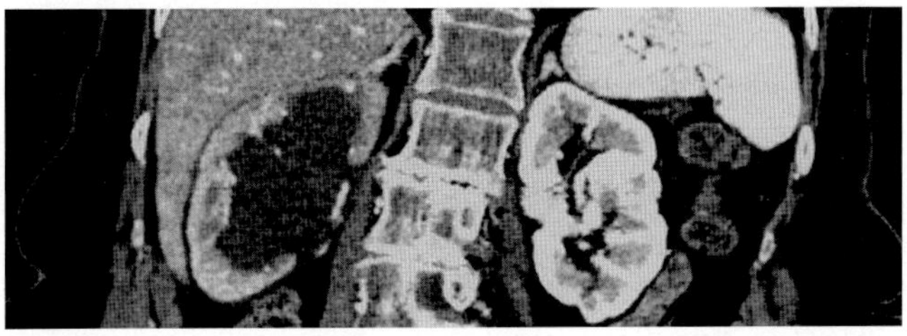

Figure 1. Case 1: CT arterial phase renal angiogram (Siemens Somatom Plus 4 Volume Zoom, Forcheim, Germany). Coronal multiplanar reconstruction image; there is clear reduction in perfusion (enhancement) of the right kidney and gross dilatation of the renal calyces.

Received 15 July 2004 and in final form 10 November 2004 and accepted, accepted 6 December 2004.

Address correspondence to Dr Jamshed B Bomanji.

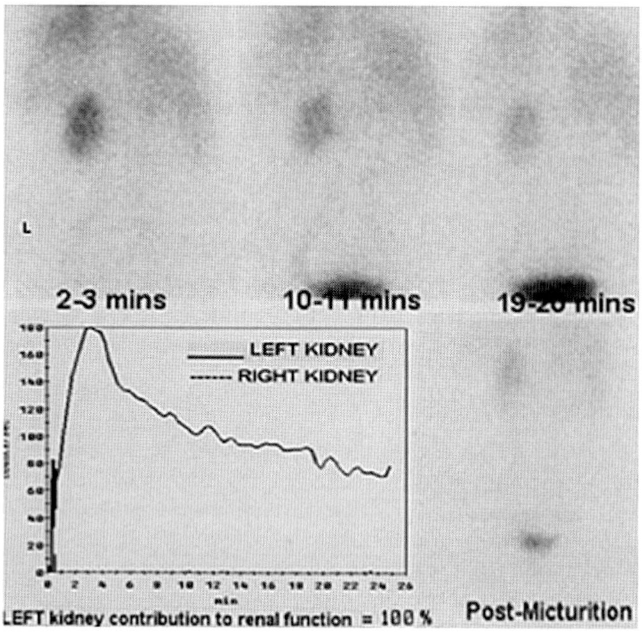

(a)

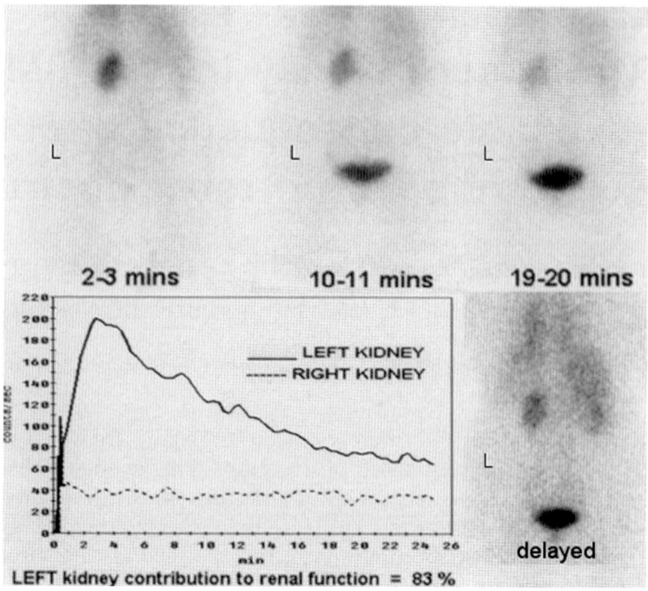

(b)

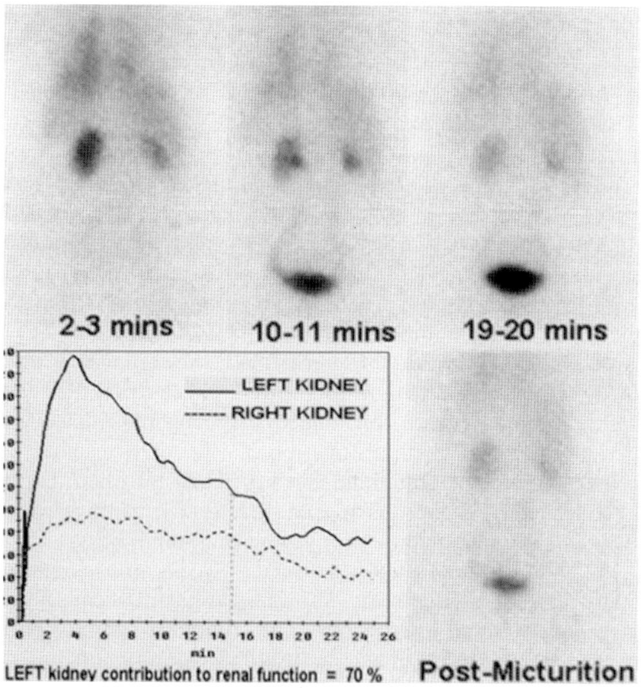

(c)

Figure 2. Case 1: (a) $^{99}Tc^{m}$-MAG3 renogram 4 days post CT angiogram. The right kidney appears to be absent, no tracer uptake can be identified in the right kidney. (b) Follow up renogram 2 days later, shows a poorly perfused right kidney with prolonged nephrogenic phase of activity. (c) $^{99}Tc^{m}$-MAG3 renogram 6 weeks later following ureteric stent placement shows good perfusion, significant recovery of function and rapid excretion of tracer.

Case two

A 61-year-old man with Parkinson's disease presented with intermittent loin pain over several weeks, microscopic haematuria and normal serum urea and electrolytes. An IVU (70 ml 300 mg ml^{-1} Iohexol) showed a left nephrogram but no left sided contrast excretion. The right renal tract was normal. A further bolus of 70 ml Iohexol 300 mg l^{-1}was given (total dose 140 ml 600 mg l^{-1}), but despite the second dose subsequent films failed to show any contrast excretion from the left kidney with a persistent left nephrogram on a delayed 72 h film. An ultrasound, performed on the same day revealed only mild pelvicalyceal dilatation (anteroposterior (AP) pelvis diameter 1.1 cm).

The patient remained clinically well but 72 h post-IVU the serum urea and creatinine rose to 148 μmol l^{-1} and 9.2 mmol l^{-1}, respectively. A $^{99}Tc^{m}$-MAG3 renogram (5 days post IVU) was performed to further evaluate the left kidney (Figure 3a). The left kidney was poorly perfused with poor uptake and virtually no excretion of tracer and a divided renal function of less than 10% in the left kidney. The right renal appearance and uptake was within normal limits.

A nephrostomy was placed in the left kidney and a subsequent contrast enhanced CT scan of the abdomen revealed retroperitoneal fibrosis as a likely cause of urinary obstruction. The fibrosis was probably induced by pergolide prescribed for Parkinson's disease. Urea and

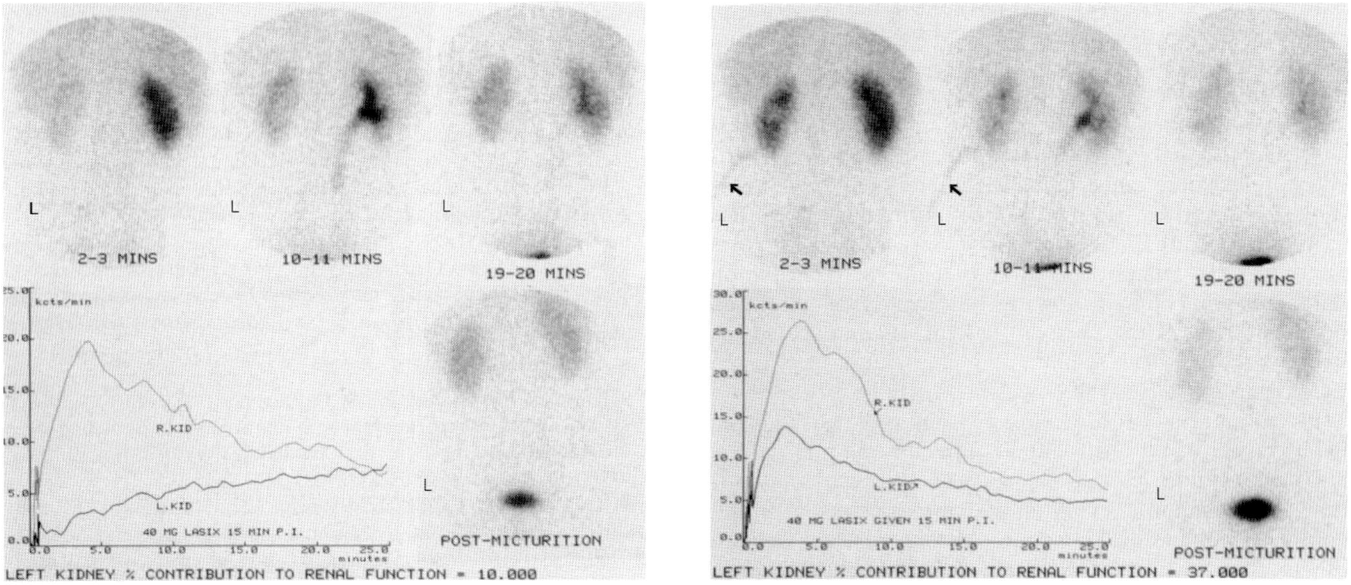

(a) (b)

Figure 3. Case 2: (a) ^{99}Tc^{m}-MAG3 renogram 5 days after high dose urography demonstrates severe reduction in perfusion and function of left kidney with no excretion of tracer. (b) Follow up renogram 6 weeks post placement of left nephrostomy (arrows); there is improved perfusion of left kidney, dramatic improvement in left renal function and normal excretion of tracer.

electrolytes normalized within 10 days of the nephrostomy and a repeat ^{99}Tc^{m}-MAG3, 6 weeks later (Figure 3b) showed good, almost symmetric perfusion of the left kidney with brisk excretion of tracer. The left kidney contributed 37% to the total renal function compared with 10% pre-nephrostomy.

The patient underwent bilateral ureterolysis (surgical release of ureter by blunt dissection). During the procedure a retroperitoneal biopsy was performed which was consistent with retroperitoneal fibrosis. Follow-up over 4 years with yearly ^{99}Tc^{m}-MAG3 renograms have shown no change in differential function or outflow pattern of tracer from the left kidney.

Discussion

Unilateral, reversible, shutdown of renal perfusion is an uncommon occurrence in clinical practice. In the two cases we describe, there were some common features, which could have caused rapid loss of renal function. Both patients were exposed to intravenous contrast and their kidneys were already incompletely obstructed secondary to a unilateral PUJ obstruction in case 1 and retroperitoneal fibrosis in case 2. It is likely that both patients had an acute on chronic renal insult, which led to virtual unilateral renal shutdown.

The one common trigger, which led to this chain of events, was the intravenous administration of a rapid and large volume iohexol contrast bolus. A number of mechanisms are responsible for contrast nephrotoxicity [5, 7, 8]. Contrast media induced diuresis leads to increased tubular and interstitial pressure leading to compression of small renal vessels. Contrast media stimulate the release of endothelin and also induce aggregation of red blood cells. The net effect of these changes is to reduce renal blood flow. In addition diuresis causes increased metabolic activity of tubular cells leading to medullary hypoxia and contrast media have a direct cellular toxic effect [5]. Contrast nephrotoxicity is exaggerated in the presence of volume depletion and pre-existing renal impairment [5, 6]. The classical pattern of contrast-induced nephrotoxicity on a ^{99}Tc^{m}-MAG3 study (which is dominantly secreted by the tubules) mimics acute tubular necrosis and involves both kidneys. The ^{99}Tc^{m}-MAG3 scan shows reduced perfusion of the kidneys coupled with tracer accumulation in the renal parenchyma and virtually no excretion of activity [9, 10]. It is uncommon to observe such a pattern in one kidney only.

It could be argued that acute renal obstruction could have caused rapid loss of renal perfusion and that it was not due to contrast in both cases. It has been shown that acute urinary obstruction is associated with reduction in medullary renal blood flow, with apoptosis of tubular cell as early as 2 h post ureteral ligation [7]. The second case illustrates the changes expected with severe obstruction (Figure 3). There was reduced perfusion and uptake of ^{99}Tc^{m}-MAG3 with non-visualization of the intrarenal and extrarenal tract and virtually no drainage from the kidney even after frusemide diuresis (40 mg IV, bolus). This was depicted graphically as a rising time-activity curve. However, reduction in perfusion does not lead to a virtual absence of activity on an isotope renogram, unless there is a second superimposed renal insult. In case two, superimposed contrast induced nephrotoxicity would explain the transient unilateral renal shutdown. The patient had undergone high dose urography a few days prior to the ^{99}Tc^{m}-MAG3 renogram and had evidence of contrast induced nephrotoxicity with a subsequent rise in serum urea and creatinine. Indeed there is experimental evidence that contrast media exacerbates medullary ischaemia in obstructed kidneys [7]. In the first case, non-visualization of the kidney on ^{99}Tc^{m}-MAG3 renogram (Figure 2a) was more extreme and beyond the changes expected with classic severe obstructive nephropathy. Interestingly, the patient had suffered no clinical symptoms in the interval between the initial $^{99}Tc^{m}$-MAG3 (done 1 month prior to the CT angiogram) and the $^{99}Tc^{m}$-MAG3 demonstrating absent right renal perfusion. It is reasonable to attribute the severe decline in renal perfusion post CT angiogram, at least in greater part to contrast induced nephrotoxicity. There were two risk factors for contrast nephrotoxicity; pre-existing renal impairment and age >70 years [11, 12]. Another possible compounding factor in this case, was the presence of urinary obstruction [7, 8]. It is also possible, that the marked renal pelvis dilation impaired renal blood flow in the overlying stretched renal arteries. These vessels have been implicated as markers of surgical failure, and can cause or worsen PUJ obstruction [13–15].

Predicting functional recovery from contrast induced nephrotoxicity and obstruction is difficult and may take a few days to several weeks. It has been suggested that it is best to allow an interval of at least 2 weeks after IV contrast medium administration to ensure changes are not due to contrast media [1]. In case two the improvement in function of the involved kidneys, 6 weeks post-stent insertion was probably due to resolution of obstruction and recovery from contrast induced nephrotoxicity. This is a more likely outcome in the context of normal renal cortical thickness demonstrated on the CT scan in both cases. Niemczyk et al [16] used the $^{99}Tc^{m}$-MAG3 renogram to evaluate patients undergoing endopyelotomy for PUJ obstruction and found no improvement in post-operative function when function prior to surgery was less than 30%. Gupta et al [15] found the success rate for open pyelotomy in PUJ obstruction reduced from 80% to 54% for patients with renal function of 25–40% versus function of less than 25%.

Our cases highlight a relatively common clinical scenario. Patients presenting with urinary obstruction often receive IV contrast media in addition to NSAIDs (non steroidal anti inflammatory drugs). There is compelling evidence that the usage of NSAIDS and IV contrast agents results in cumulative renal insult [7]. On this basis caution has been advised over the usage of contrast in patients with urinary obstruction [8]. Documented clinical cases have, however, been lacking. Our cases provide some clinical data to back up the experimental evidence and reinforce the message that caution should be exercised over the usage of contrast media in this scenario. In particular large volumes of intravenous contrast in patients with severe upper urinary tract obstruction can lead to virtually absent perfusion of the involved kidney. Fortunately the potential of significant improvement in renal function following timely treatment is good.

References

1. Brown SCW. Nuclear medicine in the clinical diagnosis and treatment of obstructive uropathy. In: Murray IPC, Ell PJ, editors. Nuclear medicine in clinical diagnosis and treatment (2nd edn). London: Churchill Livingstone, 1998:291–313.
2. Britton KE, Maisey NM. Renal disease. In: Maisey NM, Britton KE, Collier BD, editors. Clinical Nuclear Medicine (3rd edn). Cambridge: Chapman and Hall, 1998:389–24.
3. Sfakianakis GN, Cohen DJ, Braumstein RH, Leveillee RJ, Lerner I, Bird VG, et al. MAG3-F0 scintigraphy in decision making for emergency intervention in renal colic after helical CT positive for a urolith. J Nucl Med 2000;41:1813–22.
4. Barrett BJ. Contrast nephrotoxicity. J Am Soc Nephrol 1994;5:125–37.
5. Rudnick MR, Goldfarb S. Pathogenesis of contrast-induced nephropathy: experimental and clinical observations with an emphasis on the role of osmolality. Rev Cardiovasc Med 2003;4 Suppl. 5:S28–33.
6. Rudnick MR, Goldfarb S, Wexler L, Ludbrook PA, Murphy MJ, Halpern EF, et al. Nephrotoxicity of ionic and nonionic contrast media in 1196 patients: a randomized trial. Kidney Int 1995;47:254–61.
7. Heyman SN, Fuch S, Jaffe R, Shina A, Ellezian L, Brezis M, et al. Renal microcirulcation and tissue damage in during acute ureteral obstruction in the rat: effect of saline infusion, indomethacin and radiocontrast. Kidney Int 1997;51:653–63.
8. Morcos SK. Ureteric obstruction and intravascular administration of contrast media: is there a risk? Br J Radiol 2003;76:564–5.
9. Dhawan RT, Foo M, Bomanji J, Setna F, Ell PJ. Contrast nephrotoxicity and the role of radionuclide renal scan. J Nucl Med 1996;37:1828–30.
10. Oei HY. Dynamic and static renal imaging. In: Murray IPC, Ell PJ, editors. Nuclear medicine in clinical diagnosis and treatment (2nd edn). London: Churchill Livingstone, 1998:29–44.
11. Morcos SK, Thomsen HS. European society of urogenital radiology guidelines on administering contrast media. Abdominal Imaging 2003;28:187–90.
12. Morcos SK, Thomsen HS, Webb JAW. Contrast media safety committee of the european society of urogenital radiology. Contrast media induced nephrotoxicity: a consensus report. Eur Radiol 1999;9:738–40.
13. Khaira HS, Platt JF, Cohan RH, Wolf JS, Faerber GJ. Helical computed tomography for identification of crossing vessels in ureteropelvic junction obstruction-comparison with operative findings. Urology 2003;62:35–9.
14. Rigas A, Karamanolakis D, Bogdanos I, Stefanidis A, Androulakkis PA. Pelvi-ureteric junction obstruction by crossing renal vessels: clinical and imaging features. Br J Urol Int 2003;92:101–3.
15. Gupta M, Tuncay O, Smith AD. Open surgical exploration after failed endopyelotomy: a 12-year perspective. J Urol 1997;157:1613–8.
16. Niemczyk P, Kirsch EB, Zeiger L, Marmar JL. Use of diurtetic renogram in evaluation of patients before and after endopyelotomy. Urology 1999;53:271–5.

The British Journal of Radiology, *78* (2005), 353–354
DOI: 10.1259/bjr/13082711

Case report
MRI and CT findings of cryptococcal vaginitis

[1]S RANGANATHAN, MBBS, MRAD, [1]F MOOSA, MBBS, FRCR, [2]A KAMARULZAMAN, MBBS, FRACP and [3]L M LOOI, MBBS, MPath, FRCPath

Departments of [1]Radiology, [2]Medicine and [3]Pathology, University Malaya Medical Centre, Lembah Pantai, 59100 Kuala Lumpar, Malaysia

Abstract. *Cryptococcus neoformans* is a yeast like fungus, which is commonly found in bird droppings, especially pigeons. Most cases of cryptococcal infections occur in immunocompromised patients or in those who are on long term immunosuppressant therapies. Cryptococcal infection usually presents as a meningoencephalitis or a pulmonary infection. Skin, bone and genital infections are very rare. We report the second case of vaginal cryptococcossis to be reported in English literature and the first to be imaged with CT and MRI.

Case report

A 20-year-old Chinese female was referred with a history of vaginal pain and intermittent per vaginal bleeding for 5 months. Vaginal examination revealed nodularity all over the vagina which resembled adenocarcinoma and a punch biopsy and vaginal smear was taken for analysis. Biopsy revealed cryptococcal vaginitis. The vaginal smear had scanty growth of *Cryptococcus neoformans*, while serology for *Cryptococcus neoformans* antigen was positive at 1:256 dilution.

The patient was treated with oral Flucanozole for 2 months and a single course of vaginal Flucanozole. However, symptoms recurred 3 weeks after completion of treatment. Significant past history was that she had unprotected intercourse with only one partner and underwent a termination of pregnancy at 6 weeks of amenorrhoea a year prior to onset of symptoms. She was not immunocompromised.

The cerebrospinal fluid and blood investigations were negative for detection of Human Immunodeficiency Virus, Hepatitis B and C antigens, and sexually transmitted diseases. CT and MRI were performed to exclude involvement of other sites and to note the extent of the lesion. CT of the brain, chest and abdomen were normal. CT pelvis revealed a mixed attenuation necrotic soft tissue mass arising from the right lateral wall of the vagina involving the right fornix with pockets of air extending up to the lower cervical canal with no involvement of the endocervical canal. The lesion measured 6 cm × 5 cm × 3.5 cm and showed no significant enhancement (Figure 1). There was no apparent involvement of the parametrium. No free fluid was seen in the pelvis and no pelvic lymphadenopathy was present. MRI of the pelvis at 1.5 Tesla showed a high signal intensity lobulated mass within the upper right vaginal wall on the T_2 weighted sequences (Figures 2 and 3) which returned a low signal on T_1 weighted images. The lesion extended into the right lateral fornix, with extension into the lower cervix but without involvement of the endocervical canal. The uterus was normal in size with normal ovaries. The margins of this lesion were clearly demarcated. Following intravenous gadolinium, minimal enhancement of the lesion was noted. A punch biopsy of the vagina showed tissue pieces lined by stratified squamous epithelium. The underlying stroma was oedematous and lined by foamy histiocytes within which were numerous round encapsulated organisms which stained positive with periodic acid Schiff stain (PAS). Mucocarmine stain showed the mucinous capsule outlined by pink stain (Figure 4). Budding forms were noted. The findings were compatible with cryptococcal vaginitis.

The patient was discharged on long term treatment with oral Flucanozole 400 mg daily for 6 months.

Received 19 August 2003 and in final form 27 November 2004, accepted 16 December 2004.

Discussion

Cryptococcus neoformans is an encapsulated basidiomycetous yeast like fungus found commonly throughout the world in bird excreta, mainly pigeon droppings [1]. In humans, most cases of cryptococcal infection are thought

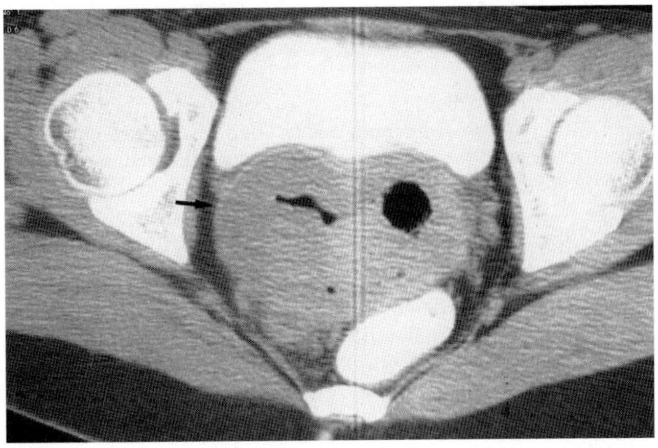

Figure 1. Axial enhanced CT image of the pelvis showing a mixed attenuation necrotic soft tissue mass measuring 6 cm × 5 cm × 3.5 cm arising from the right lateral wall of the vagina involving the right fornix (arrow) with pockets of air extending up to the lower cervical canal with no involvement of the endocervical canal and showing no significant enhancement.

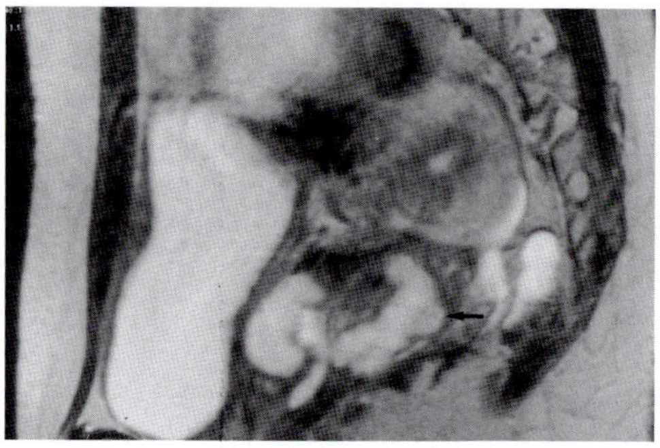

Figure 2. Sagittal T_2 MR image showing high signal intensity lobulated mass within the upper right vaginal wall (arrow) extending to the lower cervical region.

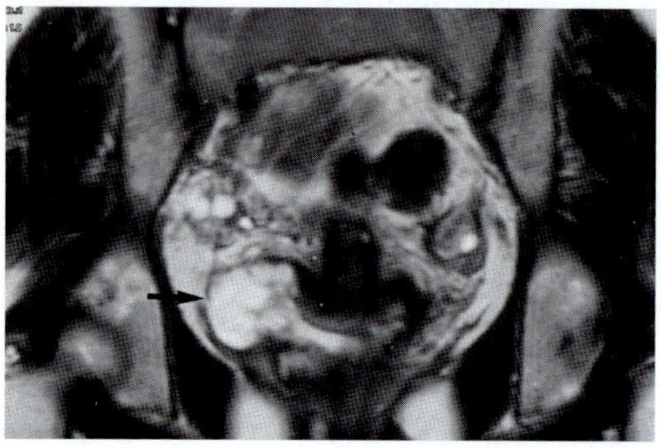

Figure 3. Coronal T_2 MR image showing high signal intensity lesion in the right side of the vaginal wall (arrow).

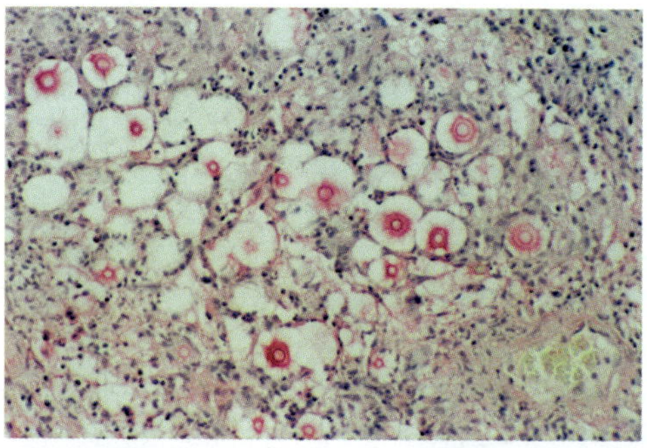

Figure 4. Histopathology of the vagina showing foamy histiocytes within which were numerous round encapsulated cryptococcal organisms the capsules of which are outlined in pink by Mucocarmine stain.

to be due to airborne particles. However, the vector is unknown [1]. Immunocompromised people are more susceptible to being infected with cryptococcosis. Skin and genital infections with *Cryptococcus neoformans* are rare. There has been only one reported case of vulval lesion, which was seen in a patient who had been on immunosuppressant therapy [2]. Only one case of cryptococcal vaginitis has been reported in the English literature. Chen et al [3] noted a suspicious vaginal lesion diagnosed histologically to be a cryptococcal infection of the vagina in a 72-year-old patient who had undergone resection of the colon for cancer [3]. However, unlike previous reported vaginal cryptococcal infection, our patient was not immunocompromised and had no exposure to pigeons. There have been no previous reports of imaging of these lesions. CT and MRI were performed after the biopsy of the lesion, which showed no specific findings except for a nodular mass in the right lateral wall of the vagina.

Differential diagnosis would include an infective process or malignant lesions such as carcinoma of the vagina, adenoma malignum or malignant melanoma.

Carcinomas of the vagina generally are ill-defined lesions that appear hypodense on CT images and usually show significant enhancement with contrast. Primary vaginal carcinoma usually returns low signal on T_1 weighted MRI, high signal on T_2 weighted sequences and demonstrates contrast enhancement. Infections too may show similar findings, however they may show more adjacent inflammatory changes compared with malignant tumour. Adenoma malignum is a special subtype of adenocarcinoma which may appear benign on histology. This lesion appears as multicystic lesions with solid components. The solid components appear isointense with muscle on T_1 weighted sequence and enhance with gadolinium [4].

Malignant melanoma of the genitalia usually presents in post menopausal women appearing as a well defined nodule which is easily diagnosed on clinical examination. On CT, malignant melanoma may appear as high attenuation mass which enhances moderately with contrast. On MRI, it may be of high signal on both T_1 weighted and T_2 weighted sequences and shows intense enhancement following contrast [5].

Although our patient was not immunocompromised, in a younger patient, a differential diagnosis of an infective process has to be considered. However biopsy is necessary to make the diagnosis.

Cryptococcus neoformans infection can be treated effectively with Flucanozole which is better tolerated than Amphotericin B, the previous mainstay of treatment [6].

Relapse may occur when treatment is discontinued and long term therapy may be needed.

References

1. Ellis DH, Pfeiffer TJ. Ecology, life cycle, and infectious propagule of Cryptococcus neoformans. Lancet 1990;336: 923–5.
2. Blocher KS, Weeks JA, Noble RC. Cutaneous cryptococcal infection presenting as vulvar lesion. Genitourin Med 1987;63:341–3.
3. Chen CK, Chang DY, Chang SC, Lee EF, Huang SC, Chow SN. Cryptococcal infection of the vagina. Obstet Gynecol 1993;81:867–9.
4. Okamoto Y, Tanaka YO, Nishida M, Tsunoda H, Yoshikawa H, Itai Y. MR imaging of the uterine cervix: imaging-pathologic correlation. Radiographics 2003;23:425–45; quiz 534–5.
5. Moon WK, Kim SH, Han MC. MR findings of malignant melanoma of the vagina. Clin Radiol 1993;48:326–8.
6. Sugar AM, Saunders C. Oral fluconazole as suppressive therapy of disseminated cryptococcosis in patients with acquired immunodeficiency syndrome. Am J Med 1988; 85:481–9.

The British Journal of Radiology, *78* (2005), 355–357
DOI: 10.1259/bjr/36150185

Case report

The reverse target sign in liver disease: a potential ultrasound feature in cirrhotic liver nodules characterization

[1]G J KRAUS, MD, [1]P SCHEDLBAUER, MD, [2]S LAX, MD, [3]D ZEBEDIN, MD and [1]F FLUECKIGER, MD

Institutes of [1]Radiology and [2]Pathology, General Hospital Graz-West, Goestingerstrasse 22, 8020 Graz and [3]Department of Radiology, University Hospital Graz, Auenbruggerplatz 1, 8036 Graz, Austria

Abstract. In patients with suspected liver disease, ultrasound is the most commonly performed initial imaging modality. We report a patient who had previously undiagnosed liver cirrhosis with target-shaped lesions interspersed throughout the liver parenchyma on ultrasound seen as multiple uniform round shaped lesions with varying isoechoic to hyperechoic centres surrounded by a hyperechoic rim. We have termed this the "reverse" target sign as there is inversion of the typical echoic pattern that is normally seen in metastatic liver disease. We suggest this ultrasound sign may represent a method for differentiating cirrhotic liver nodules from other nodular liver lesions.

Ultrasound is often the preliminary and most widely available imaging modality in evaluation of liver disease. The ultrasound and the CT appearance of metastatic liver disease and cirrhotic nodules can be quite similar. If there are no concomitant morphological imaging findings, the differential diagnosis is based on histology and clinical history.

Case report

A 55-year-old patient was referred to our institution for the liver ultrasound because of a weight loss of 17 kg over 3 months. His alanine aminotransferase (56 U l^{-1}; normal range 5–22 U l^{-1}), aspartate aminotransferase (33 U l^{-1}; normal range 5–18 U l^{-1}), alkaline phosphatase (214 U l^{-1}, normal range 60–170 U l^{-1}) and gamma glutamyle transferase (35 U l^{-1}; normal range 5–28 U l^{-1}) were elevated, and his cholinesterase (1444 U l^{-1}; normal range 5300–12 920 U l^{-1}) was below the reference value. All other laboratory values concerning the liver were within the normal range.

The prior medical history revealed that the patient suffered from pulmonary tuberculosis, as well as non insulin dependent diabetes mellitus. Serology for viral hepatitis A, B and C proved to be negative.

Ultrasound (Combison 401; General Electric Medical Systems, Milwaukee, WI) showed multiple lesions dispersed throughout the whole liver parenchyma with an isoechoic to hyperechoic centre and a hyperechoic rim (Figure 1). On colour Doppler ultrasound, there was regular hepatopetal blood flow in the portal vein.

On a triple phase CT-scan the lesions were best visible in the unenhanced phase (Figure 2), faintly visible as slightly hypodense lesions in the portalvenous phase at 70 s delay (not shown) and isodense to liver parenchyma in a delayed phase at 180 s. In the unenhanced phase the large centre was slightly hypodense to liver parenchyma imbedded in a more hypodense rim (Figure 2). There was delayed uptake of contrast media in the centre and subtle enhancement of the rim in the portalvenous phase (not shown). There was no nodularity of the liver contour and the ratio of the caudate lobe to the right lobe was within the normal range (*i.e.*<0.6). Secondary changes of cirrhosis such as ascites, varicose venous collaterals and splenomegaly were absent.

The most likely diagnosis was of metastatic liver disease. We did not perform contrast-enhanced ultrasound or MRI.

For further diagnostic work-up biopsy under ultrasound guidance was performed, and a 16 G Surecut™ biopsy needle (Boston Scientific, Natick, MA) was used. The histological specimens of two representative lesions showed features of large regenerating nodules with changes such as architectural distortion, cirrhosis and steatosis of hepatocytes (Figure 3).

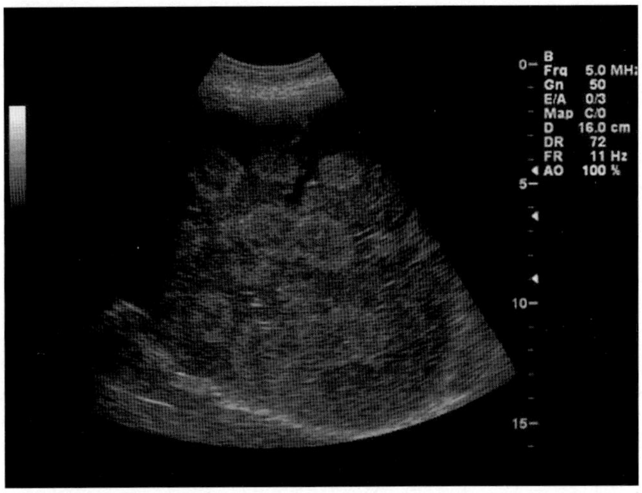

Figure 1. Ultrasound (B-mode) shows disseminated isoechoic to hyperechoic macronodular lesions with a hyperechoic rim (reverse target sign) throughout the liver parenchyma.

Received 21 June 2004 and in revised form 12 November 2004, accepted 5 January 2005.

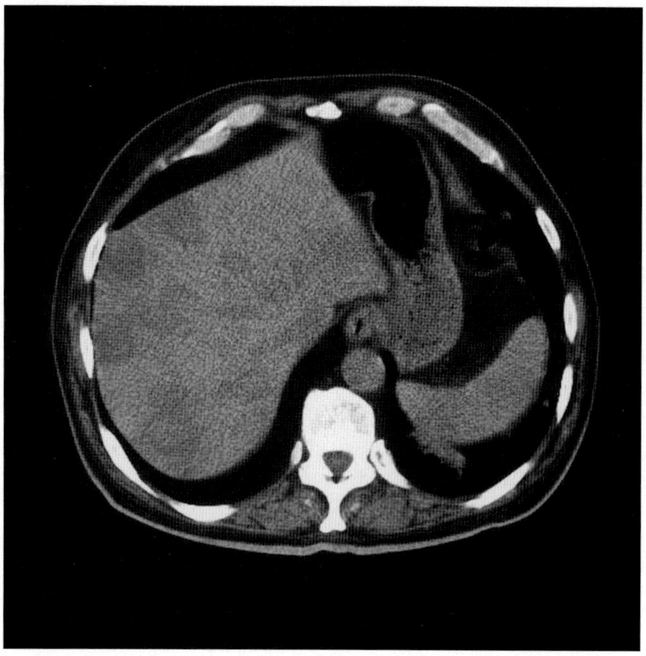

Figure 2. On an unenhanced spiral CT-scan, the lesions are isodense to liver parenchyma with a hypoattenuating rim.

Discussion

Cirrhotic nodules and dysplastic nodules (DN), with different grades of histological differentiation, are viewed as a spectrum of changes towards possible hepatocellular carcinoma [1] with up to 21.5% of nodules in cirrhotic livers proving to be dysplastic [2]. Cirrhotic or regenerative nodules (RN) and DN can show a variety of ultrasound and CT patterns [3]. Many malignant liver lesions may typically present a sonolucent halo, the so called target sign or bulls-eye lesion [4]. The histomorphological aetiology of this sonolucent halo is controversial and has been correlated with an aggressive growth pattern, although it is non-specific and can also be seen in hepatocellular carcinoma, adenoma, focal nodular hyperplasia, haemangioma, lymphoma and fungal microabscesses [4].

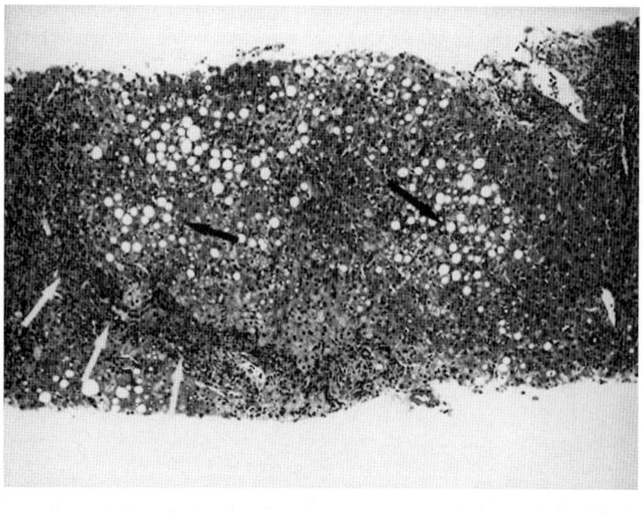

Figure 3. Histology: regenerative nodule with fibrocirrhotic changes (white arrows) surrounding partly steatotic hepatocytes (black arrows) (Chronotrop-Aniline-Blue stain, magnification 40×).

However, in our patient, the rim was hyperechoic, which is believed to correspond with a histological pattern of septal fibrosis and increased vascularity (Figure 3). Owing to this sonomorphological pattern, we have termed it the "reverse" target sign. The ultrasound patterns of metastatic liver disease are variable, and correlated with the histology of the primary tumour can be echogenic, hypoechoic, cystic, infiltrative, and may even calcify [4]. Haemangiomas larger than 3 cm can also have the sonomorphological pattern of the reverse target sign and should be considered in the differential diagnosis [5]. On CT the typical nodular dynamic contrast enhancement with "filling-in" centripetally is missing, the lesions are more radio-opaque than haemangiomas, and haemangiomas do not occur in the disseminated fashion seen in our patient.

The multiplicity of the lesions and missing signs of cirrhosis, such as contour irregularity, led us to the hypothesis of metastatic liver disease. Surface nodularity of the liver has the highest diagnostic accuracy and specificity for cirrhosis compared with caudate lobe hypertrophy and hepatic venous blood flow patterns in ultrasound [6], and it might have been useful to assess the liver surface, using a high frequency linear array probe.

The role of MRI in the diagnosis of nodular liver lesions is still uncertain [3]. Ferumoxide-particles administered intravenously are cleared by phagocytosis by Kupffer cells, and this shortens the T_2* signal [7]. DN and RN have an almost identical or even increased number of Kupffer cells compared with the surrounding parenchyma. Metastatic tumours are devoid of Kupffer cells; therefore ferumoxide-enhanced MRI can help to differentiate metastases from RN. But moderately and poorly differentiated HCC development in a cirrhotic liver are also found to have a significantly decreased number of Kupffer cells [8]. MRI is more accurate in the detection of nodular liver lesion in the cirrhotic liver than CT but tumour size is a restricting factor and small lesions can easily be missed [9].

The characterization of focal liver lesions with Gd-BOPTA and dynamic contrast enhanced MRI may be of greater importance in the future [10].

In summary, the diagnostic work-up of nodular liver lesions in some patients, even using all radiodiagnostic modalities, can be misleading and lead to misdiagnosis. Clinical and laboratory findings, as well as patient history may help in achieving the correct diagnosis. Although liver biopsy can yield false-negative results in about one-third of patients, for accurate characterization of liver nodules biopsy and histology remains the gold standard [11].

References

1. International Working Party. Terminology of nodular hepatocellular lesions. Hepatology 1995;22:983–93.
2. Terada T, Terasaki S, Nakanuma Y. A clinicopathologic study of adenomatous hyperplasia of the liver in 209 consecutive cirrhotic livers examined by autopsy. Cancer 1993;72:1551–6.
3. Lim JH, Choi BJ. Dysplastic nodules in liver cirrhosis: imaging. Abdom Imaging 2002;27:117–8.
4. Harvey CJ, Albrecht T. Ultrasound of focal liver lesions. Eur Radiol 2001;11:1578–93.

5. Leifer DM, Middleton WD, Teefey SA, Menias CO, Leahy JR. Follow-up of patients at low risk for hepatic malignancy with a characteristic hemangioma at US. Radiology 2000;214:167–72.
6. Colli A, Fraquelli M, Andreoletti M, Marino B, Zuccoli E, Conte D. Severe liver fibrosis or cirrhosis: accuracy of US for detection-analysis of 300 cases. Radiology 2003;227:89–94.
7. Stark DD, Weissleder R, Elizondo G, Hahn PF, Saini S, Todd LE, et al. Superparamagnetic iron oxide: clinical application as a contrast agent for MR imaging of the liver. Radiology 1988;168:297–301.
8. Tanaka M, Nakashima O, Wada Y, Kage M, Kojiro M. Pathomorphological study of Kupffer cells in hepatocellular carcinoma and hyperplastic nodular lesions in the liver. Hepatology 1996;24:807–12.
9. de Ledinghen V, Laharie D, Lecesne R, Le Bail B, Winnock M, Bernard PH, et al. Detection of nodules in liver cirrhosis: spiral computed tomography or magnetic resonance imaging? A prospective study of 88 nodules in 34 patients. Eur J Gastroenterol Hepatol 2002;14:159–65.
10. Schneider G, Grazioli L, Morana G, Kirchin M, Seidel R, Altmeyer K. Characterization of focal liver lesions with Gd-BOPTA: a review of imaging findings on unenhanced, dynamic, and hepatobiliary phase MR imaging. (Abstract) RSNA 2003 URL: http://rsna2003.rsna.org/rsna2003/VBK/conference/event_display.cfm?em_id=3106019 (cited 10 December 2003).
11. Poniachik J, Bernstein DE, Reddy KR, Jeffers LJ, Coelho-Little ME, Civantos F, et al. The role of laparoscopy in the diagnosis of cirrhosis. Gastrointest Endosc 1996;43:568–71.

The British Journal of Radiology, 78 (2005), 358–361
DOI: 10.1259/bjr/56095273

Case report

Re-treatment of a lung tumour using a simple intensity-modulated radiotherapy approach

[1]A W BEAVIS, PhD, [2]A ABDEL-HAMID, FRCR and [2]S UPADHYAY, MD

[1]*Department of Medical Physics, Hull and East Yorkshire NHS Trust and Clinical Biosciences Institute, University of Hull, Princess Royal Hospital, Saltshouse Road, Kingston Upon Hull HU8 9HE and [2]Department of Clinical Oncology, Princess Royal Hospital, Saltshouse Road, Kingston Upon Hull HU8 9HE, UK*

Abstract. We present a lung tumour case where, although the proximal spinal cord had already reached its dose tolerance, re-treatment was indicated. Minimization of the cord dose was defined as the main constraint for this case, however additional dose to the heart was considered. A simple (4 field) intensity-modulated radiotherapy (IMRT) treatment which proved superior to the standard conformal plan was developed using the Computerized Medical Systems (CMS) XiO treatment planning system. The IMRT plan was found to be superior to the conventional conformal plan regarding tumour coverage. It provided 100% saturation of the planning target volume (PTV) by the 95% isodose cloud, whereas the latter only provided 77% coverage. A step and shoot delivery using 10 intensity levels was developed and subsequently delivered for this patient. We considered it to be a routine application of IMRT and an important example of how it can offer benefit in individual and appropriate cases where conventional treatment is inadequate.

Case study

Recently, a patient presented with moderately to poorly differentiated squamous carcinoma recurrent lung tumour. He had responded to initial radiotherapy, however he was symptomatic with disease progression and further treatment was indicated to improve his quality of life; he declined chemotherapy. The previous treatment meant the cord had already received its dose tolerance, so any further radiotherapy required that it received "no further dose". The heart had also received the full prescribed dose. Various plans were considered, including simple two-dimensional (2D) and conformal three-dimensional (3D) plans, it became clear that the only option that could provide the homogeneous dose required to the planning target volume (PTV) whilst simultaneously avoiding giving unacceptable doses to the cord and heart was an intensity-modulated radiotherapy (IMRT) plan.

Treatment planning options

At our Cancer Centre all computerized treatment planning is performed using the XiO (previously FOCUS) treatment planning system from Computerized Medical Systems (St. Louis, MO). This system has an integrated IMRT option/inverse planning module, which essentially comprises an optimization algorithm, a leaf sequencing algorithm and quality assurance (QA) options [1]. These component parts enable the design of intensity modulated beams that satisfy a required dose be delivered to both the PTV and dose is restricted to the proximal organs at risk.

For this patient the rationale in developing the plan for this re-treatment course was simply to give "zero" dose to the spinal cord. The dose tolerance for the cord is considered to be 45 Gy when given in 2 Gy fractions, the dose it was given in the initial treatments is biologically equivalent to this. Furthermore, as a secondary consideration it was deemed desirable to minimize the dose to the heart and contralateral lung.

Initially, simple conformal options were attempted. The only way to achieve the cord goal was to ensure the organ was well shielded and no entrance or exit doses were incident to it. A two field conformal plan was developed that achieved these constraints, however the compromise was significant lack of coverage of the PTV. This trade off was not considered clinically acceptable.

An IMRT plan, following a conformal avoidance strategy, was developed using inverse planning. Four beam directions were chosen, the field portal defining collimators were manually set to totally shield the cord. Figure 1 shows the beam's eye view of these fields. Two of the beams did not irradiate the whole of the PTV, the inverse planning software was used to develop intensity modulated beams that essentially compensated for this, using the other two beams to provide a reasonable coverage through the PTV by "filling in the gaps".

The demand placed on the plan was to cover the PTV with the 95% isodose surface and to keep the volume irradiated to greater than the prescription dose as small as possible, idealistically we aim to have 0% of the PTV receiving more than 107%. A 6 MV beam set was used. Since the cord was not directly irradiated no specific dose constraints for it were defined in the optimizer. The doses in all other (non-target) tissues were controlled by a single constraint parameter in the cost-function; a maximum dose of 25 Gy was defined. This constraint was assigned a relative importance of 5% (as compared with that of the target), however the interplay between the terms in the cost function [2] is complicated and outside the scope of this manuscript.

Received 12 September 2003 and in final form 10 December 2004, accepted 5 January 2005.

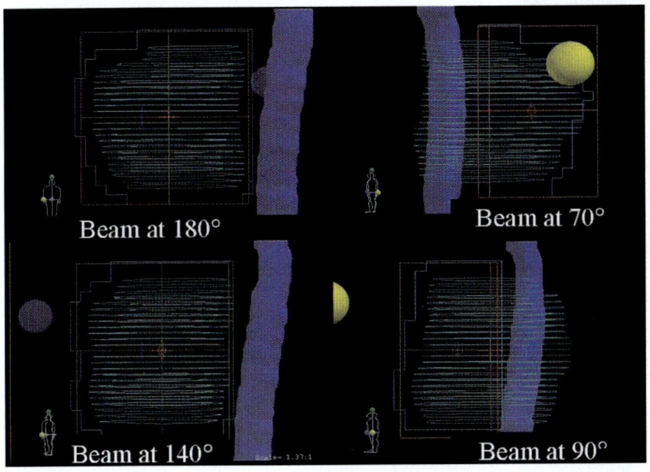

Figure 1. The rectangular outlines in each beam's eye view denotes the field defining collimators. We use a gantry angle convention where a 0 degree beam direction defines an anterior field for a supine patient and angles increase in a clockwise direction about the patients left side. We note that each beam is forced to conformally avoid the (rendered) cord. The non-uniform outline denotes the maximum irradiated area under each of the intensity modulated beams.

The resulting beams were produced using a "Bortfeld-Boyer" [3] based leaf sequencing algorithm using 10 intensity levels and 0.5 cm "steps", segments smaller than 1 cm^2 were automatically deleted before the final forward computation. The spatial resolution in the leaf travel direction is chosen to reflect the leaf widths of the multileaf collimator (MLC) used in our centre.

At this stage dose–volume histograms (DVH) are generated. The dose–volume profiles given to the PTV and organs at risk are assessed. Furthermore, the 3D dose distribution is consulted to determine the position of hot spots to assess their significance. Until an acceptable plan was obtained this entire optimization-through-DVH generation was iterated upon.

The treatment was delivered using a 600CD Clinac equipped with a Millennium 120 MLC and an aSi Electronic Portal Imaging, this equipment was manufactured by Varian Oncology Systems (Palo Alto, CA).

The "best" conventional plan, regarding cord avoidance, was not acceptable owing to spatially incomplete irradiation of the PTV. This plan utilized a wedged pair of posterior oblique fields at gantry angles of 132° and 200°. By employing the MLC to shield the cord in the beam's eye view a "zero" cord dose was obtained, however only 77% of the PTV received 28.5 Gy (95% of the prescribed dose to the isocentre) with the sub-volume proximal to the cord, receiving only approximately 13.3 Gy.

The IMRT plan that was accepted delivered 28.5 Gy to 100% of the PTV. The four field plan used fields at 70°, 90°, 140° and 180°. The maximum dose inside the PTV of 34.3 Gy was generated, a small 118% hot spot was evident lying just outside and posteriorly to the target volume. These were considered acceptable due to the absolute value of the prescription dose. The DVH curves generated for both plans are shown in Figure 2. The dose–volume profiles are displayed for the cord, heart and PTV. We note that similar distributions were achieved by either approach for the organs at risk. However, the target

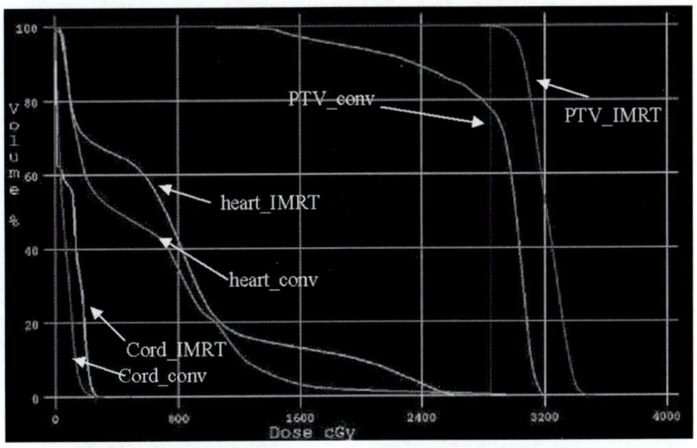

Figure 2. Dose–volume histogram showing the dose–volume profiles for the planning target volume (PTV) and organs at risk for plans: (1) the intensity-modulated radiotherapy (IMRT) solution chosen and (2) the best conventional option regarding dose to the cord.

coverage given by the conventional treatment option is clearly inferior to that offered by the IMRT plan. The curve for the conventional treatment PTV implies that re-normalization of that plan was not a serious option in any attempt to improve the high dose coverage of the PTV. The lung doses from the two plans were comparable, the V_{20} for the IMRT plan was 1% and 2% for the two field conformal plan. This result was not surprising given the prescription dose was 30 Gy, to aid comparison with other techniques we computed a V_{20} of 2% having re-normalized the IMRT plan prescription to 55 Gy and 3% for 64 Gy.

Figure 3 demonstrates the geometry of the problem posed by this patient's treatment. The dose cloud that obscures the PTV is that of the 95% isodose. The highest dose inside the "posterior protuberance" of the 90% isodose cloud was 32 Gy.

Discussion

In Figure 4 we show digital images, from our Odelft Simulator, obtained during an assessment of the patients suitability for conformal treatment. The upper row were anterior–posterior images, the lower row lateral images, those in the left column were obtained under normal

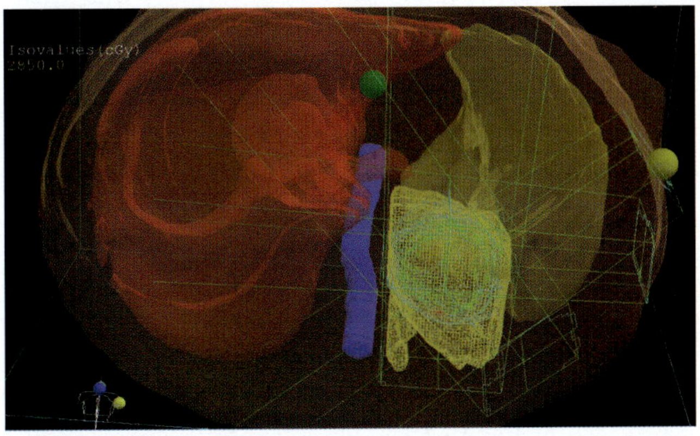

Figure 3. Shows the 95% dose cloud covering the planning target volume (PTV).

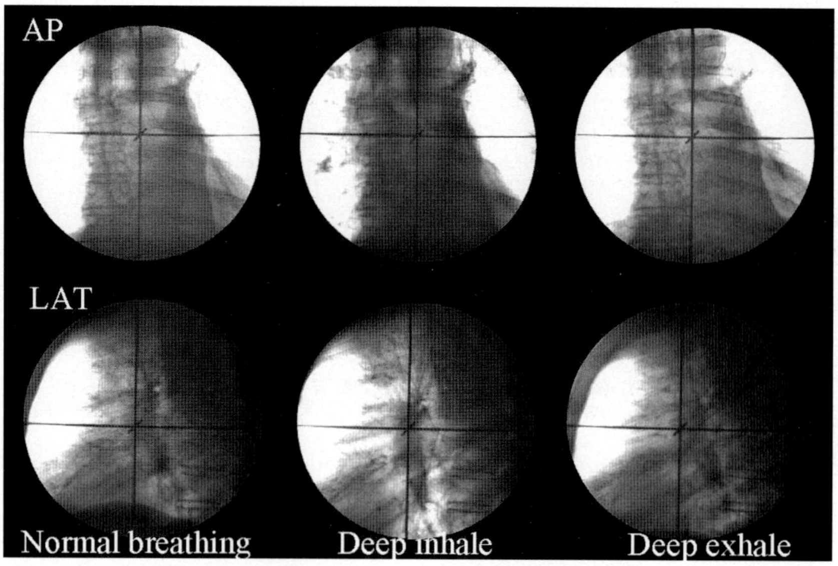

Figure 4. Digitally captured images from the simulator. The upper row were anterior–posterior (AP) images and the lower row lateral (LAT) images. The left column were obtained under normal respiration. The centre column on breath-hold at deep inhalation and the right column similarly at deep expiration.

respiration. The patient was asked to breathe deeply, then hold at deep inhalation (centre column) and again at deep expiration (right column). We note from the images that the cord–isocentre distances remain fairly constant. We did not consider tumour/organ motion a significant issue in the delivery of this treatment.

Further to this proactive analysis, we should mention that our practice is to contour the cord canal and so a protective margin of several millimetres is always assigned to our cord volumes.

The choice of dose calculation algorithms is an important consideration [4, 5] when using "high end" planning methodologies and comparing one method with another, especially so in lung treatments. We used a convolution algorithm using the FFT (fast Fourier transform) approximations [6] that require invariant dose deposition kernels, as with all our current IMRT work. There is a very strong argument that a Full, or superposition, convolution algorithm [7, 8] should be used in order to give a better approximation of the dose delivered to the lung and to lung–proximal tissue interfaces. In our department we have a guiding philosophy governing the introduction of new services, wherein we do not change too much at once. Hence, rather than introduce an algorithm not yet routinely used we elected to "stick with" the FFT-convolution algorithm.

There are a variety of studies and methods reported [9–13] using IMRT for the initial treatment of lung tumours. Our report is concerned with a different clinical situation, that being a re-treatment following initial radiotherapy where cord tolerance was reached.

A final consideration and point worth discussing in the context of our approach is the option offered by forward planned [14] multiple segmented treatments. In some cases we choose to manually add segments to "fill in cold areas" in dose distributions. These cases are usually large volumes that cover most of the thoracic region. We considered this option when planning this patient. However, having developed a good deal of experience and confidence with inverse planned IMRT we concluded that it would be quicker and more efficient to have the optimization routines deal with the problem. This is not to say that a forward planned, approach is not valid, we simply feel that our solution was a better use of resources in our clinic.

Acknowledgments

We would like to thank Computerized Medical Systems for their invaluable support, practical and financial, and enthusiasm for our research and clinical development programmes. It is also a pleasure to acknowledge the support of the Clinical BioSciences Institute of the University of Hull and that of Yorkshire Cancer Research.

References

1. Webb S. Intensity modulated radiotherapy. Bristol: IOP Publishing, 2000.
2. Xing L, et al. Fast iterative algorithms for 3D inverse treatment planning. Med Phys 1998;25:1845–9.
3. Bortfeld T, Boyer A. Realization and verification of three-dimensional conformation radiotherapy with modulated fields. Int J Radiat Oncol Biol Phys 1994;30:899–908.
4. Miften M, Beavis A, Marks L. The influence of the dose calculation model on treatment plan evaluation in conformal therapy: a three case study. Med Dosim 2002;27:51–7.
5. Jeraj R, Keall P, Siebers J. The effect of dose calculation accuracy on inverse treatment planning. Phys Med Biol 2002;47:391–407.
6. Boyer A, et al. Fast Fourier transform convolution calculations of x-ray isodose distributions in homogeneous media. Med Phys 1989;16:248–53.
7. Mackie T, Scrimger J, Battista J. A convolution method of calculating dose for 15 MV X-rays. Med Phys 1985;12:188–96.
8. Miften M, et al. Implementation of FFT convolution and multigrid superposition models in the FOCUS RTP system. Phys Med Biol 2000;45:817–33.
9. De Jaeger K, et al. Incorporating an improved dose-calculation algorithm in conformal radiotherapy of lung cancer: re-evaluation of dose in normal lung tissue. Radiother Oncol 2003;69:1–10.
10. Derycke S, et al. Non-coplanar beam intensity modulation allows large dose escalation in Stage III lung cancer. Radiother Oncol 1997;45:253–61.

11. Derycke S, et al. Conformal radiotherapy of Stage III non-small cell lung cancer: a class solution involving non-coplanar intensity modulated beams. Int J Radiat Oncol Biol Phys 1998;41:771–7.
12. Dirkx M, Heijmen BJ. Beam intensity modulation for penumbra enhancement and field length reduction in lung cancer treatments: a dosimetric study. Radiother Oncol 2000;56: 181–8.
13. Zaider M, Amols HI. A little to a lot or a lot to a little: is NTCP always minimized in multiport therapy? Int J Radiat Oncol Biol Phys 1998;41:945–50.
14. Xia P, Pickett B, Vigneault E, Verhey LJ, Roach M 3rd. Forward or inversely planned segmental multileaf collimator IMRT and sequential tomotherapy to treat multiple dominant intraprostatic lesions of prostate cancer to 90 Gy. Int J Radiat Oncol Biol Phys 2001;51:244–54.

The British Journal of Radiology, *78* (2005), 362–369
DOI: 10.1259/bjr/93120352

Pictorial review

Diseases of the submandibular gland as demonstrated using high resolution ultrasound

[1]F ALYAS, MRCP, [2]K LEWIS, [2]M WILLIAMS, FDS, FRCS, [2]A B MOODY, FDS, FRCS, [3]K T WONG, FRCR, [3]A T AHUJA, FRCR and [1]D C HOWLETT, MRCP, FRCR

[1]Department of Radiology, [2]Department of Maxillofacial Surgery, Eastbourne District General Hospital, Eastbourne, UK and [3]Department of Diagnostic Radiology and Organ Imaging, Prince of Wales Hospital, Hong Kong

Abstract. In this review the high resolution ultrasound appearances of the normal anatomy and pathology involving the submandibular gland are demonstrated. The submandibular gland is affected by a number of disease processes that may be difficult to distinguish clinically. Its superficial location makes it ideal for ultrasound evaluation and a useful adjunct to clinical examination. In the assessment of submandibular pathology ultrasound allows intraglandular and extraglandular lesions to be localized and differentiated. These lesions can be further characterized as being benign or malignant and the extent of any extraglandular extension determined. Ultrasound is the first-line investigation in the assessment of sialolithiasis due to its high specificity and sensitivity. In severe infective sialadenitis ultrasound can confirm the presence and guide drainage of abscesses. Ultrasound also has an important role in the assessment of chronic inflammatory disorders such as sarcoidosis and Sjögren's syndrome.

High resolution ultrasound is a safe, inexpensive and accurate method of assessing the extent and nature of submandibular disease, providing valuable information to guide further imaging and management. The ultrasound appearances of the normal glandular anatomy, together with common and more unusual pathologies that may involve the submandibular gland will be considered in this review.

Normal ultrasound anatomy and relations of the submandibular gland

The submandibular gland lies within the submandibular triangle in the plane of the anterior belly of the digastric muscle. The submandibular gland has a homogeneous echotexture on ultrasound which is slightly hyperechoic compared with surrounding muscle. Intraglandular ducts may be identified as small linear hyperechoic stripes (Figure 1). There is a larger superficial lobe and a smaller and more posterior deep lobe which connect around the posterior border of the mylohyoid muscle. In ultrasound evaluation of the gland isolation of pathology to a particular lobe is not relevant clinically as the surgical treatments are the same [1, 2].

Wharton's duct appears as tubular structure which may be apparent on ultrasound. It is best seen when pathologically dilated but may be demonstrable in normal subjects. The duct emerges from the hilum of the submandibular gland and passes medially around the posterior border of mylohyoid (Figure 2). It then courses medial to the sublingual gland to the papilla in the floor of the mouth. The path of Wharton's duct is best viewed in a slightly oblique plane [1, 2].

Relations to the gland are as follows. Anteriorly to the gland is a fat filled triangular space. Superomedially and deep to mylohyoid, is the lingual vein. Posteriorly lies the retromandibular vein, laterally the facial vein and inferiorly platysma and subcutaneous tissue. There are several regional lymph node groups surrounding the gland although normal lymph nodes are not found within gland, unlike the parotids, due to early glandular encapsulation. During ultrasound examination it is important to be aware of the Küttner lymph node. Its close relationship to the posterior of the submandibular gland (also just adjacent to the parotid gland) means it should not be mistaken for submandibular pathology (Figure 3).

Pathological processes involving the submandibular gland

Sialolithiasis

Salivary gland calculi most commonly occur in the submandibular glands and this reflects the more mucinous content of submandibular secretions. 90% of calculi are radio opaque [1] and they are multiple in 25% of patients [2]. Ultrasound has a high degree of accuracy (96%) in their diagnosis [3].

Most calculi (85%), occur in Wharton's duct while the remainder (15%) are found within the gland (Figure 4) or at the ductal hilum. Most commonly calculi impact at the curvature of Wharton's duct as it goes around mylohyoid (35%) [2]. Ductal stones may cause an obstruction or stricture causing dilatation of the main duct and proximal intraglandular ducts which will be visible on ultrasound. One third of Wharton's duct calculi occur at the ostium and small stones here are difficult to visualize, however

Received 27 February 2004 and in revised form 20 September 2004, accepted 26 October 2004.

Address correspondence to Dr David Howlett, Consultant Radiologist, Department of Radiology, Kings Drive, Eastbourne, East Sussex BN21 2UD, UK.

consequent main duct dilation is visible in 65% of these cases [4] (Figure 5).

On ultrasound stones appear as hyperechoic foci casting posterior acoustic shadowing (Figure 4). Those smaller than 2 mm may not cast acoustic shadows.

Ultrasound can also assess the complications of calculi, *e.g.* sialadenitis, sialocele, abscess and in chronic circumstances gland atrophy (see later).

Sialadenitis

This can be sub-divided into acute and chronic sialadenitis.

Acute sialadenitis

The majority of infections have a viral aetiology (most commonly mumps) and do not require imaging routinely. Bacterial infections are usually a result of salivary stasis allowing retrograde passage of organisms. This is common in the elderly/debilitated, following surgery, dehydration, trauma, irradiation, and in relation to obstructing lesions such as stones, tumours and strictures [2]. The most common causative organisms are *Staphylococcus aureus* or *Streptococcus viridans*.

In acute sialadenitis the gland appears enlarged and hypoechoic on ultrasound [5]. Ultrasound is useful in severe cases of bacterial infection, especially if abscess formation is suspected. Abscesses are seen as ill-defined hypoechoic foci, with intraglandular ducts passing through the lesion as opposed to ductal displacement, which would favour tumour. There may be adjacent regional lympadenopathy [2] (Figure 6). Ultrasound can also be used to guide drainage of suspected abscess.

Primary tuberculosis rarely presents in the submandibular gland and involvement usually occurs as a result of haematogenous dissemination or spread from adjacent structures and lymph nodes [2]. It can present acutely with sialadenitis or subacutely mimicking tumour [2]. Overall the imaging features are non-specific although a mixed echogenicity mass lesion may be seen (Figure 7).

Chronic sialadenitis

Infective causes Chronic sialadenitis is mainly caused by infection secondary to sialolithiasis. With recurrent infection the gland atrophies and is replaced by fibrotic tissue (Figure 8). Sonographically the gland appears atrophic and diffusely hypoechoic with irregular margins, the ultrasound appearances often simulating a "cirrhotic" liver [6]. There is an association between chronic infection, *e.g.* secondary to dental sepsis and duct stricture formation also.

Küttner tumour (chronic sclerosing sialadenitis) is a focal lesion resulting from chronic inflammation of the submandibular gland usually caused by bacterial infection or duct obstruction and these lesions may have a pseudotumour appearance. Biopsy or excision is often needed to confirm the diagnosis. Sonographically these lesions can mimic tumours appearing as a focal, hypoechoic lesion (Figure 9). Colour flow Doppler examination shows with a radial branching vascular pattern within the mass [6] (Figure 10).

Non-infective causes Sarcoidosis is a non-caseating granulomatous condition more usually affecting the parotids, with parotid involvement described in 6% of patients [1]. It may also affect the submandibular glands [2], presenting clinically with painless enlargement [1].

The ultrasound features of sarcoidosis in the submandibular gland are not well described although we have observed appearances similar to those described in the parotid gland. The appearances of sarcoidosis in the parotid are non-specific [1]. A variety of manifestations may be seen ranging from multiple hypoechoic foci to diffuse hypoechoic glandular enlargement (Figure 11) and there may be associated lymphadenopathy [1, 5]. The gland may be hypervascular on colour Doppler flow studies. Necrosis is not a feature in sarcoidosis and this may help in distinguishing it from tuberculosis [7].

Sjögren's syndrome is an autoimmune syndrome which consists of dry mucus membranes (*e.g.* eyes and mouth) and a connective tissue disorder predominantly affecting middle-aged women. Parotid or submandibular enlargement occurs in 80% of patients [2]. An appreciation of the underlying pathology is helpful in understanding the variety of ultrasound appearances. Initially there is inflammation involving the peripheral ductal system which results in intraglandular duct dilation and destruction of gland tissue predisposing to recurrent infection.

The progression of ultrasound changes reflects the various stages of this inflammatory process. Initially ultrasound of the gland may be normal, then showing diffuse gland enlargement, inhomogeneity and then sialectasis (shown in Figure 12) [8]. On colour Doppler flow assessment there is hypervascularity [9]. It is worth mentioning that the lacrimal glands are also frequently involved and are easily examined at the same time. They may often show similar ultrasound appearances to the submandibular gland (Figure 13).

As the disease progresses numerous cystic spaces are seen reflecting progressive glandular destruction and prominent intraglandular sialectasis [8, 9] (Figure 14). These appearances are similar to those recognized in the parotid in HIV infection [10]. In end stage disease the gland becomes fibrotic and atrophic [11]. As these patients are at increased risk of lymphoma development ultrasound has been advocated as a surveillance tool by some authors [11].

Tumours

The overall incidence of salivary gland tumours in the general population is 3%. They are more frequent in the parotid gland with only 14% of salivary gland tumours occurring in the submandibular gland. However there is a greater of incidence of malignancy in submandibular gland tumours (approximately half of all submandibular gland tumours are malignant [2] compared with 10% of all parotid tumours [1]) and the sonographer should be vigilant when ultrasound examination is performed in this respect. If a suspected neoplasm is identified within the gland ultrasound can then be used to guide fine needle aspiration (FNA) or core biopsy of the lesion to confirm its nature. FNA is a quick, safe and accurate technique, although core biopsy does provide an alternative with potential advantages [12].

Ultrasound will act as a guide to the need for further imaging, either CT or MRI, for sonographically malignant lesions or large lesions whose extent is difficult to access on ultrasound alone.

Benign tumours

Pleomorphic adenoma is the most common neoplasm of the submandibluar gland accounting for the majority of benign tumours [2]. On ultrasound these tumours appear as circumscribed, round, hypoechoic masses with a lobulated border, which may show posterior acoustic enhancement [2] (Figure 15). 25% of pleomorphic adenomas are associated with smaller satellite lesions [1]. Larger tumours may appear more atypical, developing areas of internal necrosis or haemorrhage and cystic changes or areas of calcification may occur [13]. Malignant transformation to adenocarcinoma is rare but should be suspected in patients with long standing tumours that become painful or grow rapidly.

Warthin's tumour (Cystadenolymphoma) although relatively common in the parotid is very unusual in the submandibular gland. Early encapsulation of the submandibular gland during fetal development prevents structures from the lymphatic, vascular and nervous system developing within the gland. This in turn makes disease of the lymphatic tissue, such as Warthin's tumour (and lymphoma), rare in the submandibular gland [2]. This is in contrast to the parotid gland which undergoes delayed encapsulation where such pathologies are relatively more common.

Oncocytoma is a rarely described tumour accounting for 1% of all salivary gland tumours, 11% of which occur in the submandibular gland. Histologically oncocytoma is composed of oncocytes derived from striated duct cells. It may relate to previous irradiation and can undergo malignant transformation. It appears similar to pleomorphic adenoma on ultrasound [1] (Figure 16).

Malignant tumours

There are several histological subtypes of primary malignant submandibular tumours, the most common being adenoid cystic carcinoma, followed by mucoepidermoid carcinoma and other sub-types such as acinic cell carcinoma and adenocarcinoma are rare [1]. Adenoid cystic carcinoma occurs in patients in their fifth or sixth decade [2], accounting for 17% of all submandibular tumours [1]. It can be multiple, has a propensity for perivascular and perineural spread and can metastasise to regional lymph nodes, lung and bone [2]. Ultrasound is able to distinguish benign from malignant tumours in 80% of cases [1]. It is also able to demonstrate extracapsular spread and any regional lymph node involvement. However it cannot distinguish between the different subtypes of malignant tumours. These appear similarly as masses of heterogeneous echotexture (Figure 17) with irregular infiltrating borders (Figure 18), and associated posterior acoustic shadowing. On colour Doppler examination malignant tumours may show multiple, irregular internal vessels, with hypervascularity and high resistance arterial flow [14]. Studies mainly performed on the parotid gland have shown that a resistive index (RI)$<$0.8 and pulsatility index (PI)$<$1.8 favours a benign over a malignant lesion [15]. It should be noted that small, low grade malignant tumours may appear benign on ultrasound and that histological confirmation should always be obtained.

Lymphoma

Primary lymphoma rarely occurs in the submandibular gland for reasons that have already been described and the gland is usually involved secondarily via haematogenous spread [7]. Primary disease may occur in patients with Sjögren's syndrome who are at significantly increased risk of developing a non-Hodgkin's lymphoma in particular [2].

The ultrasound features of lymphoma within the submandibular gland are rarely described [16] and lesions may appear as solid, hypoechoic or pseudocystic masses (Figure 19).

Metastasis

Metastases to the submandibular gland are rare, occurring mainly as a result of haematogenous spread. These are mainly from head and neck tumours or melanoma. The ultrasound features of submandibular gland metastases are not well described, although the appearances are likely to be similar to these demonstrated in parotid metastatic disease [13]. Parotid metastases can vary in appearance but tend to be hypoechoic, with heterogeneous internal architecture and poorly defined margins [13].

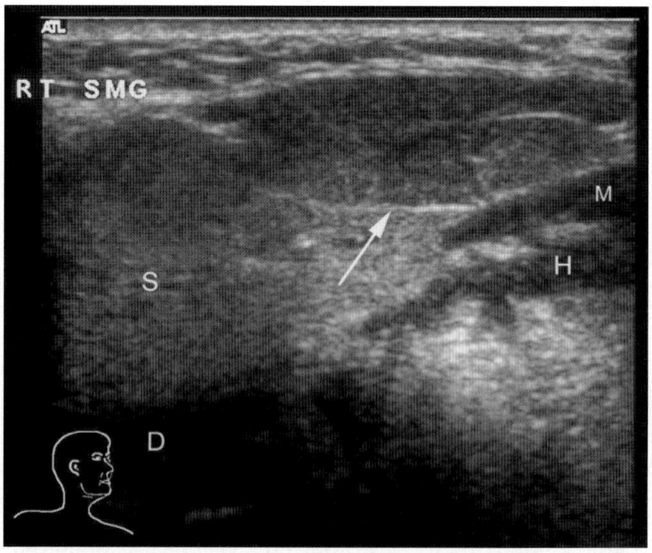

Figure 1. Axial ultrasound through a normal right submandibular gland showing its relationship to adjacent structures. S, submandibular gland; M, mylohyoid muscle; H, hyoglossus muscle; White arrow, intraglandular duct; D, posterior belly of digastric muscle.

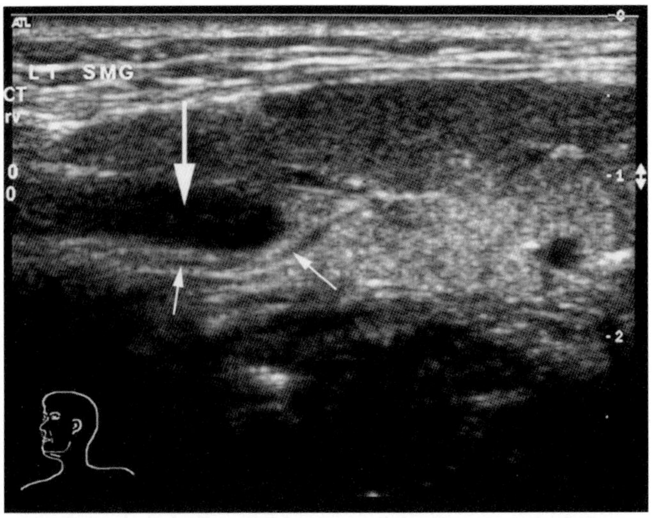

Figure 2. Oblique axial ultrasound through a normal left submandibular gland demonstrating the normal Wharton's duct. Small white arrow, Wharton's duct; Large white arrow, mylohyoid muscle.

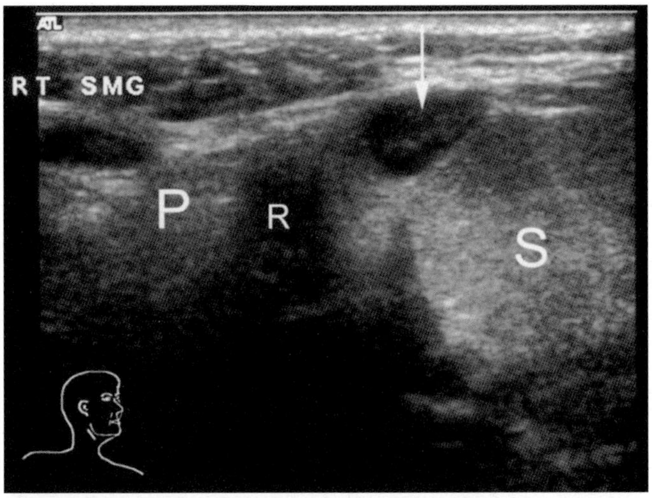

Figure 3. Oblique axial ultrasound through a normal right submandibular gland demonstrating the position of the Küttner lymph node. P, parotid gland; White arrow, Küttner lymph node; R, retromandibular vein; S, submandibular gland.

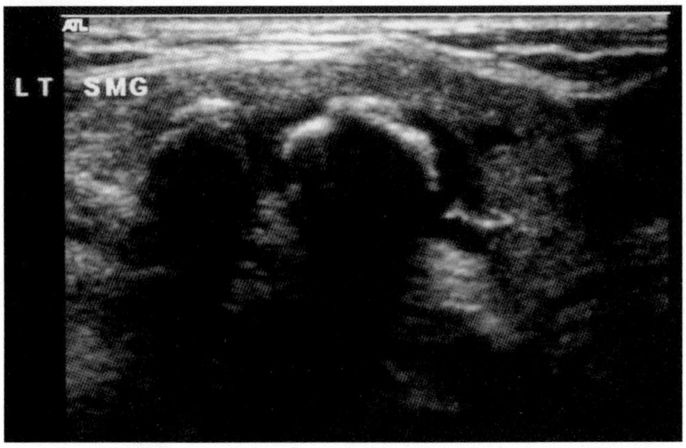

Figure 4. Ultrasound of left submandibular gland demonstrating intraglandular sialolithiasis. Note the two large hyperechoic calculi within the gland that cast acoustic shadows.

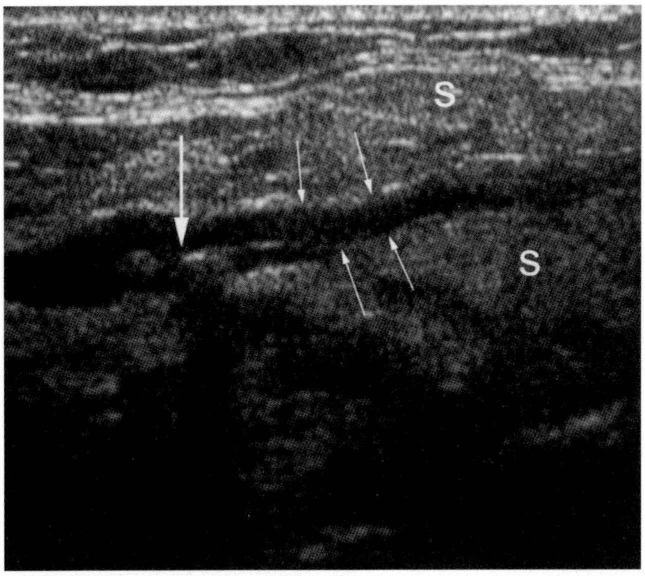

Figure 5. Ultrasound demonstrating sialolithiasis with dilatation of Wharton's duct (small white arrows) secondary to a meatal stone (not shown, see text). There is a non-obstructing intraductal calculus within Wharton's duct casting an acoustic shadow (large white arrow), together with sludge. S, submandibular gland.

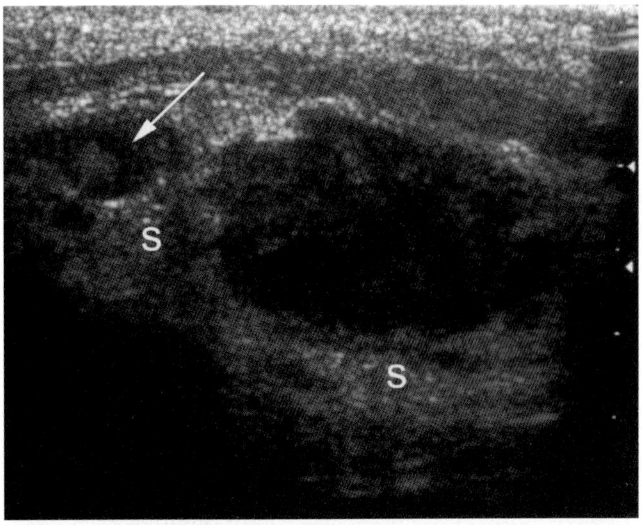

Figure 6. Ultrasound demonstrating a submandibular abscess in a man who presented with an acutely painful and enlarged gland. There is an ill-defined intraglandular hypoechoic mass and adjacent enlarged reactive lymph node (white arrow). Under ultrasound guidance pus was aspirated and subsequent culture grew *Staphylococcus aureus*. S, submandibular gland.

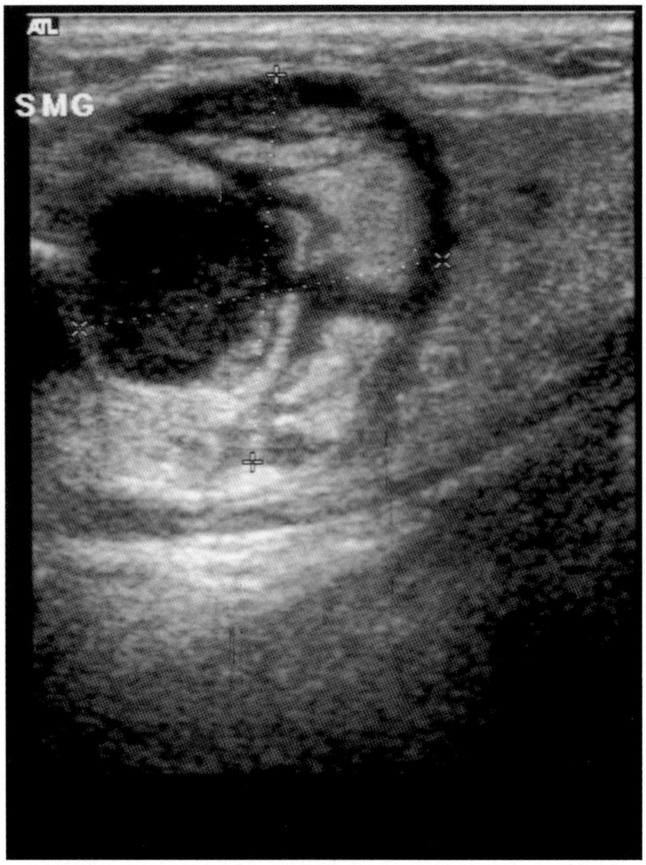

Figure 7. Ultrasound demonstrating intraglandular tuberculous abscess. There is a complex mass (callipers) in the submandibular gland with a central necrotic abscess cavity. Excision confirmed involvement of the gland with *Mycobacterium tuberculosis*.

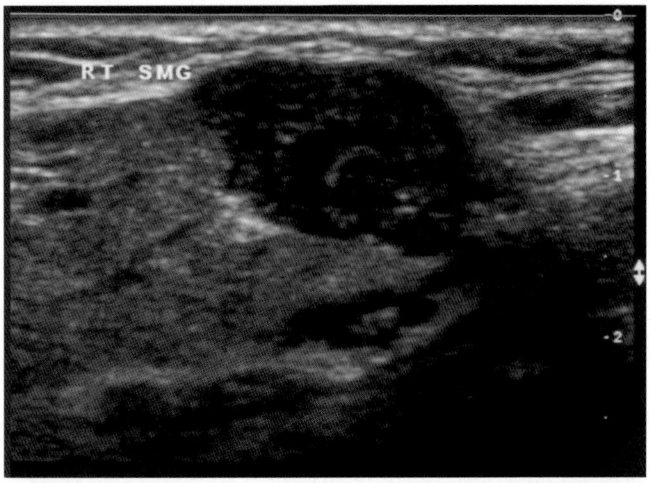

Figure 9. Ultrasound of the right submandibular gland demonstrating a Küttner tumour. There is a well-defined, hypoechoic mass in the submandibular gland, which could be mistaken, clinically and sonographically for a tumour. Diagnosis of chronic inflammation was confirmed by core biopsy and subsequent excision.

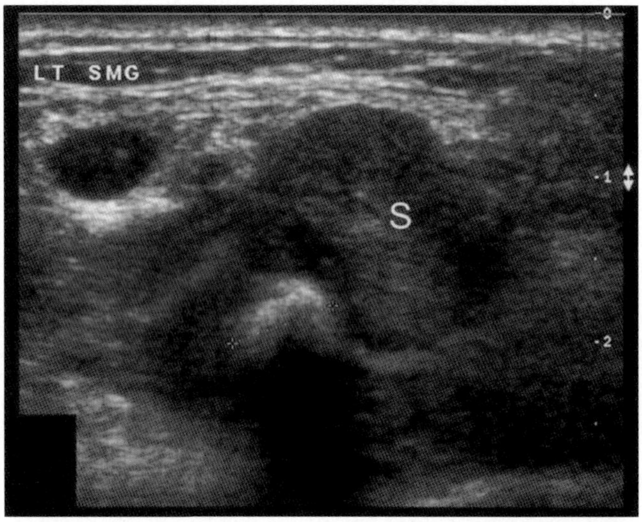

Figure 8. Ultrasound of left submandibular gland demonstrating chronic sialadenitis secondary to stone disease. S, atrophic, hypoechoic, irregular gland. Note the associated intraglandular calculus (callipers).

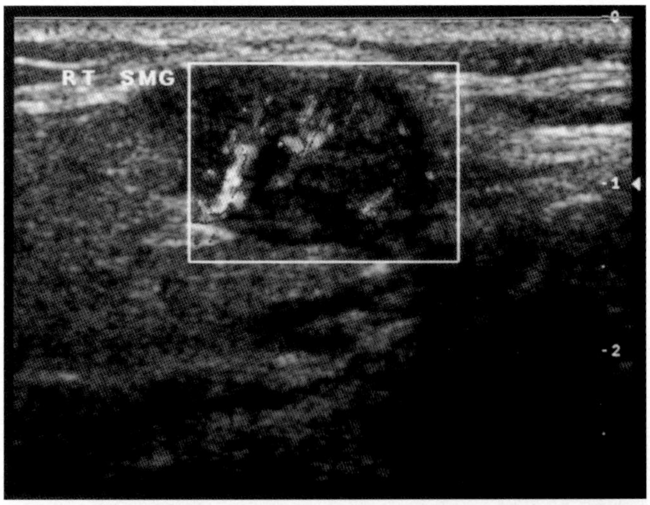

Figure 10. Ultrasound of the same patient as in Figure 9 demonstrating increased radial flow on Doppler examination within the lesion.

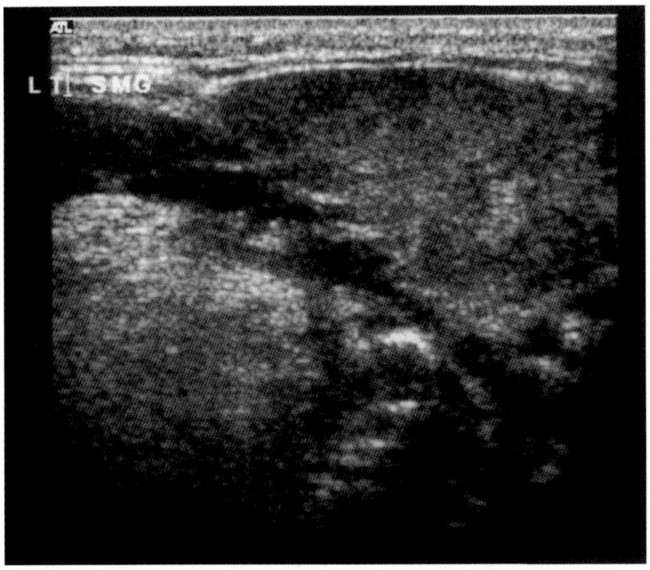

Figure 11. Ultrasound of the left submandibular gland in a patient with suspected thoracic sarcoidosis and painless salivary gland enlargement. The submandibular gland is enlarged, heterogeneous in texture and hypoechoic. Subsequent glandular biopsy confirmed the presence of sarcoid granulomata.

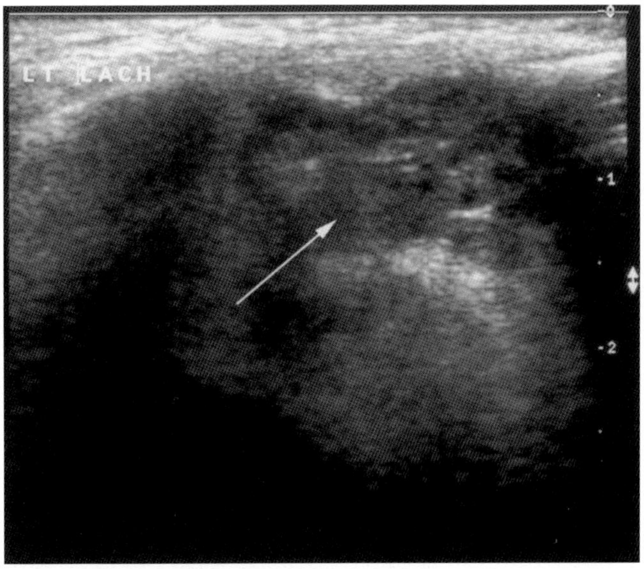

Figure 13. Ultrasound of the lacrimal gland in a patient with Sjögren's syndrome. There are hypoechoic foci present within the enlarged gland (white arrow), which has a similar appearance to the submandibular gland in Figure 12.

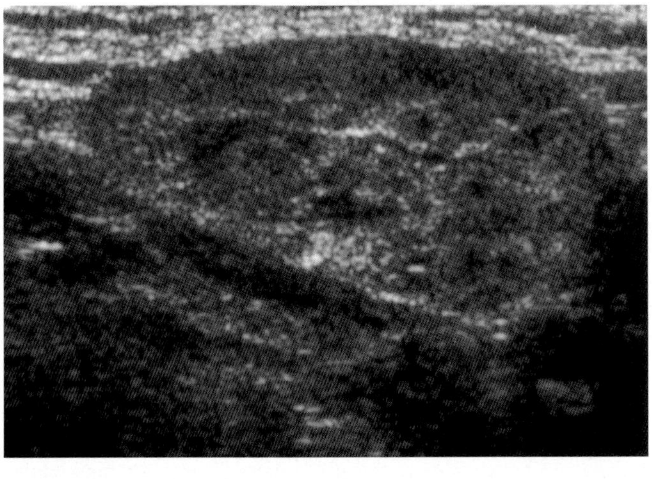

Figure 12. Submandibular ultrasound in a patient with Sjögren's syndrome. The gland is diffusely enlarged and of heterogeneous echotexture. Note the hypoechoic foci within the gland representing early sialectatic changes.

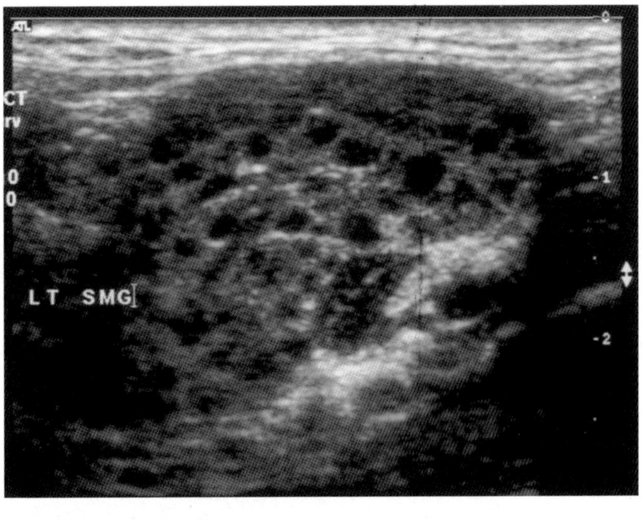

Figure 14. Ultrasound of the left submandibular gland demonstrating numerous prominent cystic spaces typical of florid sialectasis in Sjögren's syndrome. A similar appearance can occur in HIV infection.

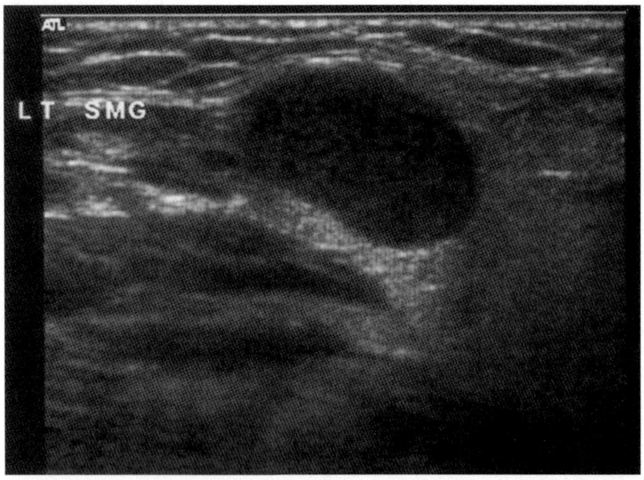

Figure 15. Ultrasound demonstrating submandibular gland pleomorphic adenoma. This lesion appears rounded, well defined and hypoechoic with distal acoustic enhancement present.

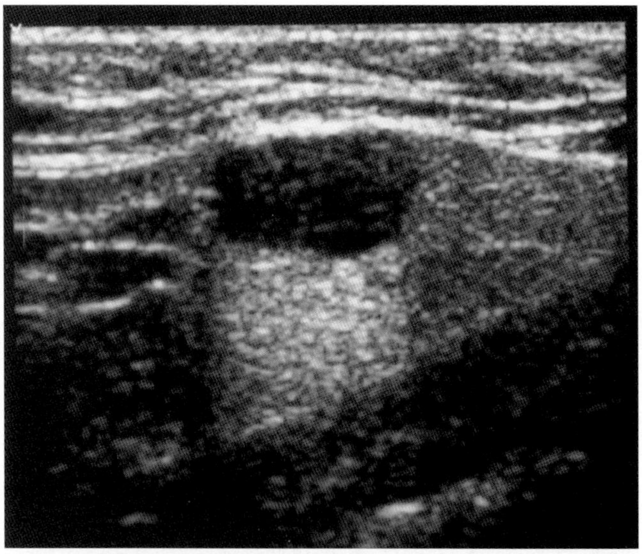

Figure 16. Submandibular ultrasound demonstrating an oncocytoma confirmed on gland excision. It has a similar appearance to pleomorphic adenoma (see Figure 15).

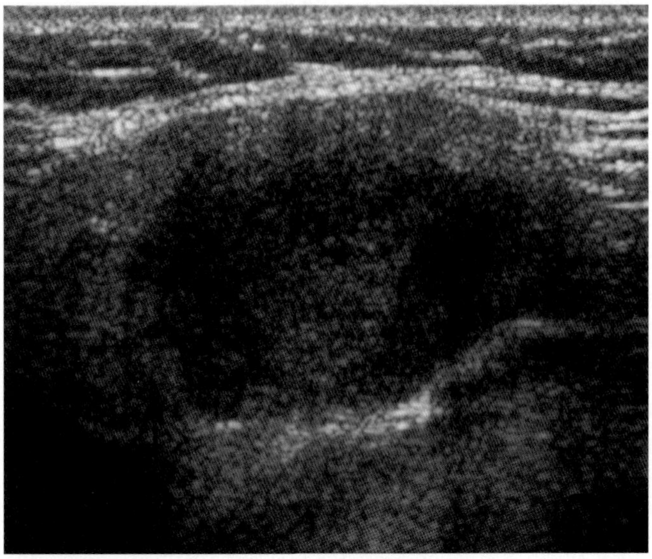

Figure 17. Submandibular ultrasound in a patient with an intraglandular adenoid cystic carcinoma. This appears as an ill-defined, hypoechoic and inhomogeneous mass.

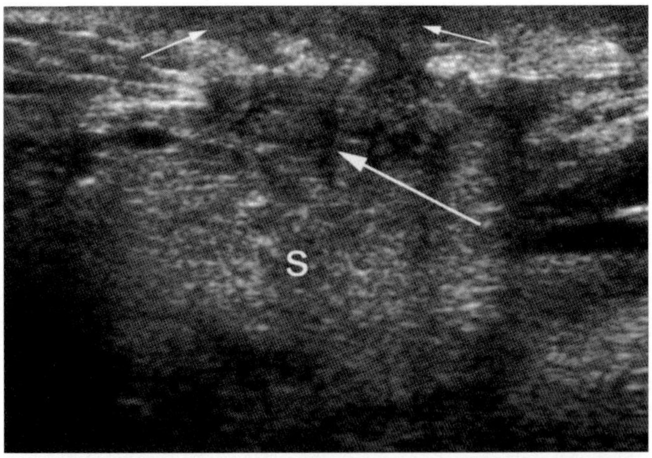

Figure 18. Submandibular ultrasound in a patient with mucoepidermoid carcinoma (large white arrow). Sonographically the features shown are similar to the adenoid cystic carcinoma in Figure 17. Note that in this case there is also extraglandular extension of tumour with invasion of the subcutaneous tissues and skin (small white arrows).

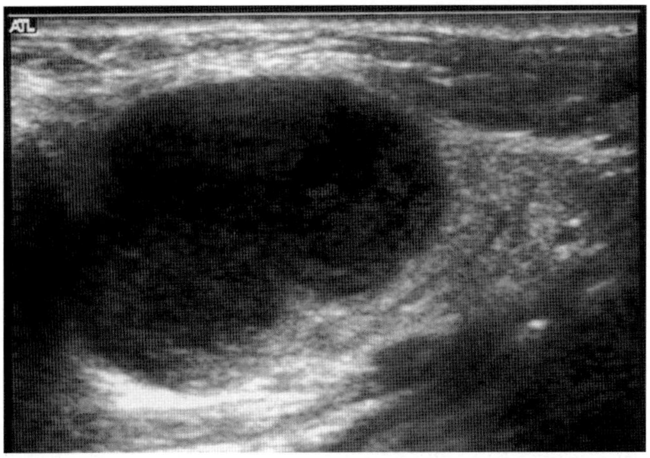

Figure 19. Ultrasound demonstrating lymphoma of the submandibular gland confirmed with biopsy. There is a large, hypoechoic intraglandular mass. This patient had known disseminated B-cell lymphoma.

Conclusion

High-resolution ultrasound is the initial imaging tool of choice for the evaluation of the symptomatic submandibular gland and adjacent structures. As well as providing information on the site, nature and extent of submandibular pathology, ultrasound can be used in the guidance of FNA, core biopsy and abscess drainage. Ultrasound is also able to act as a guide to the need for further imaging, usually with CT or MRI.

Acknowledgments

The authors would like Nick Taylor for preparation of the illustrations.

References

1. Bradley MJ. Chapter 2: Salivary glands. In: Ahuja A, Evans R, editors. Practical head and neck ultrasound. London: Greenwich Medical Media, 2000; 19–37.
2. Silvers AR, Som PM. Salivary glands. Radiol Clin N Am 1998;36:941–66.
3. Gritzmann N. Sonography of the salivary glands. AJR Am J Roentgenol 1989;53:161–6.
4. Ching ASC, Ahuja AT. High resolution sonography of the submandibular space: anatomy and abnormalities. AJR Am J Roentgenol 2002;179:703–8.
5. Koischwitz D, Gritmann N. Ultrasound of the neck. Radiol Clin N Am 2000;38:1029–43.
6. Ahuja AT, Richards PS, Wong KT, King AD, Yuen HY, Ching AS. Küttner tumour (chronic sclerosing sialadenitis) of the submandibular gland: sonographic appearances. Ultrasound Med Biol 2003;29:913–9.
7. Fischer T, Filimonow S, Petersein J, Zimmer C, Beyersdorff D, Guski H. Diagnosis of Heerfordt's syndrome by state-of-the-art ultrasound in combination with parotid biopsy: a case report. Eur Radiol 2002;12:134–7.
8. Makula E, Pokorny G, Rajtar M, Kiss I, Kovacs A, Kovacs L. Parotid gland ultrasonography as a diagnostic tool in primary Sjögren's syndrome. Br J Rheumatol 1996;35:972–7.
9. Martinoli C, Derchi LE, Solbiati L, Rizzatto G, Silvestri E, Giannoni M. Colour Doppler sonography of salivary glands. AJR Am J Roentgenol 1994;163:933–41.
10. Gooding GA, Sooy CD, Hybarger CP. Ultrasonography of cystic parotid lesions in HIV infection. Similarity of sonographic appearance with Sjögren's syndrome. J Ultrasound Med 1992;11:35–9.
11. Ahuja AT, Metreweli C. Ultrasound features of Sjögren's syndrome. Australas Radiol 1996;40:10–4.
12. Kesse KW, Manjaly G, Violaris N, Howlett DC. Ultrasound guided biopsy in the evaluation of focal lesions and diffuse swelling of the parotid gland. Br J Oral Maxillofac Surg 2002;40:384–8.
13. Howlett DC. High-resolution ultrasound assessment of the parotid gland. Br J Radiol 2003;76:271–7.
14. Martinoli C, Derchi LE, Solbiati L, Rizzatto G, Silvestri E, Giannoni M. Colour Doppler sonography of salivary glands. AJR Am J Roentgenol 1994;163:933–41.
15. Bradley MJ, Durham LH, Lancer JM. The role of colour flow Doppler in the investigation of the salivary gland tumour. Clin Radiol 2000;55:759–62.
16. Yasumoto M, Yoshimura R, Sunaba K, Shibuya H. Sonographic appearances of malignant lymphoma of the salivary glands. J Clin Ultrasound 2001;29:491–8.

The British Journal of Radiology, *78* (2005), 370–372

Correspondence

(The Editors do not hold themselves responsible for opinions expressed by correspondents)

EBM and the diagnosis of hepatocellular carcinoma

The Editor—Sir,

The recent systematic review of imaging methods for detecting hepatocellular carcinoma (HCC) in patients with cirrhosis [1] illustrates some of the reasons why the methods of evidence-based medicine (EBM) are often unhelpful and may be misleading in the evaluation of diagnostic procedures.

1. The subject material is out of date: the papers on which this review was based were published between 1995 and 2001. With the inevitable delay between acquisition of data and publication, this means that the results discussed in the review date back at least 4–5 years, possibly over 10 years in some cases. During this time there have been considerable advances in experience with multislice CT and with improved contrast-enhanced MRI techniques. Iodized oil CT is extinct and CTPA not far off being so, whilst new contrast agents have completely transformed ultrasound.

2. The approach is high selective and arbitrary: the authors detailed only 29 out of 997 papers containing relevant data. Whilst it must be accepted that much of the imaging literature is unsubstantiated and studies show major variations in diagnostic criteria and the selection of patients, an appreciative reading of the literature would seek to answer the question "what new, useful and reliable information can be gained from this study?" Using rigid and arbitrary criteria to dismiss over 97% of published material on the subject looks more like systematic neglect than systematic review, and risks throwing the baby out with the bath water.

3. The standard of reference is too variable: even amongst the 29 studies included in the review, the evidence for confirmation of the diagnosis varied from histological examination of the explanted liver – which is desirable – to "confirmatory imaging" or "rising AFP" – which is clearly inadequate. It seems perverse to exclude the vast majority of studies from consideration, but then to include some publications with inadequate verification of the true diagnosis.

4. There is no account of observer variation: it appears that in the selection of the studies for inclusion in this analysis, no account was taken of whether single or multiple observers reviewed each individual case. There is a huge amount of literature on observer variation in diagnostic imaging, all of which supports the view that studies which use a single observer for image interpretation are less reliable than those which use multiple observers. Whilst there is an argument for single observers in prospective studies – when the intention is to reflect clinical practice – retrospective studies seeking to compare different imaging methods or to measure diagnostic accuracy should certainly have multiple observers.

5. Dumbing down the detail: the Procrustean approach of bundling together studies using different patient selection, different diagnostic criteria, different modes of verification, and many variations in detail of imaging techniques, deliberately obscures the type of detail which may be critical in the proper evaluation of each study. For example, is it sensible to concatenate studies using single phase and multiphase CT, and those with different slice thicknesses? Although contrast agents in MRI do receive a brief mention, there is no discussion of the details of technique which in some cases are critical to success, and no consideration of the different virtues of tissue-specific and extracellular contrast agents.

6. The conclusion is erroneous: although the authors mentioned some of the points raised above as limitations of their review, they still came to the erroneous conclusion that "there is insufficient evidence to decide on the best imaging technique for the detection of HCC in cirrhotic patients". There is evidence – it is just that the authors' analysis is too limited and too crude to detect it. Many of the 968 studies ignored by the authors contain at least some valuable messages – for example, data on the detectability of HCCs in cirrhotic patients using dual contrast MRI with pathological correlation is given in Ward et al [2] and Bhartia et al [3], whilst a fairly recent review of the whole subject may be found in Ward and Robinson [4]. What is needed is an attempt to understand the difficulties of imaging in this context, rather than a search for a single idiot-proof method which will fit all patients.

7. It is post-modern pseudoscience: The most worrying feature of the pseudoscientific approach illustrated by this review is that it affords a cloak of apparent respectability to erroneous conclusions based on an inadequate analysis. Whilst there is a strong argument for the use of EBM methods in assessing the effects of therapeutic interventions, the case for using this approach in the assessment of diagnostic methods is very weak, largely because the outcomes are much less clearly definable. We have no diagnostic equivalent to the randomized clinical trial. In the diagnostic specialties we should really concentrate our efforts and our research on the study of patients and disease, rather than relying on an over-simplification of the literature which is closer to tabloid journalism than to erudition.

Intelligence may be defined as the ability to learn from experience, so it is unfortunate that the authors of this review – who are undoubtedly capable and dedicated professionals – give the impression that having scrutinised 997 publications relating to the diagnosis of HCC in cirrhosis, they are no nearer knowing how to go about this task than when they started.

Yours etc.,

P J A Robinson

Professor of Clinical Radiology
St James's University Hospital
Beckett Street
Leeds LS9 7TF

(Received 10 November 2004 and accepted 21 December 2004)
DOI: 10.1259/bjr/75613849

References

1. Fung KTT, et al. Systematic review of radiological imaging for hepatocellular carcinoma in cirrhotic patients. Br J Radiol 2004;77:633–40.
2. Ward J, Guthrie JA, Scott DJ, et al. Hepatocellular carcinoma in the cirrhotic liver: double-contrast MR imaging for diagnosis. Radiology 2000;216:154–62.
3. Bhartia B, Ward J, Guthrie JA, Robinson PJ. Hepatocellular carcinoma in cirrhotic livers: double contrast thin-section MR imaging with pathologic correlation of explanted tissue. AJR Am J Roentgenol 2003;180:577–84.
4. Ward J, Robinson PJ. How to detect hepatocellular carcinoma in cirrhosis. Eur Radiol 2002;12:2258–72.

Authors' reply

The Editor—Sir,
Whilst we are pleased that Prof. Robinson has taken time to both read and comment on our paper [1], we feel that most of his comments are misdirected.

1. Inevitably new papers are published which may shed new light on a topic, but our review is still valid with respect to what was evaluated. Moreover, at the time of submission only one other relevant article (fulfilling selection criteria) had been published. We do not deny that technological advances in imaging continue apace, but the purpose of our systematic review was to establish the evidence for which is the best next imaging modality following ultrasound when a suspicious nodule is detected in a cirrhotic patient. This question is still relevant as most centres still use ultrasound (without contrast agents) as a first imaging technique.

2. As detailed in our methods we specifically set out to select articles reporting the characterization of liver lesions in cirrhotics, and thus those related to assessment of therapy, small studies (<10 patients), or when it was unclear if only cirrhotics were evaluated, were excluded. This excluded most studies but this does not mean that they are not a valuable contribution to the literature, just that they did not relate to the question we set out to evaluate.

3. We agree that the gold standard for reference to validate imaging for hepatocellular carcinoma (HCC), should be the explanted liver. We did indeed use this, but this was only evaluated in 10 studies (159 patients from 918) in the 29 studies selected; only 4 studies had direct comparison of imaging techniques. If Prof. Robinson had wished us solely to use this, then only 10 of 997 studies would have been selected. Thus we used other confirmatory criteria for diagnosis of HCC that are used in daily clinical practice: rising alpha fetoprotein or radiological evidence of tumour growth or diagnostic biopsy or confirmatory imaging (as defined by the authors themselves), as reference standards "to prove the lesion" was indeed HCC. These are not inadequate criteria as he implies.

4. The observer variation is an important issue and a relevant one. Prof. Robinson states that multiple observers improve diagnostic accuracy. This is true, but in practice a single radiologist reports a single image sequence for a patient, as he acknowledges. We did not exclude multiple observer studies, but did not come across a single study in cirrhotics (in our time frame) with confirmatory imaging or with the other criteria we have listed, in which multiple observers were used.

5. To make the paper readable, we felt we grouped studies in a sensible fashion and detailed the particular imaging techniques used. The very variation between studies, that Prof. Robinson points out, favours our conclusions in the discussion. Where the authors' results were corroborated either in relation to diagnostic impact or performance, we stated it, as these details were relevant ones for our study. The absence of such information was a limitation of the data available, as pointed out by us. The value of differential MRI contrast agents (tissue specific and extracellular) is a well known research interest of Prof. Robinson [2]. His paper with explant data after liver transplantation was published in March 2003 [3], after submission of our review. It may well be, that if this form of MRI is available, then it could be the next best test following an ultrasound. However, no comparison was made with other imaging techniques to prove it was superior.

6. We disagree about his comments on our conclusions. We couched them very carefully, suggesting ways in which reporting and evaluation of diagnostic imaging could be made in a uniform manner. He quotes our one sentence summary conclusion, by which we stand, which solely relates to the data we evaluated. However, we extensively preface this sentence with comments on assessing diagnostic impact and diagnostic performance as two separate issues, and provide examples of the difficulties encountered and the reasons why these exist. This makes it clear how the summary sentence should be interpreted and read. Furthermore, we suggest that studies assessing therapeutic impact might supersede diagnostic ones – a point that we feel Prof. Robinson should agree upon, as therapeutic modalities for HCC in cirrhosis depend heavily on accurate imaging diagnosis and staging.

7. We sense the frustration that Prof. Robinson has had, but respectfully point out that the basis for it is the poor reporting, poor evaluation and lack of published evidence concerning the subject matter and not the particular evaluation we have put forward. Thus any "post modern pseudoscience" resides in the data of most, but not all, the individual studies. Many unfortunately cannot be used conclusively to answer the question we posed. We accept that Prof. Robinson can have an opinion regarding our review as "tabloid journalism", but obviously disagree with his opinion as did the reviewers. We also strongly disagree with him that diagnostic methods cannot have outcomes as well defined as therapeutic techniques. This is with respect, patent nonsense: sensitivity, specificity and accuracy are key issues (as well as cost) for any diagnostic procedure [4]. Where the limits are set depends on the clinical context: the diagnosis of HCC in cirrhotics requires the highest possible optimum in all three parameters. This is particularly so, as therapeutic decisions are based on imaging, as often histology is cannot obtained (problems with clotting, anatomical position and seeding).

No doubt Prof. Robinson will want to disprove our conclusions in the future, concerning the current literature, by further publishing his own data. We hope he will succeed. If our review has spurred him on, then it has reached one of our objectives: better papers, better evaluation in papers, and eventually more streamlined and better diagnosis (needing less imaging) for cirrhotics with suspicious nodules on ultrasound examination. Lastly we feel that if Prof. Robinson re-reads our discussion carefully, (which can be an example of learning from experience, which he has emphasised to us), he will agree with what we say, as his own research aims in this area are designed to overcome the issues we raised.

Yours etc.,

[1]A K Burroughs
[1]K T T Fung
[1]F T W Li
[1]M L Raimondo
[2]D Maudgil
[1]A Mancuso
[2]J M Tibballs
[2]A A Watkinson
[1]D Patch

[1]Liver Transplantation and Hepatobiliary Medicine and
[2]Department of Radiology
The Royal Free Hospital
Pond Street
London NW3 2QG

(Received 15 December 2004 and accepted 21 December 2004)
DOI: 10.1259/bjr/61032139

References

1. Fung KT, Li FT, Raimondo ML, Maudgil D, Mancuso A, Tibballs JM, et al. Systematic review of radiological imaging for hepatocellular carcinoma in cirrhotic patients. Br J Radiol 2004;77:633–40.
2. Ward J, Robinson PJ. How to detect hepatocellular carcinoma in cirrhosis. Eur Radiol 2002;12:2258–72.
3. Bhartia B, Ward J, Guthrie JA, Robinson PJ. Hepatocellular carcinoma in cirrhotic livers: double-contrast thin-section MR imaging with pathologic correlation of explanted tissue. AJR Am J Roentgenol 2003;180:577–84.
4. McDonald J, Feagan B, Burroughs A. Introduction: (application of a diagnostic test). In: McDonald J, Burroughs AK, Feagan B, eds. Evidence Based Gastroenterology and Hepatology. Oxford: Blackwell Publishing Ltd, 2004:1–11.

The British Journal of Radiology, *78* (2005), 373–375
DOI: 10.1259/bjr/61980420

Case of the month

An unusual cause of rectal bleeding

A M KAISER, MD, FACS and C SPANOS, MD

Department of Colorectal Surgery, Keck School of Medicine, University of Southern California, 1441 Eastlake Avenue, Suite 7418, Los Angeles, CA 90033, USA

A 62-year-old man with acute onset of rectal bleeding was admitted to the hospital where he was transfused several units of blood. Similar intermittent episodes had occurred in the past since early childhood. Some 30 years ago, portal hypertension was postulated, and a splenorenal and subsequently a portocaval shunt procedure were performed. Nevertheless, the rectal bleeding episodes continued, but the patient remained in a relatively stable condition until the present admission.

On physical examination, the patient showed mild abdominal distention and moderate jaundice. Digital rectal exam revealed gross blood, a sponge-like rectal wall but no palpable mass. Proctosigmoidoscopy showed large submucosal lesions with bluish discoloration. A CT scan with oral contrast and intravenous contrast was obtained with findings characteristic of the diagnosis (Figure 1).

What is the diagnosis? What further studies are indicated? What is the treatment?

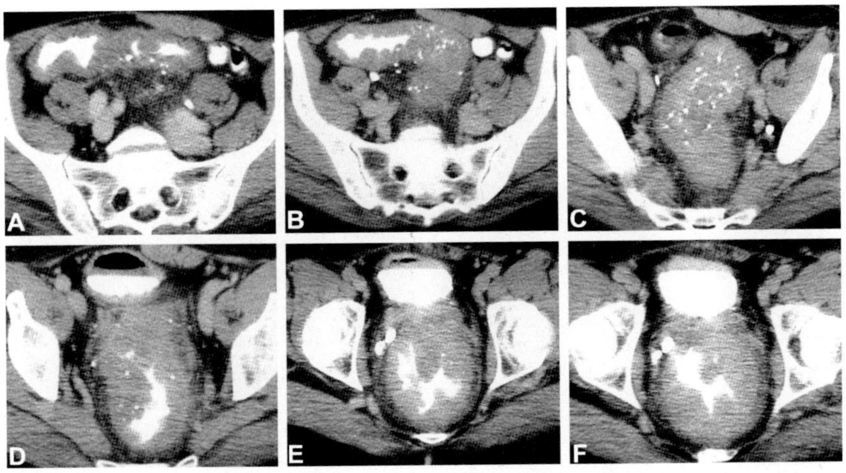

Figure 1. CT with intravenous and oral contrast. Panels moving from proximal to distal in alphabetical order.

Received 24 September 2004 and in revised form 7 December 2004, accepted 4 January 2005.

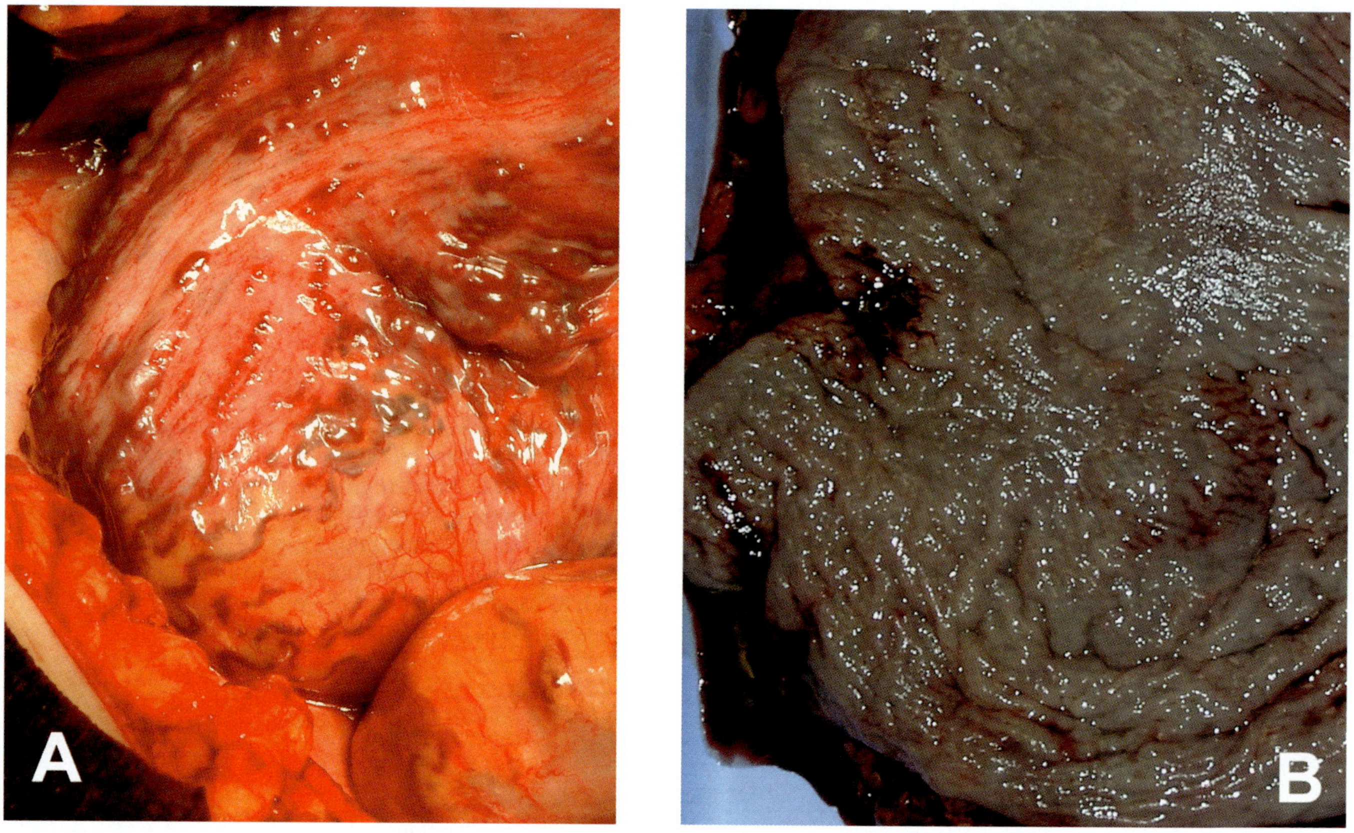

Figure 2. Macroscopic appearance. (A) Intraoperative view of the rectosigmoid with extension of venectasies into the surrounding connective tissue. (B) Opened resection specimen with bluish-greyish mucosa and network of depression of the surface in areas of the emptied vascular lakes.

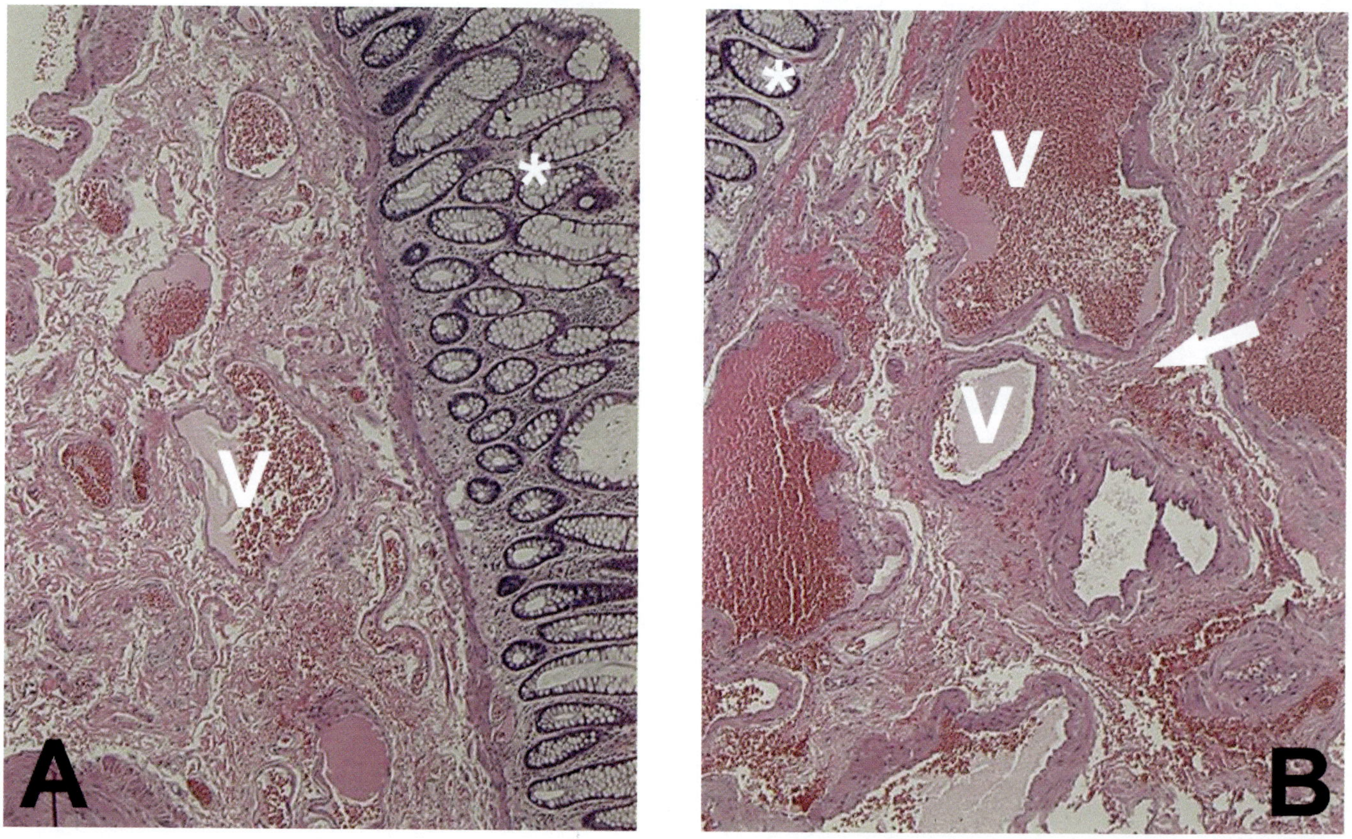

Figure 3. Microscopic appearance. Both panels showing different views with intact mucosa (asterisk) and large submucosal accumulation of thin-walled vascular lakes (V) with smooth muscle fibres and connective tissue stroma (arrow).

Diffuse cavernous haemangioma of the rectum and sigmoid colon (DCHRS) is the diagnosis.

DCHRS is a rare entity characteristically but not exclusively affecting young (male) adults. The most common site of cavernous haemangioma is the recto-sigmoid area (DCHRS), however extraintestinal sites are common and part of syndromes (Klippel-Trenaunay syndrome [1], Bean's syndrome [2]). A common symptom is intermittent painless rectal bleeding, findings may include anaemia, thrombocytopenia and consumptive coagulopathy. Misdiagnosis is the rule and includes ulcerative colitis, haemorrhoids and portal hypertension.

Morphologically, DCHRS shows an extensive network of vascular lakes (Figure 2B), involving the entire intestinal wall with extension into the surrounding connective tissue (Figure 2A). Microscopic examination reveals large, thin-walled vessels with smooth muscle fibres and connective tissue stroma, primarily in submucosal location (Figure 3).

Endoscopy (not shown) reveals bluish-purple submucosal lesions of varying size, protrusion, and extent (Figure 2A) which correlate with a full dilatation of the vascular lakes seen in Figure 3.

CT/MRI are diagnostic under the given circumstances and – in conjunction with endoscopic findings – the test of choice for this pathology (Figure 1), showing characteristic transmural thickening of the involved bowel segment, intramural phleboliths, as well as thickening and vascular engorgement of the mesentery and/or mesorectal fat [3]. The differential diagnosis includes tumour calcifications in adenocarcinoma (scirrhous-type, psammomatous-type calcifications) or lymphoma, or sclerotic alterations of medium to large vessels. The asymmetry noted on CT in the rectus muscle of our patient is not related to the DCHRS, but likely is the result of his previous transverse laparotomy.

Other tests are of lesser value but may provide indirect evidence for the presence of a cavernous haemangioma. Angiography depicts arteriovenous malformations in the majority of cases. A contrast enema (not shown) often demonstrates multilobular scalloping of the wall, similar to the appearance of the luminal contrast in the CT in Figure 1. Endorectal ultrasound may be supplemental and show a marked thickening of the rectosigmoid wall with hypoechogenic tubular lesions [3].

Treatment is either symptomatic or involves surgical resection of the involved segment, either an abdomino-perineal resection or a proctectomy with a colo-anal anastomosis [4], the latter of which was performed in our patient.

In summary, the diagnosis in our patient had been missed for 30 years. Portal hypertension was presumably suspected because of a lack of diagnostic tools and misinterpretation of the rectal pathology as rectal varices. The temporary jaundice seen at presentation was caused by the massive transfusion and the partially bypassed liver circulation (shunt) and resolved post-operatively.

References

1. Ghahremani GG, Kangarloo H, Volberg F, Meyers MA. Diffuse cavernous hemangioma of the colon in the Klippel-Trenaunay syndrome. Radiology 1976;118:673–8.
2. Moretti G, Beylot J, Faivre J, Longy M. [Cutaneous and rectosigmoid cavernous hemangiomas. Bean's syndrome]. Sem Hop 1974;50:1731–6.
3. Djouhri H, Arrive L, Bouras T, Martin B, Monnier-Cholley L, Tubiana JM. Diffuse cavernous hemangioma of the rectosigmoid colon: imaging findings. J Comput Assist Tomogr 1998;22:851–5.
4. Aylward CA, Orangio GR, Lucas GW, Fazio VW. Diffuse cavernous hemangioma of the rectosigmoid--CT scan, a new diagnostic modality, and surgical management using sphincter-saving procedures. Report of three cases. Dis Colon Rectum 1988;31:797–802.

Book reviews

Fetal radiology: a diagnostic atlas. By R Schumacher, L H Seaver and J Spranger. pp. viii+194, 2004 (Springer-Verlag, Berlin, Heidelberg, New York), £115.50
ISBN 3-540-20342-7

Skeletal dysplasias have always held a fascination for paediatric radiologists setting a challenge to aid the geneticist in their drive to come to a diagnosis in those unfortunate children born with skeletal malformations. In more recent years with the increase in antenatal ultrasound it is becoming increasingly necessary to attempt to reach a diagnosis of skeletal abnormality in the fetus either prior to termination or as a result of a post termination skeletal survey. This atlas fills a gap created by this recent development. The early part of the book is devoted to an atlas of normal skeletal development from 14 weeks to 23 weeks of fetal life. The normal appearances beyond this are well recognised from live born premature babies. The majority of the book is taken up with an atlas of abnormalities with separate sections on single skeletal defects and a large section on osteochondrodysplasias. As is traditional it is subdivided by the most obvious radiological features and examples of all the common and many of the rarer abnormalities are given. Each section gives the major radiographic features, mode of inheritance, what the prenatal appearances have been on ultrasound, a differential diagnosis, prognosis and the key references.

Obviously this atlas will have only a limited appeal but it is a very good starting point for radiologists and geneticists involved in this field where the need for an accurate diagnosis is crucial for counselling for future pregnancies.

D Pilling

Radiology of the postoperative GI tract. By BR Javors and EL Wolf. pp. xi+385, 2003 (Springer-Verlag, New York, NY), £111.50
ISBN 0-387-95200-4

This is a remarkable tome, containing as it does only 6 chapters. But what chapters! Each deals with an aspect of the gastrointestinal tract in some detail.

The initial chapter effectively discusses plain film features of the post operative abdomen, but also includes a discourse on the thorny topic of the use of barium *vs* water soluable contrast media. This is followed by an extensive section on tubes and lines, concentrating on Cantor Tubes. These appear to have many complications, which is perhaps why they do not appear to be used elsewhere.

The other chapters are formatted slightly differently, covering the accepted divisions of the GI Tract, with anatomy, surgical procedures and radiological investigative techniques to the fore.

There is extensive use of schematic line drawings to illustrate the surgical techniques used, together with their variations. Indeed a whole page is given to the variations of Billroth surgery to the stomach. This reviewer found the line drawings excellent, but unfortunately cannot say the same of the radiographic reproduction. Many features described in the captions are just not clear. While this mainly applies to analogue images, even the detail of digital CT could have been better. However the range of radiographs showing complications is quite comprehensive, which tends to make up for the reproduction failure.

Each chapter has an excellent list of references, with over 600 in total.

Despite its drawbacks, this book has a place in X-ray department libraries. It will prove essential reading for those in training as the experience available in years past of performing many barium studies is far less likely to be obtained by future generations of radiologists.

R H Corbett

Meetings & Courses

Image display workstations
12 April 2005
London, UK
Further details: The British Institute of Radiology, 36 Portland Place, London W1B 1AT.
Tel: 0207 307 1406. Fax: 0207 307 1414.
Email: registrations@bir.org.uk. Visit: www.bir.org.uk

MR angiography
15 April 2005
London, UK
Further details: The British Institute of Radiology, 36 Portland Place, London W1B 1AT.
Tel: 0207 307 1406. Fax: 0207 307 1414.
Email: registrations@bir.org.uk. Visit: www.bir.org.uk

Nuclear medicine in oncology: new perspectives and innovations in treatment
28 April 2005
London, UK
Further details: The British Institute of Radiology, 36 Portland Place, London W1B 1AT.
Tel: 0207 307 1406. Fax: 0207 307 1414.
Email: registrations@bir.org.uk. Visit: www.bir.org.uk

Prepare yourself for PACS
6 May 2005
London, UK
Further details: The British Institute of Radiology, 36 Portland Place, London W1B 1AT.
Tel: 0207 307 1406. Fax: 0207 307 1414.
Email: registrations@bir.org.uk. Visit: www.bir.org.uk

President's Conference 2005
25–26 May 2005
London, UK
Further details: The British Institute of Radiology, 36 Portland Place, London W1B 1AT.
Tel: 0207 307 1406. Fax: 0207 307 1414.
Email: registrations@bir.org.uk. Visit: www.bir.org.uk

IMRT
8 July 2005
Manchester, UK
Further details: The British Institute of Radiology, 36 Portland Place, London W1B 1AT.
Tel: 0207 307 1406. Fax: 0207 307 1414.
Email: registrations@bir.org.uk. Visit: www.bir.org.uk

International Cancer Imaging Society Meeting and 5th Annual Teaching Course
3–5 October 2005
Beurs van Berlage, Amsterdam, The Netherlands
Further details: The British Institute of Radiology, 36 Portland Place, London W1B 1AT.
Tel: 0207 307 1406. Fax: 0207 307 1414.
Email: icis@bir.org.uk. Visit: www.icimagingsociety.org.uk

BIR CORPORATE MEMBER SCHEME

The BIR Corporate Member Scheme is aimed at all companies with an interest in radiology and allied sciences. For an annual subscription member companies are offered an attractive benefits package. To find out why your company should join the leading edge companies listed below, please contact Mr Adrian C Laws, Marketing Manager, British Institute of Radiology, 36 Portland Place, London W1B 1AT. Tel: +44 (0) 20 7307 1404.

Agfa-Gevaert Ltd
Tel: 020 82314900
Contact Mr M Hill, Business Manager Medical Imaging and PACS Systems
Product Code: 1, 2, 3, 4, 6, 9, 10, 12, 13, 14, 15, 20, 22 and 23

Alliance Medical Ltd
Tel: 01295 671223
Contact Mr Charles Fox, Marketing Executive
Product Code: 1, 4, 5, 16, 20 and 21

Amersham Health
Tel: 01494 798666
Contact Mr D G Rothery, Marketing Manager
Product Codes: 1, 2, 3, 4, 5 and 6

Bard Limited
Tel: 01293 606864
Contact Ms T Empson, Product Manager
Product Code: 2

B.M.V.A.
Tel: 01483 689838
Contact Dr R Bowden, Meetings Officer
Product Codes: 1, 3, 4, 9, 10 and 21

Bracco UK Ltd
Tel: 01628 851500
Contact Mr A Quinn, Product Manager
Product Codes: 1, 2 and 5

BVM Medical Ltd
Tel: 01455 614555
Contact Jay Tailor, Managing Director
Product Codes: 2 and 18

Cerner Corporation (UK)
Tel: 01452 831533
Contact Mr C Harrison, Client Executive
Product Codes: 9, 10, 13 and 20

Clinical Press Ltd
Tel: 0117 9420256
Contact Professor Paul Goddard, Chairman
Product Codes: 17 and 21

Cook (UK) Ltd
Tel: 01462 482884
Contact Mr Iain Mackintosh, regional Manager - Diagnostic and Interventional Products
Product Code: 2

Department of Radiography & Imaging Sciences (St Martin's College, Lancaster)
Tel: 01524 384640
Contact Mr Philip Harris, Acting Head of Department
Product Code: 21

Dictaphone International
Tel:020 78785000
Contact Dr F Brabant, Director of Product Management
Product Codes: 9 and 13

E-Z-EM Ltd
Tel: 01869 366900
Contact Mr Martin Suggitt, Product Manager
Product Codes: 1, 2 and 8

Ferrania UK Ltd
Tel: 01344 312100
Contact Mr Alan Budge, General Marketing Manager
Product Codes: 1, 3, 4, 9, 10, 13, 14, 15 and 18

Fuji Photo Film (UK) Ltd
Tel: 01234 326780
Contact Mr R G Brown, Strategic Business Manager
Product Codes: 1, 3, 4, 6, 9, 10, 12, 13, 14, 15, 18 and 22

GE Medical Systems
Tel: 01753 874000
Contact Mr A Trivett, Managing Director
Product Codes: 1, 2, 3, 4, 6, 8, 9, 10, 15, 18 and 22

Guerbet Laboratories Ltd
Tel: 01908 522888
Contact Mr Trevor Furniss, General Manager
Product Code: 1 and 2

Insignia Medical Systems Ltd
Tel: 01420 540206
Contact Mr Richard Dormer, Managing Director
Product Code: 9

Kimal plc
Tel: 01895 270951
Contact Mr S Clarke, Technical Director
Product Code: 2

Kingsmoor Publications Ltd
Tel: 01371 812960
Contact Mr David Roberts, Managing Director
Product Code: 17

Kodak Ltd
Tel: 01442 844473
Contact Mr Chris Wright, Marketing Manager UK and Ireland
Product Codes: 1, 3, 4, 6, 8, 9, 10, 12, 13, 14, 15, 18, 21, 22 and 23

Landauer, Inc.
Tel: 01865 373008
Contact Dr T Finnigan, Director, European Operations
Product Code: 8

Lanmark
Tel: 01494 675535
Contact Mrs Liz Beckmann, Director
Product Codes: 6, 9, 10, 13, 17 and 20

Lodestone Patient Care Limited
Tel: 020 89449630
Contact Mrs J Hill, Director of Operations
Product Code: 1, 3 and 21

Medical Imaging Systems Limited
Tel: 020 82059500
Contact Mr P W Sykes, Director
Product Code: 1

Mirada Solutions Ltd
Tel: 01865 265500
Contact Dr Clare Jones, VP Marketing
Product Codes: 1, 4, 6, 9, 10, 13, 21 and 22

Nucletron UK Ltd
Tel: 018297 71111
Contact Mr J Banks, Managing Director
Product Codes: 6 and 8

Pantak Medical Systems Agfa NDT
Tel: 0118 9310310
Contact Mr R Howton, Managing Director
Product Codes: 1, 6, 7 and 8

Philips Medical Systems
Tel:01737 230400
Contact Ms Anita Littlechild, Marketing Communications Manager
Product Codes: 1, 2, 9, 10, 22 and 23

Samsung SDS Europe Ltd
Tel:020 83807000
Contact Mr G Wheeler, Sales Manager (Medical)
Product Codes: 1, 9, 10, 13, 15, 16 and 20

Schering Health Care Ltd
Tel: 01444 232323
Contact Mr Chris Matthews, Product Manager
Product Codes: 1, 2 and 3

Sectra Ltd
Tel: 020 86106033
Contact Jan Wolfram, Managing Director
Product Codes: 9 and 10

Siemens Medical Solutions
Tel: 01344 396317
Contact Mr Mike Bell, Manager, Advertising and Exhibitions
Product Codes: 1, 2, 3, 4, 6, 9, 15 and 22

Sony Scientific and Medical
Tel: 01932 816267
Contact R Holt, Marketing Manager
Product Code: 14

Sonosite Ltd
Tel: 01767 313117
Contact Ms Gillian Duffy, European Marketing Director
Product Codes: 3

Southern Scientific Ltd
Tel: 01903 604000
Contact Mr Stephen Adams, Sales Manager
Product Codes: 1, 3, 4, 8, 10, 12 and 22

Toshiba Medical Systems UK
Tel: 01293 653700
Contact Mr S M Weeden, Manager X-ray Products
Product Codes: 1, 2, 3, 4, 9, 10 and 15

Varian Oncology Systems
Tel: 01293 531244 (UK)
Contact Mr Rolf Stähelin (Switzerland - tel. 00 41 417498844), Marketing Manager, Europe
Product Code: 6

Vertec Scientific Ltd
Tel: 01734 817431
Contact Mr B Hipgrave, Managing Director
Product Codes: 1, 4, 6, 8 and 12

Wardray Premise Ltd
Tel: 020 83989911
Contact Mr R Beach, Sales Manager
Product Codes: 8, 18 and 20

Wolverson X-Ray
Tel: 01902 637333
Contact Mr N Bacon, Sales Director
Product Codes: 1, 8, 15, 18 and 23

Xograph Imaging Systems
Tel: 01666 501501 or 07000 for X-ray
Contact Mr N Staff, Technical Director
Product Codes: 1, 8, 12, 14, 15, 18, 22 and 23

PRODUCT CODES

1. Diagnostic X-ray including NMR and CT
2. Interventional radiology
3. Ultrasound
4. Nuclear medicine
5. Radiopharmaceuticals
6. Radiotherapy and oncology
7. Radiobiology
8. Radiation protection
9. PACS
10. Image processing
11. Nuclear fuel cycle service
12. Quality assurance
13. Radiology data management computer systems
14. Video printing
15. Equipment leasing
16. Hospital-shared services
17. Medical publishing
18. X-ray consumables distribution
19. Electricity generation
20. Medical reporting systems
21. Education
22. Mammography
23. Dental X-ray

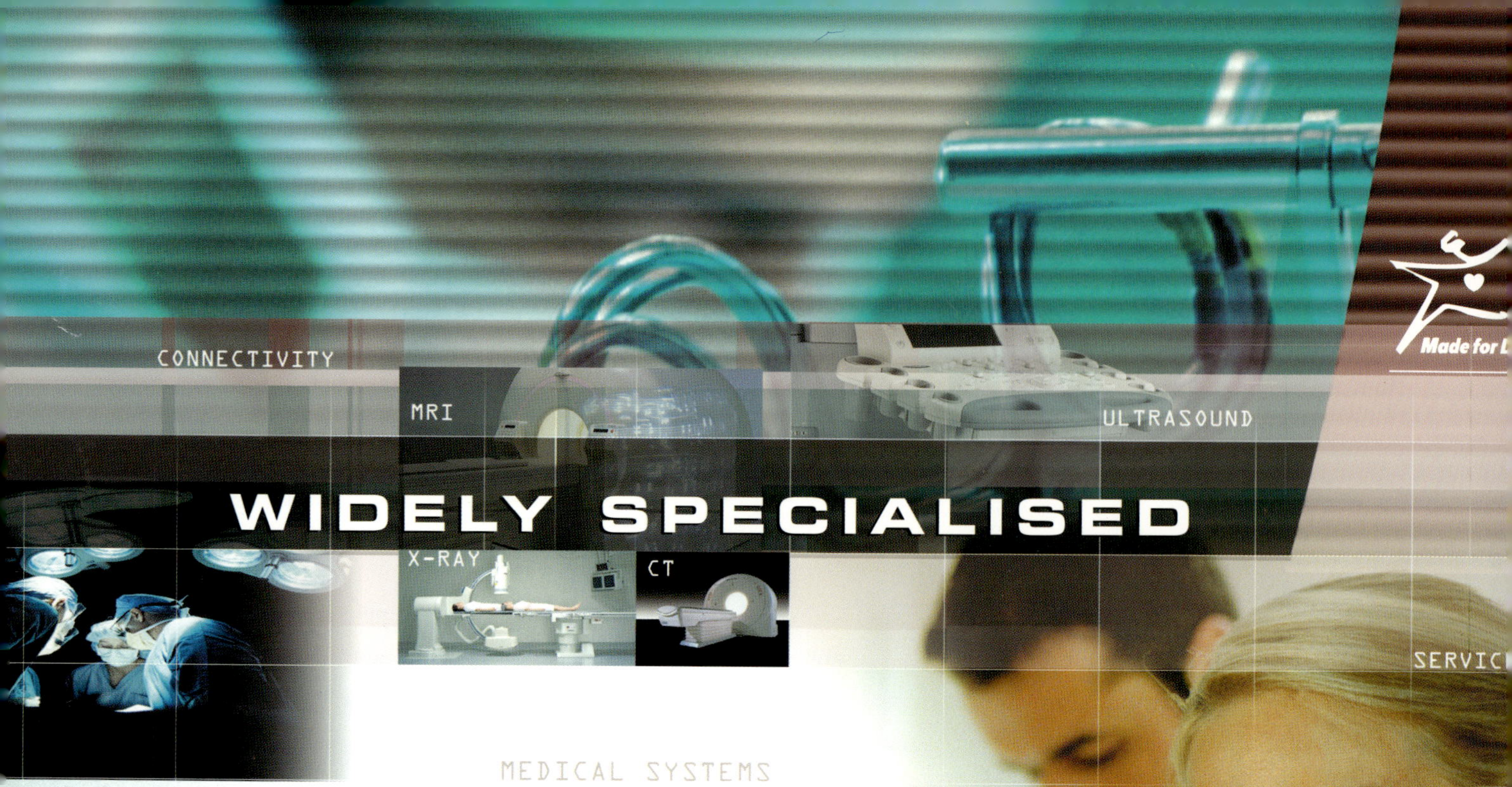

WIDELY SPECIALISED

MEDICAL SYSTEMS

Being widely specialised may seem a contradiction in terms, but it is perfectly possible, provided that your organization is big enough and that you have the required expertise in-house. Communication and proper co-operation with your clinical partners, incorporating their feed-back in the process of product development, makes this challenge achievable.

For years Toshiba has provided leadership in the technological and clinical development of CT, Ultrasound, MRI, X-ray and Connectivity Solutions. Practical developments focusing on clinical impact that bring added value to the diagnostic process. No gadgets or gimmics, but relevant and productive innovations for the realization of improved image quality, higher processing speed and advanced ergonomics.

A growing effectiveness that provides benefit for your patients, and for you ....

Like to know more?

Talk to Toshiba, serving medicine and its practitioners.

TOSHIBA
MEDICAL SYSTEMS LIMITED
www.toshiba-europe.com/medical

Manor Court, Manor Royal
Crawley, West Sussex, RH10 9PY
Tel: 01293 653700
Fax: 01293 560791

Volume 78| **May 2005**

BJR British Journal of Radiology

Full papers

Accuracy of transvaginal ultrasound in diagnosing endometrial pathology in women with post-menopausal bleeding on Tamoxifen

Normal radiographic anatomy of thoracic structures: analysis of 1000 chest radiographs in the Japanese population

Management of non-Hodgkin's lymphoma of the thyroid: the Royal Marsden Hospital experience

Transient failure of opening of the lower oesophageal sphincter on upright oesophagrams: radiographic and clinical findings

Role of ultrasound in Dengue fever

Colonic muco-submucosal elongated polyp: diagnosis with endoscopic ultrasound

Investigation of optimum energies for chest imaging using film–screen and computed radiography

A case of stunning of lung and bone metastases of papillary thyroid cancer after a therapeutic dose (3.7 GBq) of ^{131}I and review of the literature: implication for sequential treatments

Commentary
Review
Short communication
Case reports
Pictorial review
Correspondence
Case of the month
Book reviews

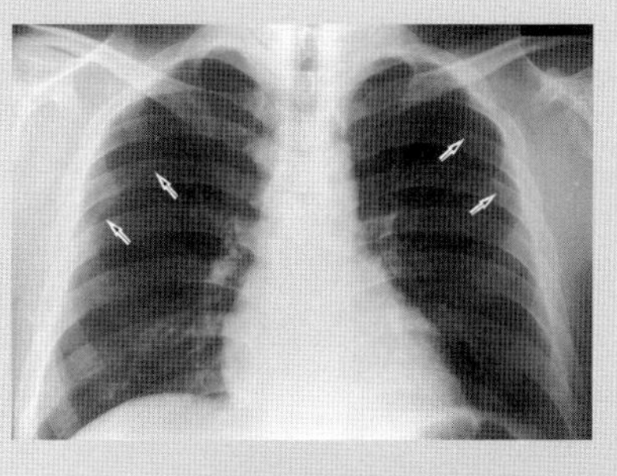

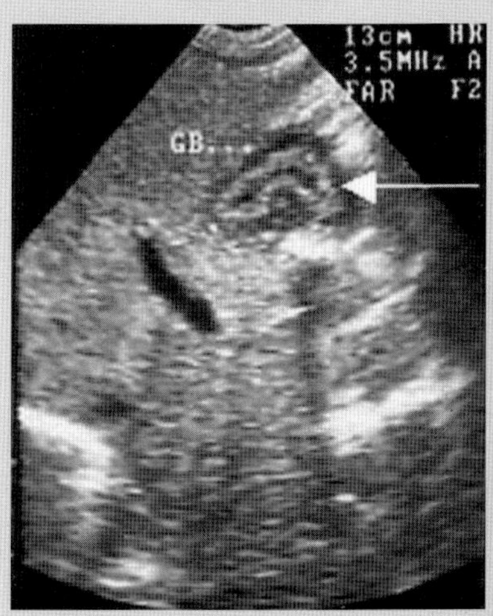

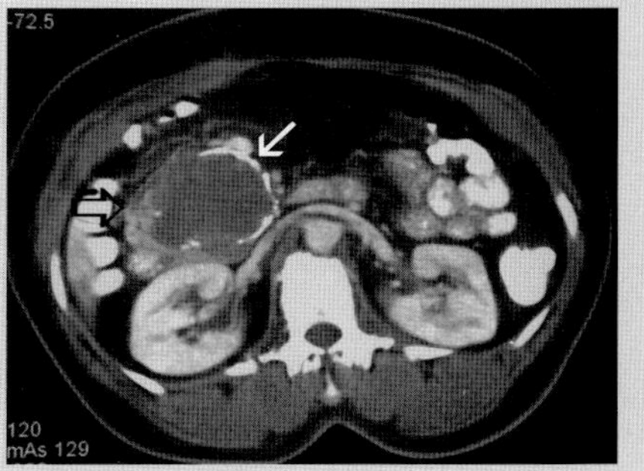

Published by

BIR The British Institute of **Radiology**

http://bjr.birjournals.org

ISSN 0007-1285

BJR

ISSN 0007 1285

THE BRITISH JOURNAL OF RADIOLOGY

Aims and Coverage

The *British Journal of Radiology* is the official peer-reviewed monthly research journal of the British Institute of Radiology. It is a multidisciplinary journal covering all clinical and technical aspects of diagnostic imaging, radiotherapy and oncology, medical physics and radiobiology. BJR is an international journal containing papers both from the UK and overseas, and is circulated to Full Members of the BIR and to libraries worldwide.

Authors are strongly advised to submit manuscripts online using Editorial Manager™, at http://bjr.edmgr.com. Online submission will expedite the peer-review process. Instructions to Authors are available on request from the Refereeing Administrator at the address given below, and are also available on the BIR's website at www.bir.org.uk

Published by the British Institute of Radiology, 36 Portland Place, London W1B 1AT, UK.
Editorial enquiries: Tel: +44 (0)20 7307 1424; Fax: +44 (0)20 7307 1414
Email: publications@bir.org.uk
Advertising sales and enquiries: please contact Gareth Liddiatt at McMillan Scott: Tel: +44 (0)20 7878 2313
Email: gareth@mcmslondon.co.uk
www.bir.org.uk www.birjournals.org bjr.edmgr.com

Subscriptions

Subscriptions fulfilment is carried out by PSP Subscriptions, BMA House, Tavistock Square, London WC1H 9JR, UK (Telephone +44 (0)20 7383 6270; Fax +44 (0)20 7383 6402; email subscriptions@bmjgroup.com). The 2005 annual subscription rate for the printed version of BJR is £524 (includes 12 issues plus two Special Issue). Subscriptions are on a calendar basis only.

Institutional BJR subscribers have free access to both BJR Online and Imaging Online, and are offered a 33% discount on a print subscription to the BJR's quarterly review journal Imaging (see http://imaging.birjournals.org).

US Mailing Agent

The British Journal of Radiology (ISSN 0007 1285) is published monthly by the British Institute of Radiology, c/o Mercury Airfreight Int. Ltd, 365 Blair Road, Avenel, NJ 07001. The Dollar price for US direct subscribers is $786. Periodicals Postage Paid at Rahway NJ. Postmaster: send address corrections to the British Journal of Radiology, c/o Mercury Airfreight Int. Ltd, 365 Blair Road, Avenel, NJ 07001.

Back Issues

Back issues can be ordered from Vine House Distribution, Waldenbury, North Common, Chailey, East Sussex BN8 4DR, UK (Telephone +44 (0)1825 723398; Fax +44 (0)1825 724188). Price is £40 per issue.

BJR Online

BJR Online, produced in association with HighWire Press, is available free of charge to BIR members and Institutional print subscribers: http://bjr.birjournals.org. Enquiries to publications@bir.org.uk

Typeset, printed and bound by The Charlesworth Group, Wakefield, UK. Telephone +44 (0)1924 204830.

BJR

VOLUME 78

Number 929

Contents

May 2005

Front cover: The illustrations used on the front cover of this issue of BJR can be found on pages 401, 417, and 442. We thank the authors for granting us permission to use their figures.

Commentary

Page

- The conventional wisdom and the activities of the middle range — 381
  A J Munro

Review article

- Stereotactic radiosurgery at St. Bartholomew's hospital: third quinquennial review — 384
  A K El Hamri, J Monk and P N Plowman

Full papers

- Accuracy of transvaginal ultrasound in diagnosing endometrial pathology in women with post-menopausal bleeding on tamoxifen — 394
  J Weaver, J M McHugo and T J Clark
- Normal radiographic anatomy of thoracic structures: analysis of 1000 chest radiographs in Japanese population — 398
  H Abiru, K Ashizawa, R Hashmi and K Hayashi
- Management of non-Hodgkin's lymphoma of the thyroid: the Royal Marsden Hospital experience — 405
  K J Harrington, V J Michalaki, L Vini, C M Nutting, K N Syrigos, R A'Hern and C L Harmer
- Transient failure of opening of the lower oesophageal sphincter on upright oesophagrams: radiographic and clinical findings — 411
  C A Raptis, M S Levine, S E Rubesin, I Laufer and D A Katzka
- Role of ultrasound in dengue fever — 416
  P M Venkata Sai, B Dev and R Krishnan
- Colonic muco-submucosal elongated polyp: diagnosis with endoscopic ultrasound — 419
  K Akahoshi, M Matsumoto, M Kimura, A Murata, H Murao, Y Sumida, M Kubokawa, K Ito and M Oya
- Investigation of optimum energies for chest imaging using film–screen and computed radiography — 422
  I D Honey, A Mackenzie and D S Evans
- A case of stunning of lung and bone metastases of papillary thyroid cancer after a therapeutic dose (3.7 GBq) of ^{131}I and review of the literature: implications for sequential treatments — 428
  A F Leger, M Pellan, F Dagousset, A Chevalier, I Keller and J Clerc

Short communication

■ Hepatic transit time: indicator of the therapeutic response to radiofrequency ablation of liver tumours 433
X Zhou, D Strobel, J Haensler and T Bernatik

Case report

■ Pulmonary blastoma: presentation of two atypical cases and review of the literature 437
R I Walker, K Suvarna and S Matthews

■ Solid-pseudopapillary tumour of the pancreas associated with dorsal agenesis 441
S Ulusan, N Bal, O Kizilkilic, F Bolat, S Yildirim, T Yildirim and E A Niron

■ Myoepithelial carcinoma of the breast: a case report with imaging and pathological findings 444
E K Woo, A D James, J Mercer, S M Allan and D C Howlett

■ Pericardial rupture and cardiac herniation after blunt trauma: a case diagnosed using cardiac MRI 448
J H Sohn, J W Song, J B Seo, K H Do, J S Lee, D K Kim, K S Song and T H Lim

■ Bilateral multilocular cystic nephromas: a rare occurrence 450
K S Sodhi, S Suri, R Samujh, K L N Rao, K Vaiphei and A K Saxena

■ Hepatic artery pseudoaneurysm after liver transplantation: definitive treatment with a stent-graft after failed coil embolisation 453
G Maleux, J Pirenne, R Aerts and F Nevens

Pictorial review

■ Imaging of pelvic injuries in athletes 457
J Brittenden and P Robinson

Correspondence

■ Second cancer risk 469
S Green and B Jones

■ Threshold-contrast detectability curves for digital acquisition 469
C J Kotre and N W Marshall

■ Author's reply 470
D S Evans, A Mackenzie, C P Lewinski and D Smith

Case of the month

■ Breast or chest? A diagnostic conundrum 471
J C Lee, S Banerjee and D M King

Book reviews 473

BIR Company Subscribers 474

Meetings and courses 476

ANNOUNCEMENT

The British Journal of Radiology
Young Investigator Award

The British Institute of Radiology is pleased to announce the introduction of a new Award to encourage young workers in the general areas of diagnostic imaging, radiotherapy and related topics to carry out research and publish it. It will be known as the BJR Young Investigator Award and the winner will receive a prize to be known as the Editors' Prize.

Terms and conditions

1. The Award is made annually to the author of the best paper by a younger investigator published in the British Journal of Radiology during the calendar year.
2. The paper must be a "Full Paper" according to the Journal's criteria - not a technical note, short communication etc.
3. The sole author, or first-named author of a multi-author paper, must be under the age of 35 when the paper is first submitted.
4. First-named authors under the age of 35 are asked to indicate that they are eligible for the Award when the paper is submitted.
5. Only papers that are accepted by both referees at the first submission, either without change or with only minimal changes (AccMin) will be eligible for consideration.
6. Short listing is by the Members of the BIR Publications Committee. The definitive choice for the award is made by the Honorary Editors, whose decision is final.
7. The value of the Award is £250. There will also be a certificate.
8. The presentation will be made at the BIR Annual General Meeting and the winner will be invited to be a guest of the Institute at the dinner which follows in the evening.

Interim arrangements

For the 2005 Award, the authors of all papers already published or provisionally accepted that meet the AccMin criterion (see paragraph 5) will be contacted with respect to the age criterion.

The British Journal of Radiology, *78* (2005), 381–383
DOI: 10.1259/bjr/19582409

Commentary

The conventional wisdom and the activities of the middle range

A J MUNRO, BSc, FRCR, FRCP(E)

University of Dundee, Department of Surgery and Molecular Oncology, Ninewells Hospital and Medical School, Dundee DD1 9SY, UK

> *"It is the duty and virtue of all knowledge to abridge the infinity of individual experience"* [1].

Just under 50 years ago, when J K Galbraith coined the phrase "The conventional wisdom", he was defining "the ideas which are esteemed at any time for their acceptability" [2]. His intention was to point out that there may be important differences between what is acceptable, the territory of the conventional wisdom, and what is true. For clinicians, the current conventional wisdom is that clinical practice must be evidence based and that randomized controlled trials provide the best evidence upon which to base practice [3]. As a result we are supposed to judge articles in medical journals according to a hierarchy of research designs, a hierarchy headed by randomized clinical trials (RCTs) and systematic reviews [4, 5]. In this world-view, observational studies and accounts of accumulated clinical experience are considered to be neither of merit nor of interest, and so, according to the conventional wisdom, they are not usually worth publishing. So why does this issue of the BJR contain a paper by El Hamri and colleagues [6] which is simply a review of the experience at one institution, St Bartholomew's Hospital, with one technique, stereotactic radiosurgery?

Galbraith's comments on the conventional wisdom apply neatly to evidence based medicine [3] in its more dogmatic incarnations.

> *"...the accepted ideas become increasingly elaborate. They have a large literature, even a mystique... ...the very vigour of minor debate makes it possible to exclude as irrelevant... any challenge to the framework itself... ...the conventional wisdom often makes vigorous advocacy of originality a substitute for originality itself.... ....deviation in the form of originality is condemned as faithlessness or backsliding... ...expounding the conventional wisdom is both necessary for, and a prerogative of, success..."*

However, the conventional wisdom is not necessarily true and we should always approach it with that healthy scepticism that is an essential component of scientific practice. One final comment from Galbraith: "the enemy of the conventional wisdom is not ideas but the march of events..." [2]. It seems, therefore, both pertinent and legitimate to ask whether or not the concept of a hierarchy of evidence will remain valid, or are events marching?

There is an increasing realisation that the issues that can be dealt with by RCTs are limited – by restriction (to certain groups of patients, or to specific types of intervention) and by level of detail (generic issues are adequately covered, but the particular cannot be accommodated) [7, 8]. Since clinical practice involves helping individual patients to make individually appropriate decisions, even when the evidence is available, we have difficulty incorporating the evidence from randomized controlled trials into our everyday practice. Simple questions from acute general medicine ("should patients with uncomplicated myocardial infarction be routinely treated with Warfarin?") are far more amenable to an evidence-based approach than more complex questions involving patients with chronic diseases ("does chemotherapy improve both quality of life and survival in patients with inoperable non-small cell lung cancer?"). We measure that which is easy to measure – survival. We find it far more difficult to measure a person's comfort, hopes and expectations, and so we have little or no evidence concerning the effects of chemotherapy on these important aspects of life. The position is even more difficult when we consider evidence-based radiation oncology. Radiotherapy is both a complex intervention and an evolving technology. Expertise-based randomization [9] is, at best, only a partial solution to these problems. Results from randomized trials using obsolete technologies can be no guide to current practice [10].

I am not advocating that we abandon the appropriate use of randomized trials, nor would I argue for a clinical practice based entirely on a mixture of anecdote, custom and personal whim. I would simply point out that there are important activities in clinical research that are neither randomized nor systematic, nor hopelessly anecdotal: to borrow an expression from sociology, we may speak of "activities of the middle range" [11]. Activities of the middle range are those that form a bridge between the general, as epitomised by randomized controlled trials and systematic reviews, and the particular, such as case reports and anecdotes. The idea that activities (and theories) of the middle range are worthy in their own right is, of course, not new. Francis Bacon was acutely aware of the importance of such activity and mischievously misquoted Plato in support of his argument: "And Plato in his Theaetatus noteth well, *That particulars are infinite, and the higher generalities give no sufficient direction: and that the pith of all sciences, which maketh the artsman different*

Received 1 February 2005 and accepted 17 February 2005.

from the inexpert, is in the middle propositions, which in every particular knowledge are taken from tradition and experience" [1] {XIII.2} p150. Hogarth took a middle range approach to the aesthetics of representative art [12]. George Orwell's journalism was an activity of the middle range, but was his journalism in any way inferior to his novels? Is West Side Story a lesser work than the Chichester Psalms? The 300 (or so) cantatas that Bach wrote for the Thomasschule were liturgically demanded, rather than divinely inspired, but that in no way diminishes their beauty or importance. Lofty purpose does not always imply high achievement, nor are everyday tasks devoid of value.

The problem we face as providers and consumers of clinical research is that the use of the concept of a hierarchy of evidence has inappropriately diminished the importance of activities of the middle range [13]. Somehow we have convinced ourselves that the talismanic words "randomized" and "systematic" are guarantees of scientific worth and that any activity to which the word "observation" is attached is of dubious merit and that the adjective "mere" should be automatically attached to it.

Observation is now, and always has been, crucial for medical progress. We need observational studies for a variety of reasons:

- They are more likely than contrived experiments, such as randomized trials, to reflect the realties of clinical practice.
- They can address issues for which randomized trials would either be unethical or impractical.
- They provide a useful historical record of clinical practice: what was done; why it was done; what it achieved.
- They provide the raw material from which hypotheses can be generated and in prospective experimental designs, tested.
- They provide the necessary checks and balances in the evolution of clinical interventions – for example the post-marketing surveillance of the results of clinical trials. Did the best intervention really work in practice?
- They are a pluralist enterprise. You do not need a vast amount of resource and infrastructure to perform and report an observational study.
- Accurate observation is a cornerstone of clinical practice.
- They are the only method whereby we can accumulate knowledge about the clinical manifestations and management of rare conditions.
- Detailed observational studies can help to identify confounders that might otherwise be hidden. The parsimonious approach to data management in large randomised trials means that important confounders are unlikely to be identified.

We ignore the fact that bad research is bad research, whether randomized or observational, and that the opposite is also true. If research based on observation has a bad name, this is a consequence of the way the research is usually carried out and reported. Many observational studies are badly designed and reported and it is extremely difficult to draw any worthwhile conclusions from them, even in aggregate [14]. This is a failure of implementation rather than a fundamental and ineluctable flaw in the approach itself. We need to set, and to achieve, higher standards in observational research. Randomized trials have their CONSORT (Consolidated Standards of Reporting for Trials) statement [15, 16], systematic reviews have their QUOROM (Quality of Reporting of Meta-analyses) statement [17]. We need similar standards for observational studies. Fortunately, such standards are now emerging for studies in epidemiology and public health [18, 19], for studies of diagnostic tests (STARD: Standards for Reporting of Diagnostic Accuracy) [20–22], and for studies of prognostic factors [23–25]. These standards should be of use and interest to both contributors and readers of the BJR.

Events overtake the conventional wisdom. Well-conducted observational research is likely to replace randomized trials as the engine of clinical progress. We are on a cusp: looking backwards towards randomized trials; looking forwards to a world of personalized medicine. A world in which we meticulously observe each individual patient, accumulating large amounts of data, and then combine the power of informatics with clinical experience to establish the optimal management for that individual. The RCT is to clinical investigation as the bicycle is to transport. We needed randomized trials because we could neither identify nor handle important confounding variables. As methods for acquiring, handling and relating data improve, we will be able to identify confounders and randomized trials will become a less important source of evidence upon which to base decisions. It is a pleasant irony to consider that increasing scientific sophistication, in molecular biology and computing will move us away from mindlessly accruing subjects for clinical trials and put clinical medicine back where it has always belonged; with the individual human being. We shall harness the power of science to put the humanity back into clinical practice. In the meantime, we should continue to report upon, and to publish, well-conducted observational studies. We should neither apologise for, nor deprecate, the activities of the middle range. It is in this spirit that we publish the article by El Hamri et al [6].

> *"The reality of much clinical research is that the starting point is a series of observations in which the astute clinical observer notices something exceptional"* [26].

References

1. Bacon F. The second book of Francis Bacon of the proficience or advancement of learning divine and human. In: Wright WA, editor. The advancement of learning (5th edn). Oxford: Clarendon Press; 1900: vii[6] p117.
2. Galbraith JK. The concept of the conventional wisdom. In: The affluent society. London: Hamish Hamilton, 1958.
3. Evidence-Based Medicine Working Group. A new approach to teaching the practice of medicine. JAMA 1992;268:2420–5.
4. Centre for Evidence Based Medicine. Levels of evidence and grades of recommendation. Accessed via http://www.cebm.net/levels_of_evidence.asp (15th January 2005).
5. Scottish Intercollegiate Guidelines Network. SIGN 50 A guideline developers' handbook Section 6: Forming guideline recommendations. 2004. Accessed via http://www.sign.ac.uk/guidelines/fulltext/50/section6.html (15th January 2005).
6. El Hamri AK, Monk J, Plowman PN. Stereotactic radiosurgery at St. Bartholomew's Hospital: third quinquennial review. Br J Radiol 2005;78:384–93.

7. Black N. Why we need observational studies to evaluate the effectiveness of health care. BMJ 1996;312:1215–8.
8. Vandenbroucke JP. In defense of case reports and case series. Ann Intern Med 2001;134:330–4.
9. Devereaux PJ, Bhandari M, Clarke M, Montori VM, Cook DJ, Yusuf S, et al. Need for expertise based randomised controlled trials. BMJ 2005;330:88–92.
10. Munro AJ. What now for postoperative radiotherapy for lung cancer? Lancet 1998;352:250–1.
11. Merton RK. On sociological theories of the middle range. In: Social theory and social structure: 1968 enlarged edition. New York: The Free Press, 1968:39–72.
12. Hogarth W. The analysis of beauty. Written with a view to fixing the fluctuating ideas of taste. London: Reeves, 1753.
13. Petticrew M, Roberts H. Evidence, hierarchies, and typologies: horses for courses. J Epidemiol Community Health 2003;57:527–9.
14. Munro AJ, Lain S, Lane DP. P53 abnormalities and outcomes in colorectal cancer: a systematic review. Br J Cancer 2005;92:434–44.
15. CONSORT. Consolidated Standards of Reporting Trials. In; 2005. Accessed via http://www.consort-statement.org/ (16th February 2005).
16. Moher D, Schulz KF, Altman DG. The CONSORT statement: revised recommendations for improving the quality of reports of parallel-group randomised trials. Lancet 2001;357:1191–4.
17. Moher D, Cook DJ, Eastwood S, Olkin I, Rennie D, Stroup DF. Improving the quality of reports of meta-analyses of randomised controlled trials: the QUOROM statement. Quality of reporting of meta-analyses. Lancet 1999;354: 1896–900.
18. Des Jarlais DC, Lyles C, Crepaz N. Improving the reporting quality of nonrandomized evaluations of behavioral and public health interventions: the TREND statement. Am J Public Health 2004;94:361–6.
19. TREND Group. Transparent reporting of evaluations with nonrandomized designs. 2005. Accessed via http://www.trend-statement.org/asp/trend.asp (15th January 2005).
20. Bossuyt PM, Reitsma JB, Bruns DE, Gatsonis CA, Glasziou PP, Irwig LM, et al. Towards complete and accurate reporting of studies of diagnostic accuracy: The STARD Initiative. Radiology 2003;226:24–8.
21. Bossuyt PM, Reitsma JB, Bruns DE, Gatsonis CA, Glasziou PP, Irwig LM, et al. The STARD statement for reporting studies of diagnostic accuracy: explanation and elaboration. Ann Intern Med 2003;138:W1–12.
22. Whiting P, Rutjes AW, Dinnes J, Reitsma J, Bossuyt PM, Kleijnen J. Development and validation of methods for assessing the quality of diagnostic accuracy studies. Health Technol Assess 2004;8:iii, 1–234.
23. Altman DG. Systematic reviews of evaluations of prognostic variables. BMJ 2001;323:224–8.
24. Riley RD, Abrams KR, Sutton AJ, Lambert PC, Jones DR, Heney D, et al. Reporting of prognostic markers: current problems and development of guidelines for evidence-based practice in the future. Br J Cancer 2003;88:1191–8.
25. Simon R, Altman DG. Statistical aspects of prognostic factor studies in oncology. Br J Cancer 1994;69:979–85.
26. Peters DK. Exceptional matters. Lancet 2004;364:2142–51.

The British Journal of Radiology, 78 (2005), 384–393
DOI: 10.1259/bjr/25963871

Review article

Stereotactic radiosurgery at St. Bartholomew's hospital: third quinquennial review

A K EL HAMRI, MSc, J MONK, MSc and P N PLOWMAN, MD, FRCR

St. Bartholomew's Hospital, London EC1, UK

Introduction and "case mix"

This manuscript describes the stereotactic radiosurgical work of one institution over a 5 year (1999–2004) period and discusses this work in the context of the changing field of radiosurgery.

In 1949, Leksell described a system, which concentrated radiation therapy on intracranial targets within the brain [1]. He conceived image guided, multiple, cross-firing, tightly collimated and small radiation portals "focusing" a high single radiotherapy dose on an intracranial target. His first clinical work was aimed at destroying intracerebral pathways in functional disorders and he coined the name stereotactic "radiosurgery" – a nickname which has endured. The early work was hampered by inadequate equipment, as only a 200 KV X-ray apparatus was available. The concept was next furthered in 1968, again in Sweden, with the introduction of a cobalt-60 gamma unit [2]. The UK's first gamma unit became operational in Sheffield in 1985 [3]. In the current machine at St. Bartholomew's/London Radiosurgical Centre (Gamma Knife; Electa Instruments AB, Linköping, Sweden) there are 201 fixed cobalt-60 sources, each a thin rod of 1 mm diameter, the long axis of which is oriented along a radius of a hemisphere – the helmet, into which the patient's head, within a stereotactic frame, fits. The centre point (or isocentre) of this hemisphere is the point at which the stereotactic co-ordinates of the mapped intracranial target are positioned. In the last decade there have been several advances in Gamma Knife technology. The introduction of the model "C" machine has brought automation to various aspects, whilst maintaining the principal design features. The biggest single change has been the introduction of the motorized automatic positioning system (APS) for targeting each shot of the therapy. The APS has been demonstrated to significantly shorten the overall time taken to deliver a treatment and by reducing the need for human intervention, to lessen the risks of treatment errors [4]. In tandem with hardware improvements, there is continual progress in software design and functionality. The most significant has been the introduction of Gamma Knife "Wizard™". This software can be used to semi or fully automate the treatment planning process. Whereas previously, a treatment plan was formulated by a skilled operator, who placed "shots" to obtain an optimal plan, the Wizard employs a computer to automatically calculate the optimal distribution and weighting of shots to best encompass the target. At present, the unit at our centre is the "B" model, although we are capable of mimicking certain "C" model/Wizard characteristics (*vide infra*).

The last decade has seen a substantial advance in the quality and accuracy of three dimensional imaging technologies. The finer detail and clarity obtained improves the accuracy in delineating target lesions (*e.g.* the excellent imaging of the trigeminal nerve by modern MRI for radiosurgical therapy of trigeminal neuralgia – a routine part of Gamma Knife practice for drug resistant patients). With the increasing availability of PET, work by a variety of groups has started to integrate PET with conventional static, anatomical CT/MRI into the Gamma Knife treatment planning process [5]. Early results suggest that these combined methods of imaging improve target definition, particularly for infiltrating tumours whose boundaries are not so certainly defined on MR alone – we illustrated this in our last quinquennial review [6] and predicted that the technique would also prove valuable to demonstrate whether abnormalities persisting on MRI/CT, after a full cancer therapy programme, remain viable and should be targeted by radiosurgery (*e.g.* after chemotherapy in the case of intracranial germ cell tumours or after whole brain radiotherapy in the case of metastases) [7].

Over the last 15 years, linear accelerators (linacs) have been adapted for stereotactic delivery of radiation therapy, initially using the isocentric mounting and rotation technology but latterly both fixed fields and dynamic arcing methods have been introduced, in combination with multileaf collimator (MLC) conformational technology. In 1989, the first UK linac based radiosurgery system commenced clinical operation at St. Bartholomew's Hospital and initially employed multiple non-coplanar arcs around the stereotactically mapped target (usually as a single iso-centre) as the treatment technique. In our last quinquennial review we described our work using that technology [6]. Since that time, the routine availability of multileaf collimation in linacs (leaf widths from 3–10 mm – either as additional accessories (mMLC) or as an integral part of a linac) has allowed improved beam shaping and now most centres practising stereotactic radiation therapy employ either multiple fixed fields or dynamic arcing together with multileaf collimation to improve the conformity of the technique.

At St. Bartholomew's, the acquisition of both Gamma Knife technology and 3 mm leaf width micro-multileaf collimation (in conjunction with our stereotactic linac technology) within the last 5 years has allowed the present

Received 14 September 2004 and in revised form 19 November 2004, accepted 6 December 2004.

Address correspondence to Dr P N Plowman, Department Radiotherapy, St. Bartholomew's Hospital, London EC1, UK.

quinquennial review to report interesting data on many aspects of practise and be in the unique UK position to make some objective, comparative observations concerning the two major photon technologies currently utilized for stereotactic radiation therapy.

The distribution of tumour types treated in the last 5 years (circa 400 patients) has been compared with those (circa 400 patients) reported in the last quinquennial review [6] (Figure 1). Differences are noteworthy.

Despite the proportionate increase in other diagnoses, arteriovenous malformations (AVM) remain the most common disease category treated by our unit, and remain the diagnosis par excellence that established the technology as a powerful force in modern therapeutics (Figure 1). The cavernous angioma is overall less common (but diagnosed incidentally more commonly now, during modern MR examinations for other reasons). We accept patients with recurrent symptomatic bleeds for focal radiation therapy. There have been several reports of higher complication rates following radiosurgery for cavernoma (size-for-size and dose-for-dose) than AVM and we have made some recent observations that we believe may explain a phenomenon that we have not encountered in our radiation series for ocular or other cavernous angiomas. We have utilized these observations to adapt our treatment methods. These are discussed below.

Meningiomas currently comprise a larger proportion than in our early series and are, for the majority, skull base tumours which have proved difficult to curatively resect (*e.g.* those involving the cavernous sinus), although parasagittal meningiomas represent another separate site group which has also grown in referral numbers. We attribute this increase in referral and treatment practice to a better awareness of the success of such therapy. In our series, atypical/aggressive meningiomas are not more heavily represented than their true incidence.

The treatment of vestibular (acoustic) neuroma (and of other intracranial neuromas) by stereotactic radiation therapy has become a standard, front-line, definitive treatment of this disease with excellent, durable, local control rates and reasonable hearing preservation results. There has been recent litigation in the UK for failing to counsel concerning such treatment by a patient who went for open resection, which was attended by complications. Not surprisingly, the representation of vestibular neuroma has risen in our latest series (Figure 1). Nowhere in stereotactic radiation therapy is the controversy between Gamma Knife and linac technology more hotly contested than in the treatment of vestibular neuroma, largely owing to the passage of the "innocent bystander", normal and radiosensitive acoustic nerve through the target volume during therapy and the desire for hearing preservation, discussed below.

Pituitary adenoma has presented an intellectual problem. On the one hand, our data and those of others have demonstrated the high efficacy of well-fractionated, moderate dose equivalent conventional radiotherapy for the long term control of pituitatry adenoma [8] and with little late morbidity (pituitary hormone endocrine deficiency being the most common late sequel). On the other hand, the adenoma is frequently a discrete and small lesion, within the fossa and well visualized on MRI; furthermore, recent radiosurgical publications suggest good tumour and endocrine control of such lesions [9]. As predicted in our last quinquennial review [6], a selective increase in the numbers of pituitary adenomas accepted onto the programme has occurred in the recent series, although conventionally fractionated radiotherapy remains the treatment recommended for the majority of patients presenting to this hospital with pituitary adenoma. Paediatric pituitary adenoma presents a particularly difficult area for us – on the one hand there is a paucity of data following radiosurgery whilst on the other hand, conventionally fractionated radiotherapy undoubtedly encompasses more hypothalamus/normal brain – even in the present conformal age – with potential attendant morbidity. This matter is further discussed below in the context of our recently reported large series of radiation treated paediatric Cushing's disease patients.

Craniopharyngioma presents a problem not dissimilar to that of vestibular neuroma in that there is a normal special sensory (radiosensitive) nerve, the optic chiasm, frequently within the target volume, and the price of harming that special sensory nerve structure is clearly devastating. Interestingly, the proportional representation of craniopharyngioma has not appreciably increased in our current series but we have reported new observations

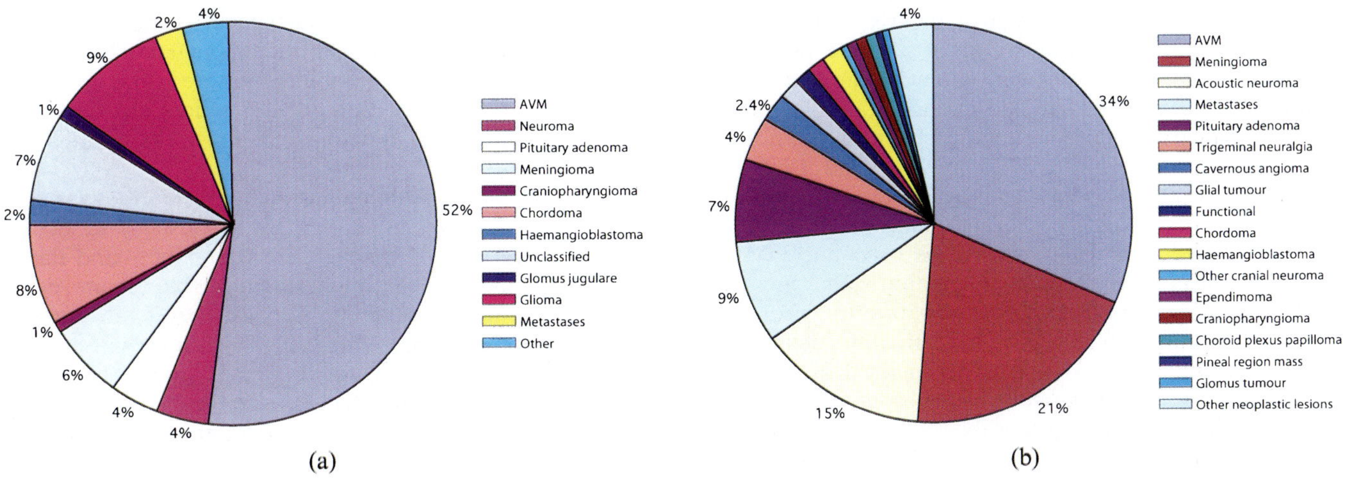

Figure 1. Pie diagrams of (a) distribution of diseases treated to 1999 and (b) 1999–2004 by radiosurgery at this centre.

on one particular subgroup (intrasellar disease) and this is discussed below.

In our last quinquennial review [6], we noted that only 2% of our treated cases had been metastatic disease to the brain and drew attention to the fact that metastases comprised up to 33% of some Gamma Knife caseloads in other radiosurgical units. We predicted that there would be an increase in the number of metastases accepted onto our programme in the future and this has proved the case (Figure 1). The literature demonstrates the high efficacy of the technique for sterilizing individual lesions [10], but we still believe that selection of cases must be vigorous (*vide infra*): patients undergo high quality and thin slice MRI scans of brain to best define the extent (number) of metastatic disease and systemic staging before acceptance onto our programme – acceptance being via a multi-disciplinary advisory group meeting for all patients (and all diagnoses). This is discussed below.

Other diagnoses accepted include haemangioblastoma (reviewed in our last quinquennial report [6]) and residual/recurrent discrete targets after conventional therapy (*e.g.* low grade glioma, central neurocytoma etc.). These are not discussed in depth here, but the point is worth making that for some other discrete and unresectable tumourous lesions, radiosurgery becomes the prime therapy choice. Similarly, the acquisition of Gamma Knife technology, with its extreme precision and ability to treat down to 4 mm collimator size portals, has led to the practice of "functional radiosurgery" (*e.g.* trigeminal neuralgia, the treatment of mesotemporal sclerosis causing refractory epilepsy), not previously represented in our last quinquennial review [6]; this will be the subject of future research.

Physics research

In the second half of the 1990s, and for linac based radiosurgery, there was a move away from multiple arcing beams using circular collimators to multiple static conformal beams. Conformality is produced by shaping each field either by custom made lead blocks or by multileaf collimation. A comparison by Adams et al [11] between stereotactic conformal radiation therapy treatment plans using a standard 10 mm leaf width multileaf (MLC) and custom made blocks had demonstrated that, for a similar planning target volume, there was worse conformality achieved by the MLC. However, the width of 10 mm of the MLC was regarded as the weak point of this comparison and 5 mm leaf width MLC were becoming available as standard equipment on our Varian linacs thus improving conformality. We had published a study on the comparative conformality of our early linac technology with that of Gamma Knife technology [12] and it became clear that we should repeat the study using the newer conformal static field conformal linac methodology. However, there had been recently released micro-MLC equipment (BrainLAB, Munich, Germany) with 3 mm leaf widths and it seemed clear that if we were to produce a definitive study on the respective conformalities achievable on linac versus Gamma Knife technologies then it would be sensible to first examine whether conformality was indeed significantly better using the micro-MLC and then use the perceived optimal linac technique. Added to this, there were some data suggesting that dynamic arcs might be better than fixed fields in conformal therapy and so we factored this into the comparison. Adding to the difficulties in the design of this study was the fact that the dosimetry of the Gamma Knife technology was also improving in the following regard: the newest model of the Gamma Knife had computer assisted planning and automated sequencing of fields which made it more practical to treat many more "shots" using the smallest (4 mm) collimator – thus enhancing conformality. To compare like with like we decided to mimic this facility in our comparison such that optimal technologies were compared.

Thus, our first study compared the 3 mm/micro-MLC with the 5 mm leaf width collimator for linac stereotactic radiation therapy: 14 patients with various irregular shaped intracranial lesions were selected for this study. All were planned for therapy using both the micro-MLC with 3 mm leaf widths (BrainLab, Munich, Germany) and the Varian Millenium MLC (5 mm leaf widths). There was a small but significant improvement in the conformality using the 3 mm leaf-MLC. For the treating clinician, the salient point was that the mean increase in the volume of adjacent critical structure enclosed within the 50% and 70% isodoses was 5.7% and 4.9%, respectively [13]. Whilst there remains debate as to whether the size of this improved conformity mandates stereotactic radiation therapy departments to acquire the micro-MLC equipment, we thereafter accepted that we should utilize the micro-MLC technology for comparison with the latest planning methodology of Gamma Knife (Electa Instruments AB, Linköping, Sweden).

Our second comparative study therefore compared fixed field and dynamic arc linac technology using the micro (3 mm)-MLC equipment with modern Gamma Knife technology [14]. We chose acoustic neuroma as the disease for the comparison, as it has generated more controversy than perhaps any other in the discussions of optimal stereotactic radiation therapy technique. Eight patients with neuromas of various sites (intracanalicular, extracanalicular and both) and sizes were selected for study and conformity indices (total volume of prescription isodose/volume of target covered at the prescription isodose level) and dose–volume histogram (DVH) (for target and brainstem) were computed. A clear difference between linac technology and gamma knife was found. Gamma Knife technology demonstrated a statistically significantly better conformity index ($p<0.02$). Additionally, when linac techniques were compared, dynamic arcing demonstrated a statistically lower conformity index ($p<0.05$) than fixed fields. Of course, conformity indices were worse for small targets in all techniques but the differences just described were true across the board, albeit most exaggerated for small targets.

Although the logical conclusion from the above is that the adjacent normal tissue (*viz.* the brainstem) should be better spared in the Gamma knife technique – and this is true, nevertheless, the highest point maximum doses received in the brainstem in our series were in patients with larger acoustic neuroma indenting/abutting the brainstem and planned for Gamma Knife. This is a feature of the higher internal dose gradient in the Gamma Knife technique, which relies on overlapping fields/shots.

The study of the minimum dose to the target (TD_{min}) has proved an interesting subject [15]. As a consequence of high conformality, the Gamma Knife technique delivered a lower TD_{min} than either linac technique. When the two linac techniques were compared, the dynamic arc still achieved a higher TD_{min} than the fixed field method notwithstanding the fact that it also achieved a slightly better conformity index over the fixed field technique – this was unexpected. The subject of TD_{min} is of potential clinical importance in that underdosing of tumourous areas may lead to treatment failure; consequently the quest for high conformity may need to be tempered when high conformity leads to a significantly lower TD_{min} (underdosed target/tumour areas).

The potential importance of our TD_{min} observations prompted the next study where the TD_{min} was held constant and differences in conformity were scrutinised. In short, we adjusted the Gamma Knife plans such that the TD_{min} on the Gamma knife plan was the same as on the linac plans and then (re-)compared the conformity index. Interestingly, the Gamma Knife plans still maintained the advantage over the linac ones. We conclude that too little attention has been made of the TD_{min} as a parameter that rates alongside conformity index in importance and this conclusion has applicability in other conformal radiotherapy planning outside the cranium [15].

Another physics contribution was the study of the need (or not) for distortion correction during the use of digital subtraction angiography (DSA) in the mapping of arteriovenous malformations (AVM) for Gamma Knife therapy [16]. DSA offers several advantages over conventional angiography, including increased contrast sensitivity (reducing the volume of contrast agent injected), easier image manipulation and "real time" viewing. However, the technique suffers from worse spatial resolution and is prone to geometric distortions, which may require individual correction. The degree of geometric distortion varies inversely with radial position and is significantly reduced at the centre of the image. In our stereotactic radiosurgery work it was clearly important to know if we should routinely employ such corrections, but it was also possible that this would be unnecessary as we deliberately fit the stereotactic frame such that the target to be treated is placed near the centre of the frame, where any distortion is least. In the study, patient and phantom images (with and without image distortion correction) were assessed. The errors measured in angiograms were compared with those of MR and CT images. All errors measured in the study were sub-millimetre. In the patient group, errors of distortion correction measured 0.13 mm (range 0–0.3 mm). Without distortion correction, errors averaged 0.34 mm (range 0.1–0.6 mm). By comparison, the average error for intracranial MRI was 0.3 mm (max. 0.6 mm). We concluded that distortion correction did not significantly reduce (*i.e.* by a factor that was clinically important) error(s) associated with the definition of the stereotactic co-ordinates in our Gamma Knife radiosurgery work for AVM [16].

A further publication related to the possible substitution of MR mapping alone rather than combined MR and conventional angiography in the mapping of AVM for stereotactic radiosurgery [17]. Current radiosurgical treatment of AVMs relies on planning protocols which integrate data from both MR and stereotactic angiography. However, angiography is invasive and carries small but not insignificant risks, whereas MR is non-invasive with multiplanar capability and can demonstrate AVM anatomical detail well. Guo et al [18] found that the delineation of the AVM nidus by MR mapping was superior to conventional stereotactic angiography particularly for medium to larger AVM. However, the authors did not believe that MR should be used alone for the mapping process because of concerns regarding geometric distortion arising from the magnetic field, inhomogeneity, MRI artefacts and the inability of MR to demonstrate the temporal sequence of vascular filling and the distribution of the feeding artery/ies. In our study, AVM planned in the conventional manner were re-planned using MR technology alone by another member of the team. In the first instance it was found that there was insignificant interindividual variation with regard to MR nidus definition on MR amongst the team – a crucial first step. There was no significant difference in the target volume between conventional dual modality planning and MR only but there was significant (random) displacement of the volume in space, that varied little between individuals. We concluded that MR mapping alone led to random displacement of the target compared with dual modality planning and such displacements could produce variation that was too large for safe radiosurgery [17].

Arteriovenous and cavernous malformation therapy research

AVM was the diagnosis for which the technique of stereotactic radiation therapy (radiosurgery) first established itself as a first line therapy and then came acceptance of the technique for other angiomas. A review of this subject was the subject of an editorial in 2002 [19] and research into the subject of AVM currently revolves around the role or otherwise of embolisation in conjunction with radiosurgery in these cases and whether there is logic, safety and efficacy in treating parts of large AVM at different radiosurgical treatment sessions over time to lessen the risks of late complications associated with treatment of large volumes.

Our major vascular malformation manuscript this last 5 years [20] has dealt with the subject of cavernous angiomas of the brain and specifically the observation in several series that there is a higher incidence of late treatment complications following radiosurgery for these angiomas than AVM (equated for size, site and dose). This has not been observed in publications on radiotherapy for cavernous angiomas elsewhere in the body and certainly not in our large ocular cavernous angioma experience [21, 22]. As we say in our manuscript [20]: "speculation that a tumour/angioma may "radiosensitise" its normal tissue environs is a foreign concept in radiation therapy and presents a novel problem". Given the safety of radiation therapy for cavernous angiomas elsewhere, our interest in the problem centred on the unique presence of the haemosiderin stained fringe of normal brain tissue that always surrounds a brain cavernous angioma, well seen on modern MRI (Figure 2). The possibility that normal brain tissue surrounding a brain cavernous angioma is sensitized to radiation by virtue of "staining" by haemosiderin is a thesis that we elaborated. Under conditions of reduced pH (*e.g.* hypoxia, inflammation) iron is liberated from haemosiderin and can act to promote both hydroxyl free radical formation in the presence of hydrogen peroxide

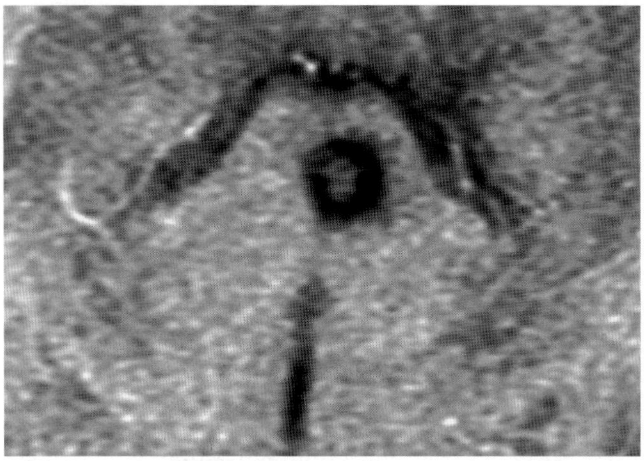

Figure 2. T_1 weighted axial MR scan in the region of the upper pons, demonstrating a small brainstem cavernous angioma. The angioma is surrounded by a haemosiderin ring (black on scan), which follows chronic blood seepage into the normal surrounding brain from the angioma over time.

and lipid peroxidation in lysosomes, quite apart from any enhancement of secondary electron flux. In situations where there is impairment of protective cellular mechanisms *e.g.* a reduction of cellular reducing metabolites, this capability of released iron to generate reactive oxygen intermediates, leading to oxidation and peroxidation of membranes and DNA, may become unchecked and result in tissue damage. We reviewed evidence that the perilesional brain is under conditions of chronic inflammation and could well fall into the situation just described. We also called on Nelson and Stevens' study in Chinese hamster ovary cells demonstrating that the presence of iron enhanced damage in this *in vitro* assay [23] and the data of Hornsey demonstrating in an *in vivo* assay of rat spinal cord that chelation of iron reduced the late effects of radiation (by reducing the production of hydroxyl free radicals) [24] to support our thesis [20]. Lastly, we called attention to the fact that the iron impregnated tissues could influence the accuracy of MR mapping due to the magnetic susceptibility effect caused by haemosiderin [20]. (Iron containing substances cause intravoxel magnetic field inhomogeneities with line broadening on MR).

Vestibular (acoustic) neuroma research

In the last 5 years, the acceptance of radiation therapy as a first line curative therapy for vestibular/acoustic neuroma, and an alternative to neurosurgery, has become standard. Long term control and morbidity results following radiation therapy compete attractively with those from microsurgical units [25]. Hereafter, the controversy as to which radiation therapy method is optimal represents the largest area of disagreement in the profession at present. On the one hand, the data from the Gamma Knife centres undoubtedly contribute the majority of the world literature concerning long term, good control rates and low morbidity, arguing strongly that this method has the best pedigree. However, the very high internal dose gradient of the Gamma Knife technique, allowing double dosing of the innocent bystander cochlear nerve (particularly in intracanalicular cases), may well prejudice hearing preservation more than a technique, which has firstly a much lower internal dose gradient and secondly allows fractionation. Here enters the linac methodology into the "fray". With a low internal dose gradient (circa 10% versus circa 100% in the Gamma Knife technique) and the capability to fractionate, there is much interest in the use of linac stereotactic methods, where hearing preservation is of prime concern. Early data appear promising [26] but longer follow up is needed to be sure that this is durable and is not at the expense of loss of tumour control. The Gamma Knife offers the better validated data on tumour ablation – after all, the integral dose within the tumour will be vastly more in a technique that has such a high internal dose gradient. Our physics contributions to this debate have been reviewed above and we discussed this topical clinical controversy in a recent editorial [27].

In 2003, we presented the first UK case of a patient experiencing the return of hearing in a "dead" ear following radiosurgery (Figure 3) [28].

Neurofibromatosis type 2 (NF-2) patients carry an oncogene in the genome and this may predispose them to oncogenesis following radiation therapy. Thus, whereas Baser et al [29] found the background rate of CNS malignancy amongst 1500 NF-2 sufferers to be 0.5%, these same authors found that of 117 neurofibromatosis patients who had received radiation therapy the incidence of late malignancy was 6% occurring within the radiation field or penumbral region – including four cases of malignant peripheral nerve sheath tumour, suggesting malignant change within the tumour itself. The very real possibility is there that the inherited loss of the NF-2 gene on the long arm of chromosome 22 leads to the loss of a critical tumour suppressor gene. As we said in our first publication on this topic: "this might well interact with radiation to lead to this higher observed incidence of late oncogenesis" [30]. We subsequently enhanced the thesis by invoking the analogy with hereditary retinoblastoma, where Knudson [31] modelled a scenario in which the first predisposition to the development of a tumour was the possession of the inherited loss of the Rb suppressor gene in the genome (the "first hit in a two hit process" in Knudson vernacular); radiation provided the second predisposition/hit by mutating the second allele. We suggested that a comparable situation applied to the NF-2 cases treated with radiation, although we called attention to the fact radiation-induced late tumours might occur either within or without the treated target (*i.e.* in the treated tumour itself or in the penumbral zone) and observed that in the NF-2 series data so far, it appeared more common that the second tumour occurred within the target/tumour volume [32].

Meanwhile, in the last 5 years, the group in Sheffield have produced good data demonstrating that acoustic neuromas which are secondary to NF-2, respond less well to radiosurgery than sporadic cases with the volume of the treated tumour being very influential in the likelihood of control [33]. Having said this, the Sheffield experience is that overall 50% of NF-2 cases will be controlled by radiosurgery and 20% will have definitely failed by 8 years, whilst 30% will have some concerns overall durable control [34].

In a disease that is bilateral and therefore threatens total hearing loss there will remain a place for radiosurgery but

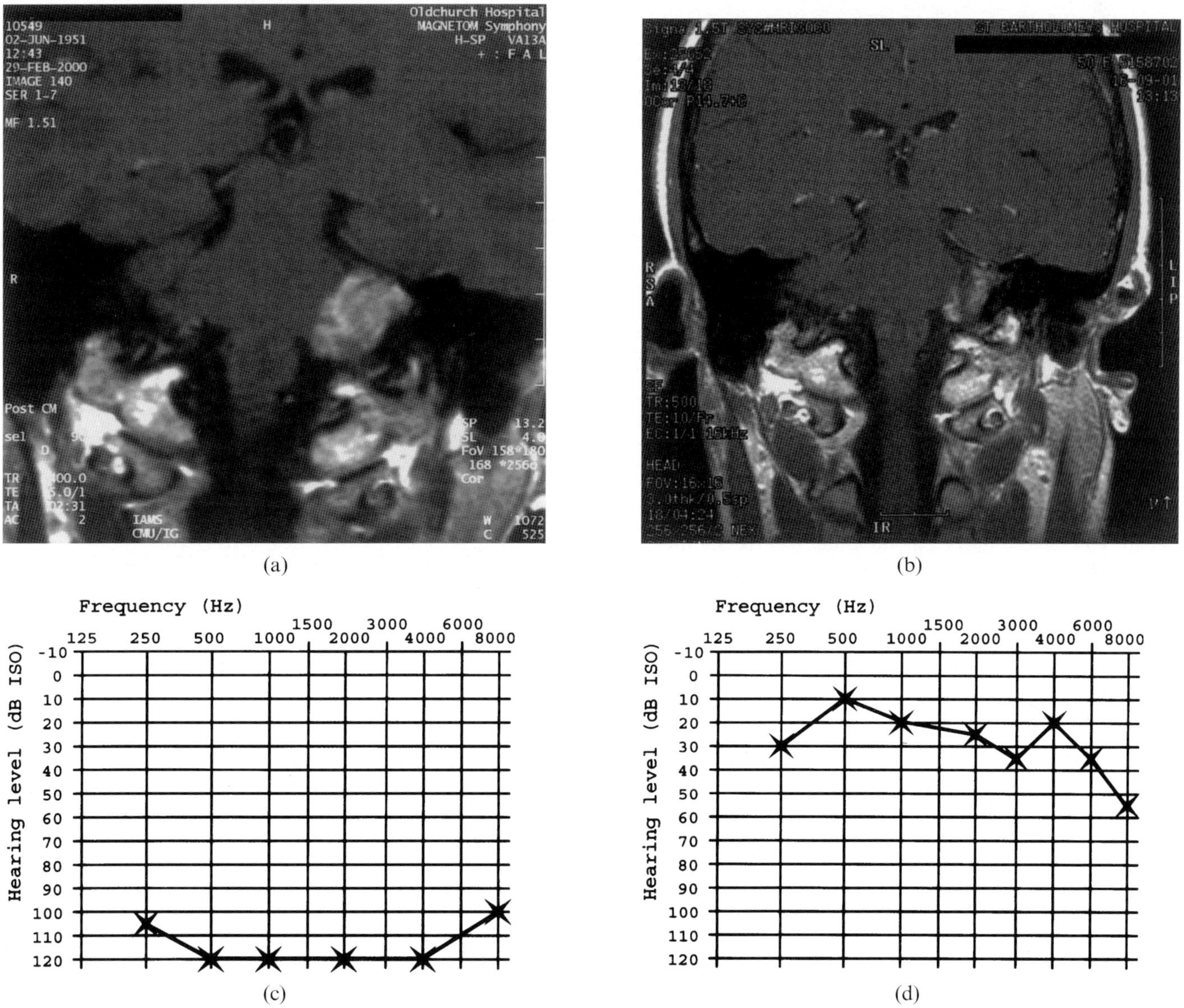

Figure 3. Gadolinium enhanced, T_1 weighted, coronal MR scans of an acoustic neuroma (a) before and (b) after radiosurgery, demonstrating unusually dramatic shrinkage. Audiograms (c) before and (d) after demonstrate the exceptionally good return of hearing in this patient following this therapy.

the last 5 years' literature has brought increasing knowledge upon which to base decisions.

Pituitary adenoma research

In our last quinquennial review [6], we outlined our intellectual problem with introducing stereotactic radiosurgery as primary definitive radiation therapy for pituitary adenoma, when conventionally fractionated radiotherapy produced excellent results and had been used in this department over decades. However, we were building up a series of patients who had failed such conventional radiation therapy. Specifically, we published the results of radiosurgery using the linac on 21 patients all of whom had undergone conventional radiotherapy to 45–50 Gy; 18 of these patients had also been operated at least once. Clearly this was a difficult population of patients in that the optic chiasm, just rostral to the target, had received the full dose of the previous radiotherapy and this prejudiced the dose of radiosurgery that could be safely be prescribed.

Swords et al [35] reported the follow-up of these 21 patients. 13 patients had somatotroph adenoma, four corticotroph adenoma, three non-functional adenoma and one prolactinoma. The radiosurgical dose varied between 8 Gy and 15 Gy (modal prescription dose 10 Gy), depending on the optic chiasmal dose; the median follow up was 33 months with a range of 3–72 months. Radiosurgery by this linac technique proved safe and effective: amongst our somatotroph ademoas, we observed a more rapid reduction in growth hormone (GH) and insulin-like growth factor (IGF-1) levels than we are accustomed after conventional radiotherapy (Figure 4), with normalization of GH and IGF-1 levels in 58%. Although Landolt et al [9] had made a previous observation regarding faster falls in GH after radiosurgery versus conventional radiotherapy, our observation was in previously irradiated patients and was therefore new.

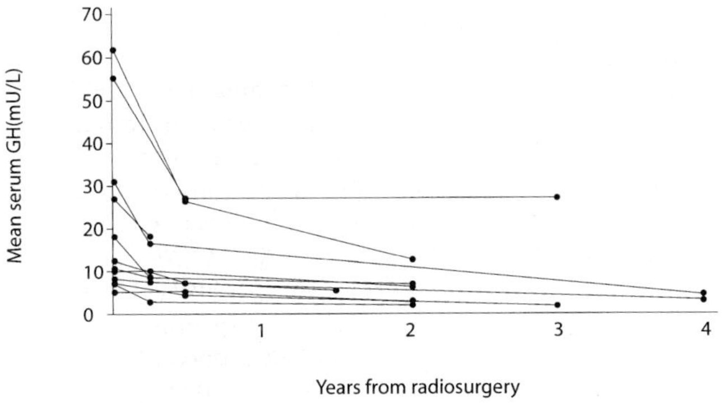

Figure 4. Mean serum growth hormone levels over time (each data point being the mean value of a five point day curve) in a population of previously irradiated (conventionally fractionated to a minimum dose of 45 Gy) patients with acromegaly, who had failed this therapy (in terms of growth hormone normalization or subsequent rise) and who were then treated by linac radiosurgery (data from Swords et al [35]).

Mean GH levels fell from 21.6 mU l^{-1} to 7.9 mU l^{-1} (Figure 4) and the mean IGF-1 level from 624 ng ml^{-1} to 384 ng ml^{-1}. In this stereotactic radiosurgical series of previously irradiated patients, there was clear cut evidence of high efficacy of stereotactic radiosurgery. The dose to the optic chiasm was limited to 3 Gy in this series and no visual complications have been observed to date. We believe that the dosimetrically superior Gamma Knife technique (with regard to sparing dose to the rostral chiasm) will take on our work in this area and we will report on this subject again, including primarily treated patients in our next review.

There is a continuing controversy as to whether stereotactic radiosurgery should supplant conventional radiotherapy in the primary therapy of pituitary adenoma. For example, it could well be argued that the dose of ionizing radiation received by adjacent structures (*e.g.* hypothalamus) would be considerably less if patients were routinely treated by radiosurgical methods. On the other hand, not infrequently pituitary adenoma is a "trans-fossa" disease and there is a necessity to fully irradiate the whole fossa and adjacent cavernous sinus up to the carotid arteries and rostrally above the diaphragma, coupled to the fact that early radiosurgical results were suboptimal [36]. These features, which remain relevant in the post-operative setting, may well argue in favour of conventional radiotherapy, which after all has an excellent pedigree of durable success/control in this disease reviewed in 1999 [36], although we are now looking at selected use of primary radiosurgery for small discrete adenomas. However, it should be born in mind that these latter cases are usually exactly the cases that do well with modern surgery.

We have recently reported on a rare form of pituitary adenoma: *viz.* paediatric Cushing's disease [37]. Here is a benign adenoma, usually small and in a vulnerable patient population with regard to late morbidity of therapy, but one in which first time cure is vital as subsequent attempts are not attended by good long term control rates. The early radiosurgical literature in this disease in adults was not persuasive [38]. Following transphenoidal surgery, we studied seven paediatric Cushing's disease children who were not cured by the surgery. All received conventionally fractionated radiotherapy and with a mean follow up of 6.9 years, all remained in endocrinological remission and probably cured [37]. The late morbidity included GH deficiency but surprisingly normal gonadotropin secretion, although one male demonstrated early puberty; adrenocorticotrophic hormone (ACTH), thyroid stimulating hormone (TSH) and interestingly prolactin axes remained normal. With these good conventional radiotherapy results we have elected to continue with conventionally fractionated radiotherapy in this patient group for the present – two children so treated in the first quarter of 2004.

Craniopharyngioma research

In our last quinquennial review we overviewed the role of radiation therapy in craniopharyngioma and illustrated good response of this disease to focal single dose radiation therapy. However, we debated the merits of focal single fraction radiation therapy versus fractionated therapy in a situation where there is a radiosensitive special sensory nerve (*viz.* the optic chiasm) running adjacent or more frequently within the target volume. For example, the case illustrated in our publication demonstrated complete response of the mass lesion after radiosurgery but the patient subsequently lost vision in the ipsilateral eye due to the radiation (Figure 4) [6]. (The situation is highly comparable with that with the radiovulnerable cochlear nerve running within the radiosurgical target volume of an intracanalicular vestibular neuroma). We concluded then that there was a real argument in favour of conventionally fractionated radiotherapy for this disease under these circumstances and that view point was highlighted when the Karolinska workers reported in 2002 on 21 consecutive patients (11 children) with craniopharyngioma who had been treated by Gamma Knife radiosurgery, with a mean of 16.8 years' follow up [39]. 13 patients received a marginal dose of 6 Gy or less to respect chiasmal single dose tolerance (which is not perceived to be a radical radiosurgical dose and certainly equates to a very much lower dose equivalent than could have been achieved by standard/conventional fractionated radiotherapy); 11 of the 13 patients had relapsed. Not only was the control rate in this series poor but there was visual deterioration in 8 of 21 patients and there was uncertainty as to the aetiology of this visual loss. The authors concluded, as have many others, that there must be a space between the chiasm and the craniopharyngioma for safe and effective radiosurgery to be indicated as a therapeutic modality; although, as in many radiosurgery papers, conventionally fractionated radiation therapy data are not reviewed as a highly effective alternative in their manuscript, highlighting the sorry divide between neurosurgeons practising (usually Gamma Knife) radiation therapy divorced from multidisciplinary teams with good radiotherapy facilities.

In 2003, we published a series of three patients who had been referred to us with recurrent craniopharyngioma entirely within the pituitary fossa and we had been safely able to deliver radical radiosurgical dosage and who had achieved complete responses [40]. We concluded that radiosurgery for intrasellar craniopharyngioma was indeed a very good treatment option.

In 1999, we published our intracystic Y-90 instillation results for cystic craniopharyngioma [41], and the only other point to highlight in this review is the combined use of intracystic Y-90 and stereotactic radiosurgery for semicystic, semisolid craniopharyngiomas for which we have only limited data at present.

The management of metastases

The optimal management of brain metastases has continued to be a controversial topic in the last 5 years, with the benefits of whole brain radiotherapy continually being questioned for some patient subgroups [42]. Undoubtedly, patient performance status/extent of disease predicts success or failure [43]. Notwithstanding the literature demonstrating increased control of brain disease by whole brain radiotherapy after neurosurgical resection of an apparently isolated brain metastasis, the delegates at a recent multidisciplinary conference reported in 2001 [44] demonstrated that all clinicians involved in the care of these patients were dissatisfied with the achievements of whole brain radiotherapy. In 1999, Kondziolka et al [10], reported a small trial of patients with two to four metastases, none greater than 2.5 cm in diameter and with a KPS of >70. These patients either received whole brain radiotherapy (WBRT) alone or WBRT with a radiosurgical boost to the established metastases. The rate of failure at 1 year was 100% after WBRT alone as compared with 8% after WBRT plus radiosurgical boost. Our "straw poll" [44] of the delegates of a multidisciplinary symposium in London reflected the views of an editorial of the time [45] *viz.* that stereotactic radiosurgery should be further explored for better prognosis patients. Since that time, an RTOG study [46] has concluded that patients with 1–3 cerebral metastases would be best treated (as judged by functional autonomy at 6 months after therapy or improved survival in the single brain metastatic cases) by WBRT and radiosurgical boost. The foregoing goes some way to explain the higher incidence of brain metastases patients in our recent cohort of treated patients (Figure 1); a trend we expect to continue.

Research into reactions to therapy

With increasing numbers of patients treated, we have observed more early and late reactions. It has been well established that in the first 24+ hours after radiosurgery for a AVM, particularly when located in the subcortex, there is an increased tendency to fit, owing to a presumed acute vasogenic reaction (comparable with primary erythema in skin). What we have once observed is a patient (who had suffered no fit for a long time) actually having such a fit during the treatment, causing cessation of therapy and immediate scanning demonstrated a vasogenic, oedematous response that had not been present on a comparable scan the previous week – representing a hyperacute reaction that we had not previously encountered [47]. We have also reported facial spasm complicating radiosurgery for acoustic neuroma and drawn attention to this unusual "stimulatory" reaction to radiation therapy [48]. Neither of these reactions fit comfortably into the classification that we published in 1999 [49], both being stimulatory in nature, and demonstrate the interesting new spectrum of radiation reactions that are being observed in this developing field of radiation therapy.

We have published one study regarding the possibility of modifying the post therapy radiation reaction. In our early linac based series of AVM treatments, using a single isocentre and rotational technology, we took on a quantity of large AVM cases, accepting a higher risk than is associated with treatment of smaller AVM. Following experimental animal evidence that essential fatty acids could modify that development of post-radiation transverse myelitis in pigs [50, 51], we introduced "post hoc" administration of gamma linolenic acid after radiosurgery for larger AVM. In the study that we reported in 2001 [52], any form of complication after radiosurgery for large (more than 10 cm^3) AVM fell from 20% to nil with the introduction of gamma linolenic administration. However, the obliteration rate of these AVM fell from 41% to 5%, suggesting to us that not only was the post hoc administration of this lipid altering the radiation response of the normal nervous system but also that it was altering it in the AVM. Now, AVM are an unusual target in radiation medicine in that we are here relying, to cure the AVM, on a late radiation reaction that is shared by normal tissue. Although our study did not achieve the desired objective of improving the therapeutic ratio for this target, we argued that the situation is very different in the treatment of neoplasms; here the kill of cancer cells occurs near instantaneously after radiation as distinct from the late radiation reaction that governs the late morbidity of the nervous system. Thus, that gamma linolenic acid works post hoc might well allow an improved therapeutic ratio in the therapy of brain tumours and further research is required [51].

Conclusions

Radiosurgery is a fast expanding field with the technique replacing some conventional neurosurgical procedures and allowing effective therapy where previously there was none. This manuscript is the third quinquennial review of work in the subject at St. Bartholomew's Hospital, London.

References

1. Leksell L. A stereotaxic apparatus for intracerebral surgery. Acta Chir Scand 1949;99:231.
2. Leksell L. Cerebral radiosurgery I. Gamma thalamotomy in two cases of intractable pain. Acta Chir Scand 1968;134:585–95.
3. Walton L, Bomford CK, Ramsden D. The Sheffield stereotactic radiosurgery unit: physical characteristics and principles of operation. Br J Radiol 1987;60:897–906.
4. Gerhard A, Horstmann MD, Shogens H, Albertus TCJ, Van Eck MD, Kreiner HJ, et al. First clinical experience with automatic position system and Leksell Gamma Knife Model C. J Neurosurg 2000;93(Suppl. 3):193–7.
5. Levivier M, Wikier D, Goldman S, David P, Metens T, Massager N, et al. Integration of the metabolic data of positron emission tomography in the dosimetry planning of radiosurgery with the Gamma Knife: early experience with brain tumours. J Neurosurg 2000;93(Suppl. 3):233–8.

6. Sims E, Doughty D, Macaulay E, Royle N, Wraith C, Darlison R, et al. Stereotactically delivered cranial radiation therapy: a ten year experience of linac based radiosurgery in the UK. Clin Oncol 1999;11:303–20.
7. St. George EJ, Plowman PN. The role of Gamma Knife and PET in neuro-oncology. CME Cancer Med 2002;1:3–8.
8. Plowman PN. Pituitary adenoma radiotherapy – when, who and how? Clin Endocrinol 1999;51:265–71.
9. Landolt AM, Haller D, Lomax N, Scheib S, Schubiger O, Siegfried J, et al. Stereotactic radiosurgery for recurrent surgically treated acromegaly: comparison with fractionated radiotherapy. J Neurosurg 1998;88:1002–8.
10. Kondziolka D, Patel A, Lunsford D, et al. Stereotactic radiosurgery plus whole brain radiotherapy versus whole brain radiotherapy alone for patients with multiple brain metastases. Int J Radiat Oncol Biol Phys 1999;45:427–34.
11. Adams EJ, Cosgrove VP, Shepherd SF, et al. Comparison of a multileaf collimator with conformal blocks for the delivery of stereotactically guided conformal radiotherapy. Radiother Oncol 1999;51:205–9.
12. Plowman PN, Doughty D. Stereotactic radiosurgery X. Clinical isodosimetry of gamma knife versus linear accelerator X-knife for pituitary and acoustic tumours. Clin Oncol 1999;11:321–9.
13. Monk JE, Perks JR, Doughty D, Plowman PN. Comparison of a micro-multileaf collimator with a 5mm leaf width collimator for intracranial stereotactic radiotherapy. Int J Radiat Oncol Biol Phys 2003;57:1443–9.
14. Perks JL, St. George EJ, El Hamri K, Blackburn P, Plowman PN. Stereotactic radiosurgery XVI. Isodosimetric comparison of Gamma Knife versus linear accelerator micro-leaf MLC stereotactic radiotherapy methods for the therapy of acoustic neuroma – potential clinical importance. Int J Radiat Oncol Biol Phys 2003;57:1450–9.
15. El Hamri AK, Blackburn P, Perks JP, Plowman PN. Relationship of conformity index (CI) and minimum target dose (min TD) for two stereotactic treatment delivery systems. Proc Eur Gamma Knife Soc (Lugo, Italy. Dec 2003) Abstr.
16. Perks J, St. George EJ, Doughty D, Plowamn PN. Is distortion correction necessary for digital subtraction angiography in the Gamma Knife treatment of intracranial arteriovenous malformations. Stereotact Funct Neurosurg 2001;76:94–105.
17. St George EJ, Butler P, Plowman PN. Can magnetic resonance imaging alone accurately define the arteriovenous nidus for gamma knife radiosurgery? J Neurosurg 2002; 97(Suppl. 5):464–70.
18. Guo WY, Nordell B, Karlsson B, et al. Target delineation in radiosurgery for cerebral arteriovenous malformations. Acta radiol 1993;34:457–63.
19. Plowman PN. Radiation therapy for vascular malformations – a changing scene. Clin Oncol 2002;14:91–6.
20. St George J, Perks J, Plowman PN. Stereotactic radiosurgery XV. The role of the haemosiderin ring in the development of adverse reactions following radiosurgery for intracranial cavernous malformations - a hypothesis. Br J Neurosurg 2002;16:385–91.
21. Madreperla SA, Hungerford JL, Plowman PN. Choroidal haemangiomas: visual and anatomic results of treatment by photocoagulation or radiotherapy. Ophthalmology 1997;104: 1773–9.
22. Plowman PN, Hungerford JL. Radiotherapy for ocular angioma. Br J Ophthalmol 1997;81:258–9.
23. Nelson JM, Stevens RG. Ferritin ion increases killing of Chinese hamster ovary cells by x-irradiation. Cell Prolif 1992;25:579–85.
24. Hornsey S, Myers R, Jenkinson T. The reduction of radiation damage to the spinal cord by post-irradiation administration of vaso-active drugs. Int J Radiat Oncol Biol Phys 1990;18:1437–42.
25. Kondziolka D, Lunsford D, McLaughlin MR, et al. Long term outcomes after radiosurgery for acoustic neuroma. N Engl J Med 1998;339:1426–33.
26. Fuss M, Debus J, Lohr F, et al. Conventionally fractionated stereotactic radiotherapy (FSRT) for acoustic neuromas. Int J Radiat Oncol Biol Phys 2000;48:1381–7.
27. Plowman PN. Post-radiation sensorineuronal hearing loss. Int J Radiat Oncol Biol Phys 2002;52:589–91.
28. Rowlands RG, Plowman PN, Millard R, Wareing M. Recovery of hearing in a dead ear following stereotactic radiosurgery for vestibular schwannoma. Proc Fourth International conference on vestibular schwannoma and other CPA lesions. (Cambridge UK, July 2003). Abstr.
29. Baser ME, Evans DGR, Jackler RK, Sujansky E, Rubinstein A. Malignant nervous system tumours, radiotherapy and neurofibromatosis. Br J Cancer 2000;82:998–1002.
30. Plowman PN, Evans DGR. Stereotactic radiosurgery XI. Acoustic neuroma therapy and radiation oncogenesis. Br J Neurosurg 2000;14:93–5.
31. Knudson AG. Mutation and cancer: a statistical study of retinoblastoma. Proc Natl Acad Sci 1971;68:820–3.
32. Blackburn TPD, Perks JR, Plowman PN. Is there a predisposition to radiation oncogenesis in NF-2 patients and is the situation comparable to hereditary retinoblastoma. Proc Europ Gamma Knife Soc Mtg. Nov 2002 (London), Abstr.
33. Rowe JG, Radatz M, Walton L, Kemeny AA. Stereotactic radiosurgery for Type 2 neurofibromatosis acoustic neuromas: patient selection and tumour size. Stereotact Funct Neurosurg 2002;79:107–16.
34. Rowe JG, Radatz MWR, Walton L, Soanes T, Rodgers J, Kemeny AA. Clinical experience with Gamma knife stereotactic radiosurgery in the management of vestibular schwannomas secondary to type 2 neurofibromatosis. J Neurol Neurosurg Psych 2003;74:1288–93.
35. Swords FM, Allan CA, Plowman PN, Evanson J, Chew SL, Grossman AB, et al. Steretactic radiosurgery XVI: a treatment for previously irradiated pituitary adenomas. J Clin Endocrinol Metab 2003;88:5334–40.
36. Plowman PN. Pituitary adenoma radiotherapy. Clin Endocrinol 1999;51:265–7.
37. Storr HL, Plowman PN, Carroll PV, Krassas GE, Afshar F, Besser GM, et al. Clinical and endocrine responses to pituitary radiotherapy in paediatric Cushing's disease: an effective second-line treatment. J Clin Endocrinol Metab 2003;88:34–7.
38. Degerblad M, Rahn T, Bergstrand G, Thoren M. Long term results of stereotactic radiosurgery to the pituitary gland in Cushing's disease. Acta Endocrinologica 1986;112:310–4.
39. Ulfarrson E, Roberts M, Rahn T, Linquist M, Thoren M, Lindquist C. Gamma Knife surgery for craniopharyngiomas: long term results of the first patients. Proc 11th Annual Meeting of the Leksell Gamma Knife Society, Prague, May 2002.
40. Jackson ASN, St. George EJU, Hayward RJ, Plowman PN. Stereotactic radiosurgery XVII. Recurrent intrasellar craniopharyngioma. Br J Neurosurg 2003;17:138–43.
41. Blackburn TPD, Doughty D, Plowman PN. Stereotactic intracavity therapy of recurrent cystic craniopharyngioma by instillation of 90-Yttrium. Br J Neurosurg 1999;13:359–65.
42. Tsao N, Sultanem K, Chiu D, Copps F, Dixon P, Easton D, et al. Supportive care management of brain metastases: what is known and what we need to know. Clin Oncol 2003;15:429–34.
43. Gaspar L, Scott C, Rotman M, et al. Recursive partitioning analysis (RPA) of prognostic factors in three Radiation Therapy Oncology Group (RTOG) brain metastasis trials. Int J Radiat Oncol Biol Phys 1997;37:745–51.
44. Marcou Y, Lindquist C, Adams C, Retsas S, Plowman PN. What is optimal therapy of brain metastases? Clin Oncol 2001;13:105–11.

45. Shaw EG. Radiotherapeutic management of multiple brain metastases: 3000 in 10 whole brain is no longer a no brainer. Int J Radiat Oncol Biol Phys 1999;45:253–4.
46. Andrews DW, Scott CB, Sperduto PW, et al. Whole brain radiation therapy with or without stereotactic radiosurgery boost for patients with one to three brain metastases: phase 111 results of RTOG 9508 randomised trial. Lancet 2004;363:1665–72.
47. Blackburn TPD, El Hanmri K, Boxhall YL, Barett S, Plowman PN, Bullock P. Acute cerebral oedema during radiosurgery – natural history or complication? Proc Eur Gamma Knife meeting (London 2002 – Abstr.).
48. Blackburn TPD, Jeanson De Damoiseau KM, Sabin HI, Plowman PN. Facial spasm complicating stereotactic radiosurgery/therapy for acoustic schwannoma. World Gamma Knife Users Meeting (Vienna, 2004) Abstr.
49. Plowman PN. Stereotactic radiosurgery VIII. The classification of post-radiosurgery reactions. Br J Neurosurg 1999;13:256–64.
50. Hopewell JW, Van den Aardweg GJM, Morris GM. Unsaturated lipids as modulators of radiation damage in normal tissues. In: Horobin DF, editor. New approaches to cancer treatment: unsaturated lipids and photodynamic therapy. London: Churchill Communication Europe, 1994; 88–106.
51. El Agamawi AY, Hopewell JW, Plowman PN, Rezvani M, Wilding D. Modulation of normal tissue response to radiation. Br J Radiol 1996;69:374–5.
52. Sims EC, Plowman PN. Stereotactic radiosurgery XII. Large AVM and the failure of the radiation response modifier gamma linolenic acid to improve the therapeutic ratio. Br J Neurosurg 2001;15:28–34.

The British Journal of Radiology, *78* (2005), 394–397
DOI: 10.1259/bjr/60976544

Accuracy of transvaginal ultrasound in diagnosing endometrial pathology in women with post-menopausal bleeding on tamoxifen

[1]J WEAVER, MSc, DCR, [1]J M McHUGO, FRCR, FRCP, FRCPCH and [2]T J CLARK, MD, MRCOG

[1]*Department of Radiology and* [2]*Academic Department of Obstetrics and Gynaecology, Birmingham Women's Hospital, Birmingham B15 2TG, UK*

Abstract. The incidence of endometrial pathology is increased in women with tamoxifen-induced post-menopausal bleeding (PMB). The aim of this study was to determine the accuracy of transvaginal ultrasound (TVS) in diagnosing endometrial pathology in symptomatic women taking tamoxifen, using endometrial thickness measurements (5 mm and 10 mm cut-offs) and morphological changes within the uterine cavity to define abnormality. The sensitivity of TVS was 97% (95% confidence interval (CI) 83% to 100%) and the specificity 35% (95% CI 17% to 56%) at a 5 mm threshold. The corresponding likelihood ratios for a positive test were 1.47 (95% CI 1.16–2.10) and a negative test were 0.09 (95% CI 0.02–0.53). The use of a higher 10 mm threshold, characterization of endometrial morphology or combining endometrial thickness and morphology did not improve overall accuracy. TVS measurement of endometrial thickness using a 5 mm cut-off is highly accurate in excluding endometrial disease in symptomatic women taking tamoxifen and may negate the need for further diagnostic testing in women unless symptoms recur. A positive TVS result is of little value, so further testing is mandatory in order to detect benign and malignant endometrial disease associated with tamoxifen and PMB.

Tamoxifen is an effective and widely used adjuvant therapy for women with breast cancer because it reduces recurrence rates and prolongs disease free survival. It is a partial oestrogen agonist in that it exhibits anti-oestrogenic activity in the breast, but has a stimulatory effect on the endometrium. This hormonal activity results in a higher incidence of post-menopausal vaginal bleeding and endometrial pathology such as endometrial polyps, hyperplasia and cancer [1–3].

Transvaginal ultrasound (TVS) measurement of endometrial thickness has been demonstrated to have high accuracy in excluding endometrial polyps, hyperplasia and cancer in women with post-menopausal bleeding [4, 5]. Several studies have examined the usefulness of endometrial thickness measurement using TVS in asymptomatic women on tamoxifen, as they are at increased risk of significant endometrial disease [6, 7]. These studies have consistently shown the accuracy of TVS to be poor, especially in detecting endometrial disease, and thereby of limited value as a screening test. This is partly because tamoxifen can induce specific morphological endometrial changes, particularly subendometrial cysts, and such appearances can make characterization and measurement of the endometrium difficult [8, 9]. Only a few studies have assessed the accuracy of TVS in symptomatic women taking tamoxifen (*i.e.* those with post-menopausal bleeding) [6, 10] and these women have represented small subgroups of larger asymptomatic populations. The role of TVS in the diagnosis of endometrial pathology in symptomatic women taking tamoxifen is thus less clearly defined. We therefore undertook a study to estimate the accuracy of TVS in post-menopausal women on tamoxifen presenting with abnormal vaginal bleeding.

Received 27 July 2004 and in revised form 25 October 2004, accepted 23 November 2004.

Address correspondence to Dr Jo McHugo.

Methods and materials

Ethical approval for the study was obtained from our hospital's Research and Development Committee. A retrospective study was undertaken, at the Birmingham Women's Hospital, using the Radiology Department computer system to identify all women receiving tamoxifen therapy who presented with post-menopausal vaginal bleeding (PMB) and were investigated with a TVS and outpatient endometrial biopsy, between April 1st 1996 and March 31st 2000. Of the 126 women consecutively investigated, data from a random sample of 56 were retrieved for further analysis. The aim was to determine the accuracy of (a) endometrial thickness and (b) morphological changes within the uterine cavity as characterized on TVS in diagnosing serious endometrial disease (endometrial polyps, hyperplasia and cancer). The endometrial thickness was measured at the double layered thickness to include sub endometrial cysts/cystic spaces if visualized. Morphological changes were characterized as normal if the endometrium was regular or subendometrial cystic spaces consistent with tamoxifen change [8, 9] were seen. Structural changes, which could not be attributed to characteristic tamoxifen effects, were considered to represent abnormal morphology (irregular endometrium, heterogeneous echotexture and indistinct endometrial borders). All TVS were performed by Departmental sonographers or radiologists using an Acuson Sequoia with an EV8C4 probes or Acuson 128XP/10 with an EC7 probe (Acuson, Mountain View, CA). Ultrasound findings were reported independently and blinded from the pathologist interpreting the subsequent endometrial biopsy sample, which was the diagnostic reference standard.

To generate measures of diagnostic accuracy, 2×2 contingency tables were constructed. Endometrial disease was defined as endometrial polyps, hyperplasia or cancer. Atrophic endometrium, functional changes and non-diagnostic endometrial samples were considered to be negative for disease. Where more than one endometrial condition was identified histologically, the more serious condition was taken as the final diagnosis (cancer>hyperplasia>polyp). Normal and abnormal test results were defined firstly on the basis of endometrial thickness measurements using two different thresholds to define abnormality (abnormal test >5 mm and >10 mm). These thresholds were chosen as the former represents a recommended cut-off for investigating PMB [4, 5] and the latter cut-off has been recommended by some [11, 12] for investigating post-menopausal women taking tamoxifen (the higher threshold accounting for expected tamoxifen induced endometrial/subendometrial changes). Abnormality was then defined on the basis of abnormal endometrial morphology (present or absent) and finally on taking into account both thickness and morphology (abnormal test >5 mm or 10 mm, respectively, and/or abnormal morphology *vs* normal test ⩽5 mm or 10 mm, respectively and normal morphology).

Sensitivity, specificity, predictive values and likelihood ratios (LRs) were derived from the 2×2 tables to enable estimation of diagnostic accuracy. The LRs indicate by how much a given test would raise or lower the probability of having pathology. An LR of >1 increases the probability of having pathology and an LR of <1 decreases the probability of having pathology with a positive and negative test result, respectively. Moderate accuracy can be achieved with LR values of 5–10 and 0.1–0.2, whereas LRs of 1–5 and 0.2–1 would be poor [13, 14].

Results

Of the 56 women undergoing TVS and endometrial biopsy, 30 of 56 (54%) had endometrial disease. There was only one case of endometrial cancer, 10 cases of endometrial hyperplasia (one with cytological atypia) and 19 endometrial polyps.

Endometrial thickness

The 2×2 contingency table using a 5 mm cut-off for abnormality on TVS is shown in Table 1. Sensitivity was 97% (95% confidence interval (CI) 83–100%) and the specificity 35% (95% CI 17–56%). Positive and negative predictive values were 63% (95% CI 48–77%) and 90% (95% CI 56–100%), respectively. The corresponding likelihood ratios for a positive test were 1.47 (95% CI 1.16–2.10) and a negative test were 0.09 (95% CI 0.02–0.53).

Increasing the cut-off for abnormality to 10 mm reduced the sensitivity to 77% (95% CI 57–90%), but increased the specificity to 54% (95% CI 33–73%). Positive and negative predictive values were 66% (95% CI 48–81%) and 67% (95% CI 43–85%) respectively (Table 2). The corresponding likelihood ratios for a positive test were 1.67 (95% CI 1.09–2.75) and a negative test were 0.43 (95% CI 0.20–0.88).

Endometrial morphology

The 2×2 contingency table for endometrial morphology on TVS is shown in Table 3. Sensitivity was 17% (95% CI 6–35%) and the specificity 81% (95% CI 61–93%). Positive and negative predictive values were 50% (95% CI 19–81%) and 46% (95% CI 31–61%), respectively. The corresponding likelihood ratios for a positive test were 0.87 (95% CI 1.30–2.55) and a negative test were 1.03 (95% CI 0.79–1.38).

Combination of endometrial morphology and thickness

The 2×2 contingency table for endometrial thickness (5 mm cut-off) and morphology combined on TVS is shown in Table 4. Sensitivity was 97% (95% CI 83–100%) and the specificity 11% (95% CI 2–30%). Positive and negative predictive values were 56% (95% CI 41–70%) and 75% (95% CI 19–99%), respectively. The corresponding likelihood ratios for a positive test were 1.09 (95% CI 0.92–1.37) and a negative test were 0.29 (95% CI 0.04–1.90).

The 2×2 contingency table for endometrial morphology on TVS is shown in Table 5. Sensitivity was 83% (95% CI 65–94%) and the specificity 50% (95% CI 30–70%). Positive and negative predictive values were 66% (95%

Table 1. Accuracy of transvaginal ultrasound (TVS) in diagnosing endometrial disease (polyps, hyperplasia or cancer) using a >5 mm cut-off to define abnormality

	Endometrial disease	No endometrial disease	Total
Positive TVS	29	17	46
Negative TVS	1	9	10
Total	30	26	56

Table 2. Accuracy of transvaginal ultrasound (TVS) in diagnosing endometrial disease (polyps, hyperplasia or cancer) using a >10 mm cut-off to define abnormality

	Endometrial disease	No endometrial disease	Total
Positive TVS	23	12	35
Negative TVS	7	14	21
Total	30	26	56

Table 3. Accuracy of transvaginal ultrasound (TVS) in diagnosing endometrial disease (polyps, hyperplasia or cancer) using abnormal endometrial morphology to define abnormality

	Endometrial disease	No endometrial disease	Total
Positive TVS	5	5	10
Negative TVS	25	21	46
Total	30	26	56

Table 4. Accuracy of transvaginal ultrasound (TVS) in diagnosing endometrial disease (polyps, hyperplasia or cancer) using a >5 mm cut-off and/or abnormal endometrial morphology to define abnormality

	Endometrial disease	No endometrial disease	Total
Positive TVS	29	23	52
Negative TVS	1	3	4
Total	30	26	56

Table 5. Accuracy of transvaginal ultrasound (TVS) in diagnosing endometrial disease (polyps, hyperplasia or cancer) using a >10 mm cut-off and/or abnormal endometrial morphology to define abnormality

	Endometrial disease	No endometrial disease	Total
Positive TVS	25	13	38
Negative TVS	5	13	18
Total	30	26	56

CI 49–80%) and 72% (95% CI 47–90%), respectively. The corresponding likelihood ratios for a positive test were 1.67 (95% CI 1.14–2.65) and a negative test were 0.34 (95% CI 0.14–0.77).

Discussion

This study shows that endometrial thickness measurement using a 5 mm cut-off to define an abnormal ultrasound is highly accurate in excluding endometrial disease in symptomatic women taking tamoxifen and is thus useful in clinical decision making. A positive test result is of little use in detecting disease. These findings are in keeping with accuracy estimated in the general PMB populations using TVS and a 5 mm cut-off [4, 5]. A 10 mm cut-off has been advocated in women on tamoxifen so that characteristic "benign" tamoxifen induced endometrial changes (*e.g.* subendometrial cysts) are accounted for, in an attempt to reduce the false positive rate and subsequent unnecessary medical intervention [11, 12]. However, by using such a cut-off in this series, the accuracy of a negative test in excluding endometrial disease was reduced with no substantial improvement in the predictive ability of a positive ultrasound. This cut-off cannot therefore be recommended in women on tamoxifen presenting with PMB. The use of morphological endometrial changes to define abnormality was not discriminative and thereby of no use to the clinician. Accuracy was not improved when morphology was combined with endometrial thickness measurements.

It is well recognized that tamoxifen-induced changes to the uterine cavity can make characterization and measurement of the endometrium difficult [6, 7, 12]. Accuracy data for TVS in symptomatic women with PMB on tamoxifen is sparse. Most available data represent small subgroups from larger asymptomatic populations [6, 10]. Our study therefore provides important information as it evaluated symptomatic women from the outset using endometrial morphology in addition to endometrial thickness measurements. TVS was conducted by several radiologists and radiographers and this may raise concerns regarding the reproducibility and accuracy of the TVS findings. However, a prospectively agreed protocol for performing and reporting endometrial findings on TVS was followed in all cases, thereby limiting any such biases.

In addition to its clinical importance, strengths of the study include complete verification of test diagnoses and blinding of reference standard interpretation. Inferences from this study are limited by the small sample size and the retrospective, non-consecutive recruitment of patients. Although a consecutive series of eligible women may be considered ideal, our findings should still be considered generalizable because a random sub-selection of all eligible women was studied [15]. Our study may also be criticised for the sole use of endometrial histology obtained using outpatient miniature endometrial biopsy as the diagnostic reference standard. However, these devices have been shown to display good accuracy in diagnosing endometrial cancer and hyperplasia [16, 17] and its use as a diagnostic reference standard is thus reasonable and indeed well-established when assessing the accuracy of TVS [4, 5] and as part of standard clinical practice. The accuracy of endometrial biopsy in diagnosing the presence or absence of endometrial polyps is however, less well established and the addition of hysteroscopy may have been useful to improve accuracy of the reference test. Despite these potential limitations, our findings are in keeping with precise estimates of accuracy derived from systematic reviews of the general PMB population [4, 5].

The findings of our study have implications for diagnostic work-up of women presenting with PMB on tamoxifen. Additional testing is required following a positive TVS (5 mm cut-off) in the general PMB population this usually constitutes an outpatient endometrial biopsy in order to exclude endometrial cancer or hyperplasia [4, 5]. However, disease prevalence is increased in women with tamoxifen induced PMB [1–3]. Our study suggests that over 80% of women will test positive if a 5 mm TVS cut-off is employed and of these, two thirds will have endometrial pathology and approximately two-thirds of this pathology will be endometrial polyps. Additional testing with blind endometrial biopsy alone is therefore inadequate as focal pathology may be missed [18]. Saline infusion ultrasound or outpatient hysteroscopy [19, 20] should therefore be employed followed by polypectomy if appropriate, in addition to endometrial biopsy, which provides tissue for histology.

In conclusion, a normal TVS (endometrial thickness ⩽5 mm) may negate the need for further diagnostic testing in women with tamoxifen-induced PMB unless symptoms recur. Characterization of endometrial morphology does not appear to usefully improve diagnostic performance of TVS. A positive TVS result is of little value, so further testing is mandatory in order to detect benign and malignant endometrial disease associated with tamoxifen and PMB. Future research should look at the use of Doppler blood flow changes [21], saline infusion ultrasound [20] and three-dimensional ultrasound in influencing the diagnostic accuracy of TVS in women with tamoxifen-induced PMB. One randomized controlled trial has compared ultrasound and outpatient hysteroscopy for screening asymptomatic women on tamoxifen

[22]. Such trial should also be conducted in symptomatic women to compare the diagnostic effectiveness of different diagnostic work up strategies.

References

1. Neven P, Vernaeve H. Guidelines for monitoring patients taking tamoxifen treatment. Drug Saf 2000;22:1–11.
2. Barakat RR, Gilewski TA, Almadrones L, Saigo PE, Venkatraman E, Hudis C, et al. Effect of adjuvant tamoxifen on the endometrium in women with breast cancer: a prospective study using office endometrial biopsy. J Clin Oncol 2000;18:3459–63.
3. Bergman L, Beelen ML, Gallee MP, Hollema H, Benraadt J, van Leeuwen FE. Risk and prognosis of endometrial cancer after tamoxifen for breast cancer. Comprehensive Cancer Centres' ALERT Group. Assessment of liver and endometrial cancer risk following tamoxifen. Lancet 2000;356:881–7.
4. Gupta JK, Chien PFW, Voit D, Clark TJ, Khan KS. Ultrasonographic endometrial thickness for diagnosing endometrial pathology in women with postmenopausal bleeding: a meta-analysis. Acta Obstet Gynecol Scand 2002;81:799–816.
5. Smith-Bindman R, Kerlikowske K, Feldstein VA, Subak L, Scheidler J, Segal M, et al. Endovaginal ultrasound to exclude endometrial cancer and other endometrial abnormalities. JAMA 1998;280:1510–7.
6. Fung MF, Reid A, Faught W, Le T, Chenier C, Verma S, et al. Prospective longitudinal study of ultrasound screening for endometrial abnormalities in women with breast cancer receiving tamoxifen. Gynecol Oncol 2003;91:154–9.
7. Love CD, Muir BB, Scrimgeour JB, Leonard RC, Dillon P, Dixon JM. Investigation of endometrial abnormalities in asymptomatic women treated with tamoxifen and an evaluation of the role of endometrial screening. J Clin Oncol 1999;17:2050–4.
8. McGonigle KF, Shaw SL, Vasilev SA, Odom-Maryon T, Roy S, Simpson JF. Abnormalities detected on transvaginal ultrasonography in tamoxifen-treated postmenopausal breast cancer patients may represent endometrial cystic atrophy. Am J Obstet Gynecol 1998;178:1145–50.
9. Goldstein SR. Unusual ultrasonographic appearance of the uterus in patients receiving tamoxifen. Am J Obstet Gynecol 1994;170:447–51.
10. Giorda G, Crivellari D, Veronesi A, Perin T, Campagnutta E, Carbone A, et al. Comparison of ultrasonography, hysteroscopy, and biopsy in the diagnosis of endometrial lesions in postmenopausal tamoxifen-treated patients. Acta Obstet Gynecol Scand 2002;81:975–80.
11. Strauss HG, Wolters M, Methfessel G, Buchmann J, Koelbl H. Significance of endovaginal ultrasonography in assessing tamoxifen-associated changes of the endometrium. A prospective study. Acta Obstet Gynecol Scand 2000;79:697–701.
12. Gerber B, Krause A, Muller H, Reimer T, Kulz T, Makovitzky J, et al. Effects of adjuvant tamoxifen on the endometrium in postmenopausal women with breast cancer: a prospective long-term study using transvaginal ultrasound. J Clin Oncol 2000;18:3464–70.
13. Jaeschke R, Guyatt GH, Sackett DL. User's guides to the medical literature: III. How to use an article about a diagnostic test: B. What are the results and will they help me in caring for my patients? JAMA 1994;271:703–7.
14. Bakour SH, Khan KS, Gupta JK. Transvaginal ultrasonography and endometrial histology in peri- and postmenopausal women on hormone replacement therapy. Br J Obstet Gynaecol 2000;107:295.
15. Bossuyt PM, Reitsma JB, Bruns DE, Gatsonis CA, Glasziou PP, Irwig LM, et al. The STARD statement for reporting studies of diagnostic accuracy: explanation and elaboration. Ann Intern Med 2003;138:W1–12.
16. Clark TJ, Mann CH, Shah N, Song F, Khan KS, Gupta JK. Accuracy of outpatient endometrial biopsy in the diagnosis of endometrial hyperplasia: a systematic review. Acta Obstet Gynecol Scand 2001;80:784–93.
17. Clark TJ, Mann CH, Shah N, Song F, Khan KS, Gupta JK. Accuracy of outpatient endometrial biopsy in the diagnosis of endometrial cancer: a systematic review. Br J Obstet Gynecol 2002;109:313–21.
18. Guido RS, Kanbour-Shakir A, Rulin MC, Christopherson WA. Pipelle endometrial sampling: sensitivity in the detection of endometrial cancer. J Reprod Med 1995;40:553–5.
19. Neven P, De Muylder X, Van Belle Y, Van Hooff I, Vanderick G. Longitudinal hysteroscopic follow-up during tamoxifen treatment. Lancet 1998;351:36.
20. Garuti G, Cellani F, Grossi F, Colonnelli M, Centinaio G, Luerti M. Saline infusion sonography and office hysteroscopy to assess endometrial morbidity associated with tamoxifen intake. Gynecol Oncol 2002;86:323–9.
21. Develioglu OH, Omak M, Bilgin T, Esmer A, Tufekci M. The endometrium in asymptomatic breast cancer patients on tamoxifen: value of transvaginal ultrasonography with saline infusion and Doppler flow. Gynecol Oncol 2004;93:328–35.
22. Timmerman D, Deprest J, Bourne T, Van den Berghe I, Collins WP, Vergote I. A randomized trial on the use of ultrasonography or office hysteroscopy for endometrial assessment in postmenopausal patients with breast cancer who were treated with tamoxifen. Am J Obstet Gynecol 1998;79:62–70.

The British Journal of Radiology, 78 (2005), 398–404 © 2005 The British Institute of Radiology
DOI: 10.1259/bjr/20497987

Normal radiographic anatomy of thoracic structures: analysis of 1000 chest radiographs in Japanese population

H ABIRU, MD, K ASHIZAWA, MD, R HASHMI, MD and K HAYASHI, MD

Division of Radiological Science, Department of Radiology and Radiation Biology, Nagasaki University Graduate School of Biomedical Sciences, 1-7-1 Sakamoto, Nagasaki 852-8501, Japan

Abstract. The purpose of this paper was to study the frequency of visualization and characteristics of normal thoracic structures on posteroanterior (PA) chest radiographs in Japanese population. 1000 consecutive normal PA chest radiographs of men and women ranging in age from 20 years to 90 years were reviewed. Frequency of visualization and configuration of structures including (1) fissure lines such as major, minor, vertical fissure line, and accessory fissures, (2) vascular structures including normal apical opacity, aortic nipple, and descending aortic interface, and (3) other structures including air in the oesophagus, aortic pulmonary stripe, and diaphragm were studied. On PA chest radiographs: (1) minor fissure, superolateral major fissure, superomedial major fissure, vertical fissure line, superior accessory fissure, and inferior accessory fissure were visualized in 74.7%, 19.7%, 15.4%, 1.6%, 2.9% and 13.1%, respectively. (2) Normal apical opacity was seen in 3.7%, while aortic nipple was seen in 0.9%. Descending aortic interface was obliterated in 13.7%. (3) Air in the oesophagus and aortic pulmonary stripe were seen in 8.9% and 17.7%, respectively. Hemidiaphragm was obliterated in 10.3% on the right, and in 32.4% on the left. Scalloping of the diaphragm was seen in 10.6% on the right, 6.5% on the left, and 4.3% bilaterally. Frequency of visualization and characteristics of various normal anatomical structures on chest radiographs in Japanese population differ from those reported previously from the West. Familiarity with these normal thoracic structures and variations is important for our daily image interpretation.

Although the use of chest CT has greatly increased over the past several years, chest radiography remains the most frequently performed imaging examination. A good understanding of normal anatomy and variations is essential for the interpretation of chest radiographs. Important normal anatomical structures on posteroanterior (PA) chest radiographs include fissure lines such as minor fissure [1], superolateral and superomedial major fissures [2, 3], vertical fissure line [4], superior and inferior accessory fissures [1, 5], and vascular structures such as normal apical opacity [6], aortic nipple [7, 8], and descending aortic interface [9].

Most of the data regarding these normal structures have been provided from the West (Europe and USA) [1–8]. There have been few reports describing the normal radiographic anatomy and variations of the thoracic structures in Japanese population [9]. Therefore we reviewed normal PA chest radiographs and analysed the radiographic anatomy in detail among Japanese population.

Methods and materials

We evaluated 1000 consecutive normal PA chest radiographs of Japanese adults obtained between January and May in 1996. The patients were 482 men and 518 women, ranging in age from 20 years to 90 years (average 49 years). There was almost the same distribution of patients in different age groups of both sexes (Figure 1).

The chest radiographs were obtained as a part of routine work-up or follow-up study for non-chest diseases. Patients with thoracic deformities such as pectus excavatum and scoliosis were excluded. The chest radiographs were obtained in erect posture with focus to film distance of 1.5 m using 90~100 kVp, 150 mA, 10~20 ms, 1.6 mm focal spot, Fuji HR4 or Fuji HGM screen, 12:1 grid with 105 lines, and Fuji UR1 film (Fuji Medical Systems, Tokyo, Japan).

All radiographs were reviewed by two chest radiologists. PA radiographs were examined for the visualization and characteristics of: (1) fissure lines including minor fissure, superolateral major fissure, superomedial major fissure, vertical fissure line, superior accessory fissure, and inferior accessory fissure (Figure 2); (2) vascular structures including normal apical opacity, aortic nipple, and descending thoracic aortic interface; and (3) other structures including air in the oesophagus, aortic pulmonary stripe and diaphragm (Figure 3).

The following is the brief explanation of each item including the definition and points of our investigation.

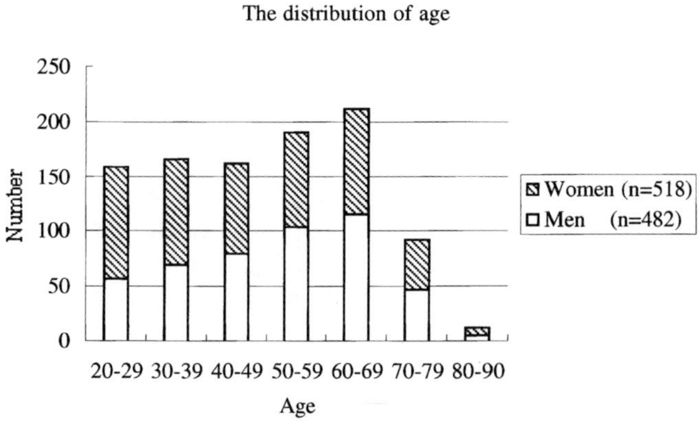

Figure 1. A bar graph showing distribution of patient's age.

Received 21 July 2004 and in revised form 11 October 2004, accepted 23 November 2004.

Address correspondence to Dr Kazuto Ashizawa.

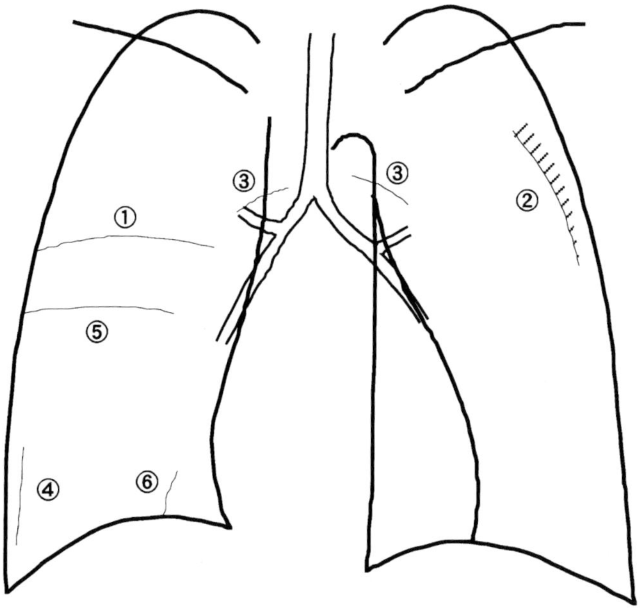

Figure 2. Schematic drawing of fissure lines. 1: Minor fissure. 2: Superolateral major fissure. 3: Superomedial major fissure. 4: Vertical fissure line. 5: Superior accessory fissure. 6: Inferior accessory fissure.

Fissure lines

Figure 2 shows schematic drawing of the 6 fissure lines.

(1) Minor fissure. When visualized, following features of the minor fissure were evaluated: number, angle (lateral side higher, medial side higher, or horizontal), shape (convex upward, convex downward, flat, or sigmoid), and length of visualization (dividing the fissure into three equal parts) [1].

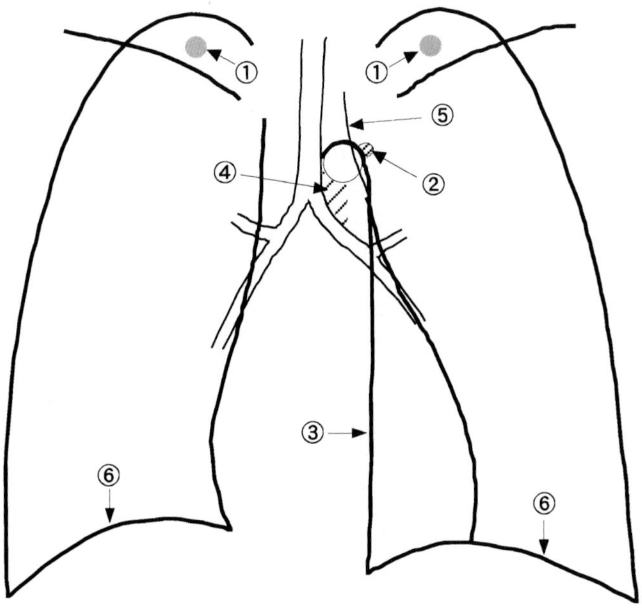

Figure 3. Schematic drawing of vascular and other structures. 1: Normal apical opacity. 2: Aortic nipple. 3: Descending thoracic aortic interface. 4: Air in the oesophagus. 5: Aortic pulmonary stripe. 6: Diaphragm.

(2) Superolateral major fissure was defined as a curving line or edge with a lateral convexity at the upper lateral right and/or left hemithorax [2].

(3) Superomedial major fissure was defined as an obliquely oriented relatively short straight line. On the right it was found in the vicinity of the right tracheobronchial angle, while on the left it was found in the vicinity of the aortic knob. When both superomedial major fissures were seen on the same PA view, the left usually extended slightly higher than the right [3].

(4) Vertical fissure line was defined as a straight or slightly curved vertical line with a lateral convexity near the right and/or left costophrenic angle [4].

(5) Superior accessory fissure was defined as a line parallel and inferior to the minor fissure. As it is difficult to distinguish between left minor fissure and left superior accessory fissure without CT, left superior accessory fissure was excluded from evaluation [1, 5].

(6) Inferior accessory fissure was defined as an oblique line near the right and/or left cardiophrenic angle [1, 5].

Vascular and other structures

Schematic drawing of vascular and other structures is shown in Figure 3.

(1) Normal apical opacity was defined as a homogeneous, round opacity with unsharp margin, approximately at the midpoint between the spine and the inner margin of the first anterior rib above the clavicle [6].

(2) Aortic nipple was defined as a small "nipple" projecting from the lateral aspect of the aortic knob [7, 8].

(3) Obliteration of the descending aortic interface was defined as non-visualization of any portion of the interface longer than 1 cm [9]. The interface was divided into three equal parts: superior, middle, and inferior portions.

(4) Air in the oesophagus was defined as collection of air below the aortic knob with triangular appearance [10].

(5) Aortic pulmonary stripe was defined as an increased density with an oblique, lateral edge that extends across the outline of the aortic knob superiorly and the left pulmonary artery inferiorly [11].

(6) Diaphragm. The difference in height between the right and left hemidiaphragm, and focal obliteration and smooth arcuate elevation (the so-called scalloping) of the diaphragm were examined. To evaluate focal obliteration, the diaphragm was divided into three equal parts (medial, middle, and lateral) [1, 12].

Results

Fissure lines

Visualization of fissure lines in our study and in reported data is shown in Table 1, and characteristics of minor fissure are shown in Table 2.

The minor fissure was visualized in 74.7%. It was visualized as one line in 49.2% (Figure 4a), as two lines in 24.2% (Figure 4b), as three lines in 1.2%, and as four lines in 0.1%. Lateral side of the fissure was higher in 24.8%, while medial side was higher in 28.2%. In 21.7% the fissure was horizontal. The fissure was convex upward in 32.3%, convex downward in 2.6%, flat in 34.5%, and sigmoid shaped in 5.3%. The minor fissure was visible for more

Table 1. Visualization of the six fissure lines

	Right	Left	Bilateral	Overall
Minor fissure	74.7 (44~56) [1]			
Superolateral major fissure	5.1 (4.0) [2]	8.5 (6.0) [2]	6.1 (4.0) [2]	19.7 (14.0) [2]
Superomedial major fissure	4.5	9.7	1.2	15.4 (8.0) [3]
Vertical fissure	0.7	0.8	0.1	1.6
Superior accessory fissure	2.9 (30.0) [5]	— (5–14) [5]	— (12.0) [5]	
Inferior accessory fissure	7.1 (5–6.6) [5]	5.2 (1.0) [5]	0.8 (0.6) [5]	13.1

Numbers are our data expressed in percentage and those in parentheses are reported data in percentage.

Table 2. Characteristics of the minor fissure

Number		Angle		Shape		Length	
1 line	49.2	Lateral side higher	24.8	Convex upward	32.3	More than two-thirds	32.0
2 lines	24.2	Medial side higher	28.2	Convex downward	2.6	One-third to two-thirds	29.6
3 lines	1.2	Horizontal	21.7	Flat	34.5	Less than one-third	13.1
4 lines	0.1			Sigmoid shape	5.3		

Numbers are expressed as percentages.

than two-thirds of its length in 32.0%, a third to two-thirds in 29.6%, and less than one-third in 13.1%.

Superolateral major fissure was visible in 19.7%, including 5.1% on the right, 8.5% on the left, and 6.1% bilaterally (Figure 5). Superomedial major fissure was seen in 15.4%, including 4.5% on the right, 9.7% on the left, and 1.2% bilaterally (Figure 6). Vertical fissure line was visible in 1.6%, including 0.7% on the right (Figure 7), 0.8% on the left, and 0.1% bilaterally. Right superior accessory fissure was visualized in 2.9% (Figure 8). Inferior accessory fissure was visible in 13.1%, including 7.1% on the right (Figure 9), 5.2% on the left, and 0.8% bilaterally.

Vascular and other structures

Visualization of normal apical opacity, aortic nipple, air in the oesophagus, and aortic pulmonary stripe in our data and in reported data is shown in Table 3.

The normal apical opacity was visible in 3.7%, including 1.2% on the right, 1.9% on the left (Figure 10), and 0.6% bilaterally. The aortic nipple was visualized in 0.9% (Figure 11). Focal obliteration of the descending aortic interface was observed in 13.7%, including 1.0% at the superior portion, 3.7% at the middle, 4.1% at the inferior portion, 0.2% at the superior to middle, and 4.3% at the middle to inferior portions (Figure 12) (Table 4). Two portions of the aortic interface were obliterated in four cases. All parts of the descending aortic interface were clearly seen in 86.3%. Air in the oesophagus was seen in 8.9% (Figure 13). The aortic pulmonary stripe was visible in 17.7% (Figure 14).

In 94.2%, the right hemidiaphragm was higher than the left, while in 1.4% the left hemidiaphragm was higher (Table 5). In the remaining 4.4%, right and left hemidiaphragms were visualized at the same level. Hemidiaphragm was obliterated in 10.3% on the right and in 32.4% on the left. In the right hemidiaphragm, focal

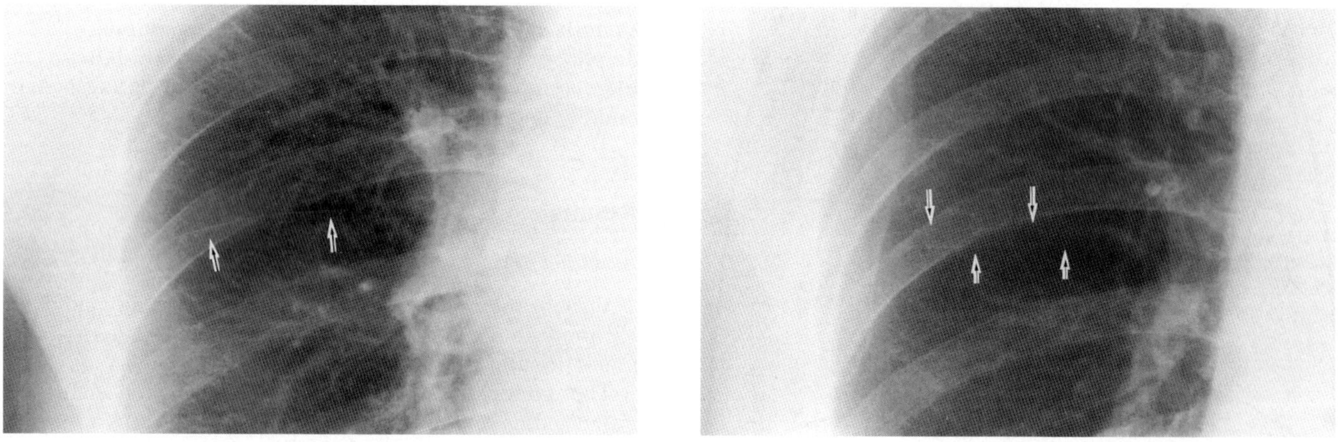

(a) (b)

Figure 4. Posteroanterior chest radiographs showing minor fissures in (a) a 67-year-old man and (b) a 54-year-old woman. (a) The minor fissure with shape of convexity upward is visible as one line (arrows). Medial side of it is higher than lateral and its length is more than two-thirds. Focal obliteration of the fissure is seen medially but outside of the pulmonary artery. (b) The minor fissure is seen as two lines running parallel to each other (arrows).

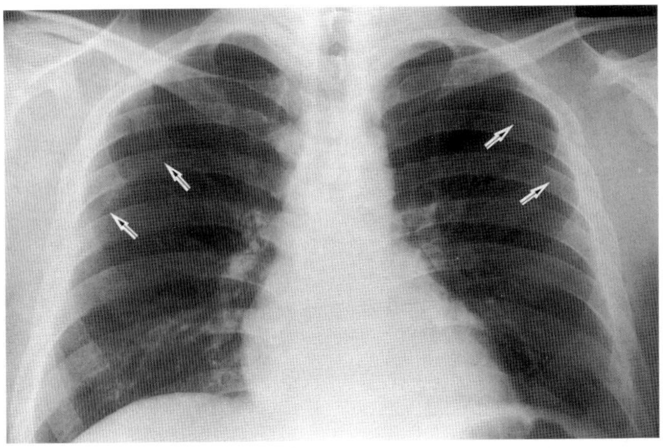

Figure 5. Posteroanterior chest radiographs showing superolateral major fissures in a 25-year-old man. Fissures are seen as curving contours with lateral opacity and medial lucency bilaterally (arrows). The left superolateral major fissure extends higher than the right.

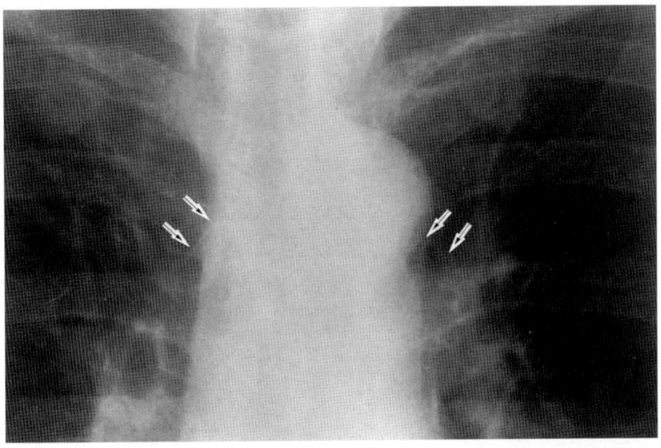

Figure 6. Posteroanterior chest radiograph showing superomedial major fissure in a 68-year-old man. Fissures appear as short straight lines bilaterally (arrows).

obliteration was seen medially in 8.8%, in middle in 0.6%, and laterally in 0.2%. In the left hemidiaphragm, focal obliteration was seen medially in 21.2%, in middle in 3.5%, and laterally in 0.7%. Smooth arcuate elevation of the diaphragm was seen in 10.6% on the right, 6.5% on the left, and 4.3% bilaterally. The number of smooth arcuate elevation of the diaphragm on the right and left were one in 11.5% and 8.3%, two in 3.2% (Figure 15) and 2.1%, three in 0.1% and 0.2%, and four in 0.1% and 0.2%, respectively.

Discussion

We evaluated 1000 consecutive normal PA chest radiographs and reported the frequency of visualization and characteristics of various normal structures among Japanese population.

There has been considerable improvement in the image quality of chest radiographs since the era when most of the papers referred to in this report were published. This improvement in image quality could be a contributing

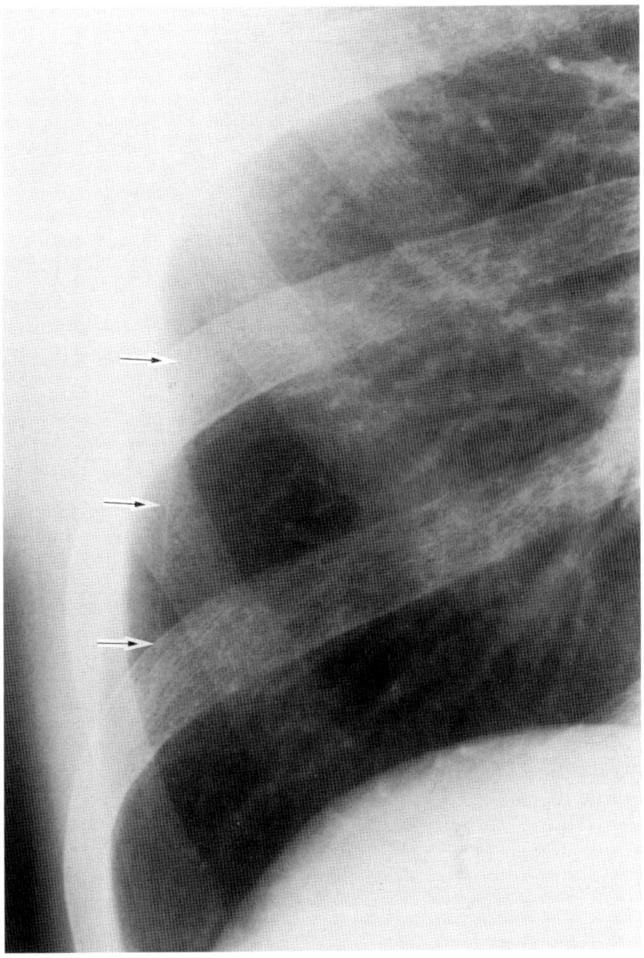

Figure 7. Posteroanterior chest radiograph showing vertical fissure line in a 30-year-old man (arrows).

factor to higher frequency of visualization of most of the fissures. According to an old study by Felson, the minor fissure was absent or poorly developed in 20% of anatomical dissections, while it was visualized in only 56% on radiograph [1]. Frequency of visualization of the minor fissure was 74.7% in our study; this approximates the data of anatomical dissection.

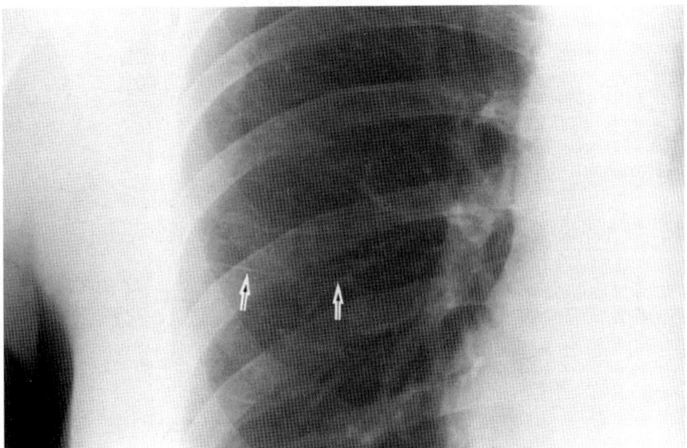

Figure 8. Posteroanterior chest radiograph showing right superior accessory fissure in a 28-year-old woman. The fissure lies inferior to and parallel to minor fissure (arrows).

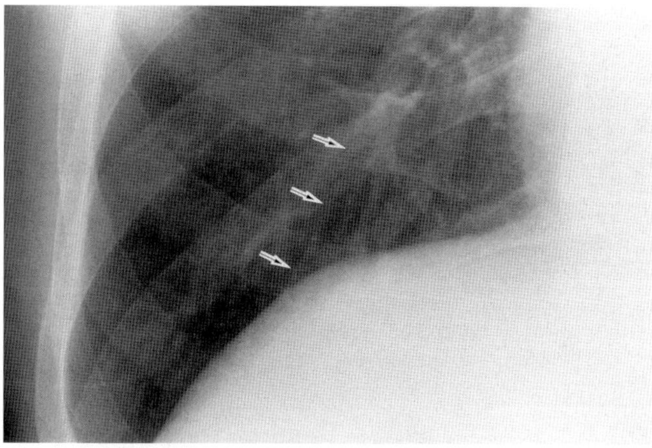

Figure 9. Posteroanterior chest radiograph showing right inferior accessory fissure in a 64-year-old man as a thin line extending from the diaphragm obliquely upward toward hilum (arrows).

Table 3. Visualization of vascular and other structures

	Right	Left	Bilateral	Overall
Normal apical opacity	1.2 (12.8) [6]	1.9 (16.8) [6]	0.6	3.7
Aortic nipple				0.9 (1.4–9.5) [7]
Air in oesophagus				8.9 (15.0) [10]
Aortic pulmonary stripe				17.7

Numbers are our data expressed in percentage and those in parentheses are reported data in percentage.

Recognition of superolateral and superomedial major fissures is essential for the daily interpretation of chest radiographs. Proto and Ball first reported these fundamental chest radiographic findings [2, 3]. Their importance is twofold. First, they should not be mistaken for some pathological condition. Second, they can serve as a landmark for the localization of intrapulmonary lesion.

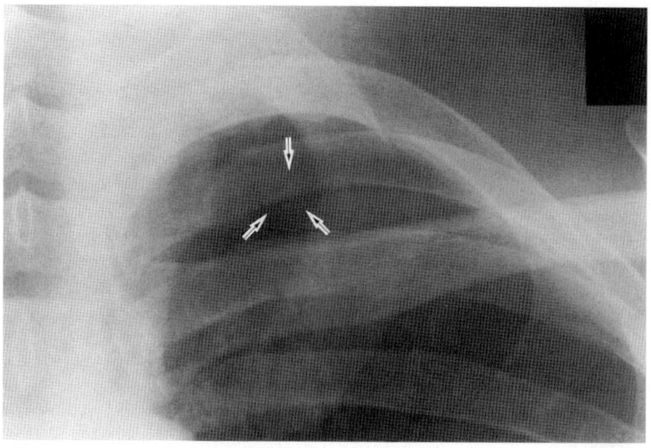

Figure 10. Posteroanterior chest radiograph showing normal apical opacity in a 41-year-old man. This opacity is seen above the clavicle and between the lateral margin of the spine and the inner margin of the first anterior rib (arrows).

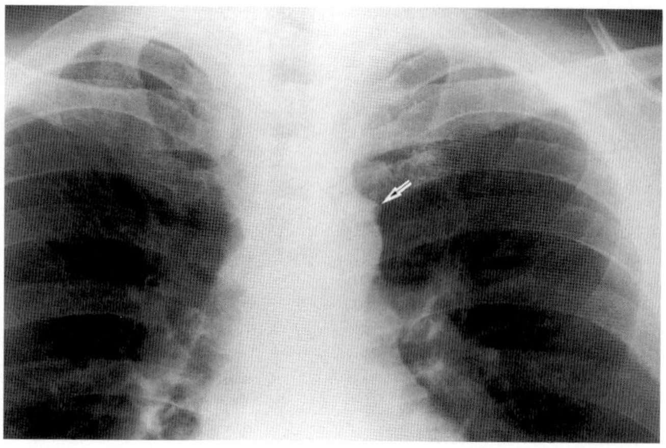

Figure 11. Posteroanterior chest radiograph showing aortic nipple in a 28-year-old man. A small nipple around the aortic knob is seen (arrow).

The apical opacity has been only reported by Proto and Challiff [6]. This is important and should be differentiated from intrapulmonary nodule, in particular early lung cancer occurring in the apical region. The visualization of the normal apical opacity in their study was astonishingly high when compared with our data. This may be due to

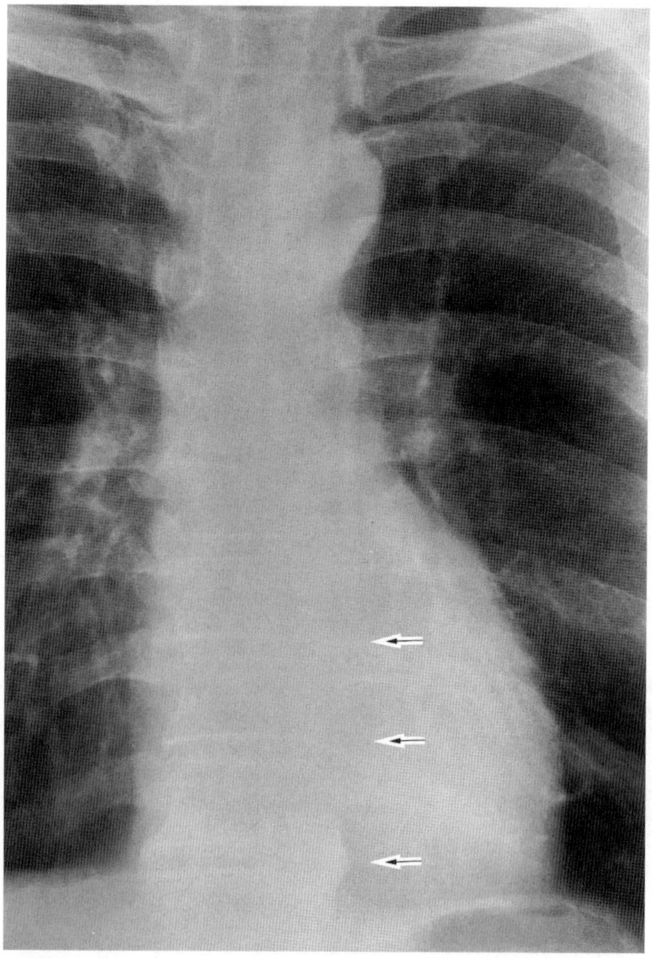

Figure 12. Posteroanterior chest radiograph showing focal obliteration of the descending aortic interface at inferior portion in a 50-year-old man (arrows).

Table 4. Rate and portion of obliterated descending aortic interface

Portion of obliteration	Obliteration rate
One portion	
Superior	1.0
Superior to middle	0.2
Middle	3.7
Middle to inferior	4.3
Inferior	4.1
Two portions	
Superior and middle to inferior	0.3
Superior and inferior	0.1
Overall	13.7

Numbers are expressed in percentage.

higher incidence of atherosclerotic tortuous subclavian artery in their patients, but may need re-evaluation.

The descending thoracic aortic interface can be obliterated in various pathological conditions. These include cardiomegaly, aortitis (such as Takayasu arteritis), and pectus excavatum. Inflammatory or neoplastic lesions adjacent to the descending thoracic aorta may also obliterate the interface. Obliterated descending aortic interface can be the first clue to the diagnosis of mediastinal lymphadenopathy or mass, mediastinal vascular disease, pleural effusion, oesophageal lesions, intrathoracic extension of retroperioneal lesions, pneumonia, and lung cancer [9]. One should be aware, however, that the similar appearance can be a normal finding. The descending aortic interface is most often obliterated at middle to inferior portion.

Smooth arcuate elevation of the diaphragm, the so-called scalloping, is one of the fundamental normal chest radiographic findings, and should not be mistaken for a mass lesion of the diaphragm or the liver. The frequency of the visualization of smooth arcuate elevation was high

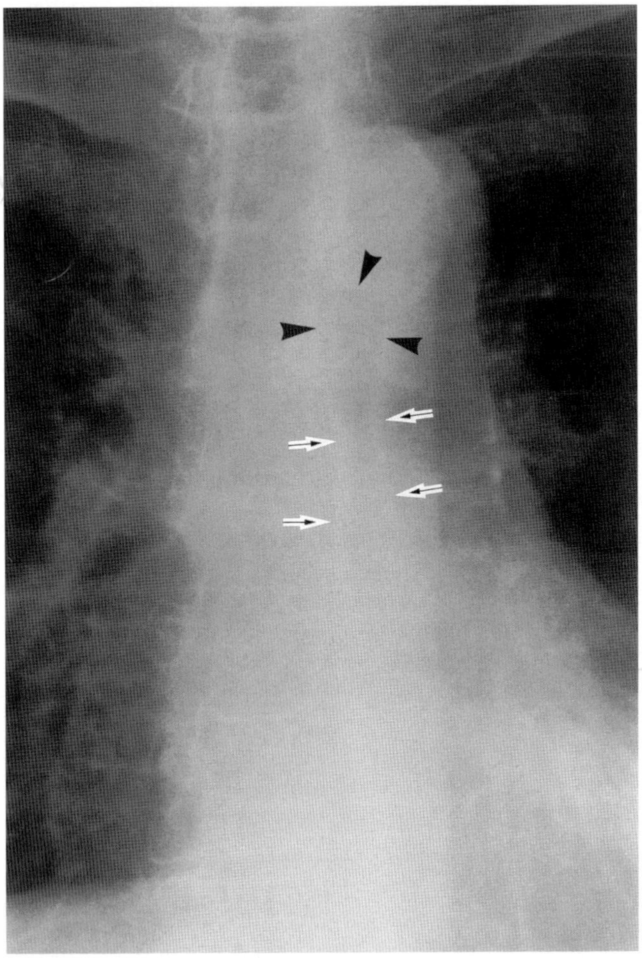

Figure 13. Posteroanterior chest radiograph showing air in the oesophagus in a 60-year-old woman. Segmental air in the oesophagus is visible as a triangular lucency below aortic knob (arrowheads). Right and left pleuroesophageal stripe are also seen (arrows).

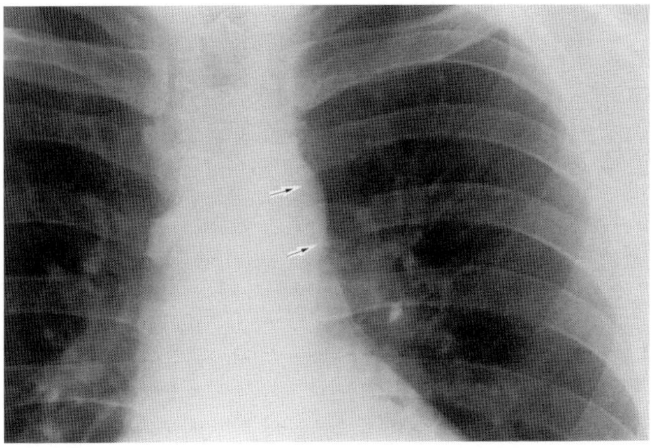

Figure 14. Posteroanterior chest radiograph showing aortic pulmonary stripe in a 23-year-old man. This stripe is seen as an oblique contour extending across the outline of the aortic knob from superior medium to the left hilum (arrows).

Table 5. Visualization and characteristics of the diaphragm

Level	Right higher	Left higher	Same
	94.2 (91) [1]	1.4	4.4

Portion of obliteration	Right	Left
Medial	8.8	21.2
Middle	0.6	3.5
Lateral	0.2	0.7
Medial to Middle	0.5	6.2
Middle to Lateral	0.1	0.2
Medial and Lateral	0.1	0.1
All portions	0.0	0.5
Overall	10.3	32.4

Scalloping	Right	Left	Bilateral	Overall
Visualization of scalloping	10.6 (4.2) [1]	6.5 (0.2) [1]	4.3 (1–1.1) [1, 12]	21.4 (5.5–10.9) [1, 12]
Number of scalloping				
1	11.5	8.3		
2	3.2	2.1		
3	0.1	0.2		
4	0.1	0.2		

Numbers are our data expressed in percentage and those in parentheses are reported data in percentage.

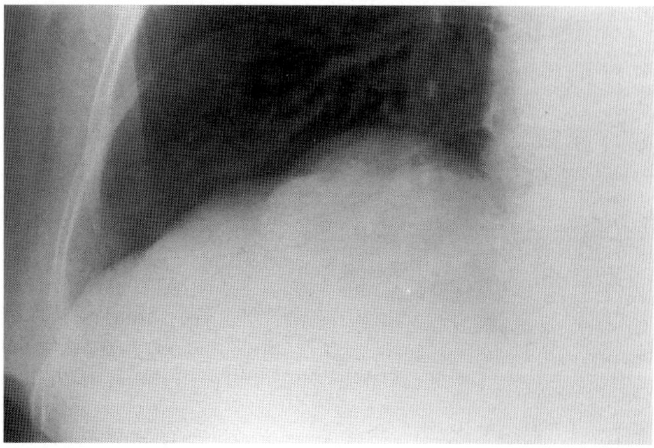

Figure 15. Posteroanterior chest radiograph showing the right diaphragm in a 77-year-old woman. The right diaphragm with two smooth arcuate elevations is seen.

in our study when compared with some others [1, 12]. In our study, hemidiaphragm was obliterated in 10.3% on the right and in 32.4% on the left. Focal obliteration was more often seen in medial portion especially on left side, probably because of obscuration by the heart. These results are in agreement with Felson's reports [1]. Although focal obliteration of the diaphragm can easily be recognized as abnormal, we should recognize that medial portion of the left as well as right diaphragm is occasionally obliterated on normal chest radiograph. The obliteration of medial portion of the right hemidiaphragm may be attributed to the phrenic nerve that descends between the pericardium and the parietal pleura, along the lateral aspect of inferior vena cava on the right side [13, 14].

In conclusion, we evaluated 1000 consecutive normal PA chest radiographs of Japanese adults, and showed frequency of visualization and characteristics of various normal anatomical structures. Our data have some differences from the data of previously published reports. It is not clear whether the differences are due to different racial and physical characteristics, different radiographic techniques or accidental. Although the number of the radiographs we evaluated may not be large, we believe our data are helpful in understanding normal thoracic structures. Familiarity with these normal structures and their variations on chest radiographs in the Japanese population is important in image interpretation in our daily work.

References

1. Felson B. Chest roentgenology. Philadelphia, PA: WB Saunders, 1973.
2. Proto AV, Ball JB Jr. The superolateral major fissures. AJR Am J Roentgenol 1983;140:431–7.
3. Proto AV. The chest radiograph: anatomic considerations. Clin Chest Med 1984;5:213–46.
4. Friedman E. Further observations on the vertical fissure line. Am J Roentgenol Radium Ther Nucl Med 1966;97:171–3.
5. Godwin JD, Tarver RD. Accessory fissure of the lung. AJR Am J Roentgenol 1985;144:39–47.
6. Proto AV, Chaliff MI. Apical opacity: a normal finding on posteroanterior chest radiographs. Radiology 1986;161:429–32.
7. Ball JB Jr, Proto AV. The variable appearance of the left superior intercostal vein. Radiology 1982;144:445–52.
8. Friedman AC, Chambers E, Sprayregen S. The normal and abnormal left superior intercostal vein. AJR Am J Roentgenol 1978;131:599–602.
9. Takahashi K, Shinozaki T, Hyodo H, Ogawa C, Ohsawa T. Focal obliteration of the descending aortic interface on normal frontal chest radiographs: correlation with CT findings. Radiology 1994;191:685–90.
10. Proto AV, Lane EJ. Air in the esophagus: a frequent radiographic finding. AJR Am J Roentgenol 1977;129:433–40.
11. Keats TE. The aortic-pulmonary mediastinal stripe. Am J Roentgenol Radium Ther Nucl Med 1972;116:107–9.
12. Kobayashi T, Watanabe T, Nakanishi F, Moriya K. Normal variants of the diaphragm: scalloping and dromedary. Rinsho Hoshasen 1979;24:361–6 [in Japanese].
13. Ojiri H, Ujita M, Ariizumi M, Tada S. CT anatomy of phrenic nerve, supradiaphragmatic inferior phrenic artery, and inferior pulmonary ligament. Rinsho Hoshasen 1993;38:47–53 [in Japanese].
14. Ujita M, Ojiri H, Ariizumi M, Tada S. Appearance of the inferior phrenic artery and vein on CT scans of the chest: a CT and Cadaveric study. AJR Am J Roentgenol 1993;160:745–7.

The British Journal of Radiology, 78 (2005), 405–410
DOI: 10.1259/bjr/31803121

Management of non-Hodgkin's lymphoma of the thyroid: the Royal Marsden Hospital experience

[1,2]K J HARRINGTON, MRCP, FRCR, [1]V J MICHALAKI, MD, [3]L VINI, FRCR, [1,2]C M NUTTING, MD, MRCP, FRCR, [1]K N SYRIGOS, MD, [4]R A'HERN, PhD and [3]C L HARMER, FRCP, FRCR

[1]*Head and Neck Cancer Unit, Royal Marsden Hospital, Fulham Road, London,* [2]*Institute of Cancer Research, Fulham Road, London,* [3]*Thyroid Unit, Royal Marsden Hospital, Fulham Road, London and* [4]*Department of Statistics, Royal Marsden Hospital, Fulham Road, London, UK*

Abstract. A retrospective review was conducted of patients treated for thyroid non-Hodgkin's lymphoma (TNHL) at the Royal Marsden Hospital between 1936 and 1996 to determine the effect of radiotherapy (RT) on outcome. 91 patients were identified from the Thyroid Unit Database. There were 77 females and 14 males with a median age of 65 years (range 22–87 years). RT was delivered according to two separate policies: (1) involved field radiotherapy (IFRT) to the thyroid bed and cervical lymph nodes; (2) extended field radiotherapy (EFRT) covering the thyroid bed, cervical and mediastinal lymph nodes. 89 patients received RT as part of definitive treatment following surgery, to a dose of approximately 40 Gy. 25 patients received IFRT and 64 patients EFRT. 27 patients received cytotoxic chemotherapy. 18 patients (72%) treated with IFRT died of TNHL with a median relapse free survival (RFS) of 10 months and a median overall survival (OS) of 21 months. In contrast, only 29 patients (46%) treated with EFRT died of TNHL with a median RFS of 76 months (p=0.01 for RFS with respect to IFRT and p=0.04 for OS). Significantly more patients treated with IFRT relapsed locally (52% *vs* 27%). There was no difference in the rates of systemic relapse (20% *vs* 22%). EFRT alone for Stage I, but not for Stage II disease, yielded acceptable rates of local control and disease free survival with doses of at least 40 Gy. These historical data strongly support the addition of combination chemotherapy to the treatment regimen in all patients with Stage II disease. Indeed, in recent years this has become the standard of care for all cases of thyroid lymphoma unless the histology is of marginal zone type (mucosa associated lymphoma tissue (MALT) lymphoma).

Thyroid non-Hodgkin's lymphoma (TNHL) is an uncommon tumour, representing 2–8% of thyroid malignancies and approximately 1–2% of extranodal lymphomas [1–4]. It occurs most frequently in elderly females and has been linked to Hashimoto's thyroiditis and prior therapeutic irradiation of the thyroid bed. Staging should include CT scanning of the neck, thorax, abdomen and pelvis, together with bone marrow aspirate and trephine [1].

There exists no universally accepted standard of care for TNHL and a number of controversies exist regarding the roles of surgery, radiotherapy (RT) and chemotherapy in the management of this disease [5–12]. Previously, surgery occupied a pre-eminent place in management and most patients underwent extensive resections. In recent years, however, the appreciation that TNHL is sensitive to RT and chemotherapy has resulted in a move towards limited surgical intervention, usually in the form of a diagnostic biopsy followed by definitive RT (or chemotherapy followed by RT). However, there are opponents of this view who recommend excision or debulking of disease followed by post-operative RT [13–22].

In spite of the controversy regarding the surgical management of TNHL, radical RT became the treatment of choice in most centres, although there has now been a shift towards using a combination of chemotherapy and RT in all cases other than mucosa associated lymphoma tissue (MALT) lymphoma of the thyroid gland. As regards therapeutic irradiation, there remain a number of unresolved issues regarding the volume of tissue that should be treated and the dose prescription required. There are two main options in the selection of radiation treatment fields: (1) involved field RT (IFRT) which aims to include the entire thyroid gland and local neck nodes; and (2) extended field RT (EFRT) which involves treating the thyroid, neck, mediastinal and in some centres, axillary nodes.

These two options have never been formally compared in a randomized study and in view of the rarity of this condition; such a study is unlikely to be conducted. A a result, the choice between IFRT and EFRT has been a matter of clinical judgement based on prior experience.

Similarly, formal evaluation of the optimal radiation dose required for local control has never been undertaken. In line with treatment of nodal and non-thyroid extranodal NHL, most patients with TNHL have received doses in the order of 40 Gy. Previous studies have suggested that there is a threshold dose below which the chance of achieving local control is small. Tupchong et al [23] reported 0% local control rated for patients who received less than 20 Gy. Therefore, in this retrospective analysis, we have attempted to address these two important questions relating to the management of TNHL by RT.

Received 27 February 2004 and in revised form 28 October 2004, accepted 6 December 2004.

Patients and methods

Data collection

A search of the Royal Marsden Hospital (RMH) Thyroid Database was undertaken for a period that spanned the years between 1936 and 1996.

This database contains a thorough summary of over 2000 patients presenting to RMH with thyroid malignancy over the last six decades. A total of 91 patients with histologically proven NHL were identified. Case notes were reviewed in order to collect demographic data, details of disease-related symptoms and tumour stage, surgical and radiotherapeutic management and standard outcome measures, including relapse free (RFS) and overall survival (OS). For the purposes of data collection, the results of staging investigations were accepted at face value and no attempt was made to re-evaluate the staging assigned to patients treated at different times. Similarly, the pathological classification of NHL has undergone a number of changes during the period of time under study [24–29]. In a previous study of 46 patients with TNHL from RMH, all of whom are included in this analysis, it was shown that the majority (91%) presented with adverse (intermediate or high grade) histology. Similar findings were apparent for this group of patients. No attempt has been made to review previous pathological specimens or re-classify cases according to the current REAL classification. Of the 91 patients who were identified, 89 were eligible for analysis of the effect of definitive RT. The two patients excluded, received primary chemotherapy without RT.

Follow up

Follow-up data were obtained for all patients treated with RT. RFS and OS times were calculated for each patient to the nearest month, taken from the time of presentation to the time of first relapse (for RFS) or death/last recorded follow-up (for OS).

Statistical analysis

Statistical analysis was performed using the Statistical Package for the Social Sciences (SPSS, Inc., Chicago, IL), statistical software. Survival curves were obtained by the Kaplan-Meier method and comparisons were made with the log-rank statistics. Factors found to be significant at univariate analysis were considered for multivariate analysis. Cox proportional hazards models were developed for the multivariate analysis of survival and any value of $p<0.05$ was considered to be statistically significant.

Results

Clinical features

Age and gender

The median age of the patients was 65 years (range 22–87 years). There was no significant difference between the median ages of the female (median 65 years, range 27–87 years) and male (median 63 years, range 22–85 years) patients. There were 77 females and 14 males, representing a female to male ratio of 5.5:1.

Table 1. Summary of patient characteristics for 91 patients with thyroid non-Hodgkin's lymphoma

Patient characteristic	No.	(%)
Female	77	(84.6%)
Male	14	(15.4%)
Stridor	30	(33.7%)
Dysphonia	28	(31.5%)
Previous goitre	31	(34.8%)
Pain	12	(14.1%)
Neck swelling	87	(97.8%)
Dysphagia	47	(53.3%)
Stage 1	35	(38.4%)
Stage 2	49	(53.8%)
Stage 3	4	(4.4%)
Stage 4	3	(3.4%)

Presenting symptoms

The presenting symptoms are documented in Table 1. For two patients, no presenting symptoms were recorded but the vast majority (98%) presented with neck swelling. Local obstructive symptoms (stridor, dysphagia and dysphonia) were frequently reported. A significant number (34%) had previously been noted to have goitre, in many cases of long-standing.

Stage

In keeping with data presented for other studies, the majority of patients presented with early stage disease. 35 had Stage I disease confined to the thyroid gland and 49 had Stage II disease. Only seven patients, were found to have more advanced Stage III or IV disease at presentation. From analysis of the database, it was apparent that these patients presented with massive thyroid enlargement and evidence of dissemination, rather than as patients with widely disseminated lymphoma with incidental involvement of the thyroid gland. Systemic B symptoms were uncommon, occurring in only two patients.

Surgery

All of the patients underwent an initial surgical procedure, the details of which are presented in Table 2.

Radiotherapy

Over the 60 year period in which patients were treated, a number of different treatment protocols were applied involving use of 220–250 kV X-rays, ^{60}Co gamma rays and 4–6 MV photons. The median tumour radiation dose was 40 Gy (range 4–72 Gy), which was delivered at a dose rate of between 1.2 Gy and 2.3 Gy per day.

Table 2. Initial surgical procedure performed on the 91 patients with thyroid non-Hodgkin's lymphoma

Surgical procedure	No.	(%)
Biopsy	43	(45.6%)
Enucleation	2	(2.2%)
Lobectomy	11	(12.0%)
Hemithyroidectomy	6	(7.6%)
Subtotal thyroidectomy	20	(22.8%)
Near total thyroidectomy	6	(6.5%)
Total thyroidectomy	3	(3.3%)

The majority (61 of 89) received a radiation dose of 40 Gy or more. Treatment was usually delivered using parallel-opposed anterior and posterior fields, although, direct anterior, anterior oblique or lateral fields were employed occasionally. Spinal cord shielding was not used. No attempt has been made to assess the effect of technique on outcome. 25 patients received IFRT to the thyroid bed and cervical lymph nodes and 64 patients received EFRT to the thyroid bed, cervical and mediastinal lymph nodes. In this latter group, there were no data detailing the number of patients in whom the superior mediastinal nodes, as opposed to all mediastinal nodes, were treated. The axillary nodes were not treated routinely.

Chemotherapy

27 patients received cytotoxic chemotherapy under a wide variety of circumstances. Two received definitive combination chemotherapy without RT. Five patients received induction chemotherapy prior to radical RT, eight received adjuvant chemotherapy following RT and 14 received chemotherapy following relapse after RT. Clearly, this experience reflects the state of what was considered optimal practice at the time that the patients presented. In current practice, it is likely that the majority of patients would receive combination chemotherapy followed by consolidation radiotherapy.

Regimens comprised cyclophosphamide, vincristine and prednisolone (COP), cyclophosphamide, doxorubicin, vincristine and prednisolone (CHOP) or prednisolone, mitoxantrone, cyclophosphamide, etoposide, bleomycin and vincristine (PMitCEBO). Analysis of the role of chemotherapy in this cohort of patients was not possible because of the small numbers and the different regimens employed. Eight of 13 patients treated initially with chemotherapy as part of a planned combined approach were long-term survivors. However, results for relapsed disease were generally poor, with only two of eight patients relapsing after RT successfully salvaged with combination chemotherapy.

Outcome and prognostic factors

The overall 5-year survival rate was 48%, with a median RFS of 34 months. Univariate analysis of OS according to patient variables and treatment factors is shown in Table 3. Adverse prognostic factors were as follows: advanced stage, surgical procedure (only biopsy *vs* more debulking procedure), extent of radiation field, radiation dose of 40 Gy or more, and the presence of stridor at diagnosis. A number of these factors have been implicated previously [29–32]. Analysis of the effect of dysphagia, dysphonia and previous goitre on the OS revealed no significant impact. Independent predictive factors obtained from multivariate analysis are shown in Table 4.

Surgical procedure

Analysis of the extent of surgical resection (biopsy alone *vs* more extensive resection), revealed that only in the last decade was there a marked change towards less extensive procedures. Thus, prior to 1990 biopsy was performed in 30 patients compared with 43 who underwent an extensive resection. After 1990, 13 patients underwent biopsy compared with only 5 who had a more extensive resection.

Table 3. Significant factors on univariate analysis of overall survival

Prognostic factors	No	(%) 5 year survival	*p*-value
Stage			
I	34	(72%)	
II	48	(36%)	
III, IV	7	(0%)	<0.001
Surgical procedure			
Biopsy	42	(26%)	
Debulking	47	(66%)	<0.001
Radiation field			
IFRT	25	32%	
EFRT	64	55%	0.04
Radiation dose			
<40 Gy	27	26%	0.002
>40 Gy	62	56%	

IFRT, involved field radiotherapy; EFRT, extended field radiotherapy.

The type of surgical procedure performed had a significant impact on the outcome of subsequent RT as demonstrated in Table 3 ($p<0.001$).

Radiation field (IFRT vs EFRT)

18 of 25 patients (72%) treated with IFRT died of TNHL. The median RFS was only 10 months and the median OS was 21 months. In contrast, only 29 of 64 patients (45%) treated with EFRT died of TNHL. The median RFS was 76 months, while the median OS has not yet been reached. The 5-year survival data according to disease stage stratified by radiation field (IFRT or EFRT) are illustrated in Figures 1 and 2. Patients who received EFRT had higher survival rates ($p<0.005$), (log rank test). For patients treated with IFRT, 52% (20% local alone and 32% combined local and distant) had evidence of loco-regional failure at the time of death, compared with only 26% (9% local alone plus 17% local and distant), of patients treated with EFRT. There was no significant difference in the rates of local control between two groups (20% for IFRT *vs* 22% for EFRT). The patterns of failure of patients dying following IFRT and EFRT are detailed in Table 5.

Radiation dose

When the survival data for patients who received <40 Gy were compared with those who received 40 Gy

Table 4. Significant independent factors on multivariate analysis of overall survival

	Hazard ratio (95% CI)	*p*-value
Stage		
I	1	
II	3.74 (1.77–7.92)	
III, IV	6.38 (2.13–19.11)	<0.001
Surgical procedure		
Debulking	1	
Biopsy	3.23 (1.72–6.06)	<0.001
Radiation field		
IFRT	1	
EFRT	0.45 (0.25–0.82)	<0.01

IFRT, involved field radiotherapy; EFRT, extended field radiotherapy.

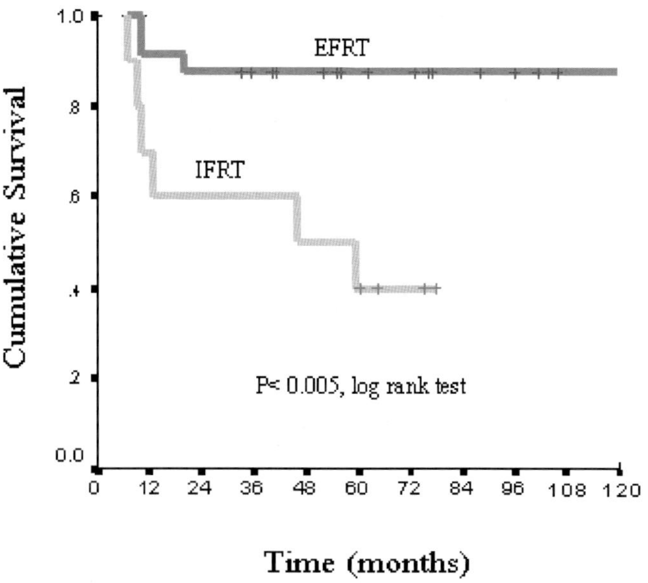

Figure 1. Kaplan-Meier curve showing overall survival of Stage I patients stratified by radiation field (extended field radiotherapy *vs* involved field radiotherapy).

or more, radiation dose was not significant in multivariate analysis of survival (hazard ratio 0.64, 95% confidence interval (CI): 0.33–1.24, $p=0.18$). However, the confidence intervals are wide and it is not possible to rule out an effect. Radiation dose was significant in multivariate analysis for local control (hazard ratio 0.42, 95% CI: 0.18–0.94, $p=0.04$). At 5 years, only 7 of 27 (26%) patients treated at the lower dose level were alive, compared with 35 of 62 (56%) treated to 40 Gy or more ($p<0.01$, log rank test). However, the first group included six patients who received doses of less than 30 Gy; none achieved local control and their maximal survival was 6 months. The effect of radiation dose on outcome is presented in Figure 3.

Table 5. Survival according to stage of disease and extent of irradiated volume

Irradiated volume	Stage I	Stage II	Stage III/IV
IFRT	4/10 (40%)	3/12 (25%)	0/3 (0%)
EFRT	22/25 (88%)	13/36 (36.1%)	0/3 (0%)
Total	26/35 (74.3%)	16/48 (33.3%)	0/6 (0%)

IFRT, involved field radiotherapy; EFRT, extended field radiotherapy.

Discussion

Analysis of the data from this large series of patients with TNHL treated over a prolonged period of time in a single centre provides valuable insights in to the management of this uncommon disease. RT has traditionally played a major role in treatment of TNHL and the findings of this study have direct bearing on its use. Multivariate analysis has highlighted the extent of radiation field as an independent prognostic factor. RFS and OS rates were significantly better for patients treated with EFRT compared with IFRT; this difference was not seen in Stage II disease. This effect seemed to be mediated at the level of the thyroid bed and adjacent lymph nodes in the neck and mediastinum because 52% of patients treated with IFRT experienced locoregional failure compared with only 27% of patients treated with EFRT. There was no difference between the two groups in terms of systemic relapse. Therefore, the poor results of IFRT in all disease stages mean that this approach should be abandoned in favour of more extensive radiation fields that encompass the mediastinal nodes. For patients with Stage I disease, definitive EFRT yielded excellent rates of local control and survival and represented the treatment of choice. However, more recently, combination chemotherapy followed by RT has become the standard of care for this disease and given the data from this study, EFRT should be considered as the standard RT technique.

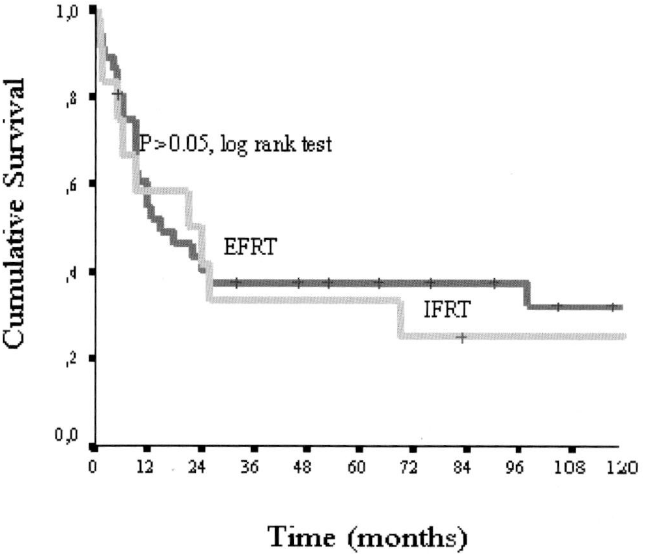

Figure 2. Kaplan-Meier curve showing overall survival of Stage II patients stratified by radiation field (extended field radiotherapy *vs* involved field radiotherapy).

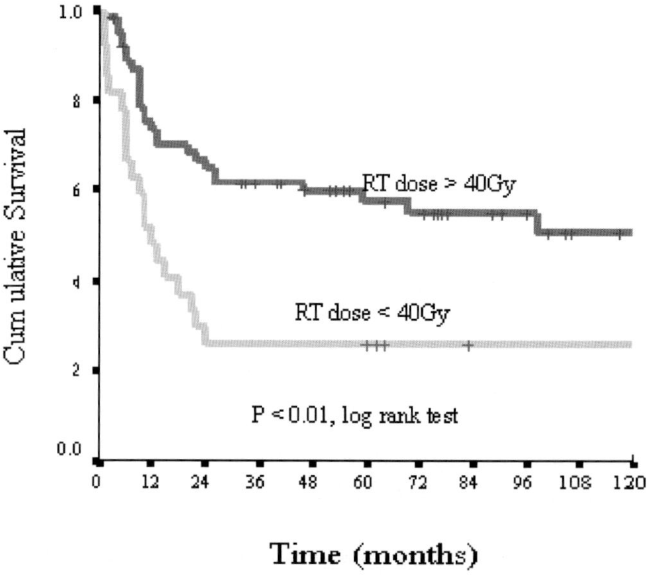

Figure 3. Kaplan-Meier curve showing overall survival of patients according to the radiation dose received (<40 Gy *vs* 40 Gy or more).

Similarly, analysis of outcomes at radiation doses below 40 Gy versus 40 Gy or more provides clear indications for clinical practice. A threshold dose of 40 Gy or more was shown to be associated with a significantly improved local control outcome. This is in keeping with previous data [23] and we suggest a standard dose of 40 Gy in 20 fractions for this disease.

The data on extent of surgical resection indicate a significantly improved outcome in patients who underwent a debulking procedure (defined as anything more than a biopsy) prior to RT and concur with those reported in previous studies [33, 34]. Patients who had total macroscopic removal of tumour had the highest rate of local control and long term survival ($p<0.001$). No significant differences were seen between lobectomy, subtotal or total thyroidectomy, although seven of nine long-term survivors (58–129 months) underwent total thyroidectomy. Despite these findings, it is unlikely that the trend towards performing open biopsy to make a tissue diagnosis will be reversed. The increasing role of combination chemotherapy and consolidating RT is likely to strengthen the move towards more conservative surgical intervention [32, 34–36].

The precise role of combination chemotherapy in TNHL remains to be defined, although in recent years it has become part of the standard management of this disease. This study demonstrates the generally poor results obtained with RT alone, even with EFRT, in patients with anything more than Stage I disease and provide strong support for the use of chemotherapy as part of the primary treatment. The ability of chemotherapy to "debulk" the tumour prior to starting RT (in an analogous fashion to surgical debulking) represents a further attraction. Indeed, despite the fact that low-grade MALT lymphomas have a low distant recurrence rate [26, 28], a review of the published literature suggests that the addition of chemotherapy to RT significantly reduces both distant and overall recurrence [37–41].

In conclusion, the following recommendations are made for the management of TNHL. IFRT yields unacceptable rates of disease free survival and OS and can not be recommended. EFRT to a dose of 40 Gy is effective for Stage I.

For Stage II–IV disease, EFRT is associated with poor outcome; these patients should receive induction chemotherapy followed by consolidation EFRT to a dose of 40 Gy.

References

1. Evans TR, Mansi JL, Bevan DH, Dalgleish AG, Harmer CL. Primary non-Hodgkin's lymphoma of the thyroid with bone marrow infiltration at presentation. Clin Oncol 1995;7:54–5.
2. Heimann R, Vannineuse A, De Sloover C, Dor P. Malignant lymphomas and undifferentiated small cell carcinoma of the thyroid: a clinicopathological review in the light of the Kiel classification for malignant lymphomas. Histopathology 1978;2:201–13.
3. Souhami L, Simpson WJ, Carruthers JS. Malignant lymphoma of the thyroid gland. Int J Radiat Oncol Biol Phys 1980;6:1143–7.
4. Vini L, Harmer C. Thyroid. Treatment of Cancer. In: Price P, Sikora K, editors. Treatment of cancer (3rd edn). London: Arnold, 2002:401–27.
5. Ansell SM, Grant CS, Habermann TM. Primary thyroid lymphoma. Semin Oncol 1999;26:316–23.
6. Bisbee AC, Thoeny RH. Malignant lymphoma of the thyroid following irradiation. Cancer 1975;35:1296–9.
7. Burke JS, Butler JJ, Fuller LM. Malignant lymphomas of the thyroid: a clinical pathologic study of 35 patients including ultra structural observations. Cancer 1977;39:1587–602.
8. Derringer GA, Thompson LD, Frommelt RA, Bijwaard KE, Heffess CS, Abbondanzo SL. Malignant lymphoma of the thyroid gland: a clinicopathologic study of 108 cases. Am J Surg Pathol 2000;24:623–39.
9. Ha CS, Shadle KM, Medeiros LJ, et al. Localized non-Hodgkin lymphoma involving the thyroid gland. Cancer 2001;91:629–35.
10. Holmes HB Jr, Kreutner A, O'Brien PH. Hashimoto's thyroiditis and its relationship to other thyroid diseases. Surg Gynecol Obstet 1977;144:887–90.
11. Pledge S, Bessell EM, Leach IH, et al. Non-Hodgkin's lymphoma of the thyroid: retrospective review of all patients diagnosed in Nottinghamshire from 1973 to 1992. Clin Oncol 1996;8:371–5.
12. Skarsgard ED, Connors JM, Robins RE. A current analysis of primary lymphoma of the thyroid. Arch Surg 1991;126:1199–203.
13. Baskal N, Erdogan G, Kamel AN, Dagci SS, Akyar S, Ekinci C. Localized non-Hodgkin's lymphoma of the adrenal and thyroid glands. Endocrinol Jpn 1992;39:269–76.
14. Butler JS Jr, Brady LW, Amendola BE. Lymphoma of the thyroid. Report of five cases and review. Am J Clin Oncol 1990;13:64–9.
15. Heimann R. Primary malignant lymphomas of the thyroid. A brief review. Acta Otorhinolaryngol Belg 1987;41:727–35.
16. Ifrah N, Rohmer V, Saint-Andre JP, Jardel H, Boasson M, Bigorgne JC. Primary lymphoma of the thyroid gland. Diagnostic and therapeutic discussion. Apropos of 4 cases. Ann Med Interne (Paris) 1988;139:344–8.
17. Kuma K, Matsuzuka F. Diagnosis and therapy of malignant thyroid lymphoma. Nippon Naika Gakkai Zasshi 1997;86: 1190–5.
18. Tennvall J, Cavallin-Stahl E, Akerman M. Primary localized non-Hodgkin's lymphoma of the thyroid: a retrospective clinicopathological review. Eur J Surg Oncol 1987;13:297–302.
19. Tsutsui K, Shibamoto Y, Yamabe H, et al. A radiotherapeutic experience for localized extranodal non-Hodgkin's lymphoma: prognostic factors and re-evaluation of treatment modality. Radiother Oncol 1991;21:83–90.
20. Friedberg MH, Coburn MC, Monchik JM. Role of surgery in stage IE non-Hodgkin's lymphoma of the thyroid. Surgery 1994;116:1061–6.
21. Rasbach DA, Mondschein MS, Harris NL, Kaufman DS, Wang CA. Malignant lymphoma of the thyroid gland: a clinical and pathologic study of twenty cases. Surgery 1985;98:1166–70.
22. Woolner LB, McConahey WM, Beahrs OH, Black BM. Primary malignant lymphoma of the thyroid. Review of forty-six cases. Am J Surg 1966;111:502–23.
23. Tupchong L, Hughes F, Harmer CL. Primary lymphoma of the thyroid: clinical features, prognostic factors, and results of treatment. Int J Radiat Oncol Biol Phys 1986;2: 1813–21.
24. Anscombe AM, Wright DH. Primary malignant lymphoma of the thyroid—a tumour of mucosa-associated lymphoid tissue: review of seventy-six cases. Histopathology 1985;9:81–97.
25. Fonseca E, Sambade C. Primary lymphomas of the thyroid gland: a review with emphasis on diagnostic features. Arch Anat Cytol Pathol 1998;46:94–9.
26. Isaacson PG. Lymphoma of the thyroid gland. Curr Top Pathol 1997;91:1–14.

27. Kossev P, Livolsi V. Lymphoid lesions of the thyroid: review in light of the revised European-American lymphoma classification and upcoming World Health Organization classification. Thyroid 1999;9:1273–80.
28. Laing RW, Hoskin P, Hudson BV. The significance of MALT histology in thyroid lymphoma: a review of patients from the BNLI and Royal Marsden Hospital. Clin Oncol 1994;6: 300–4.
29. Logue JP, Hale RJ, Stewart AL, Duthie MB, Banerjee SS. Primary malignant lymphoma of the thyroid: a clinicopathological analysis. Int J Radiat Oncol Biol Phys 1992;22: 929–33.
30. Sasai K, Yamabe H, Haga H, et al. Non-Hodgkin's lymphoma of the thyroid. A clinical study of twenty-two cases. Acta Oncol 1996;35:457–62.
31. Singer JA. Primary lymphoma of the thyroid. Am Surg 1998;64:334–7.
32. Wirtzfeld DA, Winston JS, Hicks WL, Loree TR. Clinical presentation and treatment of non-Hodgkin's lymphoma of the thyroid gland. Ann Surg Oncol 2001;8:338–41.
33. Pyke CM, Grant CS, Habermann TM, et al. Non-Hodgkin's lymphoma of the thyroid: is more than biopsy necessary? World J Surg 1992;16:604–9.
34. Tsang RW, Gospodarowicz MK, Sutcliffe SB, Sturgeon JF, Panzarella T, Patterson BJ. Non-Hodgkin's lymphoma of the thyroid gland: prognostic factors and treatment outcome. The Princess Margaret Hospital Lymphoma Group. Int J Radiat Oncol Biol Phys 1993;27:599–604.
35. Blair TJ, Evans RG, Buskirk SJ, Banks PM, Earle JD. Radiotherapeutic management of primary thyroid lymphoma. Int J Radiat Oncol Biol Phys 1985;11:365–70.
36. Kanetake H, Toda M, Kawamoto Y. Prognostic factors in primary lymphoma of the thyroid—a review of 74 cases. Nippon Jibiinkoka Gakkai Kaiho 1993;96:1105–11.
37. Belal AA, Allam A, Kandil A, et al. Primary thyroid lymphoma: a retrospective analysis of prognostic factors and treatment outcome for localized intermediate and high grade lymphoma. Am J Clin Oncol 2001;24:299–305.
38. Doria R, Jekel JF, Cooper DL. Thyroid lymphoma. The case for combined modality therapy. Cancer 1994;73:200–6.
39. Gospodarowicz MK, Sutcliffe SB, Brown TC, Chua T, Bush RS. Patterns of disease in localized extranodal lymphomas. J Clin Oncol 1987;5:875–80.
40. Leedman PJ, Sheridan WP, Downey WF, Fox RM, Martin FI. Combination chemotherapy as single modality therapy for stage IE and IIE thyroid lymphoma. Med J Aust 1990;152:40–3.
41. Vigliotti A, Kong JS, Fuller LM, Velasquez WS. Thyroid lymphomas stages IE and IIE: comparative results for radiotherapy only, combination chemotherapy only, and multimodality treatment. Int J Radiat Oncol Biol Phys 1986;12:1807–12.

The British Journal of Radiology, 78 (2005), 411–415
DOI: 10.1259/bjr/24453312

Transient failure of opening of the lower oesophageal sphincter on upright oesophagrams: radiographic and clinical findings

[1]C A RAPTIS, BS, [1]M S LEVINE, MD, [1]S E RUBESIN, MD, [1]I LAUFER, MD and [2]D A KATZKA, MD

Departments of [1]Radiology and [2]Medicine, Hospital of the University of Pennsylvania, 3400 Spruce Street, Philadelphia, PA 19104, USA

Abstract. The purpose of our study was to determine the frequency, radiographic features, and clinical importance of transient failure of opening of the lower oesophageal sphincter (LOS) on upright double-contrast views of the oesophagus. A computerized search of radiology records identified 16 patients who had transient failure of opening of the LOS on upright views from biphasic oesophagrams or upper gastrointestinal tract examinations using high-density barium but normal opening of the LOS on prone views using low-density barium. The radiographic findings were reviewed and correlated with the clinical and manometric findings. In all cases, barium studies revealed tapered, beaklike narrowing of the distal oesophagus on upright double-contrast views, with a normal-appearing distal oesophagus, normal opening of the LOS, and intact peristalsis on prone single-contrast views. Only seven patients (44%) had dysphagia. Five of these patients had clinical follow-up, and the dysphagia improved or resolved without specific treatment for LOS dysfunction in four. The remaining patient had persistent dysphagia, but this individual had polymyositis as the likely cause for his dysphagia. Manometry revealed incomplete relaxation of the LOS in two patients and normal relaxation in one. Our experience suggests that failure of opening of the LOS may be observed as a transient finding of little clinical importance on upright double-contrast views of the oesophagus using high-density barium, with normal opening of the LOS on prone single-contrast views using low-density barium. It is important to be aware of this finding, so that it is not mistaken for achalasia or other abnormalities of the distal oesophagus.

Primary achalasia is an uncommon but important oesophageal motility disorder associated with progressive dysphagia. This condition is characterized on manometry by incomplete relaxation of the lower oesophageal sphincter (LOS) with absent primary peristalsis in the body of the oesophagus [1, 2]. Other patients who do not have classic achalasia may develop dysphagia as a result of isolated LOS dysfunction with normal oesophageal peristalsis on manometry [3–5]. In our gastrointestinal radiology practice, however, we have encountered patients who had incomplete opening of the LOS on upright double-contrast views of the oesophagus using a high-density barium but normal opening of the LOS on prone single-contrast views using a low-density barium. One of these patients had previously undergone botulinum toxin injections at the gastroesophageal junction because of an oesophagram at an outside hospital in which achalasia was diagnosed on the basis of the findings on upright double-contrast radiographs. The latter case prompted us to perform a retrospective study of patients with transient failure of opening of the LOS on upright double-contrast oesophagrams in order to determine the frequency, radiographic features and clinical importance of this phenomenon.

Received 5 August 2004 and in revised form 27 October 2004, accepted 6 December 2004.

Address correspondence to Dr Marc S Levine.

Materials and methods

Patient population

A computerized search of radiology records at our university hospital revealed 29 patients in whom failure of opening of the LOS (manifested by tapered, beaklike narrowing of the distal oesophagus) was described only in the upright position on the radiographic reports from biphasic oesophagrams or upper gastrointestinal tract examinations during a 5.5-year period from January 1998 to June 2003. 10 of these 29 patients were excluded from our study because LOS dysfunction was only seen at fluoroscopy without adequate documentation on the radiological images. Three other patients were excluded because their medical records were not available. The remaining 16 patients comprised our study group.

Our institutional review board approved all aspects of the retrospective study and did not require informed consent for patients whose radiographic images or medical records were included in our study.

Examination technique

Six (37%) of the 16 patients had biphasic oesophagrams and 10 (63%) had biphasic upper gastrointestinal tract examinations that included upright, left posterior oblique (LPO) double-contrast views using an effervescent agent (Baros; Lafayette Pharmaceuticals, Lafayette, IN) and a 250% w/v high-density barium suspension (E-Z-HD; E-Z-EM Company, Westbury, NY), and prone, right anterior oblique (RAO) single-contrast views using a 50% w/v barium suspension (Entrobar; Lafayette Pharmaceuticals). The 10 patients who underwent biphasic upper gastrointestinal tract studies all received a standard dose of 0.1 mg of intravenous glucagon to optimize the double-contrast phase of the examination by producing gastric hypotonia [6]. Ideally, we would have preferred that all of the patients in our study received no pharmacological agents for their radiographic examinations. However, it has been shown that glucagon has no effect on oesophageal peristalsis [7]. Although glucagon can have a relaxant effect on the LOS [7], our patients all had incomplete opening of the LOS when swallowing high-density barium in the upright position. Because glucagon has the opposite effect on LOS relaxation, we do not believe this agent was in any way responsible for the findings in our study. As part of the examination, patients routinely were asked to take multiple discrete swallows in the prone, RAO position to evaluate oesophageal motility. All of the studies were performed by residents or fellows or one of three attending gastrointestinal radiologists, and all were interpreted by the attending radiologists.

Image and report review

The original radiographic reports and images from these 16 barium studies were reviewed jointly by two gastrointestinal radiologists without knowledge of the clinical or manometric findings. Although videotapes of swallowing are not stored by our department on a long-term basis, the radiographic reports provided a detailed assessment of oesophageal motility in these patients. In all cases, double-contrast views of the oesophagus were reviewed to determine the morphologic appearance of the distal oesophagus when the patient swallowed high-density barium in the upright, LPO position and whether or not LOS dysfunction persisted on all of the upright images. We also noted whether there was proximal oesophageal dilatation or delayed oesophageal emptying. Single-contrast views of the oesophagus were also reviewed to determine the appearance of the distal oesophagus when the patient swallowed low-density barium in the prone, RAO position and whether or not LOS dysfunction was present on prone images. The radiographic reports were also reviewed by one author to determine whether oesophageal peristalsis was normal or abnormal in the prone, RAO position. If abnormal, the nature of this dysmotility was noted.

The prevalence of transient failure of opening of the LOS in the upright position on barium studies was determined by identifying the total number of patients who had biphasic oesophagrams or upper gastrointestinal tract studies at our hospital during the same 5.5-year period. For the purposes of this study, we excluded from the denominator all patients who were known to have had surgery (*e.g.* Nissen fundoplication or surgical myotomy) or other procedures (*e.g.* oesophageal balloon dilatation) on the gastroesophageal junction.

Manometry and report review

Three (19%) of the 16 patients had manometric examinations. In all three cases, oesophageal manometry was performed using a solid-state intraluminal transducer assembly (Konigsberg Instruments, Pasadena, CA). The Konigsberg catheter was placed in the stomach via a transnasal approach. Gastric (*i.e.* intra-abdominal) positioning of the pressure transducers was confirmed by showing a rise in pressure during the inspiratory phase of respiration. The patient was then placed in a sitting position, and the LOS was identified on the distal circumferential transducer tracing, using the station pull-through technique. Catheter withdrawal was continued until the pressure inversion point was identified. LOS pressure measurements were obtained distal to the inversion point. Oesophageal body motility was then assessed after positioning the distal transducer 3 cm above the proximal border of the LOS. A series of 10 wet swallows was completed while recording pressures at 3 cm, 8 cm and 13 cm above the LOS. Measurement of LOS resting pressure and length was also performed by standard techniques, using the same transducer assembly.

One of the authors reviewed the manometry reports of these three patients to determine LOS resting pressures and LOS residual pressures on manometry. LOS resting pressure was considered high if it exceeded 45 mm Hg and LOS relaxation was considered incomplete if LOS residual pressure exceeded 8 mm Hg after swallowing. The manometry reports were also reviewed to determine whether oesophageal peristalsis was normal.

Medical records review

Medical records were subsequently reviewed by one author to determine the indications for the barium study, the nature and duration of symptoms, treatment, and patient course.

Results

Radiographic findings

All 16 patients (100%) had incomplete opening of the LOS manifested by tapered, beaklike narrowing of the distal oesophagus when swallowing high-density barium in the upright, LPO position (Figure 1a). The narrowing was severe enough that it caused delayed emptying of barium into the stomach in seven cases (44%) and proximal oesophageal dilatation in six (38%) (see Figure 1a). Although the appearance of the distal oesophagus could be mistaken for that of achalasia on individual images, the LOS intermittently opened to varying degrees in the upright position at fluoroscopy in all patients.

In contrast, all 16 patients had a normal-appearing distal oesophagus with normal opening of the LOS and normal transit of barium into the stomach when swallowing low-density barium in the prone, RAO position (Figure 1b). In all 16 cases, there was evidence of primary peristalsis in the body of the oesophagus at fluoroscopy, with normal peristalsis in 10 cases (63%), occasional non-peristaltic contractions in three (19%), and intermittently weakened peristalsis with non-peristaltic contractions in three (19%).

A total of about 4000 biphasic oesophagrams and upper gastrointestinal tract examinations were performed on

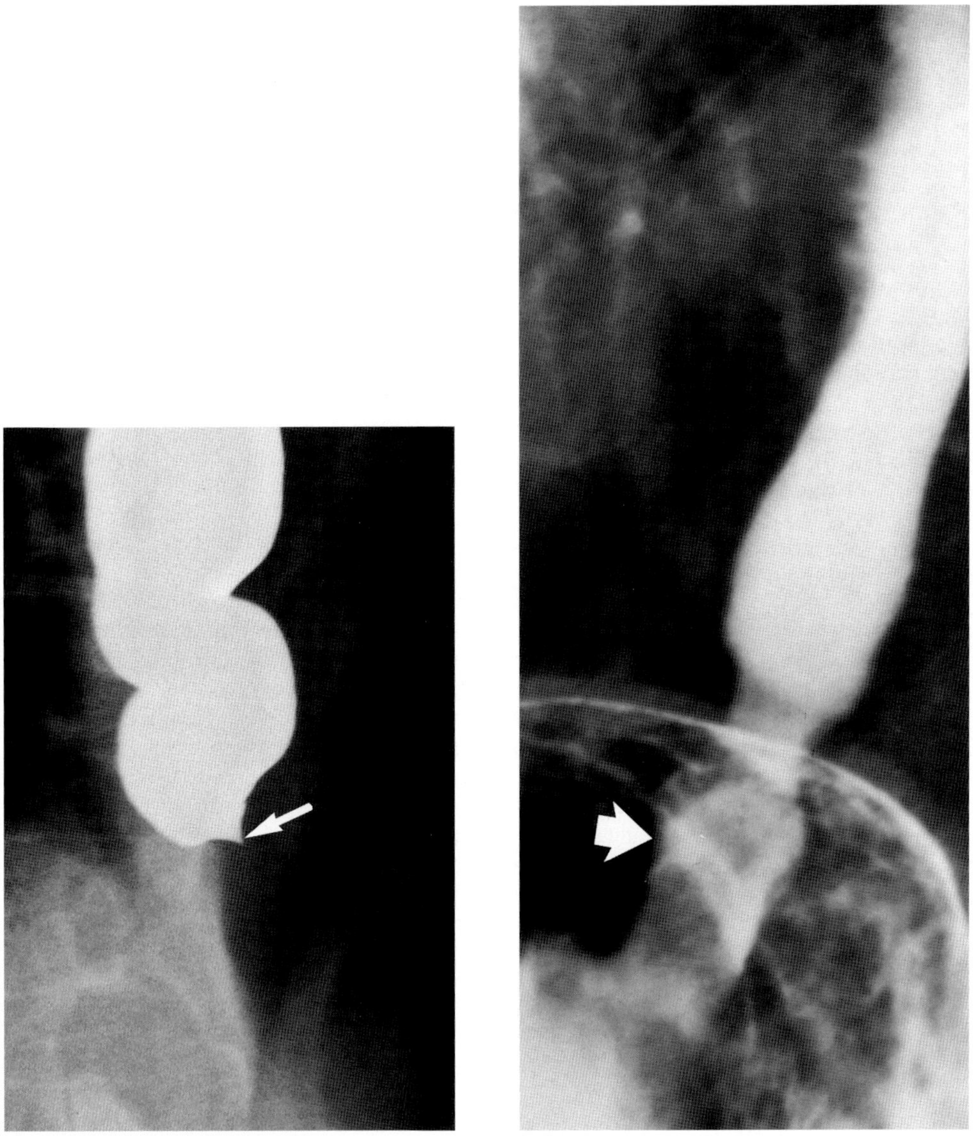

(a) (b)

Figure 1. 82-year-old man with transient failure of opening of lower oesophageal sphincter (LOS) on upright oesophagram. This patient had no history of dysphagia. (a) Initial double-contrast view of oesophagus in upright, left posterior oblique position shows tapered, beaklike narrowing (arrow) of distal oesophagus secondary to failure of opening of LOS. Note proximal dilatation of oesophagus and absence of barium in stomach. (b) Subsequent single-contrast view of oesophagus in prone, right anterior oblique position shows normal-appearing distal oesophagus with normal opening of LOS. This patient also has a small hiatal hernia (arrow).

patients who were not known to have had surgery or other procedures on the gastroesophageal junction during the 5.5-year time period of our study. In 19 of these 4000 radiographic examinations (including the three cases in which medical records were not available), transient failure of opening of the LOS was reported in the upright, LPO position on barium studies (excluding the 10 cases in which spot images failed to confirm this finding), a prevalence of 0.5%.

Clinical findings

Nine patients (56%) were women and seven (44%) were men. The average age of the 16 patients was 57.5 years (range 27–82 years). Two of the patients had a history of diabetes, one had polymyositis, one had myasthenia gravis, and one tested positive for HIV. Six patients had received calcium channel blockers, one had received nitrates, and one had received botulinum toxin injections at the LOS in the past. 14 patients (88%) had symptoms at the time of the barium study, including dysphagia in seven (44%), chest pain in six (38%), heartburn in six (38%), weight loss in five (31%), regurgitation in three (19%), cough in two (13%), vomiting in two (13%), and belching in two (13%). Four of the seven patients with dysphagia had dysphagia for solids only, two had dysphagia for solids and liquids, and one had unspecified dysphagia. The mean duration of dysphagia was 26.1 months (range 0.5–60 months).

Five (71%) of the seven patients with dysphagia had follow-up clinical data (mean duration of follow-up 19.8 months; range 7–36 months). Four (80%) of these five patients had improvement or resolution of their dysphagia without specific treatment for LOS dysfunction (*i.e.* oesophageal balloon dilatation, botulinum toxin injection, or surgical myotomy). The remaining patient had persistent dysphagia, but this individual had underlying polymyositis as the likely cause for his dysphagia.

Manometric findings

Manometry revealed LOS dysfunction in two of three patients, manifested by incomplete LOS relaxation with high LOS residual pressures (12 mm Hg and 13 mm Hg, respectively) in both patients and by a hypertensive sphincter with a high LOS resting pressure (102 mm Hg) in one. The remaining patient had normal LOS function. All three patients had normal oesophageal peristalsis.

Discussion

Primary achalasia is an uncommon oesophageal motility disorder characterized by dysphagia or, less frequently, chest pain. Most patients with this condition do not seek medical attention until they have long-standing dysphagia; the mean duration of symptoms at the time of diagnosis is approximately 5 years [8]. Achalasia is characterized on manometry by absent primary peristalsis in the body of the oesophagus and incomplete relaxation of the LOS, as defined by high LOS residual pressures [1, 2]. Similarly, barium studies may reveal absent primary peristalsis with tapered, beaklike narrowing of the distal oesophagus at or near the gastroesophageal junction as a result of incomplete opening of the LOS [9, 10].

Other patients may have isolated LOS dysfunction with a hypertensive LOS at rest or incomplete relaxation of the LOS during swallowing but no abnormalities of peristalsis in the body of the oesophagus. In a study by Vantrappen et al [3], three (2%) of 156 patients presenting for endoscopic dilatation of the LOS for impaired LOS relaxation had intact primary peristalsis on manometry. In another study by Aliperti and Clouse [5], 17 (28%) of 60 patients with incomplete LOS relaxation had normal peristalsis on manometry, and none of these cases progressed to the classic form of achalasia. In still another study by Freidin et al [4], four (25%) of 16 patients with a hypertensive LOS and normal peristalsis on manometry underwent endoscopic dilatation of the LOS for dysphagia, and all had symptomatic relief of their dysphagia. Thus, isolated LOS dysfunction has been implicated in the gastroenterology literature as a treatable cause of dysphagia with characteristic manometric features.

In contrast, we report 16 patients who had incomplete opening of the LOS manifested by tapered, beaklike narrowing of the distal oesophagus as a transient finding on upright double-contrast views of the oesophagus using a high-density barium, with a normal-appearing distal oesophagus, normal opening of the LOS, and intact primary peristalsis in the body of the oesophagus on prone single-contrast views using a low-density barium (Figure 1). The prevalence of this phenomenon on biphasic oesophagrams or upper gastrointestinal tract examinations at our hospital was 0.5%. However, this figure probably underestimates the true frequency of transient failure of opening of the LOS in the upright position on barium studies, as the three attending gastrointestinal radiologists did not always mention this finding in the radiographic reports because of uncertainty about its clinical implications.

Manometry was performed on three patients with transient LOS dysfunction in the upright position on barium studies, and impaired relaxation of the LOS was documented in two. It should be recognized that manometry routinely is performed with the patient in the sitting position at our institution. Two of our patients therefore had evidence of LOS dysfunction in the upright position both on barium studies and manometry. In the remaining patient, manometry revealed normal relaxation of the LOS despite transient LOS dysfunction in the upright position on the barium study. However, it would be unreasonable to expect perfect correlation between barium studies and manometry for evaluation of LOS function. In fact, previous studies of achalasia have shown that as many as 20–30% of patients with findings of achalasia and incomplete opening of the LOS on barium studies have normal LOS function on manometry [11, 12].

Only seven (44%) of the 16 patients with transient LOS dysfunction on barium studies were found to have dysphagia. Furthermore, the dysphagia improved or resolved without specific treatment for LOS dysfunction (*i.e.* oesophageal balloon dilatation, botulinum toxin injection, or surgical myotomy) in all but one case with clinical follow-up. If the dysphagia had been caused by the underlying LOS dysfunction, however, it would be unlikely for this symptom to improve or resolve without some form of intervention on the sphincter. Our findings therefore suggest that LOS dysfunction may be observed on upright double-contrast views of the oesophagus as a transient phenomenon of little clinical importance.

It is important for radiologists to be aware of this phenomenon on upright double-contrast oesophagrams, so that it is not mistaken for achalasia or other morphological abnormalities of the distal oesophagus. Although oesophageal motility normally is evaluated with the patient in the prone, RAO position, the fluoroscopist may fail to obtain prone views in patients with severe spasm of the LOS on upright views because of the dramatic nature of the findings or because this spasm is associated with delayed emptying of barium and proximal dilatation (as occurred in 44% and 38% of our patients, respectively), raising concern about the patient's ability to ingest barium in the prone position. In all of our cases, however, prone single-contrast views of the oesophagus using a low-density barium revealed a normal-appearing distal oesophagus with normal opening of the LOS and intact primary peristalsis in the body of the oesophagus. It therefore is important to obtain prone single-contrast views with a low-density barium when incomplete opening of the LOS is observed on upright double-contrast views with a high-density barium in order to differentiate this finding from true achalasia or isolated LOS dysfunction that persists on the prone examination.

The cause of this transient LOS dysfunction in the upright position on barium studies is uncertain. One possible explanation could be related to the temporal relationship between the pharyngeal and oesophageal phases of deglutition. Normally, a pharyngeal contractile wave precedes the onset of LOS relaxation by up to 3.2 s in order to give the swallowed bolus adequate time to reach the LOS, thereby facilitating passage of the bolus into the stomach [13]. Because of the effect of gravity, however, it is possible that swallowed barium in the upright position traverses the oesophagus ahead of the peristaltic wave, reaching the distal oesophagus before the LOS relaxes. This could result in transient failure of opening of the LOS (manifested by beaklike narrowing of the distal oesophagus) with proximal oesophageal dilatation and delayed emptying of barium into the stomach. On prone views from the same examination, however, barium might be expected to pass more slowly through the oesophagus, allowing the LOS to open as the normal contractile wave reaches the gastroesophageal junction, so the distal oesophagus appears normal on these views.

Another possible explanation could be related to the response of the LOS to increased gastric pressures. Under normal conditions, even a small increase in intragastric pressure causes LOS resting pressure to increase [14]. It is possible that administration of an effervescent agent (which is given routinely to distend the stomach before upright double-contrast views of the oesophagus are obtained) sometimes causes a brief increase in intragastric pressure with a concomitant increase in LOS resting pressure, manifested by the transient, beaklike narrowing that was observed in our patients.

It is important to recognize the inherent limitations of our retrospective study, including selection bias and possible inaccurate reporting of symptoms in medical records. We also had to rely on the original radiographic reports for characterization of the motility findings, as the videotapes from these examinations were not stored on a long-term basis. Only three (19%) of the 16 patients in our study underwent manometry, presumably because we often suggested in the radiographic reports that incomplete opening of the LOS only in the upright position was of doubtful clinical importance. Nevertheless, two of the three patients who did undergo manometry also had manometric evidence of LOS dysfunction in the upright position. Finally, no patients had follow-up barium studies, so we were unable to ascertain whether this finding persisted on serial examinations. Because of these limitations, a prospective study of a large series of patients with transient LOS dysfunction on barium studies and manometric correlation is needed to further elucidate the clinical, radiographic, and manometric features of this phenomenon.

In conclusion, our experience suggests that failure of opening of the LOS may be observed as a transient finding on upright double-contrast views of the oesophagus using high-density barium, with normal opening of the LOS on prone single-contrast views using low-density barium. Although some patients had dysphagia, their dysphagia improved or resolved without specific treatment for LOS dysfunction in all but one patient with clinical follow-up. Our experience suggests that transient LOS dysfunction on upright double-contrast views of the oesophagus is of little clinical importance in the absence of LOS dysfunction or oesophageal dysmotility on prone single-contrast views. It is important to be aware of this finding, so that it is not mistaken for achalasia or other abnormalities of the distal oesophagus.

References

1. Richter JE. Oesophageal motility disorders. Lancet 2001;358:823–8.
2. Adler DG, Romero Y. Primary esophageal motility disorders. Mayo Clin Proc 2001;76:195–200.
3. Vantrappen G, Janssens J, Hellemans J, Coremans G. Achalasia, diffuse esophageal spasm, and related motility disorders. Gastroenterology 1979;76:450–7.
4. Freidin N, Traube M, Mittal RK, McCallum RW. The hypertensive lower esophageal sphincter: manometric and clinical aspects. Dig Dis Sci 1989;34:1063–7.
5. Aliperti G, Clouse RE. Incomplete lower esophageal sphincter relaxation in subjects with peristalsis: prevalence and clinical outcome. Am J Gastroenterol 1991;86:609–14.
6. Miller RE, Chernish SM, Greenman GF, Maglinte DD, Rosenak BD, Brunelle RL. Gastrointestinal response to minute doses of glucagon. Radiology 1982;143:317–20.
7. Hogan WJ, Dodds WJ, Hoke SE, Reid DP, Kalkhoff RK, Arndorfer RC. Effect of glucagon on esophageal motor function. Gastroenterology 1975;69:160–5.
8. Eckardt VF, Kohne U, Junginger T, Westermeier T. Risk factors for diagnostic delay in achalasia. Dig Dis Sci 1997;42:580–5.
9. Laufer I. Motor disorders of the esophagus. In: Levine MS, editor. Radiology of the esophagus. Philadelphia, PA: WB Saunders, 1990:229–46.
10. Ott DJ. Motility disorders of the esophagus. In: Gore RM, Levine MS, editors. Textbook of gastrointestinal radiology (2nd edn). Philadelphia, PA: WB Saunders, 2000:316–8.
11. Katz PO, Richter JE, Cowan R, Castell DO. Apparent complete lower esophageal sphincter relaxation in achalasia. Gastroenterology 1986;90:978–83.
12. Ott DJ, Richter JE, Chen YM, Wu WC, Gelfand DW, Castell DO. Radiographic and manometric correlation in achalasia with apparent relaxation of the lower esophageal sphincter. Gastrointest Radiol 1989;14:1–5.
13. Holloway RH, Penagini R, Ireland AC. Criteria for objective definition of transient lower esophageal sphincter relaxation. Am J Physiol 1995;268:G128–33.
14. Castell DO. The lower esophageal sphincter: physiologic and clinical aspects. Ann Intern Med 1975;83:390–401.

The British Journal of Radiology, 78 (2005), 416–418 © 2005 The British Institute of Radiology
DOI: 10.1259/bjr/54704044

Role of ultrasound in dengue fever

P M VENKATA SAI, MBBS, DMRD, DNB, FICR, B DEV, MBBS, MD, DNB and R KRISHNAN, R S MBSS, MD

Department of Radiology and Imaging Sciences, Sri Ramachandra Medical College & Research Institute (DU), Porur, Chennai – 600 116, Tamil Nadu, India

Abstract. This study was performed to find out whether ultrasound is an important adjunct to clinical and laboratory profile in diagnosing dengue fever or dengue haemorrhagic fever and to further determine whether ultrasound is useful in predicting the severity of the disease. Ultrasound was performed on 128 patients (2–9 years) with clinical suspicion of dengue fever. Serological tests were performed to confirm the diagnosis. 40 patients were serologically negative for dengue fever and later excluded from the study. Of the remaining 88 serologically positive cases, 32 patients underwent ultrasound on second to third day, repeated on fifth to seventh day of fever and in 56 patients ultrasound was done only on fifth to seventh day of fever. Of the 32 patients who underwent the study on second to third day of fever, all showed gall bladder wall thickening and pericholecystic fluid, 21% had hepatomegaly, 6.25% had splenomegaly and right minimal pleural effusion. Follow-up ultrasound on fifth to seventh day revealed ascites in 53% left pleural effusion in 22% and pericardial effusion in 28%. Of the 56 patients who underwent the study on fifth to seventh day of fever for the first time all had gall bladder wall thickening, 21% had hepatomegaly, 7% had splenomegaly, 96% had ascites, 87.5% had right pleural effusion, 66% had left pleural effusion and 28.5% had pericardial fluid. To conclude, in an epidemic of dengue, ultrasound features of thickened gall bladder wall, pleural effusion and ascites should strongly favour the diagnosis of dengue fever.

Dengue is a mosquito-borne infection that in recent years has become a major international public health problem [1]. Dengue fever (DF) has been known for more than a century in the tropical areas of South East Asia and the Western Pacific regions [2]. Clinically dengue manifests with acute onset of fever, severe headache, retro-ocular pain and pain involving the muscles and joints. Haemorrhagic diasthesis and thrombocytopenia with concurrent haemoconcentration is a constant finding.

In early July 2002, there was an outbreak of dengue in Chennai, a coastal city in Southern India. Since there is no single test that can be used to diagnose the condition with a reasonable degree of accuracy and reliability, the diagnosis is based on clinical appearance in combination with serology. Serology takes approximately 7 to 10 days to give a positive result. The purpose of our study was to analyse retrospectively the ultrasound features in patients with DF, to find out whether ultrasound is an adjunct to clinical and lab profile in the diagnosis of DF and to further determine whether ultrasound is useful in predicting the severity of the disease

Materials and methods

Our institutional review board approved this retrospective study; informed consent was not required. Between June and July 2002, 128 subjects (80 male, 48 female; mean age, 5 years; age range 2–9 years) who were clinically suspected of having DF were referred for ultrasound scanning of both abdomen and thorax. Common clinical manifestations included fever (n=128), severe headache (n=104), retro-ocular pain (n=84), pain in the muscles and joints (n=80), and purpuric spots on the body (n=22). Blood laboratory investigation in 88 patients revealed thrombocytopenia (average platelet count 40 000 cells mm^{-3}) with concurrent haemoconcentration. Based on the clinical and laboratory findings 65 patients were diagnosed as classical dengue fever (CDF), 19 patients had dengue haemorrhagic fever (DHF) and 4 patients were diagnosed as dengue shock syndrome (DSS).

All ultrasound examinations were performed with a portable machine (L&T symphony model) using 3.5 MHz and 5 MHz probes. Abdominal scanning was done after 6 h of fasting to allow better distension of gall bladder (GB) [3]. GB wall thickening, which was the consistent finding in all the serologically positive cases, was measured by placing the calipers between the two layers of anterior wall [4]. Thoracic scanning was done in either sitting or supine posture. Both the pleural spaces were evaluated through an intercostal approach. Pericardial space was also evaluated for effusion subcostally. In all the patients ultrasound was performed prior to serology.

Serological tests using paired sera was performed to confirm the diagnosis in all the 128 patients which revealed 88 patients to be serologically positive for DF [5, 6]. The remaining 40 patients were serologically negative. The 88 serologically positive patients were then sorted into two groups based on the days of study. Group I (n=32) included patients who had symptoms and signs consistent with DF and in whom ultrasound was performed on the second to third day after onset of fever. These patients also had a follow up scan on fifth to seventh day. Group II (n=56) included patients who underwent ultrasound only on fifth to seventh day after onset of fever. For the 40 serologically negative patients ultrasound was performed on an average of 3.9 days (range, same day to 7 days) after admission.

Received 24 May 2004 and in final form 4 November 2004, accepted 6 December 2004.

Results (Tables 1–4)

Ultrasound findings in Group I

Of the 32 patients who underwent the study on second to third day of fever, 7 had hepatomegaly (21.8%), 32 had GB wall thickening and pericholecystic fluid (100%), 2 had splenomegaly (6.25%) and 2 had right-sided pleural effusion (6.25%). None had ascites, left sided pleural effusion or pericardial effusion. On follow-up scan (days 5–7), hepatomegaly was noted in four more patients (12.5%), splenomegaly in three more patients (9.37%) and right sided pleural effusion in 21 more patients (65.6%). GB pathology persisted in all the patients. New findings including ascites were noted in 17 patients (53.12%), left sided pleural effusion in 7 patients (21.8%) and pericardial effusion in 9 patients (28.12%).

Table 1. Profile of 88 serologically positive cases

Day of examination	Number of cases
2nd–3rd day	32
5th–7th day	56+32 (follow up cases)

Table 2. Summary of ultrasound findings in Group I

Days of examination	No. of patients (n=32)	
	2nd–3rd day	5th–7th day
Gall bladder wall thickening with pericholecystic fluid	32 (100)	32 (100)
Hepatomegaly	7 (21.8)	4 (12.5)
Splenomegaly	2 (6.25)	3 (9.37)
Right pleural effusion	2 (6.25)	21 (65.6)
Left pleural effusion	0 (0)	7 (21.8)
Ascites	0 (0)	17 (53.12)
Pericardial effusion	0 (0)	9 (28.12)

Number in parentheses are percentages.

Table 3. Summary of ultrasound findings in Group II

Features	No. of patients (n=56)
	5th–7th day
Gall bladder Wall thickening with pericholecystic fluid	56 (100)
Hepatomegaly	34 (60.9)
Splenomegaly	17 (30.35)
Right pleural effusion	55 (96.46)
Left pleural effusion	37 (66.07)
Ascites	4 (7.14)
Pericardial effusion	16 (28.57)

Number in parentheses are percentages.

Table 4. Summary of ultrasound findings in Group I and Group II

Features	No. of patients (n=88)
	5th–7th day
Gall bladder Wall thickening with pericholecystic fluid	100%
Hepatomegaly	34.3%
Splenomegaly	15.6%
Right pleural effusion	71.87%
Left pleural effusion	21.87%
Ascites	53.2%
Pericardial effusion	28.5%

Ultrasound findings in Group II

Of the 56 patients who underwent the study on fifth to seventh day of fever, GB pathology was noted in all the 56 patients (100%), 34 patients had hepatomegaly (60.9%), 17 had splenomegaly (30.35%), 4 had ascites (7.14%), 55 had right sided pleural effusion (96.46%), 37 had left sided pleural effusion (66.07%) and 16 had pericardial effusion (28.57%).

40 serologically negative patients

Of the 40 patients who were serologically negative for DF, GB pathology was present in 14 patients initially but disappeared later on follow-up scan. A clinical review of 17 other patients revealed that their symptoms were not classical of DF. Nine patients could not be followed up as they discharged themselves against medical advice.

Our study demonstrated thickened GB wall and pericholecystic fluid (Figure 1) as the most common initial ultrasound finding in all the 88 serologically positive cases (100%) followed by right sided pleural effusion (71.87%), ascites (53.2%), left sided pleural effusion (21.87%) and pericardial effusion (28.5%). Hepatomegaly and splenomegaly were noted in 34.3% and 15.6% of patients, respectively.

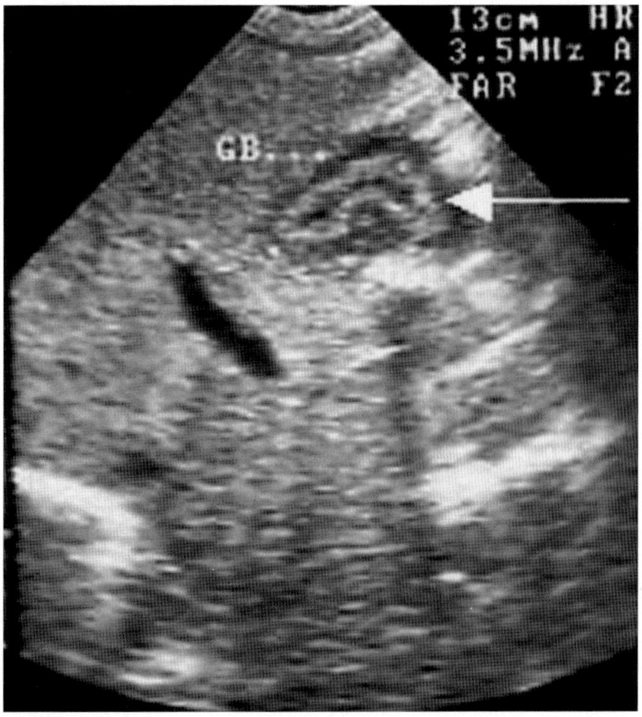

Figure 1. Ultrasound subcostal view to show gall bladder wall thickening and pericholecystic fluid.

Discussion

Dengue is an acute febrile viral disease caused by flavivirus. It occurs in two forms: DF, a milder form of the disease and DHF, the most severe form. Dengue has become a major international public health concern in recent years [2]. It is now endemic in more than 100 countries and threatens the health of 40% of the world's population. It is estimated that 50 million dengue infections occur each year with 5 000 000 cases of DHF and at least 12 000 deaths annually mainly among children [1]. The increase of DF is due to uncontrolled population growth and urbanization in the absence of appropriate water management, global spread of dengue strains via travel and trade and due to erosion of vector control programmes [7]. In India the problem is even more acute because since 1963, more than 50 outbreaks have been reported by the National Institute of Communicable diseases, New Delhi [8].

Dengue viruses are transmitted to humans through the bites of infective female Aedes mosquito. The incubation period of the disease is 3–14 days. The onset of the disease is recognized by the sudden onset of high fever, retro-orbital pain, thrombocytopenia and haemorrhagic manifestations. Common laboratory findings include pancytopenia, neutropenia, increased haemoconcentration, thrombocytopenia and prolonged bleeding time. These findings are consistent with increased vascular permeability, plasma leakage, abnormalities of haemostasis and protein losing shock syndrome, which commonly occur in DF pathogenesis.

Serology is the mainstay in the diagnosis of DF. Haemagglutination inhibition antibodies usually appear at detectable level by day 5 to 6 of febrile illness. The diagnosis of DF is often delayed owing to time taken for availability of results. The aim of our study was to evaluate the ultrasound findings in DF, to find whether ultrasound of the abdomen is an important adjunct to clinical and laboratory profile in diagnosing DF and further if ultrasound is useful in predicting the severity of the disease.

The ultrasound findings in early milder form of DF include GB wall thickening, pericholecystic fluid, minimal ascites, pleural effusion, pericardial effusion and hepatosplenomegaly. Severe forms of the disease are characterized by fluid collection in the perirenal and pararenal region, hepatic and splenic subcapsular fluid, pericardial effusion, pancreatic enlargement and hepatosplenomegaly. These findings have been demonstrated in studies carried out by the Department of Child Health in Indonesia [9] and by Joshi et al [10] in Army Hospital, Delhi Cantt. They had also found abnormal liver parenchyma, which has been attributed to intraparenchymal and subcapsular haemorrhages. In our study however we could not appreciate any significant change in the echotexture of the liver. None of these studies suggested GB wall thickening as the initial finding in DF (100%) as observed in our study, followed and pleural effusion. GB wall thickening in DF may be due to decrease in intravascular osmotic pressure. These findings may also occur in other viral infections, enteric fever and leptospirosis, but in other viral infections the historical profile, symptom complex evolution and physical findings do not mimic those of DF. Ultrasound features of enteric fever include splenomegaly, intra-abdominal lymphadenopathy, bowel abnormalities in the form of intramural thickening of the terminal ileum and caecum, renal abnormalities like arteriectasis and perinephric fluid collection in addition to GB wall thickening and polyserositis. Leptospirosis also shows gross abnormalities involving hepatic and renal parenchyma. GB wall thickening also occurs in association with other conditions such as ascites, hypoalbuminaemia, congestive cholecystopathy and in patients with cirrhosis of liver and portal hypertension. It is a very non-specific finding when considered in isolation and is therefore a major limitation of this study.

To conclude ultrasound of the abdomen is an important adjunct to clinical profile in diagnosing DF and may help to direct further confirmatory investigations. Further diagnosis can be made early in the course of disease compared with other modes of diagnosis. During an epidemic the ultrasound findings of GB wall thickening with or without polyserositis in a febrile patient should suggest the possibility of DF/DHF.

Acknowledgments

We thank Dr Uday Charan Murmu, Assistant Professor of Paediatric Medicine, Mr S Porchelvan, Department of Biostatistics and Mr S Santhosh, Department of Radiology & Imaging Sciences Sri Ramachandra Medical College & Research Institute (Deemed University), Chennai for his invaluable help in evaluation for the study.

References

1. Weekly epidemiological record. No. 36, 6th September 2002:300–2.
2. Weekly epidemiological record. No. 6, 8th February 2002: 41–3.
3. Nelson ER. Haemorrhagic fever in children: report of 69 cases. J Paediat 1960;56:101–8.
4. Shlaer WJ, Leopold JR, Scheible FW. Sonography of thickened gallbladder wall: a non-specific finding. AJR Am J Roentgenol 1981;136:337–9.
5. Bhamarapravati N. Pathology of dengue haemorrhagic fever. In: Thongcharoen P. Monograph on dengue/dengue haemorrhagic fever. WHO 1993:72–3.
6. Monograph on Dengue/Dengue Haemorrhagic fever, Compiled by Prasert Thongchroen, Regional Publication, WHO (1983); SEARO No. 22.
7. Weekly epidemiological record No 24, 16th June 2000: 193–6.
8. Health Situation in the South East Asia Region 1994–1997, Regional office for SEAR, New Delhi; WHO (1999).
9. Pramuljo HS, Harun SR. Ultrasound findings in Dengue haemorrhage fever. Pediatr Radiol J 1991;21:100–2.
10. Joshi P, Rathnam VG, Sharma S. USG findings in dengue haemorrhagic fever – our experience in the recent epidemic. Ind J Radiol Imag 1997;7:189–92.

The British Journal of Radiology, 78 (2005), 419–421
DOI: 10.1259/bjr/94407232

Colonic muco-submucosal elongated polyp: diagnosis with endoscopic ultrasound

[1]K AKAHOSHI, MD, PhD, [1]M MATSUMOTO, MD, [1]M KIMURA, MD, [1]A MURATA, MD, ^{1}H MURAO, MD, [1]Y SUMIDA, MD, [1]M KUBOKAWA, MD, [1]K ITO, MD, PhD and [2]M OYA, MD, PhD

Departments of [1]Gastroenterology and [2]Pathology, Aso Iizuka Hospital, 3-83 Yoshio, Iizuka 820-8505, Japan

Abstract. Colonic muco-submucosal elongated polyp is a new clinical entity first reported in 1998. The purpose of this report is to determine the value of endoscopic ultrasound in the diagnosis of this condition. We reviewed the endosonographic and histological findings of seven colonic muco-submucosal elongated polyps that were removed completely by endoscopic resection or surgery. The lesions appeared as pedunculated submucosal tumours, measuring 1–4 cm in maximal diameter. Endosonographically, all lesions consisted of mucosal and submucosal layers, and microcystic components were found in the submucosal layer. There were no echogenic masses or muscularis propria within the polyps. These endosonographic features corresponded to histological findings of this type of polyp which was covered with normal mucosa and composed of submucosal layer alone. The submucosal layer consisted of oedematous, loose, connective tissue and/or fibrous tissue, accompanied by dilated blood vessels and lymphatics. Endoscopic ultrasound enabled differentiation of colonic muco-submucosal elongated polyp from other submucosal lesions.

Colonic muco-submucosal elongated polyp (CMSEP) is a new clinical entity first described by Matake et al in 1998 [1]. Endoscopically, CMSEPs appear as an elongated, drumstick-shaped polyp. Histologically, the polyp is covered with normal mucosa and consists of oedematous, loose, fibrous connective tissue with a dense, fibrous submucosal layer, often showing dilation of blood vessels and lymphatics. The incidence of CMSEP was 0.39% in one endoscopic polypectomy series. Because of its rarity, the endoscopic ultrasound (EUS) features of CMSEP have been reported in only one case [2]. This report describes the characteristic EUS features of seven CMSEPs.

Patients and methods

Between June 1999 and April 2004, seven CMSEPs (in five men; age range 35–89 years) were evaluated by EUS at our institute prior to endoscopic or surgical removal. All patients were suspected of having a CMSEP at initial colonoscopy, and endoscopic biopsy revealed only non-specific findings. EUS was performed subsequently using an ultrasound catheter probe (SP-701; 12–20 MHz; Fujinon, Oomiya, Japan) with a filling technique using de-aerated water. As EUS showed all lesions to be limited to the mucosa and submucosa, with the patients' informed consent we successfully performed endoscopic resection in six of seven patients without complications. The lesion in the fifth patient was surgically resected owing to nearby advanced colonic cancer. The specimens were subjected to histological examination.

We retrospectively compared the histological features with EUS findings.

Received 19 July 2004 and in revised form 18 October 2004, accepted 6 December 2004.

Results

Patient characteristics are summarized in Table 1. The affected site was the rectum in three lesions, the sigmoid colon in two lesions, and the ascending colon in two lesions. The lesions appeared as pedunculated, submucosal tumours on endoscopy (Figure 1). All the polyps had the same endosonographic and histological features. On EUS, the first to third layers were intact in all lesions, reflecting preservation of the mucosal and submucosal layers. There

Table 1. Summary of patients characteristics

Patient no./gender/age (years)	Polyp			Symptoms	Treatment
	Location	Size (cm)	Shape		
1/m/49	Sigmoid colon	2	Pedunculated	Soft stool	Endoscopic resection
2/m/59	Ascending colon	1	Pedunculated	Occult blood in faeces	Endoscopic resection
3/m/35	Sigmoid colon	1.5	Pedunculated	Abdominal pain, diarrhoea	Endoscopic resection
4/m/88	Rectum	1	Pedunculated	Abdominal pain	Endoscopic resection
5/f/78	Rectum	1	Pedunculated	Abdominal distension[a]	Surgical resection
6/f/70	Rectum	1	Pedunculated	Bloody stool	Endoscopic resection
7/m/66	Ascending colon	4	Pedunculated	Abdominal pain	Endoscopic resection

[a]Advanced colonic cancer coexisted in this case. (Simultaneous pathologies could not be detected in the other patients.)

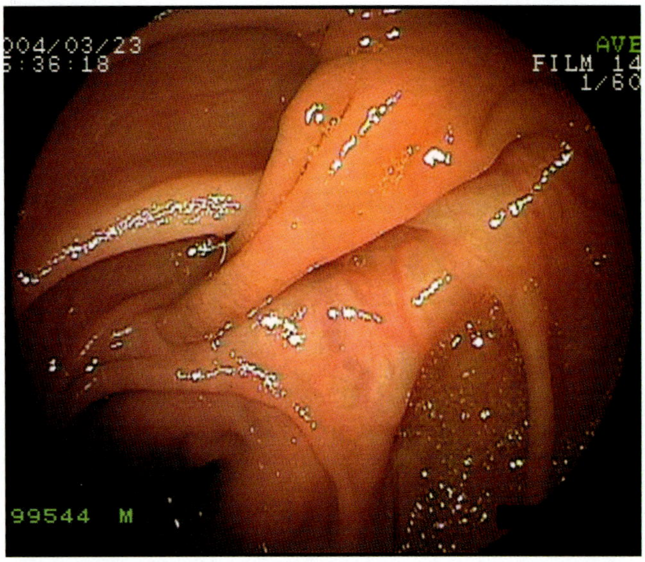

Figure 1. Patient 7. Colonoscopy of the ascending colon shows a pedunculated polypoid lesion. The surface is smooth and covered with normal colonic mucosa.

was no muscularis propria layer or echogenic mass within the polyp (Figure 2). In the third layer, microcystic components were found (Figure 3). Histologically, atypia and hyperplasia of the mucosa and lamina propria were not observed, and there was no evidence of specific inflammation (Figure 4). The submucosal layers were composed mainly of oedematous stroma with mild, chronic inflammatory infiltration. Dilated blood vessels and lymphatics were observed in all lesions (Figure 5).

Discussion

Morson and Dawson [3] divided colonic polyps into four classes: neoplastic, hamartomatous, inflammatory, and unclassified. Matake et al [1] first characterized CMSEP in 15 patients in 1998. Signs and symptoms include occult blood-positive faeces, bloody stool,

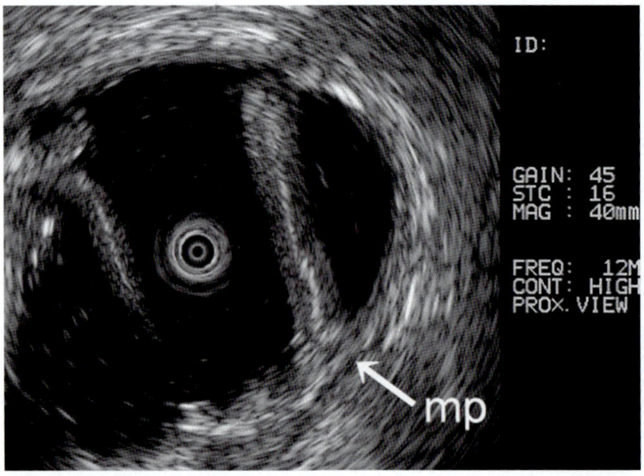

Figure 2. Patient 7. Endoscopic ultrasound shows an elongated polypoid lesion consisting of intact first to third layers, revealing mucosal and submucosal colonic layers. There is no echogenic mass or muscularis propria (arrow-mp) layer in the polyp.

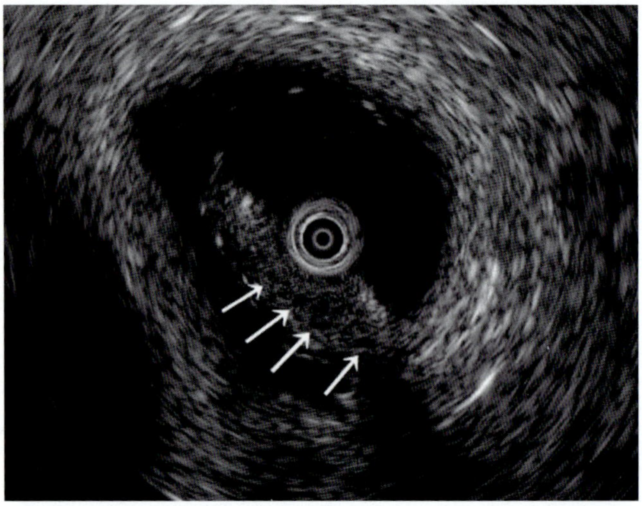

Figure 3. Patient 7. Endoscopic ultrasound of the head portion of the polyp demonstrates multiple microcystic components (arrows) in the submucosal layer.

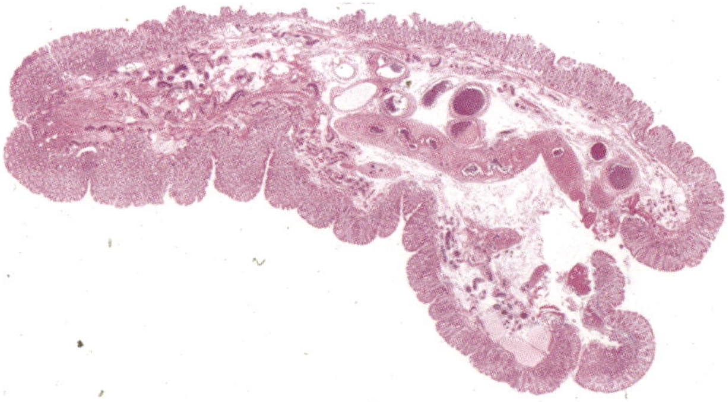

Figure 4. Patient 7. Histology showing the cross-section of a polyp consisting of mild, chronically inflamed mucosa and submucosa, with oedematous, loose, fibrous connective tissue.

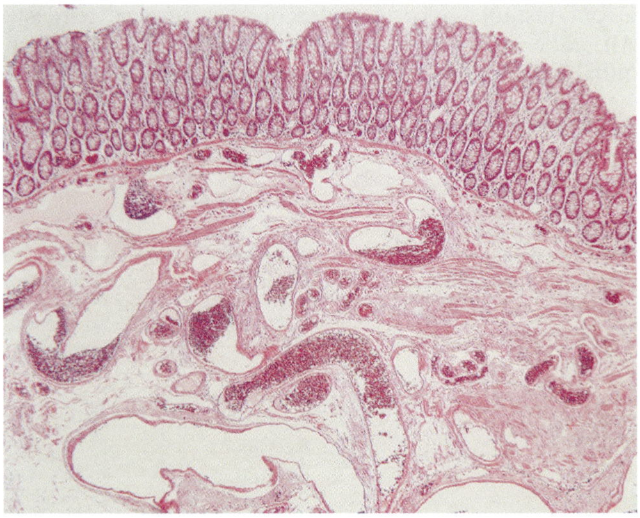

Figure 5. Patient 7. Microscopic findings of a polyp showing the submucosal oedema, with dilated vessels and lymphatics.

constipation, back pain, and abdominal pain [1, 2]. At present, the pathogenesis and treatment-of-choice of this type of polyp is undetermined [1]. Better characterization of CMSEP in future studies should help resolve these issues.

EUS is a highly accurate way of determining the characteristics of a submucosal tumour by identifying the layer of origin and echotexture [4, 5]. Catheter US probes that can be inserted through the accessory channel of standard endoscopes facilitate EUS, and the diagnosis of submucosal lesions using these devices appears to be highly accurate [5]. Although EUS has been widely used in the diagnosis of submucosal lesions, because of its rarity there has been only one case report describing the EUS findings of CMSEP in one patient [2]. In this study, we performed EUS in seven patients with endoscopic resection or surgically proven CMSEP. In this investigation, characteristic EUS features of this disease were polyps consisting of mucosal and submucosal layers. There were no echogenic masses or muscularis propria within the polyps. All lesions had multiple microcystic components in the third layer, which probably reflected submucosal dilated vessels and lymphatics. These EUS findings corresponded well to the pathological characteristic of CMSEP, as described by Matake et al [1]. Therefore, EUS can differentiate CMSEP from other submucosal lesions such as leiomyoma [5, 6], lipoma [7] and lymphangioma [8]. Pre-therapeutic endoscopic biopsy is not useful in the diagnosis of CMSEP. EUS appears to permit the definitive diagnosis of CMSEP prior to excision.

Although our study is preliminary and further investigations are necessary, we believe that the EUS features described herein are important in diagnosis of CMSEP, a benign entity, so inappropriate treatment can be avoided.

References

1. Matake H, Matsui T, Yao T, Iwashita A, Hoashi T, Yao K, et al. Long pedunculated colonic polyp composed of mucosa and submucosa. Proposal of a new entity, colonic muco-submucosal elongated polyp. Dis Colon Rectum 1998;41: 1557–61.
2. Takahashi M, Kubokawa M, Tanaka M, Sadamoto Y, Ito K, Yoshimura R, et al. Endoscopic ultrasonography features of colonic muco-submucosal elongated polyp. Endoscopy 2002; 34:515.
3. Morson BC, Dawson IM. Differential diagnosis of polyps and polyposis. In: Gastrointestinal pathology (2nd edn). London: Blackwell Scientific Publications, Ltd, 1979:607–14.
4. Byrne MF, Jowell PS. Gastrointestinal imaging: endoscopic ultrasound. Gastroenterology 2002;122:1631–48.
5. Akahoshi K, Harada N, Nawata H. The current state of endoscopic ultrasonography. In: Pandalai SG, editor. Recent research developments in radiology. Kerala: Transworld Research Network, 2003:1–22.
6. Hizawa K, Esaki M, Iwai K, Yao T, Sato H, Matsumoto T, et al. EUS in the diagnosis of diffuse esophageal leiomyomatosis. Gastrointest Endosc 2002;56:764–7.
7. Kim CY, Bandres D, Tio TL, Benjamin SB, Al-Kawas FH. Endoscopic removal of large colonic lipomas. Gastrointest Endosc 2002;55:929–31.
8. Iwakiri Y, Akahoshi K, Hamada S, Chijiiwa Y, Nawata H, Sasaki I. Endoscopic removal of a lymphangioma of the colon: case report of the diagnostic value of an endoscopic ultrasound probe. Endoscopy 1997;29:s32–3.

The British Journal of Radiology, *78* (2005), 422–427
DOI: 10.1259/bjr/32912696

Investigation of optimum energies for chest imaging using film–screen and computed radiography

I D HONEY, MSc, A MACKENZIE, MSc and D S EVANS, MSc

Kings Centre for the Assessment of Radiological Equipment (KCARE), Kings College Hospital, London SE5 9RS, UK

Abstract. The purpose of the study was to compare the image quality of film–screen (FS) and computed radiography (CR) for adult chest examinations across a range of beam energies. A series of images of the CDRAD threshold contrast detail detection phantom were acquired for a range of tube potential and exposure levels with both CR and FS. The phantom was placed within 9 cm of Perspex to provide attenuation and realistic levels of scatter in the image. Hardcopy images of the phantom were scored from a masked light-box by two scorers. Threshold contrast indices were used to calculate a visibility index (VI). The relationships between dose and image quality for CR and for FS are fundamentally different. The improvements in VIs obtained using CR at 75 kVp and 90 kVp were found to be statistically significant compared with 125 kVp at matched effective dose levels. The relative performance of FS and CR varies as a function of energy owing to the different k-edges of each system. When changing from FS to CR, the use of lower tube potentials may allow image quality to be maintained whilst reducing effective dose. A tube voltage of 90 kVp is indicated by this work, but may require clinical verification.

Introduction

Digital imaging is gradually replacing the well established technology of conventional film–screen (FS) imaging. This is primarily due to the perceived advantages of digital image processing, electronic archiving, teleradiology and the potential for optimization of image acquisition and display independently. The wide dynamic range of digital systems make them particularly attractive for imaging the widely differing attenuating structures of the chest [1]. The Ionising Radiation (Medical Exposure) Regulations (2000) [2] require that radiographic techniques be optimized for each examination type. An optimization study should investigate tube voltage and the receptor dose required to achieve the minimal acceptable level of image quality.

The Council of European Communities have published guidelines on good radiographic technique for a range of standard FS imaging examinations [3]. The suggested posteroanterior chest technique is to use 125 kVp, 180 cm focus to film distance (FDD) with an antiscatter grid in place. There is no accepted guidance for digital radiography. Fundamental differences exist between FS imaging and computed radiography (CR) and the optimum technique may not necessarily be the same. First, CR has a wide dynamic range and the ability to perform image processing operations on details in the lung and mediastinum in order to enhance their visibility. This reduces the need to minimize the contrast between signals transmitted from lung to mediastinum by selection of a high tube voltage value, as is the practice for FS which has a narrow dynamic range. With digital systems such as CR the optimum tube voltage can be obtained by maximizing the signal to noise ratio whilst maintaining an effective dose level [4–6]. Second, photo-stimulable phosphor (PSP) plates have different absorption edge characteristics to rare-earth screens owing to their different elemental compositions (see Figure 1). In the diagnostic energy range $BaF(Br_{0.85}I_{0.15})$, which is the bulk constituent of the Agfa photo-stimulable phosphor plate (Agfa, Peissenberg, Germany) [7, 8], has a k-edge at ~37 keV, whilst Gd_2O_2S (used for rare earth screens) has a k-edge at ~50 keV. It can be seen from Figure 1 that between these energies (37 keV to 50 keV) the attenuation performance of the photo-stimulable phosphor will be better relative to the FS than at other energies. For Figure 2, the fraction of the total incident transmitted beam photons, that interact with the detector, F, has been approximated using the following equation:

$$F = \frac{\sum_{\varepsilon=1}^{E} N(\varepsilon)F(\varepsilon)}{\sum_{\varepsilon=1}^{E} N(\varepsilon)} \quad (1)$$

where E=the maximum energy of the spectrum used; ε=a discrete point in the energy spectrum; $N(\varepsilon)$=the relative

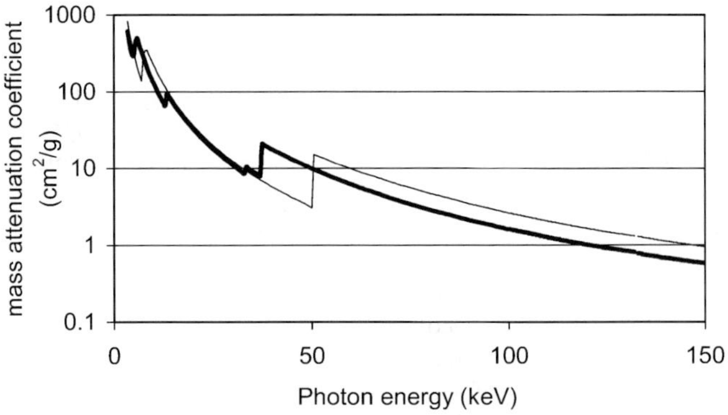

Figure 1. The mass attenuation coefficients of Gd_2O_2S (thin solid line) and $BaFB_{0.85}I_{0.15}$ (thick solid line) as a function of energy [10].

Received 30 January 2004 and in revised form 23 September 2004, accepted 1 December 2004.

Current address for D S Evans, Imaging and Medical Physics, University Hospital Birmingham NHS Trust, Birmingham, UK.

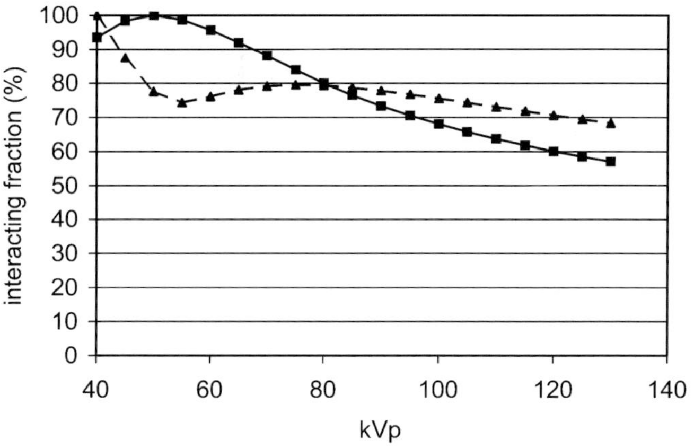

Figure 2. The fraction of photons interacting with a $BaF(Br_{0.85}I_{0.15})$ computed radiography (CR) plate (solid line) and a Gd_2O_2S phosphor screen (dashed line). The values were calculated using Equation 1, and published tables of data [9, 10]. Both curves have been normalized to their peak point.

number of photons at a discrete energy level, ε, in the primary beam after transmission through 10 cm of Perspex and 2.5 mm Al equivalent (obtained using Institute of Physics and Engineering in Medicine (IPEM) report 78 [9]); $F(\varepsilon)$=the fraction of photons of an energy, ε, that will interact within the detecting medium [10].

The relative attenuation properties of the two systems will be dependent on the thickness of material used. Since details of the effective phosphor thickness are not well known, comparison of the magnitudes of the photon interaction fractions of the two detectors in Figure 2 is not meaningful. However, the comparison of the variation of photon interaction fraction with energy for the two receptors is worthwhile. It can be seen that the variation in primary beam absorption fractions with tube voltage for the two systems is significantly different, with Gd_2O_2S maintaining its absorption efficiency better at higher energies than $BaF(Br_{0.85}I_{0.15})$.

It has been shown that for adult chest radiography, the performance of CR and FS is comparable [11–14]. It should be noted that these studies did not use FS systems of the same speed. Conversely, for paediatric chest imaging where lower tube potential is used and the scatter contribution is less, it has been shown that a dose reduction of approximately 30% is possible with CR whilst maintaining the same image quality as with FS [15].

Studies of optimum tube voltage to be used for adult chest radiography using CR have resulted in somewhat conflicting results. When assessing the visibility of low contrast opacities in human volunteers [4] and low contrast disks within a phantom [16], in the range of 80–140 kVp, it was concluded that lower tube potential would result in significantly better image quality. Conversely, using anthropomorphic chest phantoms, signal to noise ratio and image quality assessed using the Commission of the European Communities (CEC) guidelines [3] were not significantly affected by tube voltage [5, 17]. It should be noted that as well as having different methods of assessing image quality these studies have different methods of matching dose at different tube potentials.

The variation of image quality with tube potential will be a complex function of the primary beam spectrum, the scatter spectrum and the variation of receptor absorption efficiency with energy. The aims of this work were to determine the optimum tube potential for chest imaging using CR, and to assess the comparative image quality of FS and CR as a function of tube voltage.

Theory

National guidelines for the assessment of radiological equipment [18] recommend the use of threshold contrast detail detection (TCDD) for the annual routine testing of image intensifiers. TCDD has been suggested for routine testing of CR [19, 20]. A TCDD test object consists of either a series of circular holes drilled into a material, or a series of circular objects positioned on a base material. Typically the number of details of each diameter visible in the image is recorded and used to calculate values of threshold contrast index, $H_T(A)$,

$$H_T(A) = \frac{1}{(C_T\sqrt{A})} \quad (2)$$

where A is the detail area and C_T is the minimum detectable contrast. C_T must be calculated for the specific beam conditions used (energy and filtration). The threshold contrast index data can be viewed graphically, or summarized as a single quality index (QI) [21]. However, comparison of $H_T(A)$ values between images obtained at different tube potential values is not useful, since equal detail visibility would give rise to a superior $H_T(A)$ values at higher tube voltages. We propose to use a visibility index (VI) which is determined solely from the physical size of the detected objects rather than their radiographic contrasts,

$$\mathrm{VI} = \frac{1}{N}\sum_{A=1}^{N}\frac{d(A)_{\mathrm{ref}}}{d(A)_{\mathrm{image}}} \quad (3)$$

where N is the number of different groups of details with fixed diameters in the phantom used, $d(A)_{\mathrm{ref}}$ is the smallest visible depth of hole for a given detail diameter in the reference image and $d(A)_{\mathrm{image}}$ is the corresponding depth in the image of interest. Two similar depth-based image quality indices have been used in a study of chest radiographs [22]. The form of the visibility index is based on the quality index suggested by Gallacher et al [21]. The use of a reference curve taken from some "standard" image has the effect of normalizing both the quality index suggested by Gallacher and the visibility index suggested here, such that a value above 1.0 will be indicative of better-than-standard image quality.

For a quantum noise limited imaging system the detectable threshold contrast, C_T, of holes of depth, d, in an otherwise uniform background is related to receptor dose, D, as follows,

$$D^{0.5} \propto \frac{1}{C_T} \quad (4)$$

where

$$C_T \propto \exp(\mu d) - 1 \quad (5)$$

where μ is the attenuation coefficient of air in the holes in the phantom. It follows that the threshold hole depth d is proportional to $-\ln D$, and as a consequence VI must also be proportional to $-\ln D$ for a quantum noise limited detector. The mean VI value should be less affected by variations in the noise and observer performance than the individual $d(A)_{\mathrm{image}}$ values. Also, it is simpler to compare two images using a single measure of image quality, rather than compare 10–15 values of $d(A)$. However, it is still important to assess whether the system's relative performance is affected by detail size by examining the full TCDD curve.

Materials and methods

Tests were performed in a general X-ray room equipped with a Opti 150/30/50C tube and Polydoros LX50 generator (Siemens Medical Solutions, Erlangen, Germany), vertical bucky with moving antiscatter grid (focused at 1.50 m, 70 lines cm^{-1}, grid ratio 7:1), and ADC Solo CR reader with MD10 phosphor plates (Agfa Healthcare, Peissenberg, Germany). A second set of tests were performed in a general X-ray room equipped with a ROT1750 tube and Optimus 50 generator (Philips Medical Systems, Eindhoven, The Netherlands), vertical bucky with a moving antiscatter grid (focused at 1.80 m, 36 lines cm^{-1}, grid ratio 12:1), and a 400 speed HT-G film–screen cassette, processed using an Agfa CIC system.

Image quality was assessed using the CDRAD (University Hospital Nijmegen, St Radboud, The Netherlands) threshold contrast detail detectability test object. The CDRAD is a 1 cm thick Perspex plate containing circular holes of 15 different diameters (ranging from 0.3 mm to 8 mm) and 15 different depths (ranging from 0.3 mm to 8 mm) [23]. The detail depths are such that within a reasonable range of exposures some, but not all, of the details should be visible at all detail diameters.

The phantom was placed between 4 cm of Perspex (front) and 5 cm of Perspex (behind) to provide scatter and give attenuation similar to an adult chest. All exposures were made in the vertical bucky with a moving antiscatter grid, and a focal spot to detector distance of 180 cm (see Figure 3), as suggested in the CEC guidelines [3].

Images were obtained using both FS and CR at 75 kVp, 90 kVp and 125 kVp across a range of receptor doses spanning from approximately 0.5 μGy to approximately 20 μGy. The CR plates were read out using the setting 200 speed and "flat field" (without post processing). Before printing the images onto laser film, window and level were selected such that the visibility of the details appeared to be maximized and the background noise remained perceptible.

The images were scored using a masked light box and consistent low level ambient light conditions. The counting of "half visible" details was permitted, and this was accounted for in the analysis by taking a mean of the adjacent hole depths. VI values for each image were then calculated (Equation 2). The values from the 90 kVp CR automatic exposure control (AEC) images, with a receptor dose of 2.9 μGy, are used as the reference for calculating the VI values quoted throughout this report (N.B. this choice of normalization image is arbitrary). The images were scored by two experienced scorers, and the average of the two VI for each image was taken. Scoring was performed allowing variable viewing distance protocol, and standardized ambient light conditions.

Entrance surface dose was measured using a calibrated Radcal 2025 electrometer with 6 cm^3 ionization chamber (Radcal Corporation, Monrovia, CA). The entrance surface doses and beam conditions were used to calculate effective doses for each set of exposure conditions (using the "Effdose" calculation package [24, 25]).

Receptor dose with the phantom in place was measured using a Dali 120 cm^3 ion (PTW, Freiberg, Germany) chamber placed directly inside the bucky. Optical densities of the film–screen images were measured in a region away from any visible details using a Parry DT1405 densitometer (Parry, Newbury, UK).

Results

Figures 4 and 5 show the variation of VI with effective dose for the three tube potential values investigated with CR and FS, respectively. Table 1 lists the receptor doses and optical densities of the points for the FS data. Figure 6 plots the ratio of FS VI to CR VI for each tube voltage tested. With FS there is a point beyond which increasing exposure results in a decrease in detail visibility owing to optical density saturation. However, with CR at each tube potential the VI rises with exposure as lower contrast details to become more visible over the decreasing

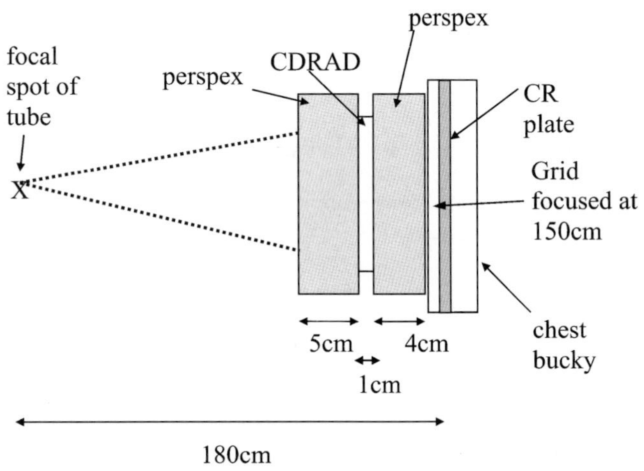

Figure 3. A schematic diagram of the experimental setup used.

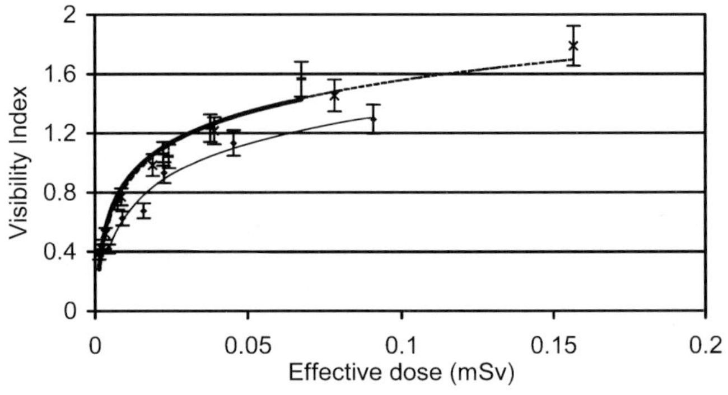

Figure 4. Plot of visibility index (VI) versus effective dose for sets of computed radiography (CR) images obtained at 75 kVp (thick solid line with data points marked by horizontal lines), 90 kVp (dashed line with data points marked by crosses) and 125 kVp (thin solid line with data points marked by diamond shapes).

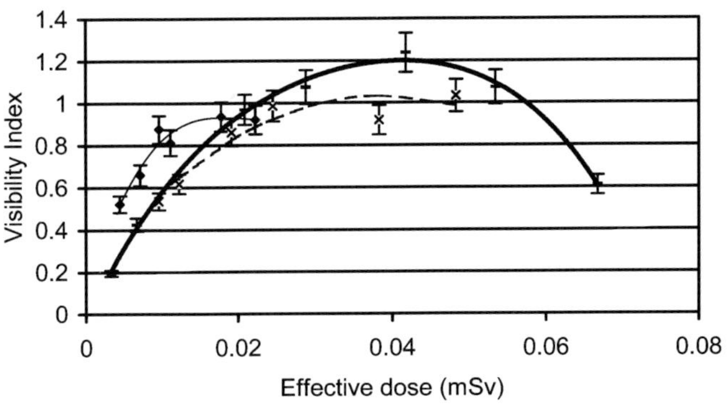

Figure 5. Plot of visibility index (VI) versus effective dose for sets of film–screen (FS) images obtained at 75 kVp (thick solid line with data points marked by horizontal lines), 90 kVp (dashed line with data points marked by crosses) and 125 kVp (thin solid line with data points marked by diamond shapes).

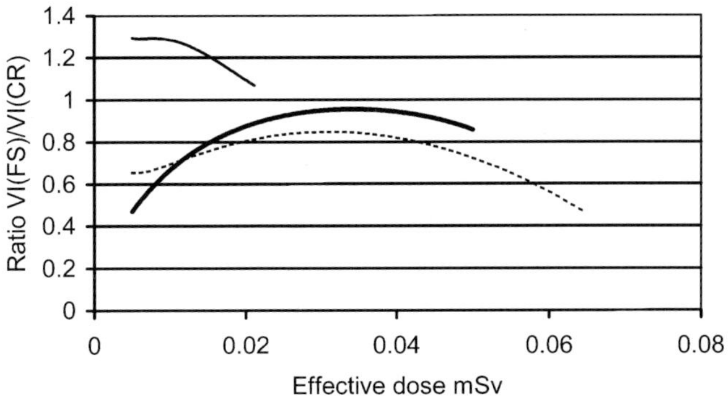

Figure 6. A plot of the ratio of film–screen (FS) visibility index (VI) trend-line to the computed radiography (CR) VI trend-line at 75 kVp (thick solid line), 90 kVp (dashed line) and 125 kVp (thin solid line).

quantum noise. Consequently the image quality performance of FS relative to CR decreases beyond the peak associated with the optimum film blackening (Figure 6).

Wilcoxen signed rank statistical tests were performed to assess the null hypotheses H_1, H_2 and H_3, defined as follows:

- H_1: The distributions of the CR VI at 125 kVp and 90 kVp are identical
- H_2: The distributions of the CR VI at 125 kVp and 75 kVp are identical
- H_3: The distributions of the CR VI at 90 kVp and 75 kVp are identical

The data were grouped into pairs of visibility indices obtained with approximately matched effective doses at different tube voltages. The data were matched such that for each pair the higher dose point was taken from the apparently lower image quality distribution (*i.e.* 125 kVp for H_1 and H_2, and 75 kVp for H_3). Differences of up to 30% in dose were accepted for matched pairs. The results are summarized in Table 2. The Wilcoxen statistical test is not appropriate for testing the film–screen data, although clearly there is a strong tube voltage dependence shown in Figure 5.

Discussion

Comparison of FS with CR for chest imaging

It can be clearly seen from Figure 6 that the difference between FS and CR is strongly dependent on beam energy. This should be considered when reviewing the results of comparative studies. For example the Hufton et al [15] study used tube voltages in the range 60–70 kVp for chest X-rays of infants, and assessed image quality against the CEC criteria. They concluded that dose reductions of the order of 30% were possible when using CR instead of 400 speed FS, whilst maintaining image quality. Conversely Cook et al [11] found no statistically significant difference between FS and CR at 125 kVp, for threshold contrast detail detectability phantoms with scatter conditions similar to an adult chest.

With FS it should be noted that the clinical details of interest in the lung and mediastinum will often not be displayed at the optimum optical density. Consequently the true performance of FS relative to CR will generally be poorer than indicated here, since CR VI improve relative to FS away from the peak of the FS curves (Figure 6).

Optimum tube voltage for CR chest examinations

Figure 4 demonstrates that the image quality for the CR system was poorest at 125 kVp across the range of effective doses investigated. This is due to a combination of the variation of detector response with photon energy (see Figures 1 and 2) and the decreased signal contrast at high tube voltage.

It can be seen from Figure 2 that over the range of beam energies investigated in this study the photostimulable phosphor suffers a much greater reduction in primary beam absorption efficiency than the gadolinium oxysulphide screen. This is in broad agreement with the results of

Table 1. The percentage difference in visibility index between film–screen (FS) and computed radiography (CR) at the dose level of the peak in FS image quality

	75 kVp		90 kVp		125 kVp	
Point	Receptor dose (μGy)	Optical density	Receptor dose (μGy)	Optical density	Receptor dose (μGy)	Optical density
1	0.45	0.29	1.38	0.58	1.00	0.44
2	0.90	0.36	1.77	0.76	1.60	0.67
3	2.8	1.12	2.77	1.2	2.16	1.06
4	3.89	1.51	3.54	1.64	2.51	1.18
5	5.6	2.13	5.54	2.12	4.01	1.70
6	7.22	2.56	6.98	2.48	5.01	2.00
7	9.02	3.28	—	—	—	—

Table 2. Results of Wilcoxen signed rank test

Null hypothesis	Sample size	p-value	Result
The distributions of the CR VI at 25 kVp and 75 kVp are identical	5	<0.001	Reject null hypothesis H_1
The distributions of the CR VI at 125 kVp and 90 kVp are identical	5	<0.001	Reject null hypothesis H_2
The distributions of the CR VI at 90 kVp and 75 kVp are identical	6	>0.2	No evidence to reject H_3

CR, computed radiography; VI, visibility index.

Fetterly and Handiandreou [26] who showed that the DQE of a Fuji CR system decreased with increasing tube voltage from 70 kVp to 95 kVp and 120 kVp. The different behaviour is due to the different k-edge positions of the two materials. The higher k-edge of Gd_2O_2S is beneficial for detecting high tube potential beams which have a greater percentage of photon energies above this threshold. It should be noted that the depth at which interactions occur in both the CR plate and intensifying screen will have some energy dependence. The efficiency of the transfer of light from the phosphors to either the film or the photomultiplier tube (in the case of CR) will be dependent on the depth of its origin. For CR, the average depth of interaction will be greater for the higher tube voltages, resulting in a greater spread of laser light and attenuation of photostimulated luminescence. For the FS system the relationship between depth of absorption and image quality is more complex owing to the dual screen geometry.

The sensitivity to the primary beam photons is a partial explanation for the comparatively poor performance of the CR system at high tube voltages. The scattered photon absorption efficiency of the two receptors should also be considered. Unfortunately this effect cannot be quantified as easily as the effect of the primary beam spectrum. Both detectors will in general be more sensitive to the scattered radiation incident on them than to the primary beam due to its lower energy. It can be seen from Figure 2 that the sensitivity of the photostimulable phosphor increases more sharply with decreasing tube potential than the Gd_2O_2S screen. The scatter spectrum can be crudely considered to the equivalent to a beam of lower tube potential than the primary beam. At the higher energies the sensitivity to scatter and primary will be broadly similar for the Gd_2O_2S screen. For the photostimulable phosphor however, the sensitivity to scatter may be significantly higher than the primary beam.

The results of this study of the optimum tube voltage for CR support the results of other investigations [4, 16]. Both these studies used Fuji CR plates which use $BaF(Br_{0.85}I_{0.15})$ phosphors similar to that used by the Agfa system investigated in this work. These studies are therefore all comparable, and all suggest an improvement in detail visibility at tube voltages lower than the 125 kVp suggested for FS imaging [3]. It should be noted that the rationale behind the choice of high tube potential for FS is to maintain an acceptable range of radiographic densities across both the lung and mediastinum, rather than to maximize detail visibility in one or other of these regions. With CR the wide dynamic range and the ability to process data post acquisition suggest that minimization of contrast between mediastinum and lung should not be necessary [4]. The use of a tube voltage lower than 125 kVp is strongly suggested. The CEC guidelines require that chest exposures should be no longer than 20 ms to minimize cardiac motion artefact. It is recommended from the results of this work that a tube voltage in the range of 75 kVp to 90 kVp is used provided that the exposure time can be limited below 20 ms. Clinical trials a required to verify this result.

Conclusions

CR and FS have inherently different imaging characteristics; for example different energy response and responses to variations in exposure. It is therefore unlikely to be appropriate to acquire images using the same exposure factors for both systems. For chest imaging the results reported here indicate that CR produces optimum image quality in the range of 75 kVp to 90 kVp, rather than the higher energies which are often used in practice.

Acknowledgments

The authors would like to acknowledge the Medicine and Healthcare products Regulatory Agency (MHRA) for funding this projects and the staff of the imaging departments for their assistance and co-operation in providing access to the imaging systems.

References

1. Goodman LR, Wilson CR, Foley WD. Digital radiography of the chest: problems and promises. AJR Am J Roentgenol 1988;150:1241–52.
2. Ionising radiation (medical exposure) regulations 2000. UK: The Stationary Office Limited, 2000.
3. Council of European Communities. European guidelines on quality criteria for diagnostic radiographic images, Rep EUR 16260 EN, 1996.
4. Nobuhiro O, Hajime N, Seiichi M, Kunihiro T, Katsumi N, Akira Y. Optimal beam quality for chest radiography. Invest Radiol 1996;31:126–31.
5. Tingberg A, Sjostrom D. Search for optimal tube voltage for image plate radiography. Prog Biomed Optics Imaging 2003;4:187–96.
6. Dobbins JT, Samei E, Chotas HG, Warp RJ, Baydush AH, Floyd CE, et al. Chest radiography: optimisation of x-ray spectrum for caesium iodide – amorphous silicon flat panel detector. Radiology 2003;226:221–30.
7. Nakano Y, Gido T, Honda S, Maezawa A, Wakamatsu H, Yanagita T. Improved computed radiography image quality from BaFI:Eu photostimulable phosphor. Med Phys 2002;29:592–7.
8. Rowlands JA. The physics of computed radiography. Phys Med Biol 2002;47:123–66.
9. Craney K, Gilmore BJ, Fogarty GWA, Desponds A, Sutton DG. Catalogue of diagnostic x-ray spectra and other data. Institute of Physics and Engineering in Medicine report 78 (CDROM), York: IPEM, 1997.

10. Boone JM, Chavez AE. Comparison of x-ray cross sections for diagnostic and therapeutic medical physics. Med Phys 1996;23:1997–2005.
11. Cook LT, Insana MF, Mcfadden MA, Hall TJ, Cox GG. Comparison of low contrast detectability of a screen film system and third generation computed radiography. Med Phys 1994;21:691–5.
12. Ganten M, Radeleff B, Kampschulte A, Daniels MD, Kauffmann G, et al. Comparing image quality of flat panel chest radiography with storage phosphor radiography and film screen radiography. AJR Am J Roentgenol 2003;181:171–6.
13. Schaefer-Prokop CM, Prokpop M, Schmidt A, Neitzel U, Galanski M. Selenium radiography versus storage phosphor and conventional radiography in the detection of simulated chest lesions. Radiology 1996;201:45–50.
14. Bacher K, Smeets P, Bonnarens K, De Hauwere A, Verstraete K, et al. Dose reduction in patients undergoing chest imaging. AJR Am J Roentgenol 2003;181:923–9.
15. Hufton AP, Doyle SM, Carty HML. Digital radiography in paediatrics: radiation dose considerations and magnitude of possible dose reduction. Br J Radiol 1998;71:186–99.
16. Dobbins JT, Rice JJ, Beam CA, Ravin CE. Threshold perception performance with computed and screen film radiography: implications for chest radiography. Radiology 1992;183:179–87.
17. Chotas HG, Floyd CE, Dobbins JT, Ravin CE. Digital chest radiography with photostimulable phosphors: signal-to-noise ratio as a function of kilovoltage with matched exposure risk. Radiology 1993;186:395–8.
18. IPEM CoR/NRPB. Recommended standards for the routine testing of diagnostic x-ray imaging systems, IPEM report 77. York: Institute of Physics and Engineering in Medicine, 1997;41–7.
19. Samei E, Seibert JA, Willis CE, Flynn MJ, Mah E, Junck KL. Performance evaluation of CR systems. Med Phys 2001;28:361–71.
20. Finch A, Bury R, Davies G, Fife I, Hufton A, Workman A. Assurance of quality in the diagnostic imaging department. London: British Institute of Radiology, 2001;67–71.
21. Gallacher DJ, Mackenzie A, Batchelor S, Lynch J, Saunders JA. Use of a quality index in threshold contrast detail detection measurements in television fluoroscopy. Br J Radiol 2003;76:464–72.
22. Soldt RTM, Zweers D, Van Den Berg L, Geleijns J, Jansen JThM, Zoetelief J. Survey of posteroanterior chest radiography in The Netherlands: patient dose and image quality. Br J Radiol 2003;76:398–405.
23. Thijssen MAO, Bijkerk KR, Van der Burght RJM. Manual CDRAD-phantom type 2.0. University Hospital Nijmegen, 1998.
24. Hart D, Jones DG, Wall BF. Estimation of effective dose in diagnostic radiology from entrance surface does and dose area product measurements. NRPB Report NRPB-R262 Chilton, UK: National Radiological Protection Board, 1994.
25. Effdose software V1.04. National Board of Health. Denmark: National Institute of Radiation Hygiene, 1995.
26. Fetterley KA, Hangiandreou NJ. Effects of the x-ray spectra on the DQE of a computed radiography system. Med Phys 2001;28:241–8.

The British Journal of Radiology, 78 (2005), 428–432
DOI: 10.1259/bjr/92548685

A case of stunning of lung and bone metastases of papillary thyroid cancer after a therapeutic dose (3.7 GBq) of ^{131}I and review of the literature: implications for sequential treatments

A F LEGER, MD, M PELLAN, MD, F DAGOUSSET, MD, A CHEVALIER, PhD, I KELLER, MD and J CLERC, MD, PhD

Department of Nuclear Medicine, Hôpital Necker–Enfants Malades, 149 rue de Sèvres, 75743 Paris Cedex 15, France

Abstract. Thyroid stunning is usually defined as the inhibition or suppression of iodide trapping by remnant thyroid tissue or by functioning metastases following a diagnostic dose of ^{131}I. The risk of stunning increases progressively with larger doses. Because the threshold above which this effect occurs in thyroid remnants seems to be between 37 MBq and 111 MBq of ^{131}I, therapeutic ^{131}I doses of 3.7 GBq may cause stunning. We describe stunning of papillary thyroid cancer lung and bone metastases after a therapeutic dose of ^{131}I (3.7 GBq). A T1 bone metastasis and bilateral lung metastases were diagnosed by post-therapeutic dose whole-body scan. Nuclear MRI detected another lesion at T4, whose ^{131}I fixation was not obvious. An additional 0.7 GBq were given after recombinant TSH, 37 days after the therapeutic dose; 24 h later, uptake by the lung and T1 metastases had disappeared, but trapping was again seen 6 months later on the post-therapeutic scan. This re-appearance is evidence in favour of the transitory and reversible character of stunning, and confirms its correspondence to the decreased ability of viable thyroid cells to trap iodine and not to their destruction. A better understanding of stunning would make it possible, in the event of rapidly progressing disease and in conjunction with recombinant thyroid stimulating hormone (TSH), to give several therapeutic doses of ^{131}I in close succession without each dose hampering the effectiveness of the subsequent one.

The treatment of differentiated thyroid cancer and the diagnosis of its metastases are based on the capacity of thyroid cells to actively trap radioactive iodine ^{131}I. Initial treatment usually combines total thyroidectomy and destruction of thyroid remnants with an ablative therapeutic dose of ^{131}I [1–3]. Post-thyroidectomy diagnostic scintigraphy with a small dose of ^{131}I (37–111 MBq) can detect cervical thyroid remnants before administration of an ablative dose of 3.7 GBq of ^{131}I. Because it is now known that the higher the diagnostic dose of ^{131}I, the better the sensitivity of scintigraphy to render visible more foci trapping radioactivity [4], the diagnostic dose has been increased up to 185 MBq.

In 1986, it was hypothesised that these high diagnostic doses of ^{131}I might be responsible for the subsequently diminished capture of "therapeutic" ^{131}I [5]. Since then, numerous studies [6–19] have confirmed the existence of stunning, usually defined as the inhibition or suppression of iodide trapping by thyroid cells, following diagnostic doses of ^{131}I, resulting in the loss of efficacy of therapeutic ^{131}I. Stunning was recently described after fractionated ablative doses of ^{131}I [20].

In the case of rapidly progressing thyroid cancer with distant metastases taking up iodide, it would be desirable to administer several successive therapeutic ^{131}I doses at close intervals. But in so doing, the possibility of one therapeutic dose blocking, by stunning, the efficacy of the subsequent one must be avoided.

We describe stunning induced by a therapeutic dose of 3.7 GBq of ^{131}I.

Received 7 July 2004 and in revised form 29 October 2004, accepted 9 December 2004.

Case report

A 16-year-old Caucasian boy (height 183 cm; weight 55 kg) had left cervical adenopathy for 3 years. Biopsy of the lesion showed it to be a metastasis of papillary thyroid adenocarcinoma. Total thyroidectomy with bilateral exeresis of the lymph nodes yielded an 8 mm diameter, non-encapsulated, papillary thyroid adenocarcinoma with numerous vascular emboli on the left, and lateral tracheal (n=8) and jugular–carotid lymph node metastases (n=5) also on the left.

A therapeutic dose (3.7 GBq) of ^{131}I was given 4 weeks after thyroidectomy. Laboratory findings are reported in Table 1. Scintigraphy, performed 7 days after ^{131}I administration, detected four cervical foci of ^{131}I uptake, and diffuse ^{131}I trapping in both lungs, estimated at 1/1000 (Figure 1a). CT scan showed micronodules at the limit of visibility in the lung bases. Thyroid hormone replacement with levothyroxine (L-T4) was initiated.

6 months later, a second therapeutic dose of ^{131}I (3.7 GBq) was administered. Scintigraphy performed 4 days later revealed the persistence of two of the cervical foci – left lower paramedian and upper external jugular–carotid – and bilateral lung uptake estimated at 6/10 000.

After a further 6 months, the third therapeutic dose of ^{131}I (3.7 GBq) was administered. Scintigraphy 4 days later showed that the upper jugular–carotid focus had disappeared, but the lower cervical and lung trapping (estimated to be 8/10 000) of ^{131}I persisted (Figure 1b). Bone scintigraphy showed that the persistent cervical uptake corresponded to the first thoracic vertebral body, T1. Nuclear MRI visualized a 10 mm lytic metastasis in the left half of T1 and a sub-centimetre lytic image in vertebral body T4 of unknown nature.

Table 1. Biological data at the times of therapeutic and diagnostic ^{131}I doses

^{131}I dose No.	GBq	TSH (mIU l^{-1})	Tg[a] (µg l^{-1})	Total serum iodine (nmol l^{-1})	Urinary iodine (nmol l^{-1})	Urinary I/C[b]
1	3.7	44.8	92.7	226	1113	65
2	3.7	251.9	116.0	197	1058	64
3	3.7	307.6	88.7	13	554	21
rTSH	0.7	32.7[c]	17.9	609	935	77
4	3.7	324.6	48.2	118	177	41
5	3.7	345.0	22.5	68	1756	73
Normal values		0.5–3	<35.0[d]	338–724	~800 in France	30–300

[a]No anti-thyroglobulin (Tg) antibodies were detected.
[b]Urinary iodine/urinary creatinine ratio.
[c]40 h after the second injection of recombinant thyroid stimulating hormone (rTSH).
[d]Normal Tg after thyroidectomy and ablative dose of ^{131}I: <1 µg l^{-1}.

Upon re-examination of the ^{131}I scintigram (posterior view), the T4 region was difficult to interpret because of bilateral ^{131}I trapping by the lungs. Prior to scheduled surgery on T1 and after administration of recombinant thyroid-stimulating hormone (rTSH), 0.7 GBq of ^{131}I were given 37 days after the third therapeutic dose and scintigraphy was performed 48 h later. To our surprise, no ^{131}I was taken up at T1, T4 or in the lungs (Figure 1c), but the physiological sites (salivary glands and mediastinum) of scintigraphic contrast were clearly visible. The absence of iodine overload was verified (Table 1). T1 was surgically removed. Radiation therapy delivered 40 Gy to the spine C6–T5.

6 months later, the fourth therapeutic dose of ^{131}I (3.7 GBq) was administered. Scintigraphy performed 5 days later revealed the re-appearance of radioactive uptake in both lungs (estimated to be 2/10 000) and weak trapping at T1 but not T4 (Figure 1d).

1 year later, the fifth therapeutic dose of ^{131}I (3.7 GBq) was administered. Scintigraphy performed 3 days later showed trace uptake at T1 and faint pulmonary uptake comparable with that of the mediastinum.

Discussion

The need for emergency surgery on the T1 metastasis and MRI discovery of a T4 lesion led us to repeat the scintigraphy with 0.7 GBq of ^{131}I. Iodine overload, with diminished iodide clearance by the thyroid, is the first hypothesis to explain the association of known metastases that trapped ^{131}I and negative scintigraphy. The increased intrathyroid concentration of iodide beyond a certain threshold decreases the sodium/iodide symporter (NIS) activity [21, 22] and increases its turnover, leading to fewer NIS complexes. An iodine overload in our patient was excluded because of normal blood and urine iodine levels. The persistence of the effect of a recent iodine overload cannot be excluded: however, an in-depth inquiry found no potential source of iodine intake for this 16-year-old teenager.

A second hypothesis raises the possibility of thyroid stunning by the 3.7 GBq of ^{131}I given 37 days before the absorption of 0.7 GBq of ^{131}I for scintigraphy.

The existence of this phenomenon remains controversial [23–27], with the results of most studies confirming that it exists *in vivo* [6–17] and *in vitro* [18, 19], but those of other studies failing to do so [28–31].

Stunning corresponds either to a partial destruction of iodine-trapping tissues by the diagnostic dose, with an irreversible phenomenon of radiation-induced cell death, or to transitory, reversible episodes, with less cellular uptake of iodide, attesting to the viability of remaining cells.

In the first case, a possible mechanism to explain stunning is the cell death resulting from early necrosis (within 24–48 h) or differed apoptosis. Guiraud-Vitaux et al [18] administered increasing ^{131}I doses to rat thyroid cells and observed morphological and ultrastructural modifications typical of necrosis with no signs of apoptosis. The number of affected cells paralleled the ^{131}I dose. Other authors found signs of apoptosis in response to ionizing radiation [32].

Postgard et al [19] used pig thyroid epithelial cells to measure transcellular transport of iodide and its accumulation in the follicular lumen. 5 days after irradiation with 3 Gy, iodide transport was diminished by almost 50% and almost 90% after 30 Gy; but no signs of cell death were observed.

Several groups studied stunning using qualitative [28, 29, 33] or quantitative methods [5, 7, 13, 17, 24]. The qualitative approaches required subjective comparison of diagnostic and post-therapeutic scintigrams, taking into account the number of foci trapping the radioelement and the intensity of the uptake. Given that the scintigraphic appearance depends on the activity of the iodine administered, the imaging technique, and the interval between iodine administration and scintigraphy, these qualitative methods are often open to criticism.

The quantitative approaches measure the reduction of iodide uptake. All the studies that used such a method confirmed the existence of stunning. Other researchers compared the effect of a diagnostic dose of ^{131}I on the effectiveness of an ablative dose, as assessed by the disappearance at the next evaluation, at least 6 months later, of iodine trapping by thyroid remnants. Successful outcomes were more frequent after a diagnostic ^{131}I dose of 37 MBq than after 111 MBq [10]. It was concluded that stunning might hinder ablative therapy. The transitory disappearance of foci known to take up radioactive iodine, although not strictly a quantitative method, appears to be a convincing argument in favour of stunning [9, 14].

Stunning has mainly been described after diagnostic doses of ^{131}I, which emits beta and gamma rays, but also after high doses of pure gamma-emitting ^{123}I [17].

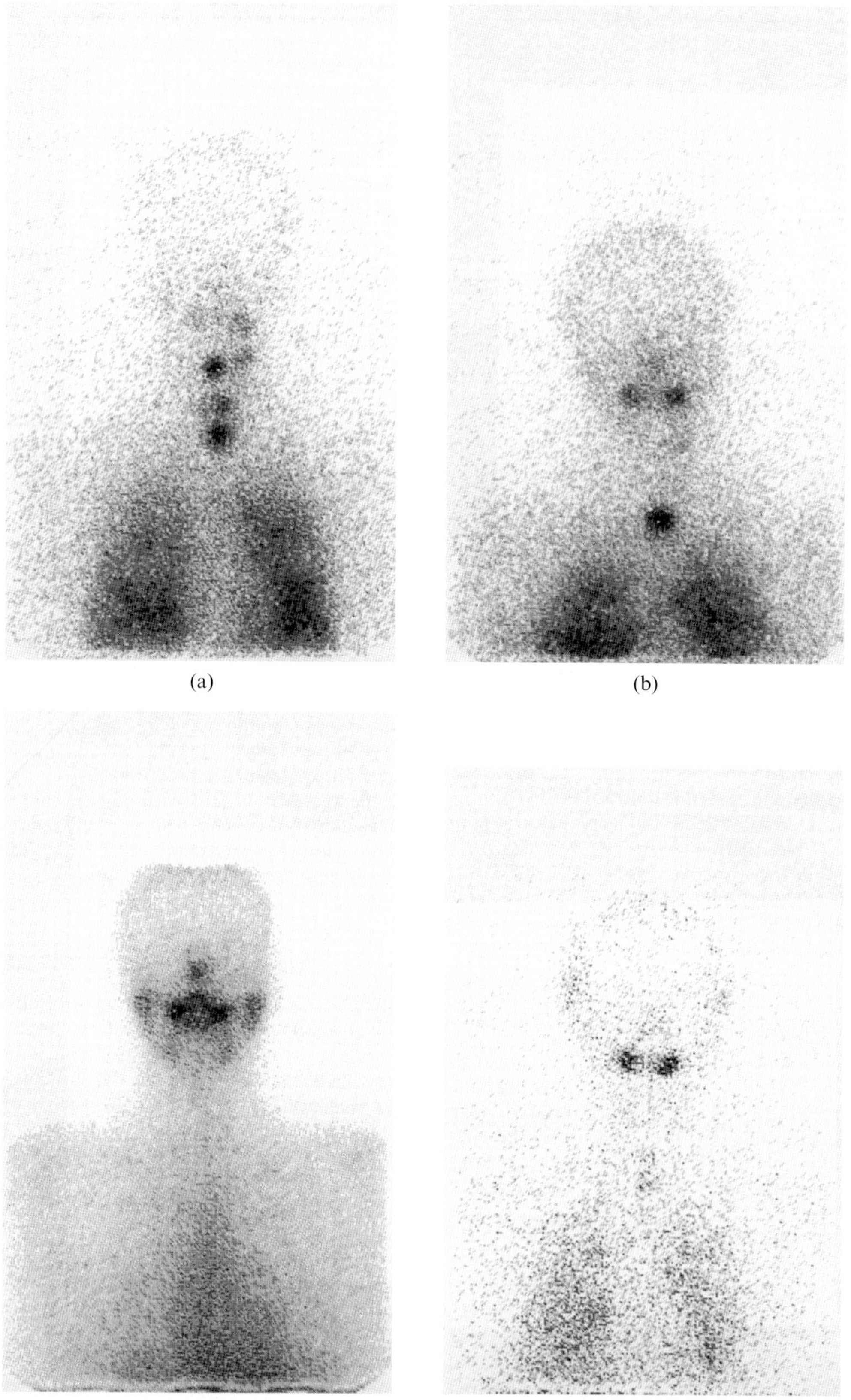

(a) (b) (c) (d)

Figure 1. ^{131}I scintigrams of the head and thorax, anterior views. (a) 7 days after the first therapeutic dose, several cervical foci of ^{131}I uptake and diffuse trapping in the lungs. (b) 4 days after the third therapeutic dose, persistence of one cervical focus and lung uptake. (c) Scintigram with 0.7 GBq of ^{131}I 37 days after recombinant thyroid stimulating hormone (rTSH) and the third therapeutic dose: disappearance of ^{131}I uptake at T1 and in the lungs, but the salivary glands and mediastinum are clearly radiolabelled. (d) 5 days after the fourth therapeutic dose: re-appearance of the radiotracer in both lungs and persistence of weak uptake in T1 despite surgery.

Stunning intensity seems to parallel the ^{131}I dose. In the literature, the threshold of ^{131}I diagnostic activities responsible for stunning was estimated to range between 74 MBq [11, 13] and 111 MBq [8, 17]. The radiation absorbed dose, estimated in Gy, and the dose rate, estimated in Gy h^{-1}, are undoubtedly more appropriate parameters than the administered dose. Jeevanram et al [5] observed stunning in remnants that had received an absorbed dose of at least 10 Gy. Muratet et al [10] found a threshold of 17.5 Gy, whereas Kao [33] reported a threshold of 35 Gy, as did Sabri et al [34], for benign thyroid diseases. However, the radiation absorbed dose is difficult to determine because the mass of the targeted tissue is most often unknown. Since thyroid stunning is dose-dependent, it seems logical that therapeutic ^{131}I doses could be responsible for more intense, more rapid and/or more prolonged stunning than that provoked by diagnostic doses.

The interval between iodine exposure and stunning has not yet been clearly established. There is an indication from some data that the degree of diagnostic stunning may increase with time up to 20–25 days, then diminish [17, 35].

It has even been suggested that the therapeutic iodine dose itself could induce immediate "intratherapeutic stunning" or "self-stunning": during the hours following the administration of a therapeutic ^{131}I dose, the high radiation dose might have a major impact on the subsequent iodide clearance rate by the thyroid [12].

The salivary glands do not seem to be affected by stunning because they remained visible on the scintigraphy. The lack of adaptative iodide clearance in the salivary glands suggests that the mechanism of active iodide transport differs from that in thyroid cells [36].

In the past few years, the presence of thyroid remnants has been quasi-constant, even after total thyroidectomy. The trend has been to administer a therapeutic ^{131}I dose of 3.7 GBq, without diagnostic scintigram [37], followed by whole-body scintigraphy to visualize the remnants and detect possible metastases. This approach could avoid diagnostic dose induction of stunning.

In contrast, therapeutic stunning raises a major practical problem. The intensity of iodide trapping by thyroid cells depends on the TSH level. The recent synthesis of rTSH now enables scintigraphy to be performed and treatments to be given after two rTSH injections without stopping L-T4 [38]. In the case of rapidly progressing disease, the availability of rTSH means that several therapeutic doses can be given in close succession without stopping L-T4. But to do so, one therapeutic dose must not interfere with the next.

Our data support the idea that stunning is a transitory inhibition of iodide uptake. Therapeutic stunning is probably more intense and more prolonged than diagnostic stunning. Better understanding of the mechanism inducing it, the time to its appearance and its duration is needed, perhaps using ^{123}I studies, to adapt treatment protocols.

References

1. Mazzaferri EL. An overview of the management of papillary and follicular thyroid carcinoma. Thyroid 1999;9:421–7.
2. Wartofsky L, Sherman SI, Gopal J, Schlumberger M, Hay ID. The use of radioactive iodine in patients with papillary and follicular thyroid cancer. J Clin Endocrinol Metab 1998;83:4195–203.
3. British Thyroid Association and Royal College of Physicians. Guidelines for the management of thyroid cancer in adults. London: Royal College of Physicians, 2002.
4. Coakley AJ, Page CJ, Croft D. Scanning dose and detection of thyroid metastases. J Nucl Med 1980;21:803–4.
5. Jeevanram RK, Shah DH, Sharma SM, Ganatra RD. Influence of initial large dose on subsequent uptake of therapeutic radioiodine in thyroid cancer patients. Int J Rad Appl Instrum B 1986;13:277–9.
6. Park HM, Perkins OW, Edmondson JW, Schnute RB, Manatunga A. Influence of diagnostic radioiodines on the uptake of ablative dose of iodine-131. Thyroid 1994;4:49–54.
7. Huic D, Medvedec M, Dodig D, Popovic S, Ivancevic D, Pavlinovic Z, et al. Radioiodine uptake in thyroid cancer patients after diagnostic application of low-dose ^{131}I. Nucl Med Commun 1996;17:839–42.
8. Park HM, Park YH, Zhou XH. Detection of thyroid remnant/metastasis without stunning: an ongoing dilemma. Thyroid 1997;7:277–80.
9. Leger FA, Izembart M, Dagousset F, Barritault L, Baillet G, Chevalier A, et al. Decreased uptake of therapeutic doses of iodine-131 after 185-MBq iodine-131 diagnostic imaging for thyroid remnants in differentiated thyroid carcinoma. Eur J Nucl Med 1998;25:242–6.
10. Muratet JP, Daver A, Minier JF, Larra F. Influence of scanning doses of iodine-131 on subsequent first ablative treatment outcome in patients operated on for differentiated thyroid carcinoma. J Nucl Med 1998;39:1546–50.
11. Hurley JR. Management of thyroid cancer: radioiodine ablation, "stunning," and treatment of thyroglobulin-positive, (131)I scan-negative patients. Endocr Pract 2000;6: 401–6.
12. Diehl M, Grunwald F. Stunning after tracer dosimetry. J Nucl Med 2001;42:1129.
13. Yeung HW, Humm JL, Larson SM. Radioiodine uptake in thyroid remnants during therapy after tracer dosimetry. J Nucl Med 2000;41:1082–5.
14. Bajen MT, Mane S, Munoz A, Garcia JR. Effect of a diagnostic dose of 185 MBq ^{131}I on postsurgical thyroid remnants. J Nucl Med 2000;41:2038–42.
15. McMenemin RM, Hilditch TE, Dempsey MF, Reed NS. Thyroid stunning after (131)I diagnostic whole-body scanning. J Nucl Med 2001;42:986–7.
16. Lees W, Mansberg R, Roberts J, Towson J, Chua E, Turtle J. The clinical effects of thyroid stunning after diagnostic whole-body scanning with 185 MBq ^{131}I. Eur J Nucl Med Mol Imaging 2002;29:1421–7.
17. Hilditch TE, Dempsey MF, Bolster AA, McMenemin RM, Reed NS. Self-stunning in thyroid ablation: evidence from comparative studies of diagnostic ^{131}I and ^{123}I. Eur J Nucl Med Mol Imaging 2002;29:783–8.
18. Guiraud-Vitaux F, Feldmann G, Vadrot N, Charles-Gupta S, Durand-Schneider AM, Colas-Linhart N, et al. Early ultrastructural injuries in the thyroid of the normal rat radioinduced by diagnostic and/or therapeutic amounts of iodine-131. Cell Mol Biol 2001;47:495–502.
19. Postgard P, Himmelman J, Lindencrona U, Bhogal N, Wiberg D, Berg G, et al. Stunning of iodide transport by (131)I irradiation in cultured thyroid epithelial cells. J Nucl Med 2002;43:828–34.
20. Wu HS, Hseu HH, Lin WY, Wang SJ, Liu YC. Decreased uptake after fractionated ablative doses of iodine-131. Eur J Nucl Med Mol Imaging 2005;32:167–73.
21. Shen DH, Kloos RT, Mazzaferri EL, Jhian SM. Sodium iodide symporter in health and disease. Thyroid 2001;11: 415–25.

22. Dohan O, De la Vieja A, Paroder V, Riedel C, Artani M, Reed M, et al. The sodium/iodide symporter (NIS): characterization, regulation, and medical significance. Endocr Rev 2003;24:48–77.
23. Coakley AJ. Thyroid stunning. Eur J Nucl Med 1998;25:203–4.
24. Medvedec M. Thyroid stunning. J Nucl Med 2001;42: 1129–31.
25. Medvedec M. Seeking a radiobiological explanation for thyroid stunning. Eur J Nucl Med 2001;28:393–5.
26. Brenner W. Is thyroid stunning a real phenomenon or just fiction? J Nucl Med 2002;43:835–6.
27. Morris LF, Waxman AD, Braunstein GD. Thyroid stunning. Thyroid 2003;13:333–40.
28. McDougall IR. 74 MBq radioiodine ^{131}I does not prevent uptake of therapeutic doses of ^{131}I (i.e. it does not cause stunning) in differentiated thyroid cancer. Nucl Med Commun 1997;18:505–12.
29. Cholewinski SP, Yoo KS, Klieger PS, O'Mara RE. Absence of thyroid stunning after diagnostic whole-body scanning with 185 MBq ^{131}I. J Nucl Med 2000;41:1198–202.
30. Morris LF, Waxman AD, Braunstein GD. The nonimpact of thyroid stunning: remnant ablation rates in ^{131}I-scanned and nonscanned individuals. J Clin Endocrinol Metab 2001;86: 3507–11.
31. Karam M, Gianoukakis A, Feustel PJ, Cheema A, Postal ES, Cooper JA. Influence of diagnostic and therapeutic doses on thyroid remnant ablation rates. Nucl Med Commun 2003;24: 489–95.
32. Baatout S, Derradji H, Petitfour O, von Suchodoletz H, Mergeay M. Mécanismes de l'apoptose radio-induite. Can J Physiol Pharmacol 2002;80:629–37.
33. Kao CH. Stunned thyroid after a diagnostic dose of I-131 for a whole body scan. Clin Nucl Med 1998;23:102–4.
34. Sabri O, Zimny M, Schreckenberger M, Meyer-Oelmann A, Reinartz P, Buell U. Does thyroid stunning exist? A model with benign thyroid disease. Eur J Nucl Med 2000;27: 1591–7.
35. Modoni S, Martino G, Valle G, Perrone E, Frusciante V. How is thyroid remnant ablation affected by former 131-I diagnostic doses and/or elapsed time? Eur J Nucl Med 2000;27:1152.
36. Wolff J. Transport of iodide and other anions in the thyroid gland. Physiol Rev 1964;44:45–90.
37. de Klerk JM, de Keizer B, Zelissen PM, Lips CM, Koppeschaar HP. Fixed dosage of ^{131}I for remnant ablation in patients with differentiated thyroid carcinoma without pre-ablative diagnostic ^{131}I scintigraphy. Nucl Med Commun 2000;21:529–32.
38. Robbins RJ, Robbins AK. Clinical review 156: Recombinant human thyrotropin and thyroid cancer management. J Clin Endocrinol Metab 2003;88:1933–8.

The British Journal of Radiology, 78 (2005), 433–436
DOI: 10.1259/bjr/62169440

Short communication

Hepatic transit time: indicator of the therapeutic response to radiofrequency ablation of liver tumours

[1,2]X ZHOU, MD, [1]D STROBEL, MD, [1]J HAENSLER, MD and [1]T BERNATIK, MD

[1]*Department of Ultrasound, Department of Medicine I, Friedrich-Alexander-University Erlangen-Nürnberg, Ulmenweg 18, D-91054 Erlangen, Germany and* [2]*Ultrasound Department, Union Hospital, Hua Zhong University of Science and Technology (HUST), Wuhan, P. R. China*

Abstract. The aim of this study was to evaluate changes of hepatic transit time (HTT) in patients treated by radiofrequency ablation (RFA). Five consecutive patients (2 females, 3 males; mean age 66 years) referred for treatment of liver neoplasm with percutaneous application of RFA were included in this study. The HTT of contrast agent (Sonovue®; Bracco International B.V., Amsterdam, The Netherlands) was measured in patients with liver metastases on the basis of time intensity curve (TIC®) before and after RFA, respectively. Changes of HTT before *vs* after RFA were compared with therapeutic response based on three-phase dynamic CT or MRI. Before RFA HTT in all 5 patients was less than 10 s (mean 6.2±1.5 s). After RFA HTT in patients with complete therapeutic response was 11.3±1.2 s, whereas two patients with incomplete treatment showed unchanged HTT below 10 s (mean 6.3±1.8 s). Successful RFA leads to a normalization in HTT. HTT using ultrasound contrast agent appears to provide a new and alternative approach in assessing the therapeutic effect of RFA in liver metastases.

Although the radiofrequency ablation (RFA) technique has been greatly improved, incomplete therapy or tumour recurrence still remains a problem [1]. Tumour recurrence rates vary depending on tumour size and remain high for tumours with a diameter above 4 cm [1]. Thus, post-procedural assessment is important for control of tumour ablation. A novel, simple and easy method using microbubble ultrasound contrast agents to measure the so-called hepatic transit time (HTT) was developed [2–4]. It has been shown that HTT is significantly shortened in patients with liver metastases [2–4]. A shortened HTT might be a potential marker to identify patients with residual or recurrent metastases after RFA. We have evaluated the changes of HTT in a series of patients treated with RFA, to test the hypothesis that HTT will lengthen with successful treatment.

Received 14 May 2004 and in final form 2 November 2004, accepted 16 December 2004.

Address correspondence to PD Dr. med. Thomas Bernatik.

Patients and methods

Five consecutive patients (2 females, 3 males; mean age 66 years) with liver metastases who were referred for percutaneous RFA using perfusable radiofrequency electrode needles (Berchtold, Tuttlingen, Germany) were included in the study. All treated lesions (Table 1) were histologically proven by ultrasound-guided biopsy. All treatments were approved by the ethical committee of Erlangen-Nuremberg University. Written informed consent was obtained from all patients at enrolment. Ultrasound examinations were performed by one experienced ultrasound specialist using Sonoline Elegra Advanced with 3.5C4H ultrasound probe (Siemens Medical Systems Inc., Issaquah, Washington) equipped

Table 1. Patient characteristics

Patient	Primary entity	Tumour size (cm[a])	Tumour number	HTT before RFA (s)	Follow-up (days)	HTT after RFA (s) Complete response[b] (n=3)	HTT after RFA (s) Incomplete treatment[b] (n=2)
1	Melanoma	3	3	7	31		5
2	Colon cancer	3.8	1	6	42	12	
3	Melanoma	3.2	1	4	46	10	
4	Uterus cancer	4.7	2	8	32		7.5
5	Hypernephroma	5.4	3	6	38	12	
Mean				6.2±1.5	37.8±6.4	11.3±1.2	6.3±1.8

[a]Maximum diameter of largest tumour.
[b]According to CT or MRI results.
HTT, hepatic transit time; RFA, radiofrequency ablation.

with phase inversion harmonic imaging (ensemble contrast imaging, ECI®) and time intensity curve (TIC®) software.

Method of the hepatic transit time (HTT) measurement

All patients included in the study underwent HTT measurement of the US contrast agent (Sonovue®; Bracco International B.V., Amsterdam, The Netherlands) before and after RFA. The ultrasound investigator was blinded for the CT or MRI results. The hepatic artery and a branch of the hepatic vein were visualized simultaneously in an intercostal section. The patient was asked to either hold his/her breath or, if this was not possible, to take small breaths with half-filled lungs. After activation of the ECI mode with a medium mechanical index (MI: 0.5) and adaptation image quality, 4.8 ml Sonovue® was administered intravenously as a bolus followed by 10 ml of 0.9% saline solution. We have not used low MI ($\leqslant$0.1) as commonly used for characterization of liver tumours. For measuring arrival of contrast media in the liver vein higher MI is needed to get a sufficient contrast. We have not used high MI ($\cong$1.0) as commonly used for Levovist on detection of liver metastases to prevent bubble destruction. Because MI of 0.5 still leads to some bubble destruction we had to use twice the standard dose of Sonovue® (4.8 ml). The entire image sequence from the entry of the ultrasound contrast agent into the hepatic artery up to its visualization in the hepatic vein was acquired (TIC® software). After rewinding the sequence to the first image (in a cine loop), two "regions of interest" (ROI) were placed over the hepatic artery and hepatic vein. The sizes of the ROI were adapted to vessel diameter. After activation of automatic movement correction, the smooth time–intensity curve of the brightness (intensity) alterations in the ROI were automatically calculated by means of the aforementioned TIC software (Figure 1).

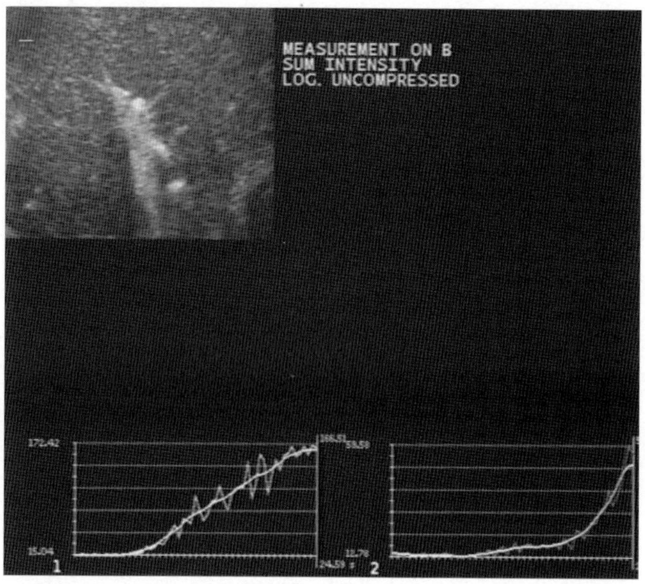

Figure 1. Hepatic transit time calculated using the time intensity curve (TIC) software in a patient with liver metastasis before radiofrequency ablation. Left curve: arrival of contrast agent in the hepatic artery; right curve: arrival of contrast agent in the hepatic vein.

Thus, an increase in brightness provides a graphic representation of the arrival of ultrasound contrast agent in the intrahepatic artery or, respectively, in the vein. The difference between the arrival times of the ultrasound contrast agent (defined as 10% rise above baseline) presents the real HTT.

Follow-up

CT or MRI results for evaluation of the therapeutic response was considered as gold standard in this study. Complete response was defined as absence of any liver metastases and complete necrosis of the treated lesion. Incomplete response was defined as either incomplete necrosis of the treated lesion or presence of further liver metastases elsewhere. At the time of follow up (Table 1) the HTT was repeated to see any changes compared with pre-treatment values.

Results

A total of 5 patients (2 females, 3 males; mean age 66 years) were enrolled in the study. Complete response was achieved in 3 of 5 patients (Figure 2). The other two patients, although showing successful local treatment, had to be classified as incomplete because both were found to have extra small metastases demonstrated by contrast-enhanced ultrasound imaging and CT and not visualized by conventional ultrasound.

Table 1 and Figure 3 show the analysis of HTT. Before RFA, the mean HTT was 6.2$\pm$1.5 s (mean$\pm$standard deviation (SD)) ranging from 4 s to 8 s. After RFA, HTT in three patients with proven complete response was 11.3$\pm$1.2 s (mean$\pm$SD) ranging from 10 s to 12 s [delay rate $\geqslant$100%, delay rate=(HTT after RFA−HTT before RFA)/HTT before RFA]. On the other hand, the mean HTT of the other two patients with incomplete treatment was 6.3$\pm$1.8 s (mean$\pm$SD). The HTT of the complete response patients increased significantly compared with unchanged HTT in incompletely treated patients (p<0.05 using a Fisher-test). There was no change in the shape of the TIC curve (rate of rise) for hepatic vein arrival after RFA.

Discussion

As RFA is becoming an increasingly accepted local treatment method for malignant liver tumours, the evaluation of the therapeutic response is extremely important for correctly deciding whether further treatment is necessary. Preferably, as most RFA are guided by ultrasound, application of ultrasound for evaluation of the therapeutic response is most suitable. Blomley et al [2] first suggested that the transit time of a contrast agent from injection to its arrival in the hepatic vein could be a simple marker for diagnosis of metastatic spread to the liver, as it was shown to be shortened in seven patients with liver metastases. Bernatik et al [3, 4] improved the method by measuring transit time from the hepatic artery to the hepatic vein directly and showing that this HTT is a reliable indicator of the presence of metastatic liver disease [4]. In our study, findings showed no difference between patients before and after RFA with incomplete treatment.

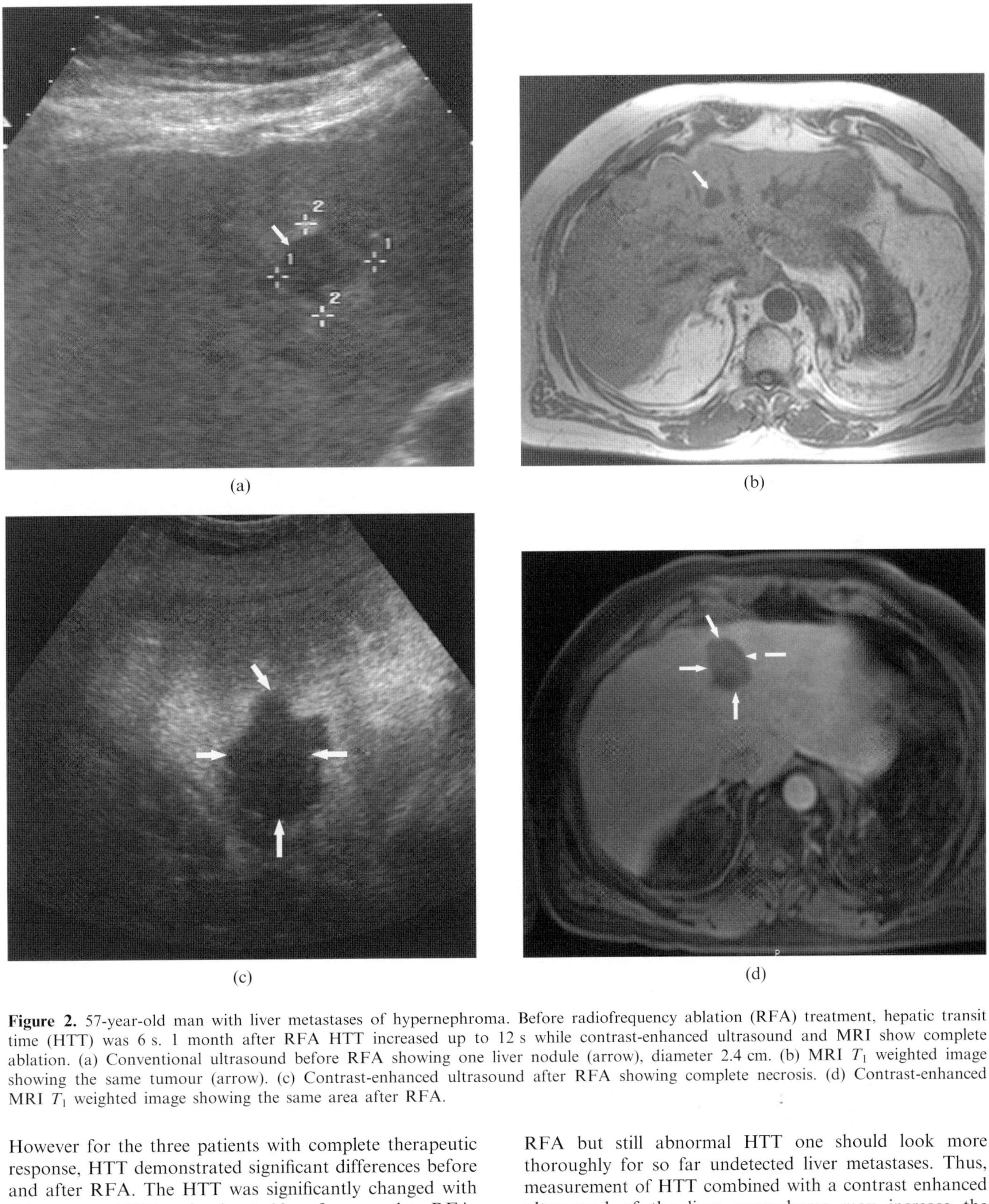

Figure 2. 57-year-old man with liver metastases of hypernephroma. Before radiofrequency ablation (RFA) treatment, hepatic transit time (HTT) was 6 s. 1 month after RFA HTT increased up to 12 s while contrast-enhanced ultrasound and MRI show complete ablation. (a) Conventional ultrasound before RFA showing one liver nodule (arrow), diameter 2.4 cm. (b) MRI T_1 weighted image showing the same tumour (arrow). (c) Contrast-enhanced ultrasound after RFA showing complete necrosis. (d) Contrast-enhanced MRI T_1 weighted image showing the same area after RFA.

However for the three patients with complete therapeutic response, HTT demonstrated significant differences before and after RFA. The HTT was significantly changed with delay rate $\geqslant$100% and value $\geqslant$10 s after complete RFA. Normal cut-off point of 10 s for HTT corresponded well with previous report, where no patient with proven liver metastases showed HTT of more than 10 s [4].

HTT may be a sensitive and practical indicator for assessing effectiveness of RFA. Achieving normalization of the HTT, might indicate the therapy being complete. On the other hand in patients with complete necrosis after RFA but still abnormal HTT one should look more thoroughly for so far undetected liver metastases. Thus, measurement of HTT combined with a contrast enhanced ultrasound of the liver parenchyma may increase the detection sensitivity for metastasis by drawing attention to patients with abnormal HTT.

This pilot study suggests that CT, MRI or contrast-enhanced ultrasound together with HTT may be a promising protocol for therapeutic assessment following liver ablation, and larger numbers are needed in future studies to evaluate the potential of the technique.

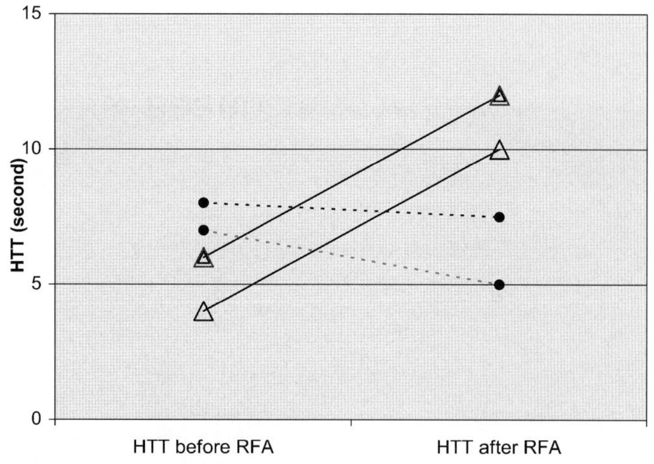

Figure 3. Diagram showing hepatic transit times (HTT) before and after radiofrequency ablation (RFA) (△ patients showing complete response after RFA, ♦ patients with incomplete response).

References

1. Solbiati L, Livraghi T, Goldberg SN, et al. Percutaneous radio-frequency ablation of hepatic metastases from colorectal cancer: long-term results in 117 patients. Radiology 2001;221:159–66.
2. Blomley MJ, Albrecht T, Cosgrove DO, et al. Liver vascular transit time analyzed with dynamic hepatic venography with bolus injections of the US contrast agent: early experience in seven patients with metastases. Radiology 1998;209:862–6.
3. Bernatik T, Becker D, Neureiter D, et al. Hepatic transit time of an echo enhancer: an indicator of metastatic spread to the liver. Eur J Gastroenterol Hepatol 2004;16:313–7.
4. Bernatik T, Strobel D, Haensler J, Hahn EG, Becker D. Hepatic transit time of an ultrasound echo enhancer indicating the presence of liver metastases – first clinical results. Ultraschall Med 2002;23:91–5.

The British Journal of Radiology, 78 (2005), 437–440
DOI: 10.1259/bjr/45172814

Case report

Pulmonary blastoma: presentation of two atypical cases and review of the literature

[1]R I WALKER, MRCP, [2]K SUVARNA, MRCP FRCPath and [1]S MATTHEWS, MRCP, FRCR

Departments of [1]Radiology and [2]Pathology, Northern General Hospital, Herries Road, Sheffield S5 7AU, UK

Abstract. Pulmonary blastoma is a relatively rare aggressive adult malignancy. The clinical and radiographic features of two cases are described and the literature reviewed. Pulmonary blastoma usually presents radiologically as a well-defined mass lesion on chest radiography, which may be large enough to completely opacify the hemithorax and cause mediastinal shift. On CT, pulmonary blastoma is seen as a mixed solid and cystic lesion with variable contrast enhancement and a necrotic centre. Pleural effusion may be present but is not the predominant abnormality. Our cases are unusual as recurrent pleural effusions in the absence of a significant lung mass were the presenting findings.

Pulmonary blastomas are a relatively rare group of primary lung neoplasms that are composed of immature malignant epithelial and/or mesenchymal tissues whose features may resemble early embryological lung tissues [1]. First described by Barnard in 1952, they have been divided into three subgroups – classic pulmonary blastoma (PB), well-differentiated fetal adenocarcinoma (WDFA) and pleuropulmonary blastoma (PPB) of childhood [1, 2]. The radiological appearance of PB is typically described as a well-circumscribed mass lesion [3, 4]. We present two cases of classic biphasic pulmonary blastoma (CBPB) which presented with pleural disease as the main abnormality.

Case reports

Case 1

A 21-year-old white Caucasian woman presented with a 3 week history of shortness of breath, non-productive cough, fever and right-sided non-pleuritic chest pain. She had received two courses of oral antibiotics without improvement in her symptoms. She was a non-smoker, who was previously fit and well. Signs of a right pleural effusion led to a clinical diagnosis of empyema. Initial investigations showed a neutrophil leucocytosis (19×10^9 l^{-1}), thrombocytosis (745×10^9 l^{-1}), reduced serum albumin (26 g l^{-1}) and mild liver impairment (AST 71 IU l^{-1}). On the chest radiograph there was complete opacification of the right hemithorax with contralateral mediastinal shift consistent with a large pleural effusion (Figure 1). A litre of blood stained pleural fluid was removed at pleurocentesis. Cytopathological examination of the pleural fluid revealed a poorly cellular specimen with mixed inflammatory cells, mesothelial cells and no evidence of malignancy. Bacterial cultures of the pleural fluid were negative. A contrast enhanced CT of the thorax confirmed a large right pleural effusion with associated mediastinal shift and almost complete collapse of the right lung. In addition, multiple ring enhancing cystic structures were identified in the pleural space. There was extensive mediastinal lymphadenopathy predominantly involving the right paratracheal, precarinal and subcarinal locations (Figure 2). No abnormality was seen in the left hemithorax or upper abdomen.

The patient was transferred to the regional cardiothoracic surgical centre for further management. Complete drainage of the pleural effusion was unsuccessfully attempted via an intercostal drain. Hence, she underwent a right thoracotomy and decortication. At surgery the pleura was extensively thickened. The pleural cavity revealed large masses of debris with adherent deposits on the diaphragm. The right middle lobe was obliterated. Large pericardial lymph nodes were found and sampled.

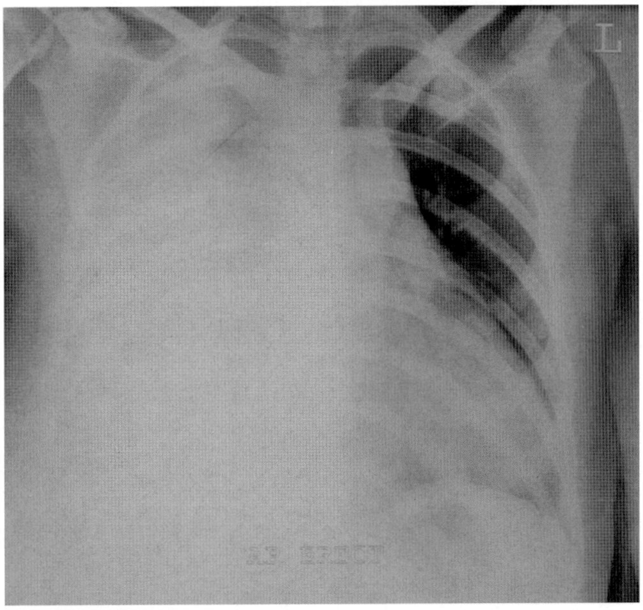

Figure 1. Case 1: Chest radiograph at presentation shows complete opacification of the right hemithorax with contralateral mediastinal shift.

Received 13 August 2004 and in revised form 12 November 2004, accepted 5 January 2005.

Address correspondence to Dr S Matthews, Consultant Radiologist.

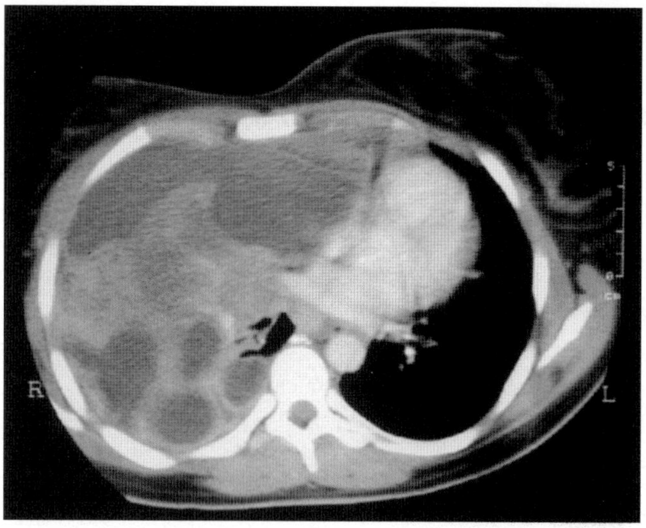

Figure 2. Case 1: Enhanced CT of the thorax showing a large right pleural effusion with contralateral mediastinal shift, mediastinal lymphadenopathy and multiple ring enhancing cystic structures within the pleural cavity.

The pathology examination revealed fragments of thickened pleural tissue with sheets of pleomorphic immature cells. Scattered mitoses were present together with widespread areas of irregular necrosis. Immunohistochemistry revealed positive pan-cytokeratin staining in addition to reactivity for BerEp4, CK7 and EMA. Negative reactions were seen with thyroglobulin, CA125, PLAP, CD45, CD56, CEA, vimentin, CD34, CD31 and CD99. The overall appearances were consistent with a PB (Figure 3).

Her post-operative course was complicated by a deep vein thrombosis in the right internal jugular vein. A subsequent CT scan revealed significant residual tumour medially within the right upper hemithorax and extensive mediastinal lymphadenopathy, features of superior vena cava obstruction (requiring stent insertion) and lymphangitis in the right upper lobe. She commenced chemotherapy but her disease progressed with the development of bone metastases. She died less than 6 months after initial presentation.

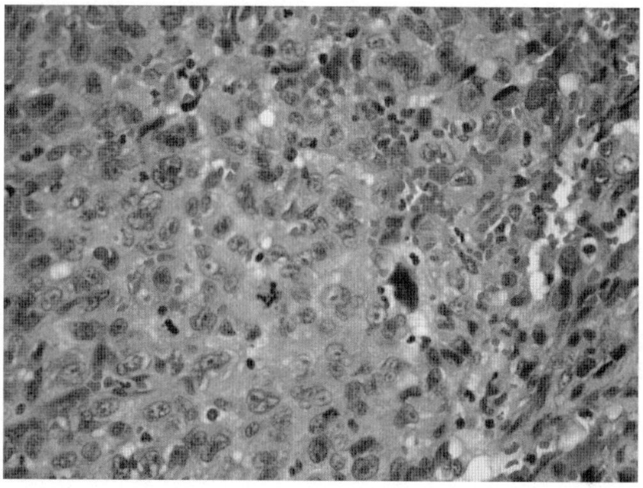

Figure 3. Case 1: Histological specimen showing highly pleomorphic polygonal cells with pronounced nuclear atypia. (Haematoxylin and eosin stain, magnification $\times 400$).

Case 2

A 41-year-old white Caucasian woman presented with a 2 month history of shortness of breath and chest pain. She was a smoker (five per day) but had no significant past medical or therapeutic history. Clinical examination was unremarkable. Investigations revealed a normocytic normochromic anaemia (Hb 7.9 g dl^{-1}), neutrophil leucocytosis ($25 \times 10^9\ l^{-1}$), thrombocytosis ($658 \times 10^9\ l^{-1}$), reduced serum albumin (30 g l^{-1}) and raised inflammatory markers (ESR 105, CRP 113). The chest radiograph showed a small left pleural effusion that was confirmed on ultrasound (Figure 4a). At diagnostic aspiration, the pleural fluid was heavily blood stained. No evidence of malignancy was detected at cytopathological examination. Culture of the pleural fluid was negative.

1 month after the initial presentation, the patient developed progressive shortness of breath owing to enlargement of the pleural effusion (Figure 4b) and complained of tingling and paraesthesia in her arms. A CT head scan showed two enhancing mass lesions in her right frontal lobe consistent with cerebral metastases. A CT of the thorax demonstrated a large left pleural effusion with contralateral shift of the mediastinum (Figures 5a,b). There was extensive diffuse pleural thickening involving the mediastinal pleural and multiple enhancing cystic structures within the pleural space. There was mild enlargement of the subcarinal lymph nodes. At bronchoscopy, there was complete obstruction to the left lower lobe bronchus but no endobronchial lesion was identified. The patient was transferred to the regional cardiothoracic surgical centre and underwent left thoracotomy and mediastinoscopy. At thoracotomy, a large quantity of organized blood clot and a partially necrotic left lower lobe was found. The haematoma was evacuated and a partial left lower lobectomy was performed.

Histology revealed irregular haemorrhagic and partly necrotic beige tissue fragments containing a high grade epithelioid neoplasm with polygonal cells showing a high nuclear: cytoplasmic ratio. Immunohistochemistry revealed positive cytokeratin, EMA and vimentin reactivity. No staining was seen with cytokeratin 5/6, calretinin, AFP, CD34, CD31, S100 protein, HMB45, PLAP, BerEp4, CA19.9, CA125, alpha-actin, desmin and AUA1. The findings were consistent with a high grade PB.

Cranial palliative radiotherapy was given. Post-operative imaging showed increasing infiltration of her lung. She was treated symptomatically, and died 4 months after the initial presentation.

Discussion

PB is a rare tumour accounting for 0.25–0.5% of malignant lung neoplasms [1, 5]. Originally termed "embryoma" by Barnard in 1952 [2], the term blastoma was introduced in 1961 by Spencer to reflect that the tumours arise from the pulmonary blastema in a similar manner to other tumours developing from fetal tissue

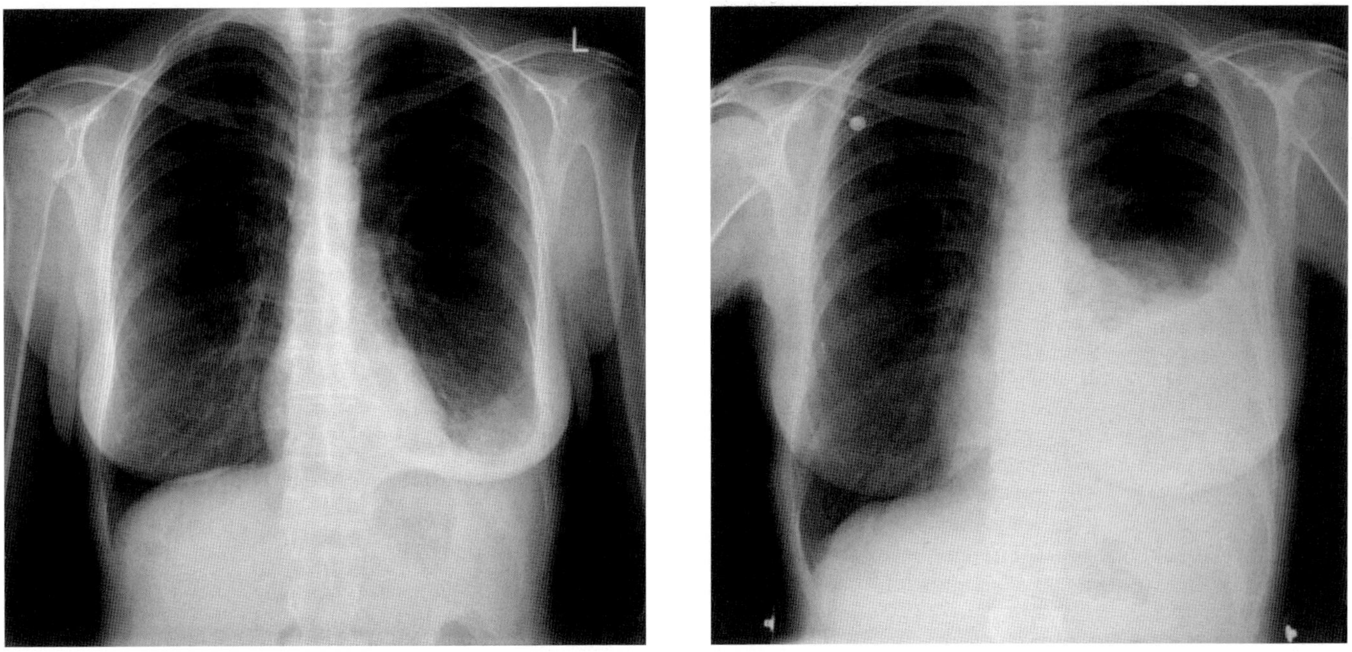

(a) (b)

Figure 4. Case 2: Serial chest radiographs demonstrating (a) the presenting chest radiograph and (b) enlargement of the left pleural effusion 1 month later.

[6]. Subsequently PB have been further subdivided by Koss et al [1] into three categories: CBPB, WDFA and PPB. CBPB is the most common of these three subtypes.

WDFA usually affects middle-aged adults, often with a tobacco smoking history, and has a pathogenesis similar to that of bronchogenic carcinoma. Prognosis is usually better than bronchogenic carcinoma. PPB are rare intrathoracic tumours, occurring predominantly in children less than 3 years old. Approximately 80% of CBPB occurs in adults [1]. However, two peaks in age are described in the first and fourth decades and cases have been reported from 0 to 80 years [5]. There is a slight male predominance. In adults there is an association with cigarette smoking and in children CBPB has been seen in association with pre-existing benign cysts of the lung [3, 5, 7]. A p53 gene mutation with or without p53 protein overproduction has been linked to both CBPB and WDFA [8]. Yousem et al consider that CBPB develop from a pluripotent blastema that gives rise to the epithelial and mesenchymal tumour components [9]. This view is supported by the observed simultaneous expression of cytokeratin and vimentin in the blastomatous component. These pluripotent cells may be stimulated through genetic and/or environmental influences to differentiate.

In general CBPB presents with non-specific respiratory symptoms that may mimic a respiratory tract infection: cough, haemoptysis, dyspnoea and chest pain [8]. 40% of cases are asymptomatic and found coincidentally on chest

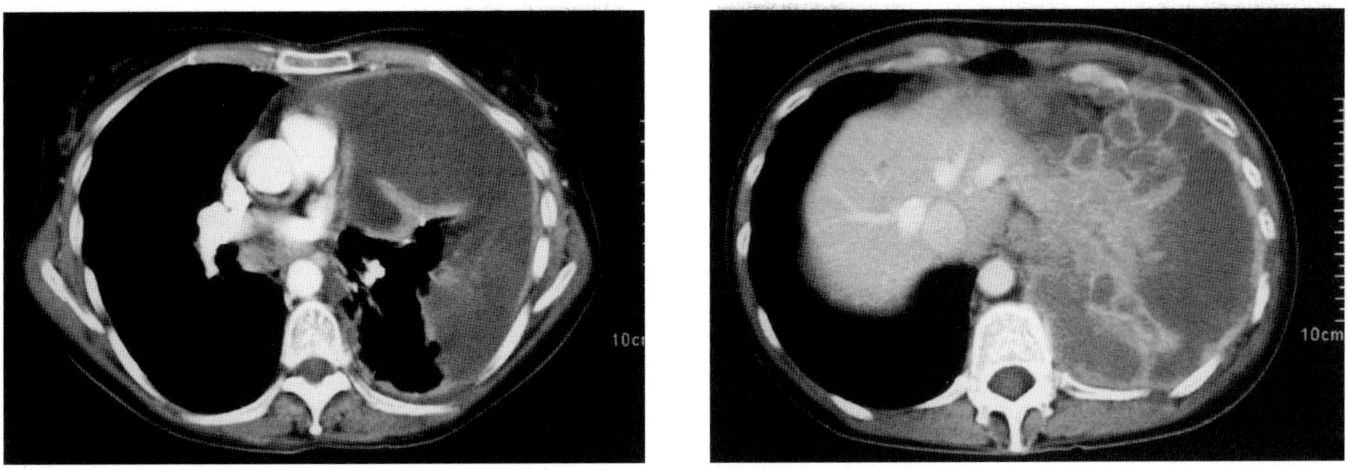

(a) (b)

Figure 5. Case 2: Contrast enhanced CT of the thorax showing (a) a left pleural effusion with mediastinal shift and diffuse mediastinal pleural thickening and (b) multiple enhancing pleural cysts with peripheral pleural thickening.

radiographs performed for other indications. The chest radiographic appearance usually consists of a well-circumscribed mass measuring 1.5 cm to 13 cm in diameter [1, 3, 4]. In children the lesion often completely fills the affected hemithorax to produce contralateral mediastinal shift [3]. In adults the lesion usually presents as a solitary peripheral nodule [3]. The tumour appears to be located either peripherally or centrally and there is no definite lobar predominance. In children pre-existing lung disease may be noted. CBPB may rarely present as a spontaneous pneumothorax [10, 11]. There has been a single case of PB presenting as a chronic lobulated pleural effusion that was initially diagnosed as pleural tuberculosis [12]. On ultrasound CBPB presents as an echogenic or mixed echogenic mass that may contain cystic areas [13]. This is comparable with the CT appearance of a partly solid/partly cystic lesion with a necrotic centre [8, 11]. The mass may have a whorled appearance and display variable contrast enhancement. The presence of pleural or mediastinal involvement is an indication of metastatic disease.

PB is an aggressive tumour associated with a poor prognosis. Surgery is the preferred treatment, often with post-operative adjuvant chemotherapy and/or radiotherapy [3]. Prognosis is worse if the tumour is larger than 5 cm at presentation. Distant metastases are frequently seen.

Our cases are unusual as in both cases pleural effusion was the predominant abnormality and a pulmonary mass lesion was not evident. In Case 1 empyema was the original working diagnosis. Ultrasound or CT of the chest ultimately revealed a more complex problem, with a multicystic enhancing intrapleural mass. The diagnosis ultimately required histology. In both cases the presentation and radiology were more in keeping with pleuropulmonary blastoma, a tumour of childhood. There have been several reported cases of PPB simulating chronic empyema [14, 15]. The CT scan in PPB has been reported to show multilocular cystic lesions in the pleural space similar to our cases [16]. These similarities may reflect the common origin from the pulmonary blastema.

These cases highlight the importance of excluding a malignant cause for a pleural effusion, even in young adults, and that PB should be considered in the differential diagnosis.

Acknowledgments

We would like to acknowledge the contributions of Mr R Vaughan and Mr D Hopkinson; the thoracic surgeons involved in managing the patients' care.

References

1. Koss M, Travis W, Moran C. Pulmonary sarcomas, blastomas, carcinosarcomas and Teratomas. Spencer's Histopathology of the Lung (5th edn). New York, NY: McGraw Hill, 1996:1092–100.
2. Barnard WG. Embryoma of lung. Thorax 1952;7:299.
3. Senac MO, Wood BP, Isaacs H, Weller M. Pulmonary blastoma: a rare childhood malignancy. Radiology 1991;179: 743–6.
4. Ohara N, Tominaga O, Oka T, et al. Pulmonary blastoma: report of a case. Surg Today 1999;29:385–8.
5. Larsen H, Sorenson JB. Pulmonary blastoma: a review with special emphasis on prognosis and treatment. Cancer Treat Rev 1996;22:145–60.
6. Spencer H. Pulmonary blastomas. J Pathol Bacteriol 1961;82:161–5.
7. Koss MN, Hochholzer L, O'Leary T. Pulmonary blastomas. Cancer 1991;67:2368–81.
8. Bini A, Ansaloni L, Grani G, Grazia M, Pagani D, Stella F, et al. Pulmonary blastoma: report of 2 cases. Surg Today 2001;31:438–42.
9. Yousem SA, Wick MR, Randhawa P, Manivel JC. Pulmonary blastoma: an immunohistochemical analysis with comparison with fetal lung in its pseudoglandular stage. Am J Clin Path 1990;93:167–75.
10. Ohtomo K, Araki T, Yashiro N, Iio M. Pulmonary blastoma in children. Radiology 1983;147:101–4.
11. Shyamkumar NK, Athyal RP, Govindarajuli G, Narayan VP, Rangad F, Govil S, et al. Pneumothorax preceding pulmonary blastoma in a child. Australas Radiol 2001;45:387–9.
12. Chin NK, Lee CN, Lee YS, Tan WC. Pulmonary blastoma in an adult presenting as a chronic loculated effusion: a diagnostic problem. Thorax 1994;49:838–9.
13. Saks AM. Case of the season. Semin Roentgenol 1995;30: 222–3.
14. Katz DS, Scalzetti EM, Groskin SA, Kohman LJ, Patel LS, Landas S. Pleuropulmonary blastoma simulating empyema in a young child. J Thorac Imaging 1995;10:112–6.
15. Merriman TE, Beasley SW, Chow CW, Smith PJ, Robertson CF. A rare tumor masquerading as an empyema: pleuropulmonary blastoma. Pediatr Pulmonol 1996;22:408–11.
16. Hill DA, Sadeghi S, Schultz MZ, Burr JS, Dehner LP. Pleuropulmonary blastoma in an adult. Cancer 1999;85:2368–74.

The British Journal of Radiology, 78 (2005), 441–443
DOI: 10.1259/bjr/91312352

Case report

Solid-pseudopapillary tumour of the pancreas associated with dorsal agenesis

[1]S ULUSAN, MD, [2]N BAL, MD, [1]O KIZILKILIC, MD, [2]F BOLAT, MD, [3]S YILDIRIM, MD, [1]T YILDIRIM, MD and [1]E A NIRON, MD

Departments of [1]Radiology, [2]Pathology and [3]Surgery Baskent University Adana Teaching and Medical Research Centre, 01250 Yuregir, Adana, Turkey

Abstract. Solid-pseudopapillary tumour of the pancreas is a rare benign or low-grade malignant epithelial tumour; its association with pancreatic dorsal agenesis has been reported only once before. We present the radiological and histological findings of a case of pancreatic solid-pseudopapillary tumour associated with total pancreatic dorsal agenesis. A 49-year-old woman presented with abdominal pain radiating to the back for several months. Radiological findings showed absence of the dorsal pancreas and an 8 cm × 6 cm diameter tumour arising from the head of the pancreas. She underwent successful complete resection of the tumour. Histopathology revealed a diagnosis of solid-pseudopapillary tumour.

Solid-pseudopapillary tumour (SPT) of the pancreas is a rare benign or low-grade malignant epithelial tumour occurring predominantly in women, accounting for 1–2% of exocrine pancreatic tumours at most institutions. It was first described by Frantz in 1959, and is also known as a solid and cystic tumour, solid and papillary epithelial neoplasm, papillary-cystic neoplasm, papillary cystic tumour and Frantz tumour. In 1996, The World Health Organization (WHO) gave a new name to this tumour as solid-pseudopapillary tumour of the pancreas [1–3]. Pancreatic anomalies are occasionally reported and association of partial agenesis of the dorsal pancreas has been reported once [4–8].

Case report

A 49-year-old woman presented with abdominal pain that radiated to the back for several months. Physical examination was unremarkable. She had non-insulin dependent diabetes mellitus diagnosed 12 months earlier. Laboratory investigations including bilirubin, aspartate transaminase, carcinoembryogenic antigen (CEA), alpha-fetoprotein (AFP), and serum glucose level were all normal. Carbohydrate antigen (CA) 19-9 was elevated at 70.42 U ml^{-1} (normal range 0–37 U ml^{-1}).

Abdominal ultrasound (US) revealed an 8 cm × 6 cm mass containing peripheral calcification in the pancreatic head. The biliary tree was not dilated. Non contrast abdominal and pelvic CT confirmed a well defined 8 cm × 6 cm mass lesion in the pancreatic head, with linear peripheral calcification, containing central cystic-necrosis. The mass displaced the adjacent superior mesenteric vein minimally and infiltrated into the second part of duodenum (Figure 1a,b). There was no normal cephalic pancreatic tissue separate from the mass and complete absence of dorsal pancreatic parenchyma anterior to the splenic vessels artery and vein was also noted (Figure 1c).

The patient was referred for surgical resection. At laparotomy, there was no body or tail of the pancreas present, and the 8 cm × 6 cm mass in the head of the pancreas appeared to have grown exophytically. Invasion into the second part of the duodenum, with adherence to the superior mesenteric and portal veins was observed. The patient underwent a pancreatoduodenectomy (Whipple's procedure). In the post-operative period she developed insulin-dependent diabetes. At post-operative follow-up her of CA 19-9 levels returned to normal.

On pathological examination; the tumour mass was greyish brown in colour and measured 6 cm × 6 cm × 8 cm in size macroscopically with a lobulated surface. The cut surface of the mass had solid, cystic, haemorrhagic and calcified areas. Microscopic examination revealed a solid, cystic and pseudopapillary growth pattern. Haemorrhage, calcification and hyalinization were seen. Tumour cells had small round nuclei with fine chromatin, inconspicuous nucleoli and moderate eosinophilic cytoplasm. The cystic areas were filled with erythrocytes and foamy histiocytes. Immunohistochemical examination revealed diffuse positivity for vimentin, and focal positivity for keratin (Figure 2), consistent with a SPT of the pancreas.

Discussion

SPT of the pancreas is a rare primary pancreatic neoplasm of unknown aetiology, occurring most commonly in young women. Its malignancy rate is low and has a good prognosis after surgical removal [1–3, 9, 10]. Grossly, these large tumours have solid, haemorrhagic, calcified and cystic areas. Histologically, they have, cystic and pseudopapillary components. Kosmahl et al [11] reported that the immunocytochemical phenotype of SPT of the pancreas were characterized by vimentin,

Received 10 August 2004 and in revised form 18 November 2004, accepted 5 January 2005.

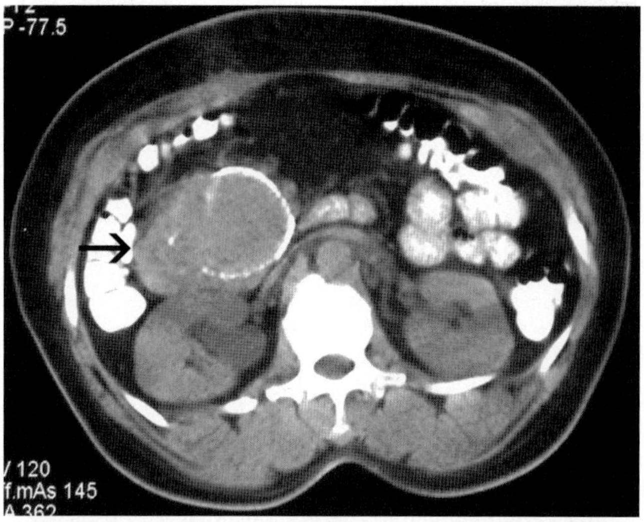

(a)

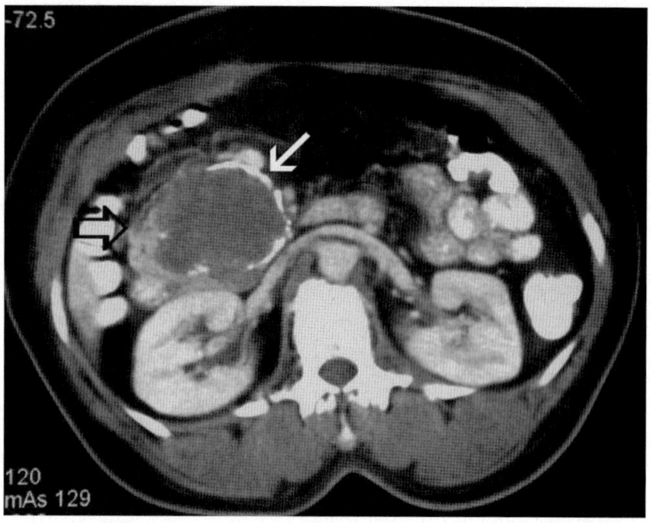

(b)

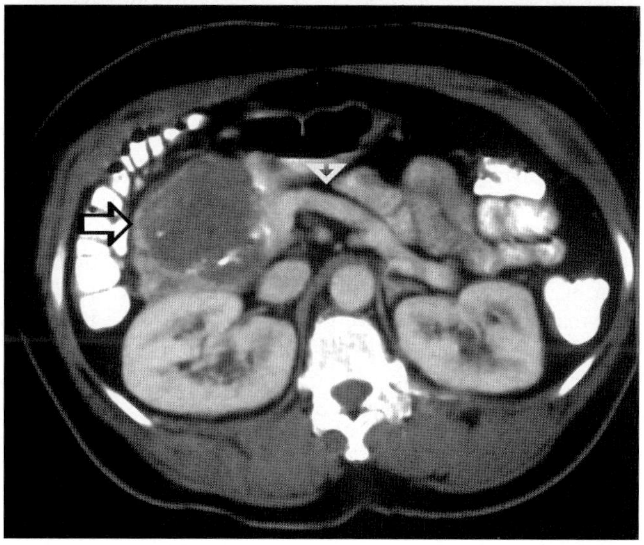

(c)

Figure 1. (a) Non-contrast enhanced CT scan shows a large mass (thin black arrow) in the head of the pancreas with characteristic solid and cystic components and peripherally calcification. (b) Contrast-enhanced CT scan shows contrast enhancement of solid component (open arrow) and peripheral calcification (thin white arrow). (c) Axial curved reformatted CT image shows the mass (open arrow) and splenic vein (arrowhead).

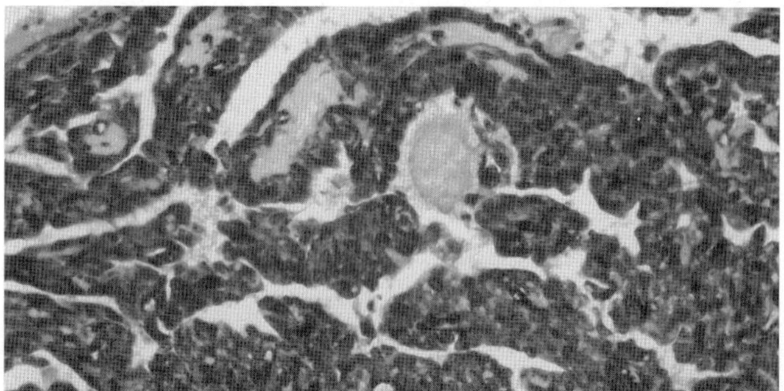

Figure 2. Vimentin positivity in tumour cells (Vimentin × 200).

neuron-specific enolase (NSE) and alpha-1 antitrypsine stain positivity in over 90% of cases, whereas cytokeratin-stains, positive in most epithelial tumours are usually negative. Our patient had all the macroscopic features and microscopic components described previously.

Embryologically the pancreas grows dorsal and ventral buds originating from the endodermal lining of the duodenum. During the seventh gestational week, the ventral buds turn posteriorly and to the left, connecting with the dorsal bud. Each of the pancreatic buds grow into a pair of branching, arborized ductal systems. The neck, body, tail and the cephalic aspect of the head of the pancreas originate from the dorsal bud. The ventral bud becomes the inferior portion of the head and the uncinate process [5–7]. The pancreas divisum is the most common anomaly of the pancreas in autopsy series with prevalence as high as 5–10% [5–7]. Other common pancreatic anomalies include an annular pancreas and agenesis of either the ventral or the dorsal bud. Complete agenesis of the pancreas is extremely rare and not compatible with life [5–7]. The exact frequency of dorsal agenesis of the pancreas is not known, and has been reported only rarely.

Since most islets cells are located in the tail and body of the pancreas, agenesis of the dorsal pancreas results in significant loss of beta-cells which impaired insulin secreting capacity [8] and as in our patient may result in the development of diabetes.

A CT diagnosis of dorsal pancreatic agenesis can be made when the presence of normal pancreatic head and absence of pancreatic tissue (body and tail) ventral to the splenic vein are demonstrated [4, 5, 7]. The CT findings of SPT of the pancreas are: non-contrast images show a well encapsulated mass with varying solid and cystic components owing to haemorrhagic degeneration, and contrast enhanced images show enhancement of solid areas peripherally, with cystic areas more centrally located [1–3, 11]. The presence of calcification in this tumour is not uncommon [1–3], as in our case.

The distribution of SPT of the pancreas are within the head in 32%, and body and/or tail of the pancreas in 68% of cases [8].

The tumour markers (CEA, CA19-9) are almost always negative in SPT of the pancreas [1–3, 8, 9], although our patient had an elevated serum levels of CA19-9. The elevation of tumour markers may be helpful diagnostically and on follow-up.

The only case of previously reported SPT of pancreas associated with pancreatic dorsal agenesis was by Nakamura et al, and as they demonstrated a pancreatic accessory duct with endoscopic retrograde cholangiopancreatography, they suggested there was partial pancreatic dorsal agenesis [8]. In contrast, our CT findings were of a calcified part solid and cystic mass with complete pancreatic dorsal agenesis.

References

1. Coleman KM, Doherty MC, Bigler SA. Solid-pseudopapillary tumour of the pancreas. Radiographics 2003;23:1644–8.
2. Klimstra DS, Wenig BM, Heffess CS. Solid-pseudopapillary tumour of the pancreas: a typically cystic carcinoma of low malignant potential. Semin Diagn Pathol 2000;17:66–80.
3. Pettinato G, Di Vizio D, Manivel C, Pambuccian SE, Somma P, Insabato L. Solid-pseudopapillary tumour of the pancreas: a neoplasm with distinct and highly characteristic cytological features. Diagn Cytopathol 2002;27:325–34.
4. Nonent M, Linard J, Leveque E, Larroche P, Bobeuf J, Senecail B. Dorsal pancreas agenesis: computed tomography appearance with three-dimensional volume rendering reconstruction. Surg Radiol Anat 2003;25:161–3.
5. Shah KK, DeRidder PH, Schwab RE, Alexander TJ. CT diagnosis of dorsal pancreas agenesis. J Comput Assist Tomogr 1987;11:170–1.
6. Macari M, Giovanniello G, Blair L, Krinsky G. Diagnosis of agenesis of the dorsal pancreas with MR pancreatography. AJR Am J Roentgenol 1998;170:144–6.
7. Soler R, Rodríguez E, Comesana ML, Pombo F, Marini M. Agenesis of the dorsal pancreas with polysplenia syndrome: CT features. J Comput Assist Tomogr 1992;16:921–3.
8. Nakamura Y, Egami K, Maeda S, Hosone M, Onda M. Solid and papillary tumour of the pancreas complicating agenesis of the dorsal pancreas. J Hepatobiliary Pancreat Surg 2001;8:485–9.
9. Potrc S, Kavalar R, Horvat M, Gadzijev EM. Urgent Whipple resection for solid-pseudopapillary tumour of the pancreas. J Hepatobiliary Pancreat Surg 2003;10:386–9.
10. Mancini GJ, Dudrick PS, Grindstaff AD, Bell JL. Solid-pseudopapillary tumour of the pancreas. Two cases in male patients. Am Surg 2004;70:29–31.
11. Kosmahl M, Seada LS, Janig U, Harms D, Kloppel G. Solid-pseudopapillary tumour of the pancreas: its origin revisited. Virchows Arch 2000;436:473–80.

The British Journal of Radiology, 78 (2005), 444–446 © 2005 The British Institute of Radiology
DOI: 10.1259/bjr/73238635

Case report

Myoepithelial carcinoma of the breast: a case report with imaging and pathological findings

[1]E K WOO, MRCP (UK), [2]A D JAMES, FRCS, [3]J MERCER, MRCPath, [2]S M ALLAN, FRCS and [1]D C HOWLETT, MRCP (UK), FRCR

Departments of [1]Radiology, [2]Breast Surgery and [3]Histopathology, Eastbourne District General Hospital, Kings Drive, Eastbourne, East Sussex BN21 2UD, UK

Abstract. We present a case of myoepithelial carcinoma of the breast together with illustrations of the imaging and pathological appearances as well as discussion on the management of this condition.

Adenomyoepithelioma of the breast is an unusual benign tumour characterized by biphasic proliferation of epithelial and myoepithelial cells. Malignant change is extremely rare and may involve both cellular components – myoepithelial carcinoma. We present a case of myoepithelial carcinoma together with illustrations of the imaging and pathological appearances as well as discussion on the management of this condition.

Case report

A 70-year-old female presented with a recent onset of a painless left-sided breast lump. Clinical examination revealed a firm mass in the outer lower quadrant with no axillary lymphadenopathy palpable. A mammogram was performed. This was technically difficult owing to the patient's immobility and only a lateral oblique view was feasible. This showed an ill-defined mass in the inferior aspect of the left breast (Figure 1). Subsequent ultrasound examination demonstrated a rounded, hypoechoic solid lesion with the margins ill-defined in part suspicious of malignancy (Figure 2). Fine needle aspiration was performed which confirmed malignant cytology. Chest radiograph and liver ultrasound did not show any evidence of metastatic disease. The patient had a significant history of coronary heart disease and therefore a decision was made to excise the lesion under local anaesthesia.

Histology showed a 15 mm × 15 mm × 10 mm well-circumscribed solid mass, which appeared pale on slicing with a central area of necrosis. It consisted of islands and tubular structures composed of epitheloid cells surrounded by a fibrous stroma. Many of the epitheloid cells had clear cytoplasm. They had moderately pleomorphic nuclei and a high mitotic rate. At the periphery of the lesion there were strands of epitheloid cells, which appeared to infiltrate the stroma (Figure 3). Immunocytochemical staining showed strong positive staining for S100 protein (Figure 4). There was positive staining for cellular adhesion molecule (CAM 5.2) and for other individual cytokeratins. These appearances were diagnostic for myoepithelial carcinoma.

Received 6 September 2004 and accepted 17 January 2005.

Address correspondence to Dr David Howlett, Consultant Radiologist.

Discussion

Adenomyoepithelioma of the breast is an unusual benign tumour, first described in 1970 [1] and is

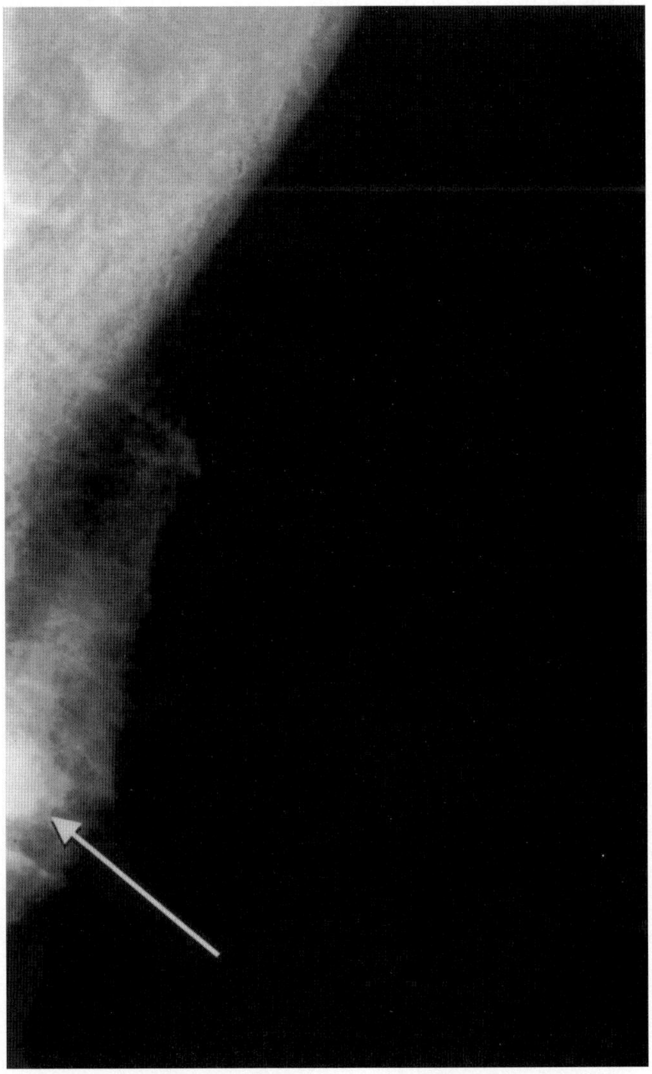

Figure 1. Lateral oblique mammogram of the left breast. An ill-defined opacity is seen inferiorly (arrow).

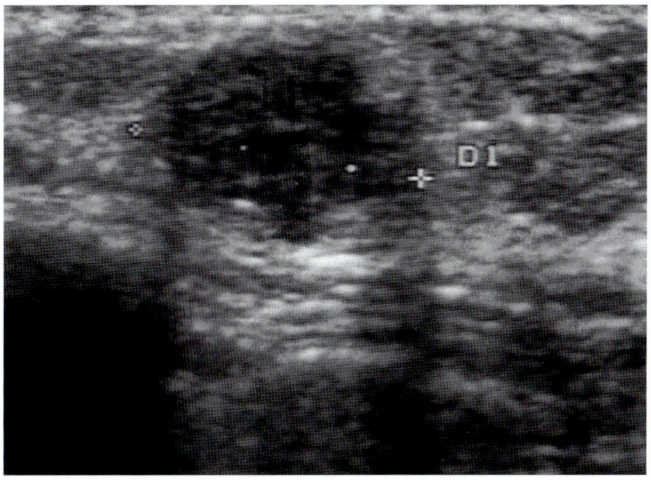

Figure 2. Left breast ultrasound shows a rounded, hypoechoic solid lesion with the borders ill-defined in part.

characterized by biphasic proliferation of epithelial and myoepithelial cellular constituents. Recent reports have indicated that one or both of the cellular constituents may undergo malignant change, myoepithelial carcinoma, although this is extremely rare [2–6]. Metastases from myoepithelial carcinoma are described and appear to be haematogenous rather than lymphatic and they also appear to be restricted to primary tumours greater than 2 cm [7–12]. These tumours are prone to local recurrence as is adenomyoepithelioma and can be predicted by narrow or incomplete excision margins [6].

Clinically, myoepithelial carcinoma presents as a rapidly enlarging mass, which may be tender and is often laterally placed in the breast [3].

The imaging findings of myoepithelial carcinoma do appear to be non-specific [2]. In our patient, as in previous cases, both mammography and ultrasound showed features suspicious for malignancy confirmed on cytology. Myoepithelial carcinoma may be difficult to diagnose specifically cytologically and core biopsy may be more accurate.

Histologically, the myoepithelial cells frequently have clear cytoplasm and immunohistochemically typically stain

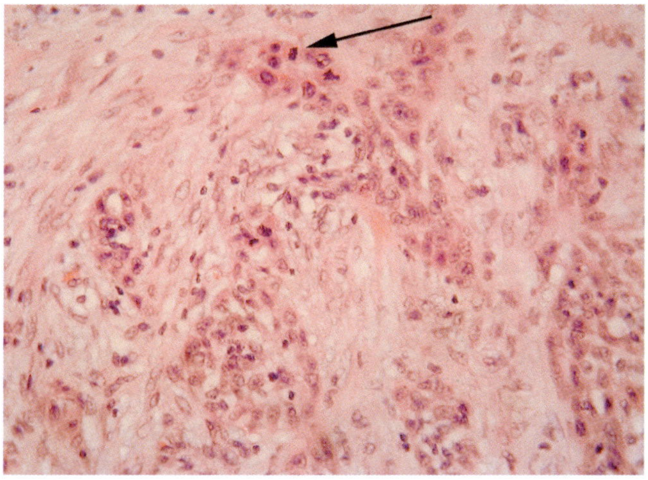

Figure 3. Haematoxylin and eosin high power view of the tumour margin showing infiltration of the stroma and mitosis (arrow).

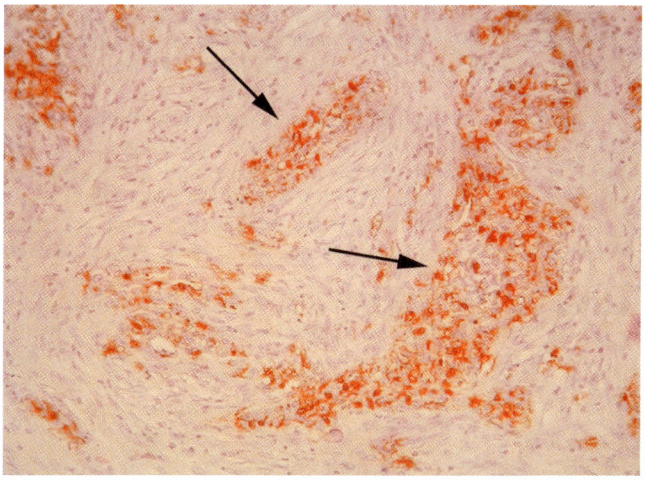

Figure 4. Positive staining for S100 (brown – arrows) in the myoepithelial component.

for S100, CAM5.2 and other cytokeratins. Malignant transformation of the cellular components indicates a carcinoma. Currently, surgical management of this rare malignant tumour is similar to that for other breast malignancy namely wide local excision or mastectomy with axillary surgery if appropriate. The response to chemotherapy and radiotherapy is unknown. If following wide local excision, the excision margin is narrow or incomplete, re-excision is advised to gain adequate margins.

In conclusion, myoepithelial carcinoma is a rare tumour, which should be considered in the differential diagnosis of a solid breast lesion. The imaging findings appear to be non-specific reflecting the malignant nature of the tumour. Surgeons and radiologists should be aware of its potential for local recurrence following wide local excision and the possibility of haematogenous rather than lymphatic metastases.

Acknowledgments

The authors would like to thank Nick Taylor for preparing the illustrations.

References

1. Hamperl H. The myothelia (myoepithelial cells): normal state; Regressive changes; hyperplasia; tumors. Curr Top Pathol 1970;53:161–220.
2. Howlett DC, Mason CH, Biswas S, Sangle PD, Rubin G, Allan SM. Adenomyoepithelioma of the breast: spectrum of disease with associated imaging and pathology. AJR Am J Roentgenol 2003;180:799–803.
3. Tavassoli FA. Myoepithelial lesions of the breast. Myoepitheliosis, adenomyoepithelioma, and myoepithelial carcinoma. Am J Surg Pathol 1991;15:554–68.
4. Rasbridge SA, Millis RR. Adenomyoepithelioma of the breast with malignant features. Virchows Arch 1998;432:123–30.
5. Pauwels C, De Potter C. Adenomyoepithelioma of the breast with features of malignancy. Histopathology 1994;24:94–6.

6. Loose JH, Patchefsky AS, Hollander IJ, Lavin LS, Cooper HS, Katz SM. Adenomyoepithelioma of the breast. A spectrum of biologic behavior. Am J Surg Pathol 1992;16:868–76.
7. Ahmed AA, Heller DS. Malignant adenomyoepithelioma of the breast with malignant proliferation of epithelial and myoepithelial elements: a case report and review of the literature. Arch Pathol Lab Med 2000;124:632–6.
8. Jones C, Tooze R, Lakhani SR. Malignant adenomyoepithelioma of the breast metastasizing to the liver. Virchows Arch 2003;442:504–6.
9. Kihara M, Yokomise H, Irie A, Kobayashi S, Kushida Y, Yamauchi A. Malignant adenomyoepithelioma of the breast with lung metastases: report of a case. Surg Today 2001;31:899–903.
10. Takahashi II, Tashiro H, Wakasugi K, Onohara T, Nishizaki T, Ishikawa T, et al. Malignant adenomyoepithelioma of the breast: a case with distant metastases. Breast Cancer 1999;6:73–7.
11. Bult P, Verwiel JM, Wobbes T, Kooy-Smits MM, Biert J, Holland R. Malignant adenomyoepithelioma of the breast with metastasis in the thyroid gland 12 years after excision of the primary tumor. Case report and review of the literature. Virchows Arch 2000;436:158–66.
12. Chen PC, Chen CK, Nicastri AD, Wait RB. Myoepithelial carcinoma of the breast with distant metastasis and accompanied by adenomyoepitheliomas. Histopathology 1994;24:543–8.

The British Journal of Radiology, 78 (2005), 447–449
DOI: 10.1259/bjr/31146905

Case report

Pericardial rupture and cardiac herniation after blunt trauma: a case diagnosed using cardiac MRI

[1]J H SOHN, MD, [1]J W SONG, MD, [1]J B SEO, MD, [1]K H DO, MD, [1]J S LEE, MD, [2]D K KIM, MD, [1]K S SONG, MD and [1]T H LIM, MD

Departments of [1]Radiology and [2]Thoracic and Cardiovascular Surgery, Asan Medical Center, University of Ulsan College of Medicine, 388-1 Poongnap-dong, Songpa-gu, Seoul 138-736, Korea

Abstract. Pericardial rupture following blunt chest trauma is rare, and is not usually diagnosed pre-operatively. If pericardial rupture is not recognized and treated promptly, it may be fatal owing to cardiac herniation. We report a case of traumatic herniation of the heart for which a CT scan and MRI made a major contribution to the diagnosis.

Pericardial rupture following blunt chest trauma is rare, and is not usually diagnosed pre-operatively, but should be suspected whenever there is severe blunt chest trauma. If pericardial rupture is not recognized and treated promptly, it may be fatal owing to cardiac herniation [1]. Few reports have emphasised the use of CT scanning as a tool for diagnosis and CT scan findings have not been well documented [2]; no report has emphasised the use of a MRI for diagnosis of the cardiac herniation. We report a case of traumatic herniation of the heart for which a CT scan and MRI made a major contribution to the diagnosis.

Case report

A 55-year-old man arrived at the emergency department following a road traffic accident. At initial examination, he was fully conscious and haemodynamically stable. The anteroposterior (AP) chest radiograph (Figure 1a) showed multiple broken ribs on both sides, pulmonary vascular congestion and a pneumomediastinum. The cardiac silhouette was enlarged mainly due to enlargement of the left ventricle.

A CT scan of the chest was performed using a General Electric Hi-speed (GE Medical Systems, Milwaukee, WI), slice thickness 7.5 mm, pitch=0.93, 0.5 s per rotation, at 140 kV and 200 mA with contrast enhancement. This CT examination confirmed bilateral haemopneumothoraces and multifocal patchy consolidations in the right upper and left lower lobes due to pulmonary contusion. The heart was displaced into the left hemithorax with clockwise rotation of the cardiac apex (Figure 2a). At the level of the ventricles, the anterior surface of the right ventricle showed a wavy and undulated contour with focal dimpling (Figure 2b). From these CT findings, a diagnosis of cardiac herniation was suggested. Clinically, there was doubt about the diagnostic suggestion of pericardial rupture with cardiac herniation because of the patient's good haemodynamic status and normal sinus rhythm on electrocardiogram. A follow-up chest radiograph showed improvement in the pulmonary contusion, however, the cardiac outline remained abnormal and there was collapse of the left lower lobe and a left pleural effusion (Figure 1b).

On the 12th day after admission, MRI of the chest was performed using a 1.5 T unit (Intera CV; Philips, DA, Netherlands). Cine MRI was performed in coronal images, using a breath-hold balanced fast field-echo sequence (repetition time/echo time (TR/TE) 3.4 ms/1.7 ms; flip angle 50°; field of view 350 mm; matrix 256×256; slice thickness 8 mm). MR examination showed clockwise rotation of the cardiac axis with compression of the left inferior pulmonary vein between the aorta and left ventricle with left lower lobe collapse. On the coronal cine MRI, there was an exaggerated up- and down-movement of the cardiac apex, separated from the left hemi-diaphragm by a left pleural effusion (Figure 3a, b). Because the separated movement between the cardiac apex and left hemi-diaphragm was distinct, pleuropericardial rupture and cardiac herniation was diagnosed.

On the 16 day after admission, the patient underwent a thoracotomy; this confirmed that the heart was dislocated from its pericardium, which was torn from the level of the left upper pulmonary vein to the left hemi-diaphragm and located within the left pleural cavity. The tear was vertical, 12 cm long, and located just behind the phrenic nerve. The heart was relocated and the pericardial tear was repaired.

Discussion

In a review of the literature, Clark et al [3] reported on 142 traumatic ruptures of the pericardium. The left pleuropericardium was injured in 71 (50%), the right pleuropericardium in 24 (17%), the diaphragmatic pericardium in 39 cases (27%) and the superior mediastinal pericardium in 6 cases (4%). A cardiac herniation was found in 31 of left and 5 of right pleuropericardial defects, and in 4 diaphragmatic tears of the pericardium. We have noted 55 additional cases of pericardial ruptures since 1987 on performing a literature search, 35 (64%) of the cases being complicated with cardiac herniation. In cases with

Received 5 August 2004 and in revised form 22 November 2004, accepted 17 January 2005.

Address correspondence to Jae-Woo Song.

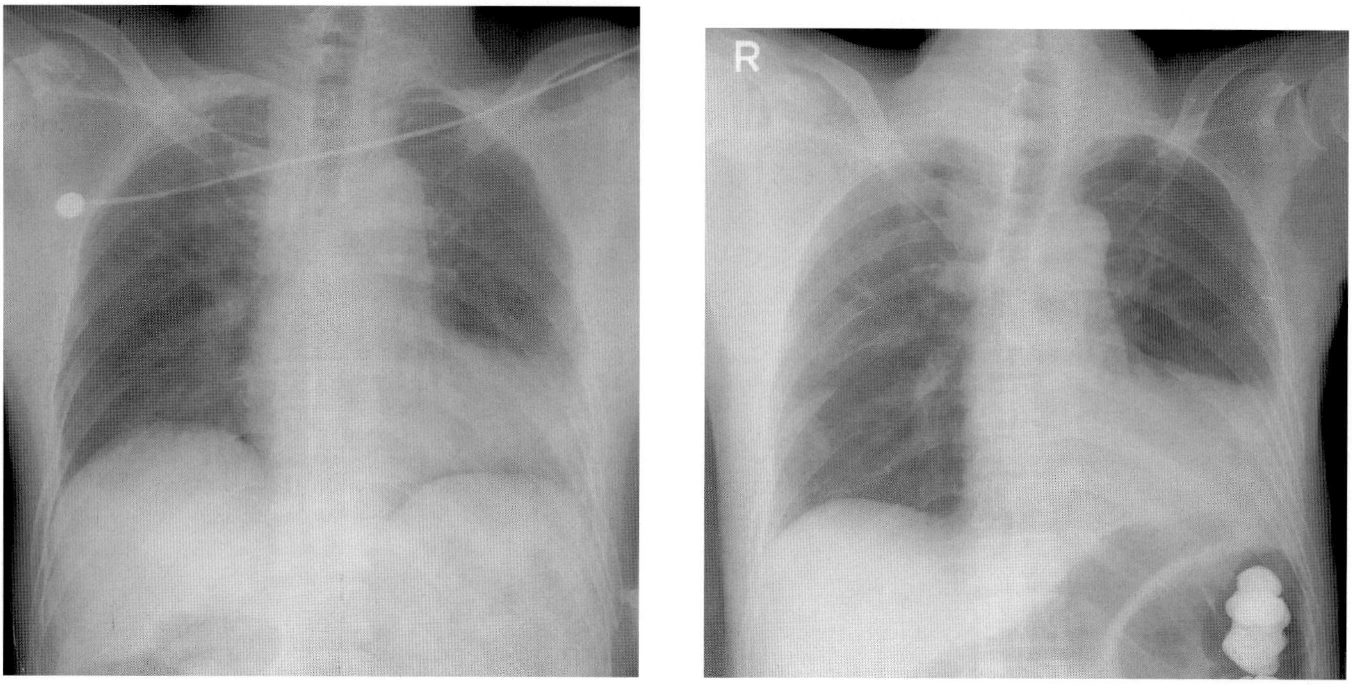

(a) (b)

Figure 1. 55-year-old man with history of road traffic accident. (a) The initial anteroposterior (AP) chest radiograph shows multiple broken ribs on both sides, pulmonary vascular congestion and pneumomediastinum. The heart shadow is enlarged mainly due to enlargement of the left ventricle. (b) On the 14th day after admission, the follow-up chest radiograph shows decreasing extent of the opacities owing to contusion and vascular congestion. However, the cardiac outline remains obliterated and there is collapse of the left lower lobe and left pleural effusion.

ruptured diaphragmatic pericardium, abdominal protrusion of viscera into the pericardial sac may occur, but cardiac herniation is rare. In ruptured pleuropericardium, the tear is most often located along the phrenic nerve and when the tear is large enough, the heart may be dislocated. Dislocation of the heart may result in a torsion along an axis made by the inferior vena cava and the great vessels with strangulation of the heart [4].

Pericardial rupture is often reported as an incidental finding at emergency thoracotomy or laparotomy in patients with multiple trauma. The survival rate of patients who reach hospital alive and are diagnosed as having pericardial rupture is poor, ranging from 36.4% to 42.9% [5, 6]. As cardiac herniation is more complicated, most of the reported survivors had stable haemodynamics on arrival and were treated promptly in hospital when cardiac herniation occurred a few days after admission. According to a report in the Japanese literature [7], a pre-operative diagnosis of cardiac herniation was made in four out of eight patients, by chest radiography in two, by cardiac angiography in one, and by chest CT in one patient. In the other four patients, the diagnosis was made incidentally at

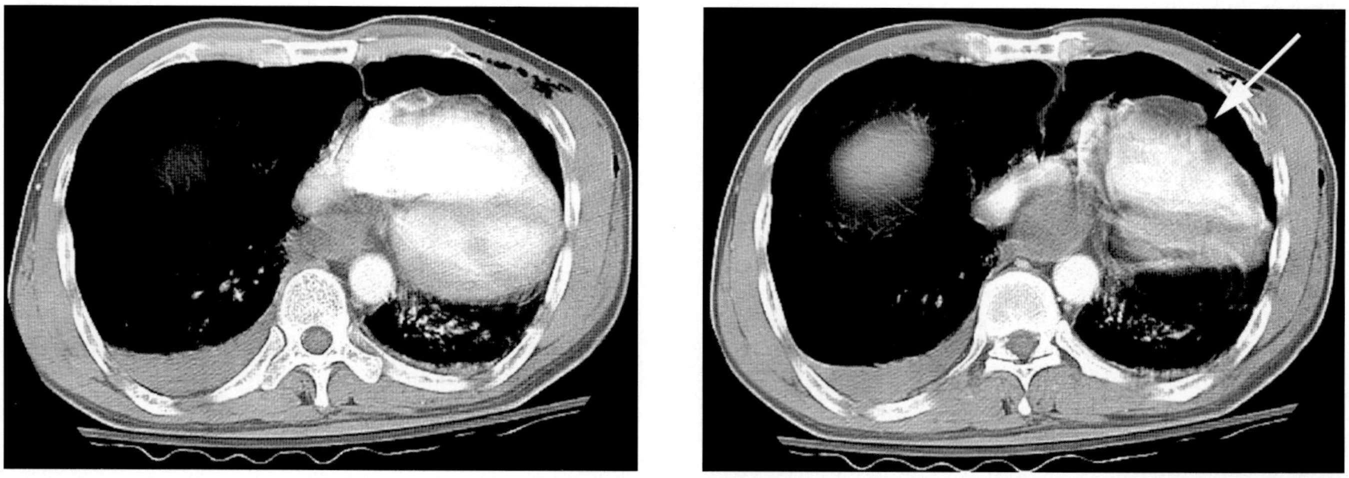

(a) (b)

Figure 2. Chest CT findings. (a, b) Chest CT scans show displacement of the heart and clockwise rotation of the cardiac apex. The anterior surface of the right ventricle shows a wavy and undulated contour with a focal dimpling (arrow in Figure 2b).

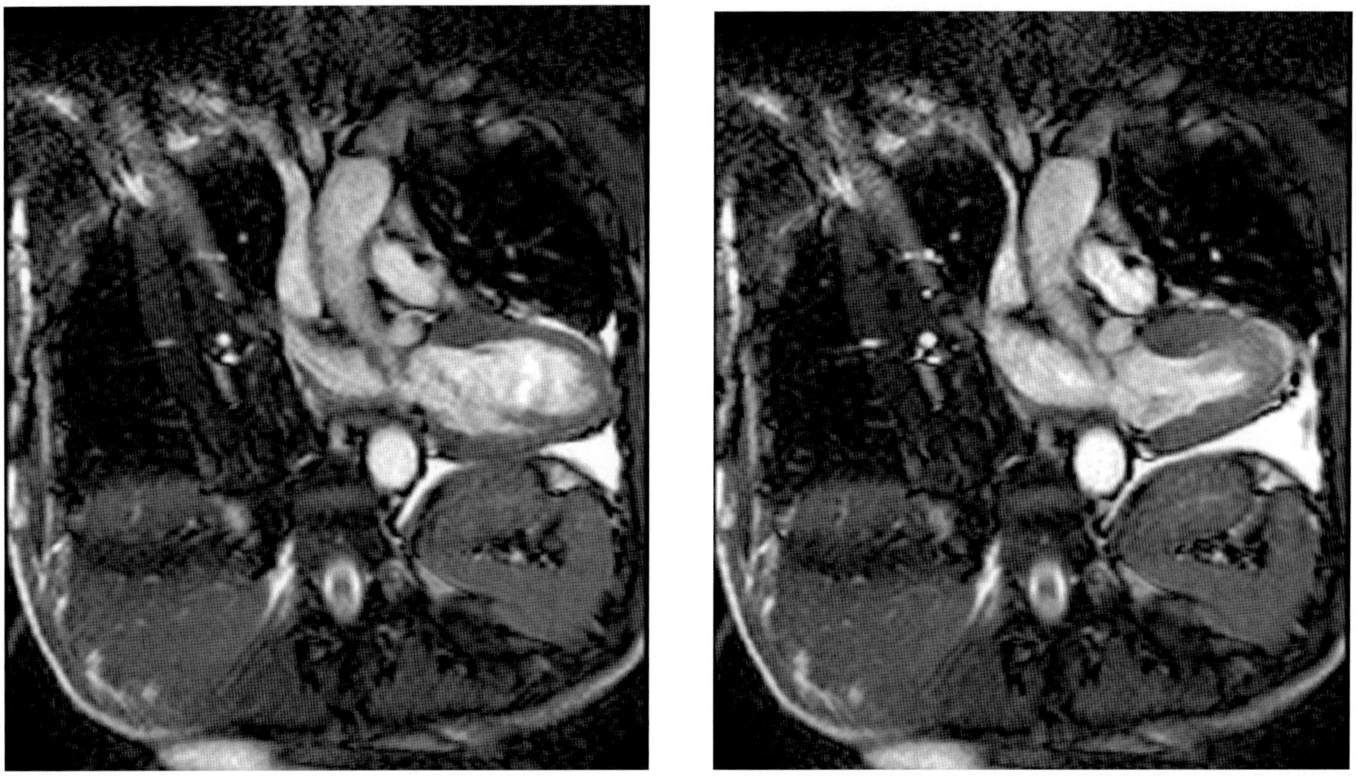

(a) (b)

Figure 3. Cardiac cine-MRI findings. (a) Coronal cine MRI at the diastolic and (b) systolic phases demonstrate an exaggerated up- and down-movement of the cardiac apex, separated from the left hemidiaphragm by pleural effusion, suggesting pleuropericardial rupture and cardiac herniation.

thoracotomy. The pericardial rupture was on the left side in six patients and on the right side in two, and all ruptures ran along the phrenic nerve.

When our patient was admitted to hospital, we suspected a pericardiac rupture with cardiac herniation on CT. This patient was a haemodynamically stable and transoesophageal echocardiogram did not find any sign of pericaridial tear or cardiac herniation, so this rare occurrence in cardiac dislocation made the diagnosis difficult. Surprisingly, haemodynamic conditions were preserved in the five cases of right cardiac herniation in report of Clark et al [3]. In our case, cardiac MRI confirmed the diagnosis of cardiac herniation. This case report describes the first known successful MRI diagnosis of cardiac herniation associated with traumatic rupture of the pericardium.

References

1. Janson JT, Harris DG, Pretorius J, Rossouw GJ. Pericardial rupture and cardiac herniation after blunt chest trauma. Ann Thorac Surg 2003;75:581–2.
2. Schir F, Thony F, Chavanon O, Perez-Moreira I, Blin D, Coulomb M. Blunt traumatic rupture of the pericardium with cardiac herniation: two cases diagnosed using computed tomography. Eur Radiol 2001;11:995–9.
3. Clark DE, Wiles C III, Lim MK, Dunham CM, Rodriguez A. Traumatic rupture of the pericardium. Surgery 1983;93:495–503.
4. Thomas P, Saux P, Lonjon T, et al. Diagnosis by video-assisted thoracoscopy of traumatic pericardial rupture with delayed luxation of the heart: case report. J Trauma 1995;38:967–70.
5. Kato K, Henmi H, Yamamoto Y, Mashiko K, Kimura A, Kushimoto Y, et al. An evaluation of blunt traumatic pericardial rupture (in Japanese with English abstract). JJAAM 1992;3:163–72.
6. Fulda G, Rodriguez A, Turney SZ, Cowlew RA. Blunt traumatic pericardilal rupture. A ten-year experience 1979 to 1989. J Cardiovas Surg 1990;31:525–30.
7. Matsuda S, Hatta T, Kurisu S, Ohyabu H, Koyama T, Kita Y. Traumatic cardiac herniation diagnosed by echocardiography and chest CT scanning: report of a case. Surg Today 1999;29:1221–4.

The British Journal of Radiology, 78 (2005), 450–452
DOI: 10.1259/bjr/62643156

Case report
Bilateral multilocular cystic nephromas: a rare occurrence

[1]K S SODHI, MD, [1]S SURI, MD, DABR, [2]R SAMUJH, MCh, [2]K L N RAO, MCh, FACS, FAMS, [3]K VAIPHEI, MD and [1]A K SAXENA, MD, DNB

Departments of [1]Radiodiagnosis, [2]Pediatric Surgery and [3]Histopathology, Postgraduate Institute of Medical Education and Research, (PGIMER), Chandigarh – 160 012, India

Abstract. We present a rare case of bilateral renal cystic tumours in an 18-month-old female child, which proved to be cystic nephromas on imaging and histopathology. Although unilateral cystic nephromas are known in children; the occurrence of bilateral tumours is rare.

Cystic nephroma, also called multilocular cystic nephroma is a rare renal neoplasm. Bilateral cystic nephromas are much rarer. In fact, unilaterality of the lesion was one of the eight initial diagnostic criteria proposed by Powell et al [1] and revised by Boggs and Kimmelstiel [2]. To the best of our knowledge, only 4 paediatric cases of bilateral cystic nephromas have been reported [3], including two cases with asynchronous involvement.

Case report

An 18-month-old female child presented with a complaint of a gradually increasing abdominal lump on the right side of the abdomen, present for the last 10 months. She had no history of fever, gastrointestinal or urinary complaints.

On examination, she was active, afebrile, well built, with a normal pulse, respiratory rate and blood pressure. Laboratory tests were normal with a creatinine of 1.0 mg dl^{-1}. Abdominal examination revealed a large, firm, smooth, mobile, cystic, non-tender mass in the right lumbar region, which crossed the midline. The left flank was normal. Ultrasound of the abdomen (Figure 1) and CT (Figure 2a,b), revealed the presence of large, well circumscribed, multiloculated, purely cystic masses, in both lumbar regions, arising from both kidneys. There was no evidence of calcification or fat within the lesions. The right sided mass compressed the head of the pancreas, the liver, gallbladder and spleen were normal, and there was no ascites or abdominal lymphadenopathy. Based on CT scan, diagnosis of cystic nephromas was made. The patient underwent bilateral partial nephrectomies. Histopathological examination of the resected tumours revealed numerous varying sized cystic structures, lined by flattened to low cuboidal cells, with intervening septae showing proliferating fibroblasts, thin walled vessels, lymphoid aggregates and few flattened tubules and glomeruli. No blastemal nodules or solid areas were seen. The histological diagnosis was of bilateral multilocular cystic nephromas.

Received 13 September 2004 and accepted 17 January 2005.

Discussion

Bilateral renal cystic tumours in children are an uncommon group of tumours and include cystic wilms tumour, renal lymphangiomatosis, tuberous sclerosis complex, cystic nephroma and cystic poorly differentiated nephroblastoma.

Of these, tuberous sclerosis complex consists of multiple angiomyolipomas and cysts, while renal lymphangiomatosis consists of multiple perirenal and parapelvic cysts. Both these entities can be easily diagnosed on imaging. The other three entities; cystic wilms tumour, cystic nephroma and cystic poorly differentiated nephroblastoma are less easily differentiated on imaging.

Cystic nephroma is an uncommon renal neoplasm, initially thought to only occur unilaterally. Powell et al [1] established eight diagnostic criteria for these lesions: unilateral involvement; solitary lesion; multilocular lesion; non-communication with the renal pelvis; non-communication of the cysts with each other; loculi lined by epithelium; intralocular septa devoid of renal parenchyma; and if residual renal tissue were present, it should be normal. Of these criteria, one was modified by Boggs and Kimmelstiel [2], several years later to include the presence of immature renal tissue in the intervening septa. These

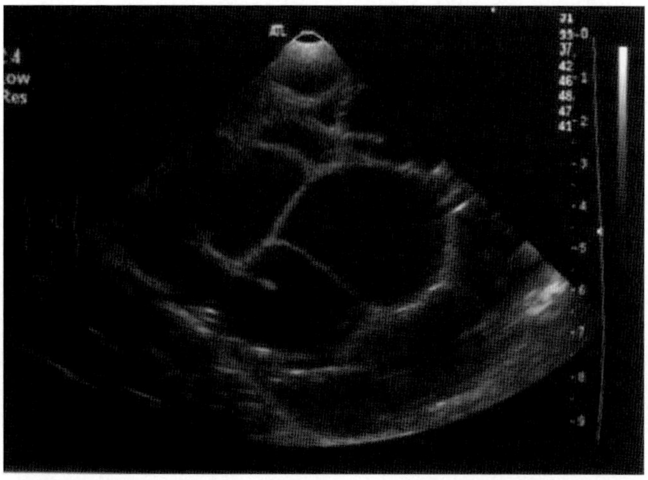

Figure 1. Ultrasound abdomen of an 18-month-old girl reveals a multiseptate cystic mass in the left hypochondrium.

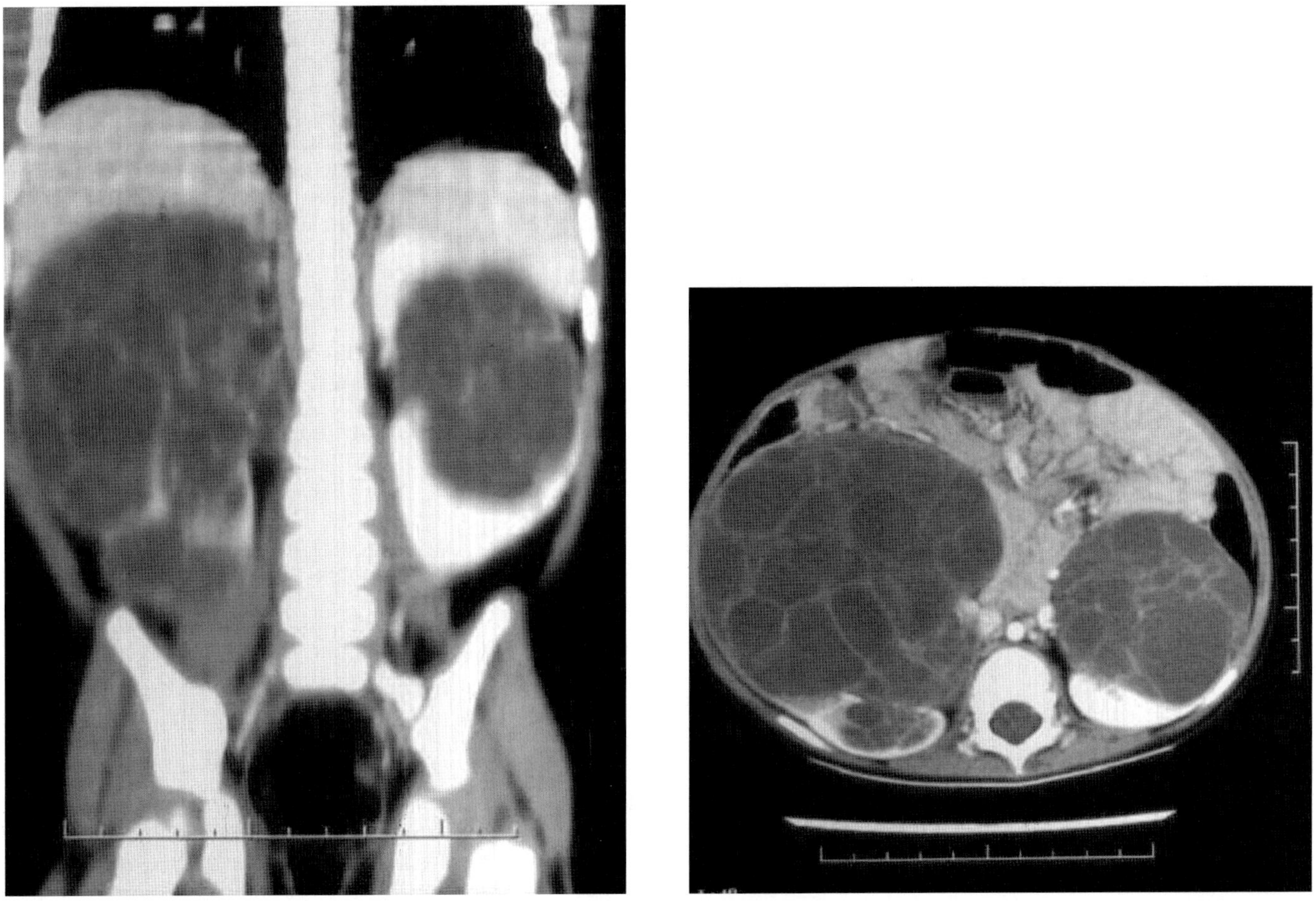

(a) (b)

Figure 2. (a) Coronal and (b) axial contrast enhanced CT abdomen of the same patient showing bilateral, cystic, multiseptate renal masses.

criteria have remained largely unchanged over the years, although more recently some authors have proposed the elimination of unilaterality as a diagnostic criteria [3].

Multilocular cystic renal tumours refer to two types of generally benign renal tumours: cystic nephroma (CN) and cystic poorly differentiated nephroblastoma (CPDN) [4, 5], although the other end of the spectrum does include cystic wilms tumours. These are well circumscribed, discrete lesions consisting entirely of cysts and septae, without solid tumour components except for the septae. These tumours generally follow a benign course; nephrectomy alone is usually curative, with rare local recurrences effectively managed by local radiation or chemotherapy.

These tumours usually present as an abdominal mass, in a young child between the ages of 3 months and 4 years [6]. The mass may slowly increase in size or may demonstrate rapid growth. Systemic symptoms are uncommon.

Cystic nephroma and cystic poorly differentiated nephroblastoma are indistinguishable on gross examination as well as on imaging. The masses are often large, averaging 8–10 cm in size and are single, unilateral, and involve only part of the kidney [4]. There is no communication between cysts or with the collecting system. Septae in CN are fibrous and may contain well-differentiated tubular structures; poorly differentiated tissues and blastemal cells are absent in the septae of CN. CPDN resembles CN in every feature except that the septae in CPDN contain blastemal cells with or without other embryonal stromal cells. It is important to note that that there are no solid elements (other than septae) in this lesion, differentiating the entity from wilms tumour and other renal neoplasms, which may contain cystic spaces owing to haemorrhage and necrosis [7].

Radiologically, plain film findings may demonstrate a soft tissue mass with displacement of bowel loops. Ultrasound demonstrates a complex intrarenal mass with acoustic enhancement. Septations, dividing the mass into discrete sonolucent locules, may be seen if the cysts are of sufficient size. When individual cysts are small however, ultrasound may demonstrate numerous internal echoes but no distinct loculations [6]. The findings of a peripheral crescentic rim of renal collecting system, is helpful to confirm the renal origin of the tumour. On CT, a sharply circumscribed, multiseptated mass is demonstrated, with cystic spaces between septae. The contents of the cysts may be similar to or slightly greater than water attenuation. In some tumours the cystic spaces are very small, resulting in the appearance of a solid soft tissue mass. Enhancement of septae may be seen following intravenous contrast; however, no filling of cystic spaces with contrast occurs [6]. MRI demonstrates an encapsulated multilocular renal mass, with the capsule showing low signal intensity on all pulse sequences, variable signal intensity of cyst contents on T_1 weighted images, and high signal intensity of cyst contents on T_2 weighted images [4]. All cases of CN follow a benign course and renal sparing surgery is the optimal treatment described for this lesion [3].

However, CPDN may demonstrate more aggressive behaviour with a potential for recurrence following resection. Since these two entities cannot be distinguished by imaging or by gross appearance, the treatment is complete surgical resection, with non-invasive imaging for follow-up if the tumour proves to be CPDN.

In conclusion, although cystic nephromas in children are more commonly unilateral, they may also rarely occur bilaterally and need to be differentiated from other cystic renal tumours of childhood.

References

1. Powell T, Shackman R, Johnson H. Multilocular cysts of the kidney. J Urol 1951;23:142–52.
2. Boggs LK, Kimmelstiel P. Beningn multilocular cystic nephroma: a report of two cases of so-called multilocular cyst of the kidney. J Urol 1956;76:530–41.
3. Ferrer FA, McKenna PH. Partial nephrectomy in a metachronous mutlilocular cyst of the kidney (cystic nephroma). J Urol 1994;151:1358–60.
4. Geller E, Smergel EM, Lowry PA. Renal neoplasms of childhood. Radiol Clin North Am 1997;35:1391–413.
5. Joshi V, Beckwith JE. Multi locular cyst of the kidney (cystic nephroma) and cystic, partially differentiated nephroblastoma. Cancer 1989;64:466–79.
6. Madewell J, Goldman S, Daris C, et al. Multilocular cystic nephroma: a radiographic pathologic correlation of 58 patients. Radiology 1983;146:309–21.
7. Agrons G, Wagner B, Davidson A, et al. Multi locular cystic renal tumour in children: radiologic-pathologic correlation. Radiographics 1995;15:653–69.

The British Journal of Radiology, *78* (2005), 453–456
DOI: 10.1259/bjr/12679319

Case report

Hepatic artery pseudoaneurysm after liver transplantation: definitive treatment with a stent-graft after failed coil embolisation

[1]G MALEUX, MD, [2]J PIRENNE, MD, PhD, [2]R AERTS, MD and [3]F NEVENS, MD, PhD

Departments of [1]Radiology, [2]Abdominal Transplantation Surgery and [3]Hepatology, University Hospitals Gasthuisberg, Herestraat 49, B-3000 Leuven, Belgium

Abstract. A 69-year-old woman presented with massive upper gastrointestinal bleeding owing to a ruptured hepatic pseudoaneurysm located at the surgical arterial anastomosis, 2 months after combined liver and kidney transplantation. Initially the pseudoaneurysm was successfully coiled but 3 weeks later recurrence of her symptoms occurred. Hepatic angiography revealed partial reperfusion of the coiled pseudoaneurysm; definitive treatment was performed by placement of an expanded-polytetrafluoroethylene (e-PTFE) covered coronary stent-graft, completely excluding the pseudoaneurysm. Radiological follow-up studies demonstrate a patent stent-graft functioning normally.

Formation of a pseudoaneurysm of the hepatic artery after liver transplantation is a rare, but potentially lethal complication. Pseudoaneurysms usually occur within the first months following transplantation and can present either with aspecific pain symptoms or massive upper gastrointestinal bleeding and haemodynamic shock. Classic treatment options include surgical resection of the pseudoaneurysm and revascularization of the injured vessel segment, ligation of the hepatic artery, retransplantation or radiological coil embolisation with preservation of the arterial flow to the graft. We report on a case of a bleeding extrahepatic pseudoaneurysm of the hepatic artery in a liver transplant patient, initially treated by coil embolisation, and definitively managed 3 weeks later by implantation of a stent-graft.

Case report

A 69-year-old woman with primary biliary cirrhosis was referred because of a rapidly progressive deterioration of liver function, jaundice, oesophageal varices, grade II encephalopathy and refractory ascites. The Child-Pugh score was C12. Additionally the patient developed irreversible hepatorenal syndrome. 4 months later, she subsequently underwent combined orthotopic liver and kidney transplantation. A standard orthotopic liver transplant was first performed through a bisubcostal incision and was followed by a classic heterotopic kidney transplant in the iliac fossa. Arterial reperfusion of the liver graft was via an end-to-end hepatic artery anastomosis, using the native hepatic artery just above the gastroduodenal artery and a patch of donor coeliac trunk. Arterial anastomosis was performed using a running suture 7-0 prolene. Portal reperfusion was via an end-to-end anastomosis between the donor and the recipient portal vein (running suture 5-0 prolene). Bile duct reconstruction was with a duct-to-duct anastomosis using running 5-0 polydioxanone. Her post transplant course was uneventful except for a biliary stricture that developed 13 days post transplant that required biliary dilatation and endoscopic placement of a polyethylene biliary stent. The patient gradually recovered and left the hospital 47 days after the combined transplantation. At day 73 post-transplantation the patient suddenly developed haemodynamic shock with massive upper gastrointestinal bleeding. After resuscitation and blood transfusion, hepatic angiography was performed, detecting a false aneurysm arising at the arterial anastomosis (Figure 1a). Superselective catheterization using a microcatheter (Prowler Plus; Cordis, Johnson & Johnson, Miami, FL) and packing of the aneurysmal lumen using microcoils (Boston Scientific Target, Fremont, CA) eventually stopped the bleeding (Figure 1b). Although the patient suffered a myocardial infarction during her hypovolemic shock, the post embolisation course was uneventful.

3 weeks later, the patient presented with recurrent symptoms of upper gastrointestinal bleeding and haemodynamic shock. Emergency visceral angiography was performed and revealed partial revascularization of the hepatic artery false aneurysm (Figure 2a). Because of the rather broad neck of the aneurysm and the rapid recurrence of bleeding, additional coil embolisation was not considered the best treatment option. Because of her moribund condition (shock, age, recent myocardial infarction), it was thought that she would not be fit enough to tolerate open surgery, and the decision to place a balloon-expandable coronary stent-graft (Jostent coronary stent-graft; Jomed, Rangendingen, Germany) was made. After insertion of a 7 French sheath (Terumo Europe, Leuven, Belgium) in the right groin, a 7 French hockey-stick guiding catheter (Cordis, Roden, The Netherlands) was placed in the hepatic artery. A stent-graft, mounted on a monorail stent-delivery catheter was constructed using a sandwich technique, whereby an ultra

Received 1 June 2004 and in final form 29 November 2004, accepted 26 January 2005.

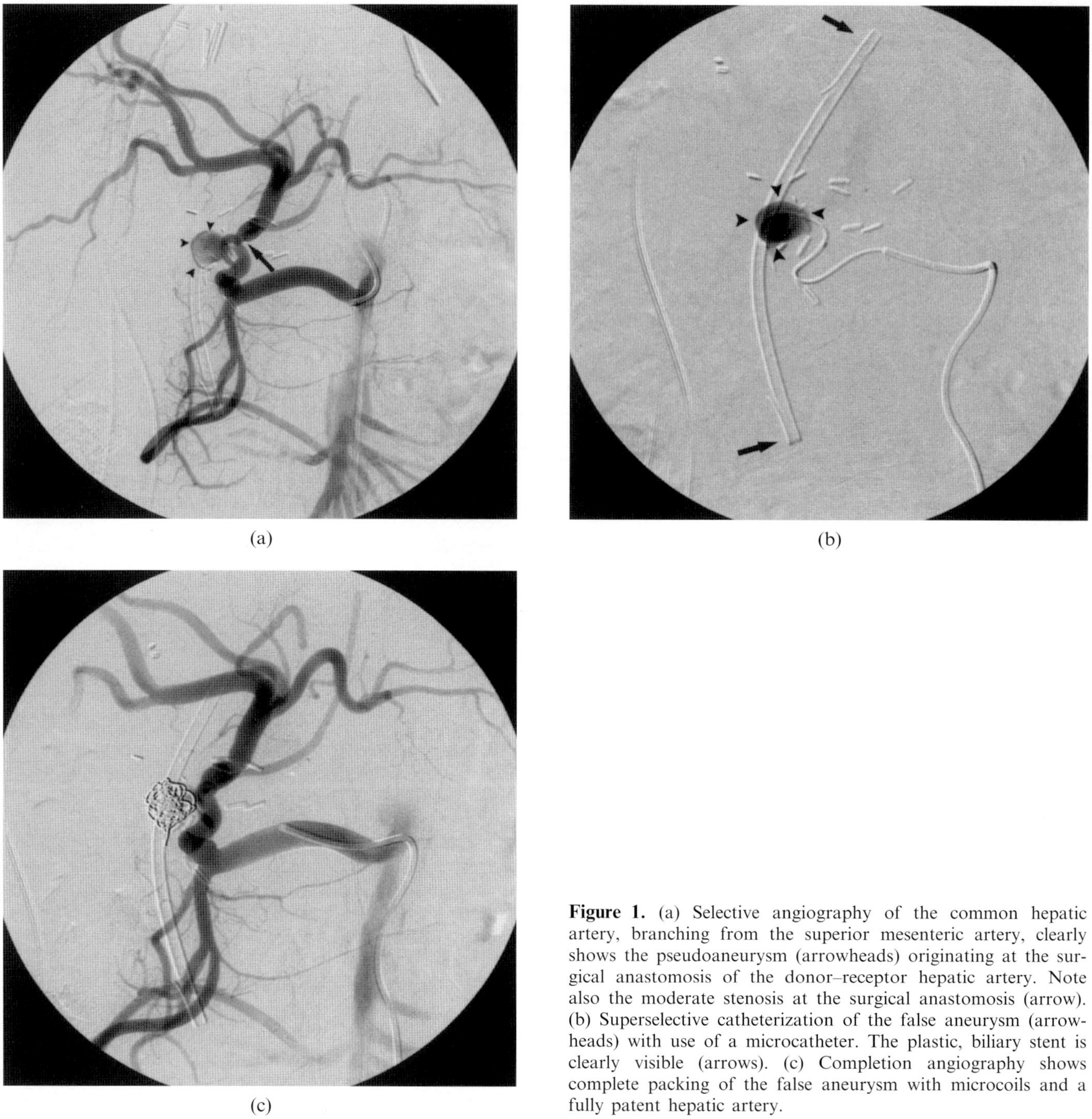

Figure 1. (a) Selective angiography of the common hepatic artery, branching from the superior mesenteric artery, clearly shows the pseudoaneurysm (arrowheads) originating at the surgical anastomosis of the donor–receptor hepatic artery. Note also the moderate stenosis at the surgical anastomosis (arrow). (b) Superselective catheterization of the false aneurysm (arrowheads) with use of a microcatheter. The plastic, biliary stent is clearly visible (arrows). (c) Completion angiography shows complete packing of the false aneurysm with microcoils and a fully patent hepatic artery.

thin layer of e-PTFE is placed between two stainless steel stents. The stent-graft having a length of 12 mm was expanded up to 5 mm diameter and placed completely covering the neck of the false aneurysm, resulting in complete exclusion of the aneurysm and preservation of the arterial blood flow to the graft. The patient became haemodynamically stable after the procedure without evidence of further bleeding and recovered well after this second episode of massive haemorrhage. For the first 2 months past stent-graft placement a daily administration of 75 mg of clopidogrel (Plavix; Sanofi Pharma, Paris, France) was prescribed to prevent early stent thrombosis. Follow-up of 20 months has shown no recurrence of bleeding. Duplex-ultrasound of the hepatic artery shows a normal arterial signal; multislice CT-angiography at 6 months and MR-angiography 9 months post-stent insertion revealed a normally patent extrahepatic and intrahepatic artery; the stented segment itself could not be adequately examined because of the major artefacts of the metallic stent-skeleton and the adjacent micro coils. At last follow-up (14 months) liver function tests were normal.

Discussion

Hepatic artery pseudoaneurysms are a rare complication after liver transplantation and have an incidence of between 0.3% and 1.3% [1]. Clinical presentation may be non-specific with unexplained fever or biliary colic, or

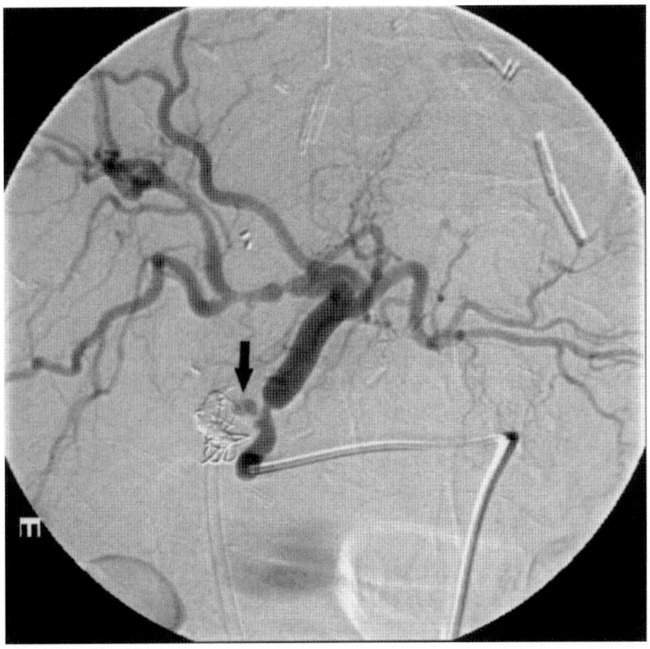

(a)

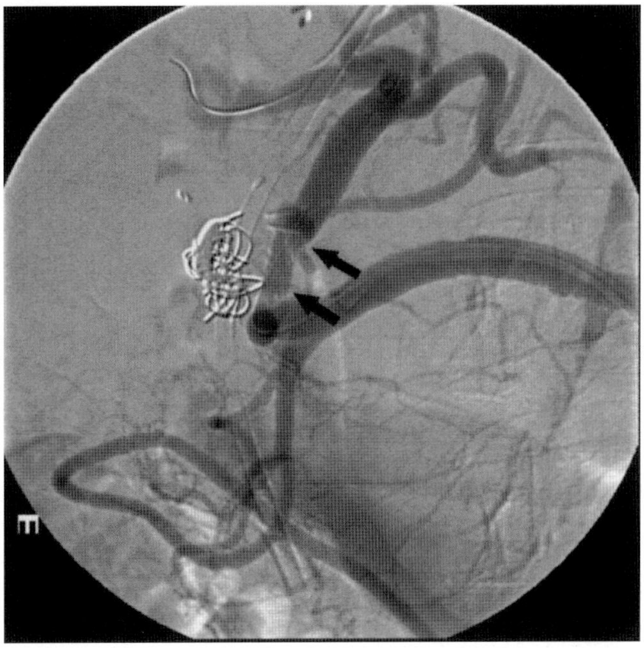

(b)

Figure 2. (a) Selective hepatic angiography 3 weeks after coiling, at the time recurrence of massive upper gastrointestinal bleeding, demonstrates the partial reperfusion of the false aneurysm (arrow). (b) Placement of a coronary stent-graft (arrows) with complete exclusion of the false aneurysm and preservation of the arterial flow.

laboratory analysis may demonstrate abnormal liver function tests. They may also present as sudden and profound haemodynamic shock with life-threatening haemorrhage into the peritoneum or gastrointestinal tract. Intrahepatic pseudoaneurysms are mostly the result of iatrogenic injury whereas extrahepatic pseudoaneurysms are commonly associated with localized infection or are due to technical, anastomotic problems [2]. In our patient no episode of localized infection or generalized sepsis was encountered although some low grade localized infection due to the transient post-operative bile duct obstruction may have occurred. Although we do not have angiographic evidence of contrast extravasation into the biliary tract or directly into the bowel, it is likely that the upper gastrointestinal bleeding occurred due to a fistula between the pseudoaneurysm and the common bile duct because of their close anatomical location and the possible pathophysiological mechanism as described above. The mortality of a bleeding hepatic pseudoaneurysm following liver transplantation is very high, 69%, owing to a combination of factors such as the poor general condition of the patient, poor graft function and medical complications in the post-operative course [1, 2]. Therefore minimally invasive treatment options have to be considered as an alternative to surgical treatment, which consists of resection of the pseudoaneurysm and creating an arterial reconstruction using an interposition graft or arterial conduit [1–5]. Radiological embolisation techniques have been described, to definitively close the pseudoaneurysm with preservation of the arterial flow to the graft: coil embolisation [6] with packing of the aneurysm or CT-guided direct percutaneous puncture of the aneurysmal lumen and injection of thrombin [7]. At first presentation we also opted for coil embolisation of the aneurysmal lumen, and although initially successful, recurrence of bleeding occurred due to partial reperfusion of the pseudoaneurysm. Additional coiling was not considered because of the broad neck of the pseudoaneurysm and potential coil migration into the distal hepatic circulation. Direct puncture also seemed to be impossible because the reperfused portion of the aneurysm was small. Therefore we decided to exclude the pseudoaneurysm with a stent-graft. This technique, which may be performed immediately following the diagnostic angiography, has the unique advantage of completely excluding the pseudoaneurysm without injecting embolic agents into the aneurysm and concomitantly preserving the arterial blood flow to the graft.

To our knowledge, successful exclusion of a bleeding, anastomotic hepatic artery pseudoaneurysm by stent-graft placement in a liver transplant patient has not been previously described.

Implantation of a stent-graft to exclude a visceral pseudoaneurysm has previously been described in patients developing a false aneurysm after Whipple's operation [8–10] and in splenic [11] and renal artery aneurysms [12, 13]. Sakai et al [13] described a similar case of a post transplant hepatic pseudoaneurysm. In their case the cause of aneurysm formation was probably an iatrogenic injury of the hepatic artery during surgery and the pseudoaneurysm was asymptomatic. The indication for treatment was a progressive increase in size of the aneurysm and the definitive treatment also consisted of placement of a coronary stent-graft. Most of the published case reports are of technical successes, but it has to be noted that stent-graft implantation in a visceral artery is not always possible. This may be due to tortuous anatomy making it impossible to negotiate some curved vessel segments by the stent catheter or due to the fact that the post interventional anticoagulation therapy, mandatory after an endovascular stent-procedure, is contraindicated. In particular, when implanting a stent-graft in the coronary arteries, an aggressive and longstanding antiplatelet therapy seems to be mandatory [14]. Additionally, placement of a stent or a graft in an infected area can provoke late graft disintegration and consequently rupture of the aneurysm [15], although some reports describe the long-term success of endovascular exclusion of a proven infected aneurysm [16].

In conclusion, placement of a stent-graft to definitively exclude a bleeding hepatic artery pseudoaneurysm following liver transplantation should be considered, in some selected cases, as an effective and minimally invasive alternative to surgery.

References

1. Marshall MM, Muiesan P, Srinivasan P, et al. Hepatic artery pseudoaneurysm following liver transplantation: incidence, presenting features and management. Clin Radiol 2001;56:579–87.
2. Leelaudomlipi S, Bramhall SR, Gunson BK, et al. Hepatic-artery aneurysm in adult liver transplantation. Transplant Int 2003;16:257–61.
3. Bonham CA, Kapur S, Geller D, Fung JJ, Pinna A. Excision and immediate revascularization for hepatic artery pseudoaneurysm following liver transplantation. Transplant Proc 1999;31:443.
4. Rudich SM, Kinkhabwala MM, Murray NG, See DM, Busuttil RW, Imagawa DK. Successful treatment of mycotic hepatic pseudoaneurysm with arterial reconstruction and liposomal amphotericin B. Liver Transpl Surg 1998;4: 91–3.
5. Fichelle JM, Colacchio G, Castaing D, Bismuth H. Infected false hepatic artery aneurysm after orthotopic liver transplantation treated by resection and reno-hepatic vein graft. Ann Vasc Surg 1997;11:300–3.
6. Ozkan OS, Walser EM, Akinci D, Nealon W, Goodacre B. Gugielmi detachable coil erosion into the common bile duct after embolization of iatrogenic hepatic artery pseudoaneurysm. J Vasc Intervent Radiol 2002;13:935–8.
7. Patel JV, Weston MJ, Kessel DO, Prasad R, Toogood GJ, Robertson I. Hepatic artery pseudoaneurysm after liver transplantation: treatment with percutaneous thrombin injection. Transplantation 2003;75:1755–7.
8. Paci E, Antico E, Candelari R, Alborina S, Marmorale C, Landi E. Pseudoaneurysm of the common hepatic artery: treatment with a stent-graft. Cardiovasc Intervent Radiol 2000;23:472–84.
9. Bürger T, Halloul Z, Meyer F, Grote R, Lippert H. Emergency stent-graft repair of a ruptured hepatic artery secondary to local postoperative peritonitis. J Endovasc Ther 2000;7:324–7.
10. Venturini M, Angeli E, Salvioni M, et al. Hemorrhage from a right hepatic artery pseudoaneurysm: endovascular treatment with a coronary stent-graft. J Endovasc Ther 2002;9:221–4.
11. Larson RA, Solomon J, Carpenter JP. Stent graft repair of visceral artery aneurysms. J Vasc Surg 2002;36:1260–3.
12. Tan WA, Chough S, Saito J, Wholey MH, Eles G. Covered stent for renal artery aneurysm. Catheter Cardiovasc Intervent 2001;52:106–9.
13. Sakai H, Urasawa K, Oyama N, Kitabatake A. Successful covering of a hepatic artery aneurysm with a coronary stent graft. Cardiovasc Intervent Radiol 2004;27:274–7.
14. Stankovic G, Colombo A, Presbitero P, et al. Randomized evaluation of polytetrafluoroethylene-covered stent in saphenous vein grafts. The randomized evaluation of polytetrafluoroethylene COVERed stent in saphenous vein grafts (RECOVERS) trial. Circulation 2003;108:37–42.
15. Chuter TA, Lukaszewicz GC, Reilly LM, et al. Endovascular repair of a presumed aortoenteric fistula: late recurrence due to recurrent infection. J Endovasc Ther 2000;7:240–4.
16. Callaert JR, Fourneau I, Daenens K, Maleux G, Nevelsteen A. Endoprosthetic treatment of a mycotic superficial femoral artery aneurysm. J Endovasc Ther 2003;10:843–5.

The British Journal of Radiology, 78 (2005), 457–468
DOI: 10.1259/bjr/73355272

Pictorial review

Imaging of pelvic injuries in athletes

J BRITTENDEN, MRCP, FRCR and P ROBINSON, MRCP, FRCR

Department of Diagnostic Radiology, Leeds Teaching Hospitals, St James University Hospital, Beckett Street, Leeds LS9 7TF, UK

The pelvis is a complex osseous anatomical region providing the origin and insertion for a number of powerful muscle groups. It performs a pivotal role in all athletic activities and forces exceeding six to eight times body weight traverse this region during even light exercise making the pelvis particularly prone to sporting injury.

The clinical features of injury within the pelvis can be non-specific and a number of diagnoses need to be considered. The location and pattern of injury depends on the sporting activity, the maturity of the athlete and whether the injury sustained is part of an acute or chronic (overuse) process. Recovery from pelvic injury can be prolonged especially if the initial diagnosis is incorrect and appropriate treatment delayed.

This article will review the spectrum of pelvic sports injuries and the imaging strategies that can be employed to diagnose and grade such injuries.

Stress reaction

Stress fractures occur when abnormal repetitive stress is applied to normal bone [1]. The muscles and soft tissues of the pelvis protect the skeleton from the effects of repeated stress explaining the greater incidence of pelvic stress fracture in female athletes, with their relatively reduced muscle bulk.

Running athletes are most commonly affected with the femoral neck and the inferior pubic ramus most frequently involved although sacral fractures are not unknown [2]. Stress fracture of the femoral neck in particular has potentially serious consequences if the diagnosis is not made promptly as the injury can progress to complete fracture, non-union and osteonecrosis [3].

Radiographic assessment of stress fracture can be insensitive, especially in the early stage of the condition and follow up films may demonstrate visible abnormalities in only 50% [3]. Bone scintigraphy has a high sensitivity but lacks spatial resolution and specificity and has been largely superseded by MRI in athletes as it can also identify alternative sources of pain such as muscle tears or joint degeneration [1]. T_1 weighted sequences provide good anatomical detail and define the low signal fracture line in stress fractures whilst fat suppressed T_2 (spectral or short tau inversion recovery (STIR)) sequences can detect periosteal, bone marrow or muscle oedema which are the early signs of osseus stress injury [4]. In advanced injury, MRI clearly depicts the findings of cortical fracture and this ability to differentiate the early changes of stress injury (Figure 1) and the later findings of stress fracture (Figure 2) are important in guiding therapy [5]. In the former a short period of rest is implemented but in overt stress fracture several months healing may be required before the athlete can return to full training.

Scintigraphy is also less useful for follow up of stress injury as abnormal uptake can persist for up to 8–10 months, although intensity usually decreases within 3–6 months [6] compared with MRI which usually demonstrates a return to normal bone marrow signal on T_2 weighted sequences at 3 months [7].

Avulsion fracture

Avulsion injuries occur in the skeletally immature athlete when forces generated within the myotendinous unit exceed the weaker attachment of the apophysis to the central skeleton [8]. During running major forces are distributed through the hip flexors and hamstrings resulting in the most frequent avulsion injuries occurring at the origin of these tendons [9, 10].

Avulsion injury of the ischial apophysis by the hamstrings is common in runners, dancers and gymnasts, with pain typically referred to the buttock region.

Avulsion injuries of the anterosuperior (sartorius) (Figure 3) and anteroinferior (rectus femoris) iliac spines are most commonly seen in the sprinting phase of running, hurdling and in kicking sports such as soccer.

The clinical findings in avulsion fractures of the pelvis are loss of function and severe localized tenderness. The diagnosis can be confirmed on plain radiographs (Figure 3a) but MRI is less specific in diagnosis because low signal cortical fragments may not contain bone marrow and can be difficult to identify. In the acute setting MRI and ultrasound may demonstrate haematoma and periosteal stripping but their main role in management is to rule out high-grade injury of the tendon (Figure 3b). Avulsion injuries should be regarded as a more serious injury than a straightforward muscle or tendon injury as it has the same implications as a fracture. Recovery from anterior pelvic avulsion typically takes approximately 5–6 weeks compared with hamstring avulsion, which may take twice as long [10]. Avulsions, if diagnosed early usually heal with conservative treatment and modification of activities. Surgical repair is undertaken if dislocation of the apophysis or bony avulsion is more than 2 cm [11]. Hamstring avulsions are also more prone to complications, because of potential involvement of the sciatic nerve by

Received 27 April 2004 and in revised form 14 September 2004, accepted 25 November 2004.

Address correspondence to Dr Philip Robinson.

direct compression from the avulsed fragment or by abundant callous formation during the healing process [12].

Muscle injury

Myotendinous strain is the most common sports related injury of the pelvis with the surrounding muscle groups performing a pivotal function in all athletic activities. The forces generated within these muscle groups exceed multiples of body weight during light jogging with major forces produced during explosive athletic activity.

The site of injury within the functional muscle unit depends on the maturity of the athlete. In young, skeletally mature athletes the main area of weakness is the myotendinous junction as well as the muscular aponeurosis [13, 14]. Conversely a similar mechanism of an injury in a skeletally immature patient will cause apophyseal avulsion (see above) while in a more mature athlete the degenerate tendon can tear.

During normal muscle contraction, the muscle belly contracts whilst the myotendinous unit lengthens. Myotendinous strain injuries typically occur in muscles that cross two joints and have a high proportion of fast twitch fibres while undergoing eccentric contraction (stretch during contraction) [14]. Specific muscles are more commonly affected than others within a synergistic group, especially rectus femoris (quadriceps), biceps femoris (hamstrings) (Figure 4), adductor longus (adductors), with less frequent involvement of the iliopsoas, gluteal and abdominal muscles.

Rectus femoris is most commonly injured at the distal myotendinous junction but proximal injuries are recognized when eccentrically resisting hip extension (*e.g.* extending the leg prior to kicking). This mechanism particularly affects the tendon of the reflected head at its junction with the straight head at the level of the acetabulum (Figure 5). The hamstrings are commonly injured in sprinting when they undergo eccentric contraction controlling knee extension. Proximal and distal myotendinous injuries occur in almost equal incidence, with biceps femoris predominantly involved [14, 15] (Figures 4 and 6).

In our experience however, proximal myotendinous tears of the hamstrings and adductor longus (Figure 7) are more common in experienced athletes presumably due to the relative weakness produced by the presence of underlying proximal tendinopathy.

Clinically, muscle strain or tear is characterized by immediate focal pain and decreased function that can be due to muscle disruption or associated muscle spasm in adjoining muscles. There is a well-established clinical grading system that has three components. Grade one injury is less than 5% loss of function, grade two injury is more severe but with some function preserved and grade three strains are complete muscle tears [16]. It is well recognized that differentiation of these clinical grades can be difficult and thus imaging has a potentially important role in these situations [17]. On ultrasound and MRI grade one muscle injuries can show normal appearances or a small area of focal disruption (less than 5% of the muscle volume) with haematoma and perifascial fluid relatively common (Figure 4) [17, 18]. Grade two injuries correspond to a partial tear with muscle fibre disruption seen (over 5%) but not affecting the whole muscle belly (Figures 6, 8 and 9). Grade three injuries (Figure 7) are complete muscle tears with frayed margins and bunching of the muscle on dynamic ultrasound assessment. Although the evaluation of muscle injury by MRI has been extensively described, ultrasound now allows demonstration of muscular architecture at a higher resolution than can currently be obtained on routine MRI. Ultrasound has a number of other advantages over MRI including dynamic muscle assessment, speed of examination, cost and the ability to perform real time intervention. However, the large muscle bulk often present in athletes means that the depth of resolution and field of view offered by ultrasound can be limiting in the pelvic area requiring familiarity with both imaging techniques (Figures 8 and 9).

During healing, ultrasound can show the development of more normal appearing muscle architecture over the following weeks (Figure 10). Once this is the predominant finding, it is suggested that more rigorous rehabilitation can occur [17]. The MRI features of healing muscle tears have not been shown to be as clinically helpful with marked signal abnormality persisting throughout the different stages of healing [15].

Another consideration in athletes is steroid misuse and this should be suspected when the extent of injury is not in keeping with the proposed mechanism or forces involved for the injury. On imaging, if the tendons seem to be predominantly involved (especially in young athletes) it should be considered unusual because steroid abuse stimulates sudden muscle growth leading to stripping of the tendons when the muscle is strained (Figure 11).

Acute complications of muscle strain include nerve irritation, especially the sciatic nerve in hamstring injury by adjacent haematoma or muscle swelling (Figure 12a). Imaging can play an important role in these cases as the referred pain can make it difficult to clinically grade and localize the injury essential for planning rehabilitation. Chronic complications such as scar tissue (Figure 12b) can be particularly debilitating in the pelvic region as the adhesions can involve adjacent nerves and limit full joint movement. Scar tissue can start to form as soon as 2 weeks post injury and as well as restricting function can reduce the contractile strength of the muscle making it more susceptible to re-injury [19].

Acetabular labral injury

The acetabular labrum is a fibrocartilaginous structure which enlarges the overall surface area for articulation with the femoral head. Until recently, labral abnormalities were thought to be only associated with major hip trauma but it is now recognized that labral tears can result from twisting injuries in athletes [20]. Labral tears in athletes can initiate or accelerate degenerative changes as the damaged labrum results in unevenly distributed loading forces over the cartilage surface, leading to development of chondral defects and osteoarthritis [21].

Labral tears can be difficult to clinically diagnose with non-specific symptoms including clicking and anterior inguinal pain. Conventional MRI and ultrasound are not sensitive for diagnosing this condition, unless an associated paralabral cyst is present. The imaging investigation of choice is MR arthrography, because the diluted paramagnetic contrast agent injected into the hip joint distends the capsule outlining the labrum and any associated abnormality (Figure 13). Studies of MR arthrography have indicated close correlation between imaging and surgical findings [22, 23]. Tears are described in relation to the four acetabular quadrants (anterior, anterosuperior, posterior and posterosuperior) with the anterior and anterosuperior components most commonly involved.

MR arthrography can also allow therapeutic injection of additional anaesthetic or steroid, which can give considerable extended symptom relief to the athlete. However ultimately, if the pain is persistent arthroscopic resection of the torn labrum relieves symptoms and may slow down the associated degenerative process [24].

Snapping hip syndrome

The "snapping hip" is a clinical entity that refers to an audible "snap" or "click" that occurs in the region of the hip joint. Internal snapping of the hip is classically associated with labral tears (see above) while external snapping occurs with the surrounding tendons. The most common cause is movement of the iliotibial band over the greater trochanter, but it is also associated with snapping of the iliopsoas tendon and gluteus maximus tendons in the region of the iliopectineal eminence and greater trochanter, respectively. It is thought that laxity of the ligaments around the hip joint allows relatively excessive movement, with subsequent local tendinous irritation [25]. Snapping usually occurs in runners and gymnasts during hip flexion and lateral rotation but is not always painful.

Imaging in this condition can be difficult, with ultrasound the method of choice for demonstrating the flicking tendon as long as the manoeuvre to reproduce symptoms allows probe contact to be maintained [26]. MRI may demonstrate fluid along the iliopsoas tendon on T_2 weighted sequences, but this is not sensitive or specific also occurring in iliopsoas tendinopathy and bursitis (Figure 14). Ultrasound can also be useful for image-guided injection of corticosteroid into any associated peritendinous inflammatory tissue if rehabilitation is unsuccessful. If non-surgical treatment is unsuccessful surgical tendon lengthening procedures can be performed [27].

Chronic groin pain

Chronic groin pain is a complex clinical problem both in diagnosis and successful management [28]. There are four main differential diagnoses to consider, namely inguinal hernias, pre-hernia complex (Sportsman's hernia), osteitis pubis and adductor dysfunction. The incidence and proposed pathology varies between different sports and clinician experience but are common to sports involving repetitive kicking or frequent change of direction (*e.g.* soccer, ice hockey, rugby and Australian rules football) [28, 29]. Accurate clinical diagnosis can be difficult because there is considerable overlap in symptoms and signs with conditions often coexisting.

Inguinal hernia

Herniography has been extensively evaluated in athletes with equivocal clinical features and studies have shown this technique to be very sensitive but relatively non-specific technique demonstrating a large number of asymptomatic hernias [30]. Although herniography has been shown to have a low complication rate the procedure is still invasive and requires ionizing radiation [30].

In our institution clinically suspected hernias in athletes are assessed with ultrasound using the inferior epigastric vessels as a landmark (as they arise from the external iliac vessels) near the deep inguinal ring. Therefore if the hernia sac arises lateral to the vessels it is indirect (passing through the deep ring) (Figure 15), but if it lies medial to the vessels it is a direct hernia (bulging through the posterior wall).

Sportsman's hernia

This is a controversial clinical area increasingly recognized as accounting for up to 5% of all groin injuries. It can be difficult to diagnose and treat effectively [31, 32] and the underlying biomechanical problem is not clearly understood but occurs more commonly in ball kicking sports [28, 29]. It is probably a chronic overuse injury, which develops insidiously with some authors postulating a chronic imbalance between the powerful adductor and the relatively weaker abdominal muscles across the symphysis pubis. The pathologies described include posterior inguinal wall weakness, aponeurosis tear and neuralgia. Although some authors [33] have proposed that posterior inguinal wall bulging on ultrasound occurs in this condition we commonly see this feature in asymptomatic athletes (Figure 16). Microtears cannot be reliably diagnosed on imaging and therefore imaging is performed to exclude other conditions that affect the groin (see above and below).

Conservative treatment involves controlled rehabilitation which can be effective but of a long duration (>6 months), whilst a number of surgical procedures have been developed predominantly involving surgery to the posterior inguinal wall, rectus abdominis and adductor muscles alone or in combination [28].

Chronic adductor strain

The adductor muscle group consists of adductor longus, brevis and magnus as well as gracilis. These muscles originate from the pubic body and inferior pubic ramus and pass distally to the femur and tibia [34]. Their main action is thigh adduction with some hip flexion and are functionally important in sports where frequent changes of direction are required [29, 35]. The tendinous origins are small and are subjected to high loads during athletic activity which accounts for the prevalence of tears and chronic tenoperiosteal injury [36].

The main clinical difficulty is differentiating adductor tendinopathy from the other causes of chronic pain as it too can present with diffuse groin pain and multiple tender areas on examination [28, 29, 37]. Additionally many athletes (professional and recreational) will have chronic adductor longus tendinopathy which can be asymptomatic [29]. Therefore detecting abnormal tendon architecture on imaging does not necessarily explain the patient's current symptoms (Figure 17a).

Ultrasound examination can evaluate the tendons looking for any specific area of focal tenderness that reproduces the patients' symptoms and evidence of superimposed acute changes within the tendon including haematoma or oedema (Figure 17b) [38]. In our institution we believe gadolinium enhanced MRI is more sensitive in detecting acute on chronic adductor enthesis changes important in athletes [39] (Figure 18). Controlled rehabilitation can successfully treat this condition but surgery involving tenotomy has been advocated in resistant cases [40].

Osteitis pubis

The symphysis pubis is a fibrocartilaginous joint of the anterior pelvis and is also the confluence for the adductors, rectus abdominis and the medial aspect of the inguinal ligament [34]. Osteitis pubis is probably a biomechanical inflammatory arthropathy across the symphysis pubis produced by an imbalance in strengths of the pelvic and abdominal muscles [32]. Again there is controversy over definition of this condition and whether this is a single entity or due to a spectrum of the processes described above. Radiographs and scintigraphy may show sclerosis and increased activity but these are non-specific features and can be seen in asymptomatic athletes.

MRI is the technique of choice in osteitis pubis demonstrating generalized and often, symmetrical symphyseal bone marrow oedema which classically extends into the soft tissues with intact adjacent muscle and tendons (Figure 19). Although oedema can be seen in asymptomatic athletes more marked changes appear to correlate with symptoms [39, 41].

Active rehabilitation used in the treatment of osteitis pubis includes a reduction in the athlete's activity level, an emphasis on strengthening the surrounding muscles and the use of non-steroidal anti-inflammatory drugs. However complete recovery can take over 6 months and an earlier return to full activity has been anecdotally reported following intra-articular corticosteroid injection [42].

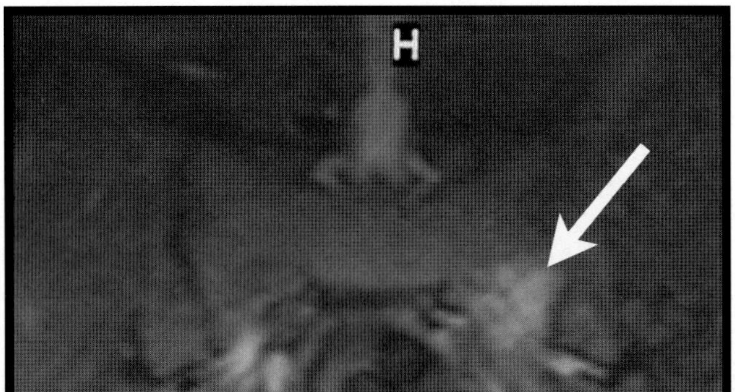

Figure 1. Sacral stress reaction in a tennis player with left sacroiliac pain and normal radiographs. Coronal short tau inversion recovery (STIR) MR image sequence shows oedema in the left sacral ala but no fracture is visible.

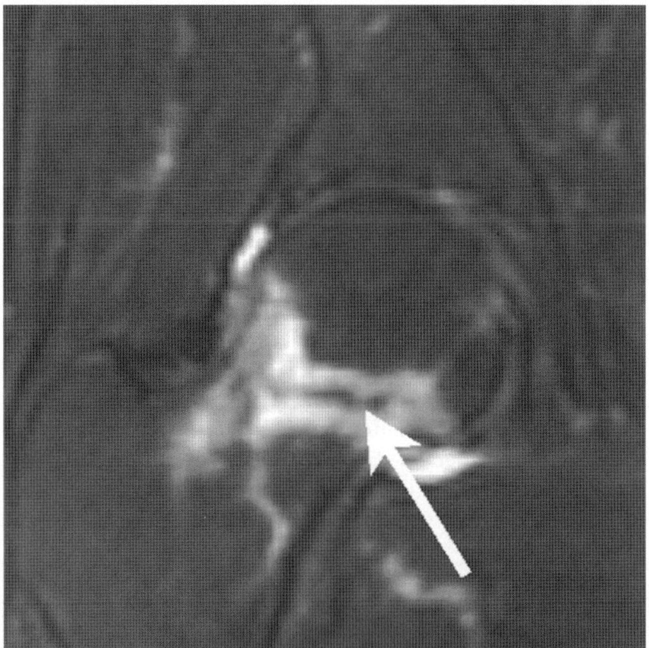

Figure 2. Runner with increasing right hip pain. Coronal T_2 weighted fat saturated MR image shows high signal within the right femoral neck with a low signal linear area (arrow) representing a fracture line. Conventional radiographs were normal.

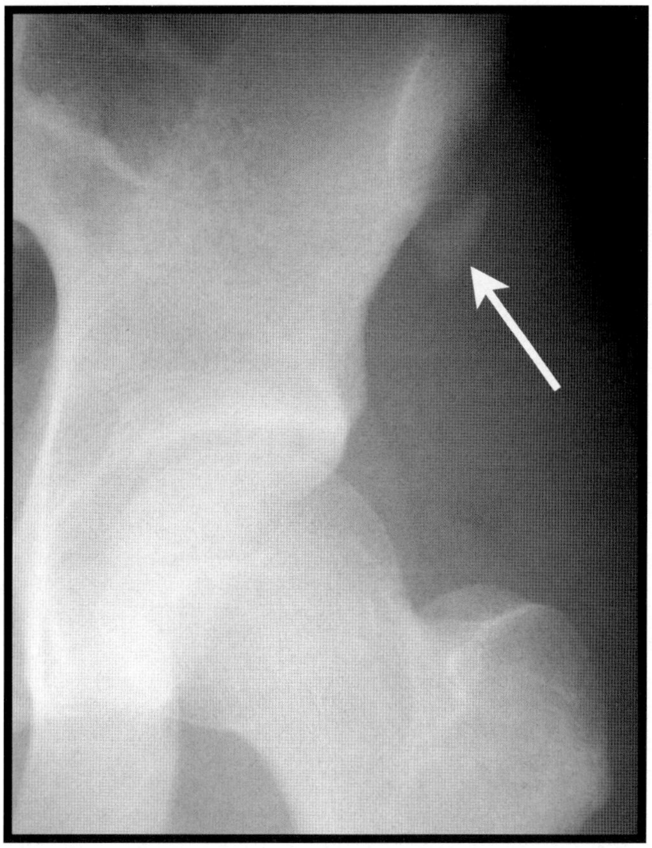

(a)

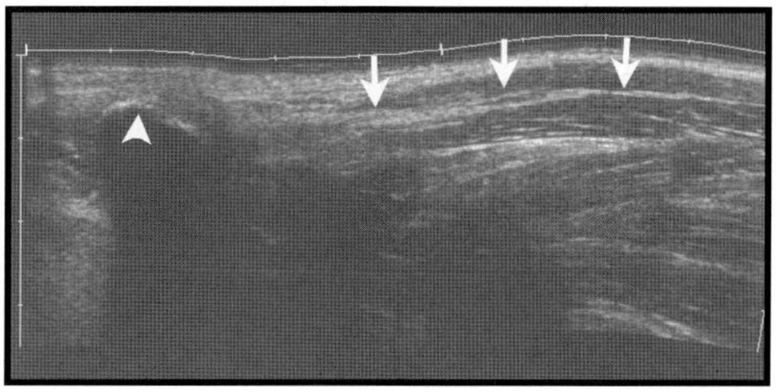

(b)

Figure 3. (a) Rugby player presenting with acute pain after kicking. Plain film shows an avulsed fragment (arrow) of bone from the anterior superior iliac spine at the site of the sartorius tendon insertion. (b) Longitudinal ultrasound in the same patient shows the avulsed fragment (arrowhead) and intact tendon and muscle (arrows).

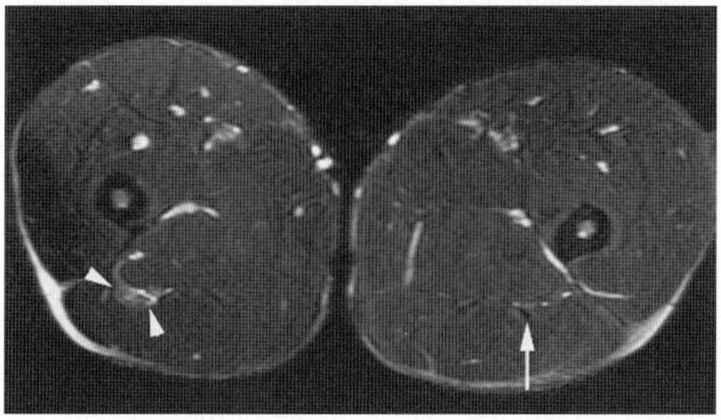

Figure 4. 100 metre sprinter with acute right thigh pain. Axial T_2 weighted fat saturated MR image of both thighs shows a normal left biceps femoris tendon (arrow). The right biceps femoris tendon can be seen as a low signal structure, but with surrounding oedema and haemorrhage (arrowheads), consistent with a grade I injury.

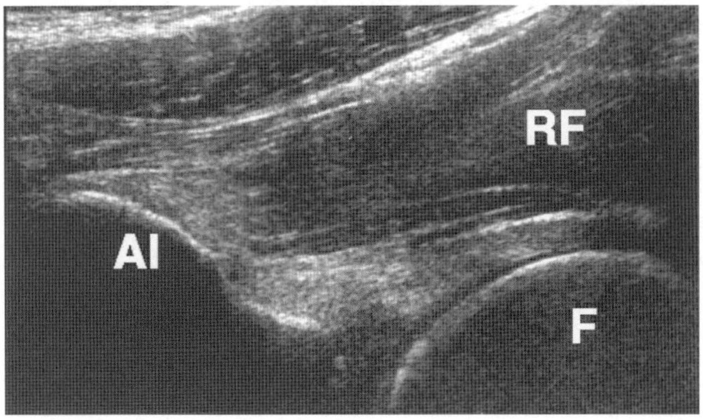

(a)

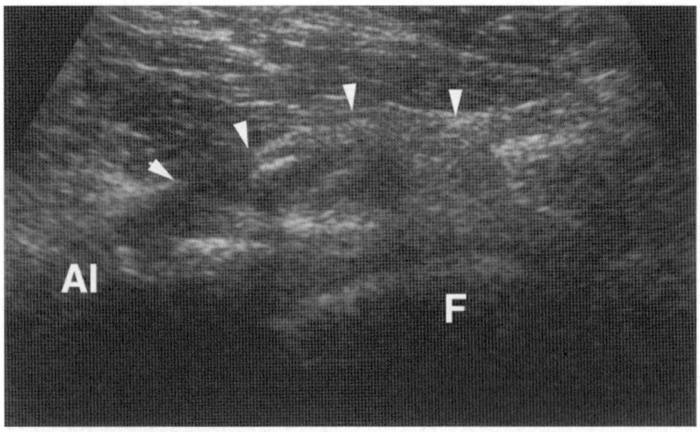

(b)

Figure 5. (a) Female discus thrower with normal proximal rectus femoris. Longitudinal ultrasound shows the origin of rectus femoris (RF) from the anterior inferior iliac spine (AI) lying anterior to the acetabulum and femoral head (F). (b) Corresponding image in a symptomatic soccer player with chronic pain on taking goal kicks. Anterior to the anterior inferior iliac spine (AI) and femoral head (F), there is an ill-defined area of chronic haematoma (arrowheads) containing echogenic scar tissue within rectus femoris, consistent with a chronic proximal tear of rectus femoris.

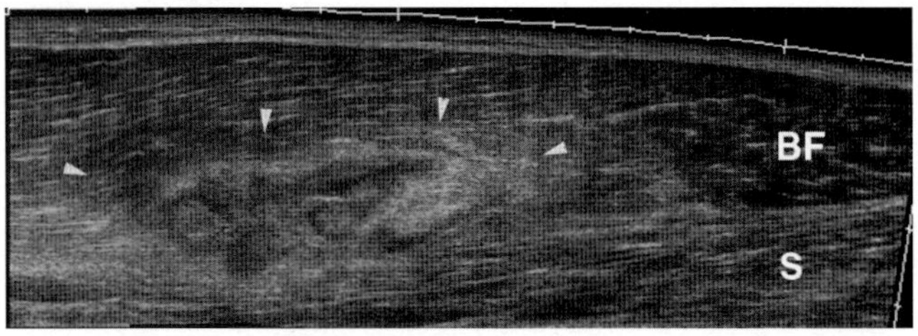

(a)

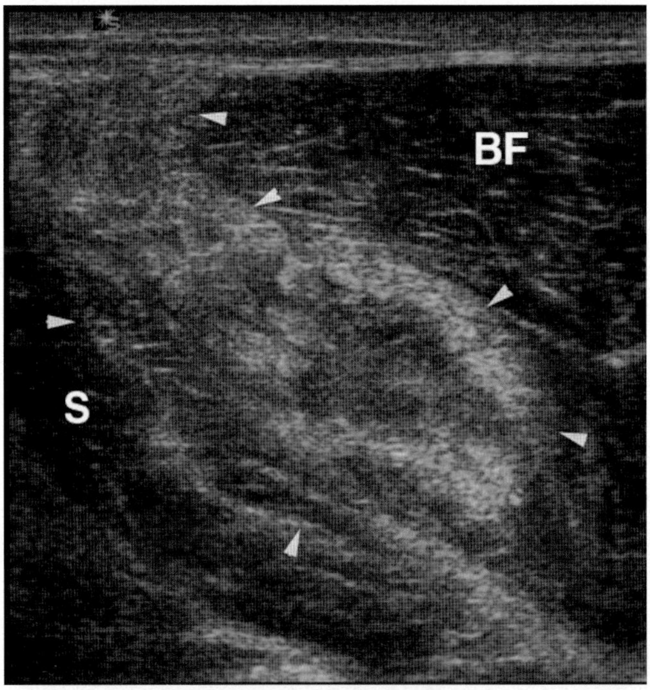

(b)

Figure 6. Male long jumper with sudden thigh pain in competition. (a) Longitudinal extended field of view ultrasound shows a grade 2 tear within biceps femoris (BF). There is a large haematoma (arrowheads) with mixed echogenicity occupying approximately 50% of the muscle and indenting the adjacent semitendinosus (S) muscle. (b) Transverse ultrasound shows the haematoma (arrowheads) extending along the aponeurosis of biceps femoris (BF) with associated mass effect indenting semitendinosus (S).

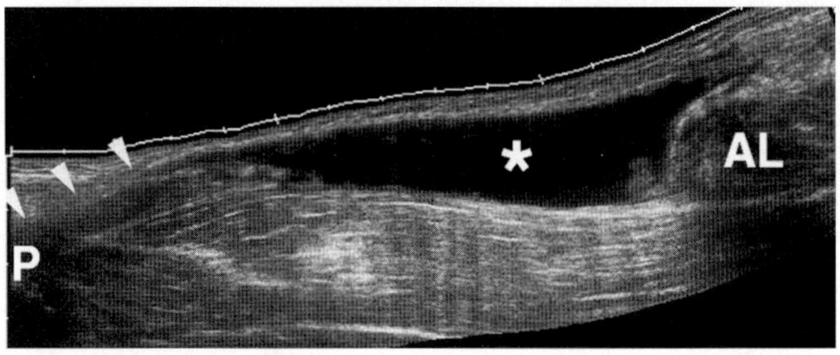

Figure 7. Professional soccer player with acute thigh pain during tackling. Longitudinal extended field of view ultrasound shows a grade 3 adductor longus (AL) tear retracted from the pubis (P) with heterogeneous but intact proximal tendon (arrowheads). Note the intervening acute hypoechoic haematoma (*).

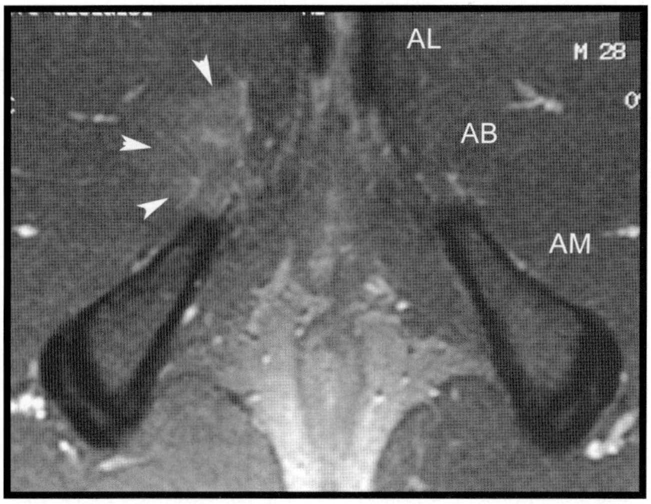

Figure 8. 110 metre hurdler with acute right groin pain during competition. Axial T_2 weighted fat saturated MR image of the pelvis shows oedema (arrowheads) within the proximal myotendinous region of right adductor brevis (AB) consistent with a grade 2 tear. (AL, adductor longus; AM, adductor magnus).

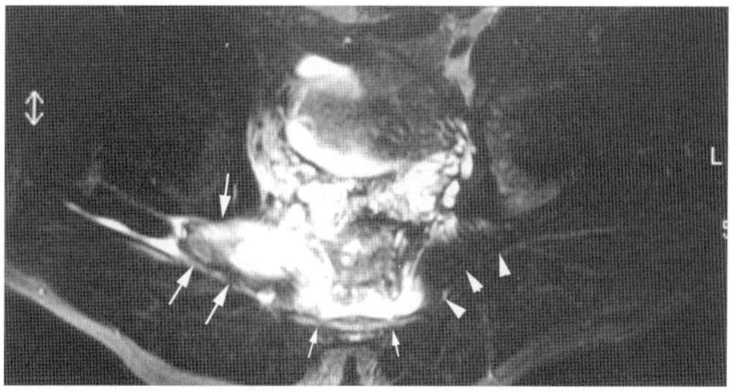

Figure 9. Professional soccer player with acute posterior thigh pain on volleying. Axial T_2 weighted fat saturated MR image of the buttock and upper thigh shows an acute grade 2 right piriformis muscle tear (large arrows). Note the low signal, intact left piriformis (large arrowheads) and the posterior sacrum (small arrows) which, along with the large buttock musculature, did not allow adequate visualization with ultrasound.

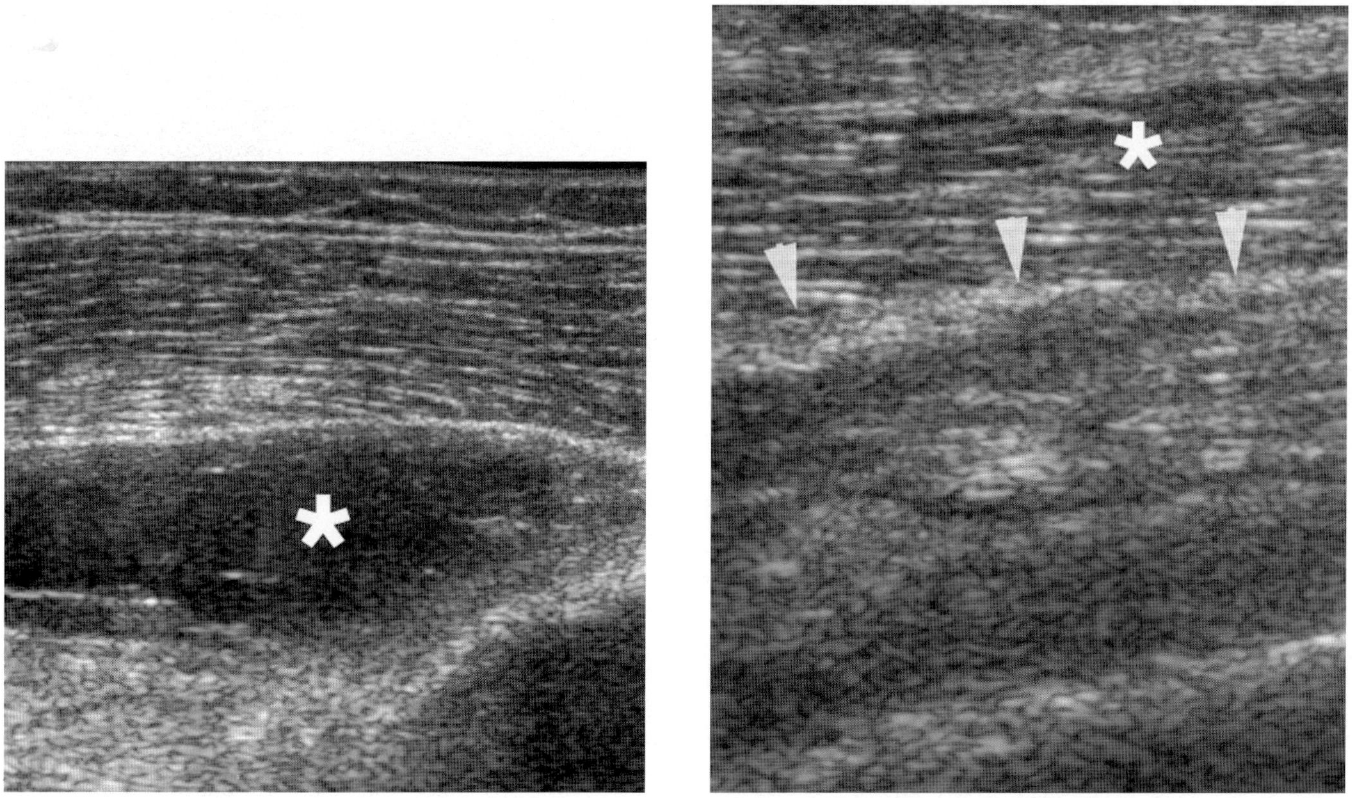

(a) (b)

Figure 10. Soccer player with proximal thigh haematoma secondary to muscle tear. (a) On day 5, there is a predominantly hypoechoic haematoma (*) with an echogenic periphery. (b) By week 2, the hypoechoic haematoma has now resolved and been replaced by connective tissue (arrowheads) which has a similar appearance to muscle (compare with intact superficial muscle (*)).

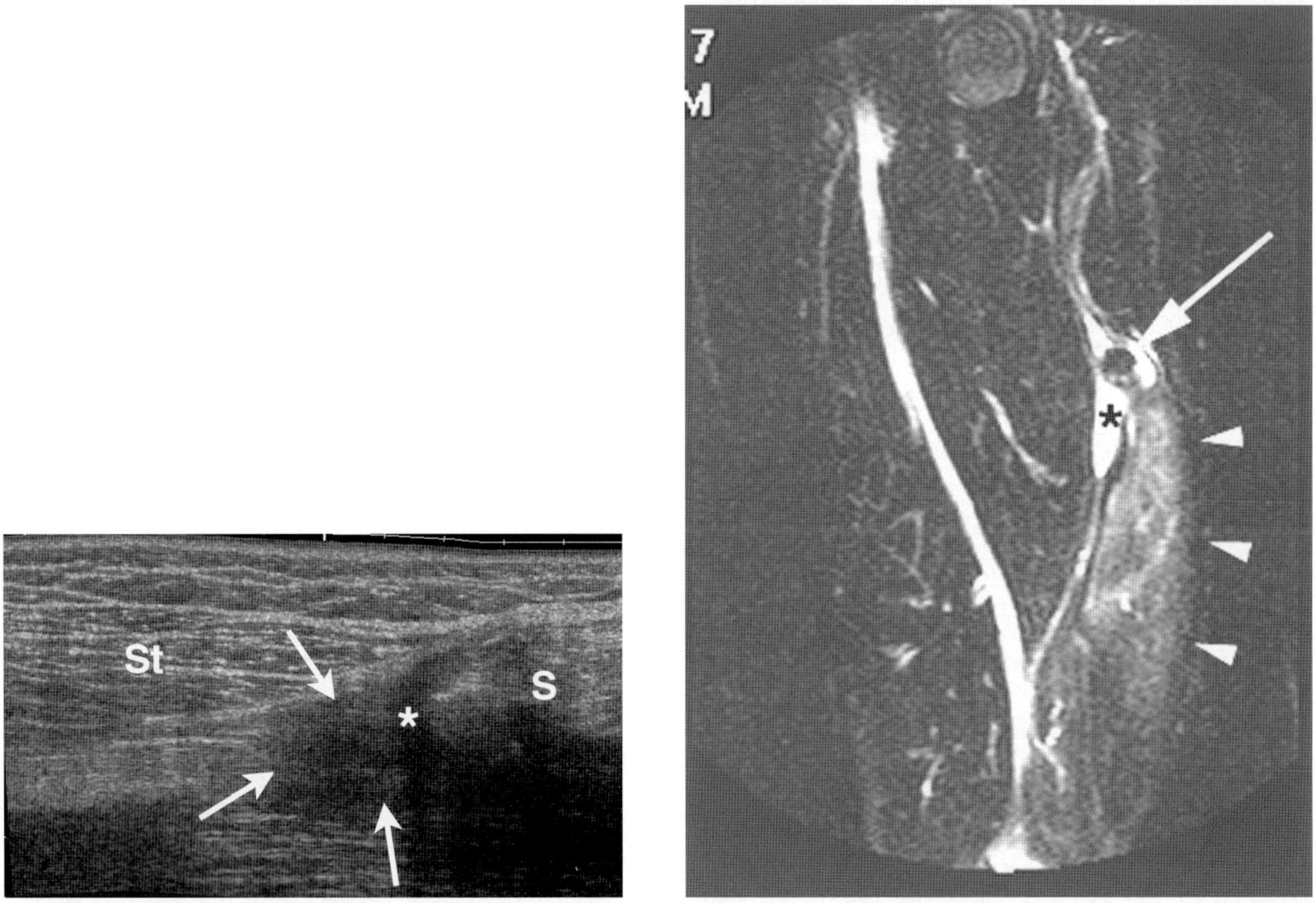

(a) (b)

Figure 11. Professional rugby player with sudden, severe thigh pain. (a) Longitudinal extended field of view ultrasound shows a proximal grade 3 semimembranosus (S) tear with a bunched up muscle belly and adjacent haematoma (arrows). The free edge of the torn muscle produces acoustic shadowing (*). (Note adjacent semitendinosus (St)). The large muscle bulk precluded complete visualization at ultrasound. (b) Sagittal short tau inversion recovery (STIR) MR image of the thigh confirms a grade 3 tear of semimembranosis with marked retraction of the muscle (arrowheads) and accompanying tendon (arrow). Because the tear occurred within the tendon and not at the myotendinous junction, with an unusual mechanism of injury, steroid abuse was suspected (see text).

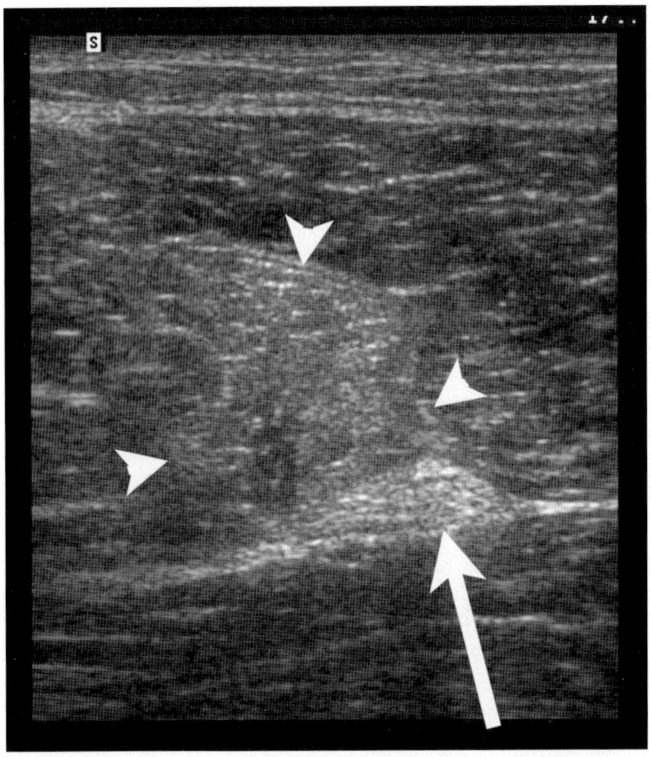

(a)

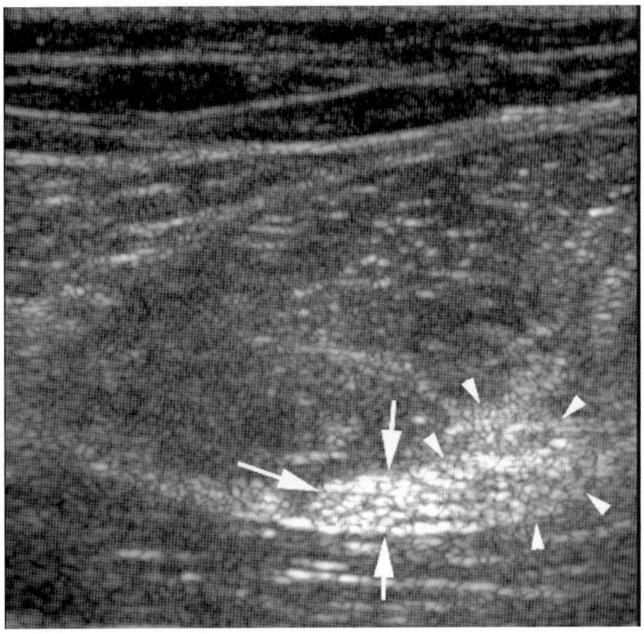

(b)

Figure 12. (a). Acute hamstring tear in a runner. Transverse ultrasound image of a grade 2 semitendinosus tear with an acute haematoma (arrowheads) impinging on the sciatic nerve (arrow). (b) Professional soccer player with recurrent posterior thigh pain on sprinting. Transverse ultrasound of the proximal thigh shows the sciatic nerve (arrows) with a large adherent nodule of echogenic scar tissue (arrowheads).

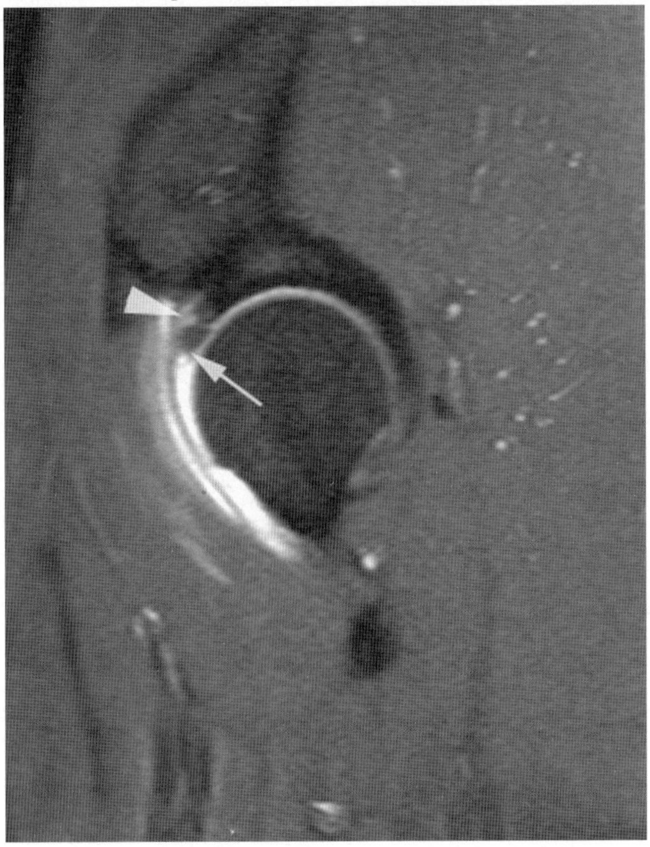

(a)

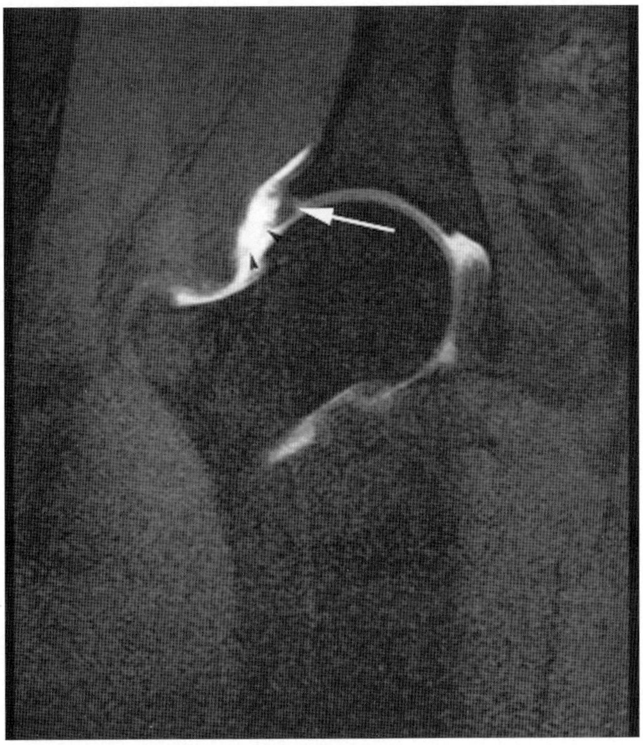

(b)

Figure 13. Acetabular labral tear in a professional footballer with right hip pain. (a) Sagittal T_1 weighted fat saturated MR arthrogram image shows a deformed anterosuperior acetabular labrum (arrow) with a proximal tear (arrowhead). (b) Coronal T_1 weighted fat saturated MR arthrogram image shows a deformed superior labrum (arrow) indented by an adjacent paralabral cyst (black arrowheads).

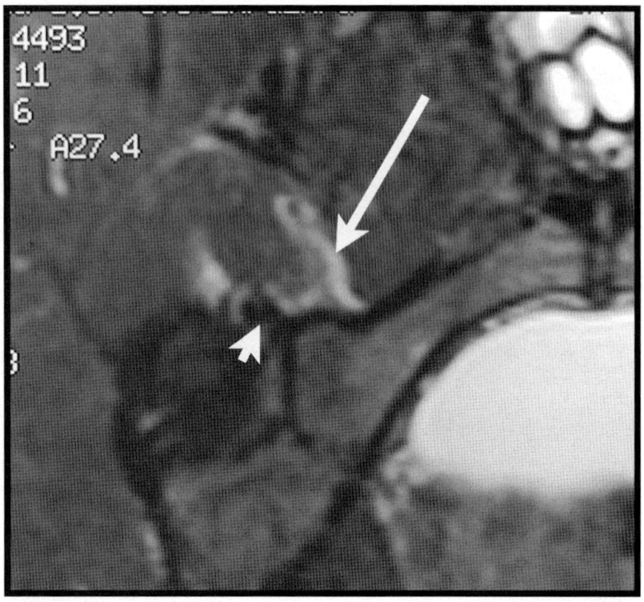

Figure 14. Triathlete with hip pain and clinically suspected snapping hip. Axial T_2 weighted fat saturated MR image at the level of the ileopectineal eminence demonstrates the normal iliopsoas tendon (arrowhead) with surrounding oedema (arrow).

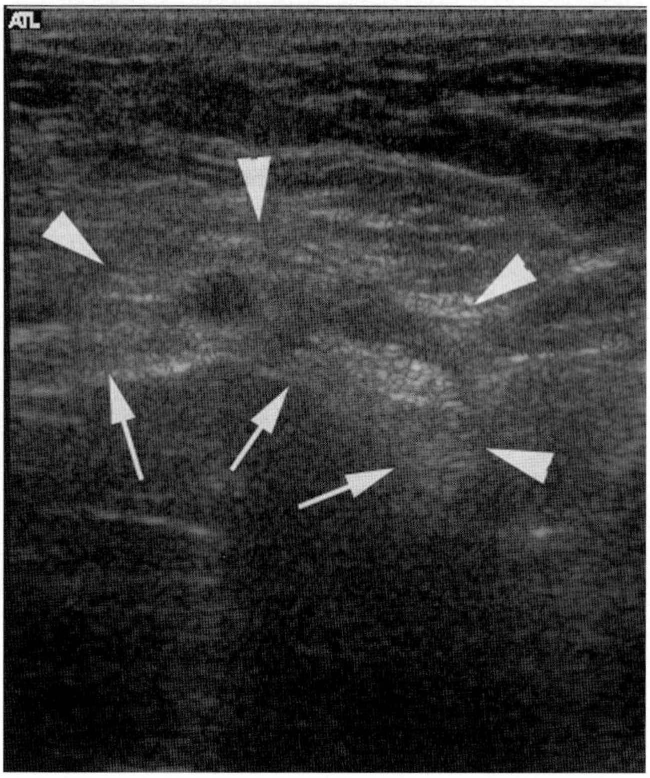

Figure 16. Demonstration of normal left posterior inguinal wall bulging on dynamic ultrasound of a patient asymptomatic in this region. On straining, the shape of the normally oval inguinal canal becomes more crescent-like (arrowheads) with distension of the vessels within the canal and pushing in ("ballooning") of the posterior wall (arrows).

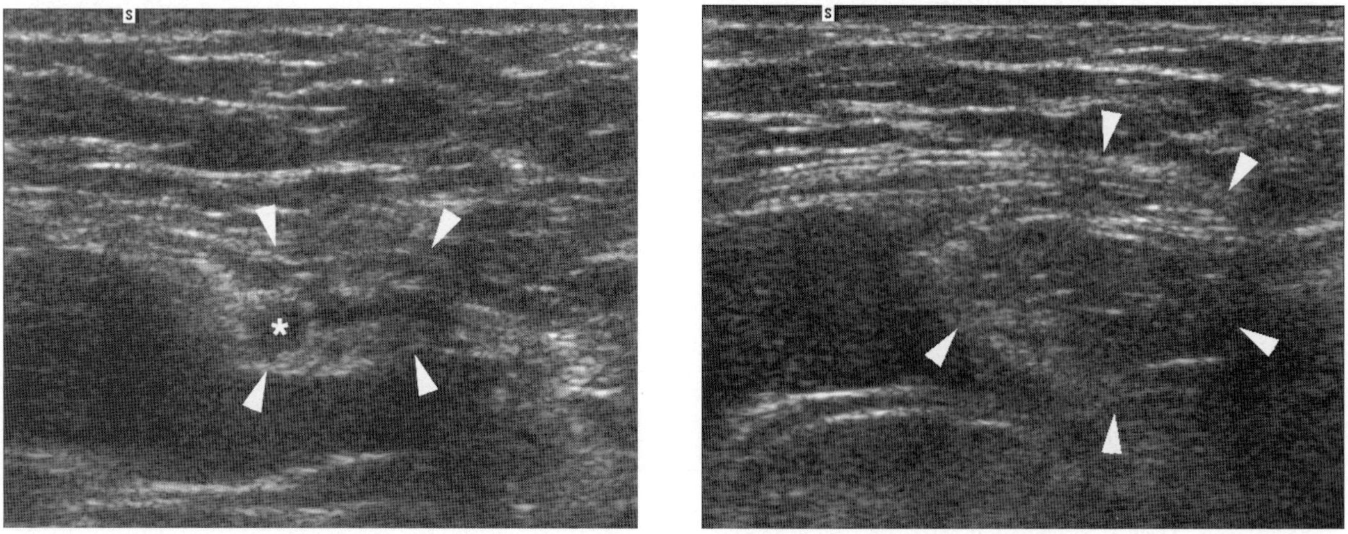

(a) (b)

Figure 15. Professional soccer player with right groin pain. (a) Sagittal ultrasound of the right groin shows the short axis of the inguinal canal (arrowheads) with a number of hypoechoic vessels and tubules (*). (b) On straining, the contents are obliterated and the canal expanded by an indirect hernia of bowel and fat (arrowheads).

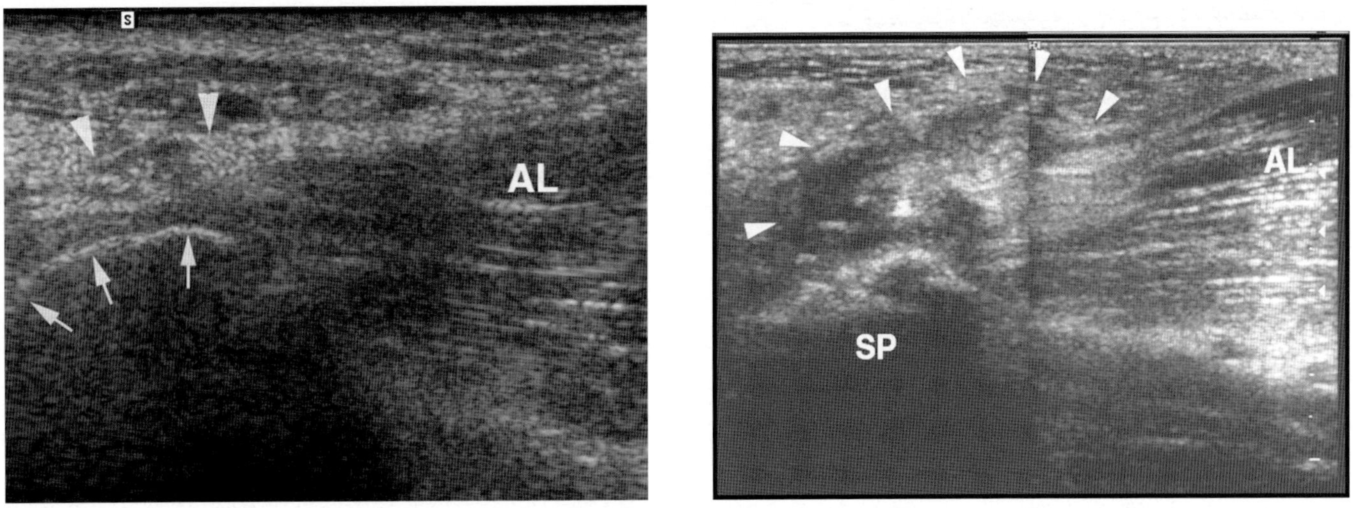

(a) (b)

Figure 17. Abnormal adductor tendon architecture in asymptomatic and symptomatic patients. (a) Professional footballer with left hip pain. Longitudinal ultrasound of the asymptomatic proximal right adductor longus (AL) (performed during assessment of the symptomatic left groin) shows the proximal tendon (arrowheads) and the pubis (small arrows). Note the tendon does not have a structured, homogeneous internal appearance consistent with chronic tendinopathy but does have a smooth defined contour. (b) Professional footballer with acute on chronic right groin pain. Longitudinal ultrasound (dual screen to extend field of view) shows marked distortion of the right adductor longus tendon which is swollen and hypoechoic (arrowheads) adjacent to the symphysis pubis (SP). The adductor longus muscle (AL) appears normal.

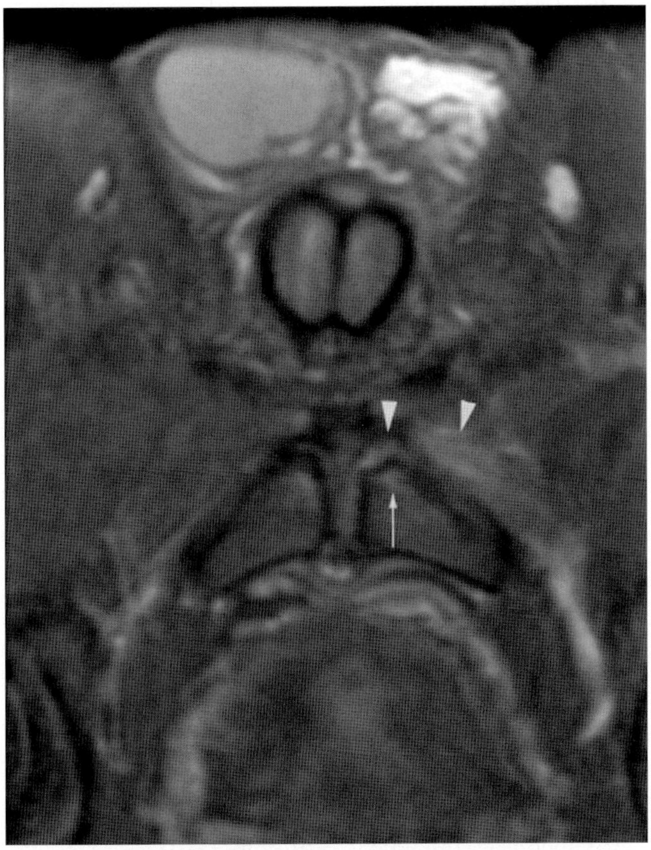

Figure 18. Professional soccer player with chronic left-sided adductor pain. Axial T_1 weighted fat saturated post-gadolinium image of the inferior symphysis pubis shows marked enhancement of the left adductor longus enthesis and adjacent myotendon (arrowheads). There is also some enhancement of the anterior subchondral bone (small arrow). Minor changes are present on the right.

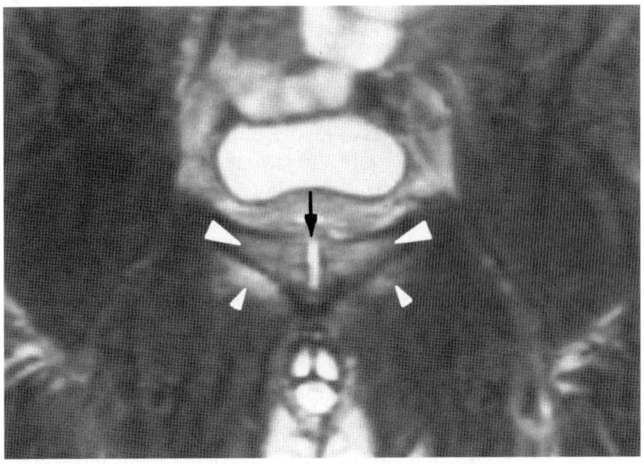

Figure 19. Professional soccer player with a clinical diagnosis of osteitis pubis. Coronal short tau inversion recovery (STIR) MR image shows diffuse symmetrical oedema throughout the pubic bodies and distal rami (large arrowheads) as well as within the adjacent soft tissues (small arrowheads). There is also fluid within the symphysis pubis (arrow).

Conclusion

The diagnosis of pelvic injuries in athletes can be difficult owing to the degree of overlap of symptoms between different injuries. Early diagnosis and injury grading is important for athletes so that appropriate treatment can be commenced to prevent the development of chronic pain or other complications. MRI and ultrasound are accurate for grading most soft tissue injuries while bone injury (the most common being stress reaction and avulsion injury) can be assessed with MRI and conventional radiographs. Chronic groin pain is a controversial clinical area and is especially difficult to diagnose and manage. In these cases we use a combination of ultrasound and MRI to try and define the origin of pain, as conventional radiographs and scintigraphy are relatively non-specific.

References

1. Anderson MW, Greenspan A. Stress fractures. Radiology 1996;199:1–12.
2. Major NH, Helms CA. Sacral stress fractures in long distance runners. AJR Am J Roentgenol 2000;174:727–9.
3. Spitz D, Newberg A. Imaging of stress fractures in the athlete. Radiol Clin N Am 2002;40:313–31.
4. Deutsch AL, Coel MN, Mink JH. Imaging of stress injuries to bone: radiography, scintigraphy and MR imaging. Clin Sports Med 1997;16:275–90.
5. Stoller DW. Magnetic resonance imaging in orthopaedics and sports medicine. Philadelphia, PA: JB Lippincott, 1993:564.
6. Rupini HD, Holder LE, Espinola DA, et al. Three-phase radionucleotide bone imaging in sports medicine. Radiology 1985;156:187–96.
7. Slocum KA, Gorman JD, Puckett ML, et al. Resolution of abnormal MR signal intensity in patients with stress fractures of the femoral neck. AJR Am J Roentgenol 1997;168:1295–9.
8. Stevens MA, El Khouray GY, Kathol MH, Brandser EA, Chow S. Imaging features of avulsion injuries. Radiographics 1999;19:655–72.
9. Peterson L, Renstrom P. Sports injuries. Their prevention and treatment. Chicago, IL: Yearbook Medical Publishers, Martin Dunitz, 1986.
10. Lynch S, Renstrom P. Groin injuries in sport: treatment strategies. Sports Med 1999;28:137–44.
11. Kujala U, Orava S. Ischial apophysis injuries in athletes. Sports Med 1993;16:290–4.
12. Spinner RJ, Atkinsons JL, Wenger DE, Stuart MJ. Tardy sciatic nerve palsy following apophyseal avulsion fracture of the ischial tuberosity: case report. J Neurosurg 1998;89:819–21.
13. Palmer WE, Kuong SJ, Elmadbouh HM. MR imaging of myotendinous strain. AJR Am J Roentgenol 1999;173:703–9.
14. Marcantonio DR, Cho GJ. Focus on muscle in orthopedic MRI. Semin Musculoskelet Radiol 2000;4:421–34.
15. Fleckenstein JL, Weatherall PT, Parkey RW, Payne JA, Peshock RM. Sports-related muscle injuries: evaluation with MR imaging. Radiology 1989;172:793–8.
16. O'Donoghue D. Principles in the management of specific injuries to athletes (4th edn). Philadelphia, PA: WB Saunders, 1984:39–91.
17. Van Holsbeeck M, Introcasco J. Musculoskeletal ultrasound 2nd edn. St Louis, MO: Mosby, 2001.
18. Steinbach L, Fleckenstein J, Mink J. MR imaging of muscle injuries. Semin Musculoskelet Radiol 1998;1:128–41.
19. Fornage BD. The case for ultrasound of muscles and tendons. Semin Musculoskelet Radiol 2000;4:375–91.
20. Byrd JW. Labral lesions: an elusive source of hip pain. Case reports and literature review. Arthroscopy 1996;12:603–12.
21. Harris WH, Bourne RB, Oh I. The acetabular labrum: a possible aetiological factor in certain cases of osteoarthritis of the hip. J Bone Joint Surg Am 1979;61:510–4.
22. Czerny C, Hoffman S, Neuhold A, Tschauner C, Engel A, et al. MR imaging arthrography of the adult acetabular capsular-labral complex: correlation with surgery and anatomy. AJR Am J Roentgenol 1999;173:345–9.
23. Leunig M, Werlen S, Ungersbock A, Ito K, Ganz R, et al. Evaluation of the acetabular labrum by MR imaging arthrography. J Bone Joint Surg Br 1997;79:230–4.
24. Santori N, Villar RN. Acetabular labral tears: result of arthroscopic partial limbectomy. Arthroscopy 2000;16:11–5.
25. Anderson K, Strickland S, Warren R. Hip and groin injuries in athletes. Am J Sports Med 2001;29:521–33.
26. Cardinal E, Buckwater KA, Capello WN, Duval N. US of the snapping iliopsoas tendon. Radiology 1998;198:52–2.
27. Gruen G, Scioscia T, Lowenstein J. The surgical treatment of internal snapping hip. Am J Sports Med 2000;30:607–13.
28. Fricker PA. Management of groin pain in athletes. Br J Sports Med 1997;31:97–101.
29. Renstrom P, Peterson L. Groin injuries in athletes. Br J Sports Med 1980;14:30–6.
30. Ekberg O. "Inguinal herniography in adults: technique, normal anatomy, and diagnostic criteria for hernias." Radiology 1981;138:31–6.
31. Peterson L, Renstrom P. Sports injuries. Chicago, IL: Year Book Medical, 1986.
32. Meyers WC, Foley DP, Garrett WE, Lohnes JH, Mandlebaum BR. Management of severe lower abdominal or inguinal pain in high-performance athletes. PAIN (Performing Athletes with Abdominal or Inguinal Neuromuscular Pain Study Group). Am J Sports Med 2000;28:2–8.
33. Orchard JW, Read JW, Neophyton J, Garlick D. Groin pain associated with ultrasound finding of inguinal canal posterior wall deficiency in Australian Rules footballers. Br J Sports Med 1998;32:134–9.
34. Agur A. Grant's Atlas of Anatomy (9th edn). Baltimore, MD: Williams and Wilkins, 1991.
35. Lovell G. The diagnosis of chronic groin pain in athletes: a review of 189 cases. Aust J Sci Med Sport 1995;27:76–9.
36. Holmich P. Adductor related groin pain in athletes. Sports Med Arthros Rev 1997;5:285–90.
37. Thomas JM. Groin strain versus occult hernia: uncomfortable alternatives or incompatible rivals? Lancet 1995;345:1522–3.
38. Kalebo P, Karlsson J, Sward L, Peterson L. Ultrasonography of chronic tendon injuries in the groin. Am J Sports Med 1992;20:634–9.
39. Robinson P, Barron DA, Parsons W, Schilders EM, Grainger AJ, O'Connor P. Adductor related groin pain in athletes. Correlation of MRI imaging with clinical findings. Skeletal Radiology 2004;33:451–7.
40. Ackermark C, Johanasson C. Tenotomy of the adductor longus tendon in the treatment of chronic groin pain in athletes. Am J Sports Med 1992;20:643–6.
41. Verrall GM, Slavotinek JP, Fon GT. Incidence of pubic bone marrow oedema in Australian rules football players: relation to groin pain. Br J Sports Med 2001;35:28–33.
42. Holt MA, Graf BK, Helwig DC. Treatment of osteitis pubis in athletes. Results of corticosteroid injections. Am J Sports Med 1995;23:601–6.

The British Journal of Radiology, 78 (2005), 469–470

Correspondence

(The Editors do not hold themselves responsible for opinions expressed by correspondents)

Second cancer risk

The Editor—Sir,
The two informative articles by Aird [1] and Harrison [2] on second cancer risks following radiotherapy are very thought-provoking. We would like to draw your attention to several additional points, namely:

1. The discussion on doses from diagnostic X-rays, CT scans and scattered radiation from megavoltage therapy assumes a radiation weighting factor (w_r) of 1.0, the standard recommended value. However there is mounting evidence of higher relative biological effect (RBE) values (around 4.0) for certain endpoints in the case of low energy photons [3–5]. While the published data are related to photon energies that are lower than those considered by Aird and Harrison, the RBE values in the complete diagnostic energy range are worthy of scientific investigation, and higher w_r values may eventually be required.
2. Repeated imaging studies associated with clinical trials are necessary for data acquisition but are sometimes unnecessary in terms of clinical management of the individual patient. However these protocols can be inadvertently continued following cessation of trials and in such cases represent unnecessary radiation exposure. Whereas there are comprehensive guidelines on optimum imaging strategies in radiotherapy treatment planning [6], similar guidance is not available for patient follow-up.
3. One clear-cut answer to some of the questions posed by Aird [1] is that a greater use of proton beams in radical treatments should reduce the incidence of second malignancy, due to the substantially reduced integral dose. The expected yield of radiation-induced secondary cancers is estimated to be reduced by a factor of between 2 and 15 when compared with either conventional megavoltage or intensity-modulated X-ray treatments [7, 8]. We gather that modern radiation-protection regulations are adding weight to the already strong clinical case for proton therapy expansion within the EU. The most important strategic decisions confronting the UK radiotherapy community are whether and when investment in a National Proton Therapy Centre or Centres should be made [9].

Yours etc.,

S Green
B Jones

University Hospital Birmingham NHS Trust
Edgbaston
Birmingham
B15 2TH
UK

(*Received 7 January 2005 and accepted 18 January 2005*)
DOI: 10.1259/bjr/89346355

References

1. Aird EGA. Second cancer risk, concomitant exposures and IRMER(2000). Br J Radiol 2004;77:983–5.
2. Harrison RM. Second cancers following radiotherapy: a suggested common dosimetry framework for therapeutic and concomitant exposures. Br J Radiol 2004;77:986–90.
3. Heyes GJ, Mill AJ. The neoplastic transformation potential of mammography x ray and atomic bomb spectrum radiation. Radiat Res 2004;162:120–7.
4. Frankenburg D, Kelnhofer K, Bar K, Frankenberg-Schwager M. Enhanced neoplastic transformation by mammography X rays relative to 200 kVp X rays: indication for a strong dependence on photon energy of the RBE(M) for various end points. Radiat Res 2002;157:99–105. Erratum in: Radiat Res 2002;158:126.
5. Goggelmann W, Jacobsen C, Panzer W, Walsh L, Roos H, Schmid E. Re-evaluation of the RBE of 29 kV x-rays (mammography x-rays) relative to 220 kV x-rays using neoplastic transformation of human CGL1-hybrid cells. Radiat Environ Biophys 2003;42:175–82.
6. Imaging for Oncology: Collaboration between Clinical Radiologists and Clinical Oncologists in Diagnosis, Staging and Radiotherapy Planning; Royal College of Radiologists, London 2004.
7. Miralbell R, Lomax A, Cella L, Schneider U. Potential reduction of the incidence of radiation-induced second cancers by using proton beams in the treatment of pediatric tumors. Int J Radiat Oncol Biol Phys 2002;54:824–9.
8. Schneider U, Lomax A, Lombriser N. Comparative treatment planning using secondary cancer mortality calculations. Phys Med 2001;17 Suppl. 1:97–9.
9. Jones B, Rosenberg I. Particle Therapy Co-operative Oncology Group (PTCOG 40) Meeting, Institute Curie 2004. Br J Radiol 2005;78:94–7.

Threshold-contrast detectability curves for digital acquisition

The Editor—Sir,
We noted with interest the findings of Evans et al [1] in the September 2004 issue of BJR, that the threshold-contrast performance for native (non-subtracted) digital acquisition on a sample of modern image intensifier systems was generally insensitive to differences in radiation doses-per-image. This result is in agreement with results we have previously published [2], and which are kindly referred to in the paper by Evans et al [1]. We are not, however, in agreement with the implication that that it is acceptable to adopt image quality standards where dose-per-image is not a consideration.

The reason that the threshold-contrast (*i.e.* signal-to-noise) performance in some digital fluorography systems is insensitive to the dose-per-image is because quantum noise is not the dominant noise source at high dose-per-image settings [1, 2]. Simplistically, the total image noise σ_T can be taken as the quadrature sum of the quantum noise σ_Q and the system noise σ_S,

$$\sigma_T = \sqrt{\sigma_Q^2 + \sigma_S^2} \quad (1)$$

where this system noise may have components of electronic and non-stochastic structural noise. In the case of digital fluorography, the static granular appearance of the image intensifier input phosphor is the main element of the system noise [3]. We have argued that the upper limit to the dose-per-image for any radiological imaging system should be that where

$$\sigma_Q = \sigma_S \quad (2)$$

so that systems are always operated within the region where quantum noise dominates. This, we would consider, is at least the first step towards optimization. One method for confirming operation within this region is by making a series of threshold-contrast measurements over a range of dose-per-frame values [2]. It is our view that where radiological images are not quantum noise limited, the dose levels are simply too high. They are not as low as reasonably achievable (ALARA), not optimized and not justified [4, 5].

Yours etc.,

[1]C J Kotre
[2]N W Marshall

[1]Regional Medical Physics Department
Newcastle General Hospital
Newcastle-upon-Tyne
NE4 6BE
UK
[2]Clinical Physics Group
St Bartholomews Hospital
London
EC1A 7BE
UK

(*Received 22 November 2004 and accepted 15 February 2005*)
DOI: 10.1259/bjr/61956631

References

1. Evans DS, Mackenzie A, Lawinski CP, Smith D. Threshold contrast detail detectability curves for fluoroscopy and digital acquisition using modern image intensifier systems. Br J Radiol 2004;77:751–8.
2. Marshall NW, Kotre CJ, Robson KJ, Lecomber AR. Receptor dose in digital fluorography: a comparison between theory and practice. Phys Med Biol 2001;46:1283–96.
3. Kume Y, Doi K, Ohara K, Giger M. Investigation of basic imaging properties in digital radiography. 10. Structure mottle of II-TV digital imaging systems. Med Phys 1986;13:843–9.
4. ICRP. 1990 recommendations of the International Commission on Radiological Protection. Oxford, UK: ICRP Publication 60, 1990.
5. The Ionising Radiation (Medical Exposure) Regulations 2000. London: HMSO, 2000.

Author's reply

The Editor—Sir,

Thank you for your correspondence. We did not intend to imply that these dose levels are acceptable for digital acquisition images. The aim of the paper [1] was to show the current level of image quality available on the systems tested and to give some baseline image quality measurements. We agree with your findings [2] and correspondence and our paper [1] confirms that optimization is still required for digital acquisition.

Yours etc.,

A Mackenzie

KCARE
Kings College Hospital
London SE5 9RS
UK

(*Received 9 February 2005 and accepted 15 February 2005*)
DOI: 10.1259/bjr/82976242

References

1. Evans DS, Mackenzie A, Lawinski CP, Smith D. Threshold contrast detail detectability curves for fluoroscopy and digital acquisition using modern image intensifier systems. Br J Radiol 2004;77:751–8.
2. Marshall NW, Kotre CJ, Robson KJ, Lecomber AR. Receptor dose in digital fluorography: a comparison between theory and practice. Phys Med Biol 2001;46:1283–96.

The British Journal of Radiology, 78 (2005), 471–472
DOI: 10.1259/bjr/77108289

Case of the month

Breast or chest? A diagnostic conundrum

[1]J C LEE, FRCR, [2]S BANERJEE, MRCP and [2]D M KING, FRCR

[1]*Chelsea and Westminster Hospital, 369 Fulham Road, London SW10 9NH and* [2]*Royal Marsden Hospital, Fulham Road, London SW3 6JJ, UK*

A 60-year-old female presented with a 3 week history of a painless swelling in the left breast. Risk factors for developing breast carcinoma were present including smoking, a 6 year history of hormone replacement therapy, and a positive family history in two second-degree relatives. The patient had a total abdominal hysterectomy and bilateral salpingo-oophorectomy 7 years earlier for fibroids. On clinical examination, a 2 cm by 2 cm soft, lobulated mass was palpated in the upper inner quadrant of the left breast. Screening mammography had been performed 2 months prior to attendance (Figure 1). Following her clinical assessment, she was referred to the imaging department for ultrasound assessment and consideration for fine needle aspiration for cytology (Figure 2). A chest radiograph was obtained after the ultrasound (Figure 3).

What abnormalities are demonstrated? What possible pathologies are responsible?

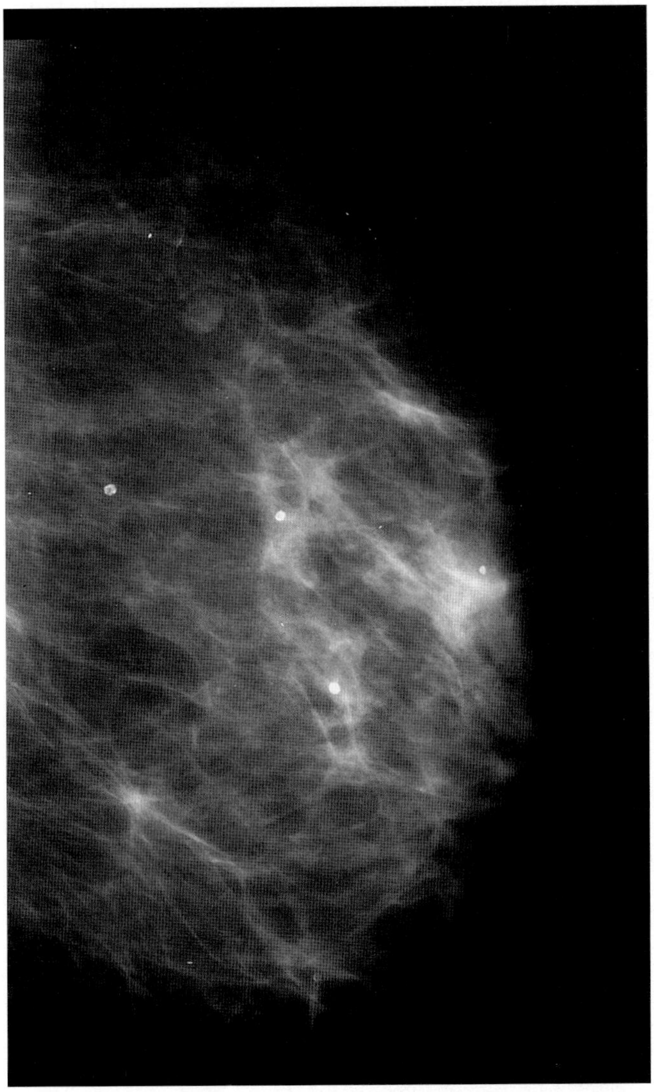

Figure 1. Left mediolateral oblique (MLO) mammogram.

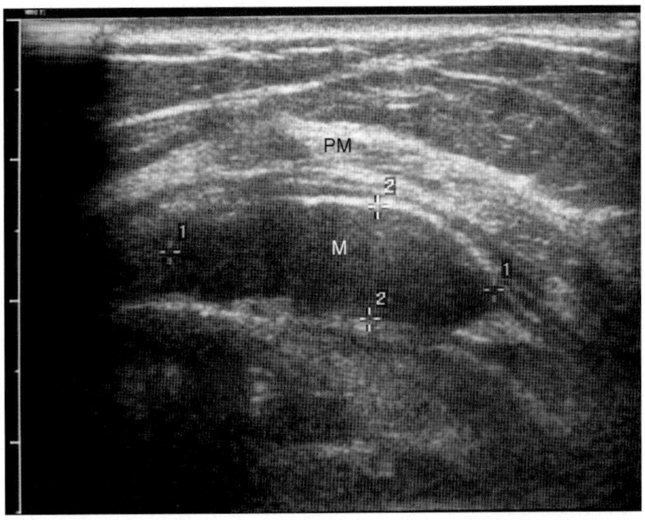

Figure 2. Transverse ultrasound image of the upper inner quadrant of the left breast.

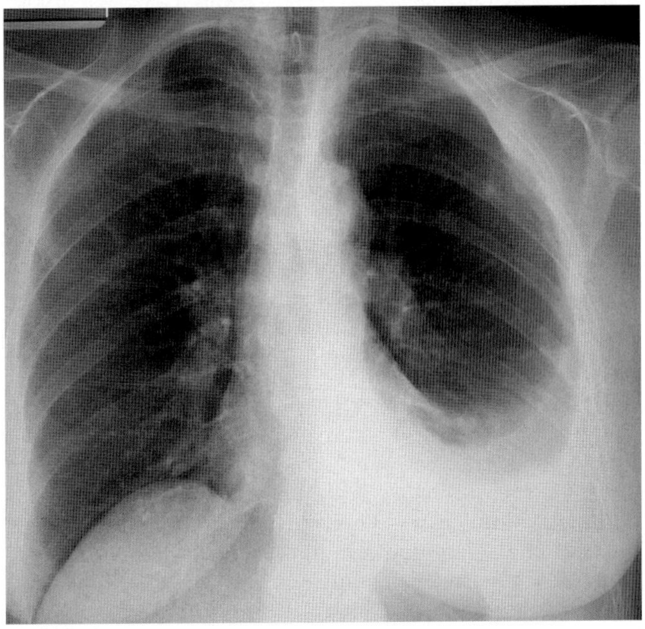

Figure 3. Frontal chest radiograph.

Received 8 November 2004 and in revised form 3 February 2005, accepted 7 February 2005.

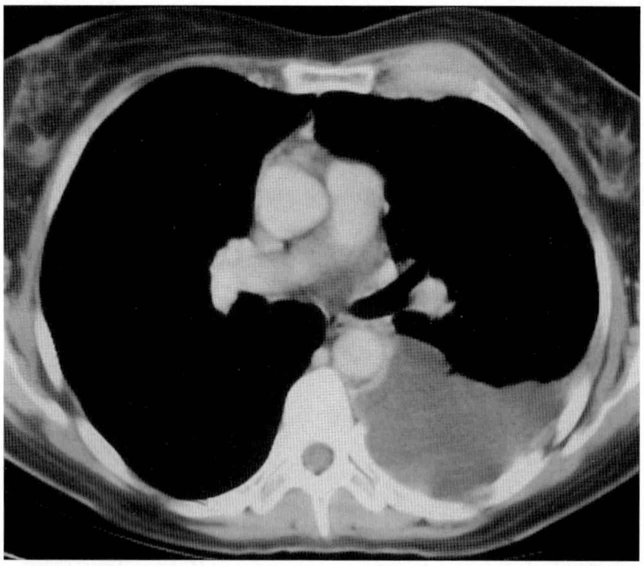

Figure 4. Axial contrast enhanced CT of the thorax at the equivalent level as the ultrasound image seen in Figure 2.

The mammogram (Figure 1) shows normal glandular architecture with several areas of benign calcification. No mass lesion is seen. The ultrasound image (Figure 2), demonstrates a well-defined, hypoechoic mass (M) deep to the pectoralis muscle (PM). The overlying breast tissue is sonographically normal. The chest radiograph (Figure 3) reveals a moderate-sized left pleural effusion with irregular pleural thickening superolaterally.

The differential diagnosis, at this point in the patient's management, included an atypical ductal/lobular carcinoma originating deep within the breast, an enlarged intramammary lymph node, or a chest wall mass such as an intramuscular lipoma, or rhabdomyosarcoma. To clarify the situation further, a CT was performed (Figure 4).

This demonstrates an infiltrating, soft-tissue density mass in the left anterior chest wall just lateral to the mid-sternum, associated with destruction of the costochondral junction. The mass arises deep to the pectoralis muscle and is associated with a large left pleural effusion. Note the enhancing thickened pleura adjacent to the descending thoracic aorta.

The initial fine needle aspirate for cytology was inadequate. Owing to the complex nature of the lesion, an excisional biopsy of the anterior chest wall mass was performed under general anaesthetic. Histopathlogy established a diagnosis of malignant pleural mesothelioma.

Discussion

90–95% of all breast masses are due to carcinoma, cysts or fibroadenomata [1]. The remaining 5–10% includes conditions arising from the ducts, *e.g.* papillomas; the glandular tissues, *e.g.* sclerosing adenosis; or from the supporting structures, *e.g.* lipomas. In a small subset of patients, breast masses may result from more unusual pathological processes. These include a variety of systemic diseases including diabetic fibrous mastopathy, amyloidosis and Wegener's granulomatosis, as well as rare primary tumours of the breast including hamartomas and haemangiomas, and malignant lesions such as lymphoma, leukaemia, and the sarcomas. Secondary haematogenous spread to the breast can occur from almost any primary malignancy of which the most common are melanoma and lung, but gastric, renal, cervical, and uterine tumours are known occasionally to metastasise [2].

However, it should be remembered that not all breast lumps represent breast disease and that tumours may arise from the chest wall beneath the breast. Primary chest wall tumours include sarcomas, fibromas, lipomas, desmoid tumours, lymphomas, osteochondromas and neurogenic tumours. Furthermore, bronchogenic carcinomas, intrathoracic lymphoma, and malignant pleural mesothelioma may involve the chest wall by direct spread from the thoracic cavity [3].

Malignant pleural mesothelioma (MPM) is a rare, aggressive tumour arising from the serosal lining of the chest and abdomen. In England and Scotland, the prevalence is 8 per 100 000 in the 40–74 year age group, with an overall incidence of 1–2 cases per million per year [4]. The link to asbestos exposure is well established. MPM principally spreads by the direct route and only rarely metastasises haematogenously. Direct spread typically results in circumferential nodular thickening of the pleural space and this process may involve the pericardium and mediastinum. Invasion by MPM through the chest wall is recognized and occurs in up to 16% of cases, although this usually occurs with advanced disease [5]. However, a review of the literature suggests that this is the first report of MPM presenting as a breast mass.

When surgical pleural resection is not possible, as in the illustrated case, recent advances in the medical management of MPM have, for the first time, demonstrated improved quality of life scores and prolonged survival in unresectable or recurrent cases [6].

From the radiologist's perspective, it is important to remember that not all breast masses arise from the breast itself. One should bear in mind that chest wall lesions and intrathoracic pathology can present as breast lesions.

References

1. Dixon JM, Mansel RE. Chapter 34 The Breast. In: Burnand KG, Young AE, editors. New Aird's companion in surgical studies. (1st edn). London, UK: Churchill Livingstone, 1994:811–44.
2. Feder JM, de Paredes ES, Hogge JP, Wilken JJ. Unusual breast lesions: radiologic-pathologic correlation. Radiographics 1999;19:11–26.
3. Glazer HS, Duncan-Meyer J, Aronberg DJ, Moran JF, Levitt RG, Sagel SS. Pleural and chest wall invasion in bronchogenic carcinoma: CT evaluation. Radiology 1985;157:191–4.
4. Montanaro F, Bray F, Gennaro V, Merler E, Tyczynski JE, Parkin DM, et al. Pleural mesothelioma incidence in Europe: evidence of some deceleration in the increasing trends. Cancer Causes Control 2003;14:791–803.
5. Ng CS, Munden RF, Libshitz HI. Malignant pleural mesothelioma: the spectrum of manifestations on CT in 70 cases. Clin Radiol 1999;54:415–21.
6. Budde LS, Hanna NH. Pemetrexed (Alimta(R)): improving outcomes in malignant pleural mesothelioma. Expert Rev Anticancer Ther 2004;4:361–8.

Book reviews

MR imaging of the spine and spinal cord. By D Uhlenbrook (Eds). pp. ix + 518, 2004 (Georg Thieme Verlag, Stuttgart, Germany), €149.00

ISBN 3-13-130941-5

This book intended for radiologists, neuroradiologists, trauma surgeons, orthopaedic surgeons and neurosurgeons is a translation from a German text first published in 2001 and revised in 2003. In general, this has been an excellent translation, but it is formal and occasionally uses unfamiliar phraseology, *e.g.* Bechterew's disease (ankylosing spondylitis).

There are nine chapters, each well referenced and relatively well indexed. There are 1305 illustrations which are generally of a high standard. All pathologies have been well demonstrated but more annotation might be welcomed from the clinical groups who would use this text. It has also been assumed that the reader is familiar with normal MR appearances.

There are 518 pages covering the outlined topics with the following clinical waiting; Embryology and Malformation (20%), Degenerative Disorders of the Spine (20%), Tumours (20%), Inflammatory Disorders (15%), Physics, Spinal Surgery, Acute Spinal Trauma, Vascular Disorders and Open MR Systems (25%)

The limited physics introduction was welcomed and I found the brief overview on artefacts helpful. The summary at the end of each chapter was useful but on one occasion, there was disparity between the detail in the main text and summary, *e.g.* location of spinal meningioma. 30 pages were allocated to discussing ageing disc, end plate changes and radial tears, which was probably excessive but comprehensive. At least one image of a sagittal lumbar spines was wrongly labelled as T_1 instead of T_2.

In conclusion, this was an excellent overview of MR imaging of the spine and spinal cord, with extensive imaging examples of all pathologies. It is relatively easy to read, is reasonably priced and will be a welcome addition to any library.

F Gardner

Multislice CT (2nd edn). By MF Reiser, M Takahashi, M Modic and CR Becker (Eds). pp. x + 280, 2004 (Springer-Verlag, Berlin, Heidelberg, New York), £92.50

ISBN 3-540-43638-3

This is another of the excellent series of medical radiology books from Springer Verlag that is edited by Professors Baert and Sartor. This book aims to provide a complete and concise overview to people using the new multislice CT systems and I have to say I think it does an extraordinarily good job of it. The first four chapters of the book deal with the concepts, theory and design of multislice CT scanners, the problems associated with radiation dose contrast delivery and the visualization of large imaging data volumes. This technical section is brief, extremely concise and very well informed and I actually greatly enjoyed reading it. It is then followed by a series of applicational sections, with four chapters on imaging the brain, three on head and neck, six on chest and eight on abdomen. Each of these appears to be written by an expert in the clinical area with significant experience in the use of multislice CT. I would not have claimed to have read all of them but have read a good number of them in detail and they appear to be uniformly well written, well laid out and knowledgeable. They are also extremely well referenced. I am currently suggesting this as the standard book on CT for our radiography students and it is sitting on my bookshelf next to the CT scanner, since I consider it to be an invaluable reference work. If you are looking for something to help you get to grips with the new multislice systems, this should definitely be on your shopping list.

A Jackson

BIR CORPORATE MEMBER SCHEME

The BIR Corporate Member Scheme is aimed at all companies with an interest in radiology and allied sciences. For an annual subscription member companies are offered an attractive benefits package. To find out why your company should join the leading edge companies listed below, please contact Mr Adrian C Laws, Marketing Manager, British Institute of Radiology, 36 Portland Place, London W1B 1AT. Tel: +44 (0) 20 7307 1404.

Agfa-Gevaert Ltd
Tel: 020 82314900
Contact Mr M Hill, Business Manager Medical Imaging and PACS Systems
Product Code: 1, 2, 3, 4, 6, 9, 10, 12, 13, 14, 15, 20, 22 and 23

Alliance Medical Ltd
Tel: 01295 671223
Contact Mr Charles Fox, Marketing Executive
Product Code: 1, 4, 5, 16, 20 and 21

Amersham Health
Tel: 01494 798666
Contact Mr D G Rothery, Marketing Manager
Product Codes: 1, 2, 3, 4, 5 and 6

Bard Limited
Tel: 01293 606864
Contact Ms T Empson, Product Manager
Product Code: 2

B.M.V.A.
Tel: 01483 689838
Contact Dr R Bowden, Meetings Officer
Product Codes: 1, 3, 4, 9, 10 and 21

Bracco UK Ltd
Tel: 01628 851500
Contact Mr A Quinn, Product Manager
Product Codes: 1, 2 and 5

BVM Medical Ltd
Tel: 01455 614555
Contact Jay Tailor, Managing Director
Product Codes: 2 and 18

Cerner Corporation (UK)
Tel: 01452 831533
Contact Mr C Harrison, Client Executive
Product Codes: 9, 10, 13 and 20

Clinical Press Ltd
Tel: 0117 9420256
Contact Professor Paul Goddard, Chairman
Product Codes: 17 and 21

Cook (UK) Ltd
Tel: 01462 482884
Contact Mr Iain Mackintosh, regional Manager - Diagnostic and Interventional Products
Product Code: 2

Department of Radiography & Imaging Sciences (St Martin's College, Lancaster)
Tel: 01524 384640
Contact Mr Philip Harris, Acting Head of Department
Product Code: 21

Dictaphone International
Tel:020 78785000
Contact Dr F Brabant, Director of Product Management
Product Codes: 9 and 13

E-Z-EM Ltd
Tel: 01869 366900
Contact Mr Martin Suggitt, Product Manager
Product Codes: 1, 2 and 8

Ferrania UK Ltd
Tel: 01344 312100
Contact Mr Alan Budge, General Marketing Manager
Product Codes: 1, 3, 4, 9, 10, 13, 14, 15 and 18

Fuji Photo Film (UK) Ltd
Tel: 01234 326780
Contact Mr R G Brown, Strategic Business Manager
Product Codes: 1, 3, 4, 6, 9, 10, 12, 13, 14, 15, 18 and 22

GE Medical Systems
Tel: 01753 874000
Contact Mr A Trivett, Managing Director
Product Codes: 1, 2, 3, 4, 6, 8, 9, 10, 15, 18 and 22

Guerbet Laboratories Ltd
Tel: 01908 522888
Contact Mr Trevor Furniss, General Manager
Product Code: 1 and 2

Insignia Medical Systems Ltd
Tel: 01420 540206
Contact Mr Richard Dormer, Managing Director
Product Code: 9

Kimal plc
Tel: 01895 270951
Contact Mr S Clarke, Technical Director
Product Code: 2

Kingsmoor Publications Ltd
Tel: 01371 812960
Contact Mr David Roberts, Managing Director
Product Code: 17

Kodak Ltd
Tel: 01442 844473
Contact Mr Chris Wright, Marketing Manager UK and Ireland
Product Codes: 1, 3, 4, 6, 8, 9, 10, 12, 13, 14, 15, 18, 21, 22 and 23

Landauer, Inc.
Tel: 01865 373008
Contact Dr T Finnigan, Director, European Operations
Product Code: 8

Lanmark
Tel: 01494 675535
Contact Mrs Liz Beckmann, Director
Product Codes: 6, 9, 10, 13, 17 and 20

Lodestone Patient Care Limited
Tel: 020 89449630
Contact Mrs J Hill, Director of Operations
Product Code: 1, 3 and 21

Medical Imaging Systems Limited
Tel: 020 82059500
Contact Mr P W Sykes, Director
Product Code: 1

Mirada Solutions Ltd
Tel: 01865 265500
Contact Dr Clare Jones, VP Marketing
Product Codes: 1, 4, 6, 9, 10, 13, 21 and 22

Nucletron UK Ltd
Tel: 018297 71111
Contact Mr J Banks, Managing Director
Product Codes: 6 and 8

Pantak Medical Systems Agfa NDT
Tel: 0118 9310310
Contact Mr R Howton, Managing Director
Product Codes: 1, 6, 7 and 8

Philips Medical Systems
Tel:01737 230400
Contact Ms Anita Littlechild, Marketing Communications Manager
Product Codes: 1, 2, 9, 10, 22 and 23

Samsung SDS Europe Ltd
Tel:020 83807000
Contact Mr G Wheeler, Sales Manager (Medical)
Product Codes: 1, 9, 10, 13, 15, 16 and 20

Schering Health Care Ltd
Tel: 01444 232323
Contact Mr Chris Matthews, Product Manager
Product Codes: 1, 2 and 3

Sectra Ltd
Tel: 020 86106033
Contact Jan Wolfram, Managing Director
Product Codes: 9 and 10

Siemens Medical Solutions
Tel: 01344 396317
Contact Mr Mike Bell, Manager, Advertising and Exhibitions
Product Codes: 1, 2, 3, 4, 6, 9, 15 and 22

Sony Scientific and Medical
Tel: 01932 816267
Contact R Holt, Marketing Manager
Product Code: 14

Sonosite Ltd
Tel: 01767 313117
Contact Ms Gillian Duffy, European Marketing Director
Product Codes: 3

Southern Scientific Ltd
Tel: 01903 604000
Contact Mr Stephen Adams, Sales Manager
Product Codes: 1, 3, 4, 8, 10, 12 and 22

Toshiba Medical Systems UK
Tel: 01293 653700
Contact Mr S M Weeden, Manager X-ray Products
Product Codes: 1, 2, 3, 4, 9, 10 and 15

Varian Oncology Systems
Tel: 01293 531244 (UK)
Contact Mr Rolf Stähelin (Switzerland - tel. 00 41 417498844), Marketing Manager, Europe
Product Code: 6

Vertec Scientific Ltd
Tel: 01734 817431
Contact Mr B Hipgrave, Managing Director
Product Codes: 1, 4, 6, 8 and 12

Wardray Premise Ltd
Tel: 020 83989911
Contact Mr R Beach, Sales Manager
Product Codes: 8, 18 and 20

Wolverson X-Ray
Tel: 01902 637333
Contact Mr N Bacon, Sales Director
Product Codes: 1, 8, 15, 18 and 23

Xograph Imaging Systems
Tel: 01666 501501 or 07000 for X-ray
Contact Mr N Staff, Technical Director
Product Codes: 1, 8, 12, 14, 15, 18, 22 and 23

PRODUCT CODES

1. Diagnostic X-ray including NMR and CT
2. Interventional radiology
3. Ultrasound
4. Nuclear medicine
5. Radiopharmaceuticals
6. Radiotherapy and oncology
7. Radiobiology
8. Radiation protection
9. PACS
10. Image processing
11. Nuclear fuel cycle service
12. Quality assurance
13. Radiology data management computer systems
14. Video printing
15. Equipment leasing
16. Hospital-shared services
17. Medical publishing
18. X-ray consumables distribution
19. Electricity generation
20. Medical reporting systems
21. Education
22. Mammography
23. Dental X-ray

Meetings & Courses

Prepare yourself for PACS
6 May 2005
London, UK
Further details: The British Institute of Radiology, 36 Portland Place, London W1B 1AT.
Tel: 0207 307 1406. Fax: 0207 307 1414.
Email: registrations@bir.org.uk. Visit: www.bir.org.uk

President's Conference 2005
25–26 May 2005
London, UK
Further details: The British Institute of Radiology, 36 Portland Place, London W1B 1AT.
Tel: 0207 307 1406. Fax: 0207 307 1414.
Email: registrations@bir.org.uk. Visit: www.bir.org.uk

IMRT
8 July 2005
Manchester, UK
Further details: The British Institute of Radiology, 36 Portland Place, London W1B 1AT.
Tel: 0207 307 1406. Fax: 0207 307 1414.
Email: registrations@bir.org.uk. Visit: www.bir.org.uk

Upper gastrointestinal cancer workshop
2 September 2005
London, UK
Further details: The British Institute of Radiology, 36 Portland Place, London W1B 1AT.
Tel: 0207 307 1406. Fax: 0207 307 1414.
Email: registrations@bir.org.uk. Visit: www.bir.org.uk

MR of the extremities
23 September 2005
Bristol, UK
Further details: The British Institute of Radiology, 36 Portland Place, London W1B 1AT.
Tel: 0207 307 1406. Fax: 0207 307 1414.
Email: registrations@bir.org.uk. Visit: www.bir.org.uk

CT PET
29 September 2005
London, UK
Further details: The British Institute of Radiology, 36 Portland Place, London W1B 1AT.
Tel: 0207 307 1406. Fax: 0207 307 1414.
Email: registrations@bir.org.uk. Visit: www.bir.org.uk

International Cancer Imaging Society Meeting and 5th Annual Teaching Course
3–5 October 2005
Beurs van Berlage, Amsterdam, The Netherlands
Further details: The British Institute of Radiology, 36 Portland Place, London W1B 1AT.
Tel: 0207 307 1406. Fax: 0207 307 1414.
Email: icis@bir.org.uk. Visit: www.icimagingsociety.org.uk

Volume 78| **June 2005**

BJR British Journal of Radiology

Full papers

Differences in bone mineral density and geometry in men and women: the Newcastle Thousand Families Study at 50 years old

The costs and effects of introducing selectively trained radiographers to an A&E reporting service: a retrospective controlled before and after study

Acute ureteric calculus obstruction: unenhanced spiral CT versus HASTE MR urography and abdominal radiograph

Real-time blood-pool images of contrast enhanced ultrasound with Definity in the detection of tumour nodules in the liver

Effectiveness of flexible noise control image processing for digital portal images using computed radiography

Comparative analyses of the dynamic properties of the bladder wall studied by repetitive CT scans of patients and cryo-sections of cadavers

Differentiation between solitary brain metastasis and high grade glioma by diffusion tensor imaging

Editorial
Commentaries
Review
Short communications
Case reports
Correspondence
Case of the month

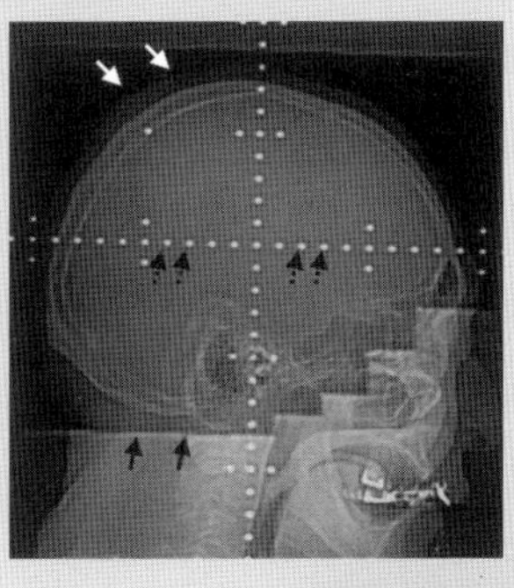

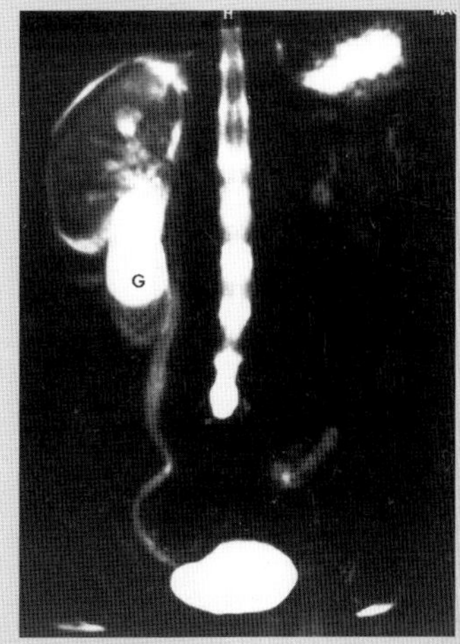

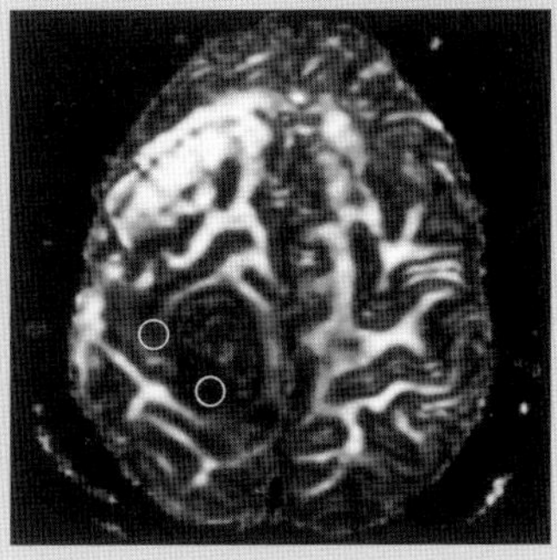

http://bjr.birjournals.org

ISSN 0007-1285

Published by

BIR The British Institute of **Radiology**

BJR

ISSN 0007 1285

THE BRITISH JOURNAL OF RADIOLOGY

Aims and Coverage

The *British Journal of Radiology* is the official peer-reviewed monthly research journal of the British Institute of Radiology. It is a multidisciplinary journal covering all clinical and technical aspects of diagnostic imaging, radiotherapy and oncology, medical physics and radiobiology. BJR is an international journal containing papers both from the UK and overseas, and is circulated to Full Members of the BIR and to libraries worldwide.

Authors are strongly advised to submit manuscripts online using Editorial Manager^{TM}, at http://bjr.edmgr.com. Online submission will expedite the peer-review process. Instructions to Authors are available on request from the Refereeing Administrator at the address given below, and are also available on the BIR's website at www.bir.org.uk

Editorial Board

Overseas Advisory Panel

Published by the British Institute of Radiology, 36 Portland Place, London W1B 1AT, UK.
Editorial enquiries: Tel: +44 (0)20 7307 1424; Fax: +44 (0)20 7307 1414
Email: publications@bir.org.uk
Advertising sales and enquiries: please contact David Lancaster at McMillan Scott: Tel: +44 (0)20 7878 2313
Email: david@mcmslondon.co.uk
www.bir.org.uk www.birjournals.org bjr.edmgr.com

Subscriptions

Subscriptions fulfilment is carried out by PSP Subscriptions, BMA House, Tavistock Square, London WC1H 9JR, UK (Telephone +44 (0)20 7383 6270; Fax +44 (0)20 7383 6402; email subscriptions@bmjgroup.com). The 2005 annual subscription rate for the printed version of BJR is £524 (includes 12 issues plus two Special Issue). Subscriptions are on a calendar basis only.

Institutional BJR subscribers have free access to both BJR Online and Imaging Online, and are offered a 33% discount on a print subscription to the BJR's quarterly review journal Imaging (see http://imaging.birjournals.org).

US Mailing Agent

The British Journal of Radiology (ISSN 0007 1285) is published monthly by the British Institute of Radiology, c/o Mercury Airfreight Int. Ltd, 365 Blair Road, Avenel, NJ 07001. The Dollar price for US direct subscribers is $786. Periodicals Postage Paid at Rahway NJ. Postmaster: send address corrections to the British Journal of Radiology, c/o Mercury Airfreight Int. Ltd, 365 Blair Road, Avenel, NJ 07001.

Back Issues

Back issues can be ordered from Vine House Distribution, Waldenbury, North Common, Chailey, East Sussex BN8 4DR, UK (Telephone +44 (0)1825 723398; Fax +44 (0)1825 724188). Price is £40 per issue.

BJR Online

BJR Online, produced in association with HighWire Press, is available free of charge to BIR members and Institutional print subscribers: http://bjr.birjournals.org. Enquiries to publications@bir.org.uk

Typeset, printed and bound by The Charlesworth Group, Wakefield, UK. Telephone +44 (0)1924 204830.

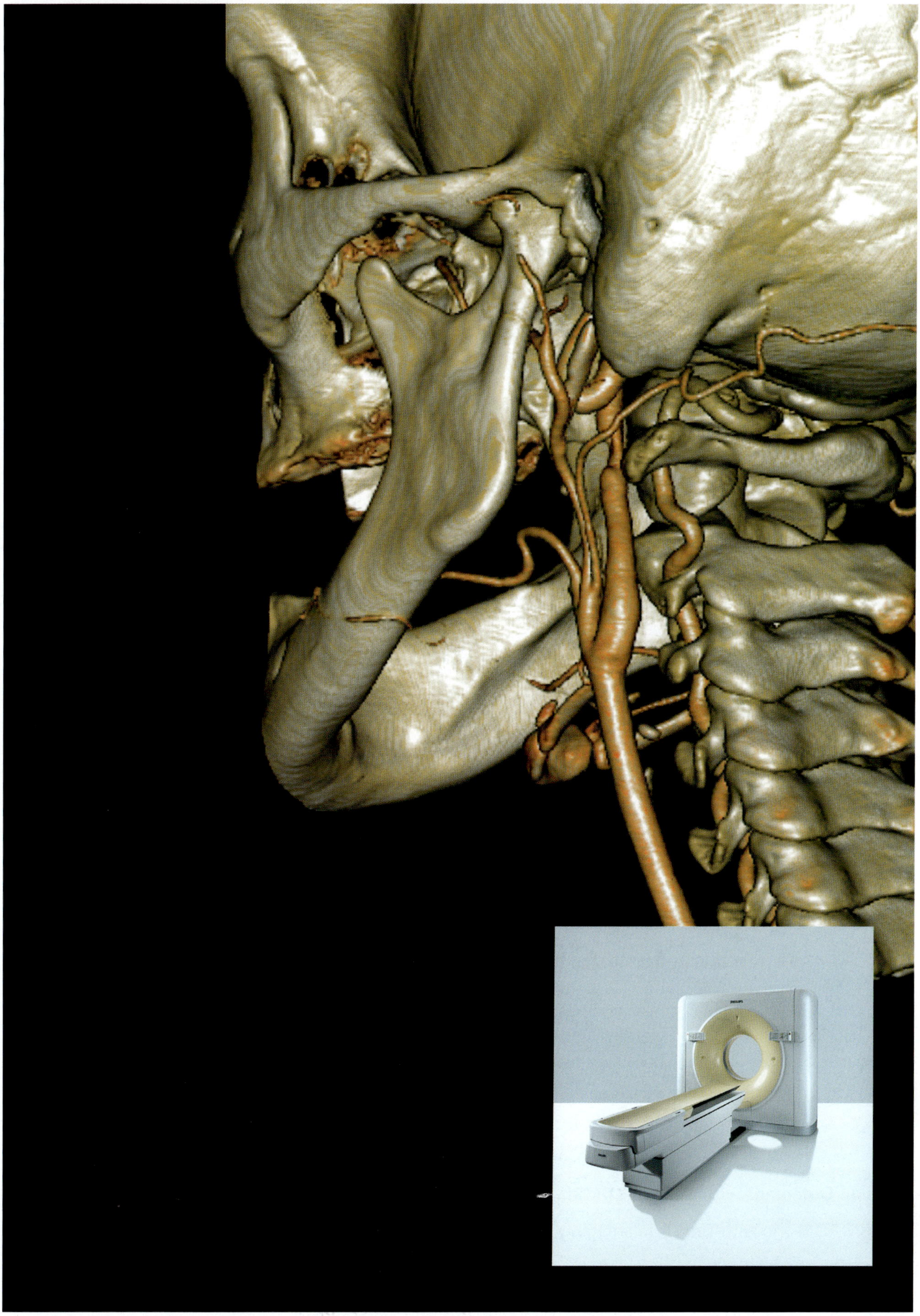

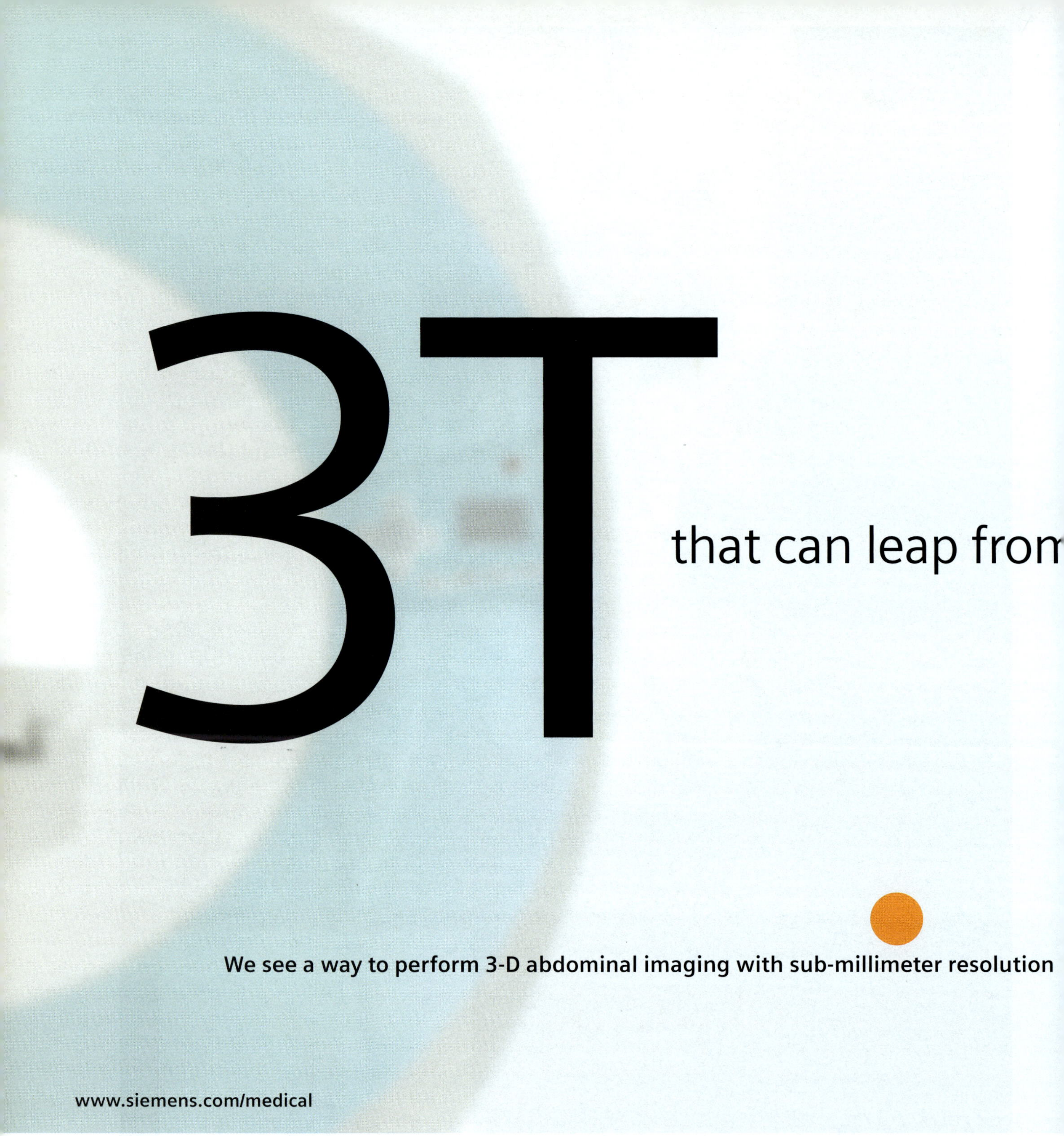
3T
that can leap from
We see a way to perform 3-D abdominal imaging with sub-millimeter resolution
www.siemens.com/medical

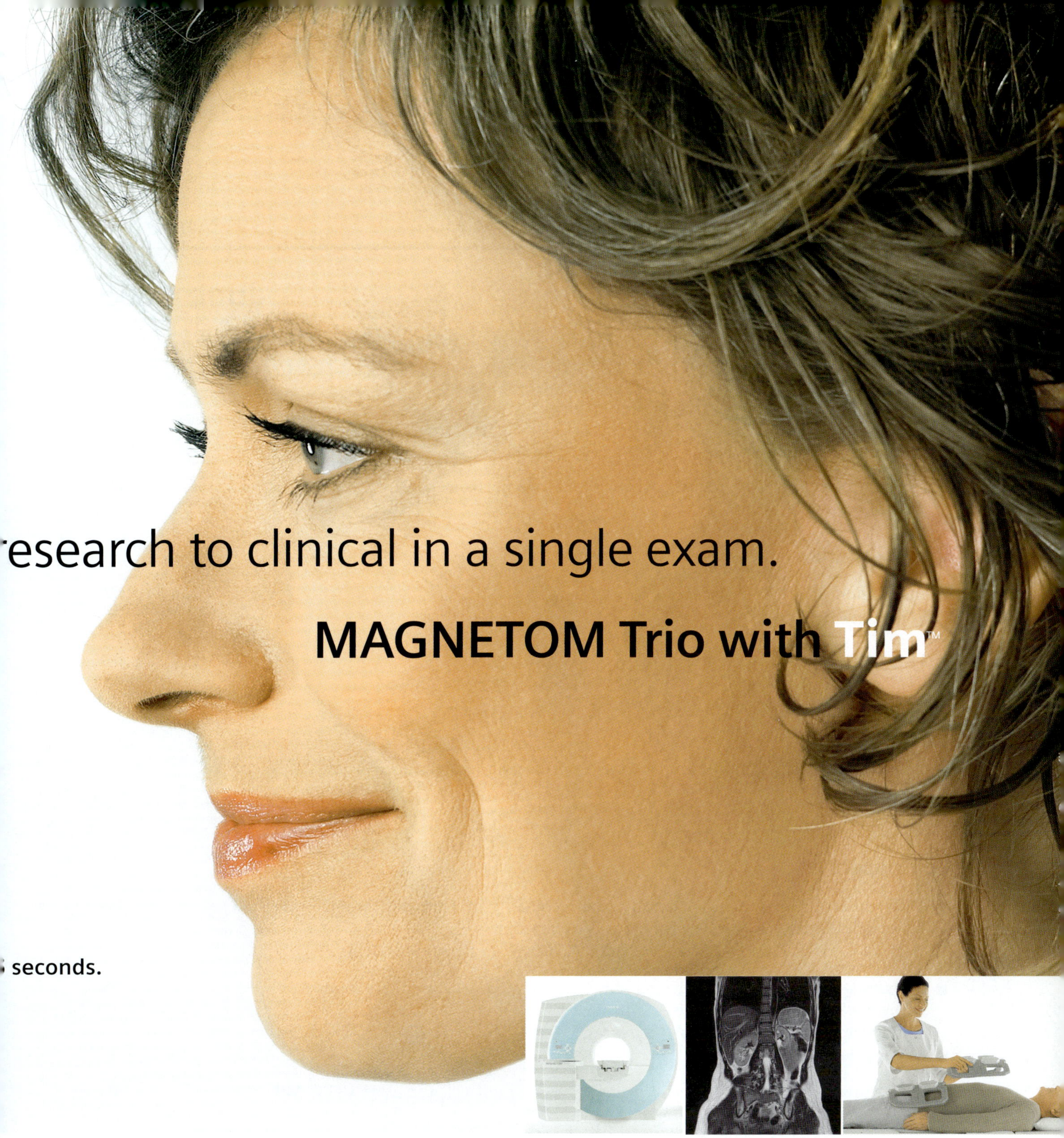

MAGNETOM Trio, A Tim System

SIEMENS
medical

BJR

VOLUME 78

Number 930

Contents

June 2005

Front cover: *The illustrations used on the front cover of this issue of BJR can be found on pages 509, 520 and 534. We thank the authors for granting us permission to use their figures.*

Editorial

Page

■ 20 years of patient dose studies: where should we go from here? 477
C J Martin

Commentaries

■ Installation of a PACS system 480
D D Dundas

■ Using PACS as a teaching resource 483
D Blunt and D O'Regan

Review

■ Rationale for using multiple antioxidants in protecting humans against low doses of ionizing radiation 485
K N Prasad

Full papers

■ Differences in bone mineral density and geometry in men and women: the Newcastle Thousand Families Study at 50 years old 493
S P Tuck, M S Pearce, D J Rawlings, F N Birrell, L Parker and R M Francis

■ The costs and effects of introducing selectively trained radiographers to an A&E reporting service: a retrospective controlled before and after study 499
S Brealey, D G King, S Hahn, C Godfrey, M T I Crowe, K Bloor, S Crane and D Longsworth

■ Acute ureteric calculus obstruction: unenhanced spiral CT versus HASTE MR urography and abdominal radiograph 506
F Regan, B Kuszyk, M E Bohlman and S Jackman

■ Real-time blood-pool images of contrast enhanced ultrasound with Definity in the detection of tumour nodules in the liver 512
H Maruyama, S Matsutani, H Saisho, Y Mine, N Kamiyama, T Hirata and M Sasamata

■ Effectiveness of flexible noise control image processing for digital portal images using computed radiography 519
S Yamada and K Murase

■ Comparative analyses of the dynamic properties of the bladder wall studied by repetitive pelvic CT scans of patients and cryo-sections of cadavers 528
E Dale, T P Hellebust, Ø S Bruland and D R Olsen

■ Differentiation between solitary brain metastasis and high-grade glioma by diffusion tensor imaging 533
K Tsuchiya, A Fujikawa, M Nakajima and K Honya

Short communications

■ The effect of introducing radiographer reporting on the availability of reports for Accident and Emergency and General Practitioner examinations: a time-series analysis 538
S D Brealey and P A Scuffham

■ The low energy X-ray response of the LiF:Mg:Cu:P thermoluminescent dosemeter: a comparison with LiF:Mg:Ti 543
C R Edwards, P J Mountford, S Green, J E Palethorpe and A J Moloney

Case reports

■ Helical tomotherapy for craniospinal radiation 548
G Bauman, S Yartsev, T Coad, B Fisher and T Kron

■ Benign external compression of the inferior vena cava associated with thrombus formation 553
R A England, I P Wells and C M Gutteridge

■ Cystic adenomyosis with florid glandular differentiation mimicking ovarian malignancy 558
I Imaoka, Y Kaji, Y Kobashi, A Wada, G Honjo, M Hayashi, M Yoshida and M Matsuo

■ Duodenal diverticulum mimicking a cystic pancreatic neoplasm 562
A Hariri, S S Siegelman and R H Hruban

■ Solitary fibrous tumour of the epididymis: MRI features 565
A Ch Tsili, C Tsampoulas, X Giannakopoulos, A Batistatou, E Arkoumani, An Silakos, N Sofikitis and S C Efremidis

■ Bilateral absence of the internal carotid artery: MR angiography and ultrasound findings 569
D W Anderson

Correspondence

■ Moderate dose rate ionizing radiation increases longevity? 573
G M Kendall and C R Muirhead

Case of the month

■ Seizures following bone marrow transplantation 575
M Bratby and D MacVicar

BIR Company Subscribers 578

Meetings and courses 580

The British Journal of Radiology, 78 (2005), 477–479
DOI: 10.1259/bjr/27292976

Editorial

20 years of patient dose studies: where should we go from here?

C J MARTIN, PhD

Department of Clinical Physics and Bioengineering, Gartnavel Royal Hospital, Health Physics, West House (Ground Floor), 1055 Great Western Road, Glasgow G12 0XH, UK

The first comprehensive survey of patient doses for a range of diagnostic X-ray examinations was published in the UK in 1986 by the National Radiological Protection Board (NRPB) [1]. Concern about the wide variation in patient doses for similar examinations revealed in the survey persuaded medical physicists and others to measure doses in their own hospitals and investigate whether changes in equipment or technique should be made when these were found to be high. The last 10–15 years has seen a regular quota of patient dose studies for radiology examinations published in the literature. There is, on average, one in each issue of the *British Journal of Radiology* at the present time. The NRPB and others have derived tables of conversion coefficients to allow effective doses to be calculated from the various dose quantities normally measured so that doses from different examinations can be compared [2]. Estimates of potential risk from developing cancer can be derived using coefficients published by the International Commission on Radiological Protection (ICRP) [3]. Much useful work has been done and there are always more things that can be investigated. However, there comes a point where the benefit is limited and more may be achieved through application of effort in other areas. We have to ask questions about the need for further studies of patient dose and the level of quantification that is justified. What should we be trying to achieve from a patient dose study? When is it appropriate to publish results from such studies? Ought we to pay more attention to the impact on image quality, and if so, how do we assess it? How far do we go in our dose calculations? Are we justified in drawing conclusions about effective dose and risk, since factors that we use in the calculations change as the state of knowledge develops?

One of the main benefits from patient dose surveys has been to provide information on doses in different hospitals for comparison, which give an indication of whether the techniques used in our own hospitals are optimized in terms of dose. The introduction of diagnostic reference levels (DRLs) through the Ionising Radiation Regulations [4] has formalized this process in the UK. The accumulation of patient dose data on which DRLs can be based is important. The NRPB (now part of the Health Protection Agency) has collated doses from hospitals throughout the UK and publishes reports presenting these data every 5 years [5]. These reports provide us with a large databank of doses for a wide range of hospitals that we can draw on, and are ideal for setting national DRLs.

Received 2 February 2005 and in revised form 15 February 2005, accepted 15 February 2005.

The time has passed when results of a patient dose survey from a particular region of the country should be published just to provide information on dose magnitudes, but independent studies can make important contributions to our knowledge. They can show how different techniques influence dose, because radiology staff and physicists can analyse techniques and identify factors contributing to larger doses, and this information is useful in optimization. However, we should review critically the aims and objectives before undertaking a study. The following are examples of the questions we might ask ourselves.

- Is the procedure to be studied representative of ones that are performed widely?
- Are there sufficient results from other studies on current dose levels for the examination(s)?
- Will the study provide new data on general dose levels in a particular country?
- Are the data going to assist others in setting DRLs?
- Will the study provide information on relative merits of different techniques?
- Are results likely to be useful in optimization?
- Does the study contribute new ideas on methods for dose measurement?

If simple studies are to present dose information that is representative of current practice, results from at least 3–4 hospitals are required and preferably 8–10. Doses for fluoroscopy equipment will be strongly influenced by the equipment performance and facilities available, as well as the radiologists' techniques, so studies on one or two units may give misleading results. If there are only one or two hospitals carrying out the procedure in an area, then a joint study with colleagues from other centres might be more appropriate. Otherwise, probably the best course of action for UK groups is to send results to the NRPB for inclusion in their next patient dose report. Some of the examinations for which there is less information available are in interventional radiology and cardiology. A problem with studies on complex procedures such as these is the difficulty in defining standard procedures, since the vessels investigated have a major influence on the dose. Categories of procedures must be worked out carefully so that like is compared with like.

So far we have considered patient dose in isolation, but this is only half of the optimization equation [6]. The most important component is ensuring that the image quality is good enough to enable the diagnosis to be made. We cannot reduce dose indefinitely without affecting image quality. The consequences of a failure to make a correct diagnosis because of poor image quality are immediate and the risks are far greater than those from the radiation exposure. There are some applications where the relative positions of structures are being assessed, such as bone alignments, where a noisy image obtained with a low dose of radiation will give all the diagnostic information required. However, for the majority of applications we need as high quality an image as the technique can provide, since it is the fine detail which allows a definitive diagnosis to be made. Some thoughts about assessment of image quality are given below.

- We should look at simple contrast to noise ratios to determine the best exposure parameters to use for imaging different parts of the body. The contrast to noise ratio is the signal to noise ratio (SNR) which can be measured for larger structures with areas covering hundreds of pixels.
- We should look at SNR as a function of spatial frequency (detail size) to determine how well our system can visualize structures of different size. This can be accomplished in terms of Detective Quantum Efficiency or Noise Equivalent Quanta, which provide objective assessments of imaging performance for an ideal observer.
- We should establish methods of image quality measurement that are linked more closely to the perception tasks involved in making diagnoses.
- We need to establish links between the sizes and attenuating properties of structures important in clinical diagnosis for different organs and tissues, and details in test objects that might be included in imaging phantoms.
- We should make use of computer simulations to evaluate imaging performance and predict optimum exposure conditions for different examinations.
- We need to understand the effects of image processing techniques on the appearance and perception of digital images.
- More ready access to data from digital imaging equipment will allow image analysis and information on the look up tables used in producing the displayed image would be advantageous.

The final question to consider in relation to patient dose studies is what information should be provided on dose? The measured quantities dose–area product, entrance surface dose, CT dose index and dose–length product are the most important as they can be used for direct comparisons. However, it has been the practice to provide information on assessment of effective dose as well. There are large uncertainties in the coefficients used to convert dose measurements to effective dose. They are based on risk coefficients for a cross-section of the population with all ages and both genders, which is clearly not applicable to the population undergoing diagnostic medical examinations. The ICRP have suggested in a draft of their future recommendations that effective dose should only be used for establishment of prospective radiation protection guidance, not for assessing risks of stochastic effects at low doses in retrospective situations. Nevertheless, effective dose is useful as a comparator for relative magnitudes of doses for different types of examination, but we must not attribute to this more certainty than is justified. This is especially true since the definition of effective dose published by ICRP will change as more information becomes available from epidemiological studies. For examinations where particular radiosensitive organs receive significant doses, it may be more appropriate to give estimates of doses to these organs in the assessment, rather than effective dose. For complex examinations, detailed analyses of dose for each projection have been undertaken. This has allowed an indication of effective dose to be obtained for particular examinations, which has been interesting. However, this level of detail requires a significant effort to provide information that is of limited value. A simple presentation of measurable dose quantities with advice on techniques may be more appropriate in future studies.

While dealing with patient dose assessments, it is worth considering what information should be given as an indication of potential harm to an individual who as a patient has received an overexposure or who is to take part in a research study. Any risk assessment is only indicative, because, not only is the dose calculation an approximation, but also the accuracy of the risk assessment depends on the validity of underlying assumptions used in making extrapolations of limited data from epidemiological studies. Placing a numerical value on the risk for a specific case suggests a degree of certainty that is not justified. The ICRP indicate in a draft of their revised recommendations that risk coefficients are intended for assessment of risks in general terms, not for retrospective assessment of risks in specific populations. In fact risk assessment calculations are based on the linear no threshold (LNT) dose–effect model, which may represent a worst case. Use of general terminology is more appropriate for conveying our state of knowledge [7]. Bearing in mind doses received from other sources such as natural background radiation (2.3 mSv per year on average in the UK), the risks derived from the LNT model, and the fact that the exact value of the excess risk of developing cancer at doses below 200 mSv is a matter of debate [8, 9], it is more appropriate to use general terms for risks associated with the low radiation doses received from diagnostic procedures. The following are offered as suggestions for describing the risks associated with effective doses in different ranges.

- <1 mSv negligible/trivial
- 1–10 mSv very low
- 10–100 mSv low

More explanation of the risk is appropriate for doses above 100 mSv.

In conclusion, a significant effort has been put into determining dose levels for radiology examinations over the last 20 years and much useful information has been obtained. We now need to be more selective in the studies that we choose to undertake and think carefully about what we want to achieve from each. Effective dose is an ephemeral quantity that evolves with time. Too much effort should not be wasted on complex calculations to derive a quantity which may be of limited value. The way forward should be through optimization involving all aspects of the imaging process in which measurement of dose is only one component. Finding the appropriate level of image quality is the most important objective. Keeping the dose low should always be secondary.

References

1. Shrimpton PC, Wall BF, Jones DG, Fisher AS, Hillier MC, Kendall GA, et al. A national survey of doses to patients undergoing a selection of routine X-ray examinations in English hospitals. NRPB-R200. Chilton: NRPB, 1986.
2. Hart D, Jones DG, Wall BF. Estimation of effective dose in diagnostic radiology from entrance dose and dose area product measurement. NRPB-R262. Chilton: NRPB, 1994.
3. International Commission on Radiological Protection. 1990 recommendations of the International Commission on Radiological Protection. ICRP Publication 60. Ann ICRP 1991;21(1–3).
4. The Ionising Radiation (Medical Exposure) Regulations. SI (2000) 1059. London: HMSO, 2000.
5. Hart D, Hillier MC, Wall BF. Doses to patients from medical X-ray examinations in the UK – 2000 Review. NRPB-W14. Chilton: NRPB, 2002.
6. Martin CJ, Sutton DG, Sharp PF. Balancing patient dose and image quality. App Radiat Isot 1999;50:1–19.
7. Harrison JR. Health of the nation. Radiation Protection Bulletin No. 184, pp 10–13. Chilton: NRPB, 1996.
8. United Nations Scientific Committee on the Effects of Atomic Radiation. Sources and effects of ionising radiation, Vol. II Effects. New York: United Nations, 2000.
9. Kellerer AB. Radiation risk – historical perspective and issues. J Radiol Prot 2002;22:A1–A10.

The British Journal of Radiology, 78 (2005), 480–482 © 2005 The British Institute of Radiology
DOI: 10.1259/bjr/91804098

Commentary

Installation of a PACS system

D D DUNDAS, FRCR

St George's Hospital, Blackshaw Road, London SW17 0QT, UK

This is a personal view of a Picture Archiving and Communication System (PACS) installation but there will no doubt be resonance with the experience of others who have gone through the process and hopefully some useful pointers for those who are about to embark on the journey.

At St George's Hospital we have been through a process of PACS procurement and implementation, which has been tortuous and at times difficult with differing demands from various NHS bodies which moulded the process over the past 5 years. This is a very individual experience but much was learned on the way. Fortunately, 18 months post implementation I can say that we would do it all again as PACS has revolutionized the way we work and has increased our organizational efficiency as nothing else could.

From late 1999 when we started out we progressed from a single Trust project to a South West London Sector Project (at the behest of the Regional Health Authority) to the installation of PACS at St George's only in June 2003. This was not because the Sector Project was problematic as six Trusts worked together in an exemplary way and unanimously selected a preferred supplier showing that a large project with mutual shared benefit can succeed. However, the establishment of the Strategic Health Authority resulted in re-evaluation of the project at a late stage and the National Programme for Information Technology (NPfIT) was looming into view. St George's implemented largely because of the imminent opening of a Neurosciences and Cardiothoracic PFI build designed to have PACS. Hopefully the remainder of the sector will now progress within NPfIT as all of the groundwork has been done.

It was, in our view, absolutely essential to appoint a member of staff to oversee the project and we appointed a Project Manager at the outset. This greatly assisted progress as other members of staff were already too busy to take on this huge extra task. The sector project also had a Project Manager which kept the entire sector on schedule. The employment of external consultants to assist with planning, consultation and outline and full business case was extremely helpful.

In the early stages clinical colleagues were involved in focus groups and later two were incorporated into the PACS Project Board, one a cardiologist and the other an orthopaedic surgeon. A neurosurgeon was involved in the final selection process of the system. It is essential to involve other disciplines and make the project a hospital project rather than a radiology one. PACS alters everyone's working environment and practices. It is, however, difficult to maintain the interest of clinicians over a lead up time as long as ours, but it is important at least to keep the PACS Board members informed of progress and consult with them when necessary.

The technical specification was drawn up partly using our own knowledge from reading, attending conferences and asking others about their experiences with PACS. We also employed an external consultant who had had involvement with other PACS installations and Medical Physics advice proved invaluable. IT upgraded the network to the satisfaction of PACS suppliers and we have a virtual local area network (VLAN) reserved for PACS. All storage is on RAID (Redundant Array of Independent Disks), which is a hard disc system, with backup on digital linear tape (DLT). The sector project specified a central DVD store with all examinations in working storage, but this aspect has not been resolved for the St George's site alone. Having everything in working storage is undoubtedly an advantage.

Resources were always to be a big issue and there were several reviews of the specification to make the project as affordable as possible. Most PACS now only include software for a web browser application as most modern PCs are capable of running the application and are usually available throughout Trusts. Standard PC screens have improved over recent years making them adequate for viewing most PACS images. Extra PCs for the wards were funded from monies to decrease junior doctors' hours and special consideration was given to A&E, intensive care areas, the chest clinic and rheumatology and orthopaedic outpatients as well as neurosurgery theatres. Viewing facilities throughout the Trust are web browsers with larger, high resolution dual monitors in the key areas. No major items were left out in looking at affordability and the system delivered has adequate numbers of CR readers, connectivity with all equipment and sufficient dedicated radiologist reporting stations (Table 1) for efficient working. The network upgrade, which was necessary regardless of PACS, was not included in the cost of the project.

Reduction in staffing to offset PACS costs is an issue which requires very careful consideration. There is a need for fewer filing clerks, but there are other tasks, such as scanning in request forms, producing CDs of images for outside hospitals and importing images and CDs from outside and allocation of reporting which will redeploy some processing technicians and clerks. Secretarial efficiency is undoubtedly improved by PACS and digital dictation.

The tendering process was managed by the sector project team who provided invaluable support. St George's expended a large amount of effort in producing the Output Based Specification which included all issues of

Received 21 December 2004 and accepted 16 February 2005.

Table 1. Distribution of radiologists reporting stations

Area	Number of radiologists reporting stations
All X-ray areas (except mammography)	11 with 2 reporting monitors
Mammography	1 with 2 reporting monitors
CT	2 with 2 reporting monitors
MRI (general)	2 with 2 reporting monitors
Nuclear medicine	1 with 2 reporting monitors
Neuroradiology	4 with 4 reporting monitors
Ultrasound	1 web browser monitor per room

performance and site-specific requirements as well as a benefits analysis. The responses from the companies were assessed and scored. The tendering process initially reduced the companies who could meet the specification from 4 to 2. Further evaluation and visits resulted in the selection of the preferred supplier. With consultant and project management support this process went smoothly.

One of the most important issues to consider as far as responsibilities of the vendor is concerned is prime contractor status, whereby the vendor takes overall responsibility for the PACS system. Interfaces, especially with existing radiology computer systems are of vital importance and there is absolute necessity for the buck to stop rather than be passed on. In our experience this was one of the most difficult technical issues and although there was some amelioration from our PACS provider having prime contractor status, some ongoing issues remain.

The convergence of the agreement that the contract could be signed and the opening of the St George's Hospital PFI building resulted in a very rapid implementation period which is not to be recommended. In the existing part of the hospital the removal of processors and building works for PACS coincided with the installation of the CR readers. This resulted in a congested, noisy and dusty environment which was good neither for the equipment nor the staff. The CR system went live in the main part of St George's Hospital 6 weeks after the commencement of the installation. During the 6 week period almost all modalities were connected to PACS. The Neuroradiology Department in the PFI building opened 2 months later with PACS and a filmless environment.

During this short implementation period training for all staff inside and outside radiology was carried out. The radiographers clearly require extensive and detailed training as theirs is the most difficult task in the change to CR. Radiologists need less training but the 1 h which most of us had left us less than proficient with some of the more subtle features of the system – learning has been ongoing. Key workers in the clinical areas of the hospital were trained initially including some who had no computer skills whatsoever. Junior doctors who have started work in the Trust more recently are given basic information by their colleagues but the system is intuitive and for every day use, anyone who is computer literate can easily navigate the system – it is very user friendly.

The plan at the time of going "live" was to print film for 6 months while building a PACS archive. This permitted a transition from film to PACS and gave the users throughout the hospital the opportunity to become familiar with PACS without being totally dependent upon it. It also allowed problems to surface after our rapid implementation. It had never been the intention to scan in historic images to provide an archive – this is expensive and time consuming and of little benefit. The film archive is pruned year on year as previously and will diminish over the next 4 years. 18 months after implementation X-ray packets are not issued automatically but only to outpatient clinics, which have positively asked to continue to have old films.

The integration of the Patient Administration System (PAS), Radiology Information System (RIS) and PACS was always regarded as a major factor in a satisfactory PACS installation, but this has been one of the most difficult issues and continues as a relatively minor difficulty in comparison with earlier problems. It has emphasised the absolute necessity for the PACS provider to have prime contractor status. Integrated RIS and PACS from one manufacturer would be the simplest solution, but that will not be the reality for most sites and this issue must be a top priority in the implementation. A demonstration that integration can work does not guarantee a fully functional system with satisfactory messaging between RIS and PACS.

Downtime for PACS has been greater than expected and has had a number of causes from Trust network and computer room problems to PACS failures and planned downtime. There have been times of great inconvenience, but no clinical disasters caused by PACS failure. A very unusual and unexpected disc failure in the RAID caused the most difficult problem, fortunately before St George's became completely filmless. Concerns regarding a high level of reliability of the system postponed the date of going filmless from December 2003 until March 2004 and the major failure occurred in January 2004. Planned downtime has significantly exceeded that stated in the contract and this remains an issue. During periods of downtime films are printed but previous imaging is not available. The examinations performed during these periods are subsequently loaded into PACS.

Overall, PACS has been well received by clinicians in the Trust as one of the major disadvantages of the old system was lack of availability of films for outpatient clinics and wards, the latter often being because the Radiology Department had the films for reporting. The system is more dependable than in the early days and at one stage there was concern regarding image availability in key areas such as neurosurgery theatres. A great deal of work has gone on in the background by members of all staff groups in the Department to make the system as good as it can be and there are now only a few remaining issues. One of the problems for the clinicians has been lack of availability of reports on PACS, part of the interface/messaging issue. This is much better, but not yet 100% reliable.

The very rapid deployment of PACS was difficult and an implementation period of 6 weeks before going "live" is definitely not to be recommended. Looking back over the past 18 months the difficulties have largely been centred around interface issues between RIS and PACS. The near catastrophic disc failure in January 2004 was a rare one-off event (hopefully). Progress in some areas has been very slow and it has been interesting to find that, when a problem is raised, there is often not an easy off the shelf solution. It appears that some difficulties have not been envisaged and a solution has to be developed. There have been a few scenarios where patient safety has been an issue, such as the attribution of examinations to the wrong patient record, and vigilance is essential. Awareness of such potential problems and their rapid remedy is vital. The addition of administrative work stations for management of workload has been vital for the safe working of PACS and these were not initially considered necessary by the vendor.

I am pleased to say that the efficiency of the Radiology Department and the Trust has improved and we are now in an excellent position with a system that, despite a few difficulties which we continue to resolve, works very well. The Department and the Trust would not go back to the days of film packets. Images are almost always available anywhere in the hospital and this enhances patient care as well as clinical meetings when all imaging is available for discussion. PACS, thanks to our chief clerical officer, has given us a system where all examinations are allocated and reported and we are reminded on a regular basis of the workload which we have not yet dealt with. St George's does not have electronic requesting and request forms are scanned into PACS. This has been of huge and unexpected benefit in speeding up reporting, such that we are almost always completely up to date with our "hot" reporting. Clinicians can form time-limited worklists of their own patients and review reports and imaging on PACS as a means of ensuring that all reports are read. These Clinical Governance aspects are not necessarily at the forefront of everyone's mind in relation to PACS installation, but they are a very helpful contribution to safe patient care.

I did not expect that a PACS installation, particularly into an existing department, would be easy but it was significantly harder than envisaged. My colleagues were hugely supportive throughout the project, with no dissent about the desirability of PACS and that helped greatly in difficult times. I can, however, end on a "high" and say that we are delighted to be working with a PACS system and even the large volumes of plain film reporting are not a chore.

The British Journal of Radiology, 78 (2005), 483–484 © 2005 The British Institute of Radiology
DOI: 10.1259/bjr/82539295

Commentary

Using PACS as a teaching resource

D BLUNT, MRCP, FRCR and D O'REGAN, MRCP, FRCR

Charing Cross Hospital, Fulham Palace Road, London W6 8RF, UK

Digital storage has become the normal accepted method of collecting images, not only within radiology departments and hospitals but, with widely available digital cameras, to the general public; the term "pixel" has now entered common usage. This widespread acceptance of digital image storage has been mirrored in radiology departments with an ever-increasing number embracing PACS (Picture Archive and Communication System). This process has also proved highly acceptable to other clinical groups [1]. Within the National Health Service there is a proposed nationwide PACS roll out programme and most large hospital departments and training departments are either filmless or have plans to become so. The possibilities of PACS on improving and assisting many aspects of training in radiology has so far received relatively little attention [2–7].

The requirements

Most large departments worldwide have a training role, both for radiologists and non-radiologists. Within the UK the Royal College of Radiologists has a requirement, during training accreditation visits, that training departments have a film museum for teaching purposes [8]. The expansion in training numbers and increasing use of district general hospitals means that the majority of UK departments are involved to some extent in radiology training, and almost all will be involved in some form of teaching. Just as PACS has quickly become far more than an electronic viewing box, it has potential to be a huge extension to the concept of a simple collection of interesting cases. A PACS based film museum should be able to provide much more than a retrieval mechanism from stored lists.

The formats in which PACS can be used as a teaching resource should include the following:

1. The ability for self directed study with retrieval of investigations in an anonymised, possibly randomised format, preferably on a topic or group of topics with hidden reports but available clinical details. This should include the complete DICOM data to simulate the real reporting experience. This will assist for preparation in examination technique and reporting and as importantly, simulate the day to day reporting experience.
2. Studies should be retrievable by key word searching, as well as being retrievable by examination/modality type or pathology searching. Good examples of any condition which has been stored on PACS should be rapidly accessible. Key word searching is an accepted part of data retrieval and bypasses the need for strict coding [4].
3. A mechanism for adding cases which does not require complex or lengthy case editing or authorship, nor coding procedures. Within a daily work pattern, the ability to highlight a case for teaching purposes needs to be rapid, easy and should not interrupt workflow significantly [6].
4. Personal archive functionality. The best teaching cases are often those which the trainer has been involved in clinically rather than anonymous cases, however well validated, from another institution.

Workflow planning

Introducing PACS into a training department has implications for many facets of daily work. The ability to make cases available for viewing on multiple workstations simultaneously can allow a trainer to teach trainees of different levels of seniority on several cases almost simultaneously. The days of trainees competing for space around a viewing box are long gone but the new model poses challenges in organising rotas, staffing levels and uninterrupted teaching time as well as posing challenges for functionality. The functionality issues are crucial and encompass the ability to co-report an examination, referencing trainer and trainee within the report as well as allowing for checking of the final written report once this has been transcribed. This has medicolegal implications in the training environment, to ensure the appropriate accreditation of a report is given accurately.

The survey

We have been greatly surprised by the failure of PACS manufacturers to appreciate the demand for archiving and case retrieval functionality in PACS systems. In response to direct questioning we were surprised to learn that such functionality had rarely been mentioned in output based specification documents when developing PACS, or if mentioned, only as a possible future development (personal communication, GE Medical Systems, Slough, UK). We conducted a postal survey of the UK departments of radiology to assess the level of demand in the UK for PACS software that provides the capability to create integrated virtual film libraries and teaching resources. It asked each department to indicate if they had already installed or intended to install PACS within 5 years; whether the availability of software to provide an integrated virtual film library and training resource

Received 21 February 2005 and accepted 1 March 2005.

would be of interest to them; and how much it would determine their future choice of PACS provider. 237 questionnaires were posted and 144 responded (response rate 61%). 44 (31%) departments had already installed PACS and a further 97 (67%) intended to install it within 5 years. 95% of responders indicated that the availability of such software would be of interest to them. Of those intending to install PACS within 5 years 65 (67%) indicated that the availability of such a resource would be either a significant or decisive factor in their choice of PACS provider, if they were in a position to make the choice.

Other approaches

There have been various attempts to realise the potential teaching possibilities of PACS [9], but the solution must not simply aim at a validated collection of images in some digital film archive. The potential for digital film collections has been recognised by the RSNA MIRC project [10]. This allows for on-line access to a verified teaching archive of cases, accrued from a wide number of teaching centres. This project has not been without its difficulties. Many attempts to streamline the authoring process have been developed. This project provides a very useful archive and incorporates some self-directed learning opportunities but it does not incorporate full DICOM file retrieval and in its current format does not simulate the experience of reporting a case in daily work practice.

The challenge

PACS manufacturers have invested a huge amount in freeing radiology from the shackles of an analogue storage medium. There is a huge potential opportunity for training and teaching, in developing robust and searchable archiving facilities. Local or regional variants could allow for the retrieval of films to simulate local examination formats (for example randomise case mix of computed radiographic images, including normal studies, to simulate a rapid reporting packet for the British FRCR examination). In other countries the radiological higher specialist examinations are in part or completely digital, offering opportunities to set practice exams in formats very similar to the real exam. It is surprising that PACS manufacturers have not perceived the huge commercial advantage that a PACS system with these sorts of facilities would give them. Almost every large hospital in the UK will be a training department and it is almost inconceivable that any such department will wish to retain a conventional archive of analogue films. The same must be true around the world in large hospital departments. Failure to rise to this challenge and recognise the very widespread need will represent one of the greatest missed opportunities in radiology training in our conversion from analogue to digital storage.

References

1. Pilling JR. Picture archiving and communication systems: the users' view. Br J Radiol 2003;76:519–24.
2. Wiggins RH, Davidson HC, Dilda P, Harnsberger HR, Katzman GL. The evolution of filmless radiology teaching. J Digit Imaging 2001;14:236–7.
3. Siegal E, Reiner B. Electronic teaching files: seven-year experience using a commercial picture archiving and communication system. J Digit Imaging 2001;14:125–7.
4. Strickland NH, Allison DJ, Gishen P. Technical note: a radiological education system — organization of an image library. Br J Radiol 1995;68:524–7.
5. Mullins ME, Mehta A, Patel H, McLoud TC, Novelline RA. Impact of PACS on the education of radiology residents: the residents' perspective. Acad Radiol 2001;8:67–73.
6. Dugas M, Trumm C, Stabler A, Pander E, Hundt W, Scheidler J, et al. Case-oriented computer-based-training in radiology: concept, implementation and evaluation. BMC Med Educ 2001;1:5.
7. Harrison M, Koh J, Tran S, Mongkolwat P, Channin DS. Research and teaching access to a large clinical picture archiving and communications system. J Digit Imaging 2001;14:121–4.
8. The Royal College of Radiologists. The Royal College of Radiologists Training Accreditation in Clinical Radiology Guidance Notes for Training Schemes. London: The Royal College of Radiologists, 2000:Appendix B.
9. Lim CC, Yang GL, Nowinski WL, Hui F. Medical Image Resource Center — making electronic teaching files from PACS. J Digit Imaging 2003;16:331–6.
10. Medical Imaging Resource Center. Available at http://www.rsna.org/mirc/ (Accessed 7 March 2005).

The British Journal of Radiology, 78 (2005), 485–492
DOI: 10.1259/bjr/87552880

Review article

Rationale for using multiple antioxidants in protecting humans against low doses of ionizing radiation

K N PRASAD, PhD

Center for Vitamins and Cancer Research, Department of Radiology, School of Medicine, University of Colorado Health Sciences Center, Denver, CO 80262, USA

Abstract. Health risks of low doses of ionizing radiation (10 cGy or less) may not be accurately estimated in humans by epidemiological study or mathematical modelling because of several inherent confounding factors including environmental, dietary and biological variables that cannot be accounted for in any radio-epidemiological study. In addition, the expression of radiation-induced damage in humans not only depends upon total dose, dose rate, linear energy transfer (LET), and fractionation and protraction of total doses, but also on repair mechanisms, bystander effects, and exposure to chemical carcinogens, tumour promoters and other toxins. It also depends upon the levels of anti-carcinogenic and anti-tumour promoting agents. Low doses of ionizing radiation should not be considered insignificant with regard to increasing the incidence of somatic mutations (neoplastic and non-neoplastic diseases) and heritable mutations in humans owing to its interaction with other toxins that can enhance damage produced by irradiation. It is very prudent to continue to support the well-established radiobiological concept that no radiation dose can be considered completely safe, and that all efforts must be made to reduce both the radiation dose and biological damage, no matter how small that damage might be, without sacrificing the benefits of radiation. Based on the results of many scientific experiments, formulations containing multiple antioxidants for biological protection against radiation damage in humans can be developed, and this strategy together with the existing physical concept of radiation protection, should further reduce potential risks of low doses of ionizing radiation in humans.

Ionizing radiation is a potent mutagen and carcinogen; however, it is also used in the diagnosis and treatment of human diseases. Diagnostic doses of radiation are generally 10 cGy or less. In the USA, background radiation at sea level is about 1 mSv year^{-1} and consists of cosmic radiation and radiation emitted from radioactive substances present in the ground or commercial sources. In addition to standard hospital-based diagnostic radiation equipment (X-ray machine, CT scan, positron emission tomography (PET), nuclear medicine procedures), new ionizing radiation-based Diagnostic Centres for heart scan, virtual colonoscopy and whole-body scan are opening at a rapid rate throughout the world, especially in the USA. Individuals at younger ages are exposed to very low doses of radiation for the early diagnosis of diseases that may help to develop effective prevention and treatment strategies. However, low doses of ionizing radiation may also increase the level of genetic defects in present and future generations if no strategy for biological protection against such damage is developed and implemented. Radiation exposure during space voyage is expected to increase health risks including cancer in astronauts after return to earth. During space flight, astronauts are primarily exposed to high atomic number and high-energy particle radiation (HZE particles). Therefore, the success of long space voyages depends upon how well our astronauts are protected against radiation damage. Frequent flyers (public), flight attendants and fight crews on commercial jets, and Air Force personnel flying at very high altitudes are also exposed to low doses of ionizing radiation. Recently, a new threat of exploding so called "dirty bombs" that may emit radiation doses varying from a few cGy to a couple of Gy (may or may not produce acute lethality) has added to the urgency for developing a strategy for biological protection against radiation damage. At present there is no effective strategy to reduce the potential risk of low doses of radiation in humans. Although some of these issues have been discussed in our recent reviews [1, 2], they did not focus on the development of scientifically rational nutritional formulations that are safe and could be effective in reducing the risk of radiation damage in humans.

This review briefly discusses the potential health risks of low doses of ionizing radiation and provides scientific data in support of developing nutritional formulations containing multiple antioxidants that are known to be safe and that could provide biological protection against radiation damage in humans.

Hypotheses for potential health risks of low doses of radiation in humans

Radiobiologists have been debating the health risks from low doses of ionizing radiation in humans for decades. This is supported by the fact that six biological effects of ionizing radiation (BEIR) reports have extensively analysed *in vitro*, animal and human studies on somatic and heritable mutations, and the incidence of cancers and birth defects following radiation exposure. Heritable mutations are of particular concern, especially

Received 30 July 2004 and accepted 18 January 2005.

among women, because the number of oocytes may be fixed at birth, and mutations, if not repaired, are cumulative and can increase health risks of future generations. At present, two opposing hypotheses on the potential risks of low dose radiation in humans are being debated. We support the hypothesis that there is no dose of ionizing radiation that can be considered completely safe, and that the use of radiation must always be determined on the basis of risk *vs* benefit [1, 2]. Another hypothesis suggests that the health risks of diagnostic doses less than 10 cGy are not measurable and may even be non-existent [3, 4]. This hypothesis ignores the effect of interaction between ionizing radiation and other carcinogens, mutagens and tumour promoters that may enhance the risk of radiation-induced cancer. Health risks include not only neoplastic diseases, but also somatic mutations that may contribute to other illnesses (including birth defects and ocular maladies) and heritable mutations that may increase the risk of diseases in future generations.

Proposed mechanisms of radiation-induced human cancer

In mammals including humans, normal cellular turnover includes proliferation, differentiation and death of cells. This process is interfered with when carcinogenic changes occur. Cancer cells can arise from any dividing cells or cells that have potential to divide owing to accumulation of multiple genetic abnormalities (over-expression of genes, deletion of genes or gene mutations), some of which must occur in critical genes that regulate proliferation and differentiation. The processes may undergo three distinct processes, initiation, immortalization (pre-malignant change) and transformation (expression of malignant phenotype). Radiation-induced human cancers have long latent periods; 10 years for leukaemia and over 30 years for solid tumours [5], and may undergo similar carcinogenic processes. During the initiation phase, radiation-induced mutations (due to gene mutations and/or chromosomal damage) are detected within 24 h of radiation exposure, but these changes can be considered initiating events and may not be directly responsible for malignant transformation, because such cells continue to divide and proliferate like unirradiated normal cells. However, radiation-induced mutations cause genetic instability in irradiated cells making these cells more sensitive to mutagenic changes. Such cells may continue to proliferate and differentiate like non-irradiated cells while accumulating additional mutations for a long time without immortalization or transformation. Immortalization of irradiated cells, the first step in carcinogenesis, occurs only when the expression of genes regulating differentiation is altered. Immortalized cells can continue to proliferate until the expression of some key cellular genes, oncogenes or anti-oncogenes is altered by exposure to mutagens, carcinogens and/or tumour promoters. These cells then become malignant [6, 7].

Radiation dose–response models to estimate human cancer risk

Two dose–response models are used to estimate cancer risk in humans. The first model proposes that cancer risk following exposure to low doses of radiation (10 cGy or less) may be best estimated by a linear no-threshold relationship, since any dose has the potential to induce cancer [8–10]. The second model suggests that there is a threshold dose below which radiation may not induce cancer in humans [3, 4, 11]. Both models have relied on mathematical modelling and human radio-epidemiological studies. Mathematical modelling may assume certain constant physical factors such as body weight [11] that may not reflect the inherent biological variations associated with radiation-induced carcinogenesis. The biological variables include differences in radiosensitivity with respect to age, organs, body mass, and differences in the efficacy of repair mechanisms. The second model also utilizes data that support hormesis [4]. "Radiation hormesis" is the name given to the putative stimulatory/adaptive effects of low level ionizing radiation generally in the range of 1–50 cGy of low-linear energy transfer (LET) radiation [12–15]. It should be noted that adaptive responses are commonly observed with tissue injuries irrespective of the source of the insult. For example, hyperthermia and acute trauma also induce adaptive responses. Unlike other injurious agents such as heat and trauma, ionizing radiation is a potent mutagen and carcinogen, and radiation-induced adaptive responses do not reflect the mutagenic changes that might occur after exposure. Therefore, adaptive responses based on certain biological criteria following exposure to low doses of radiation cannot be considered beneficial to humans. On the contrary, they simply reflect that cells have been exposed to injurious agents and that attempts are being made to repair some of the damage.

Numerous radio-epidemiological studies are available in the literature [5, 8, 16–21] and if selectively used, can support either hypothesis. Radio-epidemiological studies have so many confounding factors that it is not possible to quantify purely radiation-induced cancer risk in humans. These confounding factors include environment, diet and lifestyle-related factors that contain mutagens, carcinogens and tumour promoters as well as cancer protective substances, and cellular repair systems that may vary from one individual to another owing to variation in age, environment, and diet and lifestyle-related factors. Other confounding factors include: (a) interaction of radiation with other physical (UV light), chemical and biological mutagens and carcinogens in a synergistic manner; (b) variation in sensitivity of bystander cells to subsequent radiation exposure that depends on whether they have been pre- or post-irradiated; and (c) variation in adaptive response that depends on radiation doses and protective substances (antioxidants). Thus, humans are simultaneously exposed to varieties of mutagens, carcinogens, and tumour promoters as well as to cancer protective agents, in addition to ionizing radiation. Therefore, low dose radiation-induced cancer in humans depends upon several variables, most of which are not possible to correct for in any epidemiological study. This may explain why radio-epidemiological studies in humans have produced inconsistent results. Nevertheless, these studies are important in establishing an association between radiation doses and health risks in humans.

Radiation-induced delayed cell death, genomic instability and the bystander effect

In recent years, radiation-injuries have been observed in cells away from those that are irradiated. These include radiation-induced genomic instability, bystander effects, clastogenic factors produced in plasma from irradiated individuals that can cause chromosomal damage when cultured with non-irradiated cells, and transgenerational effects of parental irradiation that can manifest in the progeny [22, 23]. Bystander cells damaged by previous radiation doses may show increased sensitivity to subsequent damage [24]. It is likely that these processes may be important factors in determining the long-term response of populations to "sub-lethal" doses of ionizing radiation [25–29]. These data further complicate the interpretation of any radiation dose–response model for estimating human health risks.

Using microbeam technology, it was found that below 200 mGy, the survival potential was dominated by the bystander effect and at higher doses, the direct effect of radiation on cell killing becomes dominant [30, 31]. Below 200 mGy, the response after irradiation of a single cell was not significantly different from the response when all cells were irradiated. This observation is particularly significant, because at low doses certain repair mechanisms are not activated [32]. These results further support the suggestion that no dose of radiation can be insignificant or totally safe.

Effect of interaction of radiation with other carcinogens and cancer protective agents

Radiation-induced cancer in humans depends upon several factors. They include interaction with several chemical carcinogens and tumour promoters, anti-carcinogenic and anti-tumour-promoting agents. The efficacy of repair mechanisms also influences the risk of cancer. Some examples of these are given below. X-irradiation enhances chemical carcinogen-induced transformation in normal mammalian cells by about nine-fold [33] and UV-induced transformation by about 12-fold [34]. X-irradiation also enhances the level of ozone-induced [35] and viral-induced [36] transformation in cell culture. Radiation doses that alone do not transform normal fibroblasts, do so when combined with a tumour promoter [37]. Ionizing radiation in combination with tobacco smoking increases the risk of lung cancer by about 50% [5]. A low dose of radiation (2 cGy) does not produce detectable levels of mutations as measured by chromosomal damage; however, in the presence of caffeine (which inhibits repair of DNA damage), mutations become detectable [38]. Low doses of radiation (2 cGy and 5 cGy) can act as a mitogen [39], and even lower doses (about 1 mGy) do not activate double-strand DNA break repair mechanisms [32]. This lack of repair can lead to accumulation of mutations. It has been reported that γ-radiation at a dose as little as 1.5 cGy [40], and space radiation doses of 5 cGy or less enhanced the levels of oxidative stress in human cell lines and rats *in vivo* [41]. At the same time, dietary and endogenously made antioxidants are known to protect tissue against radiation damage [16, 42–44]. Thus, it is nearly impossible to estimate quantitatively the health risks of low doses of radiation alone in the human population by any dose–response models owing to the above confounding factors. However, the health risks of low doses of radiation cannot be ignored.

Epidemiological studies on cancer risk in children of women exposed to low doses of radiation before and after conception

In recent debates, issues of radiation damage to children of women who have been exposed to diagnostic doses of radiation before and after conception have been ignored. Since the number of oocytes may be fixed at birth, radiation damage to oocytes, one of the most radiosensitive cells, may be cumulative, and therefore, may be very crucial for inducing heritable genetic damage. Although radio-epidemiological studies are not considered very reliable, they have addressed these issues in women. Stewart and Kneale [20] have reported that an increase in cancer risk is directly proportional to the number of X-ray films or fetus doses received. It was estimated that 1 cGy delivered to the fetus shortly before birth would cause an increase of 300–800 deaths per million before the age of 10 years due to cancer. A significant increase [19] in malignancy has been found even after 2.0–2.5 mGy to human fetuses (relative incidence of cancer=1.25). One of the most surprising results published showed an increased cancer risk by a factor of 1.6–2.0 among the children of women who received diagnostic doses of radiation before conception [45]. Another study [21] reported that diagnostic doses (0.5–7 cGy) to the gonads before conception induced aneuploidy in 10 children (8 mongoloid and 2 trisomy) among 975 exposed women in comparison with 1 aneuploidy case among unexposed women. Gonadal exposure of 5 cGy increased eye defects [46], and of 3 cGy increased the mutation rate by 1% [18]. These epidemiological studies have the same confounding problems in quantifying radiation-induced health risks as discussed with the adults.

Determination of intermediate health risk factors and non-neoplastic diseases in children exposed to low doses of radiation

The incidence of non-neoplastic diseases and intermediate health risks measured by certain specific biochemical markers were studied in children living in radiation-contaminated areas near the Chernobyl nuclear accident site. The incidence of thyroid gland enlargement and vision disorders, mostly dry eye syndrome, was closely related to the levels of contamination [47]. Increased levels of oxidized conjugated dienes, products of lipid peroxidation, were found among these children. In another report, increased levels of spontaneous chemiluminescence, an indicator of enhanced oxygen radical activity, in leukocytes of children living in contaminated areas were observed [48]. The accuracy of these intermediate markers for predicting health risks remains unknown.

Concept of maximum permissible dose (MPD)

Because of the growing use of nuclear energy in the world, especially in developing countries for civilian and military purposes, and the potential for increased risk of somatic and heritable mutations owing to increased usage of ionizing radiation, the concept of maximum permissible dose (MPD) was developed for the two major population groups (radiation workers and general population) in order provide a certain degree of safety against radiation damage. The annual MPD value for stochastic-effects (where the probability of the biological effect is proportional to the dose: linear no-threshold effect) for the general population is about 50 times less (1 mSv) than that recommended for radiation workers (50 mSv) [49]. Although the value of MPD for radiation workers for the above effect has remained fairly constant during the last several decades, this value for the population was reduced by a factor of 5 in 1993 [50, 51]. This is due to the emergence of new data on low doses of radiation on somatic and heritable mutations in mammals and in mammalian cells in culture [5, 32, 38, 52], the synergistic effect of the interaction of radiation with other chemical [33, 35] and biological [36] carcinogens and tumour promoters [37] on cancer incidence and mutations, and epidemiological studies in humans [16]. The MPD value is never considered a safe radiation dose, although some may presume it to be the case.

Evolution of radiation protection strategy in humans

Efforts to protect normal tissue were started soon after the discovery of X-rays by Dr Roentgen in 1895. However, the observation by Dr Muller of Columbia University in 1927, that radiation causes gene mutations in *Drosophila melanogaster* (common fruit fly) provided new impetus to reduce radiation exposure. The initial concept of radiation protection involved three physical principles: (a) shielding (usually by lead) of unexposed areas, especially radiosensitive organs such as bone marrow, gonads and thyroid; (b) increased distance between the radiation source and radiation workers or patients; and (c) reduction of exposure time. Each of these factors has been very useful, but they have limitations. For example, during fluoroscopy, it may not be possible to protect the gastrointestinal tract (one of the most radiosensitive organs) against radiation damage by lead shielding. Increasing the distance between the radiation source and recipients may not be practical for many radiation workers, patients, civilian or military personnel. Reducing exposure time may also not be pertinent to all populations, except those that are involved in taking care of patients who have received γ-emitting radioisotopes for medical purposes or who are responsible for radioactive decontamination as a result of accidents or attack. To address the growing concerns of radiation-induced somatic and heritable mutations, the concept of as low as reasonably achievable (ALARA) with respect to dose was recommended by national and international radiation protection agencies for radiation workers [53]. Radiation protection based on physical factors has been successful in reducing the level of unnecessary medical exposure to patients and to radiation workers. The development of a novel strategy for biological protection may improve the efficacy of current efforts in reducing the risk of radiation injuries in humans.

Search for biological radiation protection

Identification of radioprotective agents

In order to protect normal tissues from potential radiation damage, it would be important to identify biological or chemical agents which, when given before radiation exposure, could protect all normal tissues. The search for non-toxic radioprotective agents that can protect normal tissue against radiation damage began soon after World War II. Extensive radiobiological research yielded numerous agents which, when given before radiation exposure, protected animals (primarily rodents) against radiation injury [16, 42]. Most widely studied (SH)-compounds like cysteamine, cystamine and aminoethylisothiourea dihydrobromide (AET) and a cysteamine analogue, amifostine, were toxic to humans [16, 42, 54–59].

Potassium iodide as a radioprotective agent

The increased use of radioactive iodine (^{131}I) in research, diagnosis and treatment of thyroid diseases, and the release of ^{131}I during nuclear explosion made it imperative that all radiation workers working with ^{131}I take potassium iodide pills. Since iodine selectively accumulates in the thyroid gland, and the thyroid is considered a very radiosensitive organ, it was thought that the intake of potassium iodide would saturate the thyroid gland with iodine, and thus would prevent the accumulation of radioactive iodine in the thyroid. Thus potassium iodide remains a valuable strategy for protecting the thyroid gland against damage produced by radioactive iodine. However, this agent does not protect any other radiosensitive organ against γ-radiation that is produced by radioactive iodine. In addition, potassium iodide does not protect against damage produced by other radioactive isotopes or other radiation sources such as X-irradiation or γ-irradiation. Therefore, additional non-toxic agents must be identified to protect humans against radiation damage produced by sources other than radioactive iodine.

Multiple antioxidants as radioprotective agents

Although earlier identified radioprotective SH-compounds were found to be toxic in humans, glutathione-elevating agents such as N-acetylcysteine (NAC) and α-lipoic acid, that are non-toxic (within certain concentration ranges) to humans, protect normal tissues against radiation damage [48, 60]. In addition to glutathione-elevating agents, dietary antioxidants such as vitamins E, C and β-carotene are also of radioprotective value [57, 60–82], but very little attention has been given to these agents with respect to their use in protecting normal tissue against radiation damage in humans. Based on published data on antioxidants and radiation protection, it is possible to develop a non-toxic, cost-effective mixture of antioxidants (dietary and glutathione-elevating agents) that can provide biological protection against radiation damage in humans. Indeed, such formulations, referred to as Bio-Shield, (patent pending) are available commercially (Premier Micronutrient Corporation, Nashville, TN). *In vitro* animal and human studies that support the rationale of using multiple antioxidants in reducing the risk of radiation damage in humans are described below.

In vitro studies supporting the scientific rationale for using antioxidants for radiation protection in humans

It has been reported that mitotic cells, which are most sensitive to radiation, have the lowest levels of SH-compounds, whereas S-phase cells, which are the most resistant to radiation, have the highest levels of these compounds [83]. The role of SH-compounds in radiation protection was further substantiated by the fact that an elevation of the intracellular levels of these compounds in mitotic cells makes them radioresistant to the same level as S-phase cells [83]. It has been shown that vitamin E and selenium reduced radiation-induced transformation in cell culture; the combination was more effective than the individual agents [61, 62]. Natural β-carotene protected against radiation-induced neoplastic transformation in cell culture [63]. Vitamins E and C reduced radiation-induced mutations and chromosomal damage in mammalian cells [64–71], and radiation-induced lethality [69–72].

In vivo (animal) studies supporting the scientific rationale for using antioxidants for radiation protection in humans

Alpha-lipoic acid, a glutathione-elevating agent, increases the LD_{50} in mice with a dose reduction factor (DRF) of 1.26 [84]. Vitamin E, Vitamin C and β-carotene protected rodents against the acute effects of irradiation [70–79]. Vitamin A and β-carotene protected normal tissue during radiation therapy of cancer in an animal model [78]. A combination of vitamin A, C and E protected against radiation-induced myelosuppression during radiation therapy of cancer in an animal model [79]. It has been reported that L-selenomethionine and several different types of antioxidants (vitamin C, vitamin E, glutathione, n-acetylcysteine (NAC), lipoic acid and co-enzyme Q10 and soy bean-derived Bowman-Birk inhibitor) protected human cells in culture and rats *in vivo* against oxidative stress produced by photons, protons and 1 GeV iron ions [41].

Human studies supporting the scientific rationale for using antioxidants for radiation protection

Vitamin A and NAC may be effective against radiation-induced carcinogenesis [60]. Alpha-lipoic acid treatment for 28 days lowered lipid peroxidation among children chronically exposed to low doses of radiation in the area contaminated by the Chernobyl nuclear accident [48]. In another study, β-carotene reduced cellular damage in the above population of children [47]. A combination of vitamin E and α-lipoic acid was more effective than the individual agents [48]. β-carotene also protected against radiation-induced mucositis during radiation therapy of cancer of the head and neck [80]. A combination of dietary antioxidants was more effective in protecting normal tissue during radiation therapy than the individual agents [81, 82].

Table 1. Estimated doses of ionizing radiation delivered once during various diagnostic procedures

Procedure type	Effective dose (mSv)
Chest or dental X-ray	0.01
Electron-beam CT (cardiac)	1.0–1.3
Electron-beam CT coronary angiography	1.5–2.0
Catheter coronary angiography	2.1–2.5
Electron-beam CT whole body	5.2
CT (head)	2.0
CT (abdomen)	10.0
Barium enema	7.0
Upper GI examination	3.0
IV urogram	2.5
Lumbar spine	1.3
Mammogram	7.0
Passenger from Athens to New York	0.06
Occupational annual dose limit	50.0
General public annual dose limit	1.0
Background annual dose at sea level	1.0

Occupational and general public dose limit refers to chronic exposure and does not include background radiation.
GI, gastrointestinal; IV, intravenous.

When and how to use multiple antioxidants for radiation protection in humans

Commonly used doses in diagnostic procedures are listed in Tables 1 and 2. It is suggested that patients receiving diagnostic radiation doses take orally an appropriately prepared multiple antioxidants pill once 30 min to 60 min before radiation procedure. Radiation workers are advised to keep the body level of antioxidants high at all times by taking the appropriate multiple vitamins with antioxidants, B-vitamins and appropriate minerals, but no iron, copper or manganese. They may take a booster dose antioxidant pill 30 min to 60 min before exposure to higher radiation doses is anticipated. Frequent-flyers may also follow the same dose and dose schedule as radiation workers. The proposed strategy of increasing antioxidant levels in the body can also be implemented in populations living in regions with high background radiation that show increased levels of intermediate risk markers such as increased chromosomal damage or evidence of increased oxidative damage such as lipid peroxidation. Such a strategy may reduce the levels of intermediate risk markers, and thereby, protect against long-term adverse health consequences of radiation exposure among this population. The proposed antioxidant strategy, in addition to potassium iodide, should be adopted in the event of nuclear accident or explosion of a "dirty bomb". The efficacy of antioxidant strategy for biological radiation protection in humans against low

Table 2. Estimated doses of radiation from radioactive nuclides administered once during nuclear medicine procedures

Procedure type	Effective dose (mSv)
^{18}F-Flurodeoxyglucose, 10 mCi	4.8
$^{99}Tc^{m}$-MAA lung scan, 5 mCi	0.60
$^{99}Tc^{m}$-HDP bone scan, 20 mCi	4.0
^{201}Tl Thallium scan, 3 mCi	0.60

MAA, macroaggregated albumin; HDP, hydroxyethylene diphosphonate.

doses of radiation has not been tested; however, all proposed antioxidant ingredients have exhibited radiation protection in humans and/or in laboratory experiments. Direct experiments with radioprotective antioxidant formulations cannot be performed in humans for obvious ethical reasons. However, implementation of the proposed recommendation may allow prospective studies among radiation workers to determine its efficacy in reducing health risks of low doses of radiation in present and future generations.

Toxicity of antioxidants

Dietary antioxidants (vitamins C and E, β-carotene and selenium) and glutathione-elevating agents (NAC and α-lipoic acid) have been consumed by humans for decades, and within certain dose ranges, no toxicity of these nutrients has been reported. However, higher doses of these nutrients can produce some toxicity. For example, doses of 10 g or more of vitamin C as ascorbic acid can cause upset stomach in some individuals, and may increase the risk of kidney stones after long-term consumption among those who are susceptible to develop this complication. Vitamin E at doses 2000 IU or more after prolonged consumption may induce clotting defects in some individuals. β-carotene at doses of 60 mg or more can induce bronzing of the skin that is reversible after discontinuing its intake. Vitamin A at doses 10 000 IU or more can cause birth defects in pregnant women. Higher doses of vitamin A can cause liver and skin toxicity. NAC at a daily dose of 800 mg can increase the excretion of zinc in the urine. The references for the above studies have been provided in a review [85].

In summary, following the physical principles of radiation protection and the guidelines of ALARA combined with the biological protection provided by multiple antioxidants, may further reduce the health risks of low doses of radiation no matter how small that risk might be.

References

1. Prasad KN, Cole WC, Haase GM. Radiation protection in humans: extending the concept of as low as reasonably achievable (ALARA) from dose to biological damage. Br J Radiol 2004;77:97–9.
2. Prasad KN, Cole WC, Hasse GM. Health risks of low dose ionizing radiation in humans: a review. Exp Biol Med (Maywood) 2004;229:378–82.
3. Radiation risk in perspective: position statement of the Health Physics Society. McLean, VA: Health Physics Society; 1998.
4. Cohen BL. Cancer risk from low-level radiation. AJR Am J Roentgenol 2002;179:1137–43.
5. Anonymous. Biological Effects of Ionizing Radiation BEIR V. National Academic Press: Committee on the Biological Effects of Ionizing Radiation; 1990. Report No.: V.
6. Prasad KN, Hovland AR, Nahreini P, Cole WC, Hovland P, Kumar B, et al. Differentiation genes: are they primary targets for human carcinogenesis? Exp Biol Med (Maywood) 2001;226:805–13.
7. Prasad KN, Cole WC, Yan XD, Nahreini P, Kumar B, Hanson A, et al. Defects in cAMP-pathway may initiate carcinogenesis in dividing nerve cells: a review. Apoptosis 2003;8:579–86.
8. Court-Brown W, Doll R. Leukemia and aplastic anemia in patients irradiated for ankylosing spondylitis. London: Her Majesty's Stationery Office, 1957.
9. Measurements NCRP, editor. Recommendations on limits for exposure to ionizing radiation. publication 91. Bethesda, MD: National Council Radiation Protection Measurements, 1987.
10. Snowby F, editor. Annals of the ICRP, publication 26; 1977.
11. Bond VP, Benary V, Sondhaus CA. A different perception of the linear, nonthreshold hypothesis for low-dose irradiation. Proc Natl Acad Sci USA 1991;88:8666–70.
12. Macklis RM, Beresford B. Radiation hormesis. J Nucl Med 1991;32:350–9.
13. Liu S. Multilevel mechanisms of stimulatory effect of low dose radiation on immunity. In: Suguhara T, Sagan L, Aoyama T, editors. Low dose irradiation and biological defense mechanisms. Amsterdam: Elsevier Science, 1992: 225–32.
14. Redpath JL, Antoniono RJ. Induction of an adaptive response against spontaneous neoplastic transformation in vitro by low-dose gamma radiation. Radiat Res 1998;149: 517–20.
15. Hashimoto S, Shirato H, Hosokawa M, Nishioka T, Kuramitsu Y, Matushita K, et al. The suppression of metastases and the change in host immune response after low-dose total-body irradiation in tumor-bearing rats. Radiat Res 1999;151:717–24.
16. Prasad KN. Handbook of radiobiology (2nd edn). Boca Raton, FL: CRC Press, 1995.
17. Howe GR. Lung cancer mortality between 1950 and 1987 after exposure to fractionated moderate-dose-rate ionizing radiation in the Canadian fluoroscopy cohort study and a comparison with lung cancer mortality in the Atomic Bomb survivors study. Radiat Res 1995;142:295–304.
18. Herskowitz I. Damage to offspring of irradiated women. Prog Immunol Gynecol 1957;3:374–9.
19. Newcombe HB, McGregor JF. Childhood cancer following obstetric radiography. Lancet 1971;2:1151–2.
20. Stewart A, Kneale GW. Radiation dose effects in relation to obstetric x-rays and childhood cancers. Lancet 1970;1:1185–8.
21. Uchida IA, Holunga R, Lawler C. Maternal radiation and chromosomal aberrations. Lancet 1968;2:1045–9.
22. Morgan WF. Non-targeted and delayed effects of exposure to ionizing radiation: II. Radiation-induced genomic instability and bystander effects in vivo, clastogenic factors and transgenerational effects. Radiat Res 2003;159:581–96.
23. Huang L, Snyder AR, Morgan WF. Radiation-induced genomic instability and its implications for radiation carcinogenesis. Oncogene 2003;22:5848–54.
24. Zhou H, Randers-Pehrson G, Geard CR, Brenner DJ, Hall EJ, Hei TK. Interaction between radiation-induced adaptive response and bystander mutagenesis in mammalian cells. Radiat Res 2003;160:512–6.
25. McIlrath J, Lorimore SA, Coates PJ, Wright EG. Radiation-induced genomic instability in immortalized haemopoietic stem cells. Int J Radiat Biol 2003;79:27–34.
26. Mothersill C, Seymour C. Low-dose radiation effects: experimental hematology and the changing paradigm. Exp Hematol 2003;31:437–45.
27. Mothersill C, Crean M, Lyons M, McSweeney J, Mooney R, O'Reilly J, et al. Expression of delayed toxicity and lethal mutations in the progeny of human cells surviving exposure to radiation and other environmental mutagens. Int J Radiat Biol 1998;74:673–80.
28. Evans HH, Horng MF, Ricanati M, Diaz-Insua M, Jordan R, Schwartz JL. Induction of genomic instability in TK6 human lymphoblasts exposed to 137Cs gamma radiation: comparison to the induction by exposure to accelerated 56Fe particles. Radiat Res 2003;159:737–47.

29. Lorimore SA, Wright EG. Radiation-induced genomic instability and bystander effects: related inflammatory-type responses to radiation-induced stress and injury? A review. Int J Radiat Biol 2003;79:15–25.
30. Brenner DJ, Little JB, Sachs RK. The bystander effect in radiation oncogenesis: II. A quantitative model. Radiat Res 2001;155:402–8.
31. Schettino G, Folkard M, Prise KM, Vojnovic B, Held KD, Michael BD. Low-dose studies of bystander cell killing with targeted soft X rays. Radiat Res 2003;160:505–11.
32. Rothkamm K, Lobrich M. Evidence for a lack of DNA double-strand break repair in human cells exposed to very low x-ray doses. Proc Natl Acad Sci USA 2003;100:5057–62.
33. DiPaolo JA, Donovan PJ, Popescu NC. Kinetics of Syrian hamster cells during x-irradiation enhancement of transformation in vitro by chemical carcinogen. Radiat Res 1976;66:310–25.
34. DiPaolo JA, Donovan PJ. In vitro morphologic transformation of Syrian hamster cells by U.V.-irradiation is enhanced by X-irridation and unaffected by chemical carcinogens. Int J Radiat Biol Relat Stud Phys Chem Med 1976;30:41–53.
35. Borek C, Zaider M, Ong A, Mason H, Witz G. Ozone acts alone and synergistically with ionizing radiation to induce in vitro neoplastic transformation. Carcinogenesis 1986;7:1611–3.
36. Pollock EJ, Todaro GJ. Radiation enhancement of SV40 transformation in 3T3 and human cells. Nature 1968;219: 520–1.
37. Little JB. Influence of noncarcinogenic secondary factors on radiation carcinogenesis. Radiat Res 1981;87:240–50.
38. Puck TT, Morse H, Johnson R, Waldren CA. Caffeine enhanced measurement of mutagenesis by low levels of gamma-irradiation in human lymphocytes. Somat Cell Mol Genet 1993;19:423–9.
39. Suzuki K, Kodama S, Watanabe M. Extremely low-dose ionizing radiation causes activation of mitogen-activated protein kinase pathway and enhances proliferation of normal human diploid cells. Cancer Res 2001;61:5396–401.
40. Wan XS, Zhou Z, Kennedy AR. Adaptation of the dichlorofluorescein assay for detection of radiation-induced oxidative stress in cultured cells. Radiat Res 2003;160:622–30.
41. Wan XS, Kennedy AR. Protection against space radiation adverse biological effects. Radiat Res 2004;(In Press).
42. Thomson J. Radiation protection in mammals. New York, NY: Reinhold, 1962.
43. Prasad KN, Cole WC, Kumar B, Che Prasad K. Pros and cons of antioxidant use during radiation therapy. Cancer Treat Rev 2002;28:79–91.
44. Prasad KN, Cole W, Hovland P. Cancer prevention studies: past, present, and future directions. Nutrition 1998;14:197–210; discussion 237–8.
45. Graham S, Levin ML, Lilienfeld AM, Schuman LM, Gibson R, Dowd JE, et al. Preconception, intrauterine, and postnatal irradiation as related to leukemia. Natl Cancer Inst Monogr 1966;19:347–71.
46. Awa AA, Bloom AD, Yoshida MC, Meriishi S, Archer PG. Cytogenetic study of the offspring of atom bomb survivors. Nature 1968;218:367–8.
47. Ben-Amotz A, Yatziv S, Sela M, Greenberg S, Rachmilevich B, Shwarzman M, et al. Effect of natural beta-carotene supplementation in children exposed to radiation from the Chernobyl accident. Radiat Environ Biophys 1998;37:187–93.
48. Korkina LG, Afanas'ef IB, Diplock AT. Antioxidant therapy in children affected by irradiation from the Chernobyl nuclear accident. Biochem Soc Trans 1993;21:314S.
49. Anonymous. Statement from the 1985 Paris Meeting of the ICRP. Ann ICRP 1985;15:3
50. IAEA. Guidance for regulation of underground repositories for disposal of radioactive wastes. Report No.: Safety Series No.96. Vienna, Austria: International Atomic Energy Agency; 1989.
51. IAEA. Safety principles and techinical criteria for the underground disposal of high-level radioactive wastes. Report No.: Safety Series 99. Vienna, Austria: International Atomic Energy Agency; 1989.
52. Kuo SS, Saad AH, Koong AC, Hahn GM, Giaccia AJ. Potassium-channel activation in response to low doses of gamma-irradiation involves reactive oxygen intermediates in nonexcitatory cells. Proc Natl Acad Sci USA 1993;90:908–12.
53. ICRP. 1990 Recommendations of the International Commission on Radiologic Protection. Report No.: ICRP Publication 60. Oxford: Pergammon Press, 1991.
54. Capizzi RL, Oster W. Chemoprotective and radioprotective effects of amifostine: an update of clinical trials. Int J Hematol 2000;72:425–35.
55. Murray D, Rosenberg E, Allalunis-Turner MJ. Protection of human tumor cells of differing radiosensitivity by WR-1065. Radiat Res 2000;154:159–62.
56. Orditura M, De Vita F, Roscigno A, Infusino S, Auriemma A, Iodice P, et al. Amifostine: a selective cytoprotective agent of normal tissues from chemo-radiotherapy induced toxicity (Review). Oncol Rep 1999;6:1357–62.
57. Hospers GA, Eisenhauer EA, de Vries EG. The sulfhydryl containing compounds WR-2721 and glutathione as radio- and chemoprotective agents. A review, indications for use and prospects. Br J Cancer 1999;80:629–38.
58. Allalunis-Turner MJ, Walden TL Jr, Sawich C. Induction of marrow hypoxia by radioprotective agents. Radiat Res 1989;118:581–6.
59. Anne PR. Phase II trial of subcutaneous amifostine in patients undergoing radiation therapy for head and neck cancer. Semin Oncol 2002;29(Suppl. 19)80–3.
60. Sminia P, van der Kracht AH, Frederiks WM, Jansen W. Hyperthermia, radiation carcinogenesis and the protective potential of vitamin A and N-acetylcysteine. J Cancer Res Clin Oncol 1996;122:343–50.
61. Borek C, Ong A, Mason H, Donahue L, Biaglow JE. Selenium and vitamin E inhibit radiogenic and chemically induced transformation in vitro via different mechanisms. Proc Natl Acad Sci USA 1986;83:1490–4.
62. Radner BS, Kennedy AR. Suppression of X-ray induced transformation by vitamin E in mouse C3H/10T1/2 cells. Cancer Lett 1986;32:25–32.
63. Kennedy AR, Krinsky NI. Effects of retinoids, b-carotene and canthaxanthene on U.V. and x-ray-induced transformation of C3H10T 1/2 cells *in vitro*. Nutr Cancer 1994;22:219–32.
64. Ushakova T, Melkonyan H, Nickonova L, Afanasyev V, Gaziev A, Murdrik N, et al. Modification of gene expression by dietary antioxidants in radiation-induced apoptosis of mice splenocytes. Free Radic Biol Med 1999;26:887.
65. Konopacka M, Widel M, Rzeszowska-Wolny J. Modifying effect of vitamins C, E and beta-carotene against gamma-ray-induced DNA damage in mouse cells. Mutat Res 1998;417:85–94.
66. Ni O, Pei Y. Effect of beta-carotene on ^{60}Co-gamma-induced mutation at T-lymphocyte hypoxanthine-guanine phosphoribosyl transferase locus in rats. Acta Pharmacol Sinica 1997;18:535.
67. Gaziev A, Podlutsky A, Panfilov B, Bradbury R. Dietary supplements of antioxidants reduce hprt mutant frequency in splenocytes of aging mice. Mutat Res 1995;338:77.
68. Kumar B, Jha MN, Cole WC, Bedford JS, Prasad KN. d-Alpha tocopheryl succinate (vitamin E) enhances radiation-induced chromosomal damage levels in human cancer cells, but reduces it in normal cells. J Am Coll Nutr 2002;21:339–43.
69. O'Connor MK, Malone JF, Moriarty M, Mulgrew S. A radioprotective effect of vitamin C observed in Chinese hamster ovary cells. Br J Radiol 1977;50:587–91.
70. Weiss JF, Landauer MR. Radioprotection by antioxidants. Ann NY Acad Sci 2000;899:44–60.

71. Mutlu-Turkoglu U, Erbil Y, Oztezcan S, Olgac V, Toker G, Uysal M. The effect of selenium and/or vitamin E treatments on radiation-induced intestinal injury in rats. Life Sci 2000;66:1905–13.
72. Harapanhalli RS, Yaghmai V, Giuliani D, Howell RW, Rao DV. Antioxidant effects of vitamin C in mice following X-irradiation. Res Commun Mol Pathol Pharmacol 1996;94: 271–87.
73. Narra VR, Harapanhalli RS, Howell RW, Sastry KS, Rao DV. Vitamins as radioprotectors in vivo. I. Protection by vitamin C against internal radionuclides in mouse testes: implications to the mechanism of damage caused by the Auger effect. Radiat Res 1994;137:394–9.
74. El-Habit OH, Saada HN, Azab KS, Abdel-Rahman M, El-Malah DF. The modifying effect of beta-carotene on gamma radiation-induced elevation of oxidative reactions and genotoxicity in male rats. Mutat Res 2000;466:179–86.
75. Umegaki K, Uramoto H, Suzuki J, Esashi T. Feeding mice palm carotene prevents DNA damage in bone marrow and reduction of peripheral leukocyte counts, and enhances survival following X-ray irradiation. Carcinogenesis 1997;18:1943–7.
76. Ershoff BH, Steers CW Jr. Antioxidants and survival time of mice exposed to multiple sublethal doses of x-irradiation. Proc Soc Biol Med 1960;104:274–6.
77. Londer HM, Myers CE. Radioprotective effects of vitamin E. Am J Clin Nutr 1978;31:705a.
78. Seifter E, Rettura A, Padawar J, Levenson SM. Vitamin A and β-carotene as adjunctive therapy to tumor excision, radiation therapy and chemotherapy. In: Prasad KN, editor. Vitamins, nutrition and cancer. Basel: Karger; 1984:1–19.
79. Blumenthal RD, Lew W, Reising A, Soyne D, Osorio L, Ying Z, et al. Anti-oxidant vitamins reduce normal tissue toxicity induced by radio-immunotherapy. Int J Cancer 2000;86:276–80.
80. Mills EE. The modifying effect of beta-carotene on radiation and chemotherapy induced oral mucositis. Br J Cancer 1988;57:416–7.
81. Jaakkola K, Lahteenmaki P, Laakso J, Harju E, Tykka H, Mahlberg K. Treatment with antioxidant and other nutrients in combination with chemotherapy and irradiation in patients with small-cell lung cancer. Anticancer Res 1992;12: 599–606.
82. Lamson DW, Brignall MS. Antioxidants in cancer therapy; their actions and interactions with oncologic therapies. Altern Med Rev 1999;4:304–29.
83. Sinclair WK. Cysteamine: differential x-ray protective effect on Chinese hamster cells during the cell cycle. Science 1968;159:442–4.
84. Ramakrishnan N, Wolfe WW, Catravas GN. Radioprotection of hematopoietic tissues in mice by lipoic acid. Radiat Res 1992;130:360–5.
85. Prasad KN, Cole WC, Prasad KC. Risk factors for Alzheimer's disease: role of multiple antioxidants, non-steroidal anti-inflammatory and cholinergic agents alone or in combination in prevention and treatment. J Am Coll Nutr 2002;21:506–22.

The British Journal of Radiology, *78* (2005), 493–498 © 2005 The British Institute of Radiology
DOI: 10.1259/bjr/42380498

Differences in bone mineral density and geometry in men and women: the Newcastle Thousand Families Study at 50 years old

[1]S P TUCK, BSc, MB, MRCP, [2]M S PEARCE, MSc, CStat, PhD, [1]D J RAWLINGS, BSc, MPhil, [3]F N BIRRELL, MA, MRCP, PhD, [2]L PARKER, PhD, FRCPCH, FFPHM and [1]R M FRANCIS, MBChB, FRCP

[1]*Department of Rheumatology, Musculoskeletal Unit, Freeman Hospital, Freeman Road, Newcastle upon Tyne NE7 7DN,* [2]*Sir James Spence Institute of Child Health, School of Clinical Medical Sciences, University of Newcastle, The Royal Victoria Infirmary, Queen Victoria Road, Newcastle upon Tyne NE1 4LP and* [3]*Department of Rheumatology, University of Newcastle upon Tyne, Medical School, Framlington Place, Newcastle upon Tyne NE2 4HH, UK*

Abstract. In 1947 Sir James Spence initiated the Newcastle Thousand Families study, which recruited all 1142 children born in the city between May and June that year. At the age of 50 years, 832 survivors were traced and invited to attend for measurement of bone mineral density (BMD) by dual energy X-ray absorptiometry (DXA). The aim was to compare BMD measurements of men and women in this cohort, before and after adjustment for skeletal size. The femoral neck shaft angles (NSA) were also measured manually from the DXA scan printouts. A total of 171 men and 218 women agreed to participate. As expected men had greater bone mineral content and bone area at all sites ($p<0.0001$) and were taller and heavier ($p<0.0001$) than women. Men also had significantly higher BMD than women at all regions ($p<0.0002$), except at the femoral neck or lumbar spine. After correction for skeletal size and body weight, men had statistically significantly lower volumetric BMD at all sites. The measurement of NSA had good intra/interobserver errors and precision (coefficient of variations 0.79%, 1.2% and 1.2%). Men had significantly larger NSAs (mean 130°, range 121–138°) than women (mean 128°, range 119–137°). We conclude that there are gender differences in BMD, skeletal size and geometry in middle aged men and women, which together with the subsequent rate of bone loss, may influence fracture risk in later life.

Osteoporotic fractures are a major health problem causing excess mortality and considerable morbidity, resulting in substantial cost to the health and social services. There is an inverse relationship between bone mineral density (BMD) and fracture risk, with 1 standard deviation (SD) decrease in BMD being associated with a two to threefold increase in fracture incidence [1]. The risk of fracture is not only determined by BMD, but also by skeletal geometry and morphometry. Femoral geometry, including neck shaft angle (NSA), is an independent predictor of fracture risk, with 1 standard deviation increase in femoral NSA resulting in a doubling of fracture risk in both men and women [2, 3].

Dual energy X-ray absorptiometry (DXA) generates two-dimensional or areal BMD (aBMD) measurements (g cm^{-2}), which are influenced by the size of the skeleton. Throughout life males have larger bones than females, as a result of which men have a greater bone cross-sectional area and hence a higher aBMD than women [4, 5]. Melton et al found aBMD to be 15% higher in men than women, but when correction for skeletal size was made this difference fell to only 6% [4]. Indeed, the true volumetric BMD (vBMD) has been reported to be the same in healthy age-matched men and women [5].

Received 12 December 2003 and in final form 25 November 2004, accepted 5 January 2005.

Address correspondence to Dr R M Francis, Musculoskeletal Unit, Freeman Hospital, Freeman Road, Newcastle upon Tyne NE7 7DN, UK.

The Newcastle Thousand Families cohort study was initiated in 1947 by Sir James Spence, when all 1142 children born in May and June that year to mothers resident in the city of Newcastle upon Tyne were recruited. The health, growth and development of this cohort were followed in great detail up to the age of 15 years [6]. More recently survivors were followed up when they reached 50 years of age. Results from this 50 year follow up have been published on the effects of early life and later determinants of adult disease [7], risk factors for cardiovascular disease [8], central metabolic syndrome [9] and implications of childhood obesity for adult health [10].

As part of the 50 year follow up, participants of the Newcastle Thousand Families cohort study were invited to have BMD measured by DXA. The aim of the present study was to compare BMD measurements in this well-characterized cohort of 50-year-old men and women and to examine the effect of adjustment for skeletal size. We also investigated a method for the manual measurement of the femoral NSA using the DXA scan printouts, which enabled us to make gender comparisons of femoral geometry in this cohort.

Patients and methods

Design of the Thousand Families Study

Details of the original Newcastle Thousand Families study have been described elsewhere [6, 11–13], but will be outlined briefly. A total of 967 of these children were followed through until the end of the first year. In the 1990s, 832 study members were traced, either through the NHS Central Register or by contacting the study team in response to local, national and international media publicity. Between October 1996 and December 1998 self-completion questionnaires on health and lifestyle were sent out and members invited to attend for clinical examination and to take part in further studies [7–10]. The study has local ethics committee approval and all subjects gave their informed consent.

The clinical examination measured height, weight and a number of physiological risk factors for age-related disorders [8]. In addition participants were invited to attend for DXA scanning, which was performed using a Hologic QDR 2000 machine (Hologic Instruments, Waltham, MA). This had a daily calibration check using the Hologic spine phantom and had a coefficient of variation of 0.5% throughout the period of study. The lumbar spine (L1 to L4) and all regions of the hip (total hip, femoral neck, trochanteric and intertrochanteric) were measured. This generated data on area, bone mineral content (BMC) and BMD at these sites. In order to correct for size differences, an estimate of volumetric density was made (g cm^{-3}); the bone mineral apparent density (BMAD). This was calculated using the formulae of Katzman et al [14] whereby:

$$\text{Lumbar spine BMAD} = \text{BMC}/\text{area}^{3/2}$$
$$\text{Femoral neck BMAD} = \text{BMC}/\text{area}^{2}$$

where the area at the lumbar spine or femoral neck was the projected bone area, as determined from the BMD scan. BMAD cannot be calculated for the remaining sites and so an adjustment was made by dividing the BMD by height in metres. This has previously been reported to be a useful method of reducing or eliminating the difference in BMD found between men and women owing to skeletal size [4].

Geometric measurements

No morphometric measurements were made during the BMD assessment. The DXA scanner used was of fan beam design and so magnification errors made it inappropriate to measure hip axis length or femoral neck width. However, the effect of magnification on femoral NSA was thought to be minimal. In an attempt to verify this, a cadaver femur was positioned in a tissue equivalent phantom at 2 cm intervals 0–12 cm above the DXA couch.

For both patient and phantom scans NSA was measured from the DXA scan printout using a method adapted from that of Faulkner et al [15, 16]. The femoral neck axis was identified on the printout by the DXA analysis software. A line was then drawn manually from the junction between the greater trochanter and the femoral neck down to a point in the middle of the shaft at the bottom of the scan (Figure 1). The junction of these two lines gives the femoral NSA, which was measured with a long armed protractor with 0.5° intervals (a BIOMET Inc. goniometer; Biomet, Inc., Warsaw, IN). The intraobserver and interobserver errors were determined as the average coefficient of variation of a sample of 20 scans. The precision error (reproducibility) was calculated from a further 20 subjects who had had three successive scans. All

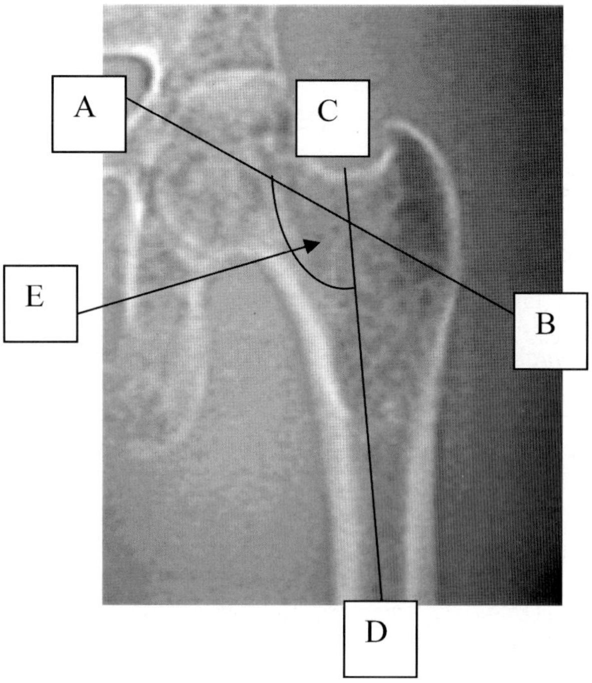

Figure 1. Measurement of the femoral neck shaft angle from the dual energy X-ray absorptiometry (DXA) scan printouts. The line AB is the hip axis marked by the scanner's software. A line is then drawn from C to D, in which C is the point at which the greater trochanter joins the femoral neck and D is the midpoint of the shaft at the bottom of the picture. E is the femoral neck shaft angle.

printouts were generated from the same printer attached to the DXA workstation.

Analysis

Statistical analysis was performed using standard statistical software packages (Graphpad Prism, SanDiego, CA) and SPSS for Windows (SPSS, Chicago, IL). Descriptive statistics were obtained and the data tested for normality. Data, which were normally distributed, were then compared using Student's unpaired *t*-tests. Associations were assessed using Pearson's correlation. The derived variables BMD/height and BMAD were compared before and after adjustment for weight using regression analysis.

Results

Response rate

Of the 832 cohort members traced, 574 (69%) completed the questionnaire and 412 (50%) attended for clinical examination [8]. A total of 389 subjects (42%) comprising 171 men and 218 women underwent DXA scanning. This sample did not differ significantly from the remainder of the original cohort of 1142 individuals in terms of birth weight and social class at birth.

DXA scan results

The results of the DXA scans are shown in Table 1, which compares men and women. All subjects were

Table 1. Comparison of anthropometric and bone mineral density (BMD) measurements by gender

	Men (n=171)		Women (n=218)		
	Mean	SD	Mean	SD	t-test p
Height (m) (range)	1.73 (1.52–1.96)	0.07	1.61 (1.48–1.75)	0.06	<0.0001
Weight (kg) (range)	81.3 (52.7–130.8)	13	69.3 (42.3–126.1)	13.96	<0.0001
Lumbar spine					
Area (cm^2)	65.7	6.49	56.5	5.31	<0.0001
BMC (g)	67.9	12.5	59.6	10.8	<0.0001
BMD (g cm^{-2})	1.03	0.13	1.05	0.14	0.08
Total hip					
Area (cm^2)	44.8	4.51	34.2	3.31	<0.0001
BMC (g)	45.4	8.26	32.6	5.47	<0.0001
BMD (g cm^{-2})	1.01	0.14	0.96	0.13	<0.0001
Femoral neck					
Area (cm^2)	5.40	0.37	4.65	0.30	<0.0001
BMC (g)	4.67	0.78	4.01	0.63	<0.0001
BMD (g cm^{-2})	0.87	0.14	0.86	0.12	0.75
Trochanteric					
Area (cm^2)	13.4	1.66	10.5	1.21	<0.0001
BMC (g)	10.5	2.28	7.71	1.42	<0.0001
BMD (g cm^{-2})	0.78	0.12	0.73	0.11	0.0001
Intertrochanteric					
Area (cm^2)	26.1	3.43	19.0	2.41	<0.0001
BMC (g)	30.3	5.82	20.9	3.86	<0.0001
BMD (g cm^{-2})	1.16	0.16	1.10	0.15	0.0002

SD, standard deviation; BMC, bone mineral content.

scanned within a few months of their 50th birthdays resulting in a mean age of 50.1 years for both men and women. The BMD was significantly higher in men than women at the total hip, trochanteric and intertrochanteric regions, but not at the lumbar spine and femoral neck.

Men had a statistically significantly greater cross-sectional area and BMC at all sites measured and were significantly taller, reflecting their larger skeletal size (Table 1). Men were also significantly heavier. The results of correction for skeletal size are shown in Table 2. Dividing the BMD by height resulted in the loss of the statistically significant difference previously seen between men and women at the total hip, trochanteric and intertrochanteric regions. However, at the femoral neck and lumbar spine, BMAD was significantly lower in the men.

Both height and weight were strongly correlated with BMD. For BMAD and BMD/height, there was no residual correlation with height, but the correlation with weight persisted. The data were therefore further adjusted to the mean weight for the entire study group (both men and women) of 74.05 kg. This resulted in men having statistically significantly lower adjusted bone mineral densities than women at all sites (Table 3).

Comparison of the BMD measurements, with those of the currently available normal reference data from NHANES III and Hologic, show them to be similar to that expected once these have been standardized to age 50 years (Table 4). The BMD means and ranges are similar, indicating that the cohort is representative of the population as a whole.

Table 2. Comparison of volumetric bone mineral density (vBMD) (bone mineral apparent density (BMAD) and BMD/ height in metres) by gender and site

	Men		Women		
	Mean	SD	Mean	SD	p-value
Lumbar spine BMAD (g cm^{-3})	0.13	0.02	0.14	0.02	<0.0001
Total hip BMD/m	0.59	0.08	0.59	0.08	0.38
Femoral neck BMAD (g cm^{-3})	0.16	0.03	0.19	0.03	<0.0001
Trochanteric BMD/m	0.45	0.07	0.45	0.07	0.58
Intertrochanteric BMD/m	0.67	0.09	0.68	0.09	0.27

SD, standard deviation.

Femoral neck shaft angles

The method described gave an intraobserver error of 0.79%, interobserver error of 1.2% and precision of $\pm$1.2%. The results are shown in Figure 2. Men had a mean femoral NSA of 130° (SD 3.3, range 121–138°). Women had a significantly (p<0.0001) smaller mean

Table 3. Comparison of volumetric bone mineral density (vBMD) (bone mineral apparent density (BMAD) and BMD/ height in metres) by gender and site after adjustment to the mean weight of 74.05 kg

	Men		Women		
	Mean	SD	Mean	SD	p-value
Lumbar spine BMAD (g cm^{-3})	0.13	0.02	0.14	0.02	<0.0001
Total hip BMD/m	0.57	0.08	0.59	0.08	0.02
Femoral neck BMAD (g cm^{-3})	0.16	0.03	0.19	0.03	<0.0001
Trochanteric BMD/m	0.44	0.07	0.46	0.06	0.0035
Intertrochanteric BMD/m	0.66	0.09	0.69	0.08	<0.0001

SD, standard deviation.

Table 4. Comparison of mean bone mineral density (BMD) (g cm^{-2}) and 95% confidence intervals (CI) between the Thousand Families study and the Hologic and NHANES III reference databases (standardized to age 50 years)

	Mean	95% CI
Male L1-4		
1000 families	1.03	0.77 to 1.29
Hologic Reference	1.05	0.83 to 1.27
Female L1-4		
1000 families	1.05	0.77 to 1.33
Hologic reference	0.97	0.75 to 1.19
Male total hip		
1000 families	1.01	0.73 to 1.29
NHANES III	0.99	0.68 to 1.29
Hologic reference	0.99	0.73 to 1.25
Female total hip		
1000 families	0.96	0.70 to 1.22
NHANES III	0.89	0.62 to 1.16
Hologic reference	0.91	0.67 to 1.15

NHANES III data relates to an American population and has only a few hundred people in each decade and consequently only a small number at any one year of age. The Hologic manufacturer's data are subject to similar constraints.

femoral NSA of 128° (SD 1.7, range 119–137°). Since the height of the femur neck above the scanning couch was not known for this group of subjects, these results take no account of possible image distortion caused by the shape of fan beam. Phantom measurements, however, indicate an apparent change in NSA of +0.27° degree per cm (Figure 3).

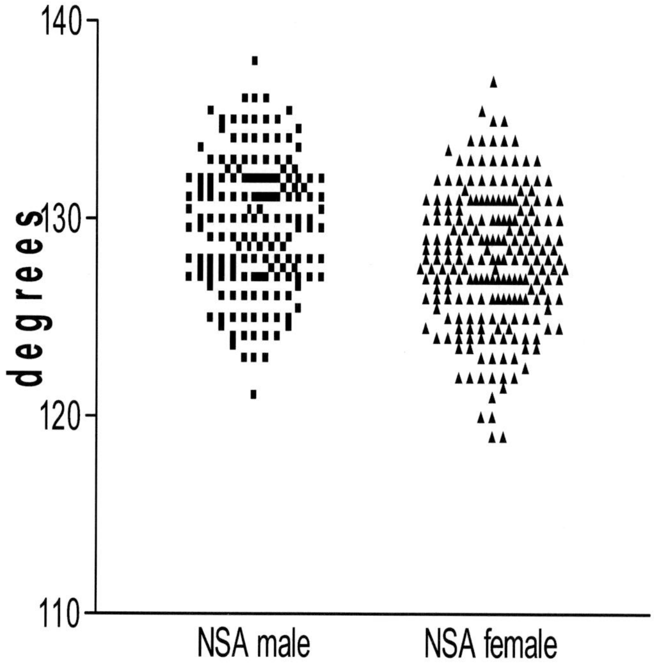

Figure 2. Scatter plot of femoral neck shaft angle (NSAs) in the men (n=171) and women (n=218).

Discussion

This paper presents the results of areal and estimated volumetric BMD and femoral geometry measurements in the Newcastle Thousand Families Study at age 50 years. Although previous studies have made gender comparisons of BMD and skeletal size [4, 5], these have included subjects with a broad age range. Our study utilizes a well-characterized cohort of men and women at the age of 50 years, before significant involutional bone loss has occurred or the confounding effect of degenerative changes on spine bone density measurements becomes a major problem.

Men had greater bone mineral content and area, indicating a larger skeletal size, consistent with them being significantly taller and heavier than women. Consistent with this finding, BMD was greater at all sites in men than women except for the femoral neck and lumbar spine. This is broadly consistent with other studies comparing men and women, which have found men to have significantly higher BMD at all sites [4, 17]. Correction for body size, either by using height or by calculation of BMAD, resulted in significantly lower size-adjusted BMD at the lumbar spine and femoral neck in men. After adjusting for weight, there was statistically

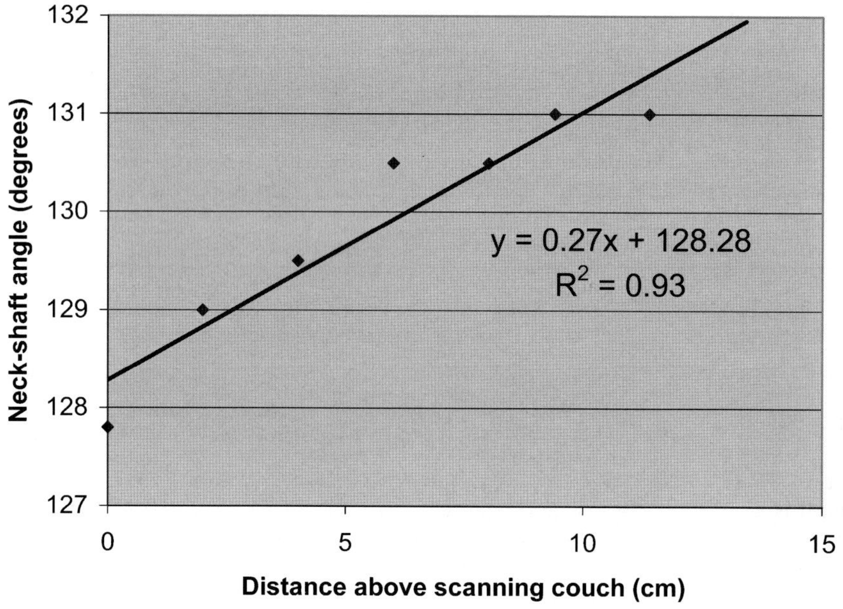

Figure 3. Measurement, from the dual energy X-ray absorptiometry (DXA) scan printout, of neck shaft angle for a single cadaver femur. The femur had been positioned, with appropriate internal rotation, at a range of distances above the DXA scanning couch to characterize image distortion caused by the fan beam.

significantly lower BMD in men at all sites. The contrasting effects of adjustment at different skeletal sites suggests that size cannot be wholly represented by a simple scaling factor. Hence, it would not be anticipated that all data might demonstrate an identical response to the adjustment for body size.

Other studies have demonstrated that correction for skeletal size resulted in a reduction in the difference in BMD between the sexes [4, 17, 18]. Duan et al found the volumetric BMD (vBMD) at the lumbar spine to be similar in young men and women aged 18–43 years, but in those aged over 60 years, vBMD was greater in men than in women [17]. Our results may be different because the subjects are all the same age and the women are perimenopausal. It may therefore represent an age group for which BMD is transitional, before menopausal bone loss results in lower vBMD in women than men. Long-term follow up of this cohort may answer this question. An alternative explanation is that this is a cohort effect. The group was born in 1947 at a time when there was post war rationing and it is possible that this and other unknown factors operating at that time could have affected the results.

Our method of femoral NSA measurement proved both reliable and precise. The precision is similar to the 0.5% and 1% quoted by Qureshi and Faulkner, respectively, [15, 16] and the intraobserver error of 1.5% and precision of 1.7% quoted by Gomez Alonso et al [2]. Furthermore, the mean values and ranges are similar to those reported in other studies [2, 3, 15, 16, 19, 20]. Using this method we were able to demonstrate that men had a larger NSA than women.

However, despite being statistically significant, this difference in NSA was small. The fan beam could have distorted the image and our phantom measurements showed an apparent change in NSA of +0.27 degree per cm from the scanning couch. Anthropometric data relating to a normal population of seated individuals are available [21]. Assuming that these translate directly to subjects lying supine on a DXA scanner then the median height above the couch for a male neck of femur is 12.0 cm (SD 0.5 cm). For a female neck of femur the median is 13.0 cm (SD 0.5 cm). Given the magnitude and direction of the measured influence of couch height on neck shaft angle, correcting patient NSA data for any such effects would have resulted in small individual changes in NSA which would have increased, rather than decreased, the significance of the above gender differences. Hence, manual assessment of NSA from fan beam DXA printouts is reliable and can be performed without additional software.

We found men to have a significantly larger NSA than women, consistent with that reported by Gomez Alonso et al [2]. This larger femoral NSA might be anticipated to predispose to an increased hip fracture risk in later life [2, 19], yet men have a lower risk than women. This is likely to be related to slower bone loss with advancing age in men, but may also be due to other gender differences in skeletal geometry. Both Karlsson et al [19] and Gomez Alonso et al [2] have demonstrated that men have larger femoral neck widths than women. Looker et al found men to have greater periosteal and cortical widths than women at all sites in the hip, even after correction for body size [22]. Furthermore, the gender differences in cortical bone size increased with age [22], suggesting that these structural differences may contribute to the lower fracture risk in men.

The study has a number of strengths and weaknesses. It is a large study with 389 subjects, all at age 50 years. Of the 1142 study members recruited at birth in 1947, 34% were included in the current study. This inclusion rate, 50 years after the study began, is higher than that reported in other studies (for example, 23% of a hospital based cohort were included in a study of fetal growth and adult hyperinsulinaemia [23] and less than 5% of a Hertfordshire birth cohort were included in a study of impaired glucose tolerance [24]).

There was no difference between the participants and the remainder of the original cohort in terms of birth weight and social class at birth. In addition, inclusion of study members no longer resident in the study region (18% of those attending a health check were resident outside of the Northern Region of England) increased how well the studied represented the population studied. Hence the study members are representative of all those born in Newcastle upon Tyne in May and June 1947.

At the time of scanning no morphometric measures were undertaken at the lumbar spine, so neither the degree of deformity nor direct measures of vertebral size were possible. Also, femoral neck geometry was not considered, which restricted analysis to neck shaft angles alone. Therefore we were unable to examine all aspects of size, structure and geometry, which may differ between men and women and affect their fracture risk.

Conclusions

In this paper we have presented the results of BMD measurements in the Newcastle Thousand Families Study. We have demonstrated that differences in areal BMD measurements between men and women are reversed following adjustment for skeletal size: vBMD is lower in men than in women at the age of 50 years. However, this may represent an age group for which BMD is transitional, before menopausal bone loss results in lower vBMD in women than men.

We have confirmed that this manual method of femoral NSA measurement is both reliable and precise and can be used retrospectively. Using this method we have shown men to have larger femoral NSAs than women, despite their lower fracture risk.

The present study did not examine the relationship between skeletal size, BMD and geometry on fracture incidence. However, post-menopausal bone loss may contribute to the increased risk of fracture in older women, when the vBMD becomes lower than men. Future studies of the pathogenesis of fracture should examine the interaction between skeletal size, BMD and skeletal geometry. Further work on the Newcastle Thousand Families study will explore the contribution of birth weight, growth, development and socioeconomic factors to adult BMD and skeletal geometry.

Acknowledgments

We would like to thank Miss Emma Scott, physics student at the University of Newcastle-upon-Tyne, for assistance and involvement in the phantom tests and the subsequent analysis of this data. We also thank the previous research teams involved in the Thousand Family Study and the study members for taking part in the present investigation. We are grateful to the Wellcome Trust, the Minnie Henderson Trust, the Sir John Knott Trust and the Special Trustees of the Newcastle Hospitals for supporting this work.

References

1. Marshall D, Johnell O, Wedel H. Meta-analysis of how well measures of bone mineral density predict occurrence of osteoporotic fractures. BMJ 1996;312:223–4.
2. Gomez Alonso CG, Diez Curiel M, Hawkins Carranza F, Perez Cano R, Diez Perez A. Femoral bone density, neck-shaft angle and mean femoral neck width as predictors of hip fracture in men and women. Osteoporosis Int 2000;11:714–20.
3. Gnudi S, Ripamonti C, Lisi L, Fini M, Giardino R, Giavaresi G. Proximal femur geometry to detect and distinguish femoral neck fractures from trochanteric fractures in post-menopausal women. Osteoporosis Int 2002;13:69–73.
4. Melton LJ, Khosla S, Achenbach SJ, O'Connor MK, O'Fallon WM, Riggs BL. Effects of body size and skeletal site on the estimated prevalence of osteoporosis in women and men. Osteoporosis Int 2000;11:977–83.
5. Seeman E. Sexual dimorphism in skeletal size, density and strength. J Clin Endocrinol Metab 2001;86:4576–84.
6. Miller FJW, Court SDM, Knox EG, Brandon S. The School years in Newcastle upon Tyne 1952–1962. London: Oxford University Press, 1974.
7. Lamont DW, Parker L, Cohen MA, White M, Bennett SMA, Unwin NC, Craft AW, et al. Early life and later determinants of adult disease: a 50 year follow-up study of the Newcastle thousand families cohort. Public Health 1998;112:85–93.
8. Lamont DW, Parker L, White M, Unwin N, Bennett SMA, Cohen M, et al. Risk of cardiovascular disease measured by carotid intima-media thickness at age 49-51: a life course study. BMJ 2000;320:273–8.
9. Parker L, Lamont DW, Unwin N, Pearce MS, Bennett SMA, Dickinson HO, et al. A lifecourse study of risk for hyperinsulinaemia, dyslipidaemia and obesity (the central metabolic syndrome) at age 49-51. Diabetic Med 2003;20:406–15.
10. Wright CM, Parker L, Lamont DW, Craft AW. Implications of childhood obesity for adult health: findings from the Newcastle thousand families cohort study. BMJ 2001;323:1280–4.
11. Spence J, Walton WS, Miller FJW, Court SD. A Thousand Families in Newcastle upon Tyne. London: Oxford University Press, 1954.
12. Miller FJW, Court SDM, Walton WS, Knox EG. Growing up in Newcastle upon Tyne. London: Oxford University Press, 1960.
13. Kolvin I, Miller FJW, Fells H. Continuities of deprivation: The Newcastle Thousand Families Study. Aldershot: Gower, 1990.
14. Katzman DK, Bachrach LK, Carter DR, Marcus R. Clinical and anthropometric correlates of bone mineral acquisition in healthy adolescent girls. J Clin Endocrinol Metab 1991;73:1332–9.
15. Faulkner KG, Cummings SR, Black D, Palermo L, Gluer CC, Genant HK. Simple Measurement of femoral geometry predicts hip fracture: the study of osteoporotic fractures. J Bone Miner Res 1993;8:1211–7.
16. Qureshi AM, McGuigan FEA, Seymoor DG, Hutchinson JD, Reid DM, Ralston SH. Association between COLIA1 Spi alleles and femoral neck geometry. Calci Tissue Int 2001;69:67–72.
17. Duan Y, Turner CH, Bonn-Taeck K, Seeman E. Sexual dimorphism in vertebral fragility is more the result of gender differences in age-related bone gain than bone loss. J Bone Miner Res 2001;16:2267–75.
18. Duan Y, Seeman E, Turner CH. The biomechanical basis of vertebral fragility in men and women. J Bone Miner Res 2001;16:2276–83.
19. Karlsson KM, Sernbo I, Obrant KJ, Redlund-Johnell I, Johnell O. Femoral neck geometry and radiographic signs of osteoporosis as predictors of hip fracture. Bone 1996;18:327–30.
20. Nelson DA, Barondess DA, Hendrix SC, Beck TJ. Cross-sectional geometry, bone strength and bone mass in the proximal femur in black and white postmenopausal women. J Bone Miner Res 2000;15:1992–7.
21. Pheasant S. Bodyspace: anthropometry, ergonomics and design. London: Taylor & Francis, 1988.
22. Looker AC, Beck TJ, Orwoll ES. Does body size account for gender differences in femur bone density and geometry? J Bone Miner Res 2001;16:1291–9.
23. Martyn CN, Hales CN, Barker DJP, Jesperson S. Fetal growth and hyperinsulinaemia in adult life. Diabet Med 1998;15:688–94.
24. Hales CN, Barker DJP, Clark PMS, Jesperson S. Fetal and infant growth and impaired glucose tolerance at age 64. Br Med J 1991;303:1019–22.

The British Journal of Radiology, 78 (2005), 499–505 © 2005 The British Institute of Radiology
DOI: 10.1259/bjr/51196310

The costs and effects of introducing selectively trained radiographers to an A&E reporting service: a retrospective controlled before and after study

[1]S BREALEY, BSc, PhD, [2]D G KING, MBChB, FRCS(Eng), FRCR, [3]S HAHN, MSc, PhD, [3]C GODFREY, BA, [4]M T I CROWE, MRCP, FRCR, [3]K BLOOR, BA, MSc, PhD, [2]S CRANE, MRCP(UK), FFAEM and [5]D LONGSWORTH, MBChB, MRCGP, FRCF Ed(A&E)

[1]*York Trials Unit, Department of Health Sciences, University of York, York YO10 5DD,* [2]*York Hospital, Wigginton Road, York YO31 8HE,* [3]*Department of Health Sciences, University of York, York YO10 5DD,* [4]*The Queen Elizabeth Hospital, Gayton Road, Norfolk PE30 4ET and* [5]*The Derwent Practice, Norton Road, Malton YO17 9RF, UK*

Abstract. The costs and effects of introducing selectively trained radiographers reporting accident and emergency (A&E) radiographs of the appendicular skeleton in a district general hospital were assessed using a retrospective controlled before and after design. Reference standard reports were compared with a random stratified sample of 200 A&E and 200 general practitioner (GP) reports before and after the intervention. GP reports were used as a non-intervention, non-equivalent control group. An A&E specialist registrar judged whether incorrect A&E reports might have a clinically important effect on patient management. The effect of incorrect A&E reports on outcome was assessed by patient re-attendance to the hospital because of missed abnormalities. The annual, average and incremental costs of radiographers and radiologists reporting A&E radiographs were calculated and a sensitivity analysis was undertaken. The introduction of the radiographers resulted in a 1% (95% CI −7.9 to 5.9) fall in A&E radiograph reporting accuracy and 11% (95% CI −33.7 to 11.3) reduction of cases in which incorrect A&E reports might have a clinically important effect on patient management. Only two A&E reports (one before and one after the intervention) affected patient outcome in that a fracture missed at the first visit resulted in patient re-attendance to the X-ray Department. There was a saving of £361 per annum to the X-ray Department. In conclusion this study provides further evidence that selectively trained radiographers can accurately report A&E plain radiographs and at no additional cost.

A shortage in doctors and the need to address increasing demand in a healthcare system with scarce resources brought about changes in government policy that promote the flexible and creative use of allied healthcare professional skills [1–4]. In X-ray departments, a national shortage of radiologists [5, 6] and a continuing rise in the level of activities undertaken [7] provided a climate that encouraged the development of radiographers in a written reporting role [8, 9]. Furthermore, reporting plain radiographs should increase radiographer job satisfaction and enhance their professional standing [10]; radiologists' time could also be freed to perform other more specialist and complex investigations [11].

There is evidence that selectively trained radiographers can accurately report Accident and Emergency (A&E) radiographs [12–14] resulting in a growing number performing this activity [15, 16]. Despite an emphasis on the clinical contribution of radiologists' reports to the management of A&E patients [17–19] this has not been evaluated for radiographer reporting; although there is evidence that radiographer reports do not adversely affect A&E patient outcome in terms of re-attendance to the X-ray Department [20]. The College of Radiographers vision was that radiographers in a reporting role should revolutionise the cost-effective management of patients [21] yet no robust cost analysis of radiographers reporting A&E plain radiographs has been performed [22].

In February 1995, following a period of postgraduate training in plain radiograph interpretation, two carefully selected radiographers in our hospital began to report A&E radiographs judged normal or insignificantly abnormal by the casualty officers. The X-ray department performs more than 7500 examinations per month, of which 29% are referred from A&E. This corresponds with a report which found that 27% of the radiology workload was generated by referral from A&E [23]. The radiographers report the appendicular skeleton, *i.e.* upper limb (shoulder girdle to fingers), lower limb (hip to toes) and foreign body examinations, but do not report the axial skeleton (pelvis, spine, head), chest, thorax and abdomen. Their introduction to the A&E reporting service was an opportunity to assess whether this skill mix initiative was an effective and efficient use of scarce resources [24]. The aim of this study was to assess the effect of introducing radiographer reporting on the accuracy of A&E reports, the subsequent effects on A&E patient management and outcome, and to examine the associated costs.

Methods

Assessment of accuracy

To assess the effect on accuracy a random sample of A&E plain radiograph reports for the period February

Received 14 July 2004 and in revised form 10 November 2004, accepted 5 January 2005.

1993 to January 1997 (2 years before and after the intervention) was selected. This was to minimize the effects of statistical regression and maturation, ensure a similar sample of reports were compared before and after the intervention, and to reflect the population of reports on A&E plain radiographs in clinical practice. To further underpin the study, so that a change in A&E radiograph reporting accuracy can be attributed to the intervention rather than other historical events, a random sample of general practitioner (GP) plain radiograph reports were selected as a non-equivalent, non-intervention control group. The GP reports are non-equivalent because these referrals are for a different type of patient with different pathology. It is a non-intervention control group as the radiographers do not report GP radiographs. The samples of A&E and GP reports were stratified by time and body area. This was to control for the effect on accuracy of reporting on different pathology at different times of the year and for radiographs that the radiographers do and do not report. The body areas that the radiographers do not report were included to capture the wider implications of introducing this intervention. For example, radiologists not reporting A&E radiographs of the appendicular skeleton might free them to spend more time reporting on the axial skeleton, which could affect the accuracy with which these radiographs were reported.

To select the reports a random sample of 3 days for each quarter were chosen. The Systems and Networks Service Department provided a list of all A&E and GP examinations performed for the selected days. A random sample of 25 A&E and 25 GP reports were selected for each quarter stratified by body area. To assess the accuracy of the reports all the radiographs were made available so that a consultant radiologist with 11 years experience in radiology and a special interest in skeletal radiology could produce a reference standard report. The radiologist reported in normal viewing conditions using the same format as during clinical practice and had access to previous radiographs but not the original and previous reports to prevent bias [25]. The arbiter who compared reports for concordance, blind to who had produced each report, was a consultant radiologist at a different hospital with 10 years experience and a special interest in skeletal radiology. Normal was defined as within normal limits, no bony injury, or a minor abnormality such as an old fracture. Abnormal was defined as all clinically relevant abnormalities. Reports were only judged concordant if they agreed on the presence, location and type of abnormality [26].

Assessment of management

For incorrect A&E reports an A&E specialist registrar decided whether this might have a clinically important effect on patient management compared with the reference standard report. Knowledge that only discordant pairs of reports were used might affect the registrar's decision about an expected difference in patient management so for every two pairs of discordant reports a convenience sample of a concordant pair of reports was included in the assessment. The concordant sample of reports was then excluded from the analysis. When comparing pairs of reports the registrar could view the plain radiographs and was provided with information from X-ray request cards, case notes, and casualty cards and chose one of the following options:

- No difference in management (treatment or advice);
- Clinically unimportant difference in management – the patient may have been treated differently but this would not affect patient outcome;
- Clinically important difference in management – the patient may have been treated differently and patient outcome would be affected.

Assessment of outcome

Patient re-attendance to A&E or the X-ray department was used as a proxy for outcome, as it may indicate that significant pathology was missed at the first visit. For A&E patients whose report was judged to be incorrect the casualty X-ray card and patient case notes were searched to identify whether a patient re-attended the A&E department within 3 months of the first visit. The Radiology department computer system was also searched to establish whether a patient re-attended for further radiographic examinations or other procedures within 1 year of the first visit. The process of searching case notes and the Radiology department computer identified three possible outcomes for patients:

- Did not re-attend A&E or X-ray department;
- Re-attended X-ray department for an unrelated examination;
- Re-attended X-ray department for a related examination.

When a patient did not re-attend A&E or the X-ray department it was assumed that any error in the report had a negligible effect on patient outcome. When a patient re-attended for a further X-ray examination that was unrelated to the same symptomatic body area as the first examination it was assumed their re-attendance was not due to an error in the report. For those patients who re-attended for a repeat X-ray examination of the same anatomical area or for a different imaging procedure it was important to establish whether an error in the report at the first visit resulted in their re-attendance. To do this a consultant radiologist compared the report from the first visit with reports of the subsequent examinations. When a discrepancy was found between the first and subsequent reports all examinations were reviewed in consensus by a group of three consultant radiologists. The reference standard radiologist or radiologist responsible for the report of radiographs under review was not included in this group to eliminate bias [25].

Assessment of costs

A cost analysis of radiographers and radiologists reporting A&E plain radiographs of the appendicular skeleton was performed from the perspective of the X-ray department. This included the capital costs of providing radiographers with the equipment and facilities to report, costs of training radiographers, and the overhead costs of the rooms used for reporting activity. There were no additional medicolegal or insurance costs. Consumable costs were excluded as they were negligible and the same

Table 1. A&E radiograph reporting accuracy

	TP	TN	FN	FP	Total	Sensitivity (95% CI)	Specificity (95% CI)	Accuracy (95% CI)
Before								
Appendicular skeleton	12	77	10	1	100	55 (35, 73)	99 (93, 100)	89 (81, 94)
Remaining body areas	11	73	13	3	100	46 (28, 65)	96 (89, 99)	84 (76, 90)
Total	23	150	23	4	200	50 (36, 64)	97 (94, 99)	87 (81, 91)
After								
Appendicular skeleton	15	74	9	3	101	63 (43, 79)	96 (90, 99)	88 (80, 93)
Remaining body areas	5	77	10	7	99	33 (15, 58)	92 (84, 96)	83 (74, 89)
Total	20	151	19	10	200	51 (36, 66)	94 (89, 97)	86 (80, 90)

TP, true positive; TN, true negative; FN, false negative; FP, false positive; CI, confidence interval.

for both professions. The cost of auditing radiographer reporting was excluded because there was already protected time to perform audits. The cost of radiographers on the rare occasion (once every 2 weeks) seeking advice from radiologists was excluded as radiologists also sometimes seek the opinion of their colleagues.

The costs were inflated to the base year 2001/2 using appropriate indices [27] and the capital costs were annuitized to produce the annual equivalent cost (AEC) [28]. When calculating the cost of radiographer and radiologist reporting it was important to estimate the time spent reporting and typing reports. The two radiographers and radiologists at the hospital were therefore asked to report again the A&E radiographs of the appendicular skeleton that the reference standard reported and record the time it took using a stopwatch. The time a radiologist spent dictating their report to tape was assumed to be the time a medical secretary spent entering the report into the computer. The radiographers also recorded the time it took to record and enter their report into the computer. To value the time spent reporting it was essential to weight for differences in the clinical productivity of the two professional groups. Radiologists and radiographers, respectively, spend 34 h and 26 h a week on clinical activity so 1 clinical minute for a radiologist is equivalent in value to 1.3 clinical minutes for a radiographer. This variation in clinical activity occurred because radiologists allocated around 15% of their time to administrative duties and clinical audit. In contrast the radiographers spend around 50% of their time on reporting, 25% on clinical activities such as general radiography and fluoroscopy, and 25% on administrative duties such as quality assurance, radiation protection, staff recruitment and organizing rotas.

A considerable number of assumptions can be made about the costs that should be included in radiographer and radiologist reporting so a series of scenarios were constructed that recognized the uncertainty of these assumptions.

Analyses

Radiograph reporting performance was presented using sensitivity, specificity, and accuracy with 95% confidence intervals (CI) around a single proportion and for the difference in proportions between two independent groups (*i.e.* before and after samples). The hypothesis tests used were the Chi-squared test or Fisher's Exact test when the total number of observations were less than 20 or any of the expected frequencies were less than 5. To analyse the effect of incorrect reports on A&E patient management the 95% CI when testing for a difference in proportions between two independent samples were calculated.

The cost analyses required the time it took in clinical minutes for radiographers and radiologists to report to be multiplied by their hourly rate. This cost was then multiplied by the number of A&E radiographs of the appendicular skeleton performed during 2001/2 (n=9713). The sum of the capital, training and overhead costs was then added to produce the annual cost of reporting. The average cost of reporting was the annual cost divided by the number of A&E radiographs of the appendicular skeleton performed during 2000/1. The incremental cost was the difference in cost between radiographer and radiologist reporting. Sensitivity analysis tested the impact of changes in assumptions about the inclusion of certain costs.

Results

Effect on accuracy

As shown in Table 1, both before and after the introduction of radiographer reporting, specificity was high in the 90s, but sensitivity only around the 50s. This indicated that normal A&E radiographs were correctly identified but nearly half of A&E radiographs judged to be abnormal by the reference standard were reported as normal. There was also more variation in sensitivity than specificity before and after the intervention. Table 2 shows that following the introduction of radiographer reporting there was a clinically insignificant difference of 1% in A&E radiograph reporting accuracy with 95% CI from −7.9% to 5.9%. For the non-equivalent, non-intervention control group there were no statistically significant differences

Table 2. Difference in A&E radiograph reporting accuracy

Statistic	Body area	% (95% CI)	p-value
Sensitivity	Appendicular skeleton	8 (−20.2, 35.1)	0.58
	Remaining body areas	−13 (−40.8, 19.5)	0.44
	Total	1 (−19.8, 22.2)	0.91
Specificity	Appendicular skeleton	−3 (−9.7, 3.5)	0.37
	Remaining body areas	−4 (−12.9, 3.7)	0.33
	Total	−3 (−8.8, 1.1)	0.17
Accuracy	Appendicular skeleton	−1 (−10.1, 8.3)	0.84
	Remaining body areas	−1 (−11.8, 9.4)	0.82
	Total	−1 (−7.9, 5.9)	0.77

before and after the intervention in GP radiograph reporting sensitivity, specificity, and accuracy for the different body areas and in total. The difference in GP radiograph reporting accuracy overall was 0% (95% CI −8.9 to 7.9). This is evidence that there were no other historical events that might have affected the accuracy with which radiographs were reported in the X-ray Department and underpins the validity of the results about the effects of this intervention on the reporting accuracy of A&E radiographs.

Effect on management

There were 56 A&E reports (27 before and 29 after the intervention) judged to be incorrect. The clinical details for two patients before and five patients after the intervention were not available so were excluded from the analyses. Table 3 shows when A&E radiographs of the appendicular skeleton were judged to be incorrect, the percentage of cases falling within the three management options was identical both before and after the intervention. In particular, there were only two incorrect reports before and after the intervention that might have a clinically important effect on patient management (95% CI −34.8 to 34.8). Table 3 also shows for incorrect reports of the remaining body areas and in total there was a 21% (95% CI −49.5 to 10.6) and 11% (95% CI −33.7 to 11.3) reduction in cases that might have a clinically important effect on patient management.

Effect on outcome

Table 4 presents the outcomes for the 56 A&E patients whose reports were discordant with the reference standard. For patients who re-attended the X-ray Department for a related examination a discrepancy was found between the first and subsequent reports for 15% (4/27) and 14% (4/29) of cases before and after the intervention. For these eight cases the consensus panel reviewed all examinations to establish the reason for re-attendance. Before the intervention there were three cases when the radiographs were not available to investigate this further, and one case when the first report missed a "subcapital fracture" diagnosed at the second visit. After the intervention there were three cases when the panel decided the first report did agree with the subsequent reports, but one case when the first report missed a "bilateral mandibular fracture" diagnosed at the subsequent visit. For both cases radiologists missed the abnormality.

Table 3. Difference in A&E patient management for incorrect reports

Body area	Management	% (95% CI)
Appendicular skeleton	No difference in management	0 (−34.8, 34.8)
	Clinically unimportant	0 (−26.8, 26.8)
	Clinically important	0 (−34.8, 34.8)
Remaining body areas	No difference in management	21 (−10.6, 49.5)
	Clinically unimportant	0 (−22.2, 23.5)
	Clinically important	−21 (−49.5, 10.6)
Total	No difference in management	12 (−11.3, 33.7)
	Clinically unimportant	0 (−13.6, 14.0)
	Clinically important	−11 (−33.7, 11.3)

Table 4. Difference in A&E patient outcome for incorrect reports

Outcome	Before (n=27) n (%)	After (n=29) n (%)
Patient did not re-attend	14 (52)	11 (38)
Re-attended for unrelated X-ray examination	8 (30)	13 (45)
Re-attended for related X-ray examination and subsequent report concordant with the original	1 (4)	1 (4)
Re-attended for related X-ray examination and subsequent report discordant with the original	4 (15)	4 (14)

Effect on costs

Table 5 presents the base, worst and best case scenarios used in the cost analyses and Table 6 presents the costs

Table 5. Scenarios used to assess cost of reporting

Scenario
Worst
• All capital costs were attributed to radiographer reporting
• Training was annuitized over 10 years
• For capital and training costs used 7% interest rate for annual equivalent cost
• All overhead costs of reporting room were attributed to radiographer reporting
• No overhead costs were attributed to radiologist reporting
• Radiographer clinical minute was 1.4
Best
• Capital costs: 50% attributed to radiographer reporting; 25% attributed to radiologist reporting; (25% attributed to general use)
• Training was annuitized over 20 years
• For capital and training costs used 5% interest rate for annual equivalent cost
• Overhead costs of radiographer reporting room: 50% attributed to radiographer reporting; 25% attributed to radiologist reporting; (25% attributed to general use)
• Overhead costs of radiologist and secretary office: 10% attributed to radiologist reporting
• No secretarial costs (they type both radiographer and radiologist reports)
• Radiographer clinical minute was equivalent to the radiologist
• Radiographer reporting time was equivalent to radiologist
Base
• Capital costs: 50% attributed to radiographer reporting
• Training was annuitized over 15 years
• For capital and training costs used 6% interest rate for annual equivalent cost
• Overhead costs of radiographer reporting room: 50% attributed to radiographer reporting
• 5% of overhead costs of radiologist and secretary floor space were attributed to radiologist reporting
• Typing reports by secretaries was an additional cost to radiologist reporting
• Radiographer clinical minute was 1.3

Table 6. Costs of plain radiograph reporting

Cost	Year	Item	Cost (£)	2001/2 (£)
Capital	1994/5	Computer terminal and bar code reader	405.38	488.47
	1994/5	Thermal Printer	988.18	1190.72
	1994/5	Worktops	750.00	903.72
	1994/5	Installation of PC and Printer	176.25	212.37
	1994/5	Installation of viewing boxes	495.00	596.46
	1994/5	Partition	965.00	1162.79
	Total		3779.81	4554.53
Training	1993/4	MSc Course – Registration	6000.00	7323.76
	1993/4	MSc Course – Travel expenses	426.42	520.50
	1994/5	MSc Course – Travel expenses	63.40	76.39
	1995/6	MSc Course – Travel expenses	14.95	17.51
	Total		6504.77	7938.16
Staff	1995/6	Basic radiographer (42 weeks pa, 35 hours pw)[a]	12376.00	16367.43
	1995/6	CSR (42 weeks pa, 35 hours pw)[b]	21002.80	27776.49
	1995/6	Radiologist – MC21 (42 weeks pa, 38 hours pw)[c]	40620.00	53720.51
	1995/6	Secretary – C3 (42 weeks pa, 35 hours pw)[d]	12788.00	16912.31
Overheads	2001/2	CSR reporting room (10.28 m^2)		3240.85
		Radiologist offices (88.64 m^2)		27944.46
		Radiologist hot reporting room (22.3 m^2)		7030.25
		Secretary office (32 m^2)		10088.25

[a]£11.13 h^{-1}.
[b]£18.90 h^{-1}.
[c]£33.66 h^{-1}.
[d]£11.50 h^{-1}.

associated with radiographer and radiologist reporting inflated to the common year 2001/2. Table 7 shows the time it took the radiographers to interpret and record a report was 47 s. This was similar to the 43 s it took consultant radiologists to dictate a report to tape. In addition the radiographers took 19 s to enter a report into the computer system, which the secretaries did for the radiologists. Table 8 presents the cost of radiographer or radiologist reporting A&E radiographs of the appendicular skeleton. Radiographer reporting for the worst case scenario could cost the X-ray department £4524 per annum, but this reflects the cost of radiographer reporting when several assumptions are made in favour of radiologist reporting. The best case scenario shows that when the assumptions are made in favour of radiographer reporting this should save the X-ray department £4528 per annum. For the base case analysis, which reflects the most realistic set of assumptions, radiographer reporting should save the X-ray department £361 per annum. Furthermore if the secretaries were to type radiographer reports, the average cost per radiograph reported would fall from £0.73 to £0.66.

Table 7. Time in seconds to report A&E radiographs of the appendicular skeleton

Body Area	Radiologist[a]	Radiographer[b]	Radiographer[c]
Upper Limb	42.6	48.0	20.8
Lower Limb	42.4	46.2	16.8
Appendicular skeleton	42.5	47.1	18.8

[a]Consultant radiologist time to dictate a report to tape.
[b]Radiographer time to interpret and record a report.
[c]Radiographer time to enter a report into the computer system.

Discussion

Introducing radiographer reporting did not have an adverse effect on A&E radiograph reporting accuracy, patient management, or outcome. The non-equivalent, non-intervention control group demonstrated no change in GP radiograph reporting accuracy. This is evidence that no other events occurred in the X-ray Department during the period of data collection that affected the accuracy with which A&E radiographs were reported. The A&E radiographs were reported less accurately than in previous studies [12, 13]; sensitivities were only in the 50s. This occurred because our study included an assessment of the effect of incorrect reports on A&E patient management so it was the A&E specialist registrar who judged the clinical importance of missed abnormalities. Therefore even when a very minor abnormality was missed the radiologist

Table 8. Cost of reporting A&E radiographs of the appendicular skeleton

Scenario	Reporting Policy	Annual Cost £	Average Cost £/radiograph reported
Worst	Radiographer	9948.91	1.02
	Radiologist	5425.02	0.54
	Increment	−4523.89	−0.48
Best	Radiographer	4886.78	0.50
	Radiologist	9414.91	0.97
	Increment	4528.13	0.47
Base	Radiographer	7137.03	0.73[a]
	Radiologist	7498.17	0.77
	Increment	−361.14	−0.04

[a]£0.66 if a secretary types radiographer reports.

arbiter classified the report as false-negative, which lowered sensitivities and accuracy.

A previous study found that the costs of introducing radiographer reporting in four NHS trusts ranged from nil to £15 000 per annum with radiographers spending around 0.5 whole time equivalent reporting [22]. The authors acknowledged that the data were limited to staff costs and were unreliable. Our analyses showed that introducing radiographer reporting saved the X-ray Department £361 per annum and further cost savings could be made as radiographers acquire the same experience as the radiologists and if secretaries type radiographers' reports. We included capital costs in the cost of radiographer reporting because it was not practical for the radiographers to use the equipment and facilities available to the radiologists so modification of an existing room and provision of additional equipment was necessary. Furthermore we included the cost of radiographer training but not radiologist training as this too was an additional cost fundamental to introducing radiographer reporting at our hospital. The cost of radiographer reporting may vary though between hospitals depending on how this change in service delivery is implemented. Excluding the capital costs (£416 per annum) and training costs (£684 per annum) from our analyses would result in a base case saving to the X-ray Department of £1461 per annum.

There were also the resource management implications and opportunity cost of radiographer and radiologist reporting. This concerns the activities that radiographers and radiologists relinquish to report A&E radiographs. To explore whether it was reasonable to assume that radiographer reporting freed radiologists to make better use of their time and expertise we conducted a retrospective assessment of different healthcare professional attitudes towards radiographer reporting [29]. The qualitative findings revealed that radiographer reporting A&E radiographs of the appendicular skeleton reduced their involvement in general radiography and they no longer worked in A&E or speciality areas such as CT or angiography. The radiographers also commented that reporting radiographs takes up "25% to 50%" of their time. In contrast the radiologists thought that radiographer reporting frees only a little of their time, possibly "about ¾ hours per week". Because this activity was shared between eight consultant radiologists, as opposed to two radiographers, this might explain why only a little of the radiologists' time appears to have been freed. These findings suggest that whereas the reporting of radiographs had a dramatic impact on activities performed by the radiographers, there was a negligible change to the radiologists' work. Not prospectively collecting data meant it was difficult to accurately establish the affect of introducing radiographer reporting on changes in staff workload and the time allocated to different activities in the X-ray department.

Another limitation of this study was the validity of a single consultant radiologist as the reference standard [30], although there was consensus in opinion among the radiologists in the X-ray Department that this radiologist was an acceptable local standard. The reference standard report was also judged to be correct for seven of the eight cases reviewed by the panel of radiologists when establishing the reason for patient re-attendance. For the other case, whereas the reference standard reported a "small bony flake adjacent to the lateral epicondyle" for a radiograph of the elbow, the consensus panel judged it to be a "fleck of calcium". This slight difference in interpretation was not clinically important, and both reports agreed there was "no convincing radial head fracture". There was also the sample size to consider. As an example, following the introduction of the intervention A&E radiograph reporting accuracy fell by 1%, which we can assume to be clinically unimportant. The wide confidence interval shows that 95% of the time the true difference ranges from −7.9% to 5.9% accuracy; a fall of 8% in accuracy might be judged clinically important. The width of the confidence interval affects our certainty about the true difference in A&E radiograph reporting accuracy before and after the intervention and whether this was clinically important.

Other limitations include the completeness and accuracy of information extracted from case notes when assessing the effect of incorrect reports on A&E patient management. Indeed, there were notes missing for two A&E patients before and five A&E patients after the intervention, although it is unlikely this affected the results. The method of assessing patient outcome was also restricted with the loss of three radiographs before the intervention preventing the consensus review. Patient re-attendance as an adverse event and proxy for patient outcome also ignores the effects of false positive reports and the morbidity of patients who suffer but do not re-attend. Furthermore patients who attended A&E may not have been local people so might have re-presented at a different hospital resulting in an underestimation of patient re-attendance as an adverse event. Because we selected a random stratified sample of A&E reports any under-estimation in re-attendance should be comparable before and after the intervention so should not affect our conclusions. The study is also only applicable to selectively trained radiographers reporting in a district hospital.

Nevertheless, this study is a valuable contribution to the evidence base as unlike previous studies it addresses accuracy, patient management and outcome, and costs [24]. It is also more pragmatic and rigorous in design, including independent reporting of radiographs by the reference standard for all radiographs and independent comparison of reports. The time period for data collection, the selection of a random stratified sample of reports, and the control group all help to eliminate threats to validity. All costs of radiographer and radiologist reporting to the X-ray department were comprehensively identified, measured and valued, and sensitivity analysis conducted acknowledging uncertainty in key assumptions. In conclusion this study provides further evidence that selectively trained radiographers can accurately report A&E plain radiographs and also at no additional cost.

Acknowledgments

The authors are very grateful to the staff in the X-ray Department for their assistance in the conduct of this study only with their support was this study feasible.

References

1. Department of Health. National Health Service and Community Care Act. London: Stationary Office, 1990.

2. Secretaries of State for Health, Wales, Northern Ireland and Scotland. Working for patients. London: Stationary Office, 1989.
3. Department of Health. The NHS Plan: A plan for investment. A plan for reform. London: Stationary Office, 2000.
4. Department of Health. Meeting the challenge. A strategy for the allied health professions. London: Stationary Office, 2000.
5. The Royal College of Radiologists. Staffing and standards in departments of clinical oncology and clinical radiology. London: Royal College of Radiologists, 1993.
6. Brindle M. Debate intensifies over non-radiologists' roles. Diagnostic Imaging Europe 1996;43–7.
7. The Royal College of Radiologists. Clinical radiology: A workforce in crisis. London: The Royal College of Radiologists, 2002.
8. The Royal College of Radiologists. Medico legal aspects of delegation. London: The Royal College of Radiologists, 1993.
9. The College of Radiographers. X-ray examination requests by nurse practitioners and radiographic reporting by radiographers. London: College of Radiographers, 1995.
10. Hughes H, Hughes K, Hamill R. A study to evaluate the introduction of a pattern recognition technique for chest radiographs by radiographers. Radiography 1996;2:263–88.
11. Craven C, Barber J. Role extension: Where are we now? Radiography Today 1995;61:12–3.
12. Robinson PJA. Plain film reporting by radiographers — a feasibility study. Br J Radiol 1996;69:1171–4.
13. Loughran CF. Reporting of fracture radiographs by radiographers: the impact of a training programme. Br J Radiol 1994;67:945–50.
14. Brealey S, King DG, Crowe MTI, Crawshaw I, Ford L, Warnock N, et al. Accident and Emergency and General Practitioner plain radiograph reporting by radiographers and radiologists: a quasi-randomized controlled trial. Br J Radiol 2003;76:57–61.
15. Paterson AM. Role development - towards 2000: a survey of role developments in radiography. London: College of Radiographers, 1995.
16. Price RC, Le Masurier SB, High L, Miller LR. Changing times: a national survey of extended roles in diagnostic radiography. Br J Radiol 1999;72:7.
17. De Lacey G, Barker A, Harper J, Wignall B. An assessment of the clinical effects of reporting accident and emergency radiographs. Br J Radiol 1980;53:304–9.
18. Snow DA. Clinical significance of discrepancies in roentgenographic film interpretation in an acute walk-in-area. J Gen Intern Med 1986;1:295–9.
19. Thomas HG, Mason AC, Smith RM, Fergusson CM. Value of radiograph audit in an accident service department. Injury 1992;23:47–50.
20. Robinson PJA, Culpan G, Wiggins M. Interpretation of selected accident and emergency radiographer examinations by radiographers: a review of 11 000 cases. Br J Radiol 1999;72:1–6.
21. The College of Radiographers. Reporting by radiographers: A vision paper. London: College of Radiographers, 1997.
22. Piper K, Paterson AM, Ryan C. The implementation of a radiographic reporting service for trauma examinations of the skeletal system, in Four National Health Service Trusts. Research & Development Directorate, South Thames Regional Office (NHSE) 1999.
23. Audit Commission. Improving your image: how to manage radiology services more effectively. London: Stationary Office, 1995.
24. Brealey S. Measuring the effects of image interpretation: an evaluative framework. Clin Radiol 2001;56:341–7.
25. Brealey S, Scally AJ. Bias in plain film reading performance studies. Br J Radiol 2001;74:307–16.
26. Robinson PJA. The nature of image reporting. In: Paterson A, Price R, editors. Current topics in radiography 2. London: W B Saunders, 1996:70–82.
27. Netten A, Curtis L. Unit costs of health and social care 2002. Kent: Personal Social Services Research Unit, 2002:187.
28. Drummond MF, Stoddart GL, Torrance GW. Methods for the economic evaluation of health care programmes. Oxford: Oxford Medical Publications, 1997.
29. Brealey S, King D, Warnock N. An assessment of different health care professionals' attitudes towards radiographers' reporting A&E films. Radiography 2002;8:27–34.
30. Brealey S, Scally AJ, Thomas NB. Methodological standards in radiographer plain film reading performance studies. Br J Radiol 2002;75:107–13.

The British Journal of Radiology, *78* (2005), 506–511
DOI: 10.1259/bjr/22314006

Acute ureteric calculus obstruction: unenhanced spiral CT versus HASTE MR urography and abdominal radiograph

[1]F REGAN, MD, FRCR, [1]B KUSZYK, MD, [1]M E BOHLMAN, MD and [2]S JACKMAN, MD

Departments of [1]Imaging and [2]Urology, Johns Hopkins Bayview Medical Center, 4940 Eastern Avenue, Baltimore, Maryland 21224, USA

Abstract. The aim of this study is to compare the performance of unenhanced spiral CT to the combination of HASTE MR urography (MRU) and plain abdominal radiography (KUB) in patients suspected of having acute calculus ureteric obstruction. 64 patients with suspected acute calculus ureteric obstruction were evaluated. The presence of perirenal fluid, presence and level of ureteric obstruction and calculi were assessed on both techniques. 44 of 64 (69%) patients had acute calculus ureteric obstruction based on clinical, radiographic or surgical findings. MRU showed perirenal fluid in acute ureteric obstruction (77%) with a greater sensitivity than CT showed stranding (45%). The combination of fluid and ureteric dilation on MRU showed a sensitivity of 93% (CT 80%), specificity of 95% (CT 85%), and accuracy of 94% (CT 81%). There were 61 findings of either fluid or ureteric dilatation on MRU in 44 acutely obstructed kidneys compared with 37 similar findings on CT ($p<0.005$). Although there was excellent reproducibility (Kappa$\geqslant$0.75) in the finding of perirenal fluid on MRU, there was only fair interobserver agreement (Kappa<0.4) regarding perirenal stranding on CT. MRU/KUB showed ureteric calculi in 21/29 (72%) of patients with calculi seen by CT. Overall, MRU/KUB revealed 2.4 abnormalities per acutely obstructed ureter compared with 1.8 abnormalities detected by CT. MRU/KUB using HASTE sequences can diagnose the presence of acute calculus ureteric obstruction with similar accuracy to spiral CT. The technique has less observer variability and is more accurate than CT in detecting evidence of obstruction such as perirenal fluid.

The clinical features of acute ureteric colic typically include severe flank pain radiating to the groin, microhaematuria and calculus retrieval from urine [1]. Although the disease is usually self limiting with the spontaneous passage of a stone, persisting pain or high grade obstruction may require hospitalization and urological intervention. As calcium stone disease has a propensity to recur with significant associated morbidity, reliable and non-invasive imaging techniques both for initial diagnosis and in follow up of the disease are required.

Intravenous urography (IVU) has traditionally been the imaging modality of choice in evaluating patients with acute ureteric calculus disease. Unenhanced spiral CT (CT) is accurate in demonstrating kidney and ureteric calculi and signs of acute obstruction such as perirenal stranding, and hydronephrosis [2–4].

Alternatively, MR urography (MRU) has been slow to gain wide acceptance in evaluating patients with ureteric obstruction. This may be explained by the limited access to fast MRI techniques, and poor detection of kidney and ureteric calculi when compared with CT. MRU using HASTE (Half-Fourier single shot turbo spin-echo) sequences can however, demonstrate both the presence and level of ureteric obstruction [5, 6], and the technique provides good urographic type images without risk of radiation or contrast media.

Received 9 February 2004 and in final form 19 November 2004, accepted 17 January 2005.

Address correspondence to Dr F Regan, Department of Radiology, Adelaide & Meath Hospital, Dublin 24, Ireland.

The goal of this study is to compare spiral CT and MRU and to determine if HASTE MRU when combined with plain radiograph of the abdomen (KUB) can be diagnostic in patients with acute ureteric colic. A secondary objective of the study was to compare interobserver variability and ease of interpretation of CT compared with MRU.

Patients and methods

A prospective evaluation of 96 patients presenting to the Emergency Department with suspected acute calculus ureteric obstruction over a 1 year period was performed. All patients had clinical evidence of acute calculus obstruction with flank pain, haematuria and/or history of stone passage.

This was a non-consecutive group of patients as MRI was performed only during weekday hours. Additionally only those patients imaged with both CT and MRU within 6 h of each other were included. Six claustrophobic patients refused imaging with MR and MRI was not available in a further six patients because of routine scanner maintenance. Five patients left the Emergency department before MRI could be performed and a further three patients who had received intravenous contrast agents were excluded from the study.

64 patients were included in the final study group and all these patients were imaged with both CT and MRU. Depending on availability at the time of referral, 42 (66%) patients underwent CT first and the remaining 22 patients underwent MRI prior to CT. KUBs were available in 45/64 (70%) patients. Informed consent was obtained in all patients.

Imaging technique

Unenhanced spiral CT (Siemens, Iselin, NJ) was carried out through both kidneys to the bladder base in three breath-hold clusters with the following imaging parameters: 130 kV, 83 mA, gantry rotation time 1.9 s. A slice thickness of 3 mm with 3 mm reconstruction was used. Depending on the size of the patient up to 120 images were generated per study.

Patients underwent HASTE MRI using a 1.5 Tesla Magnetom Vision scanner (Siemens, Iselin, NJ) in the axial, sagittal and coronal imaging planes to cover both kidneys to the bladder base. The following parameters were used: repetition time (TR) 11.9, echo time (TE) 95.0, acquisition time of 23 s for 19 slices. A slice thickness of either 4 mm (coronal and sagittal imaging) or 7 mm (axial imaging to cover the full abdomen) was applied with a variable field of view. 57 images (19×3 planes) were generated in each patient. MRU was performed using a single shot technique (TR of 2000, TE 80, single excitation and a slice thickness of 10 mm). This yielded a further 11 images per patient with a total of 68 images. A frequency selective fat suppression algorithm was used to reduce intra-abdominal fat high signal and no contrast medium was administered.

Image analysis

Images from both CT and MRU were read independently by three radiologists – a senior radiology resident (observer 1) and two attending radiologists experienced in abdominal imaging (observers 2 and 3). The readers were unaware of the final clinical outcome, results of other imaging modalities and of each other's findings. CTs and MRUs were presented in a random order to the radiologists for interpretation and read in three sessions. The KUB was read in conjunction with the patient's MRU.

The following findings were assessed on both imaging techniques: presence or absence of perirenal and periureteric stranding (CT) or fluid (MR), ureteric dilatation, and level of obstruction. A level of obstruction was determined to be either proximal, middle or distal ureter. A ureteric calculus was diagnosed as a high attenuation focus on CT or as an intraluminal signal void on MR. Calculi were documented as either kidney, proximal, middle or distal ureter in location, and their maximum diameter measured in millimetres.

The ease of interpretation was graded subjectively by each observer between 1 and 5, the most difficult interpretation being assigned a grade 1 and the easiest, grade 5. A consensus opinion was reached where there was disagreement between observers in evaluating stranding/fluid, ureteric dilation and level of obstruction.

Statistical analysis

Data from the consensus opinion of the observers was used to calculate sensitivity, specificity, positive and negative predictive values and accuracy of both techniques for detection of acute calculus obstruction. Exact confidence intervals were calculated for these results. The number of findings per acutely obstructed kidney noted by each observer and by consensus was calculated for CT and MRU/KUB techniques, and a p-value of <0.001 was considered to be significant.

Agreement between CT and MRU was measured by Kappa statistics for all three observers and for the consensus opinion. A Kappa value of $\geqslant 0.75$ denotes excellent agreement, Kappa of between 0.4 and 0.75 good agreement, and less than 0.4 marginal agreement [7]. Interobserver variability regarding findings of fluid, ureteric dilation and level of obstruction and whether the right or left kidney was affected were assessed with Kappa statistics for all possible observer combinations (observers 1 and 2, 2 and 3, and 1 and 3). The size of calculi seen on CT and KUB was compared using a two sample t-test.

A McNemar's exact test compared each finding by each observer with the presence of acute ureteric obstruction. The ability of CT and MRU/KUB in predicting disease using the combined findings of fluid, ureteric dilation and calculi was compared using the McNemar's chi-squared test. Finally, the Wilcoxon Signed rank test was applied to measure the differences in ease of interpretation of CT and MRU/KUB for all three observers.

Results

Of the 64 patients imaged with both CT and MRU, 20 (31%) showed no evidence of obstruction on any imaging modality and had a final diagnosis as follows: urinary tract infection (3), appendicitis (1), perirenal abscess (1), musculoskeletal pain (2), liver haemangioma (1), prostate carcinoma (1), prostate enlargement with urinary tract infection (1), Crohn's disease with abscess formation (1), myeloma of kidneys (1), degenerative hip or lumbar spine disease (3). No definite diagnosis was made in a further five patients. 44 of 64 (69%) patients had a final diagnosis of acute calculus obstruction. In addition to the findings on CT and KUB, there was additional confirmation of calculus disease as follows: imaging studies in 35 patients, including intravenous pyelography (14), retrograde pyelography (12), and documented movement of a calculus on sequential KUBs (8); surgery was performed in 11 patients, including urethroscopy and stone retrieval, and a further 10 patients reported passing calculi.

All CT and MR studies were considered technically adequate. No significant breathing or misregistration artefacts were noted. The sensitivity, specificity, and overall accuracy of fluid and ureteric dilatation to predict disease were 80%, 85%, and 81%, respectively, for CT (Table 1 and Figure 1), compared with 93%, 95%, and 94% for MRU. There were 61 findings of either fluid or ureteric dilatation on MRU in 44 acutely obstructed kidneys. This compared with 37 abnormalities per obstructed kidney on CT if the same parameters of fluid and dilatation were used ($p<0.005$). If fluid, dilatation and stone detection were assessed, the MRU/KUB combination showed 66 abnormalities in 27 acutely obstructed kidneys where all imaging modalities were available for evaluation, compared with 76 in 43 abnormalities per obstructed kidney on CT ($p<0.005$).

Using consensus data, there was complete correlation between CT and MRU in 48 of 64 (75%) patients. MR demonstrated perirenal or periureteric fluid in 14 patients not seen on CT scanning (Figure 2). There was only one patient where CT demonstrated stranding not shown by

Table 1. Analysis of the consensus opinion of three radiologists in evaluating acute ureteric calculus obstruction with CT and MRU. Data are number of patients and percentages. 95% confidence intervals are in parentheses

	Sensitivity[a]	Specificity[b]	PPV	NPV	Accuracy
MRU: Fluid	34/44=77 (62, 88)	20/20=100 (0.86, 1)	34/34=100 (0.92, 1)	20/30=66.7 (0.47, 0.83)	54/64=84.4 (0.73, 0.92)
CT: Stranding	20/44=45 (0.30, 0.61)	20/20=100 (0.86, 1)	20/20=100 (0.86, 1)	20/44=45 (0.277, 0.56)	40/64=63 (0.5, 0.74)
MRU: Dilation	39/44=89 (0.75, 0.96)	19/20=95 (0.75, 0.99)	39/40=98 (0.87 0.99)	19/24=79 (0.58, 0.93)	58/64=91 (0.81, 0.96)
CT: Dilation	31/44=70 (0.55, 0.83)	17/20=85 (0.62, 0.97)	31/34=91 (0.76, 0.98)	17/30=57 (0.37, 0.74)	48/64=75 (0.63, 0.85)
MRU: Fluid or Dilation	41/44=93 (0.81, 0.99)	19/20=95 (0.75, 0.1)	41/42=98 (0.87, 0.1)	19/22=86 (0.65, 0.97)	60/64=94 (0.85, 0.98)
CT: Stranding or Dilation	35/44=80 (0.65, 0.91)	17/20=85 (0.62, 0.96)	35/38=59 (0.78, 0.98)	17/26=65 (0.44, 0.82)	52/64=81 (0.69, 0.89)
MRU: Fluid or Dilation or Calculi[c]	29/31=94 (0.79, 0.99)	5/8=63 (0.25, 0.92)	29/32=91 (0.75, 0.98)	5/7=71 (0.29, 0.96)	34/39=87 (0.73, 0.96)
CT: Stranding or Dilation or Calculi	41/44=93 (0.81, 0.98)	10/14=71 (0.41, 0.91)	30/34=88 (0.73, 0.97)	10/13=77 (0.46, 0.95)	40/47=85 (0.72, 0.94)

[a]True positive cases/true positive and false negative cases. [b]True negative cases/true negative and false positive cases. [c]Although plain abdominal radiographs (KUBs) were available in 45 of the 64 patients, only 39 KUBs taken at the time of MRU were included.

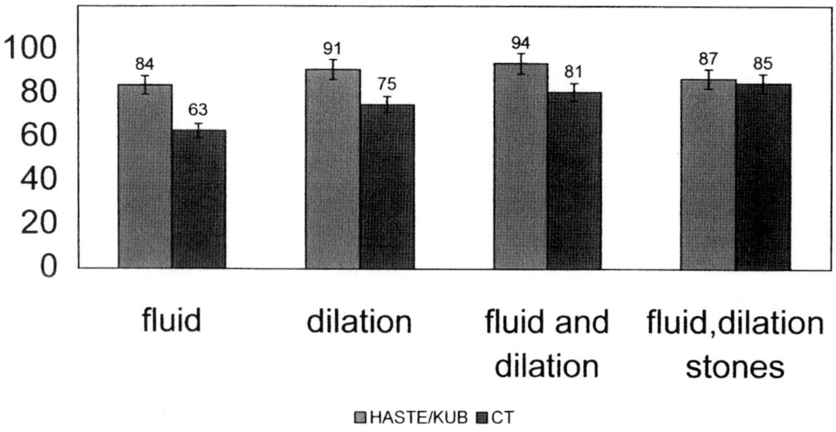

Figure 1. Accuracy of half-Fourier single shot turbo spin-echo (HASTE) MR urography/plain abdominal radiograph (MRU/KUB) compared with spiral CT in acute calculus ureteric obstruction.

MRU. The observers missed perirenal stranding on CT in four patients who had minimal intra-abdominal fat including two patients with HIV. In five further patients with acute ureteric obstruction, proximal ureteric stranding was missed by observers 2 and 3.

In one patient with bilateral pelvic kidneys, bilateral hydronephrosis was incorrectly diagnosed on CT. The correct diagnosis of multiple parapelvic cysts, without obstruction was diagnosed by MRU. In another patient, with the benefit of coronal imaging, MR identified a distal left ureterocoele, not identified on CT. There was overall good agreement between CT and MRU regarding ureteric dilation (k=0.6), level of obstruction (k=0.49) and which kidney was the affected one (k=0.69) (Table 2).

Interobserver variability

Case statistics demonstrated good overall concordance between the individual observers regarding the presence or absence of acute disease on MRU and CT (Table 3). There was strong agreement between all observers as to which kidney was acutely obstructed although interobserver agreement was generally greater for MRU than for CT. There was also good agreement between all observers in assessing the presence or absence of perirenal fluid on MRU but significant deviations ($p<0.001$) occurred between all observers in assessing perirenal stranding on CT (Table 4). Similarly there was stronger, but not statistically significant, agreement between all three interobserver combinations in the depiction of the level of obstruction on MRU.

In the obstructed kidneys, a level of obstruction was suggested by the presence of dilatation or calculi on CT in 32 patients as follows: proximal ureter 9, mid ureter 2 and distal ureter 21. Similarly, MRU/KUB demonstrated a level of obstruction in 40 patients: proximal ureter 5, mid ureter 7 and distal ureter 28.

The location and size of ureteric calculi detected by CT and KUB/MRU are shown in Table 4. CT detected 29 ureteric calculi ranging in size from 1 mm to 12 mm in length (mean 3.7 mm). Using CT as the gold standard KUB/MRU detected 21/29 (72%) ureteric calculi (size 2–14 mm) in patients with evidence of obstruction. MRU alone demonstrated calculi in only three patients, all of whom had calculi greater than 10 mm diameter in dilated systems and there was a significant difference (p=0.0001) in the mean size of calculi detected by CT (3.7 mm) and MRU/ KUB (5.1 mm).

There was no significant difference between CT and MRU in the probability of predicting acute calculus ureteric obstruction (McNemar's chi-squared=0, degrees of freedom (df)=1, p-value=1) when the combination of all three parameters (fluid, dilatation and calculi) was used

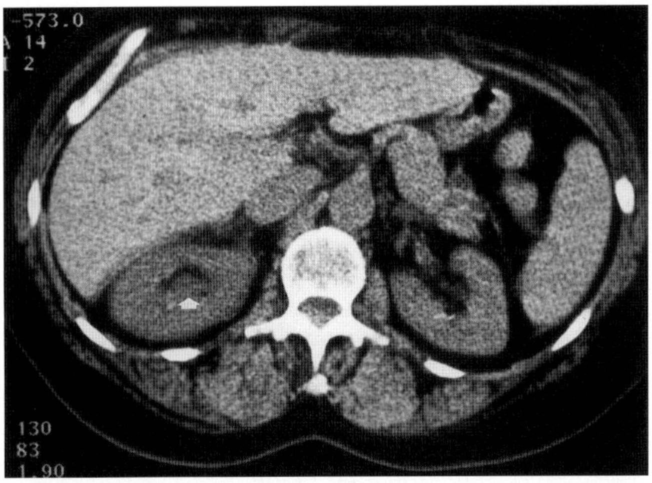

(a)

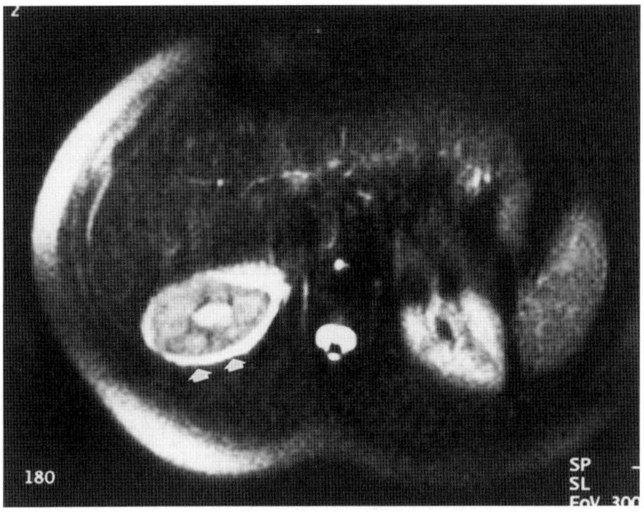

(b)

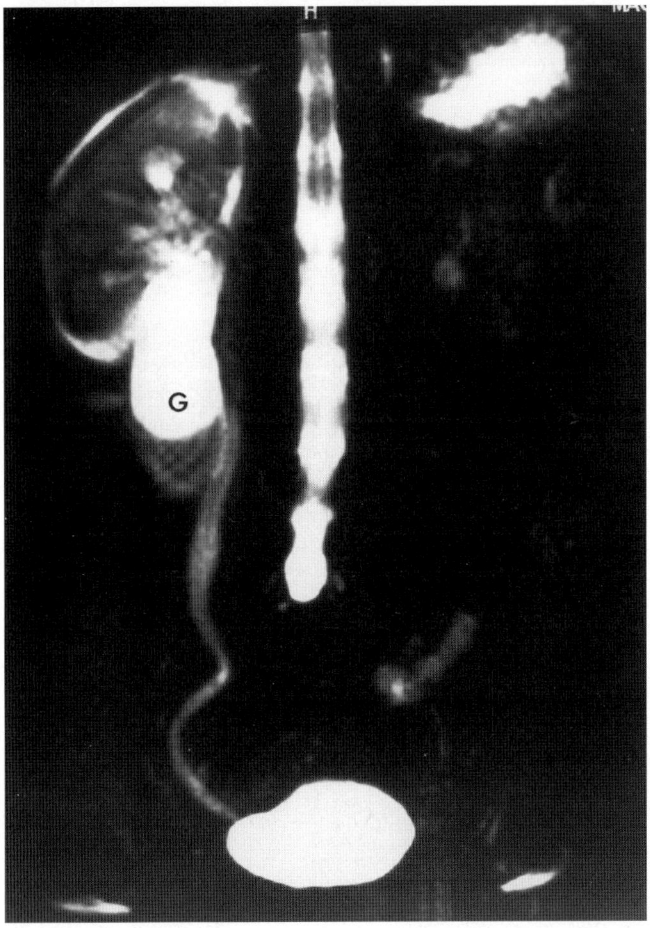

(c)

Figure 2. A 56-year-old female presented with acute right-sided flank pain caused by a right vesicoureteric junction calculus. (a) Axial CT shows evidence of hydronephrosis with but no evidence of significant stranding. (b) Axial MR, shows significant perirenal fluid (arrows). (c) MR urogram shows a dilated ureter to the level of the bladder. Gallbladder (G).

and the combination of fluid and ureteric dilatation on both techniques was significantly more predictive of disease ($p<0.001$) than the individual finding of either dilatation or fluid.

Finally, the difficulty in interpreting CTs was assigned by the three radiologists an average grade of 4, 3.5, and 3.3, respectively, and 4.4, 4.4 and 4.2, respectively, for MRU. All three interpreters found the median score significantly larger (*i.e.* easier to interpret), for MRU than CT ($p=0.001$, $p=0.000$, $p=0.000$, respectively), although the least experienced radiologist (observer 1) showed less difference in difficulty between the two imaging modalities.

Discussion

In this prospective study we found that MRU when interpreted with a plain film of the abdomen (KUB) was as accurate as unenhanced spiral CT in acute calculus ureteric obstruction. MRU was superior to acute CT in detecting perirenal fluid as a sign of obstruction. There

Table 2. Kappa statistics for the agreement between MRU and CT for all subjects as determined by the three observers and for their consensus opinion

	Observer 1	Observer 2	Observer 3	Consensus
Fluid/Stranding:	0.59	0.19*	0.28†	0.45
Dilation	0.56	0.53	0.59	0.56
Level	0.56	0.43	0.49	0.49
RLB[a]	0.66	0.67	0.69	0.69

* $p=0.106$, † $p=0.008$.
[a]Agreement between all observers regarding which kidney (right, left or both) was acutely obstructed.

Table 3. Interobserver agreement on findings by MR urography/plain abdominal radiograph (MRU/KUB) and CT in acute ureteric obstruction

	Observers 1 and 2		Observers 1 and 3		Observers 2 and 3	
	MRU/KUB	CT	MRU/KUB	CT	MRU/KUB	CT
RLB	0.88	0.88	0.81	0.77	0.86	0.78
Fluid/stranding	0.72	0.29*	0.78	0.38†	0.75	0.34‡
Dilation	0.86	0.64	0.80	0.53	0.87	0.75
Level	0.63	0.53	0.63	0.48	0.74	0.55
Calculi	0.63	0.76	0.46	0.76	0.44	0.71

*p-value=0.012. †p-value=0.004. ‡p-value=0.006, ($p<0.005$ is significant) RLB, right, left or both kidneys abnormal.

Table 4a. Calculus detection and location as demonstrated by CT and MR urography/plain abdominal radiograph (MRU/KUB). Mean stone size (mms) are in parentheses

	CT	MRU/KUB
Prox	3 (7)	3 (4.6)
Mid	4 (6.4)	3 (8.5)
Distal[b]	22 (3.1)	15 (4.4)
Total	29[a] (3.7)	21[a] (5.1)

[a]17 additional intra renal calculi were seen on CT and 6 on KUB.
[b]These included two bladder calculi.

Table 4b. Number of calculi detected by CT and MRU in the <5 mm, 6–10 mm and >10 mm mean size groups.

	CT	MRU/KUB
⩽5 mm	21 (72%)	13 (62%)
6–10 mm	6 (20%)	6 (29%)
⩾10 mm	2 (7%)	2 (10%)
Total	29	21

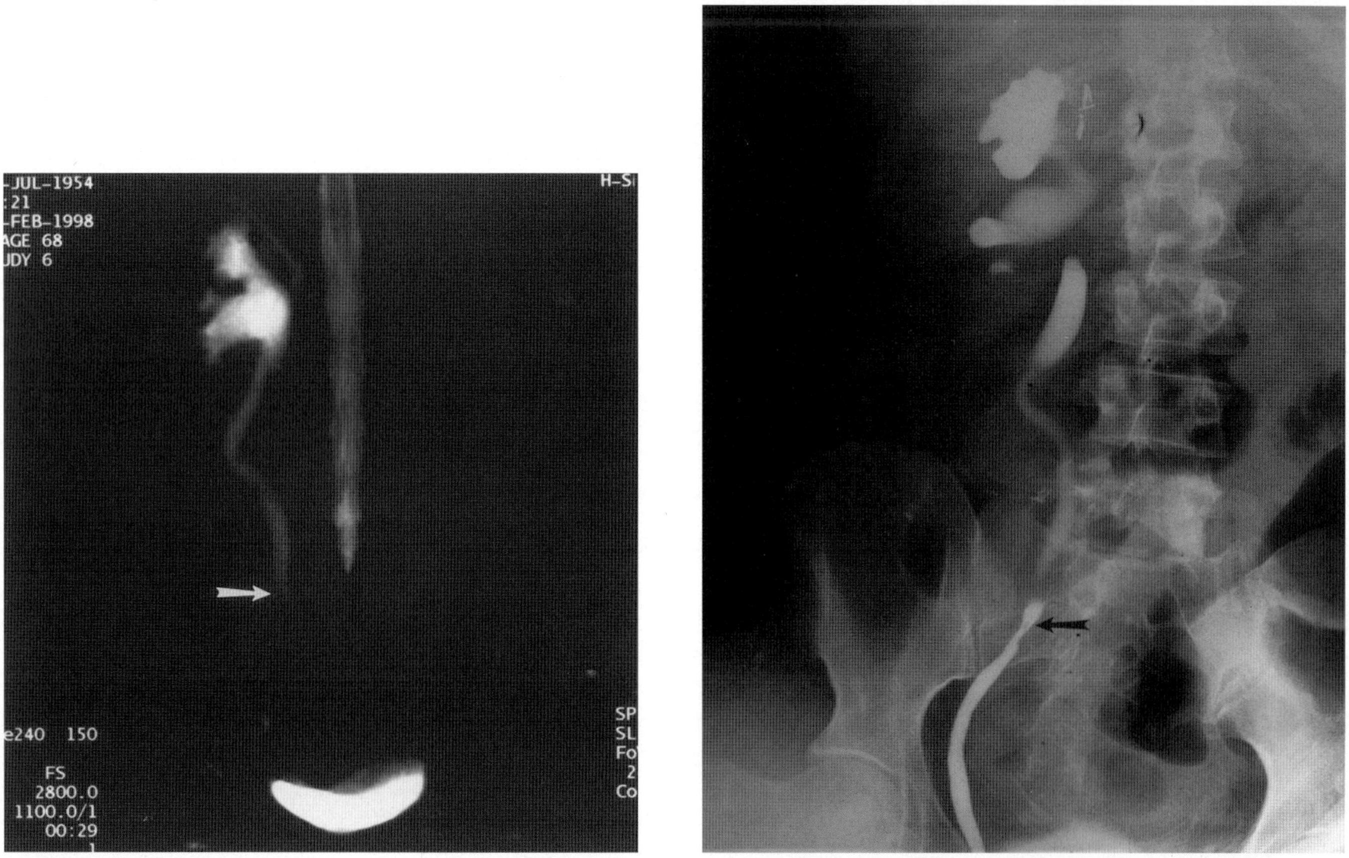

(a) (b)

Figure 3. A 46-year-old female patient with Crohn's disease presenting with acute right flank pain. (a) MR urogram shows a level of obstruction at the mid/distal third of the right ureter, and axial CT confirmed a distal ureteric calculus. (b) Retrograde pyelography demonstrates a calculus (arrow) above a distal ureteric stricture, and removed at ureteroscopy.

was less interobserver variability with MRU than with CT and our observers found MRU/KUB easier to interpret.

There have been many recent papers describing the utility of unenhanced CT in acute calculus obstruction [2–4]. Small calculi can be detected and secondary signs of obstruction such as perirenal stranding are seen without the need for administered contrast media [7, 8]. At this institution however, referring urologists were initially more comfortable at interpreting and making management decisions based on intravenous urography than CT, and interpretation difficulties may limit the value of CT in acute ureteral obstruction. Distal ureteric calculi may be difficult to distinguish from pelvic phleboliths or arterial calcifications. Although calculi have higher attenuation values than phleboliths, these values may be inaccurate if targeted views of the distal ureter are not obtained. Although analysis of calculi and reformatted images of obstructed ureters from data on the console is more accurate than hard copy images [8, 9], this is time consuming and probably inappropriate in a busy department. Signs of obstruction such as perirenal and periureteric stranding can be difficult to see on CT and this is especially true in patients with a paucity of intra-abdominal fat. Perirenal stranding is not specific to acute ureteric obstruction and occurs in diseases such as renal infection and tumour and periureteral vessels and lymphatics can be confused with stranding on CT. Numerous CT images are generated per study (up to 120 axial images compared with an average of 54 images for MRU), and these require time consuming interpretation.

Alternatively, MRU shows the effects of acute obstruction, *i.e.* perirenal fluid with greater sensitivity and less interobserver variability than CT shows stranding. The clarity with which this fluid is seen may be partly explained by the use of fat suppression and the fluid sensitive T_2 weighting of the HASTE sequences. For the same reasons, MRU clearly shows the ureter and level of obstruction, increasing the confidence whereby ureteric calculi can be diagnosed on KUB.

Although we used a simple and subjective grading system, all three radiologists found MRU easier to interpret than CT, with more robust interobserver agreement. Although MRU fails to demonstrate most kidney and ureteric calculi, if combined with a KUB, a more confident diagnosis of ureteric calculus can be made. While MRU/KUB misses small calculi, (7 mm or less), these usually pass spontaneously [1], and do not require intervention.

There are potential design flaws in this study. Patients were imaged in a non randomized fashion, and most underwent CT first. It could therefore be argued that the delay in scanning with MR allowed further accumulation of perirenal fluid. It could also be argued however, that in this time interval, a ureteric calculus may have passed and the amount of perirenal fluid would have diminished between the two studies. Second, our CT technique used multiple acquisitions rather than a single long spiral and a stone may be missed due to misregistration, and the tube current we employed could further reduce the stone detection rate due to beam hardening artefact.

In summary, MRU using HASTE sequences is a more accurate alternative to unenhanced spiral CT in detecting signs of obstruction (perirenal fluid and ureteric dilatation) without the risk of radiation. The technique shows no statistically significant difference in predicting the presence of acute calculus obstruction, demonstrates less interobserver variability, and is easier to interpret than CT.

References

1. Drach GW. Urinary lithiasis; etiology, diagnosis and medical management. In: Walsh PC, Staney TA, Vaughan ED, editors. Campbell's urology (6th edn). Philadelphia, PA: Saunders, 1992:2085–156.
2. Smith RC, Rosenfield AT, Kyuran AC, Kirk RE, Verga M, Glickman MG, et al. Acute flank pain: comparison of non-contrast-enhanced CT and intravenous urography. Radiology 1995;194:789–94.
3. Smith RC, Verga M, Dalrymple N, McCarthy S, Rosenfield AT. Acute ureteral obstruction: value of secondary signs on helical unenhanced CT. AJR Am J Roentgenol 1996;167:1109–13.
4. Heneghan JP, Dalrymple NC, Verga M, Rosenfield AT, Smith RC. Soft tissue "rim" sign in the diagnosis of ureteral calculi with use of unenhanced helical CT. Radiology 1997;202:709–11.
5. Regan F, Bohlman ME, Khazan R, Rodriguez R, Haakh H. MR urography using half-fourier acquisition single shot turbo spin-echo [HASTE] in the assessment of ureteric obstruction. AJR Am J Roentgenol 1996;167:1115–20.
6. Aerts P, Van Hoe L, Bosmans H, Oyen R, Marchal G, Baert AL. Breath-hold MR urography using the HASTE technique. AJR Am J Roentgenol 1996;166:543–5.
7. Rosner B. Fundamentals of biostatistics (4th edn). Boston, MA: Duxbury Press, 1995.
8. Phelan JS, Rochester MN, King BF, Ali AT, Welch TJ, Ilstrup DM, et al. Spiral CT in the detection of urinary stone disease: a prospective blinded comparison of soft copy vs hard copy interpretations. Radiology 1998;209[P]:452.
9. Bell TV, Fenlon HM, Davison BD, Ahari HK, Hussain S. Unenhanced helical CT criteria to differentiate distal ureteral calculi from pelvic phleboliths. Radiology 1998;207:363–7.
10. Kawashima A, Sandler CM, Boridy IC, Takahashi N, Benson GS, Goldman SM. Unenhanced helical CT of ureterolithiasis; value of the tissue rim sign. AJR Am J Roentgenol 1997;168:997–1000.

The British Journal of Radiology, *78* (2005), 512–518 © 2005 The British Institute of Radiology
DOI: 10.1259/bjr/59648297

Real-time blood-pool images of contrast enhanced ultrasound with Definity in the detection of tumour nodules in the liver

[1]H MARUYAMA, MD, [1]S MATSUTANI, MD, ^{1}H SAISHO, MD, [2]Y MINE, PhD, [2]N KAMIYAMA, PhD, [3]T HIRATA, PhD and [3]M SASAMATA, PhD

[1]*Department of Medicine and Clinical Oncology, Graduate School of Medicine, Chiba University, 1-8-1, Inohana, Chuou-ku, Chiba, 260-8670,* [2]*Toshiba Corporation, Medical Systems Company, 1385, Shimoishigami, Otawara-shi, Tochigi, 324-8550 and* [3]*Pharmaceutical Laboratories, Institute for Drug Discovery Research, Yamanouchi Pharmaceutical Co. Ltd., 21, Miyukigaoka, Tsukuba-shi, Ibaraki, 305-8585, Japan*

Abstract. Lower mechanical index (MI) technique with newer microbubble agents has been introduced into clinical practice as a newer ultrasound (US) imaging. However, the efficacy in detecting tumour nodules has not been proven scientifically. The aim of this study was to elucidate the efficacy of a blood-pool image of real-time contrast-enhanced US under low MI in detecting liver tumours. 15 rabbits with VX-2 tumour were used; the number of implantations was none in two rabbits, one in four, two in five and three in four. US equipment was APLIO (Toshiba) with linear probe (3.5/7.0 MHz). The number, location and size of tumour nodules were examined by non-contrast tissue harmonic imaging (NC-US) or contrast-enhanced pulse subtraction harmonic imaging (C-US) under extra-low MI (MI 0.065) with the injection of Definity (30 μl kg^{-1}). The number of tumour nodules detected by both NC-US and C-US were consistent with the histopathological results in five rabbits – two with none, two with one nodule and one with two nodules. In the other 10 rabbits, C-US showed all the implanted tumours and small daughter nodules around them that were confirmed by histopathology. However, NC-US failed to demonstrate two implanted nodules and all the daughter nodules. On the basis of the histopathological results, detectability of implanted tumour was not significantly different between NC-US (24/26, 92.3%) and C-US (26/26, 100%). However C-US was superior to NC-US in delineating the nodules and in detecting small daughter nodules. The sizes of the implanted tumour nodules measured by histopathology correlated closely with those measured by C-US. Real-time blood-pool images by pulse subtraction harmonic imaging under extra-low MI with Definity will contribute to the improvement of the ultrasound delineation and detection of liver tumours.

Contrast-enhanced ultrasound (US) can demonstrate the vascularity and haemodynamics of liver tumours precisely [1–3]. With this background, contrast enhancement technology can be expected to improve the US diagnosis of liver tumours in terms of detection, differentiation and therapeutic effect [4–15].

Some kinds of microbubbles such as Levovist and Sonazoid show accumulation in the liver, and the enhanced US images with those agents have been reported to be useful for detecting liver tumours [16–24]. However, some other microbubbles such as Definity and Sonovue exhibit this behaviour, though the mechanism has not been clarified [25–27]. The possible efficacy for the detection of liver tumours with these US contrast agents has not yet been widely investigated.

Definity, a recently developed US contrast agent with perfluoropropane gas-filled lipid stabilized microbubbles, provides a continuous and remarkable enhancement of the liver and tumours under extra-low mechanical index (MI) harmonic imaging [28, 29]. This agent is reported to be a blood-pool contrast agent that does not have a late liver-specific parenchymal phase with accumulated microbubbles [25, 26]. For this reason, it has not been clear whether contrast-enhanced blood-pool images with Definity could improve the US detection of small tumour nodules in the liver.

The purpose of the present study was to evaluate the efficacy of real-time blood-pool images with contrast-enhanced US in detecting tumour nodules in the liver. In this study, we examined the detectability of tumour nodules with non-contrast tissue harmonic imaging and contrast pulse subtraction harmonic imaging under extra-low MI with Definity in the rabbit liver.

Materials and methods

Animals

15 New Zealand White male rabbits weighing 2.0–2.4 kg (2.1 $\pm$ 0.1 kg, mean $\pm$ standard deviation (SD)) were used in this study. 13 rabbits were implanted VX-2 tumour tissue cubes of approximately 2 mm^3 from carrier rabbits; the number of implanted VX-2 tumour tissue cubes was one in four rabbits, two in five rabbits and three in four rabbits. The other two rabbits did not receive an implantation, but incisions were made on the abdomen similar to the rabbits with implanted VX-2 tumours. The US examination was conducted 4–5 weeks after the implantation.

The animals were anaesthetized with pentobarbital at a dose of 30 mg kg^{-1} by bolus injection followed by continuous infusion at 3.0 mg kg^{-1}h^{-1} into the auricular

Received 3 August 2004 and in revised form 6 December 2004, accepted 19 January 2005.

vein. The skin of the abdomen was shaved after the animal was stabilized, and US examination was performed at the body surface in a supine position. A 3 Fr 1.35 mm catheter was inserted into the right femoral vein and a three-way stopcock was applied at the end of the catheter, with one branch being used for administration of a contrast agent and another for the saline flush after its administration. A 4 Fr 1.0 mm plastic tube was inserted into the femoral artery to monitor and record arterial pressure and pulse rate during the examination. All studies were conducted in compliance with the regulations of the Animal Ethics Committee of Yamanouchi Pharmaceutical Co. Ltd.

Equipment

US images were obtained with SSA-770A (APLIO; Toshiba, Tokyo, Japan) with a linear probe that transmits and receives centre frequencies of 3.5/7.0 MHz. Imaging methods in this study were tissue harmonic imaging (THI) for non-contrast enhanced ultrasound (NC-US) and pulse subtraction harmonic imaging (PHI) for contrast enhanced ultrasound (C-US). All the images were taken by continuous scan at a frame rate of 48–49 Hz for THI and 15 Hz for PHI with the dynamic range at 50–60 dB throughout the examination. Gain and sensitivity time control (STC) were set at optimal levels and the focus point was set at the bottom level of the liver.

The mechanical index (MI) level used in this study was as follows; 1.0 for NC-US, a maximum level, 0.065 for C-US, a suitable level for obtaining a real-time enhancement image in liver parenchyma [29].

Contrast agent

The contrast agent used in this study was Definity™ (a perfluoropropane gas-filled lipid-stabilized microbubble, Bristol-Myers Squibb, North Billerica, MA). The contrast effect in this study was evaluated at a dose of 30 μl kg^{-1}, which is three times the recommended dose for cardiac imaging [28–30]. After shaking with an agitation machine for 45 s, the agent was injected into the rabbits via a cannula inserted into the femoral vein by manual injection at a rate of about 0.1 ml s^{-1}, followed by a 2.0 ml of saline solution flush. The images were recorded on digital videotape before and after enhancement.

Experimental procedure

Eight rabbits were examined by HM and seven rabbits by SM, both experienced in the use of US, and they were blinded to the information of the implanted VX-2 tumours. After NC-US examination, the operator investigated tumour nodules by continuous scan during a blood-pool image in the liver, which was obtained several seconds after the beginning of contrast enhancement effect. The location, number and size of the tumour nodules were examined and noted in each rabbit before and after enhancement. After US examination, all rabbits were killed with an overdose of pentobarbital (5.0 g). Histopathological examination of the liver was conducted by TH, who was blinded to the US findings. KM, who was neither the operator of US examination nor the conductor of histopathological examination, compared the histopathological results with the US results concerning the location, number and size of the tumour nodules.

Statistical analysis

The results were compared by Student's *t*-test and Pearson's correlation coefficient. Probability values less than 0.05 were considered significant.

Results

Non-contrast tissue harmonic images (NC-US) of VX-2 tumour nodules

Tumour nodules were detected in 13 of 15 rabbits by NC-US (Table 1); the number of tumour nodules was none in two rabbits, one in five rabbits, two in five rabbits and three in three rabbits. All the nodules were visualized with an isoechoic pattern with heterogeneous appearance, ranging in size from 9.2 mm to 26.9 mm (14.7±5.1 mm).

Contrast-enhanced blood-pool images (C-US) of VX-2 tumour nodules with Definity

After the injection of Definity, the liver image became distinct, with homogeneous enhancement of the liver parenchyma in all rabbits, and tumours were visualized as unenhanced nodules with or without peripheral enhancement. The size of the tumour nodules measured by C-US included the peripheral enhancement area in those cases with the enhancement. The deepest depth of the examined liver was 42 mm from the body surface.

The blood-pool phase of contrast enhancement with Definity lasted more than 4 min, long enough to examine real-time images of a whole liver. In seven of the 15 rabbits, however, shadowing phenomenon disturbed the observation of the deep area in the early phase of contrast enhancement. This phenomenon disappeared gradually after 30 s from the beginning of contrast enhancement.

Table 1. Number of tumour nodules; implanted nodules, detected by ultrasound and histopathological examination

Animal	Implanted	NC-US	C-US	Histopathological examination
1	2	2	2	2
2	3	3	3[a]	3[a]
3	1	1	1[a]	1[a]
4	2	1	2[a]	2[a]
5	0	0	0	0
6	1	1	1	1
7	3	3	3[a]	3[a]
8	2	2	2[a]	2[a]
9	2	2	2[a]	2[a]
10	1	1	1	1
11	3	2	3[a]	3[a]
12	2	2	2[a]	2[a]
13	3	3	3[a]	3[a]
14	0	0	0	0
15	1	1	1[a]	1[a]

[a]Multiple small tumour nodules were observed around the main (implanted) tumour nodules. NC-US, non contrast-enhanced ultrasound; C-US, contrast-enhanced ultrasound.

Comparison of the detection of tumour nodules between US and pathology (Table 1) (Figures 1 and 2)

Pathological examination showed large tumour nodules of a size greater than 10 mm in 13 of 15 rabbits, and the number of tumour nodules agreed with the implanted number in each rabbit. The number of these nodules detected by C-US was also consistent with the number on pathology. However, NC-US failed to detect two of the nodules (14.4 mm, 17 mm). There was no false-positive detection of nodules either by NC-US or C-US.

Pathology showed multiple satellite nodules smaller than 10 mm around the implanted tumours in 10 rabbits. These satellite nodules were thought to be daughter nodules because of the distribution of these nodules around the main implanted tumour nodules. Although NC-US did not show any of these daughter nodules, C-US demonstrated them as unenhanced areas in all 10 rabbits.

Comparison of the size of tumour nodules between US and pathology

The maximum sizes of the implanted tumour nodules were 14.7±5.1 mm (9.3–26.9 mm) on NC-US, 15.9±4.6 mm (11.1–25.5 mm) on C-US, and 16.1±4.6 mm (11–26 mm) on histopathological examination. The correlation coefficients for the comparison with the histopathological measurements were 0.751 (p=0.002) for NC-US and 0.996 (p<0.0001) for C-US. Thus, the measurement by C-US showed a close correlation with the size of tumour nodules by histopathological examination. Furthermore, the distribution of daughter nodules on C-US was similar to the pathological findings, and the smallest size of daughter nodule detected by C-US measured 2.0 mm on histopathological examination in case 11 (Figure 3).

Discussion

Detection of tumour nodules in the liver is of major importance for formulating therapeutic strategy and predicting a prognosis in malignant disease. Diagnosis of small liver tumours has always been the greatest concern in imaging diagnosis [10–19, 31].

Levovist, a popular US contrast agent, is a galactose-based microbubble for use by intravenous injection [5–10, 16–18, 20, 23]. As Levovist accumulates in the liver, a metastatic liver tumour appears as an unenhanced nodule in a late liver-specific parenchymal phase of contrast enhanced ultrasound [16, 17], and this phase is reported to be useful for detection of metastatic liver tumours. (However, some contrast agents with a different structure and chemical nature from Levovist apparently do not

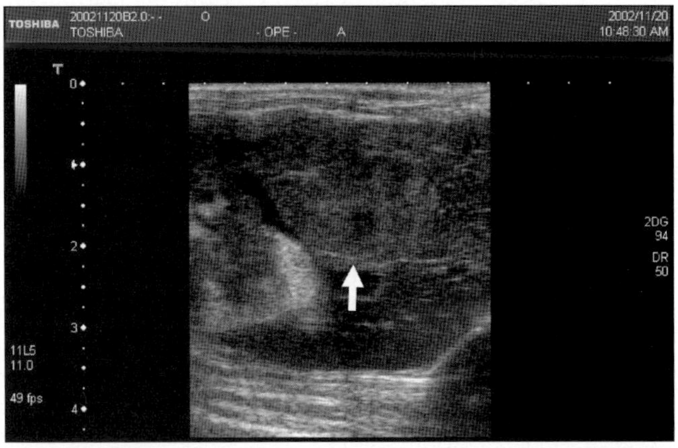

(a)

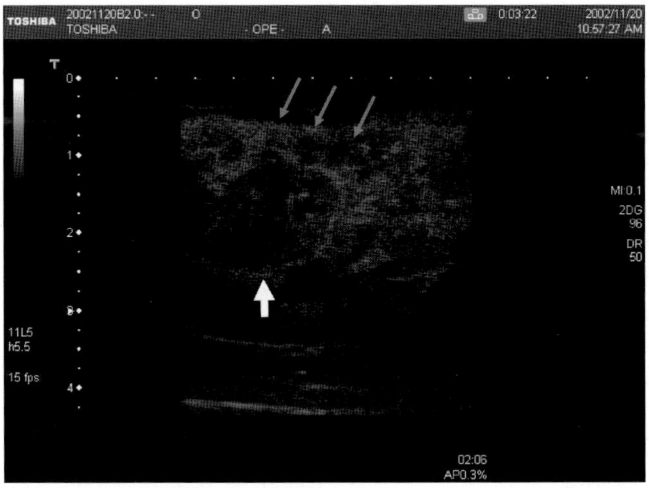

(b)

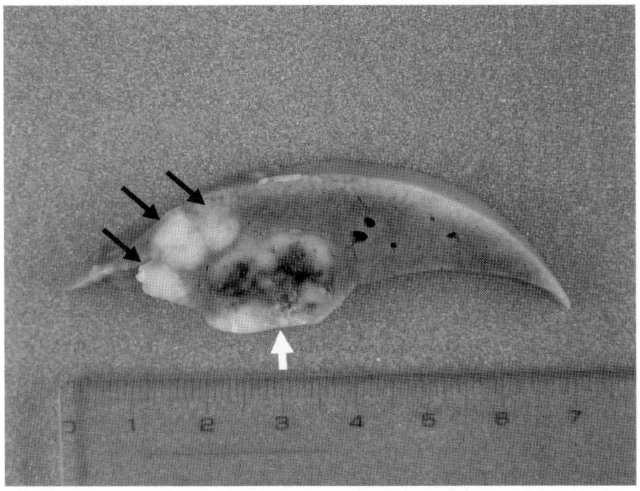

(c)

Figure 1. VX-2 tumour in the rabbit liver, Case 11, right lobe. (a) Non-contrast tissue harmonic image. One tumour nodule with heterogeneous ultrasound pattern was observed (arrow). The margin of the tumour nodule was not clear. Other tumour nodules were not detected. (b) Contrast-enhanced pulse subtraction harmonic image with Definity. One tumour nodule was observed as an unenhanced nodule with peripheral enhancement (arrow, white), and small tumour nodules were demonstrated as unenhanced nodules around this nodule (arrows, grey). All the tumour nodules were delineated clearly with homogeneous enhancement of the surrounding liver parenchyma. (c) Histopathological findings. One implanted tumour nodule 18 mm in size (arrow, white) and daughter tumour nodules (arrows, black) were observed. The implanted tumour was hypervascular in the peripheral area, corresponding to the peripheral enhancement in (b) and it was necrotic in the central area.

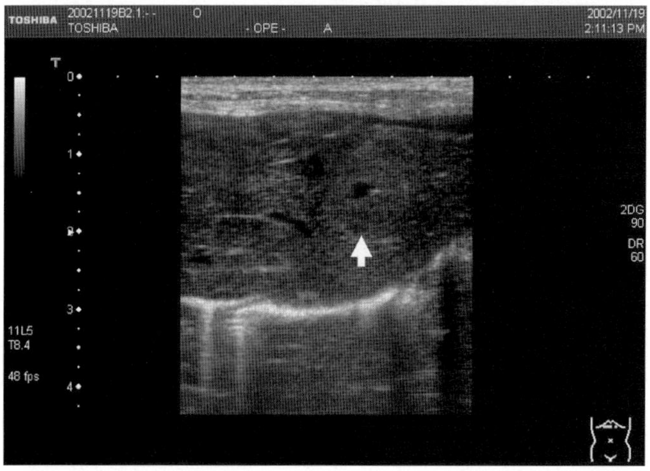

(a)

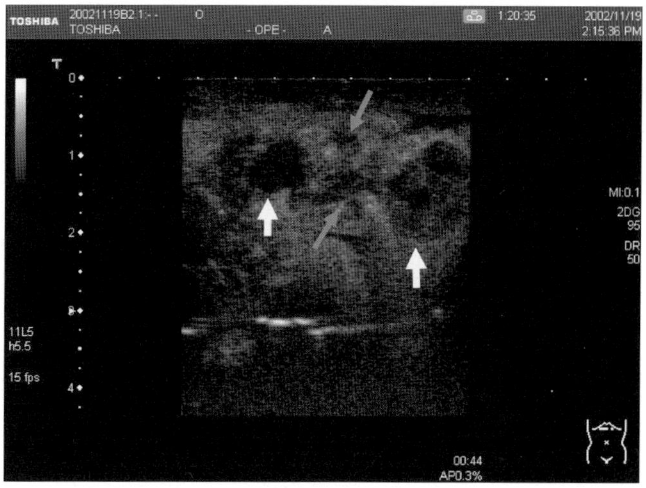

(b)

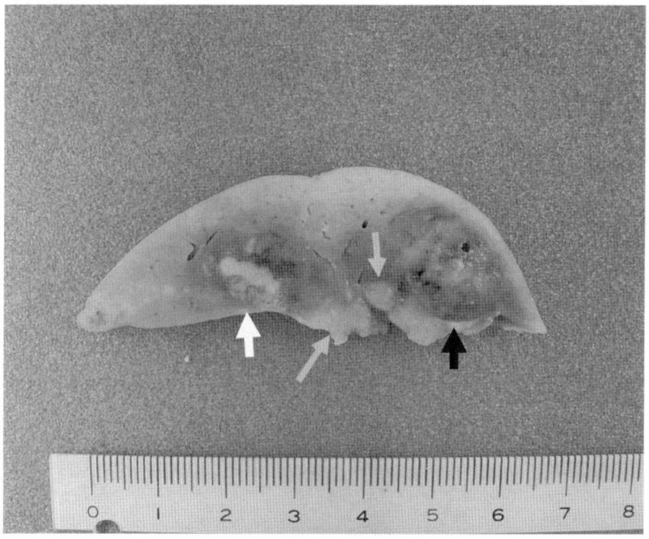

(c)

Figure 2. VX-2 tumour in the rabbit liver, Case 4. (a) Non-contrast tissue harmonic image. The one detected tumour nodule had an isoechoic appearance with a central hypoechoic area (arrow, white). The ultrasound pattern of the liver parenchyma was heterogeneous, but other tumour nodules were not clear. (b) Contrast-enhanced pulse subtraction harmonic image with Definity. Homogeneous enhancement was seen in the liver parenchyma. Two tumours were observed as unenhanced nodules with clear delineation, with one of them (right side) showing peripheral enhancement (arrows, white). Small tumours were demonstrated as unenhanced nodules around the two tumour nodules (arrows, grey). (c) Histopathological findings. There were two implanted tumour nodules, 14.4 mm and 19 mm, in the liver (arrows, white and black). Small tumour nodules were observed around the implanted tumours, and were believed to be metastatic tumour nodules (arrows, grey). The tumour tissues were necrotic, but one of them (arrow, black) had tumour vessels in the peripheral area corresponding to the peripheral enhancement in (b).

possess this phase with the accumulation of microbubbles in the liver.)

A newly developed US contrast agent, Definity, allows real-time observation with homogeneous and stable enhancement of the liver parenchyma under an extra-low MI level [28, 29]. This microbubble agent is reported to be a blood-pool contrast agent [25, 26]. So far, there has been little discussion of whether a real-time blood-pool image with circulating microbubbles is suitable for detecting tumour nodules in the liver. In this study, we evaluated the ability of real-time contrast-enhanced blood-pool images with Definity to detect a VX-2 tumour in rabbit liver as a metastatic liver tumour model.

As shown in the present study, pulse subtraction harmonic imaging under extra-low MI with Definity was superior to non-contrast tissue harmonic imaging in detecting small tumour nodules. Furthermore, C-US was superior to NC-US in delineating the nodules in all rabbits because a correlation with the tumour size by histopathological examination was closer in C-US result than in NC-US. The enhanced liver image originating from microbubble signals provided a continuous and stable enhancement of the liver parenchyma, giving the tumour nodules a more distinct appearance than on non-contrast US.

There have been some studies regarding the improvement of the detection of occult hepatic metastases with enhanced ultrasound using Levovist. However, those studies have not fully compared the results with the histopathological findings [16, 17]. According to Harvey et al the evidence of these lesions detected on a late liver-specific parenchymal image with Levovist was difficult to confirm with biopsy, because the images appeared on only a few ultrasound frames [18]. Meanwhile, the blood-pool imaging in this study has advantages for real-time and repeated observation of a whole liver with sufficient duration, which improves the reproducibility of detecting small tumour nodules in the liver. Further studies will be necessary to conclude whether the real-time blood-pool imaging under extra-low MI with newer US contrast agents is comparable with late liver specific parenchymal imaging with Levovist in detecting liver tumours.

Tissue harmonic imaging is more sensitive than fundamental grey-scale imaging in detecting focal liver lesions [32, 33], as it provides better delineation of tumours due to improved lateral resolution and signal-to-clutter ratio, and

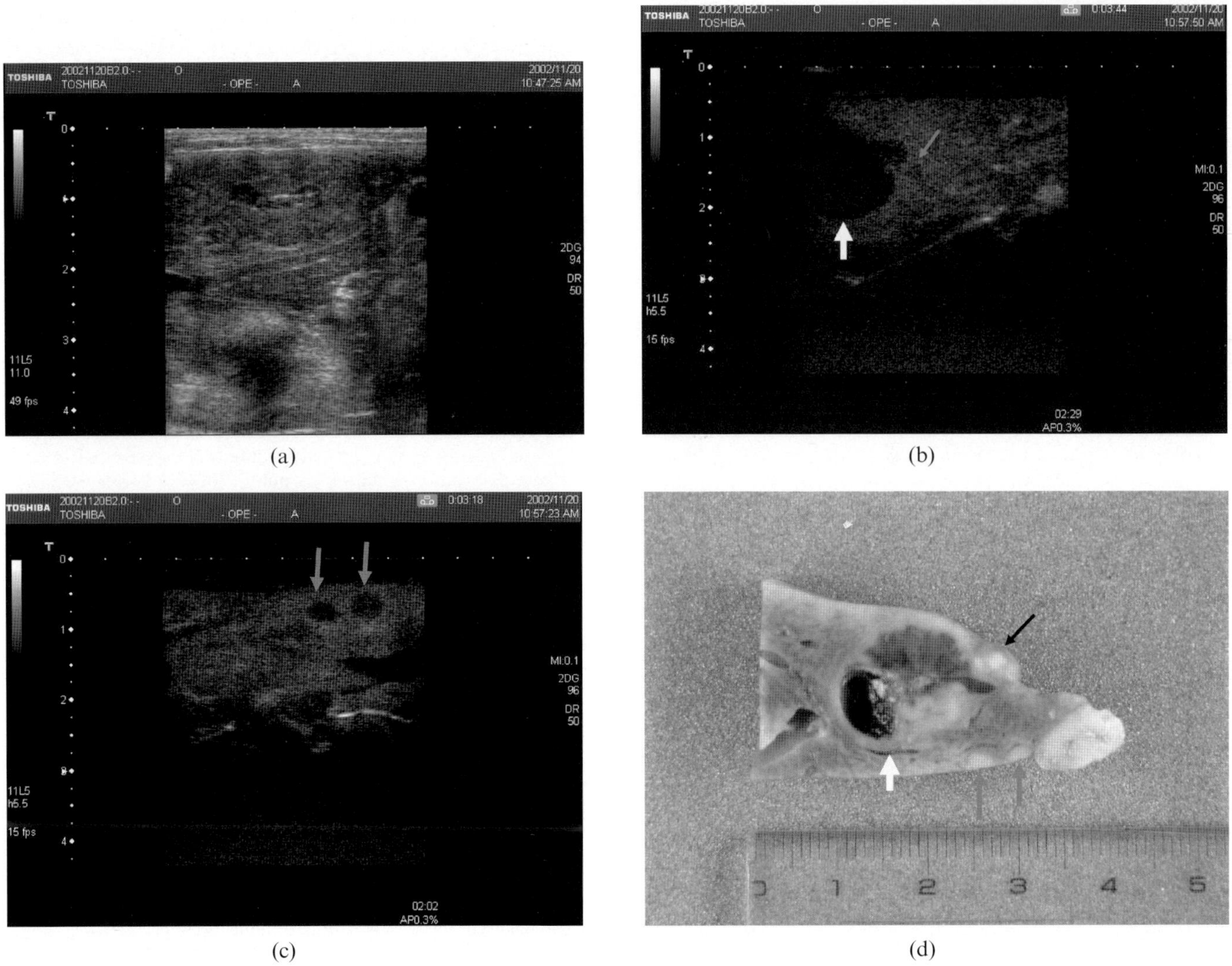

Figure 3. VX-2 tumour in the rabbit liver, Case 11, left lobe. (a) Non-contrast tissue harmonic image. No tumour nodules were recognized with non-contrast ultrasound in this case. (b) Contrast-enhanced pulse subtraction harmonic images with Definity. One tumour nodule (arrow, white) and small nodule (arrow, grey) were observed as unenhanced focal lesions. (c) Near the same tumour as in (b), two other small tumours were demonstrated as unenhanced nodules in the surface area of the liver. (d) Histopathological findings. One implanted tumour nodule 17 mm in size was found in the liver (arrow, white). Small tumour nodule was observed around the implanted tumour (arrow, black), and was thought to be metastatic tumour nodules. Two tumour nodules 2 mm in size were seen in the surface area of the liver (arrows, grey).

also reduces near-field artefacts [31, 34–36]. In the present study, however, tissue harmonic imaging failed to demonstrate a few of the implanted main tumour nodules and all the small metastatic tumour nodules, and pulse subtraction contrast harmonic imaging under extra-low MI with Definity was superior to tissue harmonic imaging in the detection of tumour nodules in the liver. One of the reasons for the poor detectability of tumours with NC-US may be that the US field in this study was too near the body surface to generate harmonic signals by non-linear propagation of a sound wave. Furthermore, the tumour nodules in rabbit liver showed an isoechoic appearance and were very small. However, the US pattern and tumour size did not disturb the detection with contrast harmonic imaging.

The present results have several shortcomings in terms of their application to the human clinical setting. As the enhanced findings were evaluated in rabbit liver with implanted VX-2 tumours, the MI level employed for this study may not be optimal for humans [28, 29]. In addition, whether the detection of tumour nodules deeply located in human liver is possible with observation under extra-low acoustic power levels remains to be elucidated.

Shadowing phenomenon caused by excessive enhancement around the surface level of the liver was observed at the beginning of echo-enhancement in seven of 15 rabbits, disturbing deep-area observation in the liver. Although the long duration time of the blood-pool phase with contrast enhancement allowed sufficient assessment of the whole liver, missing the early arterial phase of enhanced liver images is unfortunate. Continuous injection of contrast agent by drip infusion may reduce this artefact [37]. Furthermore, improvement of US equipment to reduce these phenomena may be necessary, perhaps by a modulation of the focus point and/or auto-regulation of the transmit/receive echo signals.

In conclusion, the real-time blood-pool phase of contrast-enhanced ultrasound with Definity improves the delineation and detection of liver tumours in rabbit livers. However, the translation of these results to human liver still remains to be determined.

References

1. Goldberg BB, Liu JB, Forsberg F. Ultrasound contrast agents: a review. Ultrasound Med Biol 1994;20:319–33.
2. Burns PN. Harmonic imaging with ultrasound contrast agents. Clin Radiol 1996;51 (Suppl. 1):50–5.
3. Burns PN, Wilson SR, Simpson DH. Pulse inversion imaging of liver blood flow. Invest Radiol 2000;35:58–71.
4. Schneider M, Broillet A, Bussat P, Giessinger N, Puginier J, Ventrone R, et al. Gray-scale liver enhancement in VX2 tumor-bearing rabbits using BR14, a new Ultrasonographic contrast agent. Invest Radiol 1997;32:410–7.
5. Bartolozzi C, Lencioni R, Ricci P, Paolicchi A, Rossi P, Passariello R. Hepatocellular carcinoma treatment with percutaneous ethanol injection: evaluation with contrast-enhanced color Doppler US. Radiology 1998;209:387–93.
6. Maruyama H, Matsutani S, Sato G, Nakano Y, Mitsuhashi O, Yoshikawa M, et al. Enhanced color flow images in small hepatocellular carcinoma. Abdom Imaging 2000;25:164–71.
7. Kim TK, Choi BI, Han JK, Park SH, Moon SG. Hepatic tumors: contrast agent-enhancement patterns with pulse-inversion harmonic US. Radiology 2000;216:411–7.
8. Wilson SR, Burns PN, Muradali D, Wilson JA, Lai X. Harmonic hepatic US with microbubble contrast agent: initial experience showing improved characterization of hemangioma, hepatocellular carcinoma and metastasis. Radiology 2000;215:153–61.
9. Numata K, Tanaka K, Kiba T, Saito S, Isozaki T, Hara K, et al. Using contrast-enhanced sonography to assess the effectiveness of transcatheter arterial embolization for hepatocellular carcinoma. AJR Am J Roentgenol 2001;176: 1199–205.
10. Meloni MF, Goldberg SN, Livraghi T, Calliada F, Rossi P, Pallavicini D, et al. Hepatocellular carcinoma treated with radiofrequency ablation: comparison of pulse inversion contrast-enhanced harmonic sonography, contrast-enhanced power Doppler sonography, and helical CT. AJR Am J Roentgenol 2001;177:375–80.
11. Girard MS, Kono Y, Sirlin CB, Backer KG, Deiranieh LH, Mattrey RF. B-mode enhancement of the liver with microbubble contrast agent: a blinded study in rabbits with VX2 tumors. Acad Radiol 2001;8:734–40.
12. Watanabe R, Matsumura M, Chen CJ, Kaneda Y, Ishihara M, Fujimaki M. Gray-scale liver enhancement with Sonazoid (NC100100), a novel ultrasound contrast agent; detection of hepatic tumors in a rabbit model. Biol Pharm Bull 2003;26:1272–7.
13. Albrecht T, Oldenburg A, Hohmann J, Skrok J, Hoffmann CW, Schettler S, et al. Imaging of liver metastases with contrast-specific low-MI real-time ultrasound and SonoVue. Eur Radiol 2003;13: Suppl. 3:N79–86.
14. Bernatik T, Becker D, Neureiter D, Hansler J, Frieser M, Schaber S, et al. Detection of liver metastases-comparison of contrast-enhanced ultrasound using first versus second generation contrast agents. Ultraschall Med 2003;24:175–9.
15. Liu JB, Goldberg BB, Merton DA, Rawool NM, Needleman L, Forsberg F. The role of contrast-enhanced sonography for radiofrequency ablation of liver tumors. J Ultrasound Med 2001;20:517–23.
16. Blomley MJK, Albrecht T, Cosgrove DO, Patel N, Jayaram V, Butler-Barnes J, et al. Improved imaging of liver metastases with stimulated acoustic emission in the late phase of enhancement with the US contrast agent SH U 508A: early experience. Radiology 1999;210:409–16.
17. Harvey CJ, Blomley MJK, Eckersley RJ, Cosgrove DO, Patel N, Hechemann RA, et al. Hepatic malignancies: improved detection with pulse-inversion US in late phase of enhancement with SH U 508A-Early experience. Radiology 2000;216:903–8.
18. Harvey CJ, Blomley MJK, Eckersley RJ, Heckemann RA, Butler-Barnes J, Cosgrove DO. Pulse-inversion mode imaging of liver specific microbubbles: improved detection of subcentimetre metastases. Lancet 2000;355:807–8.
19. Forsberg F, Liu JB, Merton DA, Rawool NM, Johnson DK, Goldberg BB. Gray scale second harmonic imaging of acoustic emission signals improves detection of liver tumors in rabbits. J Ultrasound Med 2000;19:557–63.
20. Von Herbay A, Vogt C, Haussinger D. Late-phase pulse-inversion sonography using the contrast agent Levovist: differentiation between benign and malignant focal lesions of the liver. AJR Am J Roentgenol 2002;179:1273–9.
21. Forsberg F, Piccoli CW, Liu JB, Rawool NM, Merton DA, Mitchell DG, et al. Hepatic tumor detection: MR imaging and conventional US versus pulse-inversion harmonic US of NC100100 during its reticuloendothelial system-specific phase. Radiology 2002;222:824–9.
22. Kono Y, Steinbach GC, Peterson T, Schmid-Schonbein GW, Matterey RF. Mechanism of parenchymal enhancement of the liver with a microbubble-based US contrast medium: an intravital microscopy study in rats. Radiology 2002;224:253–7.
23. Kitamura H, Kawasaki S, Nakajima K, Ota H. Correlation between microbubble contrast-enhanced color Doppler sonogaphy and immunostaining for Kupffer cells in assessing the histopathologic grade of hepatocellular carcinoma: preliminary results. J Clin Ultrasound 2002;30: 465–71.
24. Bryant TH, Blomley MJ, Albrecht T, Sidhu PS, Leen EL, Basilico R, et al. Improved characterization of liver lesions with liver-phase uptake of liver-specific microbubbles: prospective multicenter study. Radiology 2004;232:799–809.
25. Barr R. Seeking consensus: contrast ultrasound in radiology. Eur J Radiol 2002;41:207–16.
26. Maruyama H, Matsutani S, Saisho H, Mine Y, Yuki H, Miyata K. Different behaviors of microbubbles in the liver: time-related quantitative analysis of two ultrasound contrast agents, Levovist and Definity. Ultrasound Med Biol 2004;30:1035–40.
27. Lim AK, Patel N, Eckersley RJ, Taylor-Robinson SD, Cosgrove DO, Blomley MJ. Evidence for spleen-specific uptake of a microbubble contrast agent: a quantitative study in human volunteers. Radiology 2004;231:785–8.
28. Maruyama H, Matsutani S, Saisho H, Kamiyama N, Yuki H, Miyata K. Grey-scale contrast enhancement in rabbit liver with DMP115 at different acoustic power levels. Ultrasound Med Biol 2000;26:1429–38.
29. Maruyama H, Matsutani S, Saisho H, Mine Y, Yuki H, Miyata K. Extra-low acoustic power harmonic images of the liver with perflutren: novel imaging for real-time observation of liver perfusion. J Ultrasound Med 2003;22:931–8.
30. Kitzman DW, Goldman ME, Gillam LD, Cohen JL, Aurigemma GP, Gottdiener JS. Efficacy and safety of the novel ultrasound contrast agent perflutren (definity) in patients with suboptimal baseline left ventricular echocardiographic images. Am J Cardiol 2000;86:669–74.
31. Harvey CJ, Albrecht T. Ultrasound of focal lesions. Eur Radiol 2001;11:1578–93.
32. Hann LE, Bach AM, Cramer LD, Siegel D, Yoo HH, Garcia R. Hepatic sonography: comparison between tissue harmonic and standard sonography techniques. AJR Am J Roentgenol 1999;173:201–6.
33. Tanaka S, Oshikawa O, Sasaki T, Ioka T, Tsukuma H. Evaluation of tissue harmonic imaging for the diagnosis of focal liver lesions. Ultrasound Med Biol 2000;26: 183–7.

34. Ward B, Baker AC, Humphrey VF. Nonlinear propagation applied to the improvement of resolution in diagnostic ultrasound. J Acoustic Soc Am 1997;101:143–54.
35. Lencioni R, Cioni D, Bartolozzi C. Tissue harmonic and contrast-specific imaging: back to gray scale ultrasound. Eur Radiol 2002;12:151–65.
36. Shapiro RS, Wagreich J, Parsons RB, Stancato-Pasik A, Yeh HC, Lao R. Tissue harmonic imaging sonography: evaluation of image quality compared with conventional sonography. AJR Am J Roentgenol 1998;171:1203–6.
37. Albrecht T, Urbank A, Mahler M, Bauer A, Dore CJ, Blomley MJK, et al. Prolongation and optimization of Doppler enhancement with a microbubble US contrast agent by using continuous infusion: preliminary experience. Radiology 1998;207:339–47.

The British Journal of Radiology, 78 (2005), 519–527
DOI: 10.1259/bjr/26039330

Effectiveness of flexible noise control image processing for digital portal images using computed radiography

[1,2]S YAMADA and [2]K MURASE, MD, PhD

[1]*Department of Radiology, Kurashiki Central Hospital, 1-1-1 Miwa, Kurashiki, Okayama 710-8602 and* [2]*Department of Medical Physics and Engineering, Division of Medical Technology and Science, Course of Health Science, Graduate School of Medicine, Osaka University, 1-7 Yamadaoka, Suita, Osaka 565-0871, Japan*

Abstract. The purpose of this study was to evaluate the clinical efficacy of flexible noise control (FNC) image processing in off-line computed radiography (CR) portal images. An observer study was designed to compare FNC with multiobjective frequency processing (MFP) in images acquired using a CR portal imaging device (CRPID). The image processing of MFP and FNC used the same data and required no additional irradiation of patients, and all images were printed on 10-bit grey-level dry laser film. Four radiation technologists and one oncologist served as observers and evaluated 40 sets of images for three different treatment sites: brain, lung and pelvis. Six to 10 anatomical landmarks were selected from each treatment site. Each observer was asked to rate each landmark in terms of its clinical visibility and rate the ease of making the pertinent verification in the MFP- and FNC-processed images. In the ratings of the visibility of landmarks and for the verification of treatment ports, FNC-processed images were more visible than MFP-processed images except for several landmarks in the anteroposterior (AP) pelvis such as the pubic symphysis. The visibility of landmarks in FNC-processed images was comparable with that in MFP-processed images. The verification of treatment ports using the CRPID with FNC was generally achievable. In conclusion, this study suggests that FNC is effective for image processing of CR portal images.

Portal imaging is a widely used procedure in radiotherapy for verifying that a tumour has been irradiated and that the surrounding healthy tissue has been spared. It is important to irradiate the prescribed targets accurately, and if it is possible to use a verification system that gives high quality images and can be used frequently, the planned target volume can be minimized, providing high quality treatment. Until now, radiographic film has commonly been used for the verification images, but electronic portal imaging devices (EPID) have recently become widely used. In Japan, as well as EPID systems, computed radiography (CR) systems, by which good image quality can be obtained, are widespread. In this study, we examined techniques to improve the quality of portal images obtained by using CR.

The CR system was marketed as a diagnostic radiographic device by Fujifilm Medical Co., Ltd. (Tokyo, Japan) in 1983 [1]. There were only two methods for image processing in the initial CR apparatus, gradation processing and frequency processing [2, 3]. Gradation processing was developed to control the density of image signals, whereas frequency processing was based on the unsharp mask technique. Figure 1a shows an unsharp masked sample image. Low frequency components are enhanced when the mask size is large, while high frequency components are enhanced when the mask size is small. Image distortion occurs at the edges of the radiation field by a combination of longitudinal and horizontal unsharp mask processing. To improve the accuracy, it was necessary to restrict the degree of enhancement of frequency processing [4]. This restriction greatly hinders attempts to improve the quality of CR portal images with a low density contrast.

Received 12 December 2003 and in final form 18 November 2004, accepted 6 January 2005.

An image-processing algorithm with improved frequency processing was developed by Fujifilm Medical Co., Ltd. in 1998. This has been called multiobjective frequency processing (MFP). When MFP is used the degree of enhancement of signals with high-density contrast can be reduced, and that of signals with low-density contrast can be increased. Figure 1b shows the improvements in an MFP image, when compared with the un-sharp mask image, where the black-framed artefacts seen in Figure 1a (indicated by the black arrows) have been reduced, and low density contrast (white arrows in Figure 1a) has been improved.

MFP is now established as the most suitable processing method for portal imaging in Japan. However, there is no established processing method for removing noise from images, and this has been recognized as a problem [5].

To address this problem, six variable image processing parameters [2, 3], that can be changed according to different circumstances, have been introduced. For example, one parameter may be changed to suppress selectively the enhancement of images in low-density areas that have a high level of noise. These parameters are listed in Appendix 1, together with a brief indication of which aspects of the processing they control. Another effective method of addressing the noise problem is to absorb backward scattered radiation efficiently by attaching a lead plate to the back surface of the cassette, and this has led to the development of a commercially available cassette for portal imaging [6]. However, these methods reduced effective signals which could detract from image quality in some regions, such as near to bone edges [7].

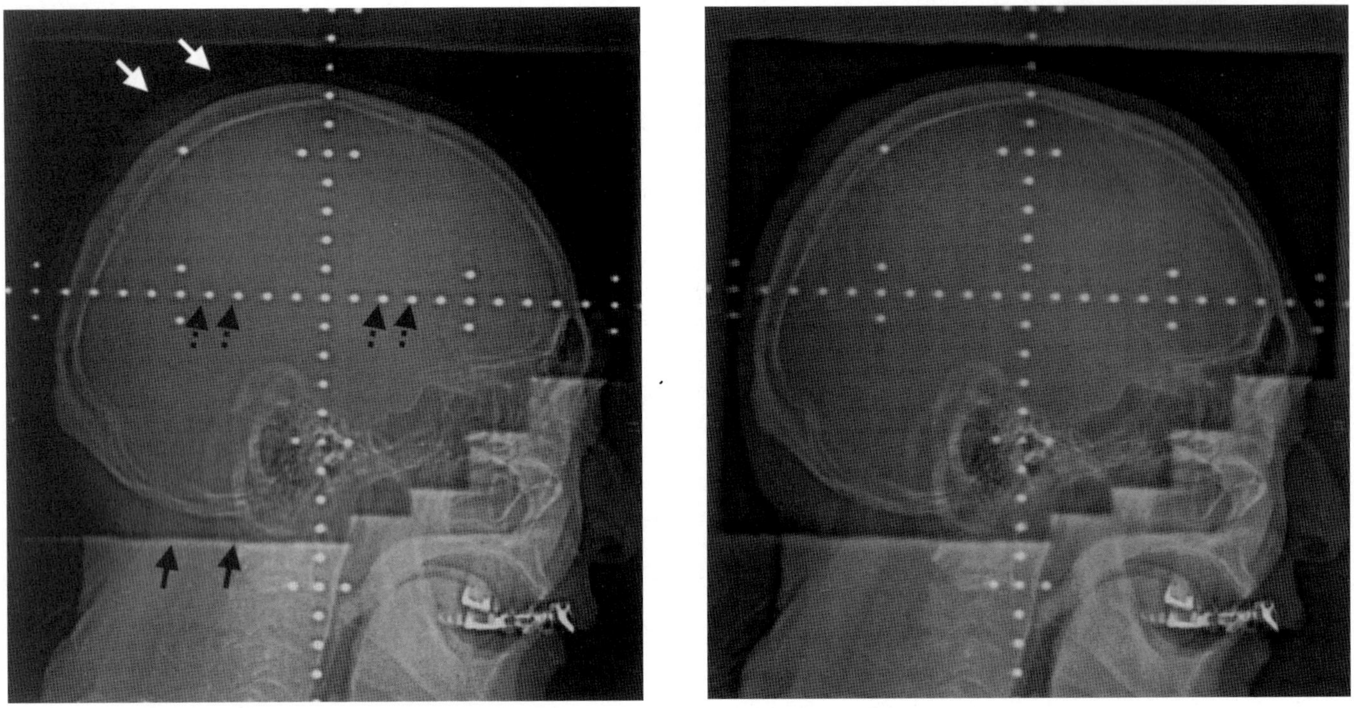

(a) (b)

Figure 1. Computed radiography (CR) portal images of the head. (a) Examples of an un-sharp mask image. Black-framed artefacts were observed around the irradiation field (black arrows) and around the scale (black arrows on the broken line). The skin boundary around the head was unclear (white arrows). (b) Examples of an multiobjective frequency processing (MFP) image. Black-framed artefacts were reduced, and the skin boundary became clear.

Recently, a new image-processing algorithm for CR has been developed by Fujifilm Medical Co., Ltd., called flexible noise control (FNC) [8]. This separates the noise and effective signals of linear structures, such as bone edges, by optimizing their different shapes, and was developed mainly to reduce the effects of noise in low-dose diagnostic radiography. There are four parameters for FNC and these are listed, together with a brief description of their purpose, in Appendix 1.

This study was designed to investigate the clinical efficacy of FNC processing, in comparison with MFP, for digital portal images obtained using CR.

Methods and materials

Images

The CR portal-imaging device used was an FCR-5000R (Fujifilm Medical Co., Ltd.), and a ST-V imaging plate with a 1 mm thick frontal metal screen cassette was used in the study. This cassette, with a rubber sheet containing 43% tungsten by volume, was placed in front of the imaging plate with a sponge on the back [9]. The CR system has an effective area of 350 mm × 350 mm for a 3520 × 3520 matrix size (0.1 mm pixel^{-1}). The acquired image undergoes conventional processing, such as gradation processing and frequency processing [2, 3]. MFP and FNC image processing were carried out using a general-purpose personal computer running the image-processing software. The image can also be printed out life size using a dry laser printer (Fuji DP-L) with 10-bit grey levels. 40 sets of images for four treatment sites (brain, lung, anteroposterior (AP) pelvis, and lateral pelvis were selected. Six to 10 landmarks were selected as references, as in the study by Yin et al [10], for each treatment site. All images were obtained using a Mitsubishi ML-15MDX linear accelerator (Mitsubishi Electric Co., Ltd., Tokyo, Japan) operating at nominal beam energy of 4 MV photons with the system in linac-graphy (LG) mode. The dose rate in LG mode is a factor of 10 lower than that in therapy mode, so 1 monitor unit (MU) in LG mode is equivalent to approximately 1 mGy.

45 MU were required to produce a conventional double-exposure portal image (15 MU for the blocked field and 30 MU for the open field) for all treatment sites except the lateral pelvis, which required 90 MU: 30 MU for the blocked field and 60 MU for the open field. Image processing by both MFP and FNC used the same data.

Image processing

Multiobjective frequency processing (MFP)

MFP has two functions: a frequency enhancement function and a dynamic range compression function [2]. Figure 2 shows the steps involved in MFP. Band-pass filter images with various frequency components are produced by determining differences between the original and unsharp mask images (step b). Processing of each band-pass filter image for enhancement corresponding to the level of contrast is performed, and an image is produced by a combination of the enhanced images (step c). An MFP-processed image is obtained by superimposing the combined image onto the original image (step d).

In enhancement processing corresponding to the level of contrast, the degree of enhancement of each band-pass

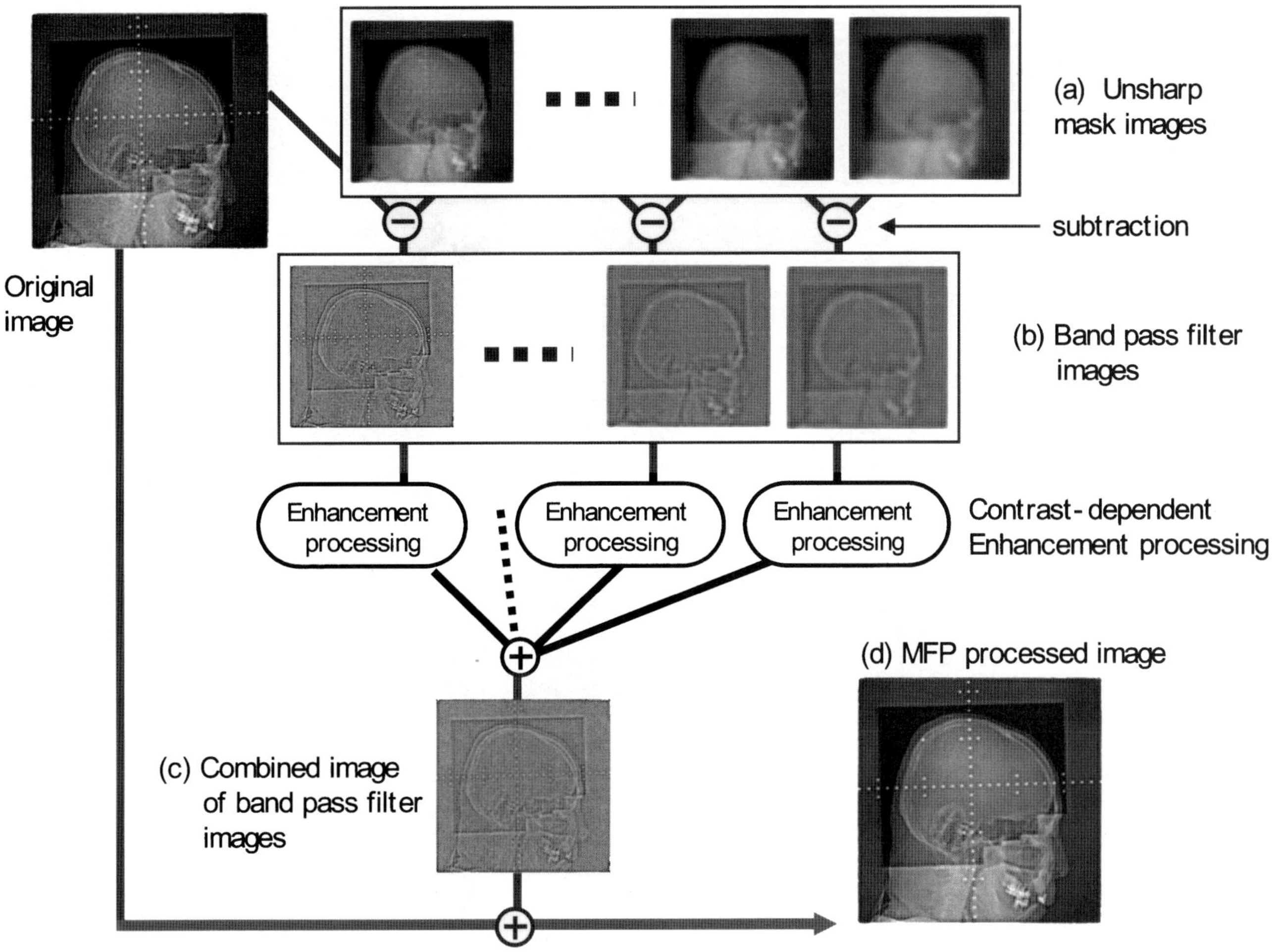

Figure 2. Outlines of multiobjective frequency processing (MFP). The original image and several unsharp mask images were prepared (step a). Several band-pass filter images were produced (step b) by subtraction processing of unsharp mask images with a similar frequency band. A combined image was produced (step c) by multiplying each band-pass filter image by each enhancement coefficient. An MFP image was obtained (step d) by adding the original image to the combined image.

signal is determined in the following way. If the input signal intensity is very much lower than the standard level, the output signal is produced by linear enhancement processing. If the input signal intensity is higher, processing with a non-linear coefficient that suppresses enhancement is performed. The enhancement in the periphery of the irradiation field, in which the contrast of portal imaging is sufficient, can be suppressed by MFP.

Dynamic range compression (DRC) widens the visible range. It compresses the dynamic ranges in areas with both low and high densities while maintaining the density contrast of images in intermediate ranges. DRC was used in conventional methods, but processing was restricted to either white areas or black areas. In MFP, DRC in both areas is possible, and so this processing method is now the most widely used for CR portal imaging in Japan.

The MFP parameters for portal imaging used for the observer study are briefly described in Appendix 1 (Table A1). These parameters are recommended for portal imaging in Japan by the manufacturers.

Flexible noise control processing (FNC)

FNC suppresses image noise whilst retaining diagnostically important contrast in anatomical structures. Figure 3 shows the steps involved in FNC processing. Band-pass filter images with various frequency components are produced (step b) by determining differences between the original and unsharp mask images (step a), as in MFP. Subsequently, noise components are extracted from each band-pass filter image. In the extraction of noise components, blur signals that exist in the periphery of linear structures are suppressed from linear structures in the direction of the lines. For the signals from dotted structures, those with low contrast below a fixed threshold are regarded as noise, and are suppressed. Signals with high contrast over a fixed threshold are maintained. Differences between images with only signal components extracted from the dotted and linear structures and the band-pass filter image are determined, providing an image with noise components alone. This processing is performed in each band-pass filter image. An image is produced (step d) by superimposing the images with only noise components in each frequency band. A noise-suppressed image is obtained (step e) by subtracting the combined noise components image from the original image. Routinely, the combined noise component image is subjected to MFP as described above.

In FNC processing it is necessary to define the noise level in order to distinguish between noise and signals from linear and dotted structures. In conventional diagnostic radiology the noise level is low for relatively high X-ray

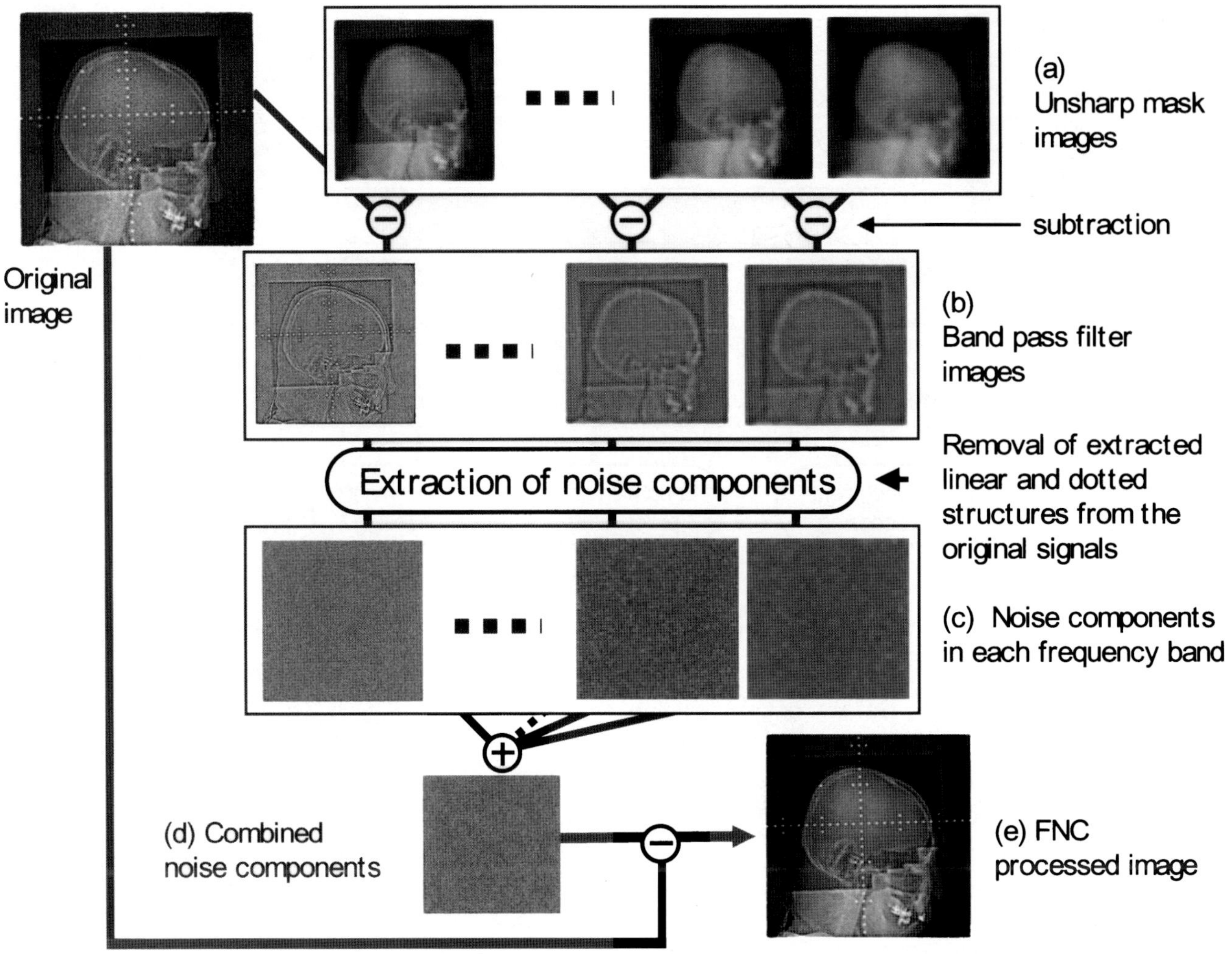

Figure 3. Outlines of flexible noise control processing (FNC). Several band-pass filter images were produced (step b) using several unsharp mask images, as in multiobjective frequency processing (MFP). Subsequently, images with extracted noise components alone were produced (step c), and an image with combined noise components was produced (step d). An FNC-processed image was obtained (step e) by subtracting the image with combined noise components from the original image. Routinely, the FNC-processed image was regarded as the original image, and was subjected to MFP.

doses, but increases as the dose decreases, and hence, for FNC processing in these circumstances, the noise level is defined for each incident dose. Noise suppression is then a function of the dose. In portal imaging, since noise will occur at any X-ray dose, we have established a method whereby noise can be suppressed irrespective of the incident dose. Table A1 (Appendix 1) also shows the parameters used for FNC processing, and again these parameters are briefly described in Appendix 1. These parameters were not optimized to improve the quality of portal images, but are the minimum parameters necessary in order to examine whether further improvement of the portal image quality can be obtained by the most commonly used MFP with additional FNC processing.

Observer study setup

Four treatment sites (brain, lung, AP pelvis, and lateral pelvis) with 40 sets of images (10 sets per site) were selected for the study. Each set was placed on a viewing box. Six to 10 landmarks were chosen for each treatment site. Of the observers, A and B were radiological technologists with more than 5 years of radiotherapy experience. Observers C and D were technologists with less than 3 years of radiotherapy experience but more than 5 years of experience in diagnosis, and observer E was an experienced radiation oncologist. With unlimited viewing time, each observer evaluated each set of images on the viewing box, and provided ratings in response to two questions.

The first question asked for a direct comparison of the MFP and FNC processed portal images of each landmark:

Question 1: Comparing the MFP and FNC-processed images, is the quality of the FNC-processed images higher than that of the MFP images? FNC processing is (1) much better, (2) slightly better, (3) comparable, (4) slightly worse, or (5) much worse.

The second question asked for a direct comparison of the ease of the overall verification of MFP and FNC processed portal images:

Question 2: Comparing the MFP and FNC-processed images, is the verification of the treatment areas easier on the FNC-processed images compared with that on the MFP images (overall impression)? The FNC processing is (1) much easier, (2) easier, (3) the same, (4) harder, or (5) much harder.

To summarize the data, the ratings were treated as quantitative scores, and the means were computed for each observer for each question. For question 1 the effects of FNC processing is indicated as better (score<3), comparable (score=3), and worse (score>3).

Question 2 data were used to compare the proportions of rates that were "much easier", "easier", and "the same" (score<4) for the ease of verification. These ratings indicate the possibility that FNC-processed images can be clinically used instead of MFP images. These questions and the selected landmarks were determined following the method of Yin et al [10] who conducted an observer study on the direct comparison of clinical efficacy.

Results and discussion

Figure 4 shows examples of MFP-processed images on the left and corresponding FNC-processed images on the right. Figure 5 is similar but shows parts of the images after magnification. The results of the observer study in respect of the image quality for each landmark are shown in Table 1. In the brain (Figure 4a and 4b), the image quality in all anatomical parameters other than peripheral skin was judged to be improved by FNC processing. The contrast on the peripheral skin was adequate on the MFP images and this is why a high proportion was judged to be comparable. Figure 5a and 5b show the pituitary fossa region after magnification. The quality of the FNC-processed image of the pituitary fossa was judged to be better in 60% of cases.

Table 1. Proportion of images for which flexible noise control (FNC) was rated "better", "comparable" or "worse" than multi-objective frequency processing (MFP), by site and landmark

Site	Landmark	Better	Comparable	Worse
Brain	Peripheral skin	0.36	0.62	0.02
	Skull brim	0.68	0.22	0.10
	Frontal sinus	0.56	0.24	0.20
	Spheroid sinus	0.64	0.22	0.14
	Maxillary sinus	0.72	0.16	0.12
	Mastoid air cells	0.70	0.10	0.20
	Pituitary fossa	0.60	0.24	0.16
	Vertebral bodies	0.68	0.12	0.20
Lung	Lung airspace	0.84	0.12	0.04
	Trachea	0.56	0.32	0.12
	Bronchi-carina	0.44	0.34	0.22
	Clavicle	0.58	0.40	0.02
	Lung apex	0.70	0.18	0.12
	Ribs	0.42	0.20	0.38
	Aortic arch	0.38	0.48	0.14
	Vertebral bodies	0.60	0.08	0.32
AP pelvis	Pelvic brim	0.60	0.16	0.24
	Ilio-pectineal line	0.34	0.40	0.26
	Pubic symphysis	0.20	0.56	0.24
	Ischial-tuberosity	0.60	0.12	0.28
	Sacroiliac joint	0.62	0.10	0.28
	Acetabulum	0.62	0.16	0.22
	Femoral head	0.70	0.16	0.14
Lateral pelvis	Pubic symphysis	0.46	0.38	0.16
	Acetabulum	0.64	0.08	0.28
	Femoral head	0.58	0.12	0.30
	Sacrum	0.74	0.12	0.14

In the lung (Figure 4c and 4d), high scores for "better" were obtained with the anatomical parameters of lung space and lung apex (Figure 5c and 5d). However, in the ribs, the rates of "better" and "worse" were 0.42 and 0.38, respectively, indicating that opinion was almost equally divided. The image quality of regions with low frequency signals, such as the bone edges of ribs, was improved by FNC processing, but the image quality of regions with high frequency signals, such as the trabeculae of ribs, was not improved because signals were attenuated together with the noise. The divided opinion may, therefore, have been because different observers focused on different features.

In the AP pelvis, the rating of "better" generally had a high proportion showing a preference for FNC processing. In this study, images of prostate patients were mainly used. For anatomical landmarks in high-density areas of the irradiation field, such as the pubic symphysis (Figure 5e and 5f) and iliopectineal line, the comparable ratings were 0.56 and 0.40, respectively, indicating no particular improvement by FNC processing. In the lateral pelvis, the usefulness of FNC processing was observed in the sacrum, in which a high level of noise was present in MFP images (Figure 4e and 4f).

Table 2 summarizes the overall evaluation of each treatment site. The rates of "much easier", "easier", and "the same" (score <4) in question 2 are shown for each observer. These ratings indicate that FNC-processed images may be used clinically instead of MFP images. Observers A, B, and E with significant experience of radiotherapy answered that the verification of treatment areas was easier on the FNC-processed images. However, observers C and D with longer experience of diagnostic radiography than radiotherapy indicated higher rates of difficulty in evaluating the treatment areas on FNC-processed images than those encountered by the other observers.

The large differences in evaluating the effectiveness of FNC processing between the observers were not considered to have been caused by differences in the experience of radiotherapy, but the observers with long experience in diagnostic radiology considered that CR portal imaging was diagnostically important and were uncomfortable when diagnostic information was diminished. However, for treatment verification purposes the ability to recognize outlines is generally considered to be more important, and so the processing in this study was primarily intended to enhance the outlines of bones and tumours. If the

Table 2. Proportion of images for which flexible noise control (FNC) was rated "much easier", "easier", and "the same" for the ease of making a verification compared with that with multi-objective frequency processing (MFP), by site and reader

Site	Reader A	Reader B	Reader C	Reader D	Reader E
Brain	1.00	1.00	0.70	0.70	1.00
Lung	1.00	1.00	0.70	0.40	1.00
AP pelvis	1.00	1.00	0.80	0.20	1.00
Lateral pelvis	1.00	0.90	0.50	0.60	1.00

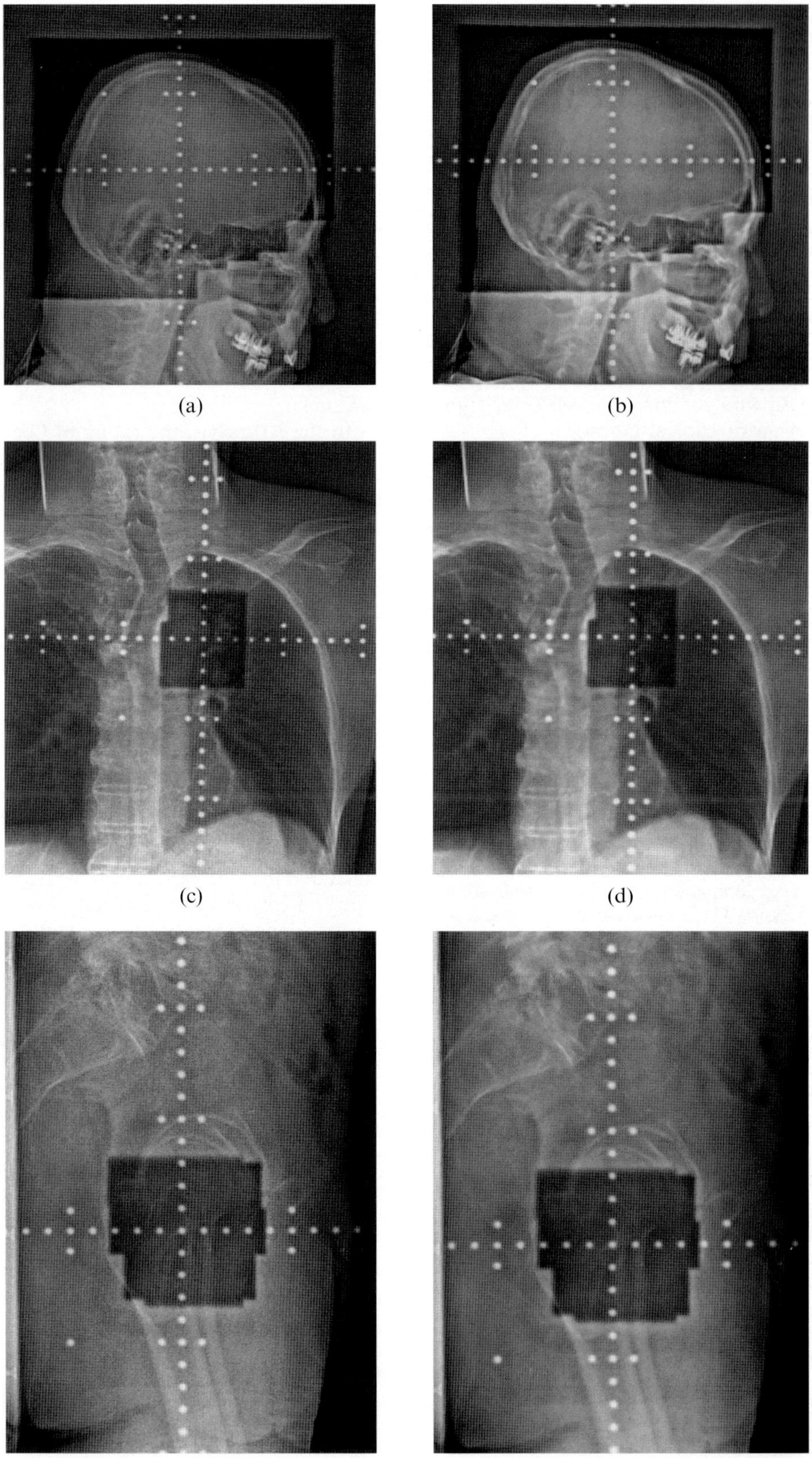

Figure 4. Sample images of multiobjective frequency processing (MFP) and flexible noise control (FNC). The upper panels (a, b) show the head, the middle panels (c, d) show the chest, and the lower panels. (e, f) show the lateral pelvis. The left panels (a, c, e) are MFP images, and the right panels (b, d, f) are FNC images.

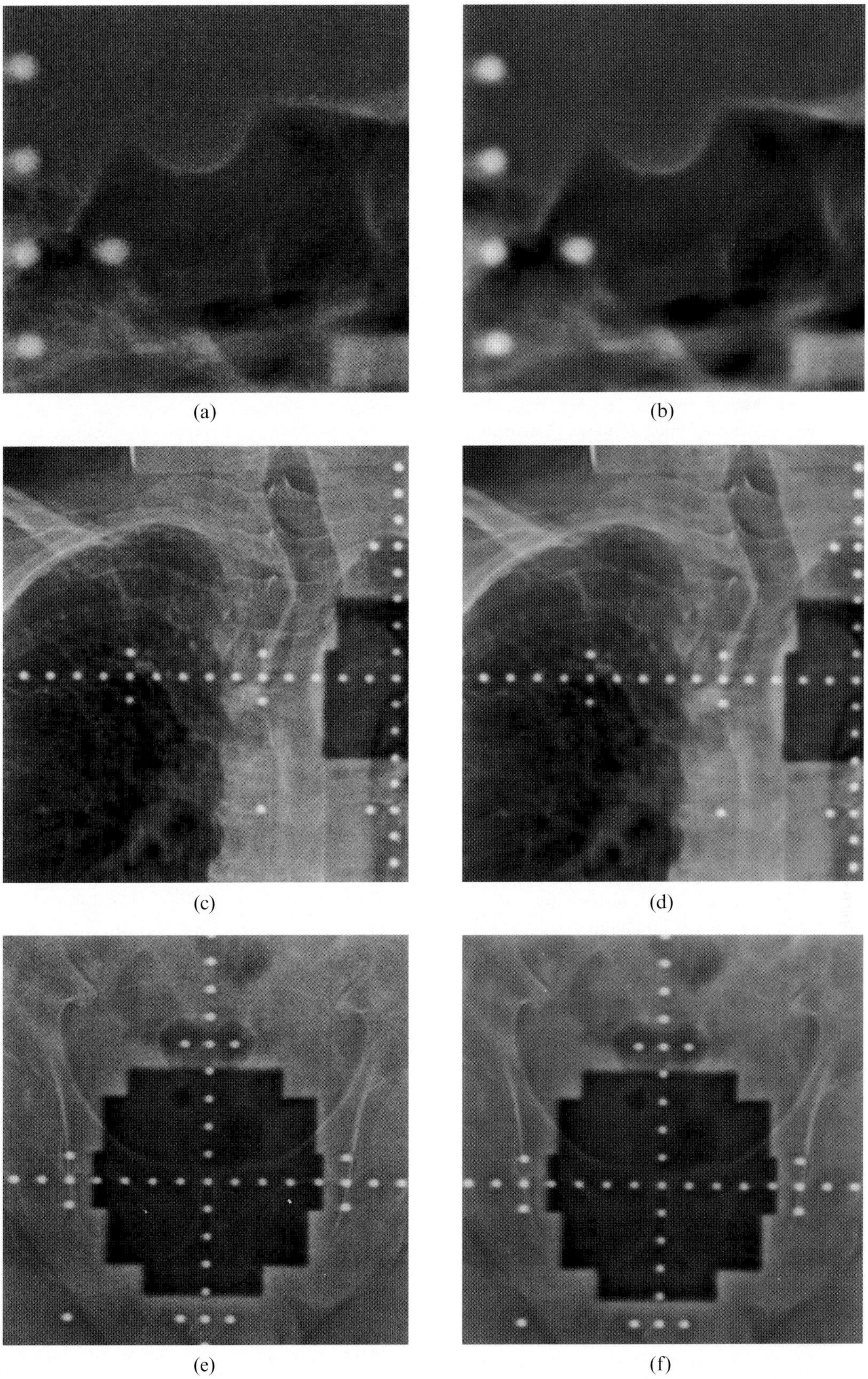

Figure 5. Parts of the multiobjective frequency processing (MFP) and flexible noise control (FNC) images after magnification. The upper panels (a, b) show the pituitary fossa, the middle panels (c, d) show the lung apex, and the lower panels (e, f) show the pubic symphysis. The left panels (a, c, e) are MFP images, and the right panels (b, d, f) are FNC images.

Table A1. Parameters of image processing used for the observer study

Parameters used for multiobjective frequency processing (MEP)						
	MRB	MRT	MRE	MDB	MDT	MDE
ALL MFP Images	C	F	5.0	G	P	0.4
Parameters used for flexible noise control image processing (FNC)						
	FFC	FNB	FNT		FNE	
ALL FNC Images	M (for portal images)	C	A		0.7	

outlining information is adequate then images that retain more diagnostic information may be regarded as better. The observer study therefore, becomes very subjective and we must clarify definitions to improve image quality.

The parameters of MFP images used in this study were adjusted to optimize the image quality by MFP alone, taking the level of noise on the images into consideration. In future studies, variable MFP parameters should be adjusted to show each anatomical parameter with the highest signal intensity without taking noise distributed on the image into consideration, and then FNC processing should be performed, which will markedly improve the image quality of the AP pelvis, where the contrast is low.

In this study, FNC processing at a certain level of suppression was performed in all density areas on the images. However, the effect of FNC processing on the improvement of the image quality was poor in high-density areas, and therefore, it would be better to select variable parameters by which the degree of noise-suppression is low in these areas. With regard to the risk of suppression of useful signals by FNC processing, it would also be useful to evaluate the threshold for the distinction between signals and noise.

Conclusion

Where the use of portal imaging is for treatment verification purposes, additional FNC processing, which provides clear bone edge signals, is considered worthwhile as the image quality is increased in the lung airspace and bone edges. The performance of FNC in the brain was especially good.

We hope that the CR system will become more widely used and replace the film method, and a future aim is to develop a portal imaging system that provides image quality equivalent to the CR system and convenience similar to the EPID.

Acknowledgments

We sincerely thank Mr Ryoji Sasada and other staff of Fujifilm Medical Co., Ltd. in Miyanodai, Japan.

References

1. Wilenzick RM, Merritt CR, Balter S. Megavoltage portal films using computed radiographic imaging with photo stimulable phosphors. Med Phys 1987;14:389–92.
2. Iwasaki N. Image processing. In: Iwasaki N. Fuji computed radiography. Japan: Fujifilm Medical Co., Ltd Press, 2000:29–51.
3. Ishida M. Image processing. In: Tateno Y, Iinuma T, Takano M. Computed radiography. Japan: Springer-Verlag, 1987:25–30.
4. Yabutani T, Endo Y, Suzuki S, Kato H, Kitazawa H, Sawada T. Effect of frequency processing on portal imaging in computed radiography. Jpn J Radiol Technol 1997;53:380–5.
5. Yamada S, Murase K. Analysis of frequency components of CR portal images and application to multi-objective frequency processing. Jpn J Radiol Technol 2003;59:864–71.
6. Sasagaki M, Matsumoto M, Mori Y. CR portal imaging –A linac graphy using storage phosphor imaging systems. Jpn J Radiol Technol 1992;48:984–90.
7. Sato H, Yokozawa M, Nishizawa M. Study of intensifying metallic plate for linac graphy using computed radiography. Jpn J Radiol Technol 1997;53:1479–86.
8. Iwasaki N. Flexible noise control. Fuji Medical Review, 2004;12:25–32.
9. Sato H, Yokozawa M, Tanaka K, Sakai H. Study of cassette system for linacography using computed radiography: application of a heavy metallic sheet to the metallic plate. Jpn J Radiol Technol 1999;55:198–204.
10. Yin FF, Rubin P, Schell MC, Wynn R, Raubertas RF, Uschold G, et al. An observer study for direct comparison of clinical efficacy of electronic to film portal images. Int J Radiat Oncol Biol Phys 1996;35:985–91.

Appendix 1

Parameters used in the two processing methods. The six parameters used in multiobjective frequency processing are:

1. Multi-frequency balance type (MRB)

MRB determines the frequency characteristics of enhanced images. Six types are available. Type A mainly enhances lower frequency and type F, higher frequency. In this study, type C was used.

2. Multi-frequency enhancing type (MRT)

MRT is a parameter of the enhancement factor function. MRT determines the shape of the function when the maximum degree of enhancement is normalized to 1.0. Eleven types are available. In this study, type F was used. With type F, the maximum degree of enhancement is performed irrespective of the image density.

3. Degree of multi-frequency enhancement (MRE)

MRE determines the degree of enhancement. Value ranges from 0.0 to 9.9 and 10 to 16.

4. Multi-DRC balance type (MDB)

MDB determines the frequency characteristics of smoothed images. Seven balance types are available.

With type G, it is possible to obtain smoothed images with the best edge images.

5. Multi-DRC enhancing type (MDT)

18 types are available. With type P both high-density areas and low-density areas were appropriately corrected.

6. Degree of multi-DRC enhancement (MDE)

MDE determines the degree of enhancement. Value ranges from 0.0 to 1.0.

Parameters used for FNC processing

The four parameters used in FNC processing are:

1. Filter control type of FNC (FFC)

FFC determines the degree of noise-suppressive processing depending on the radiation dose. FFC has modes A and M. With mode A, noise-suppressive processing becomes higher with decreases in the dose. This was intended for use in diagnostic radiography. With mode M, noise-suppressive processing is performed at a fixed level irrespective of the dose. This was developed for CR portal imaging. In this study, mode M was used.

2. Balance type of FNC (FNB)

FNB determines the degree of noise-suppressive processing in relation to frequency components. FNB has modes A to F. With mode A, noise is suppressed in all ranges from low-frequency components to high-frequency components. With modes in alphabetical order, noise-suppressive processing is performed in higher frequency components. In this study, mode C was used. With mode C, noise suppression is performed in a frequency range of over 0.4 cycles mm^{-1}.

3. Type of FNC (FNT)

FNT determines the degree of noise-suppressive processing in relation to the image density. FNT has modes A, B, and C. With mode A, noise-suppressive processing is constant irrespective of the image density. With mode B, the degree of noise-suppressive processing becomes low with increasing density, while with mode C, it becomes high with decreasing density. In this study, mode A was used.

4. Enhancement of FNC (FNE)

FNE determines the degree of noise-suppressive processing in the range of 0.0–1.0. Noise-suppressive processing is highest at 1.0, and processing is not performed at 0.0. In this study, FNE was performed at 0.7.

The British Journal of Radiology, 78 (2005), 528–532 © 2005 The British Institute of Radiology
DOI: 10.1259/bjr/82990907

Comparative analyses of the dynamic properties of the bladder wall studied by repetitive pelvic CT scans of patients and cryo-sections of cadavers

[1]E DALE, PhD, [1,2]T P HELLEBUST, MSc, [1,3]Ø S BRULAND, MD, PhD and [1,2]D R OLSEN, PhD

[1]*Centre for Training and Research in Radiotherapy,* [2]*Department of Medical Physics and* [3]*Department of Oncology, The Norwegian Radium Hospital, University of Oslo, Box 20, N-0310 Oslo, Norway*

Abstract. In radiotherapy planning systems, delineation of hollow normal tissue organs, such as the bladder, is time-consuming. Automated delineation may presuppose two assumptions: (1) the bladder resembles a spherical shell and (2) the volume of bladder tissue is preserved regardless of the volume of urine (luminal volume) inside. The purpose of the present study was to test these assumptions. 22 CT scans from 7 patients were studied retrospectively. Transverse cross-sectional areas enclosed by the outer contour (A_{out}) and inner contour of the bladder (A_{in}) were recorded from the images. Hence, the transverse cross-sectional area of the wall, $A_{wall}=A_{out}-A_{in}$, and the volume of bladder tissue at various luminal volumes, could be calculated. To quantify the method uncertainty, the same procedure was applied on three spherical plastic phantoms. The results were also compared with data from the Visible Human Project's photographs of cadaver cryo-sections. Assumption no. 1 stated above, implies that A_{wall} is constant regardless of the level of intersection of the sphere. The data from cryo-sections revealed a positive correlation for A_{wall} and A_{out}, in contradiction to assumption no. 1 ($p<0.001$). The corresponding association derived from the repetitive CT scans of patients was also statistically significant ($p<0.001$) although linear regression revealed a less steep slope. A relationship was found between the volume of bladder tissue and luminal volume, hence contradicting assumption no. 2 ($p<0.001$). In conclusion the cross-sectional wall areas of the bladder, measured from patient CT scans, increase slightly with luminal cross-sectional areas in contradiction to expected values derived from a simplistic spherical shell model. In addition, the volume of bladder tissue is related to the luminal volume. Our results may be of practical value when developing automated delineation tools in radiotherapy planning systems.

In modern three-dimensional (3D) radiotherapy planning, based on serial CT scans, accurate definition of normal tissue organs surrounding a tumour, as well as the tumour itself, is of paramount importance. Dose–volume histograms (DVH) are obtained from the CT volumes by delineating contours around the involved structures, and calculating the dose to each subvolume within the contour. The DVHs can be used to assess the normal tissue complication probability (NTCP) and tumour control probability (TCP) associated with the dose plan in question [1]. Organs of the human body that are hollow represent special challenges. The materials filling hollow organs are irrelevant from a clinical point of view and should be excluded from the DVH [2]. The luminal subvolumes may be removed from the DVH by delineating both an outer contour enclosing the external organ border as well as an inner contour demarcating the wall tissue from the lumen. Only subvolumes between the outer and inner contours are included in the DVH calculations. However, one has to delineate the double number of contours. This makes it a time-consuming task to obtain the DVH of a hollow organ structure. Meijer et al have reported a strategy to delineate the rectal inner contours automatically, based on manually drawn outer contours [3]. They proposed a cylindrical shell model for the rectum with an elastic wall undergoing changes in shape and size as a response to variable local luminal volume. The cylinder comprised thin transverse slices, each assumed to have the same constant wall volume regardless of luminal volume. Hence, knowing the location of the outer contour only, enabled the authors to calculate the position of the inner contour assuming a constant slice (annulus) volume [3]. In a recent study, Dale et al found that the rectal wall volume has a more complex dependence with luminal volume [4]: the rectal wall volume within a fixed longitudinal length of the rectum was not constant but increased with luminal volume.

The present study expands on this observation investigating another important dose-limiting hollow organ in pelvic radiotherapy, namely the urinary bladder. Located retroperitoneally and attached to the musculature of the pelvic floor, the bladder may expand relatively freely towards the peritoneal cavity with increased luminal volume. The shape of the bladder varies with the volume of urine inside, resembling a spherical shell when distended, but more like a tetrahedron with rounded edges at smaller volumes of urine [5].

The aim of the present study was to investigate whether (1) a spherical shell model may adequately model the bladder's shape and (2) the total bladder tissue volume is preserved regardless of total luminal volume. For this purpose, repetitive CT examinations of cervix cancer patients were applied, supported by area and volume measurements from CT studies of spherical hollow phantoms of relevant size. In addition, measurements

Received 5 May 2004 and in revised form 16 November 2004, accepted 13 January 2005.

from digital photographs (and corresponding CT images) of transverse cryo-sections of a male and female cadaver (US National Library of Medicine's Visible Human Project) were included (Figure 1).

Methods and materials

Repetitive CT scans of patients

22 repetitive CT examinations of 7 cervix cancer patients enrolled in a previous clinical study [6], were analysed. Two patients had two CT scans, three patients had three CT scans, and two patients had four and five CT scans each. Patients were included after informed consent was obtained, and the study was approved by a local research ethics committee. In the present report, the patient material was used to investigate the variation of cross-sectional areas and volumes of the bladder at different time points. Variations in bladder volumes were random. The CT scanner was a helical single detector, Siemens Emotion (Siemens, Erlangen, Germany), and the examinations were performed without contrast and with 3–5 mm slice thickness with an image resolution of 0.8–0.9 mm pixel^{-1}. Minimum time interval between the first and last CT scan was 1 day and maximum was 24 days. Bladder contours were delineated by one of the authors (ED) on the radiotherapy dose planning system (PLATO, Nucletron BV) using a Silicon Graphic workstation. In each image the following data were found (Figure 2):

- A_{out}=The transverse cross-sectional area enclosed by the outer contour of the organ, *i.e.* including wall tissue and lumen.

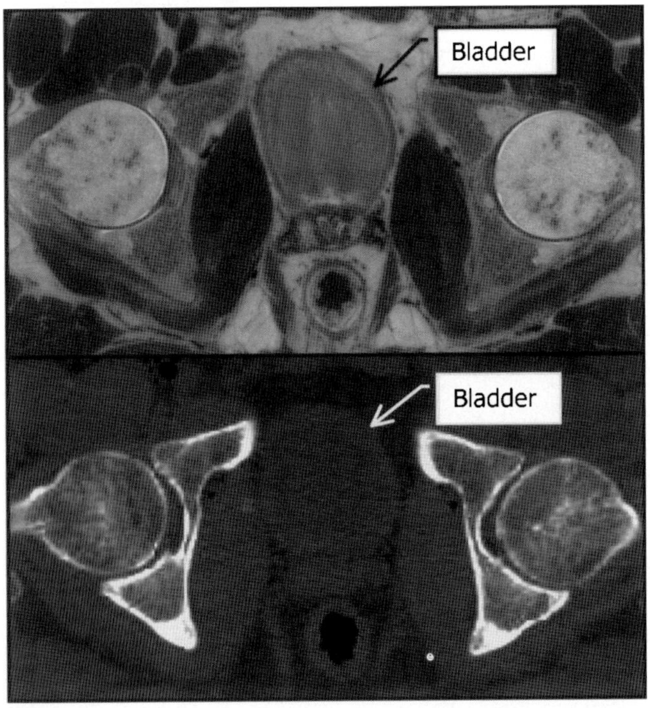

Figure 1. Example of a photograph of a cadaver cryo-section (US National Library of Medicine's Visible Human Project) from a male pelvis (top) compared with the corresponding CT image (bottom).

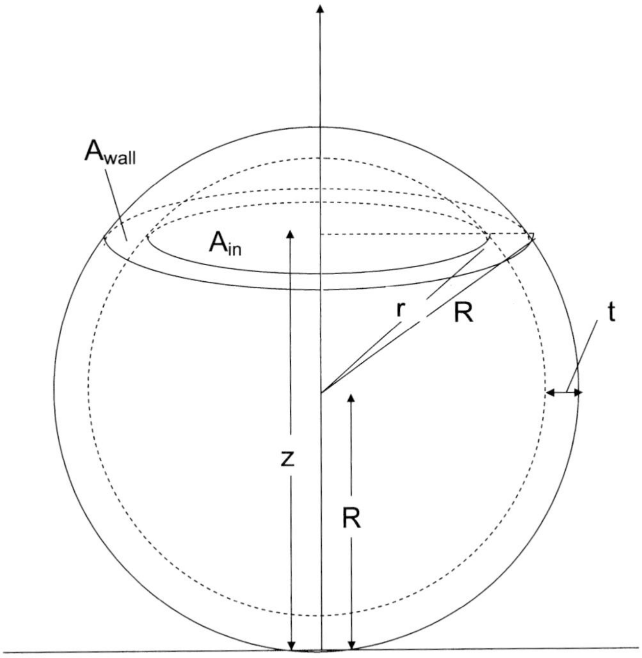

Figure 2. The spherical shell model for bladder. Symbols are explained in Appendix 1.

- A_{in}=The transverse cross-sectional area enclosed by the inner contour of the organ, *i.e.* the transverse area of the lumen.
- $A_{wall}=A_{out}-A_{in}$, the transverse cross-sectional area of the organ wall.

The theoretical formulas for the cross-sectional areas, A_{out}, A_{in} and A_{wall}, of a spherical shell as function of position along an axis through the sphere's centre, are outlined in Appendix 1. The main point in this model is that A_{wall} is constant and independent of A_{out}, assuming the cavity of the sphere is included in the cross-section.

Volume calculations based on delineation of all bladder contours were also performed with PLATO:

- V_{out}=The total volume of the bladder (outer volume).
- V_{in}=The total volume of lumen (inner volume).
- $V_{wall}=V_{out}-V_{in}$=The total bladder tissue volume.

CT scans of spherical phantoms

The purpose of the phantom study was to estimate the uncertainties in the results from the patient study. Three spherical, hollow toy balls (36 cm^3, 109 cm^3 and 380 cm^3) made of relatively rigid plastic (1.3 g cm^{-3}) were used. Two small holes were made in each ball. Water was instilled through one hole, and air removed through the other hole. An attempt was made to measure the volume of instilled water, but this proved to be too difficult due to water leakage during instillation. After complete water instillation, the holes were sealed and the balls (phantoms) were put into a water tank, fixed with nylon threads and CT scanned (3 mm slice thickness). The inner and outer contours of the phantoms were delineated on the CT images by the same author as above (ED) using PLATO. Thus, the same procedure used to obtain areas and volumes from the urinary bladders of patients, was performed to obtain areas and volumes of the plastic phantoms. The three phantoms were delineated three times each in order to acquire nine sets of measurements. These CT volume data were compared with values obtained by immersing the phantoms in water and measuring the displaced volume of water. The latter volume determination method was repeated five times for each phantom with water inside. Afterwards, the phantoms were cut into pieces (the water inside was removed) and total wall volumes of each phantom were determined, again using the displacement of water principle.

Photographs of cadaver cryo-sections

Digital photographs of cadaver slices (1 male and 1 female) and corresponding CT images obtained from the US National Library of Medicine's Visible Human Project, were imported into GNU Image Manipulation Program v1.2 (GIMP – freeware by P Mattis and S Kimball) on a personal computer (PC). Outer and inner contours of the bladder were delineated every 1 mm and every 3 mm for cadaver and CT images, respectively. The delineation was performed by the same author as above (ED) and reviewed by an experienced oncologist (ØSB). The number of image pixels within each contour was obtained. The cadaver image resolution was 0.33 mm pixel^{-1}, CT image resolution 1.0 mm pixel^{-1}, and the area within each contour could thus be calculated. Bladder volumes were determined from the sum of the areas from all contours multiplied by image slice thickness.

Statistics

The analysis was performed with univariate linear regression using Microsoft Excel 97. A significant correlation between two variables was revealed by testing if the slope parameter differed significantly from zero comparing the appropriate statistics with the *t*-distribution of $n-2$ degrees of freedom [7]. Only two-sided tests were performed and *p*-values less than 0.05 were considered statistically significant.

Results

Cross-sectional area and volume measurements from repetitive CT scans of patients

Area measurements from repetitive CT scans of one patient is shown in Figure 3. The area within the outer bladder contour (A_{out}) varied substantially with caudocranial position (explained by the shape of the bladder) and from scan to scan (explained by variable filling).

To compare area measurements from different scan days and patients in the same diagram, all area data were normalized by dividing by the mean area of each scan. The area of the wall tissue (A_{wall}) increased slightly with A_{out}, although statistically significantly (R^2=0.18, $p<0.001$, Figure 4). Also, the wall volume (V_{wall}) as a function of total volume (V_{out}) yielded a significant association (R^2=0.72, $p<0.001$, Figure 5).

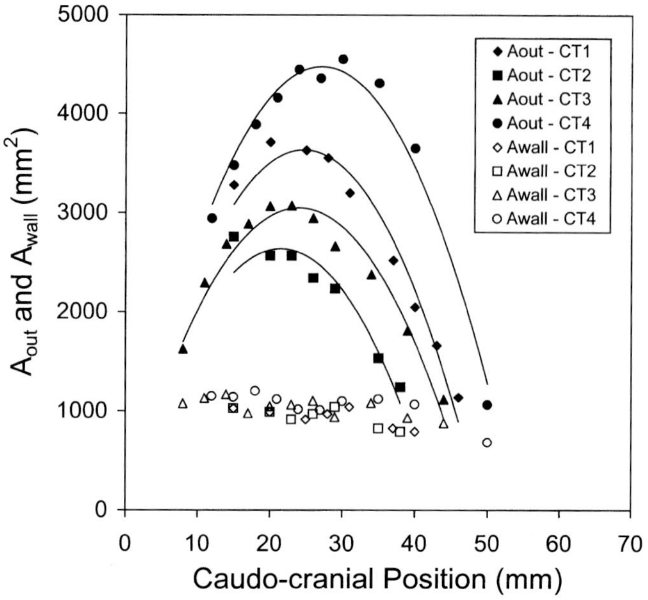

Figure 3. Transverse cross-sectional areas of the urinary bladder as a function of caudocranial position as determined from four repetitive CT scans of the same patient. Second order polynomials have been fitted to the A_{out} data in agreement with theory (Appendix 1).

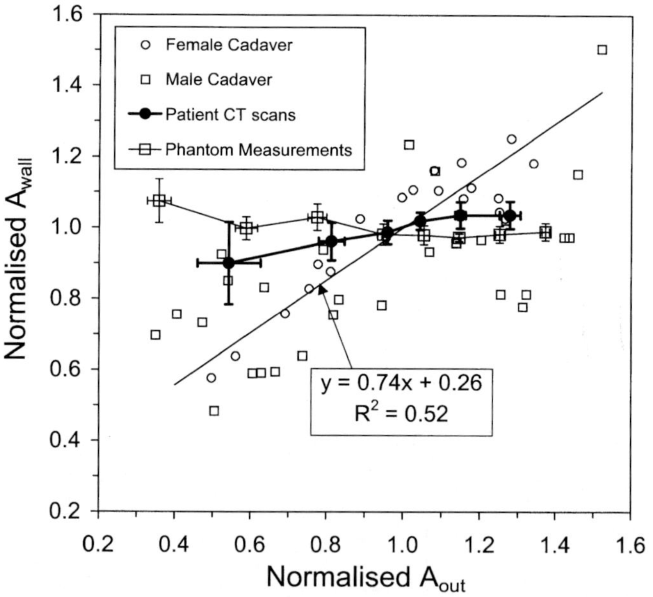

Figure 4. Normalized A_{wall} (transverse cross-sectional area of the wall tissue divided by the mean A_{wall} of each CT scan) as a function of normalized A_{out} (transverse cross-sectional area enclosed by the outer contour of the bladder divided by the mean A_{out} of the same CT scan). A linear regression line has been fitted to the cryo-section data while the patient and phantom data have been pooled (for clarity) showing mean values with 95% confidence intervals. Bin size was chosen to achieve a bin width of 0.15–0.20 along the abscissa. Linear regression analysis applied on the patient CT scan data gave y=0.21x+0.79 (R^2=0.18, $p<0.001$, n=123), *i.e.* a considerably smaller, although statistically significant slope compared with the slope of the line fitted to the cryo-section data: y=0.74x+0.26 (R^2=0.52, $p<0.001$, n=52). Linear regression applied on the phantom study provided a slight negative association: $y=-0.076x+1.08$ (R^2=0.11, $p<0.001$, n=171).

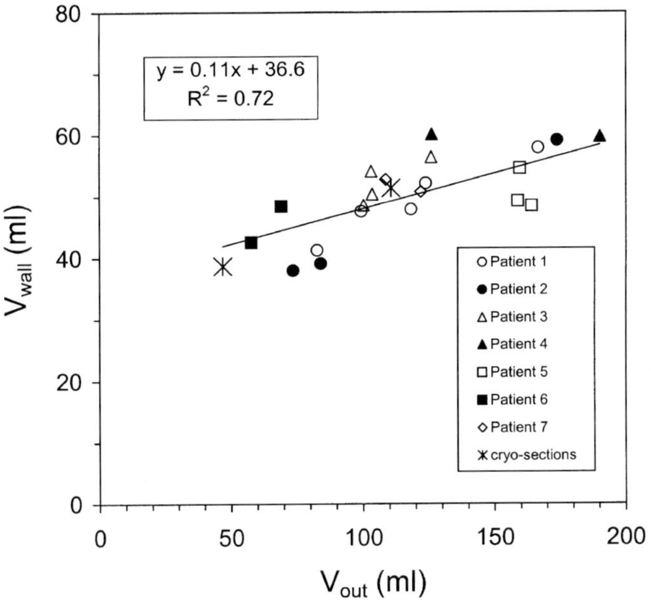

Figure 5. Volume of bladder wall (V_{wall}) as a function of total bladder volume (V_{out}) from repetitive CT examinations on our own patients and from cadaver cryo-sections. Linear regression gave a statistically significant association between V_{out} and V_{wall} (R^2=0.72, p<0.001, n=24).

Cross sectional area and volume measurements from CT scans of spherical phantoms

To validate the data from CT scans of patients, similar measurements via outlining on CT were performed on three hollow plastic spheres of different sizes. The measurements were repeated three times for each phantom to quantify the uncertainties involved. In accordance with the spherical shell model there is no positive correlation between A_{wall} and A_{out} in contrast to the results from CT scans of patients (Figure 4). On the contrary, there was a slight negative association, probably explained by a delineation artefact (R^2=0.11, p<0.001).

The outer volume and wall volume of the plastic spheres were determined by the displacement of water principle. Within acceptable uncertainty, these volumes were in agreement with corresponding values obtained from measurements from CT images. No systematic trends in the errors between water and CT measurements (size of the objects or outer versus inner volumes) were observed (Table 1).

Cross-sectional area measurements from cadaver cryo-sections

Area measurements from The Visible Human cadaver cryo-sections corresponded well with measurements obtained from the CT images of the same cadavers (R^2 in the interval 0.94–0.98 for A_{out} and A_{in}, and 0.83 for A_{wall}), thus supporting the use of CT to measure areas and volumes of the human bladder (Table 1). Diagrams of area measurements as a function of caudocranial location were comparable with the results obtained from patient CT scans (data not shown). Linear regression applied on the relationship between A_{wall} and A_{out} yielded a linear function with a steeper slope (0.74±0.20, slope coefficient±95% CI) compared with the slope obtained from the patient CT scan data (0.21±0.08, slope coefficient±95% CI) (Figure 4).

Table 1. Results from all volume measurements. Water: V_{in} has been calculated from $V_{in}=V_{out}-V_{wall}$. CT/cryo-photos: V_{wall} has been calculated from $V_{wall}=V_{out}-V_{in}$. NA: Not available. The bladder of the female cadaver was almost empty (V_{in}=8.1 ml), and it was not possible to delineate the inner contour on the CT images because of inferior contrast between wall tissue and lumen. Hence, V_{in} and V_{wall} were NA for this particular case. n=number of measurements

		Water/cryo-photos (ml)	CT (ml)
Patients (n=22)	V_{out}	NA	130±52
	V_{in}	NA	79±55
	V_{wall}	NA	52±8
Phantom 1	V_{out}	35.6±0.2	36.2, 36.2, 37.7
(Water: n=5)	V_{in}	22.5±0.3	23.3, 23.0, 23.2
(CT: n=3)	V_{wall}	13.1±0.2	12.9, 13.2, 14.5
Phantom 2	V_{out}	106.9±1.1	108, 109, 109
(Water: n=5)	V_{in}	78.0±1.1	81.0, 81.0, 80.7
(CT: n=3)	V_{wall}	28.9±0.2	27.0, 28.0, 28.3
Phantom 3	V_{out}	380.4±1.1	377, 380, 383
(Water: n=5)	V_{in}	321.9±1.2	322, 318, 317
(CT: n=3)	V_{wall}	58.5±0.5	55, 62, 66
Cadaver ♀	V_{out}	46.8	47.2
(n=1)	V_{in}	8.1	NA
	V_{wall}	38.7	NA
Cadaver ♂	V_{out}	110.6	112.6
(n=1)	V_{in}	59.2	61.3
	V_{wall}	51.4	49.3

Discussion

The aim of this study was to investigate the variation of urinary bladder wall volume as a function of variable luminal volume, both locally in transverse cross-sections, and globally looking at the whole bladder. Theoretical calculations of cross-sectional wall areas (A_{wall}) of a spherical shell showed that A_{wall} is independent of the cross-sectional area enclosed by the outer contour (A_{out}). Measurements on CT scans of human bladders revealed a slight but detectable relationship between A_{wall} and A_{out} in theoretical disagreement with the sphere model. A similar relationship was found from measurements on photographs of cadaver cryo-sections, although with a steeper slope. The explanation may be a larger heterogeneity in the patient study data, yielding a lower slope.

The validity of the method of delineating contours on computer images to measure cross-sectional areas is not obvious. Our findings could have been explained by a delineation artefact. Therefore, cross-sectional areas of three spherical phantoms similar to the human bladder, were measured repeatedly using the same methodology. The results from the phantom experiments show that the normalized A_{wall} is approximately unity for all normalized A_{out}. This is in reasonable agreement with the spherical shell model, indicating that the delineation method is not significantly biased. However, this method is limited by the improved contrast between plastic and water compared with the contrast between bladder tissue and urine.

The measured area data from the patient CT scans were not in agreement with the spherical shell model.

Correspondingly, a relationship between wall volume and luminal volume was obtained employing the CT scans of individuals with variable bladder volume at different times. The reason for variable bladder tissue volume at variable luminal volume is not evident. Dale et al have reported similar results for the rectum in a previous study using the same methodology [4]. Generally, the bladder detrusor muscle consists of smooth muscle cells with tonic activity. As the bladder is filled, intermittent micturition contractions appear, with higher frequency and force at larger luminal volumes [8]. Kershen et al found an increased blood flow in the detrusor muscle as the bladder was filled [9]. The enlarged tissue volume with increased luminal volume, found in the present study, may be explained by raised blood perfusion. This reflects the metabolic demands of the detrusor at larger luminal volumes [10].

In conclusion, we have found that the cross-sectional wall areas of the bladder differ slightly but significantly from expected values derived from a simplistic spherical shell model. The bladder tissue volume is related to luminal volume. Our results may be of practical value, for instance when developing hollow organ delineation tools in radiotherapy planning systems.

Acknowledgment

The authors are indebted to Professor Hans Hedlund and Consultant Urologist Trygve Talseth at Department of Urology, Rikshospitalet University Hospital for valuable discussions on bladder blood flow studies.

References

1. Lyman JT. Complication probability as assessed from dose-volume histograms. Radiat Res 1985;104:S13.
2. Lu Y, Song PY, Li S, Spelbring DR, Vijayakumar S, Haraf DJ, et al. A method of analyzing rectal surface area irradiated and rectal complication in prostate conformal radiotherapy. Int J Radiat Oncol Biol Phys 1995;33:1121.
3. Meijer GJ, Van den Brink M, Hoogeman MS, Meinders J, Lebesque JV. Dose wall histograms and normalised dose surface histograms for the rectum. A new method to analyze the dose distribution over the rectum in conformal radiotherapy. Int J Radiat Oncol Biol Phys 1999;45:1073.
4. Dale E, Hellebust TP, Bruland ØSB, Olsen DR. Comparative analyses of the dynamic properties of the rectum studied by cryo-sections of human cadavers and pelvic CT scans of patients. Br J Radiol 2003;76:104–8.
5. Moore KL, Dalley AF. Pelvis and perineum. In: Clinically oriented anatomy (4th edn). Philadelphia, PA: Lippincott, 1999:331–430.
6. Hellebust TP, Dale E, Skjønsberg A, Olsen DR. Inter-fraction variations in rectum and bladder volumes and dose distributions during high dose rate brachytherapy treatment of the uterine cervix investigated by repetitive CT-examinations. Radiother Oncol 2001;60:273–80.
7. Larsen RJ, Marx LM. An introduction to mathematical statistics and its applications (2nd edn). New Jersey: Prentice-Hall, 1986.
8. Guyton AC, Hall JE. Micturition, diuretics and kidney diseases. In: Textbook of Medical Physiology (9th edn). Philadelphia, PA: W. B. Saunders Co., 1996:405-24.
9. Kershen RT, Azadzoi KM, Siroky MB. Blood flow, pressure and compliance in the male human bladder. J Urol 2002;168:121–5.
10. Guyton AC, Hall JE. Local control of blood flow by the tissues, and humoral regulation. In: Textbook of medical physiology (9th edn). Philadelphia, PA: W. B. Saunders Co., 1996:199–208.

Appendix 1

Inspecting Figure 2, A_{out} can be calculated from the outer radius, R, of the spherical shell and the caudocranial position, z, of A_{out}:

$$(1)A_{\text{out}} = -\pi \cdot z^2 + 2\pi R \cdot z, \quad 0 < z < 2R$$

Similarly, the transverse cross-sectional area of the lumen of the spherical shell is:

$$(2)A_{\text{in}} = -\pi \cdot z^2 + 2\pi R \cdot z - (\pi R^2 - \pi r^2), \quad R - r < z < R + r$$

where r is the inner radius of the spherical shell. By subtracting A_{in} from A_{out}, A_{wall} is obtained:

$$(3)A_{\text{wall}} = \pi(R^2 - r^2)$$

which is independent of the location, z, of the area. A_{out} and A_{in} are second order polynomials in z (Figure 3). Please note that A_{wall} is constant for one specific luminal volume of the spherical shell. If the sphere size is increased, and the wall is made of an elastic material, it is fair to expect that A_{wall} will decrease, since the wall of the sphere is stretched. This means that A_{wall} will vary between different CT scans of the same patient if the volume of urine inside the bladder varies.

The British Journal of Radiology, 78 (2005), 533–537
DOI: 10.1259/bjr/68749637

Differentiation between solitary brain metastasis and high-grade glioma by diffusion tensor imaging

K TSUCHIYA, MD, A FUJIKAWA, MD, M NAKAJIMA, MD and K HONYA, MD

Department of Radiology, Kyorin University School of Medicine, 6-20-2, Shinkawa, Mitaka, Tokyo 181-8611, Japan

Abstract. We tested our hypothesis that fractional anisotropy (FA) maps of diffusion tensor imaging could be used to differentiate between a solitary brain metastasis and a high-grade glioma. In seven patients with a solitary metastasis and seven patients with a high-grade glioma, FA values of enhancing and non-enhancing parts of the tumour were compared. Additionally, we visually assessed FA maps. No significant difference in the FA values of either the enhancing or non-enhancing part was found between the two groups. In the visual assessment, displacement of subcortical white-matter fibres was found in five of the seven metastasis patients, but in only one glioma patient. Additionally, discrimination between tumour and oedema was possible in three of the seven metastasis patients, but not in any glioma patient. Although FA values are not helpful in differentiating between the two groups, visual differences in FA values can allow the differentiation. Displacement of white-matter fibres is another finding suggestive of metastasis.

Metastases and high-grade gliomas are the most common intra-axial brain tumours. In many clinical settings, especially in patients with multiple lesions, the diagnosis of brain metastasis is usually straightforward and uncomplicated. However, it is often difficult to differentiate a solitary brain metastasis from a high-grade glioma based on the imaging findings alone, and applied MRI techniques, such as MR spectroscopy [1] and perfusion imaging [2], have been reported to be of value in this regard.

Diffusion tensor imaging (DTI) is an MRI technique that is capable of visualizing the anisotropy of proton motion. Water proton diffusion can be quantified in several ways by using such parameters as fractional anisotropy (FA), mean diffusivity (MD), and eigenvalues of the diffusion tensor ($\lambda1$, $\lambda2$, and $\lambda3$) [3, 4]. The advent of DTI has also made it possible to depict major white matter tracts by means of fibre tracking. We hypothesized that changes on FA maps, which are more easily obtained compared with diffusion tensor tractograms and provide information on changes in anisotropy in an objective manner, can be used to make the differential diagnosis between a solitary brain metastasis and a high-grade glioma.

Materials and methods

Study subjects

Seven patients with a solitary brain metastasis (four men and three women; age range 55–70 years; mean age 60 years) and seven patients with a histologically proved grade III or IV glioma according to the WHO classification (four men and three women; age range 17–70 years; mean age 49 years) examined during a 24 month period by MRI that included DTI were retrospectively entered into this study. We excluded two patients examined during the same period who had intratumoural or peritumoural haemorrhage that may have introduced measurement errors. This was done because a haematoma could have its own FA value different from that of tumour and peritumoural tissue. As the number of excluded patients was rather small, we considered that this did not significantly affect this study. Metastatic lesions were diagnosed as solitary on the basis of the post-contrast T_1 weighted MRI findings. The diagnosis of the brain metastasis was confirmed pathologically in five patients and was made clinically in the other two patients based on the history and MRI findings. The primary lesions responsible for the metastases included lung cancer (four patients), colon cancer (one patient), and uterus cancer (one patient). The remaining patient's lesion was adenocarcinoma of unknown primary. The diagnosis of high-grade glioma was made pathologically in every patient. There were four patients with glioblastoma, two with anaplastic astrocytoma, and one with anaplastic oligodendroglioma. The DTI was performed prior to therapy in all of the metastasis and high-grade glioma patients.

Received 29 July 2004 and in revised form 13 December 2004, accepted 17 January 2005.

MRI techniques

All MR examinations were performed with a 1.5 T clinical imager (EXCELART XP SPIN Edition; Toshiba Medical Systems, Tochigi, Japan) equipped with a self-shielding gradient system (30 mT m^{-1} maximum gradient strength and 130 T m^{-1} s^{-1} slew rate). Each MR examination consisted of fast spin-echo T_2 weighted and fluid-attenuated inversion-recovery (FLAIR) sequences, pre- and post-contrast spin-echo T_1 weighted sequences, and DTI. To obtain the post-contrast T_1 weighted scans, we injected each patient with a standard dose (0.1 mmol kg^{-1}) of gadolinium-based contrast material.

DTI was performed using an inversion-recovery-prepared single-shot echo-planar diffusion-weighted (DW) sequence. Axial DW images were collected with identical section position and thickness (5 mm) by applying diffusion gradients (b=0 and 1000 s mm^{-2}) sequentially in six directions (xx, yy, zz, xy, xz, and yz). Other parameters for DTI were a repetition time/echo time/inversion time (TR/TE/TI) of 8400/120/2200 ms, a field-of-view of 260 mm $\times$ 260 mm, an acquisition matrix of 128 $\times$ 128, twenty 5 mm sections with 1.5 mm gap, and three excitations. We generated FA maps from the data thus obtained by using software incorporated in the MR imager.

Image assessment

We measured the FA values of the enhancing part and the surrounding region with T_2 prolongation that probably included oedema and/or tumour infiltration on the FA maps. We applied a region-of-interest (ROI) consisting of more than 10 pixels to each of the two regions on an image display screen (Figure 1). The ROI was placed within the white matter carefully comparing the FA maps with conventional T_2 weighted, FLAIR, and pre- and post-contrast T_1 weighted images of the identical section. In the same manner, we also measured the FA values of the white matter of the centrum semiovale on the contralateral side of the lesion. The measurement was repeated three times by different observers and the values were averaged. The statistical analysis was performed by using the unpaired Student's *t*-test with statistical significance set at $p<0.05$.

We also visually assessed the FA maps in regard to the following: (1) intensity of the enhancing part and non-enhancing surrounding part of the tumour on FA maps; (2) changes in subcortical white-matter fibres and other major tracts adjacent to the tumour; and (3) other prominent findings. The assessment was performed independently by two neuroradiologists, and when there was disagreement between them, the final judgment was made by consensus.

Results

Measurement of FA values

The results of the FA measurements in the enhancing and non-enhancing parts of the tumour are summarized in Table 1. Measurements of the two parts were not performed in one patient with brain metastasis (brain metastasis case 4) because the tumour was cystic and associated with little oedema. The FA values in both the solitary brain metastasis group and high-grade glioma group were lower in both the enhancing part and non-enhancing part than in normal white matter. The FA values of the enhancing part was smaller in the brain metastases (0.14 ± 0.05) than in the gliomas (0.16 ± 0.05), but the difference was not statistically significant ($p=0.23$). The difference between the FA values of the non-enhancing part of brain metastases (0.16 ± 0.05) and glioma (0.20 ± 0.09) was also not significant ($p=0.18$). Nor was the difference in FA values between the enhancing part and non-enhancing part significant in either the brain metastases or the gliomas ($p=0.56$ and $p=0.16$, respectively).

Visual assessment of FA maps

The results of the visual assessments of the FA maps of the two groups are summarized in Tables 2 and 3. All of the metastases were located supratentorially. Subcortical white-matter fibres displaced by tumour and/or oedema were depicted in five of the seven patients with brain metastasis (Figure 2). In three of the seven patients, the tumour and oedema showed diffuse hypointensity owing to decreased FA values. However, the tumour and oedema could be discriminated in three patients, because the tumour was clearly hyperintense (brain metastasis case 5)

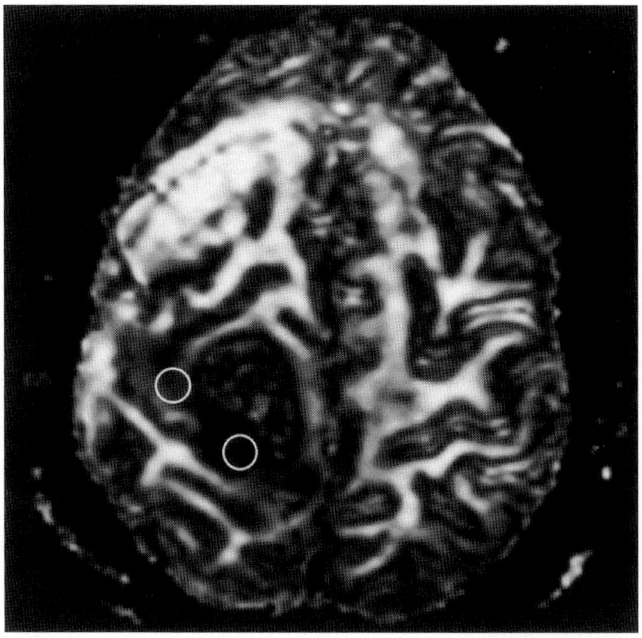

(a)

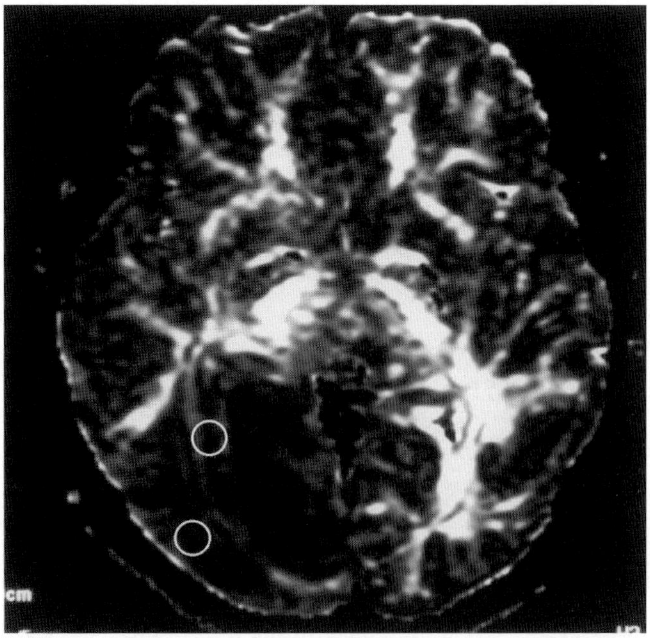

(b)

Figure 1. (a) Fractional anisotropy (FA) map shows regions of interest (ROIs) placed in an enhancing part and a surrounding region in a patient with metastatic adenocarcinoma. This image is identical to Figure 2c. (b) FA map shows two ROIs placed similarly in Figure 1a in a patient with glioblastoma. This image is identical to Figure 3c.

Table 1. Fractional anisotropy (FA) values of the tumour, peritumoural region, and normal white matter in 14 patients with solitary metastasis or high-grade glioma

Case no.	Brain metastasis				Case no.	High-grade glioma			
	Age/Sex	Enhancing part	Non-enhancing part	Normal white matter		Age/Sex	Enhancing part	Non-enhancing part	Normal white matter
1	58/M	0.11	0.19	0.62	1	64/F	0.12	0.15	0.62
2	58/F	0.17	0.13	0.57	2	70/F	0.19	0.17	0.57
3	57/M	0.15	0.12	0.5	3	61/M	0.17	0.25	0.51
4	70/M	NA	NA	0.51	4	51/M	0.2	0.37	0.64
5	55/F	0.22	0.12	0.64	5	17/M	0.07	0.12	0.6
6	60/F	0.08	0.18	0.62	6	47/F	0.2	0.15	0.59
7	65/M	0.09	0.22	0.62	7	30/M	0.16	0.17	0.56
Average ± SD		0.14 ± 0.05	0.16 ± 0.05	0.58 ± 0.06			0.16 ± 0.05	0.20 ± 0.09	0.58 ± 0.04

NA, indicates not available owing to cystic nature and lack of oedema. SD, standard deviation.

Table 2. FA map findings in seven patients with solitary metastasis

Case no.	Age/Sex	Location	Diagnosis	Findings
1	58/M	Temporal lobe	Lung carcinoma	Displacement of white matter-fibres and corticospinal tract
2	58/F	Frontal lobe	Lung carcinoma	Diffusely decreased FA
3	57/M	Frontal lobe	Colon carcinoma	Diffusely decreased FA, displacement of white matter-fibres
4	70/M	Parietal lobe	Lung carcinoma	Displacement of white matter-fibres
5	55/F	Parietal lobe	Uterus carcinoma	Diffusely decreased FA, discrimination between tumour and oedema
6	60/F	Frontal lobe	Adenocarcinoma of unknown origin	Displacement of white matter-fibres, discrimination between tumour and oedema
7	65/M	Parietal lobe	Lung carcinoma	Displacement of white matter-fibres and corpus callosum fibres, discrimination between tumour and oedema

FA, fractional anisotropy.

Table 3. FA map findings in 7 patients with high-grade glioma

Case no.	Age/Sex	Location	Diagnosis	Findings
1	64/F	Frontal lobe	AA	Diffusely decreased FA
2	70/F	Pareital lobe	GBM	Diffusely decreased FA
3	61/M	Frontal lobe	GBM	Diffusely decreased FA
4	51/M	Brainstem	GBM	Diffusely decreased FA
5	17/M	Temporal lobe	AA	Diffusely decreased FA
6	47/F	Occipital lobe	GBM	Diffusely decreased FA, optic fibres passing through
7	30/M	Frontal lobe	AO	Diffusely decreased FA, displacement of white matter-fibres

FA, fractional anisotropy; AA, anaplastic astrocytoma; GBM, glioblastoma; AO, anaplastic oligodendroglioma.

or hypointense (brain metastasis cases 6 and 7) compared with the oedema (Figure 2). By contrast, in all seven patients with glioma the enhanced part and surrounding region showed diffuse hypointensity owing to decreased FA values. Thus, the tumour and surrounding oedema could not be discriminated visually in any of the glioma patients (Figure 3). Displacement of the white-matter fibres was noted in only one glioma patient (high-grade glioma case 7).

Discussion

DTI has been applied to the imaging of brain tumours in several ways. Some groups have used FA and MD maps to assess involvement of white matter tracts by gliomas and suggested that they were useful for surgical planning [5–8]. More recently, one of the clinical applications of DTI, fibre tracking, has been reported to be of value for demonstrating the relationship between the tumour and major white matter pathways, such as the corticospinal tract [9]. In contrast to these studies, the present study was performed to determine whether DTI is capable of being useful for differential diagnosis between a solitary brain metastasis and a high-grade glioma. Most previous studies on the clinical use of DTI employed FA and MD, which represent the directionality and magnitude, respectively, of proton anisotropy. We thought that FA would be an effective index, because FA maps not only quantitatively reflect anisotropy changes but also visualize white matter pathways that may be affected by brain neoplasms.

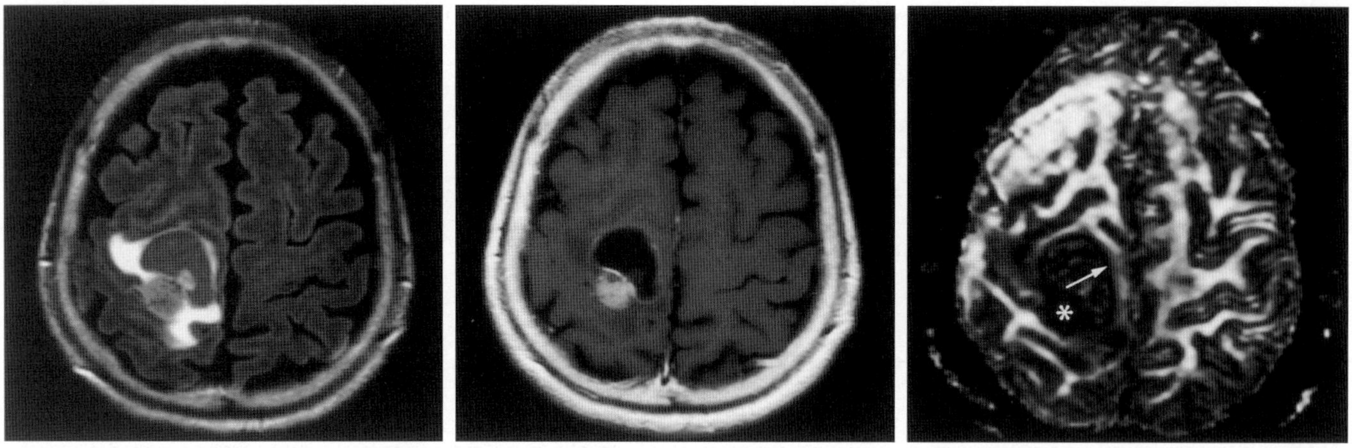

(a) (b) (c)

Figure 2. A 60-year-old woman with surgically confirmed adenocarcinoma of unknown origin (brain metastasis case 6). (a) Axial fluid attenuated inversion recovery (FLAIR) image (8000/120/2300/1 [repetition time/echo time/inversion time/number of excitations (TR/TE/TI/NEX)]) shows a hyperintense mass with cystic component surrounded by moderate degree of oedema. (b) Axial post-contrast T_1 weighted image (540/15/1.4 [TR/TE/NEX]) shows enhancement of the solid part as well as that of the cyst wall. (c) Fractional anisotropy (FA) map shows lower FA of the solid part (*, 0.08) than that of the peritumoural oedematous part (0.18). Displaced white-matter fibres are also visible (arrow).

The same as in previous reports [10–13], the FA values in both tumour tissue and peritumoural region were lower than in normal white matter. However, we found no significant difference in FA values between the enhancing tumour regions of brain metastases and high-grade gliomas. Sinha et al [10] explained the decrease in FA values within brain tumour by a loss of structural organization, while Beppu et al [12] pointed to a positive correlation between FA values and both the cellularity and vascularity of tumours. Although no histopathological analysis was performed in our study, we think that such changes are present in tumour tissue and may be responsible for the decrease in the FA values. Our study, however, showed that such FA changes are not reliable for making the differential diagnosis between brain metastasis and high-grade glioma. Tumour infiltration is thought to be present in the peritumoural areas that show hyperintensity on T_2 weighted images of high-grade gliomas. Areas adjacent to metastatic brain tumours show vasogenic oedema and are usually well demarcated from the tumour. We, therefore, speculated that there might be a difference in the FA values of the peritumoural region between the two types of tumours, but, again, no significant difference was found. Lu et al [11] conducted a study similar to our own and also found no difference in FA values but stated that the MD in the peritumoural region was significantly greater in brain metastases than in high-grade gliomas. They attributed the difference between the two parameters to possible representation of tumour infiltration by the FA. However, both the study by Lu et al [11] and our own found that the FA in the peritumoural region is unreliable as a means of differentiating between brain metastases and high-grade gliomas. The MD in the peritumoural tissue of primary

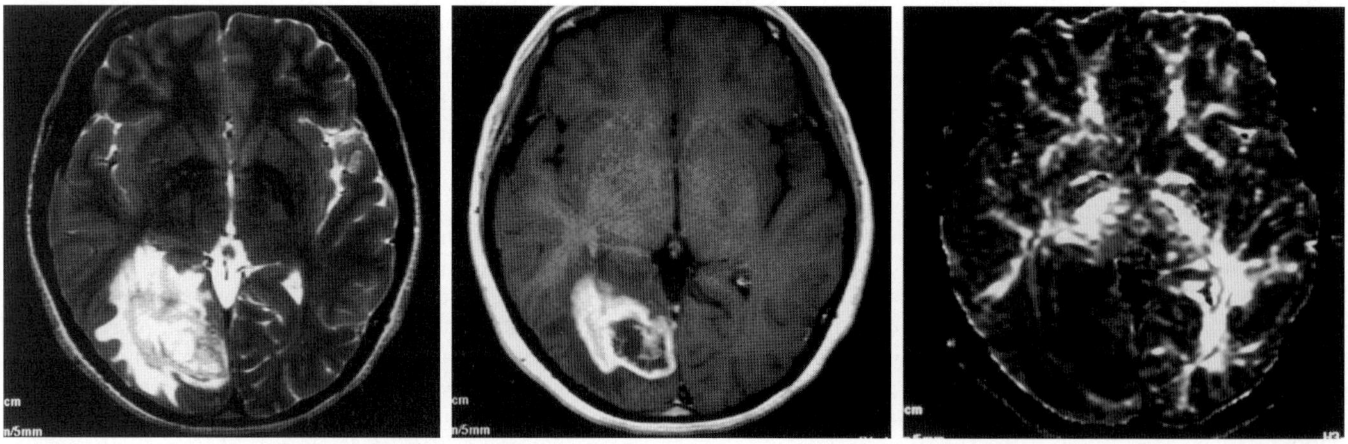

(a) (b) (c)

Figure 3. A 47-year-old woman with pre-treatment glioblastoma (high-grade glioma case 6). (a) Axial T_2 weighted image (4240/105/1 [repetition time/echo time/number of excitations (TR/TE/NEX)] shows a heterogeneously hyperintense mass surrounded by a hyperintense region. (b) Post-contrast T_1 weighted image (540/15/1.4 [TR/TE/NEX]) shows enhancement of the solid part. (c) Fractional anisotropy (FA) map shows diffuse hypointensity due to decreased FA. The enhancing part (0.2) and non-enhancing part (0.15) are hard to discriminate.

brain tumours has been reported to decrease after dexamethasone treatment [14], and the difference between the two kinds of tumours in this respect seems worthy of evaluation.

The visual assessment revealed that both the enhancing and peritumoural non-enhancing regions of both kinds of tumours showed hypointensity owing to decreased FA in most cases. Interestingly, the two regions could be discriminated on the FA maps of three patients with metastasis, but not in any of the patients with glioma. Although there were no significant quantitative differences, there seemed to be a larger variance in the FA between the two regions in metastatic tumours. On the other hand, FA maps clearly visualize subcortical white-matter fibres and adjacent fibre tracts, and they revealed displacement of the fibres in five of the seven patients with brain metastasis, but in only one of the seven patients with glioma. In the other glioma patients, hypointensity owing to decreased FA was observed in the subcortical white matter and it extended to the cortex. Metastatic brain tumours arise within the brain parenchyma and usually grow by expansion, displacing the surrounding brain tissue, whereas high-grade gliomas extend by infiltration. We think that these differences in tumour growth may be a cause of the difference in findings on FA maps.

There are several limitations to this study. First, the patient population was relatively small. Second, our results may also have been influenced by the size and location of the tumours. The visual assessment and the placement of the ROIs for the measurements of FA values were subjective, and we did not set clear criteria for ROI placement to measure the FA values in the peritumoural region. The reasons for selecting FA as the index in this study have been stated above. To overcome these issues, we are continuing this study in a larger series including other parameters such as MD as quantitative indices.

In conclusion, solitary brain metastases and high-grade gliomas cannot be reliably differentiated either visually or quantitatively on the basis of FA changes. However, a diagnosis of brain metastasis is suggested when FA maps outline the tumour or when they demonstrate displacement of adjacent white-matter fibres. Future improvements in spatial resolution may increase the diagnostic capability of FA maps in this regard.

References

1. Ishimaru H, Morikawa M, Iwanaga S, Kaminogo M, Ochi M, Hayashi K. Differentiation between high-grade glioma and metastatic brain tumor using single-voxel proton MR spectroscopy. Eur Radiol 2001;11:1784–91.
2. Cha S, Knopp EA, Johnson G, Wetzel SG, Litt AW, Zagzag D. Intracranial mass lesions: dynamic contrast-enhanced susceptibility-weighted echo-planar perfusion MR imaging. Radiology 2002;223:11–29.
3. Pierpaoli C, Basser PJ. Toward a quantitative assessment of diffusion anisotropy. Mag Reson Med 1996;36:893–906.
4. Basser PJ, Mattielo J, LeBihan D. MR diffusion tensor spectroscopy and imaging. Biophys J 1994;66:259–67.
5. Wieshmann UC, Symms MR, Parker GJ, Clark CA, Lemieux L, Barker GJ. Diffusion tensor imaging demonstrates deviation of fibres in normal appearing white matter adjacent to a brain tumour. J Neurol Neurosurg Psychiatry 2000;68:501–3.
6. Mori S, Frederiksen K, van Zijl PC, Stieltjes B, Kraut MA, Solaiyappen M, et al. Brain white matter anatomy of tumor patients evaluated with diffusion tensor imaging. Ann Neurol 2002;51:377–80.
7. Witwer BP, Moftakhar R, Hasan KM, Deshmukh P, Haughton V, Field A, et al. Diffusion-tensor imaging of white matter tracts in patients with cerebral neoplasm. J Neurosurg 2002;97:568–75.
8. Price SJ, Burnet NG, Donovan T, Green HA, Pena A, Antoun NM, et al. Diffusion tensor imaging of brain tumours at 3T: a potential tool for assessing white matter tract invasion? Clin Radiol 2003;58:455–62.
9. Clark CA, Barrick TR, Murphy MM, Bell BA. White matter fiber tracking in patients with space-occupying lesions of the brain: a new technique for neurosurgical planning? Neuroimage 2003;20:1601–8.
10. Sinha S, Bastin ME, Whittle IR, Wardlaw JM. Diffusion tensor MR imaging of high-grade cerebral gliomas. AJNR Am J Neuroradiol 2002;23:520–7.
11. Lu S, Ahn D, Johnson G, Cha S. Peritumoral diffusion tensor imaging of high-grade gliomas and metastatic brain tumors. AJNR Am J Neuroradiol 2003;24:937–41.
12. Beppu T, Inoue T, Shibata Y, Kurose A, Arai H, Ogasawara K, et al. Measurement of fractional anisotropy using diffusion tensor MRI in supratentorial astrocytic tumors. J Neurooncol 2003;63:109–16.
13. Lu S, Ahn D, Johnson G, Zagzag D, Grossman I. Diffusion-tensor MR imaging of intracranial neoplasia and associated peritumoral edema: introduction of the tumor infiltration index. Radiology 2004;232:221–8.
14. Bastin ME, Delgado M, Whittle IR, Cannon J, Wardlaw JM. The use of diffusion tensor imaging in quantifying the effect of dexamethasone on brain tumours. Neuroreport 1999; 10:1385–91.

The British Journal of Radiology, *78* (2005), 538–542
DOI: 10.1259/bjr/13870613

Short communication

The effect of introducing radiographer reporting on the availability of reports for Accident and Emergency and General Practitioner examinations: a time-series analysis

[1]S D BREALEY, PhD and [2,3]P A SCUFFHAM, PhD

[1]*York Trials Unit, Department of Health Sciences, University of York, York YO10 5DD,* [2]*York Health Economics Consortium Ltd, University of York, York YO10 5NH, UK and* [3]*School of Population Health, University of Queensland, Brisbane, Australia*

Abstract. This study explores whether the introduction of selectively trained radiographers reporting Accident and Emergency (A&E) X-ray examinations of the appendicular skeleton affected the availability of reports for A&E and General Practitioner (GP) examinations at a typical district general hospital. This was achieved by analysing monthly data on A&E and GP examinations for 1993–1997 using structural time-series models. Parameters to capture stochastic seasonal effects and stochastic time trends were included in the models. The main outcome measures were changes in the number, proportion and timeliness of A&E and GP examinations reported. Radiographer reporting X-ray examinations requested by A&E was associated with a 12% ($p=0.050$) increase in the number of A&E examinations reported and a 37% ($p\leqslant0.001$) decrease in the time taken to report on these examinations. Radiographer reporting of A&E X-ray examinations was also associated with a 14% ($p=0.067$) decrease in the time taken for GP examinations to be reported. That is, radiographer reporting A&E X-ray examinations allowed an increase in the time available to radiologists to report on examinations requested by GPs. An increase in the proportion of GP examinations reported by radiologists was associated with longer reporting times for A&E examinations. In conclusion, selectively trained radiographers reporting on A&E X-ray examinations significantly improved the availability of reports for A&E and GP examinations.

A shortage of doctors and the need to address increasing demand in a healthcare system with scarce resources has brought about changes in Government policy that promote a more flexible and creative use of allied healthcare professional skills [1, 2]. In X-ray departments, a national shortage of radiologists [3, 4] and a continuing rise in workload [5] provide a climate that has encouraged the development of radiographers in a written reporting role [6, 7]. This skill mix initiative was seen to be a natural extension of what radiographers were already doing in normal clinical practice such as marking Accident and Emergency (A&E) radiographs with a red dot to alert casualty officers to the possible presence of an abnormality [8] or the triage of A&E radiographs as normal, insignificantly abnormal, or significantly abnormal [9]. There is now evidence that selectively trained radiographers can provide accurate written text reports describing A&E radiographic appearances [10–12] resulting in a growing number of radiographers performing this task [13, 14].

In recent years, one criticism of reporting services has been clinicians' dissatisfaction with reports not being provided for all examinations and not received in time to influence patient management [15]. Therefore, not only is it important that radiographs are interpreted accurately but that they are all reported promptly. This is repeatedly emphasised as quality standards by the Royal College of Radiologists (RCR) [3, 16]. The standards suggest that all A&E examinations are reported before the patient leaves the X-ray department [3] and all general practitioner (GP) examinations should be reported within 24 h of the arrival of the patient [13, 17]. In practice, a recent survey has shown that of 110 X-ray departments, A&E examinations were not reported in 13 (15%) of the 87 hospitals that responded [18]. In a further study of 102 hospitals, only 50% of GP examinations were reported after 22 h [19]. Delays in the availability of a report may affect patient outcomes and lead to an increase in other more expensive investigations. The deployment of selectively trained radiographers in an A&E written reporting role might help X-ray departments to ensure that all A&E examinations are reported promptly. Furthermore, if this alleviates radiologists' workload, it may free their time to improve the availability of reports for other examinations, such as those requested by GPs. Can this potential be achieved?

In February 1995, following a period of training, two radiographers at a typical district general hospital began to report A&E X-ray examinations of the appendicular skeleton judged normal or insignificantly abnormal by the casualty officers. This provided an opportunity to assess whether the introduction of radiographer reporting could help to ensure that all A&E examinations were reported promptly and how this affected the reporting of GP examinations.

Received 11 February 2004 and in revised form 1 December 2004, accepted 5 January 2005.

Methods

A time-series study was undertaken to assess whether the introduction of the radiographers in a reporting role affected the availability of reports for examinations requested from A&E or general practice. The X-ray department performs more than 7500 examinations per month, of which 29% are referred from A&E and 25% from general practice. This corresponds with the findings from a recent national report which indicated that 27% of radiology workload is generated by referral from A&E and 21% from GP referrals [15].

The Systems and Network Services department provided monthly data on numbers of examinations taken, reported, the time taken to report the examinations, the profession responsible for reporting the examinations, and the referral source. This was for the period February 1993 (2 years before the intervention) to January 1998 (3 years after the intervention). A total of 418 362 examinations were performed over this 5 year period and 325 902 were reported (78%).

Radiographers were trained to report on examinations for patients referred from A&E; therefore, the primary analysis was restricted to A&E. The primary hypothesis was that reporting on A&E examinations by radiographers had no effect on the number and timing of A&E reports. Indirect effects from radiographer reporting may be present; for example, radiologists may reduce their time spent reporting A&E examinations and may have more time to report on GP examinations, and therefore, more GP examinations may be reported. This is a factor we tested in the analyses, with the hypothesis that reporting on A&E examinations by radiographers had no effect on the time taken to report GP examinations. Descriptive data for these groups are shown in Table 1.

Three statistical models for time-series regression analysis were specified: the number of A&E examinations reported (Model 1); the time to report A&E examinations (Model 2); and the time to report GP examinations (Model 3). Independent variables included total A&E and total GP examinations performed and the intervention variable. These factors were included in all models for two reasons – radiologists may substitute their time away from reporting on A&E examinations to reporting GP examinations, and when demands for examinations are high (either A&E or GP examinations), radiologists may have less time to report A&E examinations. The intervention variable used for all models was the proportion of A&E examinations reported by radiographers. In the time to report models (Models 2 and 3), the proportions of A&E and GP examinations reported were also included as explanatory variables.

Time-series data often contain trends that, without proper control, can violate the statistical properties of normality, and thus, the usual inference procedures to test hypotheses are invalid. Trends and seasonal variations can be incorporated explicitly and efficiently through structural time-series models (STSM), and thus, with a correctly specified model, the usual statistical inferences apply [20, 21]. The STSM is a general form of the Box-Jenkins autoregressive integrated moving average (ARIMA) models [22]; however, trends and seasonal components can be allowed to vary stochastically over time in response to disturbances rather than being omitted from the modelling process as occurs in ARIMA models. Therefore, valuable information can be retained in the model as the data do not require differencing, detrending or deseasonalising [20]. The seasonal component was specified as a smooth sine-wave that was allowed to vary over time.

To capture any delayed effects in the variables, three lags of each variable were included in the models. (For example, the dependent variables may respond to the explanatory variables after a time lapse; in these models, one lag, denoted $t-1$, is 1 month and so forth.) To obtain parsimonious models (*i.e.* models with all non-significant factors omitted), an iterative testing-down procedure was used where the variable with the least significance was omitted and the model re-estimated. This process was continued until the variables retained in the final models had a statistical significance of at least 90%. Similarly, the stochastic trend or seasonal component could be replaced with a deterministic component when there was no variation to the component over time. All models were subjected to tests for normality, including tests on the error terms for zero mean, constant variance, skewness, kurtosis, and importantly, serial correlation. Goodness of fit was based on the usual R^2 and an R^2 around seasonal differences (Rs^2).

Results

The fit was reasonable for all three models, with Rs^2 between 0.55 and 0.93. In all models a stochastic trend was retained owing to variation in the disturbances affecting the trend; however, the stochastic seasonal component showed no variation in all models (*i.e.* the seasonal pattern was constant). Therefore, the stochastic seasonality was reduced to deterministic seasonality in all models.

Table 1. Annual descriptive statistics

Year	Total A&E examinations (*n*)	A&E examinations reported (*n*)	A&E examinations reported (%)	Radiographer reports (% of reported examinations)	Mean time to report A&E examinations (hours)	Total GP examinations (*n*)	GP examinations reported (*n*)	GP examinations reported (%)	Mean time to report GP examinations (hours)
1993	22986	17089	74.3	—	94.6	19613	18813	95.9	34.0
1994	25778	18885	73.3	—	115.1	19232	18328	95.3	46.5
1995	24646	19367	78.6	32.7	112.3	20641	18934	91.8	41.5
1996	25318	21976	86.8	33.6	155.6	21094	19647	93.0	41.0
1997	25524	19841	77.7	44.7	100.8	22780	21584	94.7	38.2

A&E, accident and emergency; GP, general practitioner.

Table 2. Parameter estimates for the three models

	Model 1 Number of A&E examinations reported[a]		Model 2 Time to report A&E examinations[b]		Model 3 Time to report GP examinations[c]	
	Coefficient	p-value	Coefficient	p-value	Coefficient	p-value
Total A&E examinations taken	0.699	<0.001				
Proportion of reported A&E examinations reported by radiographers	477.81	0.050	−229.58	<0.001		
Proportion of reported A&E examinations reported by radiographers $t-1$					−21.561	0.067
Proportion of GP examinations reported	4018.90	<0.001	392.08	0.040		
Proportion of GP examinations reported $t-1$	−1949.60	0.013				
Reporting time for GP examinations $t-1$					0.206	<0.001

[a] R^2=0.880; Rs^2=0.856; standard deviation (SD) of disturbance to irregular component (*i.e.* noise)=69.92; SD of disturbance to the level component (*i.e.* noise around the trend)=45.20; Ljung-Box Q (LB-Q) statistic (8, 6)=5.275 (p=0.51); Normality (Bowman-Shenton χ^2 non-normality test statistic, 2 df)=0.202 (p=0.904). A dummy variable was included to control for a significant outlier in 1996, month 11, coefficient=−514.57 (p<0.001).
[b] R^2=0.670; Rs^2=0.553; SD of disturbance to irregular component=18.05; SD of disturbance to level component=8.97; LB-Q statistic (7, 6)=4.815 (p=0.57); Normality=0.036 (p=0.98). A dummy variable was included to control for a significant mean shift in 1994, month 12, coefficient=97.94 (p<0.001).
[c] R^2=0.938; Rs^2=0.928; SD of disturbance to irregular component=6.50; SD of disturbance to level component=1.34; LB-Q statistic (7, 6)=6.464 (p=0.37); Normality=4.018 (p=0.13). Dummy variables were included to control for significant outliers in 1995 month 1, coefficient=126.13 (p<0.001), 1996 month 1, coefficient=81.75 (p<0.001).
A&E, accident and emergency; GP, general practitioner.

For the number of A&E examinations reported (Model 1), the total number of examinations and the proportion reported by radiographers were significant factors (Table 2). Radiographer reporting was associated with an increase in the number of A&E examinations reported, after controlling for increases in total A&E examinations taken, by 12% per month (p=0.050). Interestingly, an increase in the proportion of GP examinations reported was associated with an increase in A&E examinations reported in the same month but a decrease in the next month. This oscillation suggests reporting is undertaken in batches with some storing of work. The parameter estimates were used to predict the number of A&E examinations reported in the absence of the intervention (Figure 1).

The time taken to report A&E examinations (Model 2) was dependent on the proportion of A&E examinations reported by radiographers and the proportion of GP examinations reported. An increase in the proportion of A&E examinations reported by radiographers reduced A&E reporting times by 36.8% (p<0.001). An increase in GP examinations reported was associated with increased A&E reporting times. The effect on A&E reporting times from radiographer reporting is illustrated in Figure 2 where the observed time to report A&E examinations is

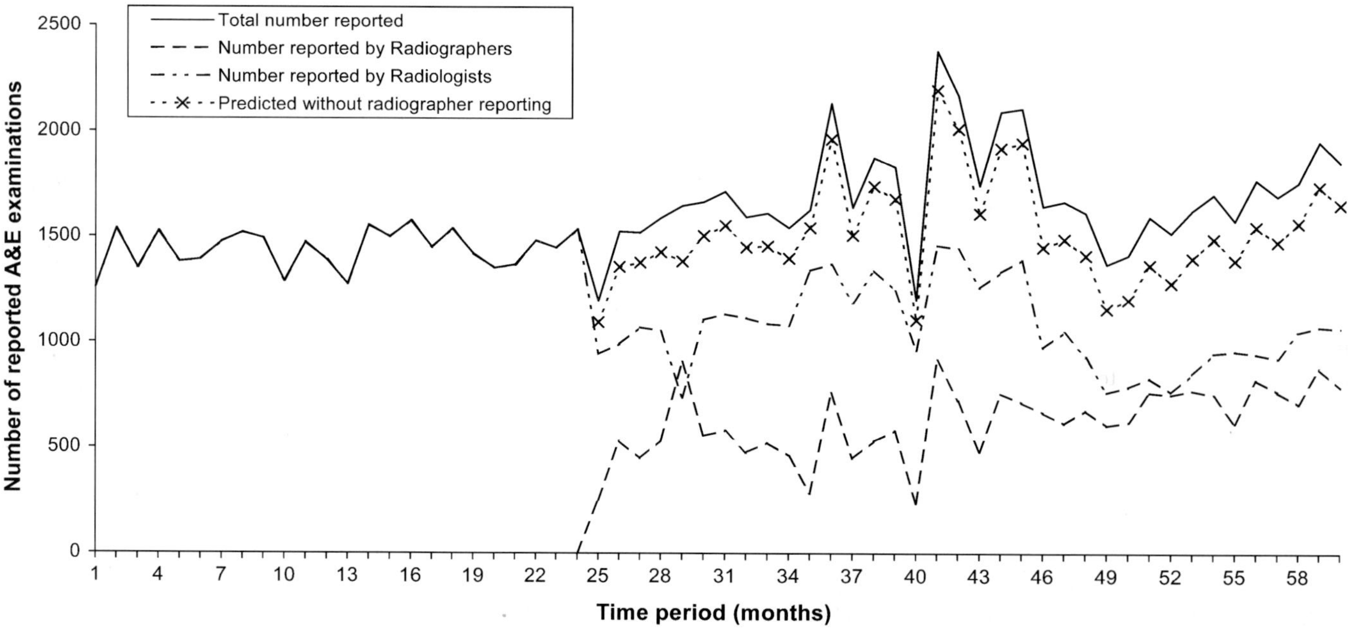

Figure 1. Number of accident and emergency (A&E) examinations reported by staff and predicted number of examinations reported in the absence of radiographer reporting.

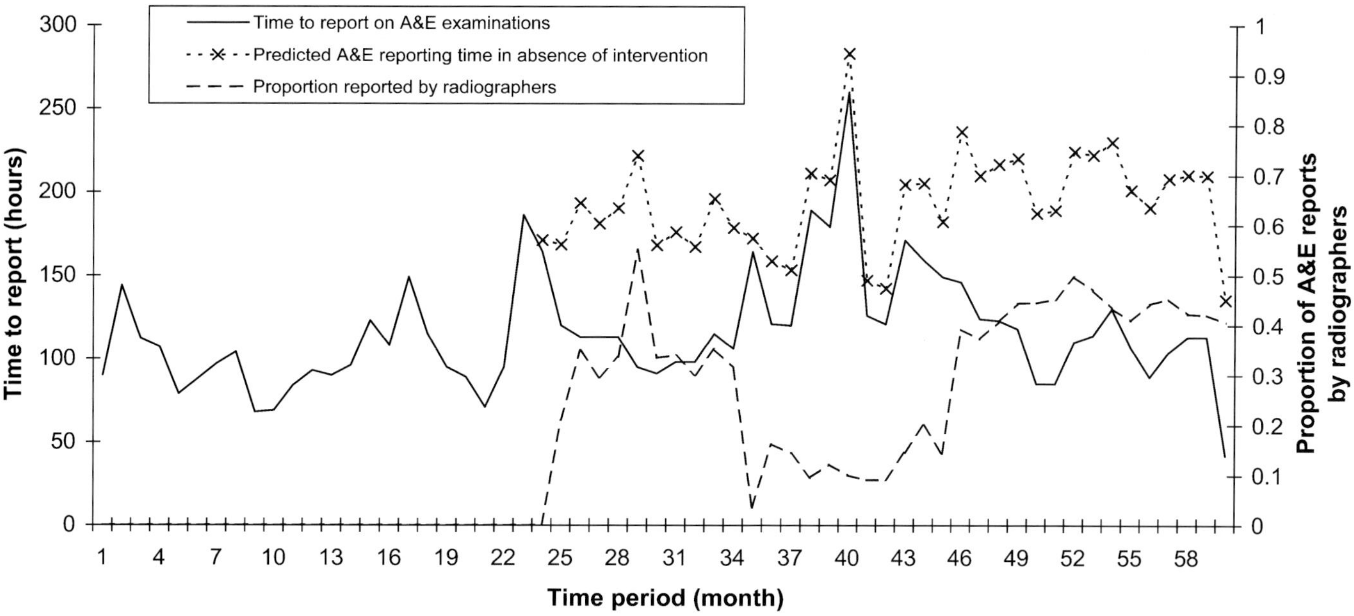

Figure 2. Observed time to report accident and emergency (A&E) examinations and predicted time in the absence of radiographer reporting.

contrasted against the longer predicted time in the absence of the intervention.

Similarly, radiographer reporting on A&E examinations significantly reduced the time taken by radiologists to report GP examinations (Model 3), but this effect was delayed by 1 month. That is, increased radiographer reporting in 1 month reduced the reporting time of GP examinations (by 14%, $p=0.067$) in the next. In addition, an increase in reporting times of GP examinations in 1 month was associated with an increase in reporting time in the next, suggesting backlogs could build up.

In the time to report models (Models 2 and 3), the total number of A&E examinations taken, the total number of GP examinations and the proportion of A&E examinations reported had no statistically significant effect on the time taken to report either A&E or GP examinations.

Discussion

A policy of both the American College of Radiology [23] and the RCR [16] is that all images should be accompanied by a written report. The Ionising Radiation (Medical Exposure) Regulations are also integral to ensuring that patients are not unnecessarily exposed to potentially harmful radiation without the benefit of the image being reported. The RCR recommends the need for images to be reported promptly; notably that A&E examinations are reported before the patient leaves the X-ray department [3] and all GP examinations are reported within 24 h of the arrival of the patient [13, 17]. In practice, surveys have shown considerable variation in the proportion of A&E examinations reported by radiologists and their timeliness [24–27]. The conclusion of a recent national audit of 102 hospitals in the UK was that X-ray departments are often unable to meet targets set for providing GPs with a prompt reporting service [19]. The availability of a report is important for influencing the referring clinician's decision-making and in turn may affect patient outcome and the need for other more expensive investigations.

A shortage of radiologists and changes in Government policy over the last decade have resulted in relaxation of restrictions on who should provide written text reports. There is now substantial evidence that selectively trained radiographers can report A&E X-ray examinations to a similar level of accuracy as radiologists [10–12]. Our analyses show that the intervention of radiographer reporting was associated with an increase in the number of A&E examinations reported. Before the introduction of radiographer reporting there were occasions when it was not feasible for the radiologists to report some A&E examinations because of excessive workloads, but subsequent to the intervention this has not occurred. Radiographer reporting also decreased times taken to report both A&E and GP examinations.

There were interactions between reporting times for A&E and GP examinations. Increases in the proportion of GP examinations reported increased reporting times for A&E examinations; and increased reporting of A&E examinations by radiographers decreased GP examination reporting times. That is, when radiologists increase GP reporting, the time taken to report A&E examinations increased as the availability of radiologists for reporting A&E examinations was reduced; and when radiographers reported A&E examinations, the radiologist's time available to report GP examinations increased and thus reduced the reporting times for GP examinations. These features show radiologists substitute their time from reporting on A&E examinations to GP examinations (and vice versa) and reporting is undertaken in batches with occasional backlogs.

Whether the results from this study are generalizable to different hospital settings and other selectively trained radiographers remains to be tested. Furthermore, the data were provided by the hospital's information management database. Problems such as duplicate records of patients' attendance for examinations or inaccurate allocation of patients' to a referral source may limit the data quality. Our findings complement those from a similar study that found the introduction of radiographer reporting in four NHS Trusts brought about a significant increase in the proportion of A&E skeletal X-ray examinations reported and timeliness of report availability [28]. However, the findings were limited by the short pre- and post-intervention study periods and the chi-squared test used for analysis. These factors meant that the apparent effect of radiographer reporting could have been due to seasonal effects alone.

In conclusion, whilst taking into consideration the possible limitations of the data available, this study provides evidence that with appropriate training and careful supervision the introduction of radiographers in a reporting role can improve the availability of reports for A&E and GP examinations, and therefore, help X-ray departments meet quality standards. This is important not only for referring clinicians' decision-making and ultimately patients' health but also the future development of radiographers' professional status and practice and addressing the shortage in radiologists.

Acknowledgments

The authors are extremely grateful for the help of the staff at the hospital for providing the data and in particular Mr Ian Crawshaw.

References

1. Department of Health. The NHS Plan: A plan for investment. A plan for reform. London: Stationary Office, 2000.
2. Department of Health. Meeting the challenge. A strategy for the allied health professions. London: Stationary Office, 2000.
3. The Royal College of Radiologists. Staffing and standards in departments of clinical oncology and clinical radiology. London: Royal College of Radiologists, 1993.
4. Brindle M. Debate intensifies over non-radiologists' roles. Diagnostic Imaging Europe 1996;11:43–7.
5. The Royal College of Radiologists. Clinical Radiology: a workforce in crisis. London: The Royal College of Radiologists, 2002.
6. The Royal College of Radiologists. Medico legal aspects of delegation. London: The Royal College of Radiologists, 1993.
7. The College of Radiographers. X-ray examination requests by nurse practitioners and radiographic reporting by radiographers. London: College of Radiographers, 1995.
8. Berman L, de Lacey G, Twomey E, Twomey B, Welch T, Eban R. Reducing errors in accident department; a simple method using radiographers. Br Med J 1985;290:421–2.
9. Renwick IGH, Butt WP, Steele B. How well can radiographers triage X-ray films in the accident and emergency department? Br Med J 1991;302:568–9.
10. Robinson PJA. Plain film reporting by radiographers — a feasibility study. Br J Radiol 1996;69:1171–4.
11. Loughran CF. Reporting of fracture radiographs by radiographers: the impact of a training programme. Br J Radiol 1994;67:945–50.
12. Brealey S, King DG, Crowe MTI, Crawshaw I, Ford L, Warnock N, et al. Accident and Emergency and General Practitioner plain radiograph reporting by radiographers and radiologists: a quasi-randomized controlled trial. Br J Radiol 2003;76:57–61.
13. Paterson AM. Role development - Towards 2000: a survey of role developments in radiography. London: College of Radiographers, 1995.
14. Price RC, Le Masurier SB, High L, Miller LR. Changing times: a national survey of extended roles in diagnostic radiography. Br J Radiol 1999;72:7.
15. Audit Commission. Improving your image: how to manage radiology services more effectively. London: Stationary Office, 1995.
16. The Royal College of Radiologists. Statement on reporting in Departments of Clinical Radiology. London: Royal College of Radiologists, 1995.
17. The Royal College of Radiologists. Clinical radiology quality specification for purchasers. London: The Royal College of Radiologists, 1995.
18. Piper K. Clinical reporting in radiography. 75th Anniversary Conference - The Society and College of Radiographers, SCoR Programme Abstract, 16, 1995.
19. The Royal College of Radiologists. Two national audits of radiographic reporting services. London: The Royal College of Radiologists, 2000.
20. Harvey AC, Durbin J. The effects of seat belt legislation on British road casualties: a case study in structural time series modelling. J R Stat Soc 1986;149:187–227.
21. Cuthbertson K, Hall SG, Taylor MP. Applied econometric techniques. Hertfordshire: Philip Allan, 1995.
22. Box GEP, Jenkins GM. Time series analysis, forecasting and control. San Francisco: Holden-Day, 1970.
23. American College of Radiology. ACR standard for communication: diagnostic radiology. Reston: American College of Radiology, 1993.
24. James MR, Bracegirdle D, Yates DW. X-ray reporting in accident and emergency departments - an area for improvements in efficiency. Arch Emerg Med 1991;8:266–70.
25. Berman L, de Lacey G, Craig O. A survey of accident and emergency reporting: results and implications. Clin Radiol 1985;36:483–4.
26. Beggs I, Davidson JK. Accident and Emergency reporting in UK teaching departments. Clin Radiol 1990;41:264–7.
27. Rose J, Gallivan S. Plain film reporting in the UK. Clin Radiol 1991;44:192–4.
28. Piper K, Paterson AM, Ryan C. The implementation of a radiographic reporting service for trauma examinations of the skeletal system, in four National Health Service Trusts. Research & Development Directorate, South Thames Regional Office (NHSE) 1999.

The British Journal of Radiology, 78 (2005), 543–547 © 2005 The British Institute of Radiology
DOI: 10.1259/bjr/73133162

Short communication

The low energy X-ray response of the LiF:Mg:Cu:P thermoluminescent dosemeter: a comparison with LiF:Mg:Ti

[1]C R EDWARDS, PhD, MIPEM, [1]P J MOUNTFORD, PhD, FIPEM, [2]S GREEN, PhD, FIPEM, [2]J E PALETHORPE, HND, IIPEM and [1]A J MOLONEY, BSc, MIPEM

[1]*Medical Physics Directorate, University Hospital of North Staffordshire, Princes Road, Hartshill, Stoke-on-Trent, Staffordshire ST4 7LN and* [2]*RRPPS, University Hospital Birmingham, Edgbaston, Birmingham B15 2TH, UK*

Abstract. LiF:Mg:Cu:P thermoluminescent dosemeters (TLD) can be used for the same X-ray dosimetry applications as LiF:Mg:Ti, with each type having the disadvantage of a response dependent on energy, particularly at low energies. Measurements were made of the response per unit air kerma of LiF:Mg:Cu:P and LiF:Mg:Ti to nine quasi-monoenergetic X-ray beams with mean energies from 12 keV to 208 keV. Each measurement was normalized to the value produced by 6 MV X-rays. LiF:Mg:Cu:P was found to under-respond to a majority of these radiations whereas LiF:Mg:Ti over-responded to a majority. Their smallest relative measured response was produced by the lowest energy beam, and the maximum measured relative response of 1.15 ± 0.07 and 1.21 ± 0.07 for LiF:Mg:Cu:P and LiF:Mg:Ti, respectively, occurred at 33 keV. Energy response coefficients were derived from these measurements to estimate the error introduced by using either type of TLD to measure the dose from an X-ray spectrum different to that used for its absolute response calibration. It was calculated that if the response of either type of TLD was calibrated at 100 kVp, then an error of no more than $\pm 2\%$ would be introduced into measurements of tube output at potentials of 50–130 kVp. LiF:Mg:Cu:P was found to introduce a larger error (up to 30%) into the measurement of body exit dose than LiF:Mg:Ti at tube potentials of 40–150 kVp, if its absolute response was calibrated using the corresponding body entrance beam. The method should allow this type of error to be estimated in other dosimetry applications for either type of TLD.

The LiF:Mg:Cu:P thermoluminescent dosemeter (TLD) can be used as an alternative to LiF:Mg:Ti for several diagnostic radiology and radiotherapy dosimetry applications. Both types of TLD have the disadvantage of a non-uniform response to low energy X-rays [1, 2] which may be significant in applications where the energy spectrum differs from that used to calibrate the absolute response of the TLD. However, there are limitations to the methods that have been used to investigate the low X-ray energy response of LiF:Mg:Cu:P such as a limited range of energies (10.0–99.6 keV) [2, 3], and the use of heteroenergetic sources [1] which will yield a less representative variation of the response than that produced by monoenergetic sources [4].

The purpose of this study was to measure the relative response of LiF:Mg:Cu:P to low energy quasi-monoenergetic X-ray sources over a wider range of energies than had been derived already using monoenergetic sources [2], and to compare this response with that of LiF:Mg:Ti. Although the measurement technique had already been used to derive the low X-ray energy response of LiF:Mg:Ti TLDs [5], these measurements were repeated in order to provide a direct comparison with the LiF:Mg:Cu:P measurements. The results were then used to derive energy response coefficients which allowed a comparison to be made between the potential errors introduced by each type of TLD when used for two dosimetry applications where the X-ray energy spectrum differed from that used to calibrate the absolute TLD response.

Received 9 July 2004 and in revised form 25 November 2004, accepted 13 January 2005.

Material and methods

Energy response measurements

Fifty LiF:Mg:Cu:P chips (0.45 cm × 0.45 cm × 0.06 cm) and 50 LiF:Mg:Ti TLDs cylindrical rods (0.1 cm diameter, 0.5 cm length) were annealed five times by the procedure recommended by the manufacturer (QADOS Ltd., Camberley, UK) to reduce the risk of sensitivity variations. Each chip and rod was then positioned in a Perspex phantom at the depth of maximum dose produced by a Varian 2100C linear accelerator (Varian Oncology Systems, CA, USA) with a 6 MV 10 cm × 10 cm field. A dose of 100 cGy (absorbed dose to water) was delivered to the TLD and its thermoluminescent response was recorded. This process was repeated three times before 30 TLDs of each type, whose response did not vary by more than $\pm 2.5\%$, were selected for the energy response measurements. Each TLD was then encased individually in black polyvinyl chloride.

Three TLDs of each type were attached to a 2 cm thick Styrofoam block to minimize backscatter (attenuation $<0.5\%$) [5] and were irradiated in the central 0.003 m^2 of a 0.025 m^2 circular field by one of the quasi-monoenergetic radiations generated by a filtered Pantak HF-320 X-ray unit (Pantak, Inc., CT, USA) with a stabilized output (Table 1). More detailed information regarding the

Table 1. Characteristics of the quasi-monoenergetic X-ray sources [6] and the relative response per unit air kerma to quasi-monoenergetic X-rays of LiF:Mg:Cu:P and LiF:Mg:Ti thermoluminescent dosemeters (TLD) normalized to that produced by 6 MV X-rays

Potential (kVp)	Mean energy (keV)	FWHM (keV)	Relative response[a]	
			LiF:Mg:Cu:P	LiF:Mg:Ti
15	12	±3.9	0.39±0.02	0.70±0.04
25	20	±6.2	0.73±0.04	1.08±0.06
30	24	±8.2	0.81±0.05	1.18±0.07
40	33	±10.7	1.15±0.07	1.21±0.07
60	48	±19.1	0.95±0.06	1.20±0.07
80	65	±19.5	0.89±0.05	1.15±0.07
100	83	±23.7	0.83±0.05	1.15±0.07
150	118	±43.7	0.76±0.05	1.02±0.06
250	208	±58.2	0.87±0.05	1.01±0.06

FWHM, full width half maximum.
[a]All uncertainties are ±1 standard deviation.

characteristic of this X-ray unit has been reported by Green et al [6]. The dose received by each TLD ranged from 24 cGy to 58 cGy depending upon the dose rate at each energy and the irradiation time available. The 6 MV calibration reference was converted from absorbed dose-to-water to air kerma following the method outlined in an earlier study by Edwards et al [5]. The response per unit air kerma of a TLD at each X-ray energy relative to that produced by 6 MV X-rays was derived from the mean value of the three measured responses for each TLD type using the method described in the previous study [5].

Energy response coefficients

Energy response coefficients were derived to estimate the potential error in the two following diagnostic X-ray dosimetry applications: first, for dose output measurements over the typical range of beam qualities produced by a diagnostic X-ray unit (Table 2), but where the absolute response of the TLD had been calibrated just at one beam quality; and second, for body exit dose measurements (*e.g.* in high dose fluoroscopy examinations) where the TLD absolute response had been calibrated using the corresponding entrance beam. The energy response coefficient α_d for each TLD type d was calculated from Equation 1 [7, 8]:

$$\alpha_d = \frac{\sum_{i=0}^{i=\infty} r_d(E_i)\cdot\phi_x(E_i)\cdot\kappa(E_i)}{\sum_{i=0}^{i=\infty} r_d(E_i)\cdot\phi_{\mathrm{cal}}(E_i)\cdot\kappa(E_i)} \cdot \frac{\sum_{i=0}^{i=\infty} \phi_{\mathrm{cal}}(E_i)\cdot\kappa(E_i)}{\sum_{i=0}^{i=\infty} \phi_x(E_i)\cdot\kappa(E_i)} \qquad (1)$$

where $r_d(E_i)$ was the variation with X-ray energy E_i of the relative response per unit air kerma for each TLD type d, obtained by fitting a curve to the results of the above measurements using the method of cubic splines. The variation with X-ray energy E_i of the fluence-to-air kerma conversion factor $\kappa(E_i)$ was obtained from the electronic version of IPEM Report 78 [9]. In the first application, $\phi_x(E_i)$ was the spectral variation of the fluence of X-rays with energy E_i for a beam quality x, and it was assumed that the absolute TLD response had been calibrated with a 100 kVp X-ray spectrum $\phi_{\mathrm{cal}}(E_i)$. In the second application, $\phi_x(E_i)$ was the body exit X-ray energy spectrum for each of the above range of beam qualities incident on a body thickness consisting of 16 cm of tissue and 2 cm of bone, and it was assumed that for each beam quality, the absolute TLD response had been calibrated with the incident X-ray spectrum $\phi_{\mathrm{cal}}(E_i)$. Each X-ray energy spectrum and its mean energy were calculated using the IPEM Spectrum Processor for a tungsten target and a 3 mm thick aluminium filter [9, 10]. As defined by Equation 1, an energy response coefficient of more or less than unity will be produced by a TLD over or under responding, respectively, to an X-ray spectrum compared with its response to the calibration spectrum.

Results

The variation in relative response per unit air kerma of each type of TLD with X-ray energy showed the same

Table 2. Characteristic properties of the X-ray sources and body exit X-ray beams and the energy response coefficients α_d calculated for two dosimetry applications

Potential (kVp)	X-ray source		Energy response coefficient[a]		Body exit X-ray beam		Energy response coefficient[b]	
	Mean energy (keV)	HVL (mm of Al)	LiF:Mg:Cu:P	LiF:Mg:Ti	Mean energy (keV)	HVL (mm of Al)	LiF:Mg:Cu:P	LiF:Mg:Ti
40	28.5	1.48	1.06±0.09	1.01±0.08	35.9	3.43	1.3±0.1	1.03±0.09
50	32.7	1.89	1.00±0.08	1.01±0.08	42.6	4.99	1.11±0.09	1.02±0.09
60	36.5	2.26	0.99±0.08	1.00±0.08	48.7	6.21	1.00±0.08	1.01±0.08
70	40.0	2.60	0.99±0.08	1.00±0.08	54.2	7.36	0.95±0.08	1.00±0.08
80	43.6	2.98	0.99±0.08	1.00±0.08	59.4	8.41	0.93±0.08	0.99±0.08
90	47.0	3.39	0.99±0.08	1.00±0.08	63.8	9.27	0.91±0.08	0.98±0.08
100	50.0	3.80	1.00±0.08	1.00±0.08	67.8	9.99	0.90±0.08	0.98±0.08
110	53.7	4.53	1.01±0.09	1.00±0.08	71.9	10.67	0.89±0.08	0.97±0.08
120	56.3	4.98	1.02±0.09	1.01±0.08	75.8	11.27	0.88±0.08	0.97±0.08
130	58.8	5.44	1.02±0.09	1.01±0.08	79.7	11.83	0.87±0.07	0.96±0.08
140	61.2	5.88	1.03±0.09	1.02±0.08	83.6	12.37	0.87±0.07	0.95±0.08
150	63.5	6.33	1.04±0.09	1.02±0.08	87.6	12.88	0.87±0.07	0.94±0.08

HVL, half value layer.
[a]Calibrated at 100 kVp (first application).
[b]Calibrated with the body entrance beam (second application).

overall shape, with the smallest value at the lowest X-ray energy measured of 12 keV (Table 1 and Figure 1). Above this energy, their relative response reached a maximum measured value of 1.15±0.07 and 1.21±0.07 for LiF:Mg:Cu:P and LiF:Mg:Ti, respectively, at an energy of 33 keV. LiF:Mg:Cu:P showed the smallest value of minimum measured relative response (0.39±0.02), and the largest overall change in relative response at energies above its maximum measured value (1.15–0.76).

The calculated values of the energy response coefficient are given in Table 2. If the response of both types of TLD was calibrated at 100 kVp, the relative response of LiF:Mg:Ti to X-rays generated at a tube potential of 40 kVp to 150 kVp did not vary by more than ±2%. However, the response of LiF:Mg:Cu:P remained within the range of ±2% over a slightly narrower tube potential range of 50–130 kVp and outside this range, it increased by more than 2% above the calibration value at 100 kVp. The ratio of the response of each type of TLD to a body exit X-ray beam spectrum compared with its calibration response to the entrance beam spectrum decreased continuously with tube potential over the range 40–150 kVp, passing through a value of unity for LiF:Mg:Cu:P and LiF:Mg:Ti at a tube potential of 60 kVp and 70 kVp, respectively. The response of a LiF:Mg:Ti TLD to a body exit beam was 3% above and 6% below its entrance beam calibration response at a tube potential of 40 kVp and 150 kVp, respectively, whereas the response of LiF:Mg:Cu:P to the exit beam was about 30% above and 13% below its entrance beam calibration response at a tube potential of 40 kVp and 150 kVp, respectively.

Discussion

The average fractional uncertainty in the relative response per unit air kerma for each LiF:Mg:Ti and LiF:Mg:Cu:P TLD was approximately ±6% (1 standard deviation (SD)). Systematic errors produced the greatest contribution to these overall uncertainties, and these errors arose from calibration of the NE2250 Secondary Standard Ionisation Chamber (±2%) used to determine the air kerma output from the Pantak HF-320 X-ray unit, the reproducibility of the response of the TLDs (±2.5%), and from the variation in the X-ray unit's output owing to fluctuations in beam flatness, current and timing (±2%) [5]. However, variation of these uncertainties with energy will have had little effect on the variation of each detector's response with energy.

The LiF:Mg:Ti TLD produced a peak sensitivity of 1.2 at 30 keV when its stopping power ratio had been compared with water [11–13]. The synchrotron radiation studies by Kron et al [2, 3] found a peak sensitivity of 1.47 at an incident energy of 26.8 keV. In the previous quasi-monoenergetic study of the response of LiF:Mg:Ti, a maximum measured relative sensitivity of 1.31±0.09 was produced for an incident energy of 33 keV [5], which overlapped within one standard deviation of the value of 1.21±0.07 found in this later study at that energy (Figure 1). A paired *t*-test, used to compare these two sets of results showed that there was no statistically significant difference in the mean response ($p>0.5$), despite the fact that this type of test does not consider the experimental uncertainties. Since the time of the first study, these TLD rods had been in continual routine use and handling of the rods may have resulted in surface

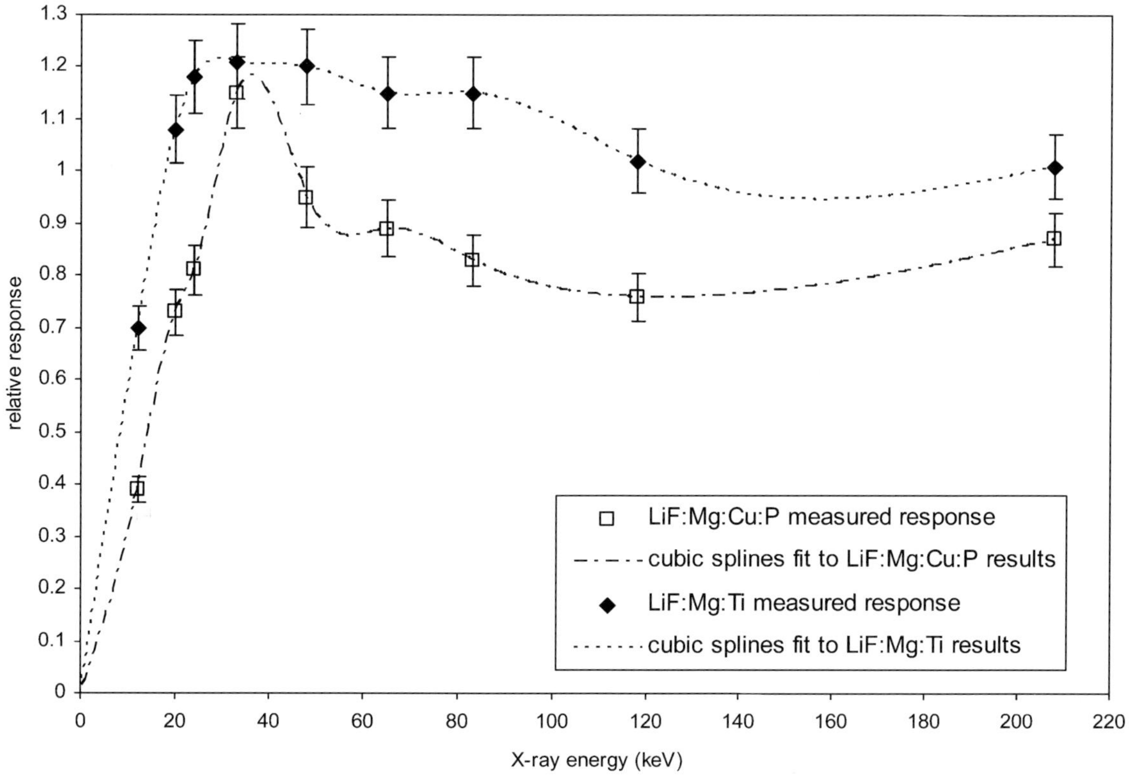

Figure 1. The relative response per unit air kerma to low energy quasi-monoenergetic X-rays of LiF:Mg:Cu:P and LiF:Mg:Ti thermoluminescent dosemeters normalized to that produced by 6 MV X-rays (error bars are ±1 standard deviation).

damage. This is one factor that could have affected their thermoluminescent properties.

The study by Kron et al [2] using synchrotron radiation to produce monoenergetic X-rays from 10.0 keV to 99.6 keV suggested a peak sensitivity of 1.05 when LiF:Mg:Cu:P was irradiated at an energy of 24 keV, compared with its response when irradiated by 6 MV photons. Cai [1] found a peak sensitivity of 1.13 for this type of TLD when irradiated by a heteroenergetic source whose mean energy was 39 keV, compared with its response when irradiated by a ^{60}Co source. The maximum measured relative response for LiF:Mg:Cu:P in this study of 1.15 ± 0.07 occurred at 33 keV (Figure 1 and Table 2), which was the source energy nearest to that of the maximum response found by Cai [1]. At energies above the peak sensitivities, both of these previously published studies gave a detector under-response, with a minimum sensitivity of 0.8 at 122 keV found by Cai [1] and approximately 0.75 at 165 keV found by Kron et al [2]. These under-responses were consistent with the minimum measured value found here of 0.76 at 118 keV. Within their statistical uncertainty, the results have demonstrated a uniform response for LiF:Mg:Cu:P above the maximum monoenergetic energy of 99.6 keV used by Kron et al [2].

LiF:Mg:Cu:P had a smaller value of maximum measured relative response to the quasi-monoenergetic radiations than LiF:Mg:Ti, and in general it tended to under-respond over the range 12–208 keV, whereas LiF:Mg:Ti tended to over-respond across this range. However, when either type of TLD is used to measure the dose from an X-ray source with a spectrum different from that used to calibrate the TLD response, the error introduced by these effects will depend on the difference between the shape of the two spectra over this range of X-ray energies, as well as on the variation in the TLD response with energy. The energy response coefficients derived in this study have been used as a simple and convenient method of estimating and comparing these potential errors for each type of TLD in two dosimetry applications for a typical range of beam qualities.

In the first application, the results indicated that for both types of TLD, there was only a small difference between their response to X-rays generated at 50–130 kVp and their response to 100 kVp radiation. Hence there would be little error introduced if the response of either type of TLD was calibrated at 100 kVp and then used for dose output measurements at other values of tube potential within that range. However, LiF:Mg:Ti would produce a smaller error than LiF:Mg:Cu:P at tube potentials above and below this range.

In the second application, the results indicated that the response of LiF:Mg:Ti to the exit beam transmitted by an 18 cm thick body (16 cm tissue, 2 cm bone) would vary from its calibration response to the entrance beam by much smaller differences than that produced by LiF:Mg:Cu:P at every value of tube potential listed in Table 2. Calibration of the response of LiF:Mg:Ti with a body entrance beam over 40–120 kVp was found to introduce an error into the corresponding body exit dose measurement which was similar in magnitude to the variation in the response to repeat irradiations ($\pm 2.5\%$), but less than the average fractional uncertainty in its measured relative response per unit kerma ($\pm 6\%$) to the quasi-monoenergetic radiations. The incident calibration spectrum always had a lower mean energy than the body exit spectrum in the second application (Table 2). Tissue backscatter was omitted from the calculation of the incident spectrum by the IPEM Spectrum Processor [10], but the effect of its inclusion would have been to reduce the mean energy of the incident spectrum and therefore to increase further the difference between the mean energy of the incident spectrum and the body exit spectrum. The actual effect of tissue backscatter on the energy response coefficient could be explored by a Monte Carlo calculation, and included in a study of the differences between the TLD response at a depth in a tissue equivalent phantom and the response to the incident calibration spectrum. In this case, its effect would be to reduce the mean spectral energy at both positions.

Finally, the results of this study suggest that a similar comparison should be made between the response of LiF:Mg:Cu:P and LiF:Mg:Ti when used for tissue surface *in vivo* dosimetry outside the main treatment field of a linear accelerator X-ray beam. The normal practice would be to calibrate the TLD absolute response with the central axis beam. However, it has been shown that the near surface X-ray spectrum outside the main field has a large peak over the energy range 25–500 keV where both types of TLD have a non-uniform response, but which is absent in the central axis spectrum [8].

Conclusions

The measurements have confirmed that both types of TLD have a non-uniform relative response to low energy X-rays, with LiF:Mg:Cu:P tending to under-respond to quasi-monoenergetic radiations from 12 keV to 208 keV, whereas LiF:Mg:Ti tended to over-respond. Derivation of an energy response coefficient based on these measurements will allow the potential errors to be estimated in dosimetric applications where the X-ray energy spectrum differs from that used to calibrate the absolute TLD response. This method could be used for a preliminary investigation before a series of experimental measurements, or to assist with the choice of the most suitable TLD for a particular application. However in the latter case, the decision should also be based on the other physical characteristics of the TLD types.

Acknowledgments

The authors would like to express their gratitude to Mr Simon Evans for use of the equipment in the Medical Physics Department at the Derby Royal Infirmary to measure the thermoluminescence of the LiF:Mg:Cu:P chips, and to the Radiology Physics staff at the University Hospital of North Staffordshire for their advice.

References

1. Cai G. The influence of the grain size of LiF:Mg:Cu:P thermoluminescent material on photon energy response and dose response. J Phys D Appl Phys 1995;28:1259–62.

2. Kron T, Duggan L, Smith T, Rosenfeld A, Butson M, Kaplan G, et al. Dose response of various radiation detectors to synchrotron radiation. Phys Med Biol 1998;43: 3235–60.
3. Kron T, Smith A, Hyodo K. Synchrotron radiation in the study of the variation of dose response in thermoluminescence dosimeters with radiation energy. Australas Phys Eng Sci Med 1996;19:225–36.
4. Thompson IMG. International Standard Reference Radiations and Their Application to the Type Testing of Dosimetric Apparatus (Proc. IAEA Symposium on National and International Standardization of Radiation Dosimetry). Vienna: IAEA, 1977:343–65.
5. Edwards CR, Green S, Palethorpe JE, Mountford PJ. The response of a MOSFET, p-type semi-conductor and LiF TLD to quasi-monoenergetic X-rays. Phys Med Biol 1997;42: 2383–91.
6. Green S, Palethorpe JE, Peach DE, Bradley DA. Development of a calibration facility for test instrumentation in diagnostic radiology. Radiat Prot Dosim 1996;67:41–7.
7. Yin Z, Hugtenburg RP, Beddoe AH. Response of silicon diode dosimeters to scattered radiation from megavoltage photon beams. Radiat Prot Dosim 2002;101:415–8.
8. Edwards CR, Mountford PJ. Near surface photon energy spectra outside a 6 MV field edge. Phys Med Biol 2004;49: N293–N301.
9. Cranley K, Gilmore BJ, Fogarty GW, Desponds L. IPEM Report 78 - Catalogue of diagnostic X-ray spectra and other data. York: The Institute of Physics and Engineering in Medicine, 1997.
10. Reilly AJ, Sutton D. IPEM Report 78 – Spectrum processor. York: The Institute of Physics and Engineering in Medicine, 1997.
11. McKinlay AF. Thermoluminescence dosimetry. Bristol: Adam Hilger Press, 1981.
12. Mobit PN, Mayles P, Nahum AE. The quality dependence of LiF TLD in megavoltage photon beams: Monte Carlo simulation and experiments. Phys Med Biol 1996;41:387–98.
13. Williams JR, Thwaites DI. Radiotherapy physics. New York: Oxford University Press Inc., 1993:231–8.

The British Journal of Radiology, 78 (2005), 548–552
DOI: 10.1259/bjr/53491625

Case report
Helical tomotherapy for craniospinal radiation

[1]G BAUMAN, MD, [2]S YARTSEV, PhD, [2]T COAD, BSc, CMD, [1]B FISHER, MD and [2]T KRON, PhD

Departments of [1]Radiation Oncology and [2]Clinical Physics, London Regional Cancer Centre, 790 Commissioners Road East, London, Ontario, N6A 4L6, Canada

Abstract. Helical tomotherapy (HT) plans for craniospinal radiation were generated for the case of a 4-year-old boy with disseminated ependymoma. The HT plans demonstrated excellent target coverage, homogeneity and organ sparing compared with a conventional linear accelerator based craniospinal radiation plan. On the basis of this case study, further evaluation of HT for craniospinal radiotherapy seems justified.

Patients with brain tumours at risk for dissemination through the cerebrospinal fluid often require craniospinal axis irradiation. Comprehensive irradiation of the craniospinal space is technically demanding [1–5]. Craniospinal radiation typically utilizes prone positioning of the patient combined with careful junctioning between opposed lateral cranial fields and a posterior spine field. In larger patients, an additional junction between upper and lower spine fields may be required [4]. Periodic junction shifts are introduced throughout the treatments to address the potential risk of underdose or overdose at the field junctions. Many of the patients requiring craniospinal radiotherapy are paediatric patients who may have difficulty cooperating with prone positioning for treatment and also may require daily anaesthesia for treatment. In these cases, supine positioning may be preferable depending on the institution preference. With either supine or prone positioning, the challenge of setting and verifying multiple field junctions and the maintenance of a homogeneous dose over a long treatment volume remains [2, 3].

Helical tomotherapy (HT) is a novel approach to the delivery of radiation for cancer treatment [6, 7]. It relies on a 6 MV linear accelerator mounted on a ring gantry that rotates around the patient as they advance slowly through the ring. During treatment delivery, the radiation fan beam is defined using a 64-leaf collimator. Each leaf projects a shadow of 0.625 mm width at the isocentre 85 cm away from the target and the fan beam width is adjustable from 0.5 cm to 5 cm. The alteration of leaf positions as a function of the gantry position while the patient advances slowly through the gantry allows great flexibility in sculpting a sophisticated target dose distribution while sparing critical normal structures. In addition, the smooth, helical delivery of the intensity-modulated fan beam allows the treatment of extended volumes in the cephalo–caudad direction in either the prone or supine position without the need for junctioning. We sought to model the potential advantages of HT delivery for craniospinal radiation for the case of a paediatric patient with disseminated ependymoma.

Received 1 June 2004 and in revised form 26 July 2004, accepted 25 January 2005.

Materials and methods

Patient presentation and treatment

The patient was initially diagnosed with a well-differentiated ependymoma of the posterior fossa at age 18 months. The tumour recurred despite multiple surgical resections and once the child reached 4 years of age, a decision was made to treat the child with craniospinal irradiation under general anaesthesia. At the time of treatment, the child had gross tumour remaining in the 3rd and 4th ventricular regions in close proximity to brainstem and optic apparatus as well as a gross tumour deposit in the spine at L4. Given the potential risk of neurocognitive side effects in a 4-year-old child and the proximity of the gross tumour to brainstem, optic apparatus and spinal cord it was decided to limit the total gross tumour volume dose to 45 Gy with a craniospinal dose of 36 Gy. For radiation treatment planning CT images from the vertex of the skull to the ischial tuborosities was acquired with uniform slice thickness and spacing of 3 mm. For clinical treatment the patient was planned and treated with a linear accelerator (LINAC) based technique. The LINAC treatment utilized a half-beam blocked technique to match the cranial and upper spinal fields. A second, lower spinal field was placed using a fixed longitudinal displacement from the superior junction using the exact bed positioning system. Field width for the posterior spine field was 6 cm with the lateral field borders extending to the edge of the transverse processes of the vertebrae. Three junction shifts of 0.5 cm were introduced using asymmetric jaws to maintain the matchline. For the final phase of treatment, reduced size, opposed lateral fields were used to boost the gross disease within the cranium while a single posterior spine field was used to boost the cauda equina disease. For this case study the archived CT planning dataset used for the LINAC treatment was re-planned at a later date using the HT system to explore potential benefits and limitations of this form of intensity-modulated radiation delivery for craniospinal treatment.

Helical tomotherapy planning

For generation of a comparison HT plan CT datasets and structures were transferred to the tomotherapy planning workstation (TomoTherapy Inc., Madison, WI)

using the DICOM RT protocol. The tomotherapy station re-samples the CT datasets in 256×256 voxels with the slice thickness re-sampled to the smallest slice separation in the original CT dataset. In the present study uniform slice thickness and separations of 3 mm were used. The planning system uses an inverse treatment planning process based on iterative least squares minimization of an objective function as described by Shepard [8]. Prior to optimization, dose volume constraints, precedence, importance and penalty factors for target and critical structures were assigned. Target constraints were a minimum of 45 Gy to the gross tumour in the brain and spinal cord and 36 Gy to the remainder of the craniospinal axis. Additional critical organ constraints for eyes (Dmax 8 Gy; D5 20%), lung (Dmax 40 Gy; V10 10 Gy), liver (Dmax 25 Gy, V10 10 Gy), bowel (Dmax 25 Gy, V10 10 Gy), heart (Dmax 30 Gy, V10 10 Gy), and kidneys (Dmax 20 Gy, V20 10 Gy) were specified. As part of the optimization the dose is calculated using a superposition convolution approach [9, 10]. Parameters specified as part of the optimization/dose calculation process are pitch, fan beam thickness (FBT) and modulation factor. These factors are similar to those specified for diagnostic CT scanning with the exception of modulation factor (which determines the range of intensity levels that can be achieved). By increasing the FBT and reducing the pitch and modulation factor one can significantly reduce the treatment time. For optimum dose conformality, small FBT and pitch and high modulation factors should be employed, at the expense, however, of longer treatment times. In clinical practice, the selection of slice width, pitch and modulation factors is unique to the clinical site being treated and represents a compromise between excessively long treatment times (with highly conformal delivery) and shorter treatment times (with some loss of conformality and/or dose homogeneity). While most diagnostic CT scanners allow a mixture of slice separations to be specified over a given volume to be scanned, the current HT unit allows only one set of delivery parameters to be specified per plan. For the current case, two HT plans were generated. The first plan used a 25 mm fan beam for delivery in order to produce a treatment that could be delivered in a reasonable length of time ($\leqslant$15 min). The second plan used a 10 mm fan beam width for the cranial component that would allow optimum conformality and dose modulation around the eyes and cribiform plate. Dose–volume histograms for both the conventional and helical tomotherapy plans were compared.

Results

Dose–volume histograms are illustrated in Figure 1 for the LINAC based plan. The gross tumour volume with margin in the brain and spine receives the prescription dose of 45 Gy while the remainder of the craniospinal axis receives 36 Gy. Inspection of the dose–volume histogram reveals considerable heterogeneity in the gross target volume (GTV) and clinical target volume (CTV) target doses, particularly in the spine (a consequence of the use of a single posterior field with prescription at depth as well as the junctions between fields). Organ at risk doses are also quite heterogeneous with some organs receiving doses close to the CTV dose, albeit to small volumes.

Dose–volume histograms for the 25 mm fan beam HT plan are illustrated in Figure 2 with a sagittal dose distribution illustrated in Figure 3. With the 25 mm fan beam an overall estimated treatment time of approximately 15 min could be realised. Inspection of the dose–volume histogram reveals excellent conformality for the CTVcord, GTVbrain and GTVcord as well as the critical structures. In addition, excellent homogeneity in dose delivery to CTV and GTV volumes is evident and doses to the organ at risk are uniformly low. Not indicated on the dose–volume histogram but of potential concern would be dose to the teeth and dose variation across the vertebral body as this could affect growth and development of these structures. Inspection inset 1 of Figure 3 indicates point doses to the individual teeth ranging from 9 Gy to 10 Gy (over 25 fractions). With regards to the vertebral bodies, with HT delivery, the dose falls off in all directions from the target volume (in this case the spinal canal) in the axial plane. This fall off is uniform in all directions and ranges from 36 Gy to 24 Gy over the width of the vertebral body (as can be seen in the sagittal view of Figure 3). Thus, the actual dose to bone will vary depending on the distance from the spinal canal but will be relatively symmetric. In comparison, with the LINAC plan the dose to the

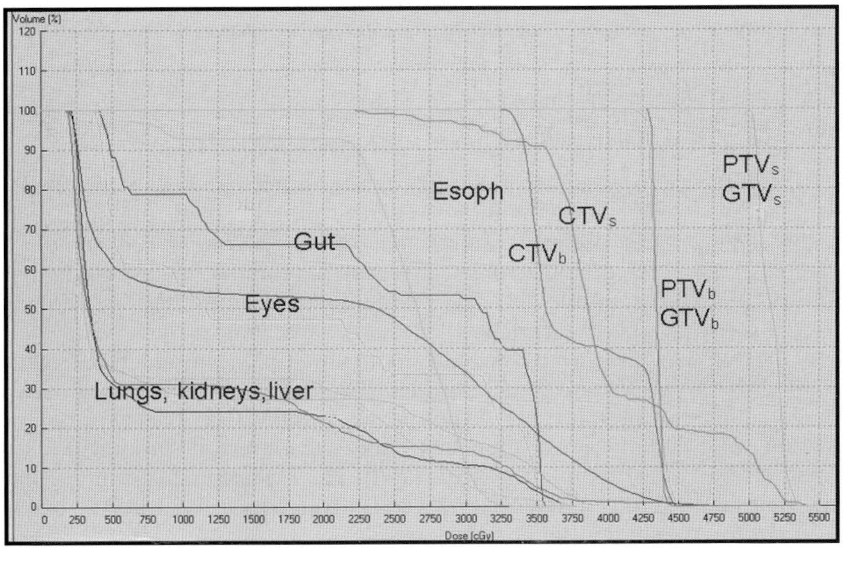

Figure 1. Dose–volume histogram for LINAC craniospinal treatment. Esoph: oesophagus; Gut: small/large bowel; CTVb/CTVs: clinical target volume brain and spine; GTVb/GTVs: gross tumour volume brain and spine; PTVb/PTVs: planning target volume for GTV boost brain and spine.

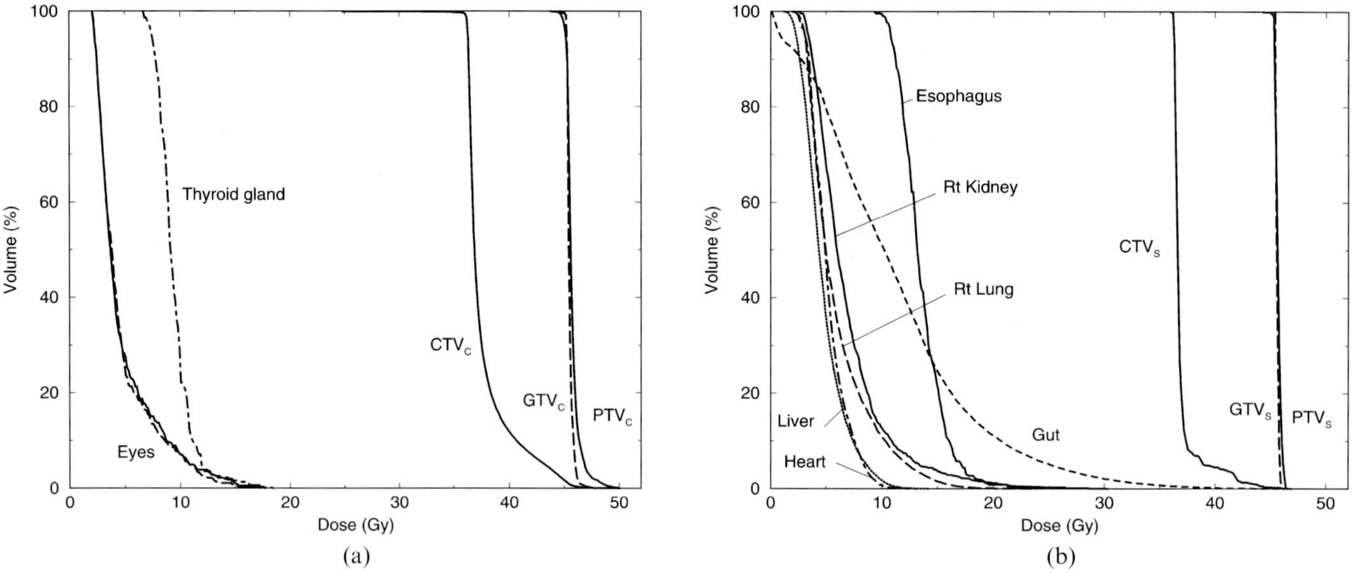

Figure 2. Dose–volume histogram (DVH) for the 25 mm fan beam plan. Excellent coverage of the clinical target volume (CTV) (craniospinal axis) with 36 Gy and the gross tumour in the cord and brain (gross target volume (GTV) with 45 Gy. Doses to critical structures (OAR) are below specified limits. Compared with the DVH for LINAC treatment (1b), variation within the GTV and CTV for brain and spine is much less and OAR doses are overall much lower. For paired organs (Lung, Kidney) only the side with the higher (*i.e.* least favourable) DVH is illustrated.

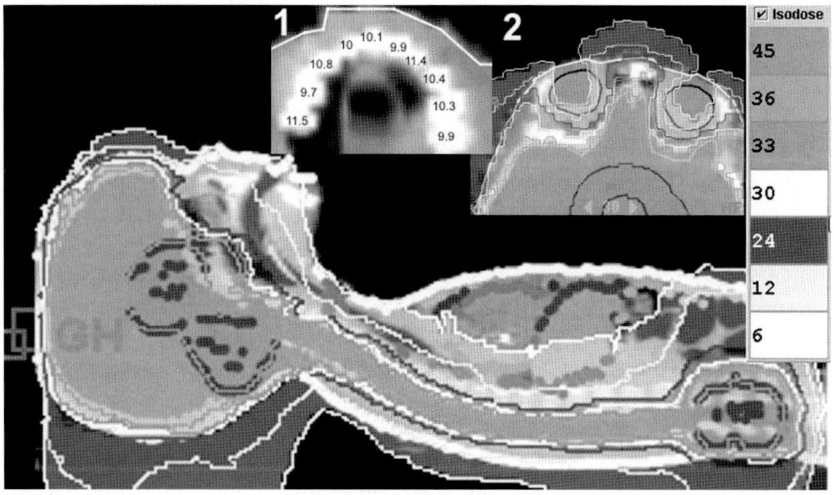

Figure 3. 25 mm helical tomotherapy plan demonstrating excellent conformality in sagittal plane. The chosen fan beam width thickness results in compromises in cribiform plate coverage in order to respect eye dose volume constraints (Inset 2).

vertebral body ranged from 40 Gy at the posterior surface to approximately 34 Gy at the anterior surface creating a non-symmetric dose gradient (and possibly a higher chance of growth plate development asymmetry as a consequence).

Inspection of a central axis slice through the level of the cribiform plate and eyes reveals an inability to achieve acceptable coverage with the necessary ocular sparing with the 25 mm fan beam (Figure 3 inset 2). An alternate plan using a 10 mm width fan beam is illustrated in Figure 4. Examination of the central axis dose distribution at the level of the eyes for this plan demonstrates excellent coverage of the cribiform plate with concomitant sparing of the retina and lens. Of concern with the 10 mm FBT plan however was the estimated delivery time. For the patient concerned, a total treatment time of 40 min was estimated if the whole brain and spine was going to be treated with the small FBT. This treatment time is significantly longer than that of the actual time for treatment experienced on the LINAC and use of the narrow fan beam for the entire craniospinal treatment would not be practical clinically.

Discussion

Craniospinal irradiation is often required in the treatment of common paediatric primary brain tumours such as primary central nervous system germ cell tumours, medulloblastoma and other primitive neuroectodermal tumours [11, 12]. Traditional craniospinal irradiation (CSI) techniques on linear accelerators have employed the prone position with multiple photon fields with junction matches. Supine positioning may be used as an alternative to the prone position at the expense of additional complexity and uncertainty in the junctioning of the photon fields [2, 3]. The HT technique examined in this study offers several advantages over LINAC based craniospinal techniques:

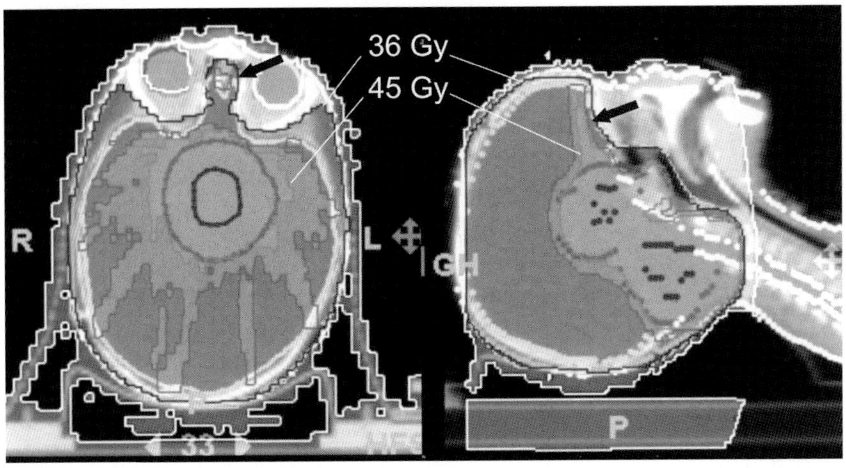

Figure 4. Helical tomotherapy plan using 10 mm fan beam width for cranial treatment. Improved coverage of the cribiform plate area is evident.

1. Helical delivery allows the treatment of extended treatment volumes without the need for field junctioning.
2. A localization pre-treatment megavoltage CT scans (MVCT) with correction for any detected shifts can be acquired prior to treatment in order to precisely align the patient each day [13].
3. Highly conformal treatments can be efficiently delivered without the need for discontinuous couch and gantry movements as employed by non-coplanar LINAC IMRT techniques.
4. The absence of beam modifiers such as blocks and attenuators reduces the chance for treatment error and speeds up the treatment process.

Clinical implementation of an optimal HT plan that realises all these advantages is limited by constraints inherent in the current HT unit. The use of a narrower fan beam and pitch as well as an increased modulation factor would facilitate improved conformality, especially around the cribiform plate, but the clinical use of these parameters would result in estimated treatment times in excess of 40 min. For children requiring general anaesthesia, remote monitoring without access to the patient for this length of time may be of concern.

Use of a wider treatment fan beam of 25 mm allows for treatment of the craniospinal volume in this case with an estimated treatment time of 15 min, similar to the treatment time on a linear accelerator. However, one consequence of this fan beam width selection, is less "resolution" for dose shaping, especially around the cribiform plate and reduction in the sharpness of the superior inferior dose gradients. The simplest way to address this concern could include treatment with variable fan beam width between the cranial and spinal fields, however the current tomotherapy unit does not provide this option. Alternative strategies include treatment of separate cranial and spinal fields with different fan beam widths but with introduction of a junction, however this obviates some of the benefits of tomotherapy delivery. Alternatively, treatment of the whole craniospinal axis with the wider fan beam width with a subsequent "dose patch" with a fine fan beam to top up dose within the cribiform plate could be considered [5]. The use of a "dose patch" with tomotherapy has been proposed for dealing with sub-optimal brachytherapy implants [14]. In the case of the craniospinal treatment the large fan beam thickness could be used to achieve a short overall delivery time to the craniospinal axis, accepting under dose in some parts of the target. The areas of underdose in the cribiform plate region would then subsequently be boosted or "patched" during the same treatment session using the fine resolution afforded by the smaller fan beam thickness and a small pitch factor. In this approach the patient position is not altered and different dose levels can be given in highly non-uniform fashion to make up exactly for the imperfection of the initial delivery. As well the overall treatment time would be kept short by restricting the use of the narrow beam to the cribiform region only. Currently, the dose patch approach cannot be performed with the current version of planning software as it is neither possible to plan on previous isodose surfaces as structures nor to add plans but may be available as a therapeutic strategy in the future.

In terms of the boost field for treatment, HT is ideally suited for the conformal irradiation of gross tumour residual or the post-operative bed. Reduced volume irradiation of the posterior fossa with conformal techniques for patients with medulloblastoma has been described [15, 16]. A potential benefit of the HT plan is the ability to easily deliver a synchronous, field-in-field boost to a target sub-volume. A synchronous in-field boost to the tumour bed may offer an opportunity to improve tumour control without an increase in normal tissue side effects. In addition, with a synchronous boost, overall treatment times can be shortened, for improved disease control [17]. For those children requiring sedation for treatment a shorter overall treatment time could also mean fewer general anaesthesia sessions. The use of a synchronous boost has implications for surrounding normal tissues in terms of fraction size in adjacent structures. Modelling of synchronous versus sequential boost in the context of head and neck treatments suggests radiobiological advantages to this approach [18]. The application of this approach in paediatric patients requires careful evaluation in the context of clinical trials where normal tissue toxicity is tracked.

In addition to technical issues, biological questions with regards to HT delivery for craniospinal radiation also exist. There may be concern regarding the potential of tumour cells within the cerebrospinal fluid to circulate in and out of a moving fan treatment beam. However, good results have been achieved with scanning electron field radiation of the posterior spine field suggesting this may not be clinically important [19]. An additional biological concern is the integral dose to the body resulting from helical delivery of the craniospinal treatments. While individual organ tolerances are incorporated in the delivery, a significant volume of tissue receives dose in the 3–10 Gy range. While these doses are unlikely to cause late tissue effects there remains a concern regarding potential for second malignancies or effects on normal tissue/organ development with larger treatment volumes in paediatric patients. Despite this concern, the paediatric radiotherapy community is starting to embrace technologies (radiosurgery, 3DCRT and IMRT) for the precision irradiation of intracranial targets that deliver relatively large low dose regions in the brain [16, 20–22]. Finally, many paediatric brain tumour patients are now treated with concurrent and/or adjuvant chemotherapy. The toxicity of a rotational *vs* a fixed field radiation technique when combined with chemotherapy for craniospinal radiation is not known. Evaluation of IMRT treatments for paediatric patients clearly will require long term follow-up to assess the possible long-term consequences on growth and development as well as second malignancy, particularly in organs that may not have been exposed to significant radiation with previous techniques.

Conclusions

A sample case of a 4-year-old boy planned for HT treatment of the craniospinal axis illustrates potential advantages and some practical implementation issues. Further development of HT techniques for craniospinal radiation seems justified and ideally, the implementation of this technique should be in the context of clinical protocols where toxicity and outcome for patients can be carefully tracked.

References

1. Mah K, Danjoux CE, Manship S, Makhani N, Cardoso M, Sixel KE. Computed tomographic simulation of craniospinal fields in pediatric patients: improved treatment accuracy and patient comfort. Int J Radiat Oncol Biol Phys 1998;41:997–1000.
2. Michalski JM, Klein EE, Gerber R. Method to plan, administer, and verify supine craniospinal irradiation. J Appl Clin Med Phys 2002;3:310–6.
3. Thomadsen B, Mehta M, Howard S, Das R. Craniospinal treatment with the patient supine. Med Dosim 2003;28:35–8.
4. Van Dyk JJD, Leung PMK, Cunningham JR. Medulloblastoma: treatment technique and radiation dosimetry. Int J Radiat Oncol Biol Phys 1977;2:993–1005.
5. Halperin EC. Impact of radiation technique upon the outcome of treatment for medulloblastoma. Int J Radiat Oncol Biol Phys 1996;26:233–9.
6. Olivera GH, Shepard D, Ruchala K, Aldridge KS, Kapatoes J, Fitchard EE, et al. Tomotherapy. In: Van Dyk J, editor. The modern technology of radiation oncology. Madison, WI: Medical Physics Publishing, 1999:521–87.
7. Mackie TR, Balog J, Ruchala K, Shepard D, Aldridge S, Fitchard E, et al. Tomotherapy. Sem Radiat Onc 1999;9:108–17.
8. Shepard DM, Olivera GH, Reckwerdt PJ, Mackie TR. Iterative approaches to dose optimization in tomotherapy. Phys Med Biol 2000;45:69–90.
9. Papanikolaou N, Mackie TR, Meger-Wells C, Gehring M, Reckwerdt P. Investigation of the convolution method for polyenergetic spectra. Med Phys 1993;20:1327–36.
10. Mackie TR, Olivera GH, Reckwerdt PJ, Shepard DM. Convolution/superposition photon dose calculation. In: Shui AS, Mellenberg DE, editors. General practice of radiation oncology physics in the 21st century. Madison, WI: Medical Physics Publishing, 2000:39–56.
11. Packer RJ VG. Pediatric glial neoplasms including brain-stem gliomas. Semin Oncol 1994;21:260–72.
12. Pollack IF. Brain tumors in children. New Engl J Med 1994;331:1500–7.
13. Ruchala KJ, Olivera GH, Kapatoes JM, Schloesser EA, Reckwerdt PJ, Mackie TR. Megavoltage CT image reconstruction during tomotherapy treatments. Phys Med Biol 2000;45:3545–62.
14. Lewis C, Kron T, Chen J, D'Souza D. Helical tomotherapy or IMRT to boost a "suboptimal" prostate brachytherapy implant: a feasibility study. AAPM 2002;29:1941.
15. Merchent TE, Happersett L, Finlay JL, Leibel SA. Preliminary results of conformal radiation therapy for medulloblastoma. Neuro-oncol 1999;1:177–87.
16. Wolden S, Dunkel IJ, Souweidane MM, PHappersett L, Khakoo Y, Schupak K, et al. Patterns of failure using a conformal radiation therapy tumor bed boost for medulloblastoma. J Clin Oncol 2003;21:3079–83.
17. Taylor RE, Bailey CC, Robinson K, Weston CL, Ellison D, Ironside J, et al. Results of a randomized study of preradiation chemotherapy versus radiotherapy alone for nonmetastatic medulloblastoma: The International Society of Paediatric Oncology/United Kingdom Children's Cancer Study Group PNET-3 Study. J Clin Oncol 2003;21:1581–91.
18. Dogan N, King S, Emami B, Mohideen N, Mirkovic N, Leybovich LB, et al. Assessment of different IMRT boost delivery methods on target coverage and normal-tissue sparing. Int J Radiat Oncol Biol Phys 2003;57:1480–91.
19. Gaspar L, Dawson DJ, Tilley-Gulliford SA, Benerjee P. Medulloblastoma: long-term follow-up of patients treated with electron irradiation of the spinal field. Radiology 1991;180:867–70.
20. St Clair WH, Adams JA, Bues M, Fullerton BC, Shell S, Kooy HM, et al. Advantage of protons compared to conventional X-ray or IMRT in the treatment of a pediatric patient with medulloblastoma. Int J Radiat Oncol Biol Phys 2004;58:727–34.
21. Merchant TE, Mulhern RK, Krasin MJ, Kun LE, Williams T, Li C, et al. Preliminary results from a phase II trial of conformal radiation therapy and evaluation of radiation-related CNS effects for pediatric patients with localized ependymoma. J Clin Oncol 2004;22:3156–62.
22. Saran FH, Baumert BG KV, Adams EJ, Garre ML, Warrington AP, Brada M. Stereotactically guided conformal radiotherapy for progressive low-grade gliomas of childhood. Int J Radiat Oncol Biol Phys 2002;53:43–51.

The British Journal of Radiology, 78 (2005), 553–557
DOI: 10.1259/bjr/21010811

Case report

Benign external compression of the inferior vena cava associated with thrombus formation

[1]R A ENGLAND, MRCP, FRCR, [1]I P WELLS, FRCP, FRCR and [2]C M GUTTERIDGE, MRCP, FRCR

[1]*Department of Clinical Imaging, Derriford Hospital, Plymouth, Devon PL6 8DH and* [2]*Department of Radiology, Royal Cornwall Hospital, Truro, Cornwall TR1 3LJ, UK*

Abstract. Malignant and benign causes of inferior vena cava (IVC) occlusion and compression are recognized. Cases of benign IVC compression with associated distal thrombus formation have not however been frequently described. We present two cases of benign external IVC compression associated with distal thrombus formation; one resulting from a giant, benign, hepatic cyst, and another due to pelviureteric junction obstruction, resulting in massive hydronephrosis.

Occlusion of the inferior vena cava (IVC) is a well recognized complication of malignancy, be this indirectly through an increased tendency to thrombus formation, or directly due to tumour thrombus extension as in the case of renal cell carcinoma. Benign causes of IVC obstruction are less frequently encountered and may also be due to external compression or internal occlusion. Benign occlusions may be membranous, a condition of disputed aetiology more frequently encountered in the Far East that predisposes to hepatocellular carcinoma, or may be due to congenital segmental deficiency. There are however few reports of benign cases of external compression of the IVC. We have found reports in the literature of three cases of benign, external IVC obstruction secondary specifically to bladder distension, two of which were in neonates. An association between IVC compression by polycystic kidneys resulting in infrarenal IVC thrombus formation and pulmonary embolus has been described [1, 2]. A single case of IVC obstruction specifically due to an enlarged renal pelvis has been reported [3]. This case was due to bladder outflow obstruction secondary to benign prostatic hypertrophy, and was not complicated by thrombus formation. External IVC compression by other uncommon causes such as hydatid cyst [4], haematoma due to blunt liver trauma [5], and ruptured abdominal aortic aneurysm [6] have been described, again with no thrombotic complications. The two cases presented here are unusual in the combination of the causes of IVC obstruction, and associated distal thrombus formation.

Case 1

A 70-year-old woman, who had an asymptomatic benign hyperplastic colonic tumour was noted on a pre-operative CT study to have a large simple cyst arising from within the right lobe of her liver. She had a medical history of ischaemic heart disease, atrial fibrillation, transient ischaemic attacks, anaemia and mild, chronic renal impairment.

Received 15 January 2004 and in revised form 22 July 2004, accepted 26 January 2005.

Prior to resection of her colonic tumour, and 12 days following coronary artery angioplasty and stent insertion for lesions in the left anterior descending and right coronary arteries, she presented with pain and swelling of the right leg. The arterial puncture had been via the right groin (size 6 French catheter) and there was no documented puncture of the femoral vein. Duplex ultrasound demonstrated echogenic material within the right common femoral vein with no evidence of femoral artery puncture complications such as haematoma or false aneurysm. She was subsequently commenced on warfarin. At this time she had been vomiting and was both clinically and biochemically dehydrated on a background of chronic renal impairment (urea 26, creatinine 209). 1 week later, with an International Normalized Ratio (INR) of 3.4, she passed a moderate amount of blood per rectum. Warfarin therapy was ceased and a repeat CT arranged to assess the upper limit of thrombus and re-assess the hepatic cyst. Both common iliac veins were occluded and the thrombus extended within the IVC to a level 3 cm below the renal veins. The cyst, which measured 17 cm in maximum diameter, significantly compressed the IVC (Figure 1a).

A Tulip filter (Cook, UK) was placed within the infrarenal IVC above the distal thrombus via a right-sided jugular approach. Venography at the time had confirmed 90% caval compression by the hepatic cyst (Figure 1b). With the filter in a satisfactory position the cyst was drained percutaneously with the aspiration of 2 l of fluid, in the knowledge that the risk of embolising thrombus, owing to the rapid increase in venous flow rate, would not result in significant pulmonary embolus. Further venography immediately following the drainage procedure demonstrated a normal appearance in the upper IVC with free flow of blood to the right atrium (Figure 1c). The drainage procedure was complicated by a localized sub-hepatic haematoma resulting in a fall in haemoglobin. This was a self-limiting problem and did not require transfusion.

Repeat ultrasound 3 weeks later demonstrated some recollection of fluid within the cyst that now measured 10 cm in diameter. Flow within the hepatic portion of the IVC was of normal characteristics and no echogenic

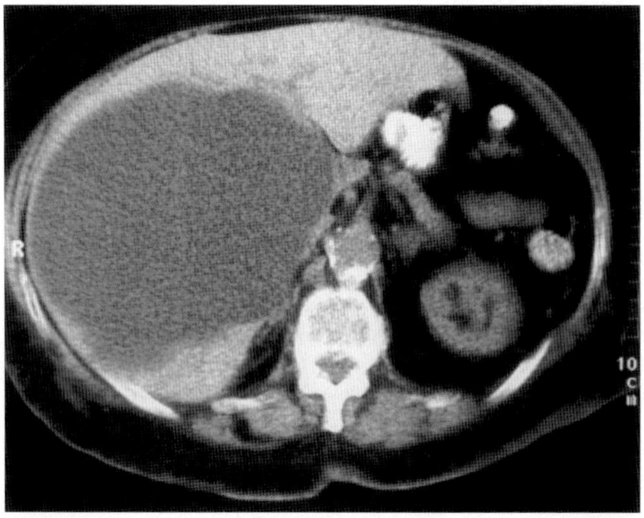

(a)

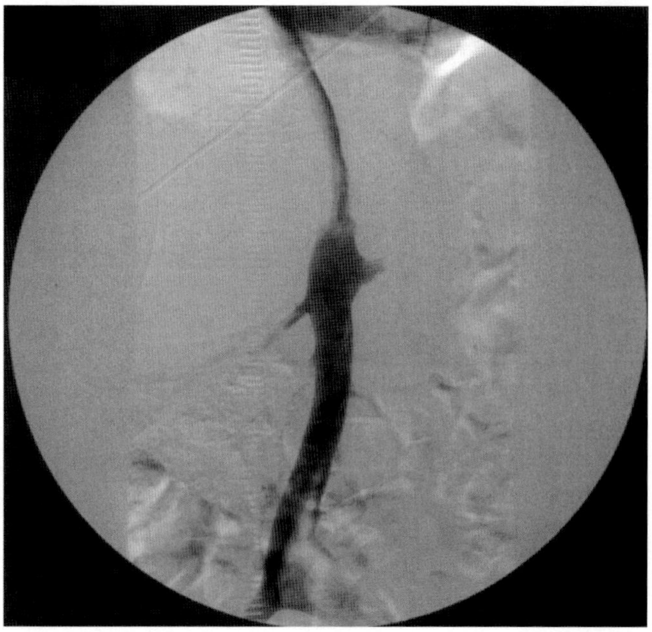

(b)

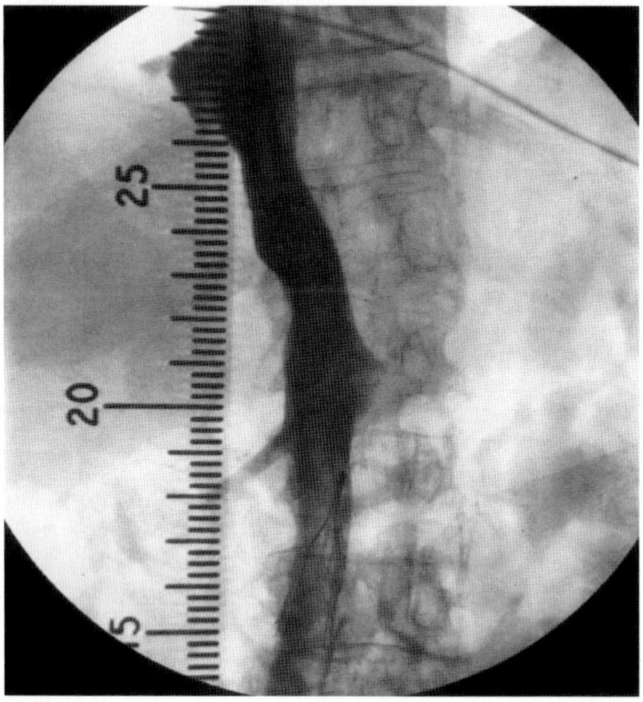

(c)

Figure 1. (a) CT of the abdomen showing a simple, but very large cyst within the right lobe of the liver. The inferior vena cava (IVC) is barely visible as it is compressed to near total occlusion. (b) Initial inferior vena cavogram showing both the extent of luminal narrowing of the IVC, and the cephalic extent of the thrombus within. (c) Following deployment of the Tulip filter, and subsequent cyst aspiration, the hepatic IVC lumen has now returned to normal appearances.

material was seen within. Following resection of the benign hyperplastic colonic polyp, the presumed source of her bleeding per rectum, she was recommenced on warfarin and there have been no further complications.

Case 2

A 45-year-old man presented as an emergency with sudden increasing shortness of breath associated with chest pain. He had a 5-week history of anorexia and weight loss, with a 2-week history of shortness of breath. He had a past medical history of hepatitis C infection secondary to intravenous drug abuse, and a right sided pelviureteric junction obstruction diagnosed 2 years previously. Dynamic renography with frusemide performed within 3 months of diagnosis had demonstrated an obstructed kidney that contributed 1% to divided renal function (PATLAK analysis). Renal biochemistry on admission was normal. He denied ever injecting into veins in either leg and claimed to have not injected for several years however this was later corrected to 6 weeks previously.

A contrast enhanced CT study performed urgently on admission revealed thrombus in the right atrium extending from the IVC (Figure 2a), and within both pulmonary arteries extending into the lower lobe vessels. The right

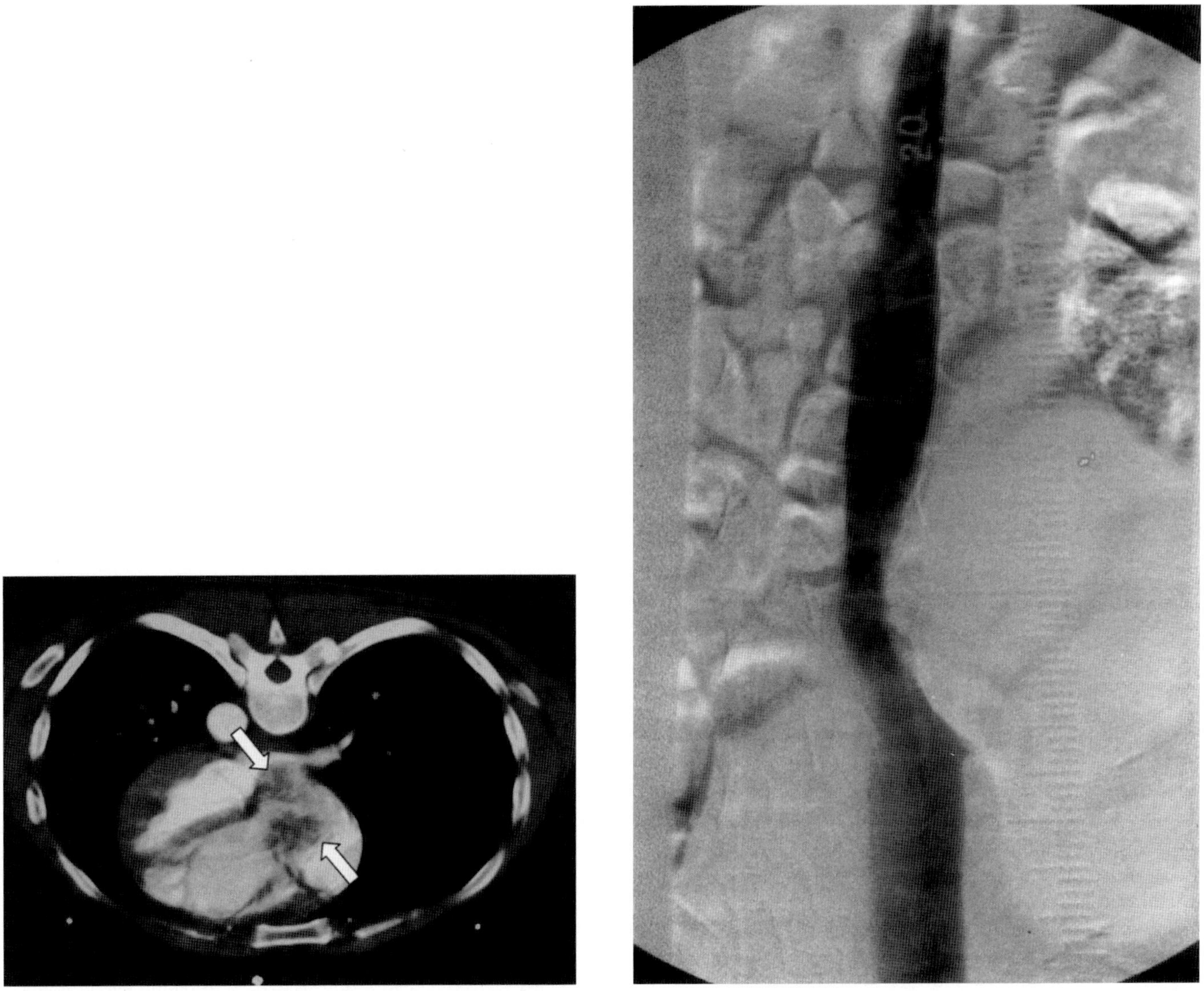

(a) (b)

Figure 2. (a) CT pulmonary angiogram showing a filling defect due to thrombus within the right atrium (arrows) and enlarged right heart chambers. (b) Post operative inferior vena cavogram demonstrating the degree of inferior vena cava (IVC) luminal compression at the level of the renal veins.

atrium and IVC were distended. The right kidney was markedly hydronephrotic with only a thin rim of cortex, and the adjacent IVC was filled with thrombus. He was transferred to the regional cardiothoracic centre for surgical consideration. Transthoracic echo again demonstrated an enlarged right atrium containing thrombus extending from the IVC. He underwent open exploration of the right atrium and main pulmonary trunk. Systolic pulmonary arterial pressure measured 70 mmHg prior to removal of thrombus from the right atrium, main pulmonary trunk, left pulmonary artery, and vena cava.

Post-operative duplex ultrasound demonstrated echogenic material within the left popliteal and superficial femoral veins to the mid thigh level. The intrahepatic and sub-hepatic portions of the IVC now appeared clear; the thrombus having presumably migrated. His post-operative recovery was complicated by a wound infection resulting in septicaemia necessitating a protracted course of antibiotics. Nephrectomy was therefore postponed and performed electively at a later date. Femoral venography performed 9 days post-operatively did not demonstrate any thrombus within the IVC, but did reveal a reduction in lumen calibre at the level of the renal veins by 70% (Figure 2b). The degree of distortion of the caval anatomy, along with the complication of sepsis, precluded the deployment of a filter and the patient remained on warfarin whilst awaiting nephrectomy. The hydronephrosis was drained percutaneously via nephrostomy 3 weeks after initial presentation with the aspiration of 850 ml of fluid. Repeat ultrasound performed 6 weeks later demonstrated no recurrence of hydronephrosis. When right nephrectomy was performed 5 months later the hydronephrosis had recollected. Factor V Leiden and prothrombin gene mutations were excluded.

Discussion

Compression of the lumen of a vein results in decreased flow caudally which, with time, may predispose to thrombus formation. In both cases presented, the external

IVC obstruction was of a chronic nature, inferred from the size of the giant hepatic cyst in case 1, and the longstanding hydronephosis in the second case. It is reasonable to postulate that the marked narrowing of the IVC with resultant flow disturbance was one factor which predisposed to the thrombosis, and in one case embolism, seen in our cases. Other factors however may well have contributed. The patient in case 1 had been vomiting for 2 days and was dehydrated, which is widely accepted as a risk factor for thrombus formation. Deep vein thrombosis (DVT) following cardiac catheterization is an uncommon but recognized complication [7] although more frequently associated with venous cannulation and multiple attempts. There was no documented venous cannulation and no ultrasound evidence of arterial puncture complication in this case.

Injection into the groin veins is the most likely compounding risk factor in an intravenous drug abuser [8, 9]. This however was denied by our patient. Hepatitis C is associated with the increased incidence of anticardiolipin antibodies, however studies have failed to show any significant increase in thrombotic tendency or anti-cardiolipin syndrome [10, 11]. There is a recognized association between advanced hepatic fibrosis secondary to Hepatitis C and an increased incidence of thrombotic risk factors [12, 13], although it is not yet clear whether this risk extends to the larger veins. Our patient did not have hepatic fibrosis, however we cannot fully exclude all associated thrombotic risk factors.

There are certain signs that should alert to the possibility of IVC flow interruption such as bilateral limb swelling in the absence of cardiac impairment, and collateral formation in the absence of chronic liver disease. In the case presenting with massive pulmonary embolus, imaging by both contrast enhanced CT and echocardiography had demonstrated thrombus extending from the IVC to the right atrium prior to surgery. At surgery later that day, the thrombus had migrated proximally from the IVC, underlining the serious and unstable nature of this condition.

Various means of imaging were employed in the diagnosis and management of these cases. Ultrasound, CT and lower limb venography all have roles to play, and vary slightly in the information that they can offer. Traditionally venography has been considered the gold standard in venous assessment, however it can have limitations, particularly in the assessment of the proximal veins, and ultrasound and CT are now often thought to be advantageous [14, 15]. Femoral venography will provide accurate information about the IVC lumen calibre, the caudal extent of narrowing or occlusion, and will demonstrate any functioning collateral vessels. Intervening bowel gas is not usually a concern when using digital subtraction, unlike with ultrasound when it may seriously compromise the image quality. It may not be possible however to define accurately the cephalad extent of complete obstruction by femoral venography alone. Both ultrasound and CT have been shown to demonstrate accurately the cephalad extent of the thrombus, although parasagittal imaging in ultrasound achieves this more definitively [15]. Both ultrasound and CT also allow further assessment of the cause of IVC flow interruption, be this detection of primary malignancy or the cause of external compression as in our cases.

Benign intra-abdominal causes of external IVC compression as a predisposition to DVT have not been widely described in the literature. Given the incidence of gross hydronephrosis and large hepatic cysts, it is surprising that associated thromboembolism has not been described more frequently. Often a pelvic ultrasound examination is requested in a hunt for malignancy, yet the abdominal viscera and IVC are usually not routinely examined in such cases. It may be postulated therefore, that some similar cases remain undetected. Ultrasound is a reliable way of assessing the upper extent of the thrombus, which is often not demonstrated on venography alone, and allows assessment of other viscera. It remains the safest and most accessible means of follow-up. When transluminal, interventional therapy is considered, such as filter insertion or venoplasty, venography remains essential.

References

1. O'Sullivan DA, Torres VE, Heit JA, Liggett S, King BF. Compression of the inferior vena cava by right renal cysts: an unusual cause of IVC and/or iliofemoral thrombosis with pulmonary embolism in autosomal dominant polycystic kidney disease. Clin Nephrol 1998;49:332–4.
2. Leimenstoll G, Loose G, Harder T, Herrmann G, Papadopoulos I, Burck HC, et al. Inferior vena cava compression syndrome in cystic kidney. Duplex ultrasonic diagnosis. Dtsch Med Wochenschr 1991;116:1583–7.
3. Davis GC, Aronson NE, Moul JW. Inferior vena cava compression due to massive hydronephrosis from bladder outlet obstruction. Tech Urol 2000;6:226–7.
4. Rajagopal KV, Bishwas R. Hydatid cyst of the liver presenting as an inferior cava obstruction. J Clin Ultrasound 2002;30:114–6.
5. Markert DJ, Shanmuganathan K, Mirvis SE, Nakajima Y, Hayakawa M. Budd-Chiari syndrome resulting from intrahepatic IVC compression secondary to blunt hepatic trauma. Clin Radiol 1997;52:384–7.
6. Ohno A, Nishimura T, Uehara T, Shimonagata T, Kumita S, Ogawa Y, et al. Interesting finding of RI venogram in a case with obstruction of inferior vena cava due to compression by the ruptured abdominal aortic aneurysm. Kaku Igaku 1993;30:557–61.
7. Zahn R, Fromm E, Thoma S, Lotter R, Zander M, Wagner S, et al. Local venous thrombosis after cardiac catheterisation. Angiology 1997;48:1–7.
8. Roszler MH, McCarroll KA, Donovan KR, Rashid T, Kling GA. The groin hit: complications of intravenous drug abuse. Radiographics 1989;9:487–508.
9. McColl MD, Tait RC, Greer IA, Walker ID. Injecting drug use is a risk factor for deep vein thrombosis in women in Glasgow. Br J Haematol 2001;112:641–3.
10. Harada M, Fujisawa Y, Sakisaka S, Kawaguchi T, Taniguchi E, Sakamoto M, et al. High prevalence of anticardiolipin antibodies in hepatitis C virus infection: lack of effects on thrombocytopenia and thrombotic complications. J Gastroenterol 2000;35:272–7.
11. Ordi-Ros J, Villarreal J, Monegal F, Sauleda S, Esteban T, Vilardell M. Anticardiolipin antibodies in patients with chronic hepatitis C virus infection: characterisation in relation to antiphospholipid syndrome. Clin Diagn Lab Immunol 2000;7:241–4.
12. Poujol-Robert A, Rosmorduc O, Serfaty L, Coulet F, Poupon R, Robert A. Genetic and acquired thrombotic factors in chronic hepatitis C. Am J Gastroenterol 2004;99:527–31.

13. Papatheodoridis GV, Papakonstantinou E, Andrioti E, Cholongitas E, Petraki K, Kontopoulou I, et al. Thrombotic risk factors and extent of liver fibrosis in chronic viral hepatitis. Gut 2003;52:404–9.
14. Park JH, Lee JB, Han MC, et al. Sonographic evaluation of inferior vena caval obstruction: correlative study with vena cavography. AJR Am J Roentgenol 1985;145:757–62.
15. Didier D, Racle A, Etievent JP, Weill F. Tumour thrombus in the inferior vena cava secondary to malignant abdominal neoplasms: US and CT evaluation. Radiology 1987;162:83–89.

The British Journal of Radiology, 78 (2005), 558–561
DOI: 10.1259/bjr/82283833

Case report
Cystic adenomyosis with florid glandular differentiation mimicking ovarian malignancy

[1]I IMAOKA, MD, [1,2]Y KAJI, MD, [3]Y KOBASHI, MD, [1]A WADA, MD, [3]G HONJO, MD, [4]M HAYASHI, MD, [4]M YOSHIDA, MD and [1]M MATSUO, MD

[1]*Department of Radiology, MR Division, Tenri Hospital, 200 Mishima, Tenri, 632-8552,* [2]*Department of Radiology, Kobe University School of Medicine, 7-5-2 Kusunoki, Chuo-ku, Kobe, 650-0017,* [3]*Department of Pathology, Tenri Hospital, 200 Mishima, Tenri, 632-8552 and* [4]*Department of Obstetrics and Gynaecology, Tenri Hospital, 200 Mishima, Tenri, 632-8552, Japan*

Abstract. We report a case of cystic adenomyosis, presenting as a huge exophytic cystic mass with florid glandular differentiation. MR findings of the mass mimicked ovarian carcinoma associated with endometriosis. The presence of signal voids bridging the uterus and tumour should suggest a mass of uterine origin. Hyperintense protuberance in a hypointense loculus on T_2 weighted images may suggest benign disease. However, surgical exploration and resection is still required to exclude an ovarian malignancy.

Adenomyosis is a common gynaecological disorder with a reported incidence ranging from 5% to 70%, with a mean of 20–30% [1]. It is characterized as ectopic endometrial glands and stroma extending into the myometrium. MRI shows diffuse or focal thickening of the junctional zone as an area of low signal intensity compared with outer myometrium on T_2 weighted images. Ectopic glands and haemorrhage in adenomyosis are usually small and punctate. Cystic adenomyosis (adenomyotic cyst) is a rare form of adenomyosis with extensive glandular cystic changes and haemorrhage.

The purpose of this report is to present MRI characteristics in a case of cystic adenomyosis, which presented as a huge exophytic cystic mass with florid glandular differentiation. MR findings of the mass mimicked ovarian carcinoma associated with endometriosis.

Case report

A 41-year-old woman (gravida 2) presented with dysmenorrhoea and hypermenorrhoea lasting for 16 years. Pelvic endometriosis had been previously diagnosed and she received gonadotropin releasing hormone (GnRH) analogue therapy from the age of 39 years. She presented with elevated serum levels of CA125 and CA19-9 of 673 U ml^{-1} and 846 U ml^{-1}, respectively. Transvaginal ultrasound showed adenomyosis and a left ovarian tumour of cystic and solid appearance. Left ovarian carcinoma was suspected and MRI was performed with a 1.5 T magnet (Magnetom Vision; Siemens Medical Systems, Erlangen, Germany) to confirm the diagnosis and for a staging. A multiloculate cystic mass of 8 cm × 8 cm × 6 cm was demonstrated abutting the left side of the uterus. The cystic loculi showed high signal intensity on T_1 weighted images and variable signal intensity on T_2 weighted images, which suggested chocolate-like haemorrhage (Figure 1a–c). The solid component within the mass contained foci of high and low T_2 signal intensity (Figure 1b,c). On T_1 weighted images, the solid structure demonstrated isosignal intensity compared with the myometrium, and markedly enhanced after intravenous administration of Gadoteridol (0.1 mmol kg^{-1}) (Figure 1d). In the uterus, adenomyosis was demonstrated on T_2 weighted images, and the interface between the solid component of the mass and myometrium with adenomyosis was irregular and unclear. Signal voids bridged the mass and the uterus, suggesting a hypervascular ovarian tumour invading the uterus. Our pre-operative diagnosis was adenomyosis and a left malignant ovarian tumour associated with endometriosis (*i.e.* endometrioid carcinoma or clear cell carcinoma) invading the uterus (stage IIA). Total abdominal total hysterectomy and bilateral salpingo-oophorectomy were performed.

Macroscopic histology showed a fist-sized tumour adhering to the uterine myometrium with adenomyosis (Figure 1e). Microscopically, the tumour was encapsulated by the hypertrophic myometrium and filled with haemorrhage. The solid protuberance within the tumour consisted of florid endometrioid glands that varied in size and haemorrhagic cellular stroma (Figure 1f). This was consistent with simple endometrial hyperplasia without malignant transformation. Microscopic examination with Berlin blue staining revealed the wall of the cyst contained haemosiderin-laden macrophages. The final pathological diagnosis was cystic adenomyosis. The patient has remained well for 2 years after surgery.

Discussion

Adenomyosis usually presents as diffuse or focal thickening of the junctional zone on MRI. Myometrial hyperplasia, a feature of adenomyosis, demonstrates low signal intensity compared with the outer myometrium on T_2 weighted images. It manifests as increased junctional

Received 13 May 2004 and in revised form 4 January 2005, accepted 26 January 2005.

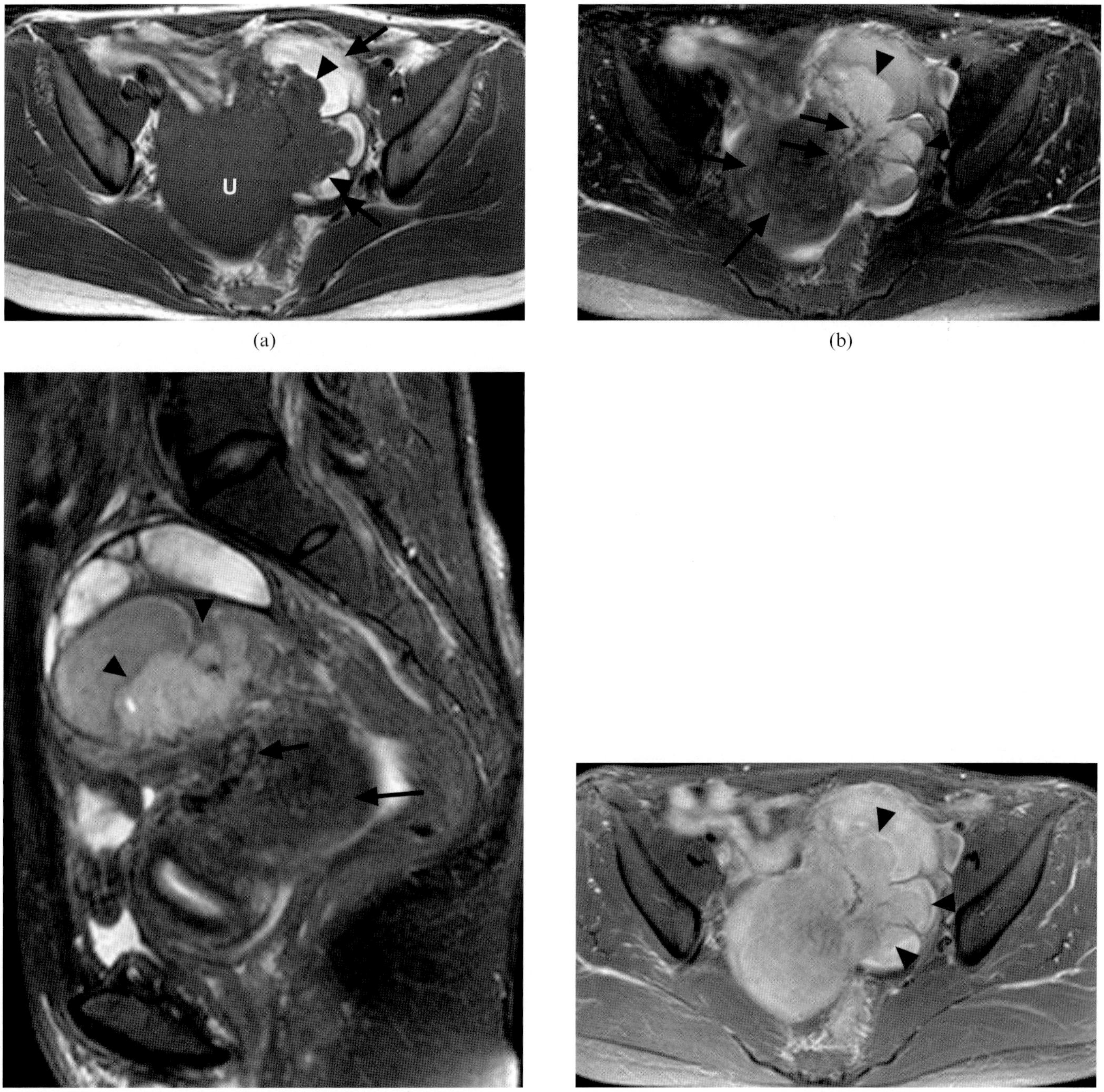

Figure 1. A 41-year-old woman with cystic adenomyosis. (a) Axial T_1 weighted MR image shows hyperintense cystic mass (arrows) abutting left side of the uterus (U). Solid structure (arrowheads) with small hyperintense foci was seen within the mass. (b) Axial and (c) sagittal T_2 weighted images with fat saturation shows hyperintense solid structure (arrowheads) in the hypointense loculus. The interface between the mass and uterus was irregular and unclear. Note that signal voids bridge between the uterus and the mass (short arrows). Adenomyosis is recognized in the uterus (long arrows). (d) Axial contrast-enhanced T_1 weighted image with fat saturation shows marked enhancement in the solid structure (arrowheads). (*Continued*)

zone thickness with unclear margins [2, 3]. Ectopic endometrial glands correspond to high signal intensity foci on T_2 weighted images, some of which are haemorrhagic [3, 4]. Ectopic endometrial glands in adenomyosis are characterized by a predominance of zona basalis and it does not respond to cyclic hormonal stimulation, whereas the zona functionalis does in endometriosis [5, 6]. Therefore haemorrhagic lesions in adenomyosis are usually small and punctate. The cystic form of adenomyosis with extensive glandular cystic changes and haemorrhage is rare [7, 8]. Haemosiderin deposits in the wall of adenomyotic cyst may explain that haemorrhage has occurred several times in the cyst as does in endometriotic cyst. A few MRI reports presented the cases of myometrial and subserosal cystic adenomyosis as prominent high intensity cysts on both T_1 and T_2 weighted images [7, 8]. The cysts were surrounded by low intensity tissue [7, 8]. Our MR findings differed from those of other reports. In our case, abundant solid structure within the mass led to misdiagnoses of ovarian carcinoma associated

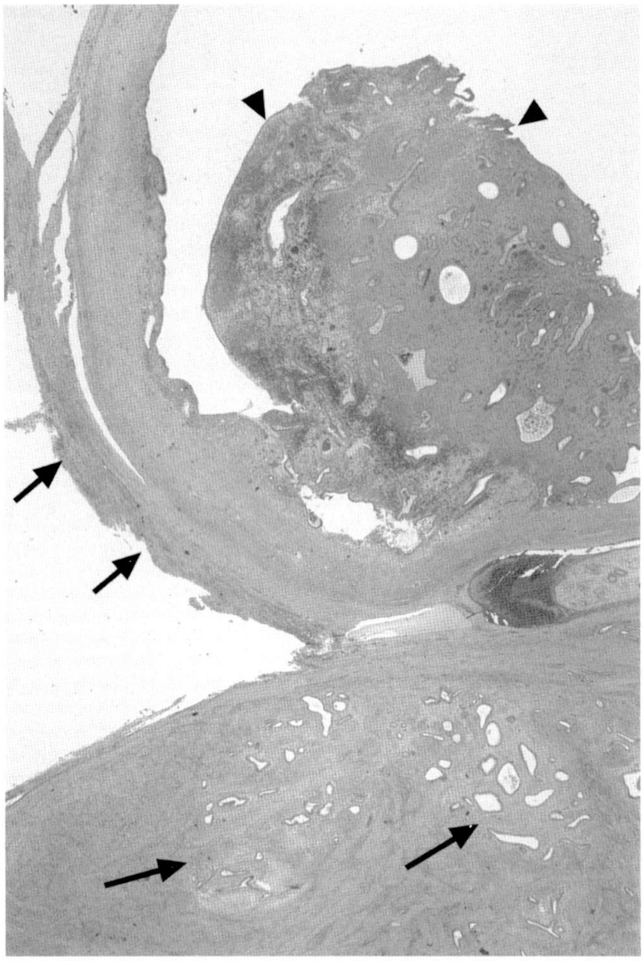

(e)

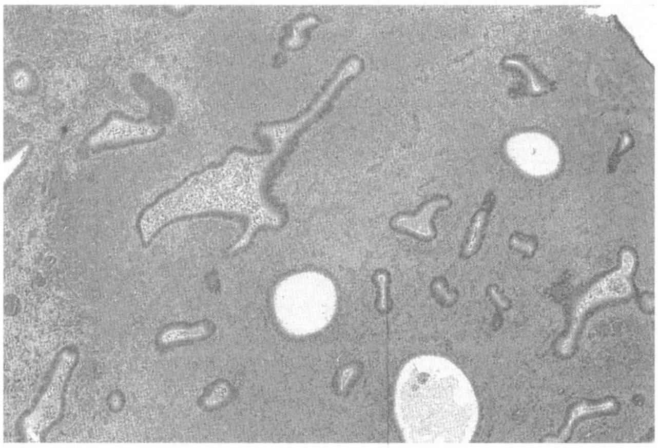

(f)

Figure 1. (*Cont.*) (e) Photomicrograph of the cystic adenomyosis (haematoxylin and eosin, ×10). The cystic adenomyosis (arrows) includes the protuberance with florid glandular differentiation (arrowheads). Adenomyosis noted in the uterine myometrium (long arrows). (f) Photomicrograph of the glandular protuberance within the cystic adenomyosis (haematoxylin and eosin, ×40). Endometrioid glands vary in size lie in haemorrhagic cellular stroma with no malignant transformation. Therefore they were considered as simple endometrial hyperplasia.

with endometriotic cyst. The interface between the solid structure and myometrium was diffuse. Signal voids bridging the uterus and tumour were demonstrated and should have suggested a mass of uterine origin. However, we interpreted these findings as invasion of the uterus by an ovarian carcinoma.

The spectrum of epithelial abnormalities including epithelial metaplasia, hyperplasia, atypia, and adenocarcinoma (*i.e.* endometrioid carcinoma and clear cell carcinoma) have been described in ovarian endometriotic cysts [9]. A report showed that endometriotic cyst with malignant transformation seldom shows low signal intensity on T_2 weighted images and usually has enhancing mural nodules [10]. The authors speculated that adenocarcinomas in endometriosis may produce some fluid that can dilute dense haemorrhagic material. In contrast, in our case of cystic adenomyosis, the loculi showed variable intensity and the enhancing solid structures were in the hypointense loculus on T_2 weighted images.

There have been few reports of adenocarcinomas arising from adenomyosis. The adenocarcinomas were present in the myometrium without involvement of the eutopic endometrium. Koshimaya et al [11] reported four cases of adenocarcinoma arising form adenomyosis, including a transition from benign adenomyotic to carcinomatous glands. In these cases, MRI and ultrasound did not detect the disease correctly and pre-operative diagnoses were ovarian carcinoma in two cases, adenomyosis in one case, and leiomyoma or leiomyosarcoma in one case. In two cases mimicking ovarian malignancy, tumours showed 7–7.5 cm solid and cystic appearance.

The process of the florid endometrioid glands (endometrial hyperplasia, simple) induced within the cystic adenomyosis remains unclear. The previous use of GnRH analogue might modify the glandular differentiation, since it is known that adenomyosis recurs when hormonal therapy is discontinued. MRI demonstrated this glandular protuberance high signal intensity on T_2 weighted images and marked enhancement. It is interesting that the same has been experienced for simple endometrial hyperplasia of the uterine endometrium [12].

In conclusion, in our patient with huge subserosal cystic adenomyosis, a confident differentiation of uterine versus ovarian mass, and of benign versus malignant tumour could not be made. Signal voids bridging the uterus and tumour should suggest a diagnosis of a mass of uterine origin. Hyperintense protuberance in the hypointense loculus on T_2 weighted images may be an atypical appearance of malignant ovarian tumour associated with endometriosis. However, surgical exploration and resection is still required to exclude an ovarian malignancy.

References

1. Vercellini P, Ragni G, Trespidi L, Oldani S, Panazza S, Grosignani PG. Adenomyosis: a deja vu? Obstet Gynecol Surv 1993;48:789–94.
2. Outwater EK, Siegelman ES, Deerlin VV. Adenomyosis: current concepts and imaging considerations. AJR Am J Roentgenol 1998;170:437–41.
3. Reinhold C, Tafazoli F, Mehio A, et al. Uterine adenomyosis: endovaginal US and MR imaging features with histopathologic correlation. Radiographics 1999;19:S147–S160.
4. Togashi K, Ozasa H, Konishi I, Itoh H, Nishimura K, Fujisawa I, et al. Enlarged uterus: differentiation between adenomyosis and leiomyoma with MR imaging. Radiology 1989;171:531–4.
5. Silverberg SG, Kurman RJ. Tumor-like lesions. In: Atlas of tumor pathology 3rd series, fascicle 3 tumors of the uterine corpus and gestational trophoblastic disease. Washington DC: AFIP, 1992:191–218.
6. Braly PS. Diseases of the uterus. In: Soutt JR, Di Saia PJ, Hammond CB, Spellacy WN, editors. Danforth's obstetrics and gynecology (8th edn). Philadelphia, PA: Lippincott, 1999:837–55.
7. Troiano RN, Flynn SD, McCarthy S. Cystic adenomyosis of the uterus: MRI. JMRI 1998;8:1198–202.
8. Kataoka ML, Togashi K, Konishi I, Hatabu H, Morioka K, Kojima N, et al. MRI of adenomyotic cyst of the uterus. J Comput Assist Tomogr 1998;22:555–9.
9. Prefumo F, Todeschini F, Fulcheri E, Venturini PL. Epithelial abnormalities in cystic ovarian endometriosis. Gynecol Oncol 2002;56:997–9.
10. Tanaka YO, Yoshizako T, Nishida M, Yamaguchi M, Sugimura K, Itai Y. Ovarian carcinoma in patients with endometriosis: MR imaging findings. AJR Am J Roentgenol 2000;175:1423–30.
11. Koshiyama M, Suzuki A, Ozawa M, et al. Adenocarcinomas arising from uterine adenomyosis: a report of four cases. Int J Gynecol Pathol 2002;21:239–45.
12. Imaoka I, Sugimura K, Masui T, Takehara Y, Ichijo K, Naito M. Abnormal uterine cavity: differential diagnosis with MR imaging. Magn Reson Imaging 1999;17:1445–55.

The British Journal of Radiology, 78 (2005), 562–564
DOI: 10.1259/bjr/52543195

Case report

Duodenal diverticulum mimicking a cystic pancreatic neoplasm

[1]A HARIRI, BSc, [1]S S SIEGELMAN, MD and [2]R H HRUBAN, MD

Departments of [1]Radiology and [2]Pathology, The Johns Hopkins Hospital, Baltimore, Maryland, USA

Abstract. Duodenal diverticula occur very commonly, with a prevalence as high as 22%. They are most frequently located in the second or third portions of the duodenum, and by nature of their proximity to the head of the pancreas, can be mistaken for cystic pancreatic neoplasms by diagnostic imaging. Patients with presumed cystic neoplasms of the pancreas often receive pancreaticoduodenectomies, which at high volume medical centres carry mortality and morbidity rates of 2–4% and 29–44%, respectively. Although most duodenal diverticula are recognized in single or repeat CT scans by the presence of air or contrast medium within the diverticula, we present a case in which serial CTs failed to yield any clue to the diverticulum's true nature and pancreaticoduodenectomy was performed. For presumed cystic lesions adjacent to the duodenum, barium studies, endoscopy, and/or endoscopic ultrasound-guided aspiration should therefore be pursued in addition to all available CT evidence prior to surgery.

Diverticula of the duodenum occur very commonly. Autopsy studies have revealed their prevalence to be as high as 22% [1]. Although they can cause diverticulitis, perforation, obstruction, or haemorrhage, the majority of duodenal diverticula are asymptomatic [2].

Most duodenal diverticula occur in the second or third portions of the duodenum, within 2.0 cm of the ampulla of Vater [3]. Owing to their proximity to the head of the pancreas, fluid-filled duodenal diverticula can be confused with cystic pancreatic neoplasms by diagnostic imaging [1]. We report such a case in which the patient underwent a Whipple resection for a putative cystic pancreatic neoplasm. Serial CT scans over 3 years failed to yield any clue to the diverticulum's true nature.

Case report

A 77-year-old woman with an ascending aortic aneurysm presented with a 2.0 cm cystic mass closely associated with the pancreas. The mass was identified by CT and presumed to be a cystic pancreatic lesion. Her thoracic aortic aneurysm, 5.4 cm in diameter, had been diagnosed by echocardiography. The decision was made to follow her with serial CT scans. During the first of those CT scans, the cystic lesion within the head of the pancreas was detected.

CT scans were obtained approximately every 6 months for 3 years (Figure 1). There was a perception that the mass had increased in size from 2 cm to 4 cm. The cystic lesion never filled with orally administered contrast medium. At no point was gas seen within the lesion. The diagnosis of duodenal diverticulum was never considered. The patient was asymptomatic. Her abdominal examination was benign and she was not jaundiced. Laboratory findings were normal. On the basis of an enlarging mass presumed to be in the head of the pancreas, the patient received a pylorus preserving pancreaticoduodenectomy. At pathological examination, the lesion proved to be a duodenal diverticulum embedded in the head of the pancreas (Figure 2).

Discussion

While the majority of cystic lesions of the pancreas are post-inflammatory pseudocysts, a wide spectrum of other cystic pancreatic lesions with varying prognoses are regularly encountered during imaging [4, 5]. Cystic pancreatic neoplasms occur in 0.7% of people and range from benign to malignant in nature. Owing to the difficulty of ascertaining the malignant potential of a

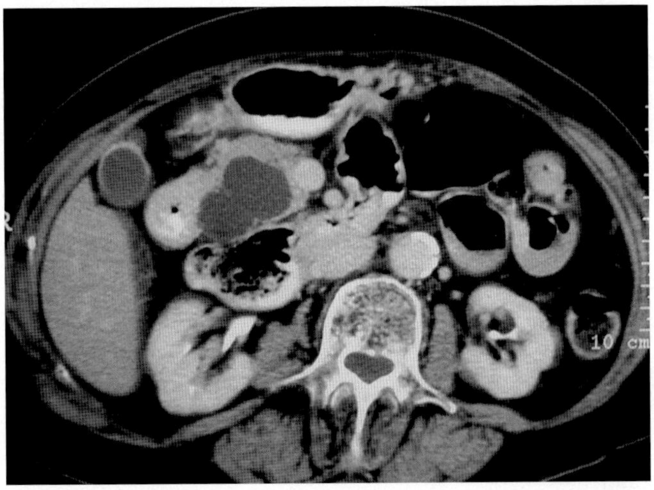

Figure 1. Duodenal diverticulum embedded in pancreatic head of a 77-year-old woman. Axial enhanced CT scan of abdomen shows a multiloculated cystic mass within the head of the pancreas, measuring 4.1 cm by 3.1 cm. The lesion is thin-walled, does not fill with oral contrast medium, and contains no gaseous densities.

Received 22 October 2004 and in revised form 19 December 2004, accepted 31 January 2005.

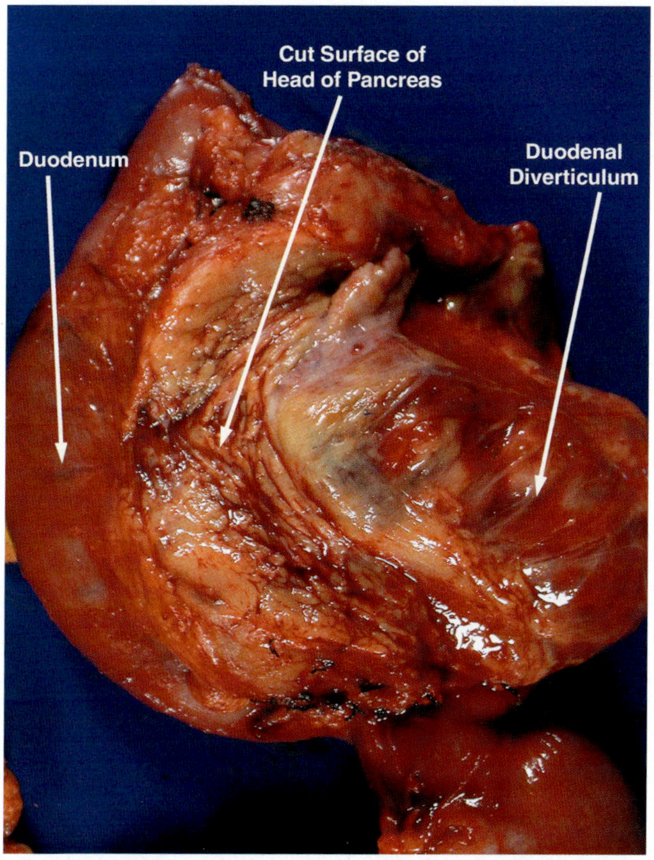

(a)

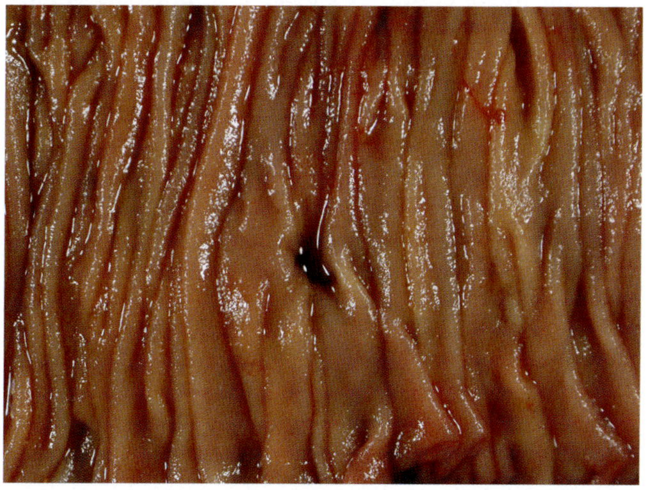

(b)

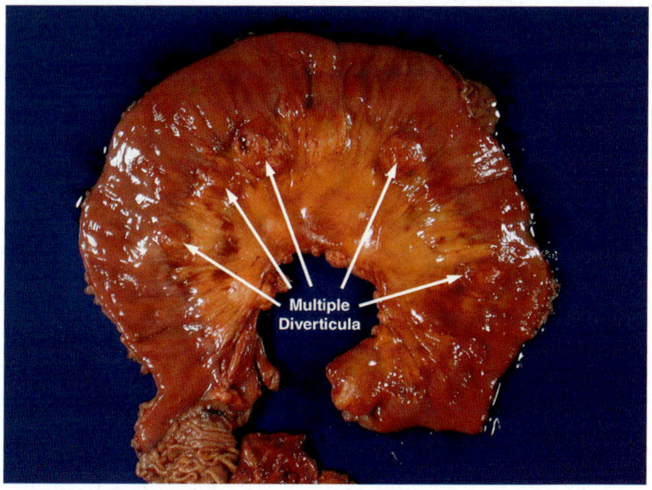

(c)

Figure 2. Gross pathology of the lesion demonstrating: (a) duodenal diverticulum embedded in the head of the pancreas; (b) diverticular orifice, which possesses a very small diameter relative to the diverticulum; (c) duodenum with multiple additional diverticulae.

cystic pancreatic lesion, some have advised surgery in patients who have radiological evidence of increasing cyst size, are symptomatic, or are fit, older patients (60% of cystic lesions in patients over 70 years are malignant) [6]. Clinical history, biopsy, and fluid aspiration can aid in narrowing the differential diagnoses of lesions. However, challenges associated with the pre-operative diagnosis and management of cystic pancreatic lesions have prompted others to advocate resection of all cystic lesions other than pseudocysts [5].

In the case presented, examination of the specimen following surgery revealed a benign lesion, a duodenal diverticulum. Pancreaticoduodenectomy, or Whipple resection, for a condition which proves to be benign is not unusual. Surveys from high-volume medical centres have shown that 9.2% of pancreaticoduodenectomies are performed for benign disorders where there is pre-operative suspicion of malignancy [7]. This is not insignificant given a mortality rate of 2–4%, and morbidity rate ranging from 29–44% depending on whether a standard or radical pancreaticoduodenectomy is performed [8]. Proper diagnosis and recognition of benign entities that could masquerade as cystic pancreatic neoplasms is therefore of paramount importance.

Our case report demonstrates one such entity: a duodenal diverticulum embedded in the head of the pancreas. A recent Finnish study of 1735 patients who had an indication for endoscopic retrograde cholangiopancreatography identified duodenal diverticula in 123 of them, with an equal male to female ratio [9]. After the colon, the duodenum is the second most common location for diverticulae; most are actually pseudodiverticula, resulting from increased intraluminal pressure causing herniation of the mucosa through the muscularis at weak points in the wall, usually where mesenteric vessels enter [2].

In the first study of duodenal diverticula mimicking cystic pancreatic neoplasms, Macari et al [1] looked at seven patients with diverticula ranging in size from 10 cm to 25 cm. MRI or CT was used to identify the lesions. Owing to their small size and benign appearance by imaging, clinical observation was deemed appropriate for six of the seven lesions. The seventh patient, whose CT demonstrated bile and pancreatic duct dilatation, received a pancreaticoduodenectomy. Notably, all diverticula – including the one for which surgery was performed – were correctly identified in imaging studies. Four were identified by the presence of gas in follow-up CT scans, one by gas and another by gas and barium in previous CT scans, and the last in a follow-up upper gastrointestinal barium exam. Even retrospectively, with the knowledge that all seven of these lesions were duodenal diverticula, Macari et al [1] found that with only a single examination, and without the benefit of past or future scans, it was not possible to definitively identify four of the diverticula.

The duodenal diverticulum in this case report presented a diagnostic dilemma. It was only 4.1 cm by 3.1 cm at its maximum size, small enough that both surgery and continued observation were considered plausible options. Despite serial CT scans performed every 6 months for 3 years, at no point did the diverticulum fill with oral contrast or gas. This was likely due to the small diameter of the diverticular orifice (Figure 2b). Although duodenal diverticula can be symptomatic – most often causing abdominal pain or bleeding [10] – the majority are asymptomatic, as in our case. While 38% of patients with cystic pancreatic neoplasms present with pain and 8% with nausea or fullness, the majority of these patients (51%) are also asymptomatic [6]. Therefore, history and physical exam did not yield a clue to the nature our patient's mass. Fluid aspiration would have been non-specific, as it is impossible to distinguish duodenal contaminants from the true composition of a presumed cyst. Nonetheless, endoscopic ultrasound-guided fluid aspiration can be useful in evaluating cystic pancreatic masses, as aspiration of mucin and mucinous fluid suggests a neoplasm (intraductal papillary mucin producing neoplasm or mucinous cystic neoplasm) that may require surgical excision.

Clinicians should therefore be aware that although most duodenal diverticula will be observed to fill with oral contrast medium or gas upon repeat imaging, there are exceptions to this rule. In addition, a diverticulum may appear to increase in size, further raising questions of malignancy. Owing to the morbidity and mortality associated with pancreaticoduodenectomy, careful review of prior imaging studies should always be performed. If previous studies do not demonstrate gas or contrast medium within a cystic lesion adjacent to the duodenum, barium studies, endoscopy, and/or endoscopic ultrasound-guided fluid aspiration should be pursued prior to surgery.

References

1. Macari M, Lazarus D, Israel G, Megibow A. Duodenal diverticula mimicking cystic neoplasms of the pancreas: CT and MR imaging findings in seven patients. AJR Am J Roentgenol 2003;180:195–9.
2. Lipsett P. Diverticular disease of the small bowel. In: Cameron JL, editor. Current surgical therapy (6th edn). St. Louis, MO: Mosby, 1998:148–50.
3. Jayaraman MV, Mayo-Smith WW, Movson JS, Dupuy DE, Wallach MT. CT of the duodenum: an overlooked segment gets its due. Radiographics 2001;21:S147–60.
4. Hammond N, Miller FH, Sica GT, Gore RM. Imaging of cystic diseases of the pancreas. Radiol Clin North Am 2002;40:1243–62.
5. Demos TC, Posniak HV, Harmath C, Olson MC, Aranha G. Cystic lesions of the pancreas. AJR Am J Roentgenol 2002;179:1375–88.
6. Spinelli KS, Fromwiller TE, Daniel RA, Kiely JM, Nakeeb A, Komorowski RA, et al. Cystic pancreatic neoplasms: observe or operate. Ann Surg 2004;239:651–7.
7. Abraham SC, Wilentz RE, Yeo CJ, Sohn TA, Cameron JL, Boitnott JK, et al. Pancreaticoduodenectomy (Whipple resections) in patients without malignancy: are they all 'chronic pancreatitis'? Am J Surg Path 2003;27:110–20.
8. Yeo CJ, Cameron JL, Lillemoe KD, Sohn TA, Campbell KA, Sauter PK, et al. Pancreaticoduodenectomy with or without distal gastrectomy and extended retroperitoneal lymphadenectomy for periampullary adenocarcinoma, part 2: randomized controlled trial evaluating survival, morbidity, and mortality. Ann Surg 2002;236:355–68.
9. Leivonen MK, Halttunen JA, Kivilaakso EO. Duodenal diverticulum at endoscopic retrograde cholangiopancreatography, analysis of 123 patients. Hepatogastroenterology 1996;43:961–6.
10. Chiu EJ, Shyr YM, Su CH, Wu CW, Lui WY. Diverticular disease of the small bowel. Hepatogastroenterology 2000;47:181–4.

The British Journal of Radiology, 78 (2005), 565–568
DOI: 10.1259/bjr/31560902

Case report

Solitary fibrous tumour of the epididymis: MRI features

[1]A Ch TSILI, MD, [1]C TSAMPOULAS, MD, [2]X GIANNAKOPOULOS, MD, [3]A BATISTATOU, MD, [1]E ARKOUMANI, MD, [2]An SILAKOS, MD, [2]N SOFIKITIS, MD and [1]S C EFREMIDIS, MD

Departments of [1]Clinical Radiology, [2]Urology and [3]Pathology, University Hospital of Ioannina, Greece

Abstract. We present a case of a solitary fibrous tumour, located at the epididymis, in a 65-year-old man, presented with a scrotal mass. Ultrasound and MRI of the scrotum revealed a paratesticular mass, with rich vascularity, arising in the left epididymis. Radiological findings were non-specific and the patient underwent surgery.

Solitary fibrous tumour (SFT) is a rare mesothelial tumour that was first described as a pleural lesion. Over the past 15 years SFTs have been recognized in many extrathoracic sites, including the orbit, upper respiratory tract, salivary glands, thyroid, peritoneum, retroperitoneum, liver, adrenal, kidney, urinary bladder and prostate [1–3], spermatic cord [4, 5], paratesticular area [6–8], soft tissue, abdominal wall, spinal cord, and meninges. In this article we present a case of SFT arising in the epididymis, which to our knowledge is a location not previously reported in the English literature. We present the ultrasound and MRI findings, with emphasis on the latter. Additionally, a review of the literature on the MRI features of the various paratesticular masses is presented, although there is limited experience on this topic.

Case report

A 65-year-old man admitted to the Urology department for a mass in the left hemiscrotum, noticed during self-examination, 3 months prior. He reported an episode of treated epididymoorchitis on the same side, 36 months previously. Clinical examination revealed a tender, firm mass, probably arising outside the testis. The other hemiscrotum was normal. Serum markers for germ cell tumours (alpha fetoprotein, b-human chorionic gonadotropin, lactate dehydrogenase) were all negative.

Ultrasound examination showed a paratesticular mass in the left hemiscrotum. The mass was well circumscribed, ovoid, appeared solid and hypoechoic, compared with the testicular parenchyma. Colour Doppler assessment revealed rich tumour vascularity (Figure 1). The left testis appeared slightly hypoechoic compared with the other testis. The examination of the right hemiscrotum was normal.

Scrotal MRI was performed using fast spin echo T_2 weighted images in the axial, coronal and sagittal planes; unenhanced and contrast-enhanced T_1 weighted images were also obtained. A paratesticular ovoid mass was seen in the left hemiscrotum. The mass had signal intensity similar to and slightly lower than that of testicular parenchyma on T_1 and T_2 weighted images, respectively (Figure 2a–c). It was well demarcated, surrounded by a low signal intensity capsule. Its relationship with the epididymis was clearly seen on sagittal images. The left testis was slightly inhomogeneous and the tunica albuginea appeared intact. The right testis was normal. After intravenous administration of gadolinium chelate the mass enhanced strongly and homogeneously (Figure 2d). A CT scan of the abdomen and thorax was performed and showed no evidence of metastases.

At left inguinal exploration a hard mass was seen in the paratesticular region. Enucleation of the lesion was impossible, and an orchiectomy was performed. At gross histological examination, a fairly well circumscribed, firm, grey-white mass, with whirling and fasciculation was seen on cut sections of the epididymis. The mass was separated from the tunica albuginea with a thin fibrous capsule. Microscopically a circumscribed lesion with variable cellularity was found in the epididymis. It consisted of a tangled network of fibroblast-like cells, with deposition of abundant collagen fibres. The nuclear atypia was slight/moderate and the maximum number of mitoses was 3/10 high power fields (HPF). Necrosis was not evident. On immunohistochemical studies the neoplastic cells stained strongly for vimentin and CD34. The left testis showed signs of atrophy. Based on the morphological and immunohistochemical characteristics, the diagnosis of SFT was made.

The patient had an uneventful recovery and remains well, 10 months now after surgery.

Discussion

SFTs, regardless their site of origin, usually follow a benign clinical course; however they can recur and metastasize after surgical resection The rate of local recurrence or distant metastases to liver, lung, retroperitoneum, or bone is approximately the same for intrathoracic and extrathoracic SFTs, and it is about 10% [6]. Histological features associated with local or distant recurrence include a high cellularity, mitotic activity >4/10 HPF, nuclear pleomorphism, presence of necrosis and positivity for p53 [4, 6]. These features individually do not inevitably imply malignant clinical behaviour, since up to 60% of benign cases may show at least one such feature. Our patient is free of recurrence or

Received 2 November 2004 and in final form 15 January 2005, accepted 31 January 2005.

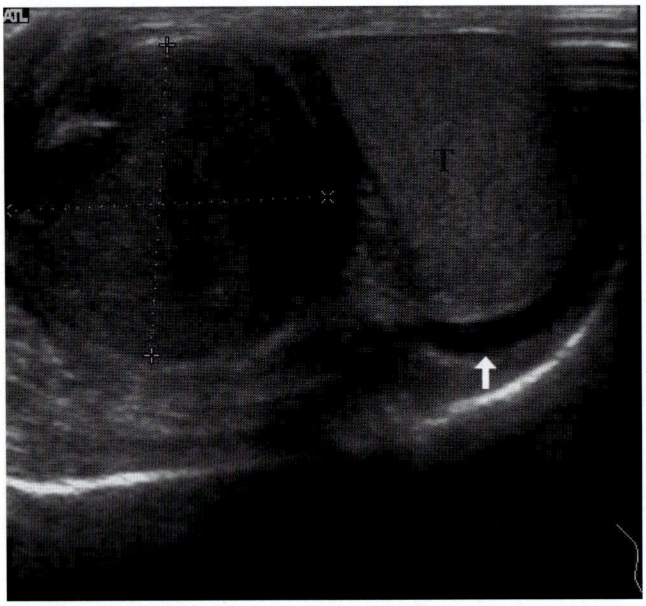

(a)

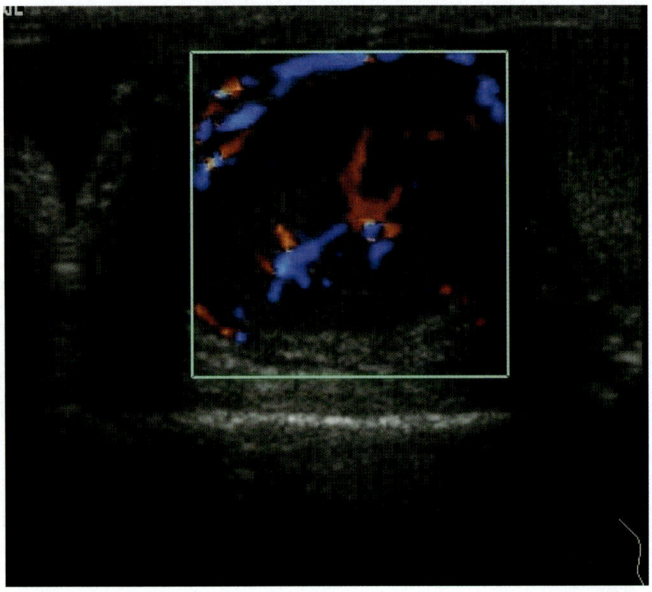

(b)

Figure 1. (a) Transverse ultrasound of the left hemiscrotum shows an ovoid, sharply demarcated, hypoechoic mass, measured 1.8 cm × 1.9 cm (cursors), located outside the testis (T). A small hydrocele is also seen (white arrow). (b) Colour Doppler examination shows rich tumour vascularity in the centre and at the periphery.

distant metastases for 10 months now after surgery. However a careful, long-term follow-up is required in all these cases.

The diagnosis of SFT is made on the basis of its histological features, supported by immunohistochemical studies, as in our case. Radiographic findings are non-specific and the pre-operative diagnosis is difficult.

In our patient MRI study showed a lesion involving the epididymis. The mass had intermediate signal intensity on T_1 weighted images and signal intensity slightly lower than that of testicular parenchyma on T_2 weighted images. The tumour was surrounded by a low signal intensity halo, corresponding to the fibrous capsule, seen on histology and enhanced after gadolinium administration, due to its high vascularity.

MRI allows the precise demonstration and localization of scrotal masses, including the anatomical relationship to the surrounding structures, as in our case. The literature concerning the MRI characteristics of paratesticular tumours is limited [9, 10]. The vast majority of paratesticular masses are benign lesions of the epididymis, like cysts or spermatoceles, scrotal fluid collections, like hydroceles and pyoceles, inflammatory lesions and hernias. The MRI findings of the spermatocele may be diagnostic. The lesion may be seen as a unilocular or multilocular paratesticular mass, of low signal intensity on T_1 weighted images and high signal intensity on T_2 weighted images, not enhancing after gadolinium administration [11, 12]. But this is not always the case, and differentiation from tumours may not be possible [10]. In cases of epididymitis MRI shows enlargement of the epididymis, which appears heterogeneous, of medium signal intensity on T_1 weighted images and of slightly high signal intensity on T_2 weighted images. The spermatic cord is enlarged, oedematous, with increased vascularity [13]. Imaging findings are non-specific and differentiation between non-specific and specific inflammations, like tuberculosis or sarcoidosis is not possible [14, 15]. Hashiguchi et al [16] described the MRI findings of a case of isolated polyarteritis nodosa of the epididymis. MRI showed an enlarged epididymis, of low signal intensity on T_1 weighted images and of mixed high and low signal intensities on T_2 weighted images. After gadolinium administration the affected epididymis enhanced strongly. The findings resemble closely to those of inflammation. On T_2 weighted images there were also multiple small nodular or tubular structures within the epididymis, with an inner high signal intensity and an outer low signal intensity. Some of the lesions showed a flow void centrally. The above findings corresponded histologically to the remarkably thickened arterial walls and may be considered specific for the diagnosis of polyarteritis nodosa.

Lipoma is the most common benign neoplasm of the paratesticular tissues and of the spermatic cord, accounting for 45% of paratesticular tumours. The tumour is easily recognized on MRI, owing to its characteristic signal intensity, bright on T_1 weighted images [9] and low signal intensity on fat-suppressed T_1 weighted images. Adenomatoid tumour is the most common tumour of the epididymis, followed by leiomyoma. Pre-operative diagnosis of these tumours, based on MRI features is difficult. Patel et al [17] described the MRI findings of an adenomatoid tumour of the tunica albuginea, appeared as a mass slightly hypointense to testicular parenchyma on unenhanced images. The tumour showed internal enhancement less than that of the normal testis, after gadolinium administration. Fibrous pseudotumour is not a true neoplasm but a reactive proliferation of paratesticular tissues. The mass may have low signal intensity on both T_1 and T_2 weighted images, because of fibrosis [10] and does not enhance after gadolinium chelate administration [9]. In the adult patients the differential diagnosis of paratesticular tumours should include sarcomas, like leiomyosarcoma, fibrosarcoma and liposarcoma. These neoplasms are

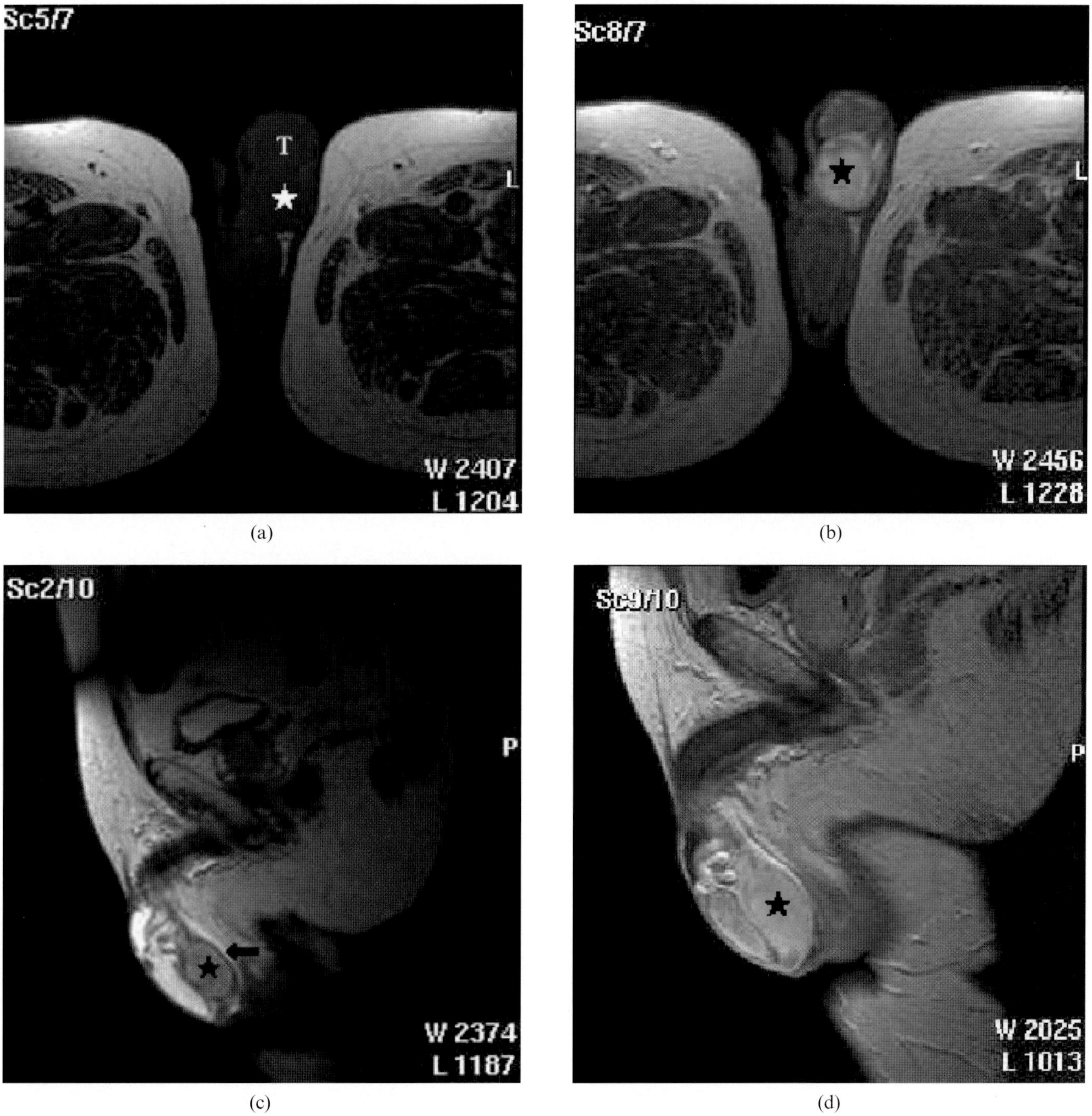

Figure 2. (a) Transverse T_1 weighted image (repetition time/echo time (TR/TE), 650/15) shows a paratesticular mass (asterisk) in the left hemiscrotum, with signal intensity similar to that of testicular parenchyma (T). (b) Transverse and (c) sagittal T_2 weighted fast spin-echo MR images (TR/TE, 4000/100) show the mass (asterisk) clearly as extra testicular, located at the area of the epididymis. It has lower signal intensity, compared with that of testicular parenchyma and surrounded by a low signal intensity capsule (arrow). (d) Sagittal post-contrast T_1 weighted image. The mass (asterisk) enhances strongly and homogeneously.

very rare and the diagnosis based on imaging findings is difficult. Finally metastases, most commonly from testicular, prostatic, renal and gastrointestinal primary neoplasms should be considered, especially if there is a history of primary malignancy.

In conclusion the pre-operative diagnosis of paratesticular tumours is difficult. In some cases, however the MRI findings, always interpreted in conjunction with ultrasound features with respect to tumour location, morphology and tissue characteristics may help narrow the differential diagnosis.

References

1. Corti B, Carella R, Gabusi E, et al. Solitary fibrous tumor of the urinary bladder with expression of bcl-2, CD34 and insulin-like growth factor type II. Eur Urol 2001;39:484–8.

2. Westra WH, Grenko RT, Epstein J. Solitary fibrous tumor of the lower urogenital tract; a report of five cases involving the seminal vesicles, urinary bladder and prostate. Hum Pathol 2000;31:63–8.
3. Grasso M, Blanco S, Franzoso F, et al. Solitary fibrous tumor of the prostate. J Urol 2002;168:1100.
4. Gold JS, Antonescu CR, Hajdu C, et al. Clinicopathologic correlates of solitary fibrous tumors. Cancer 2002;94:1057–68.
5. Fischer C, Bisceglia M. Solitary fibrous tumor of the spermatic cord. Br J Urol 1994;74:799–801.
6. Vallat-Decouvelaere A, Dry S, Fletcher C. Atypical and malignant fibrous tumors in extrathoracic locations: evidence of their comparability to intra-thoracic tumors. Am J Surg Path 1998;22:1501–11.
7. Jones MA, Young RH, Scully RE. Benign fibromatous tumors of the testis and paratesticular region: a report of 9 cases with a proposed classification of fibromatous tumors and tumor-like lesions. Am J Surg Path 1997;21:296–305.
8. Parveen T, Fleischmann J, Petrelli M. Benign fibrous tumor of the tunica vaginalis testis: report of a case with light, electron microscopic and immunohistochemical study, and review of the literature. Arch Pathol Lab Med 1992;116:277–80.
9. Akbar SA, Sayyed TA, Jafri SZ, Hasteh F, Neil JS. Multimodality imaging of paratesticular neoplasms and their rare mimics. Radiographics 2003;23:1461–76.
10. Rubenstein RA, Dogra VS, Seftel AD, Resnik MI. Benign intrascrotal lesions. J Urol 2004;171:1765–72.
11. Tartar VM, Trambert MA, Balsara ZN, Mattrey RF. Tubular ectasia of the testicle: sonographic and MR imaging appearance. AJR Am J Roentgenol 1993;160:539–42.
12. Meyer DR, Huppe T, Lock U, Hodek E, Friedrich M. Pronounced cystic transformation of the rete testis: MRI appearance. Invest Radiol 1999;34:600–3.
13. Trambert MA, Mattrey RF, Levine D, Berthoty DP. Subacute scrotal pain: evaluation of torsion versus epididymitis with MR imaging. Radiology 1990;175:53–6.
14. De Backer AI, Mortele KJ, De Roeck J, et al. Tuberculous epididymitis associated with abdominal lymphadenopathy (2004: 1b). Eur Radiol 2004;14:748–51.
15. Kodama K, Hasegawa T, Egawa M, et al. Bilateral epididymal sarcoidosis presenting without radiographic evidence of intrathoracic lesion: review of sarcoidosis involving the male reproductive tract. Int J Urol 2004;11:345–8.
16. Hashiguchi Y, Matsuo Y, Torri Y, et al. Polyarteritis nodosa of the epididymis. Abdom Imag 2001;26:102–4.
17. Patel MD, Silva AC. MRI of an adenomatoid tumor of the tunica albuginea. AJR Am J Roentgenol 2004;182:415–7.

The British Journal of Radiology, *78* (2005), 569–572
DOI: 10.1259/bjr/22072424

Case report

Bilateral absence of the internal carotid artery: MR angiography and ultrasound findings

D W ANDERSON, MBBS(hons), FRANZCR

Monash Medical Centre, 246 Clayton Road, Clayton, Victoria, Australia 3168

Abstract. Presented is a case of congenital absence of the internal carotid arteries (ICAs) in a 13-year-old boy. This condition has been rarely reported in the literature and presented are our imaging findings, including descriptions of findings with MRI, MR angiography and ultrasound.

A case of our imaging findings is presented demonstrating bilateral agenesis of the internal carotid arteries (ICAs) in a 13-year-old male. Bilateral absence of the ICA (congenital) is a very rare abnormality [1, 2]. Most cases have been demonstrated by catheter angiography or dissection studies [1]. This case describes the appearances on MRI and MR angiography (MRA) of the intracranial circulation together with the appearances of the cervical arterial vasculature on ultrasound.

Case report

A 13-year-old Caucasian male presented to a local emergency department with severe generalized headache. This followed a minor head injury sustained 6 h earlier whilst playing cricket. Onset of headache was while straining at toilet. On examination the patient appeared neurologically intact and had a Glasgow coma score of 15. There was no neck stiffness. Headache resolved over 90 min and he was subsequently discharged. Further similar headache, onset again with straining at toilet occurred 5 days later, prompting representation with subsequent CT examination performed to exclude subarachnoid haemorrhage. This revealed a large calibre basilar artery without evidence of recent subarachnoid haemorrhage. Lumbar puncture was not performed.

Given the clinical suspicion of subarachnoid haemorrhage and the appearance of the basilar artery, MRI was performed after transfer to our hospital. Routine aneurysm imaging (axial T_1, T_2, fluid attenuated inversion recovery (FLAIR), sagittal T_1, diffusion weighted imaging (DWI) and 3D time of flight (TOF) MRA) was performed which demonstrated absence of the bilateral internal carotid arteries (Figures 1–4). Both anterior circulations were supplied by large posterior communicating arteries via an intact circle of Willis. No further vascular abnormality was seen and in particular there was no evidence of aneurysm or focal stenosis. There was no identifiable intracranial bleeding or infarction. A cavum septum pellucidum et vergae was seen as a normal variant. Review of the prior CT examination demonstrated bilateral absence of the bony canal for the ICA within the skull base. Presented for comparison are the same projections of normal MRA images from a 14-year-old patient (Figures 5 and 6) as well as axial T_2 weighted images from the same normal patient (Figures 8 and 9).

Subsequent ultrasound examination of the neck arteries revealed large calibre vertebral arteries (R=4.0 mm L=4.3 mm; Figure 9), with bilateral small calibre common carotid arteries (R=2.9 mm L= 3.3 mm; Figure 10). There was no identifiable ICA, either at its expected origin or elsewhere within the neck. Vertebral flow velocities were 90/40 cm s^{-1} bilaterally. This is within the reported normal range of vertebral artery velocities for a patient of this age [3]. The patient was uneventfully discharged and remains well at 1 year post discharge.

Discussion

Absence of the ICA may be the result of acquired disease (common), congenital hypoplasia (uncommon) or congenital aplasia (very rare). This is more commonly seen unilaterally [4–8]. Most reported cases of bilateral absence have been recorded prior to 1980 [1]. There is most

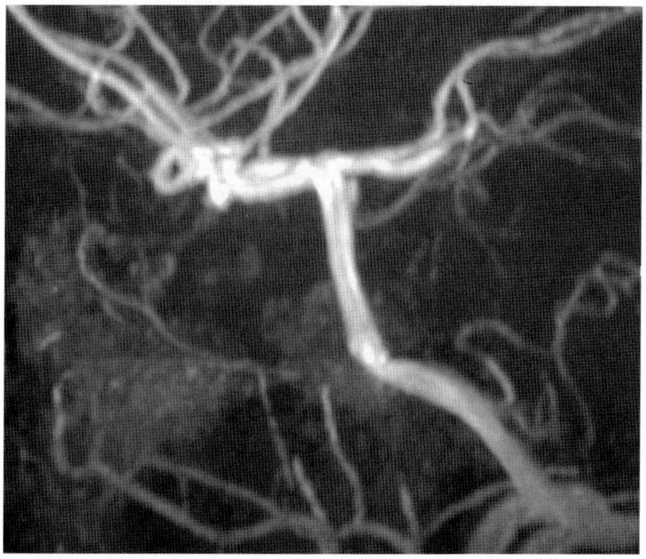

Figure 1. Lateral MR angiography projection showing absent anterior circulation below the circle of Willis.

Received 13 October 2004 and in final form 23 December 2004, accepted 31 January 2005.

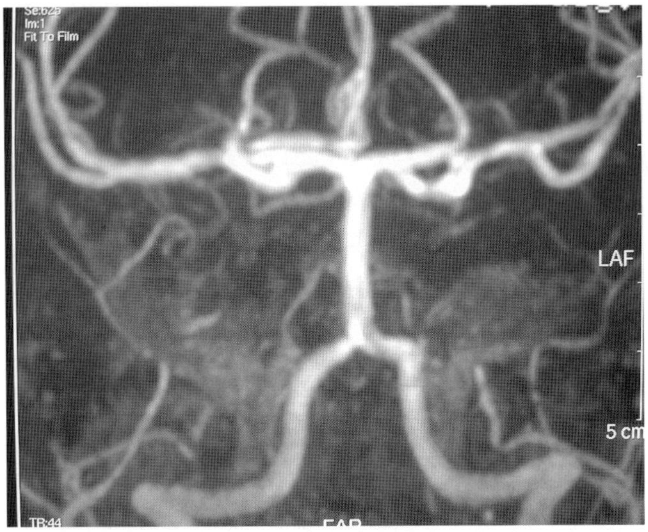

Figure 2. Anteroposterior MR angiography projection showing absent anterior circulation below the circle of Willis.

experience with catheter angiography, the first case report in 1965, where review of 1407 angiograms revealed a single case of bilateral ICA absence with supply to the anterior circulation via multiple ophthalmic and petrous collaterals [9]. Earlier case reports rely on dissection studies (4 cases) [10, 11]. This case reports the findings demonstrable with MRI, MRA and ultrasound. The developmental nature of our patient's bilateral ICA absence was confirmed by CT examination showing absence of the bony ICA canal within the skull base [12]. Several case reports have discussed the MRI and MRA findings in unilateral aplasia or hypoplasia of the ICA, including children [4–8]. Several authors have commented on the utility of MRA in providing a non invasive assessment of both the absence of vessel as well as the associated collateral circulation [4–8]. Kidooka et al believed the MRA assessment in their

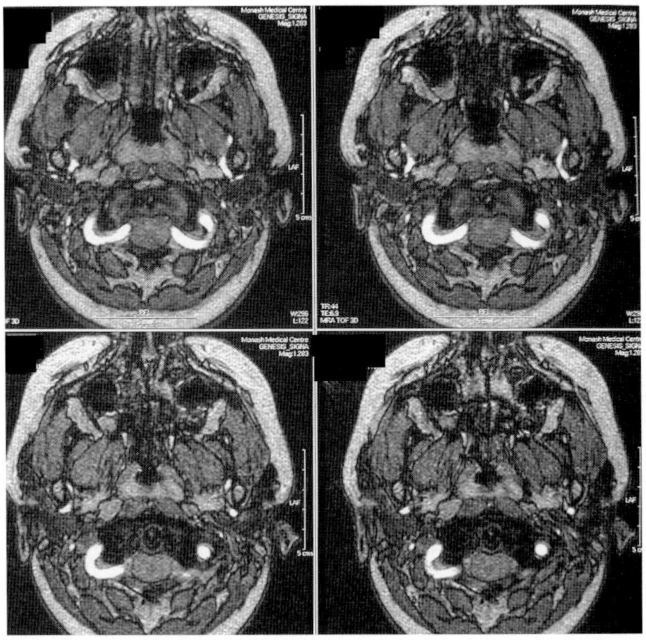

Figure 3. Axial MR angiography at C1 level showing absent internal carotid artery flow voids.

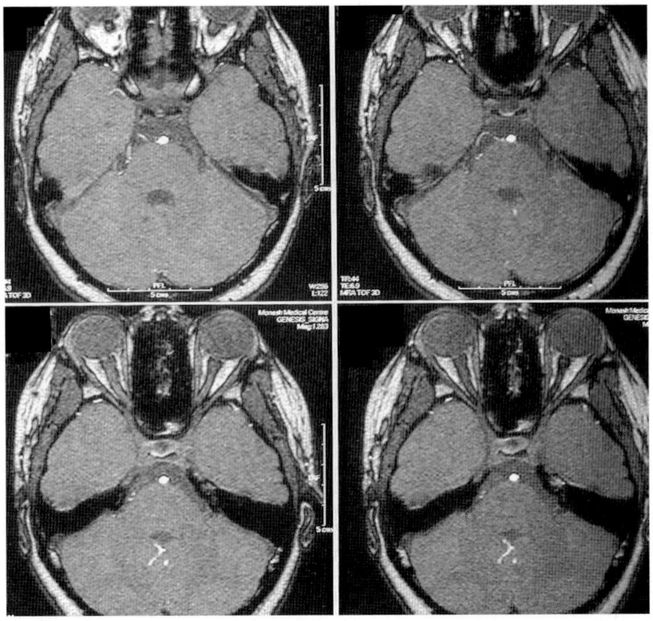

Figure 4. Axial MR angiography at level of cavernous sinuses showing absent internal carotid artery flow voids.

case was equivalent to that provided by the catheter angiography [5].

The MRA in this case demonstrated supply to the anterior circulation via enlarged posterior communicating arteries, the most commonly seen collateral arrangement (12 of 18 cases) [1]. Other recognized collateral arrangements include persistent trigeminal arteries (2 cases), ophthalmic artery (2 cases) and maxillary derived collaterals (2 cases) [1]. Petrous anastomoses and accessory meningeal supply have also been described [12, 13].

An aneurysm was not demonstrated in our patient on MRA. Correlative catheter angiography was not performed. MRA is recognized to have a limited sensitivity for the detection of small aneurysms [14–18]. This is variably stated to be as low as 54% for aneurysms <5 mm [15] and 55% for aneurysms <3 mm [17]. Whilst much

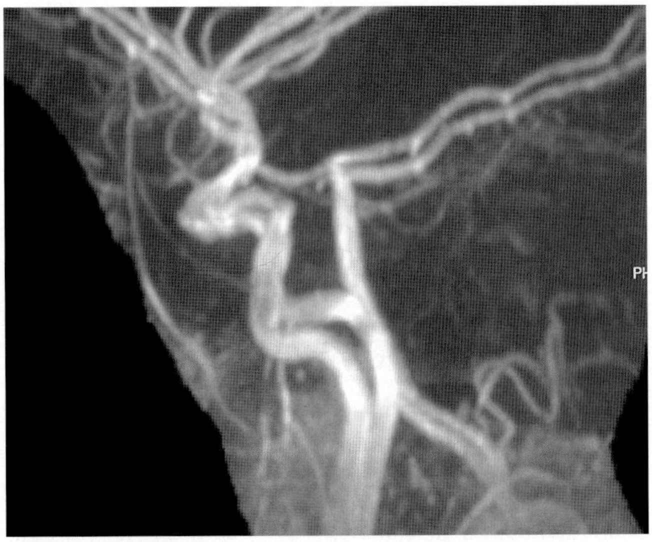

Figure 5. Normal MR angiography lateral projection from a 14-year-old patient.

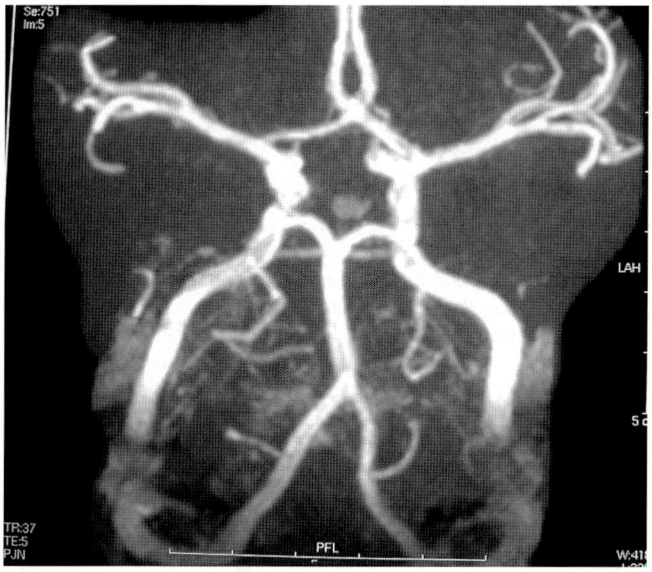

Figure 6. Normal MR angiography anteroposterior projection from a 14-year-old patient.

ongoing debate exists regarding screening for aneurysms with MRA [13, 14] it does seem that absence of the ICA is associated with a greatly increased incidence of aneurysm. This has been variably stated as 25% (9 of 36 patients) [19] and 24–36% for patients with unilateral agenesis of the ICA [18]. This is presumed the result of altered/abnormal haemodynamic stressors. Other authors have argued that unilateral ICA agenesis may be regarded as an incidental or non clinically significant finding [7]. The current available case reports of bilateral ICA absence suggest that it is unlikely to represent an incidental finding of no diagnostic or prognostic value [1].

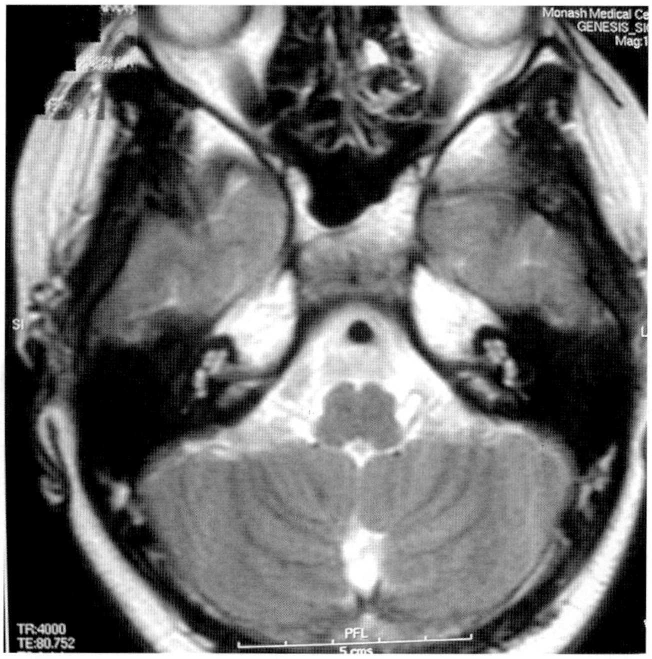

Figure 7. Axial T_2 weighted image showing large calibre basilar artery and absent internal carotid artery flow voids.

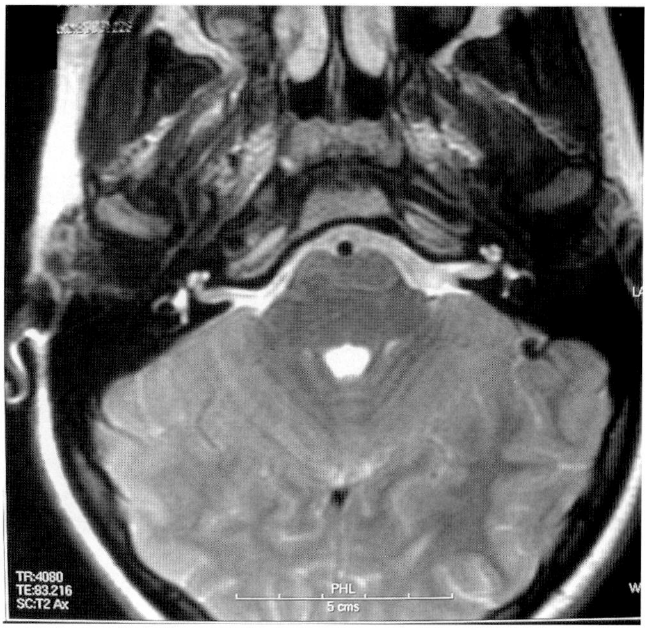

Figure 8. Axial T_2 weighted image in a normal patient demonstrating normal calibre basilar artery and internal carotid artery flow voids.

Conclusion

Bilateral absence of the ICA is a very rarely reported abnormality. Our case report suggests that MRA is able to successfully demonstrate ICA absence and common collateralisation in a non invasive fashion, in agreement with others who have described its use in unilateral ICA agenesis. There also exists the potential for aneurysm screening, of which it is likely these patients have a significantly increased incidence. We have also provided description of the ultrasound findings in the vertebral and common carotid arteries, with our case demonstrating a significantly larger calibre vertebral system in comparison with the common carotid artery.

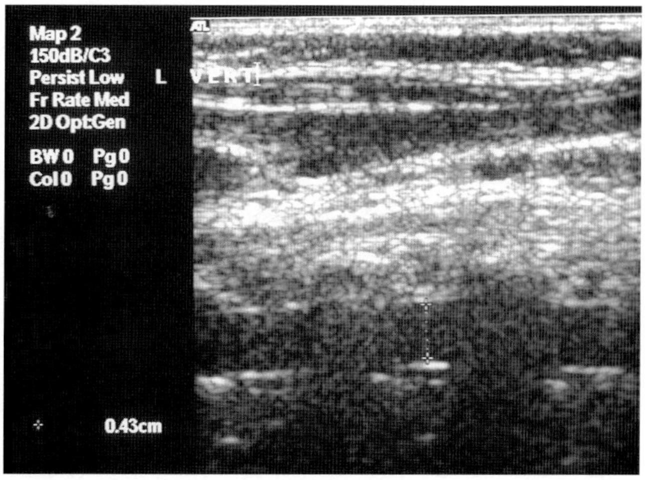

Figure 9. Ultrasound of left vertebral artery showing diffuse increased calibre.

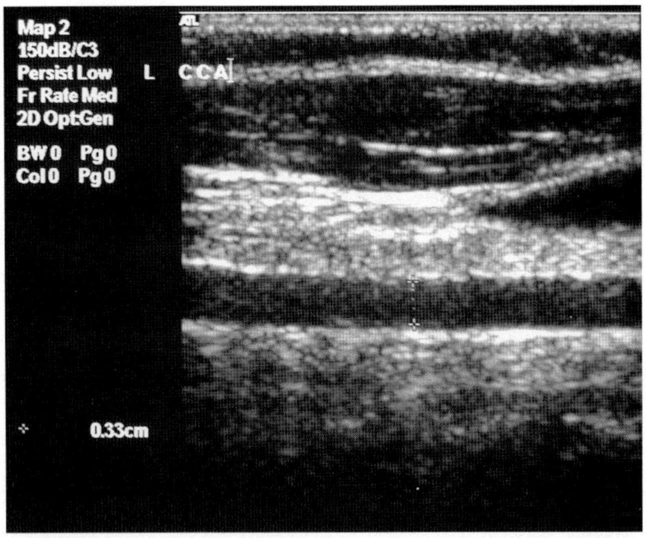

Figure 10. Ultrasound of left common carotid artery showing diffuse reduced calibre.

References

1. Cali RL, Berg R, Rama K. Bilateral internal carotid artery agenesis: a case study and review of the literature. Surgery 1993;113:227–33.
2. Owada Y, Sakuta Y. Bilateral carotid artery agenesis with corpus callosum hypogenesis - a case report. No-To-Shinkei 1995;47:589–94.
3. Schoning M, Niemann G, Hartig B. Transcranial color duplex sonography of basal cerebral arteries: reference data of flow velocities from childhood to adulthood. Neuropediatrics 1996;27:249–55.
4. Mellado JM, Merino X, Ramos A, Salvado E, Sauri A. Agenesis of the internal carotid artery with a trans-sellar anastomosis: CT and MRI findings in late onset congenital hypopituitarism. Neuroradiology 2001;43:237–41.
5. Kidooka M, Okada T, Handa J. Agenesis of the internal carotid artery – report of a case combined with arachnoid cyst in a child. No To Shinkei 1992;44:371–5.
6. Slaba SG, Zafatayeff SN, Chelala AS. Complete imaging study of internal carotid artery agenesis with intercavernous anastomosis. Neurochirurgie 2002;48:35–8.
7. Lee JH, Oh CW, Lee SH, Han DH. Aplasia of the internal carotid artery. Acta Neurochirurgica 2003;145:117–25.
8. Inaml Y, Harada K. Agenesis of the internal carotid artery and congenital pituitary hypoplasia: proposal of a cause of congenital hypopituitarism. Eur J Pediatr 2003;162:610–2.
9. Fields WS. Collateral circulation to the brain. Baltimore: Williams and Wilkins, 1965:211–2.
10. Dilenge D. Bilateral agenesis of the internal carotid artery. J Can Assoc Radiol 1975;26:91–4.
11. Hills J. Bilateral agenesis of the internal carotid artery associated with cardiac and other anomalies. Neurology 1968;18:142–6.
12. Given CA, Huang-Hellinger F, Chepuri NB, Morris PP. Congenital absence of the internal carotid artery: case reports and review of the collateral circulation. AJNR Am J Neuroradiol 2001;22:1953–9.
13. Smith R. Agenesis of the internal carotid artery with an unusual primitive collateral. J Neurosurg 1972;37:460–2.
14. International study of unruptured aneurysms (ISUIA) Investigators. Hemorrhage rates in patients with unruptured intracranial aneurysms. Stroke 1998;29:273.
15. White PM, Lindsay KW, Teasdale E, Teasdale GM. Should we screen for familial intracranial aneurysm? Stroke 1999;30:2238–48.
16. Korogi Y, Takahashi M, Mabuchi N, Nakagawa T, Fujiwara S, Horikawa Y. Intracranial aneurysms: diagnostic accuracy of MR angiography with evaluation of maximum intensity projection and source images. Radiology 1996;199:199–207.
17. White PM, Wardlaw JM. How reliable is the non invasive imaging of intracranial aneurysms? An objective assessment of the quality of the published literature. Cerebrovasc Dis 1999;9(Suppl. 1):51.
18. Okahara M, Kiyosue H, Yamashita M, Nagatomi H, Hata H, Saginoya Y, et al. Diagnostic accuracy of magnetic resonance angiography for cerebral aneurysms in correlation with 3D digital subtraction angiographic images. Stroke 2002;33:1803–8.
19. Servo A. Agenesis of the left internal carotid artery associated with an aneurysm on the right carotid siphon. J Neurosurg 1977;46:677–80.

The British Journal of Radiology, *78* (2005), 573–574

Correspondence

(The Editors do not hold themselves responsible for opinions expressed by correspondents)

Moderate dose rate ionizing radiation increases longevity?

The Editor—Sir,

In the January 2005 issue of BJR, Cameron [1] suggests that moderate doses of radiation increase longevity. His main arguments are from epidemiological studies of ecological design and also from cohort studies of workers.

It is well known that ecological studies, which lack data on individual causes of death and individual exposures to the putative risk factors, are prone to statistical problems such as confounding [2]. Cameron quotes an ecological study [3] which compared three Rocky Mountain States (Idaho, Colorado, New Mexico) with three Gulf States (Louisiana, Mississippi, Alabama) in the USA. Cancer mortality was about 26% higher in the Gulf States, while natural background was lower by a factor of about three. Cameron argues that these differences are too extreme for confounding to be a plausible explanation. But this is based on the assumption that natural background radiation is a dominant cause of cancer. This is very far from the truth.

Radiation is a minor factor in determining overall cancer rates. The importance of factors such as smoking and urban/rural lifestyle was pointed out by Archer [4] in a critique of the Jagger paper. Jagger [5] accepted that the differences in cancer rates between the Rocky Mountain and the Gulf States was probably due to these factors. He regarded the lesson to be drawn as no more than that natural background radiation is not an important cause of cancer.

It is certainly true that natural background radiation does not account for a large proportion of cancers and that it would not be expected that the effects of natural radiation could be detected in ecological studies. Consider a hypothetical study in which the highly exposed population received about twice the radiation exposure of the control population, say an extra 3 mSv pa. Over a lifetime, the extra dose would be about 200 mSv, very roughly equating to an increased risk of cancer mortality of 1% [6]. It is highly unlikely that this excess could be detected above the normal background cancer mortality of 20–25%.

Natural background radiation is thus not a dominant cause of cancer. However, it is important to remember that factors which may have a relatively minor impact on mortality are not unimportant if they are controllable. Part of the natural background radiation is almost impossible to avoid, but the component from radon, which can give very significant doses, can and should be controlled. A large pooling of case/control studies from Europe [7] has demonstrated a risk of lung cancer down to exposures of 100–199 Bq m^{-3}. There was no evidence for a threshold and if one exists it must lie below 150 Bq m^{-3}. The present Action Level in the UK is 200 Bq m^{-3}, but it is being reviewed [8].

Cameron also points to cohort studies of US shipyard workers [9, 10] and British radiologists [11]. Cohort studies are less subject to confounding than are ecological studies. However, it is a common observation that strong selection effects apply and make it difficult to interpret comparisons between the group being studied and reference populations. This frequently manifests itself as the well known "Healthy Worker Effect" [12].

Matanoski et al [9, 10] studied workers at US nuclear shipyards. They reported significantly lower standardized mortality rates (SMRs) in those overhauling nuclear-powered ships with cumulative effective doses greater than 5 mSv than in those with lower doses, and in the latter group compared with non-radiation shipyard workers. However, the authors of the study did not suggest that these results provide evidence for a beneficial effect of radiation but instead regarded selection bias as a more likely cause. It would be perverse to try to override this interpretation and suggest instead that radiation increases longevity.

Cameron also cites a study of British radiologists [11] in which it was reported that those employed after 1920 had lower SMRs than other contemporary medical doctors. However, a large proportion of these other doctors would have been General Practitioners who are known to have smoked more than other doctors [13]. In their paper, Berrington et al [11] focused on internal trends in mortality risks with time since entry into the radiology profession (as an indication of cumulative dose), rather than relying solely on external comparisons of SMRs with other groups of doctors or the more general population. Thus they found evidence for an increasing trend in risk of cancer mortality with time since first registration with a radiological society; for example, there was a 41% excess risk among those registered for more than 40 years.

Cameron also argues that life evolved in the presence of significant levels of natural background radiation and must be adapted to repair the damage that it causes. He draws the conclusion that "It is illogical to suggest that radiation damage to one cell may cause cancer". But it is indisputable that radiation is a cause of cancer and it is hard to see why a mechanism involving a rare kind of damage to a single cell should be less "logical" than any other.

Yours etc.,

G M Kendall
C R Muirhead

National Radiological Protection Board
Chilton
Didcot
Oxon OX11 0RQ
UK

(*Received 8 March 2005 and accepted 22 March 2005*)
DOI: 10.1259/bjr/27387164

References

1. Cameron JR. Moderate dose rate ionising radiation increases longevity. Br J Radiol 2005;78:11–3.
2. NCRP Report 136. Evaluation of the linear nonthreshold dose-response model for ionizing radiation. Bethesda, MD: NCRP, 2001.
3. Jagger J. Natural background radiation and cancer death in Rocky Mountain States and Gulf Coast States. Health Physics 1998;75:428–30.
4. Archer VE. Cancer death rates and background radiation. Health Physics 1999;76:692–4.
5. Jagger J. Response to Archer. Health Physics 1999;76:694–5.
6. NRPB. Risk of radiation-induced cancer at low doses and low dose rates for radiation protection purposes. Doc of NRPB 1995;6(1).
7. Darby SC, et al. Radon in homes and risk of lung cancer: collaborative analysis of individual data from 13 European case-control studies. BMJ 2005;330:223–6. See BMJ website at http://bmj.bmjjournals.com/cgi/content/abstract/bmj.38308.477650.63v1 (Accessed 23 March 2005).
8. Response Statement by the National Radiological Protection Board http://www.nrpb.org/press/response_statements/2004/response_statement_4_04.htm (Accessed 23 March 2005).
9. Matanoski GM. Health effects of low-level radiation in shipyard workers: final report. DOE contract no. DE-AC02-79 EV10095. Baltimore, MD. 1991.
10. Matanoski GM. Nuclear shipyard workers study. Radiat Res 1993;133:126–7.
11. Berrington A, Darby SC, Weiss HA, Doll R. 100 years of observation on British radiologists: mortality from cancer and other causes 1897–1997. Br J Radiol 2001;74:507–19.
12. Monson RR. Occupational epidemiology. Boca Raton: CRC Press,1980.
13. Doll R, Peto R. Mortality among doctors in different occupations. Br Med J 1977;1:1433–6.

Since receiving this letter from the NRPB we are very sorry indeed to learn of the death of Professor John Cameron.

The British Journal of Radiology, *78* (2005), 575–577
DOI: 10.1259/bjr/85140104

Case of the month

Seizures following bone marrow transplantation

M BRATBY, MA, MB BS, MRCP and D MACVICAR, MA, MRCP, FRCR

Royal Marsden NHS Foundation Trust, Downs Road, Sutton, Surrey SM2 5PT, UK

A 19-year-old male presented to our institution for bone marrow transplantation (BMT) from a matched unrelated donor. 5 years previously he had been diagnosed with acute lymphoblastic leukaemia, treated with chemotherapy according to a high-risk protocol. Remission was achieved, but CNS relapse was confirmed 2 years later. Further treatment included craniospinal irradiation. A further 2 and a half years had elapsed when further relapse was confirmed by the presence of blasts in the peripheral blood. Over the following 6 months, further remission was achieved, and the patient was referred for BMT.

Conditioning chemotherapy of busulphan, cyclophosphamide and Campath (an anti-lymphocyte monoclonal antibody) was given. Following transplantation, cyclosporin A and methotrexate were commenced for graft versus host disease prophylaxis. Immediately post-transplant, neutropenic sepsis developed and was treated with anti-microbial agents. At day 30 post-transplant he suffered tonic–clonic seizures and subsequently a reduced level of consciousness. CT scan was performed which was within normal limits. MRI of the brain was subsequently undertaken (Figures 1 and 2).

What abnormality is shown? What is the diagnosis? What is the advice to the clinical team and prognosis of the condition?

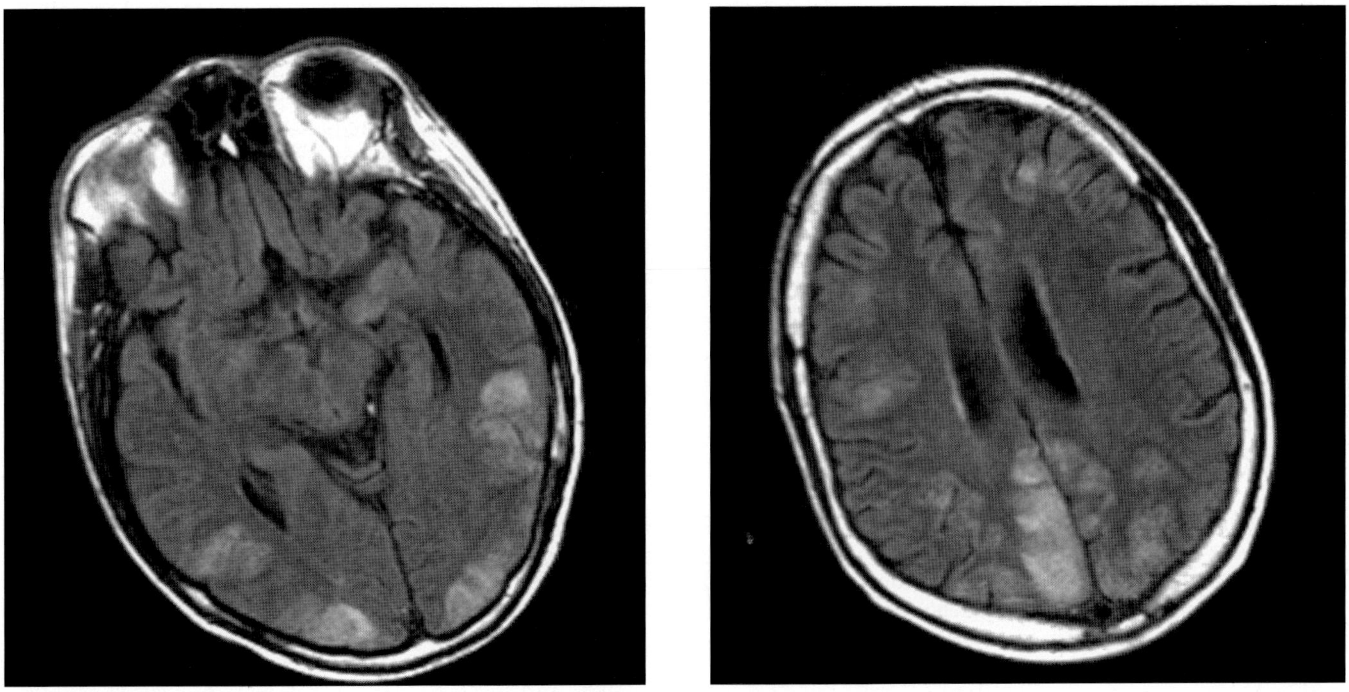

(a) (b)

Figure 1. Axial fluid attenuated inversion recovery (FLAIR) sequences of brain at level of (a) pons and (b) lateral ventricles.

Received 1 February 2005 and accepted 25 February 2005.
Address correspondence to Dr David MacVicar, Consultant Radiologist.

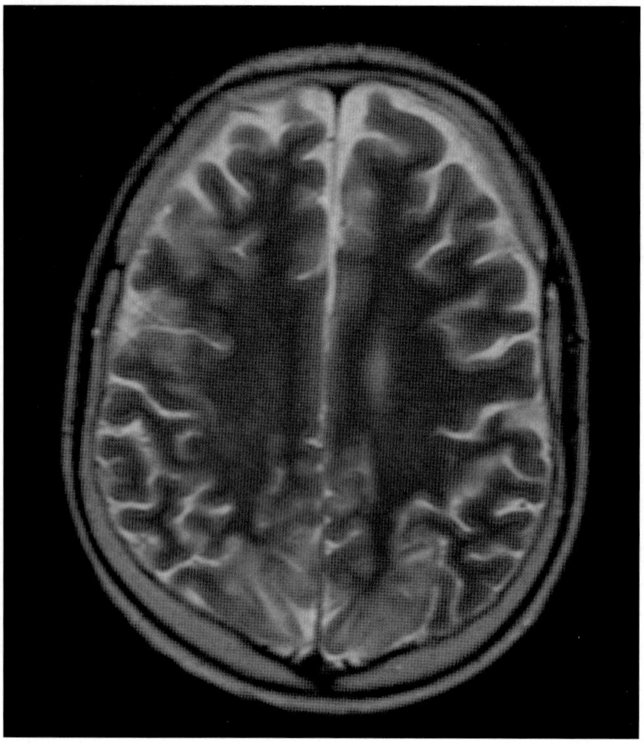

Figure 2. Axial T_2 weighted spin-echo image of brain at level of corona radiata.

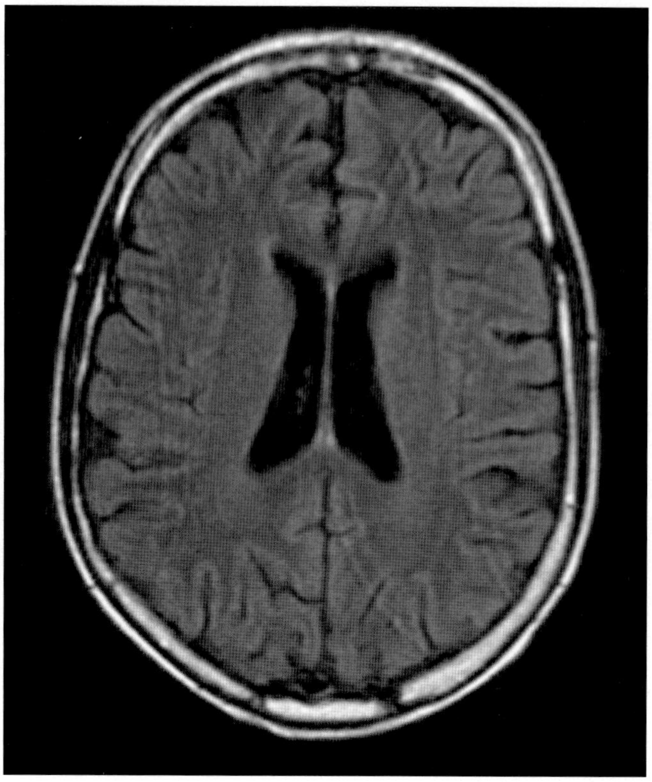

Figure 3. Follow-up MRI study. Fluid attenuated inversion recovery (FLAIR) sequence shows no abnormality in previously affected areas.

Diagnosis

Axial fluid attenuated inversion recovery (FLAIR) images (Figure 1a, b) demonstrate symmetrical abnormal high signal most marked in the parietal and occipital regions. Abnormal signal is present in both grey and white matter and the changes are predominantly in the posterior part of the brain. Asymmetrical focal areas of abnormal signal can also be detected in the left frontal lobe and the posterior part of the right frontal lobe. The T_2 weighted sequence (Figure 2) also demonstrates high signal in the posterior part of the brain, although the changes are less conspicuous on this pulse sequence.

From the clinical presentation and the MRI study a diagnosis of reversible posterior leukoencephalophathy syndrome (RPLS) was made. The likely aetiological factor was identified as cyclosporin A, and the patient was converted to mycophenylate. The neurological syndrome recovered over a 2-week period. Follow-up MRI scan (Figure 3) showed complete resolution of the high signal abnormalities.

Discussion

RPLS was described in a series of patients in 1996 [1]. The clinical findings include headache, decreased level of consciousness and seizures, and focal neurology including cortical blindness and paralysis. The imaging findings in our patient were typical of RPLS. CT may show hypodensity in white and grey matter of the parietal and occipital lobes, but is frequently considered normal. MRI is more sensitive, and the observed changes appear to reflect oedema in certain areas of the brain. Focal and diffuse areas of high signal intensity are observed on T_2 weighted and FLAIR imaging, while abnormal areas are of low signal on T_1 weighted imaging, do not enhance following contrast and do not exhibit mass effect. Abnormalities are predominantly posterior, especially involving parietal and occipital lobes, but the cerebellum, brain stem, basal ganglia, subcortical white matter and frontal lobes may also be affected [2, 3]. Diffusion-weighted imaging [4, 5] can help to distinguish between areas of vasogenic oedema (free diffusion), which is potentially reversible, and areas of established infarction, which will show cytotoxic oedema (restricted diffusion). Diffusion-weighted imaging was performed in our patient and was interpreted as showing no evidence of restricted diffusion. In many cases, as in our patient, MRI changes resolve completely, but it is well recognised that clinical and imaging abnormalities can persist.

Neurological presentations following BMT are not uncommon, and cyclosporin A has increasingly been identified as a major aetiological factor. Cyclosporin related neurotoxicity was first identified in 1984 in a patient post-BMT [6]. The mechanism by which cyclosporin causes neurotoxicity is less well known. The distribution of the lesions suggests a vascular process. In many patients with the clinical syndrome of RPLS a transient or sustained increase in blood pressure is noted, and hypertensive encephalopathy associated with renal disease and eclampsia gives similar imaging findings. Our patient experienced a blood pressure rise to a level of 160/100 from a baseline of 110/70. This rise in blood pressure resolved on withdrawal of cyclosporin. The diagnosis of RPLS is presumed in the presence of a characteristic history and imaging findings, and biopsy is rarely undertaken. Resolution of abnormalities following withdrawal of cyclosporin is usually considered confirmatory. RPLS may be seen following transplantation of liver and kidney, but appears especially frequent following BMT. In this clinical context, there is a wide differential diagnosis, given that neurological complications are frequent following BMT. The differential diagnosis includes cerebral infarction, of which the main pattern to be differentiated is that of bilateral posterior cerebral artery infarction secondary to basilar tip embolism. Immunosuppressed patients are also susceptible to acute encephalomyelitis and progressive multifocal leukoencephalopathy. The distribution of abnormalities on MRI may help to discriminate these entities [7]. An autopsy study of neuropathological findings after BMT in 180 patients identified intraparenchymal brain haemorrhage and subarachnoid haemorrhage as the most common observed abnormalities. In all, neuropathological abnormalities were demonstrated in over 90% of patients dying following BMT [8]. The incidence of severe neurological complications appears slightly higher in patients receiving transplants from matched unrelated donors compared with matched sibling donors [9]. A cerebral vasculopathy characterized by increased cerebral blood flow velocities has been proposed as a cause of cyclosporin related toxicity [10].

Despite the uncertainty surrounding the causation, RPLS comprises a recognisable set of clinical and imaging findings. Following transplantation, it is important for the radiologist to recognise these findings as patients on High Dependency Units following seizures may be attended by a variety of clinicians including anaesthetists and others without direct experience of BMT. Treatment is conservative and should include control of blood pressure and withdrawal or reduction of cyclosporin dose, which should result in resolution of abnormalities and a favourable outcome.

References

1. Hinchey J, Chaves C, Appignani B, Breen J, Pao L, Wang A, et al. A reversible posterior leukoencephalopathy syndrome. New Engl J Med 1996;334:494–500.
2. Casey SO, Sampaio RC, Michel E, Truwit CL. Posterior reversible encephalopathy syndrome: utility of fluid-attenuated inversion recovery MR imaging in the detection of cortical and subcortical lesions. AJNR Am J Neuroradiol 2000;21:1199–206.
3. Jarosz JM, Howlett DC, Cox TC, Bingham JB. Cyclosporine-related reversible posterior leukoencephalopathy: MRI. Neuroradiology 1997;39:711–5.
4. Mukherjee P, McKinstry RC. Reversible posterior leukoencephalopathy syndrome: evaluation with diffusion-tensor MR imaging. Radiology 2001;219:756–65.
5. Coley SC, Porter DA, Calamante F, Chong WK, Connelly A. Quantitative MR diffusion mapping and cyclosporine-induced neurotoxicity. AJNR Am J Neuroradiol 1999;20:1507–10.
6. Atkinson K, Biggs J, Darveniza P, Boland J, Concannon A, Dodds A. Cyclosporin-associated central nervous system toxicity after allogeneic bone marrow transplantation. Transplantation 1984;38:34–7.
7. Port JD, Beauchamp NJ Jr. Reversible intracerebral pathologic entities mediated by vascular autoregulatory function. Radiographics 1998;18:353–67.
8. Bleggi-Torres LF, de Medeiros BC, Werner B, Neto JZ, Loddo G, Pasquini R, et al. Neuropathological findings after bone marrow transplantation: an autopsy study of 180 cases. Bone Marrow Transplant 2000;25:301–7.
9. de Brabander C, Cornelissen J, Sillevis Smitt PAE, Vecht Ch J, van den Bent MJ. Increased incidence of neurological complications in patients receiving an allogenic bone marrow transplantation from alternative donors. J Neurol Neurosurg Psychiatry 2000;68:36–40.
10. Shbarou RM, Chao NJ, Morgenlander JC. Cyclosporin A-related cerebral vasculopathy. Bone Marrow Transplant 2000;26:801–4.

BIR COMPANY SUBSCRIBER SCHEME

The BIR Company Subscriber Scheme is aimed at all companies with an interest in radiology and allied sciences. For an annual subscription member companies are offered an attractive benefits package. To find out why your company should join the leading edge companies listed below, please contact Mr Adrian C Laws, Marketing Manager, British Institute of Radiology, 36 Portland Place, London W1B 1AT. Tel: +44 (0) 20 7307 1404.

Agfa-Gevaert Ltd
Tel: 020 82314900
Contact Mr M Hill, Business Manager Medical Imaging and PACS Systems
Product Code: 1, 2, 3, 4, 6, 9, 10, 12, 13, 14, 15, 20, 22 and 23

Alliance Medical Ltd
Tel: 01295 671223
Contact Mr Charles Fox, Marketing Executive
Product Code: 1, 4, 5, 16, 20 and 21

Amersham Health
Tel: 01494 798666
Contact Mr D G Rothery, Marketing Manager
Product Codes: 1, 2, 3, 4, 5 and 6

Bard Limited
Tel: 01293 606864
Contact Ms T Empson, Product Manager
Product Code: 2

Cerner Corporation (UK)
Tel: 01452 831533
Contact Mr A Fowles, Sales Manager
Product Codes: 9, 10, 13 and 20

Cook (UK) Ltd
Tel: 01462 482884
Contact Mr Iain Mackintosh, regional Manager - Diagnostic and Interventional Products
Product Code: 2

Dictaphone International
Tel:020 78785000
Contact Ms R Richardson-Aitken, Marketing Manager
Product Codes: 20

E-Z-EM Ltd
Tel: 01869 366900
Contact Mr Martin Suggitt, Product Manager
Product Codes: 1, 2 and 8

Ferrania UK Ltd
Tel: 01344 312100
Contact Mr Alan Budge, General Marketing Manager
Product Codes: 1, 3, 4, 9, 10, 13, 14, 15 and 18

Fuji Photo Film (UK) Ltd
Tel: 01234 326780
Contact Mr R G Brown, Strategic Business Manager
Product Codes: 1, 3, 4, 6, 9, 10, 12, 13, 14, 15, 18 and 22

GE Medical Systems
Tel: 01753 874000
Contact Mr A Trivett, Managing Director
Product Codes: 1, 2, 3, 4, 6, 8, 9, 10, 15, 18 and 22

Guerbet Laboratories Ltd
Tel: 01908 522888
Contact Mr Trevor Furniss, General Manager
Product Code: 1 and 2

Kimal plc
Tel: 01895 270951
Contact Mr S Clarke, Technical Director
Product Code: 2

Kingsmoor Publications Ltd
Tel: 01371 812960
Contact Mr David Roberts, Managing Director
Product Code: 17

Kodak Ltd
Tel: 01442 844473
Contact Mr Chris Wright, Marketing Manager UK and Ireland
Product Codes: 1, 3, 4, 6, 8, 9, 10, 12, 13, 14, 15, 18, 21, 22 and 23

Landauer, Inc.
Tel: 01865 373008
Contact Dr T Finnigan, Director, European Operations
Product Code: 8

Lister InHealth
Tel: 0113 2523722
Contact Mr N Mayhew, Sales and Marketing Director
Product Code: 1, 3, 4, 15, 16 and 23

Mirada Solutions Ltd
Tel: 01865 265500
Contact Dr Clare Jones, VP Marketing
Product Codes: 1, 4, 6, 9, 10, 13, 21 and 22

Nuclear Associates
Tel: 00 1 516 8700100
Contact Ms S Felner, Director of Marketing
Product Codes: 1, 3, 4, 6, 8, 9, 10, 12, 13, 21, 22 and 23

Nucletron UK Ltd
Tel: 018297 71111
Contact Mr J Banks, Managing Director
Product Codes: 6 and 8

Philips Medical Systems
Tel:01737 230400
Contact Ms Clair Daynes, Marketing Communications Manager
Product Codes: 1, 2, 9, 10, 22 and 23

Schering Health Care Ltd
Tel: 01444 232323
Contact Mr Chris Matthews, Product Manager
Product Codes: 1, 2 and 3

Sectra Ltd
Tel: 020 86106033
Contact Jan Wolfram, Managing Director
Product Codes: 9 and 10

Siemens Medical Solutions
Tel: 01344 396317
Contact Mr Mike Bell, Manager, Advertising and Exhibitions
Product Codes: 1, 2, 3, 4, 6, 9, 15 and 22

Sonosite Ltd
Tel: 01767 313117
Contact Ms Gillian Duffy, European Marketing Director
Product Codes: 3

Southern Scientific Ltd
Tel: 01903 604000
Contact Mr Stephen Adams, Sales Manager
Product Codes: 1, 3, 4, 8, 10, 12 and 22

Toshiba Medical Systems UK
Tel: 01293 653700
Contact Mr S M Weeden, Manager X-ray Products
Product Codes: 1, 2, 3, 4, 9, 10 and 15

Varian Oncology Systems
Tel: 01293 531244 (UK)
Contact Mr Rolf Stähelin (Switzerland - tel. 00 41 417498844), Marketing Manager, Europe
Product Code: 6

Vertec Scientific Ltd
Tel: 01734 817431
Contact Mr B Hipgrave, Managing Director
Product Codes: 1, 4, 6, 8 and 12

Wardray Premise Ltd
Tel: 020 83989911
Contact Mr R Beach, Sales Manager
Product Codes: 8, 18 and 20

Wolverson X-Ray
Tel: 01902 637333
Contact Mr N Bacon, Sales Director
Product Codes: 1, 8, 15, 18 and 23

Xograph Imaging Systems
Tel: 01666 501501 or 07000 for X-ray
Contact Mr N Staff, Technical Director
Product Codes: 1, 8, 12, 14, 15, 18, 22 and 23

PRODUCT CODES

1. Diagnostic X-ray including NMR and CT
2. Interventional radiology
3. Ultrasound
4. Nuclear medicine
5. Radiopharmaceuticals
6. Radiotherapy and oncology
7. Radiobiology
8. Radiation protection
9. PACS
10. Image processing
11. Nuclear fuel cycle service
12. Quality assurance
13. Radiology data management computer systems
14. Video printing
15. Equipment leasing
16. Hospital-shared services
17. Medical publishing
18. X-ray consumables distribution
19. Electricity generation
20. Medical reporting systems
21. Education
22. Mammography
23. Dental X-ray

Meetings & Courses

IMRT - the shape of things to come
7 July 2005
London, UK
Further details: The British Institute of Radiology, 36 Portland Place, London W1B 1AT.
Tel: 0207 307 1406. Fax: 0207 307 1414.
Email: registrations@bir.org.uk. Visit: www.bir.org.uk

Upper gastrointestinal cancer workshop
2 September 2005
London, UK
Further details: The British Institute of Radiology, 36 Portland Place, London W1B 1AT.
Tel: 0207 307 1406. Fax: 0207 307 1414.
Email: registrations@bir.org.uk. Visit: www.bir.org.uk

MusculoSkeletal MRI (2) Pelvis, Spine and Small Joints
23 September 2005
Bristol, UK
Further details: The British Institute of Radiology, 36 Portland Place, London W1B 1AT.
Tel: 0207 307 1406. Fax: 0207 307 1414.
Email: registrations@bir.org.uk. Visit: www.bir.org.uk

CT PET
29 September 2005
London, UK
Further details: The British Institute of Radiology, 36 Portland Place, London W1B 1AT.
Tel: 0207 307 1406. Fax: 0207 307 1414.
Email: registrations@bir.org.uk. Visit: www.bir.org.uk

International Cancer Imaging Society Meeting and 5th Annual Teaching Course
3–5 October 2005
Beurs van Berlage, Amsterdam, The Netherlands
Further details: The British Institute of Radiology, 36 Portland Place, London W1B 1AT.
Tel: 0207 307 1406. Fax: 0207 307 1414.
Email: icis@bir.org.uk. Visit: www.icimagingsociety.org.uk

Head and Neck Cancer
7 October 2005
London, UK
Further details: The British Institute of Radiology, 36 Portland Place, London W1B 1AT.
Tel: 0207 307 1406. Fax: 0207 307 1414.
Email: registrations@bir.org.uk. Visit: www.bir.org.uk

Clinical Imaging of the Colon
10 October 2005
London, UK
Further details: The British Institute of Radiology, 36 Portland Place, London W1B 1AT.
Tel: 0207 307 1406. Fax: 0207 307 1414.
Email: registrations@bir.org.uk. Visit: www.bir.org.uk